RANG AND DALE'S
Pharmacology

RANG AND DALE'S
Pharmacology

NINTH EDITION

JAMES M. RITTER DPhil FRCP HonFBPhS FMedSci
Emeritus Professor of Clinical Pharmacology, King's College London
Fellow Commoner, Trinity Hall, Senior Physician Advisor CUC (GSK), Addenbrooke's Hospital
Cambridge, United Kingdom

ROD FLOWER PhD LLD DSc HonFBPhS FMedSci FRS
Emeritus Professor of Pharmacology
Bart's and the London School of Medicine
Queen Mary, University of London
London, United Kingdom

GRAEME HENDERSON PhD, FRSB, HonFBPhS
Professor of Pharmacology
University of Bristol
Bristol, United Kingdom

YOON KONG LOKE MBBS MD FRCP FBPhS
Professor of Medicine and Pharmacology
Norwich Medical School, University of East Anglia
Norwich, United Kingdom

DAVID MacEWAN PhD FRSB FBPhS SFHEA
Professor of Molecular Pharmacology/Toxicology & Head of Department
Department of Molecular and Clinical Pharmacology
University of Liverpool
Liverpool, United Kingdom

HUMPHREY P. RANG MB BS MSc MA DPhil HonFBPhS FMedSci FRS
Emeritus Professor of Pharmacology
University College London
London, United Kingdom

For additional online content visit **StudentConsult.com**

ELSEVIER   Edinburgh   London   New York   Oxford   Philadelphia   St Louis   Sydney   2020

ELSEVIER

First edition 1987
Second edition 1991
Third edition 1995
Fourth edition 1999
Fifth edition 2003
Sixth edition 2007
Seventh edition 2012
Eighth edition 2016

The right of James M. Ritter, Rod Flower, Graeme Henderson, Yoon Kong Loke, David MacEwan, and Humphrey P. Rang to be identified as authors of this work has been asserted by them in accordance with the Copyright, Designs and Patents Act 1988.

Potential Competing Financial Interests Statements for Rang and Dale 9E (2014–2018)

HPR: has no competing financial interests to declare.
JMR: has received salary from Quintiles and GSK.
GH: has no competing financial interests to declare.
YKL: has received funding from Polpharma and Thame Pharmaceuticals.
DJM: has no competing financial interests to declare.
RJF: serves as a board member for Antibe Therapeutics.

Notices

ELSEVIER your source for books, journals and multimedia in the health sciences

www.elsevierhealth.com

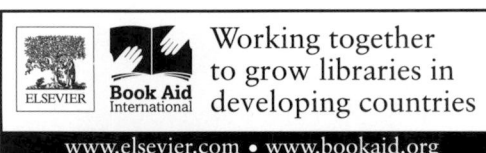

Working together to grow libraries in developing countries

www.elsevier.com • www.bookaid.org

The publisher's policy is to use paper manufactured from sustainable forests

ISBN: 978-0-7020-7448-6

Printed in China

Last digit is the print number: 9 8 7 6 5 4 3 2 1

Content Strategist: Alexandra Mortimer
Content Development Specialists: Trinity Hutton, Sam Crowe
Project Manager: Joanna Souch
Design: Renee Duenow
Illustration Manager: Nichole Beard
Marketing Manager: Deborah Watkins

Contents

Section 3 **Drugs affecting major organ systems**

Section 6 **Special topics**

Self-assessment questions compiled by Dr. Christine Edmead, University of Bath, are available through https://studentconsult. inkling.com

Rang and Dale's Pharmacology Ninth Edition Preface

In this edition, as in its predecessors, we set out to explain what drugs do in terms of the mechanisms by which they act. This entails analysis not only at the cellular and molecular level, where knowledge and techniques are advancing rapidly, but also at the level of physiological mechanisms and pathological disturbances. Pharmacology has its roots in therapeutics, where the aim is to ameliorate the effects of disease, so we have attempted to make the link between effects at the molecular and cellular level and the range of beneficial and adverse effects that humans experience when drugs are used for therapeutic or other reasons. Therapeutic agents have a high rate of obsolescence. In the decade 2008 to 2017, 301 new drugs gained regulatory approval for use as therapeutic agents. The majority exploit the same molecular targets as drugs already in use. Knowledge of the mechanisms of action of the class of drugs to which a new agent belongs provides a good starting point for understanding and using a new compound intelligently.

Significantly, however, one-third of these new arrivals are 'first-in-class' drugs. That is, they act on novel molecular targets not previously exploited for therapeutic purposes, and are therefore likely to produce effects not previously described. Not all will succeed clinically, but some will stimulate the development of improved follow-up compounds of the same type. Furthermore, about a quarter of the new compounds are 'biopharmaceuticals' – mainly proteins produced by bioengineering rather than synthetic chemistry. These are growing in importance as therapeutic agents, and generally have characteristics somewhat different from conventional drugs and are covered in a revised chapter. The very high rate of innovation in drug discovery is a recent – and very welcome – change, due in large part to the rapid advances in molecular and cell biology that have stemmed from the sequencing of the human genome in 2003. We have tried to strike a balance between the need to keep up with these modern developments and the danger of information overload. Our emphasis is on explaining the general principles underlying drug action, which apply to old and new alike, and to describe in more detail the actions and mechanisms of familiar, established drugs, while including references that cover modern and future developments.

Pharmacology is a lively scientific discipline in its own right, with an importance beyond that of providing a basis for the use of drugs in therapy, and we aim to provide a good background, not only for future doctors but also for scientists in other disciplines who need to understand how drugs act. We have, therefore, where appropriate, described how drugs are used as probes for elucidating cellular and physiological functions, to improve our understanding of how the human body functions normally and what goes wrong with it in disease, even when the compounds have no clinical use. Besides therapeutic applications, drugs have other impacts on society, which we cover in chapters on psychoactive drugs, drug abuse, and the use of drugs in sport.

Names of drugs and related chemicals are established through usage and sometimes there is more than one name in common use. For prescribing purposes, it is important to use standard names, and we follow, as far as possible, the World Health Organization's list of recommended international non-proprietary names (rINN). Sometimes these conflict with the familiar names of drugs (e.g. the endogenous mediator prostaglandin I_2 – the standard name in the scientific literature – becomes 'epoprostenol' – a name unfamiliar to most scientists – in the rINN list). In these cases, we generally adopt conventional scientific nomenclature. Sometimes English and American usage varies (as with adrenaline/epinephrine and noradrenaline/norepinephrine). Adrenaline and noradrenaline are the official names in EU member states and are used in this book.

Drug action can be understood only in the context of what else is happening in the body. So, at the beginning of most chapters, we briefly discuss the physiological and biochemical processes relevant to the action of the drugs described in that chapter. We have included the chemical structures of drugs only where this information helps in understanding their pharmacological and pharmacokinetic characteristics, since chemical structures are readily available for reference online.

The overall organisation of the book has been retained, with sections covering: (1) the general principles of drug action; (2) the chemical mediators and cellular mechanisms with which drugs interact in producing their therapeutic effects; (3) the action of drugs on specific organ systems; (4) the action of drugs on the nervous system; (5) the action of drugs used to treat infectious diseases and cancer; and (6) a range of special topics such as adverse effects, non-medical uses of drugs, etc. This organisation reflects our belief that drug action needs to be understood, not just as a description of the effects of individual drugs and their uses, but as a chemical intervention that perturbs the network of chemical and cellular signalling that underlies the function of any living organism. In addition to updating each chapter, we have added new material on biopharmaceuticals, and on personalised medicine, topics of particular current interest. Additional current material on cognition-enhancing drugs has been included in Chapter 48.

Despite the fact that pharmacology, like other branches of biomedical science, advances steadily, with the acquisition of new information, the development of new concepts and the introduction of new drugs for clinical use, we have avoided making the ninth edition any longer than its predecessor by cutting out dated and obsolete material, and have made extensive use of small print text to cover more specialised and speculative information that is not essential to understanding the key message, but will, we hope, be helpful to students seeking to go into greater depth. In selecting new material for inclusion, we have taken into account not only new agents but also recent extensions of basic knowledge that presage further drug development. And, where possible, we have given a brief outline of new treatments in the pipeline. Reference lists are largely restricted to guidance on further reading, together with review articles that list key original papers.

Finally, we hope that we have conveyed something of our own enthusiasm for the science and importance of pharmacology in the modern world.

ACKNOWLEDGEMENTS

We are grateful to many colleagues who have helped us with comments and suggestions, and would particularly like to thank the following for their help and advice in the preparation of this edition: Dr Steve Alexander, Professor Emma Baker, Dr Barbara Jennings, Professor Eamonn Kelly, Professor Munir Pirmohamed and Professor Emma Robinson. We would also like to thank Dr Christine Edmead for her work on the self-assessment questions which are available as additional material on the online edition of this book.

We would like to put on record our appreciation of the team at Elsevier who worked on this edition: Alexandra Mortimer (content strategist), Trinity Hutton (content development specialist), Joanna Souch (project manager), Nichole Beard (illustration manager).

London, 2018
Humphrey P. Rang
James M. Ritter
Rod Flower
Graeme Henderson
David MacEwan
Yoon Kong Loke

What is pharmacology?

OVERVIEW

In this introductory chapter we explain how pharmacology came into being and evolved as a scientific discipline, and describe the present-day structure of the subject and its links to other biomedical sciences. The structure that has emerged forms the basis of the organisation of the rest of the book. Readers in a hurry to get to the here-and-now of pharmacology can safely skip this chapter.

WHAT IS A DRUG?

For the purposes of this book, a drug can be defined as *a chemical substance of known structure, other than a nutrient or an essential dietary ingredient,*[1] *which, when administered to a living organism, produces a biological effect.*

A few points are worth noting. Drugs may be synthetic chemicals, chemicals obtained from plants or animals, or products of biotechnology (biopharmaceuticals). A *medicine* is a chemical preparation, which usually, but not necessarily, contains one or more drugs, administered with the intention of producing a therapeutic effect. Medicines usually contain other substances (excipients, stabilisers, solvents, etc.) besides the active drug, to make them more convenient to use. To count as a drug, the substance must be administered as such, rather than released by physiological mechanisms. Many substances, such as insulin or thyroxine, are endogenous hormones but are also drugs when they are administered intentionally. Many drugs are not used commonly in medicine but are nevertheless useful research tools. The definition of drug also covers toxins, which again are not usually administered in the clinic but nonetheless are critical pharmacological tools. In everyday parlance, the word *drug* is often associated with psychoactive substances and addiction – unfortunate negative connotations that tend to bias uninformed opinion against any form of chemical therapy. In this book we focus mainly on drugs used for therapeutic purposes but also describe psychoactive drugs and provide important examples of drugs used as experimental tools. Poisons fall strictly within the definition of drugs, and indeed 'all drugs are poisons… it is only the dose which makes a thing poison' (an aphorism credited to Paracelsus, a 16th century Swiss physician); conversely, poisons may be effective therapeutic agents when administered in sub-toxic doses. Botulinum toxin (Ch. 14) provides a striking example: it is the most potent poison known in terms of its lethal dose, but is widely used both medically and cosmetically. General aspects of harmful effects of drugs are considered in Chapter 58. Toxicology is the study of toxic effects of chemical substances (including drugs), and toxicological testing is undertaken on new chemical entities during their development as potential medicinal products (Ch. 60), but the subject is not otherwise covered in this book.

ORIGINS AND ANTECEDENTS

Pharmacology can be defined as the study of the effects of drugs on the function of living systems. As a science, it was born in the mid-19th century, one of a host of new biomedical sciences based on principles of experimentation rather than dogma that came into being in that remarkable period. Long before that – indeed from the dawn of civilisation – herbal remedies were widely used, pharmacopoeias were written, and the apothecaries' trade flourished. However, nothing resembling scientific principles was applied to therapeutics, which was known at that time as *materia medica.*[2] Even Robert Boyle, who laid the scientific foundations of chemistry in the middle of the 17th century, was content, when dealing with therapeutics (*A Collection of Choice Remedies*, 1692), to recommend concoctions of worms, dung, urine and the moss from a dead man's skull. The impetus for pharmacology came from the need to improve the outcome of therapeutic intervention by doctors, who were at that time skilled at clinical observation and diagnosis but broadly ineffectual when it came to treatment.[3] Until the late 19th century, knowledge of the normal and abnormal functioning of the body was too rudimentary to provide even a rough basis for understanding drug effects; at the same time, disease and death were regarded as semi-sacred subjects, appropriately dealt with by authoritarian, rather than scientific, doctrines. Clinical practice often displayed an obedience to authority and ignored what appear to be easily ascertainable facts. For example, cinchona bark was recognised as a specific and effective treatment for malaria, and a sound protocol for its use was laid down by Lind in 1765. In 1804, however, Johnson declared it to be unsafe until the fever had subsided, and he recommended instead the use of large doses of calomel (mercurous chloride) in the early stages – a murderous piece of advice that was slavishly followed for the next 40 years.

---

[1]Like most definitions, this one has its limits. For example, there are a number of essential dietary constituents, such as iron and various vitamins, that are used as medicines. Furthermore, some biological products (e.g. **epoietin**) show batch-to-batch variation in their chemical constitution that significantly affects their properties. There is also the study of pharmaceutical-grade nutrients or 'nutraceuticals'.

[2]The name persists today in some ancient universities, being attached to chairs of what we would call clinical pharmacology.
[3]Oliver Wendell Holmes, an eminent physician, wrote in 1860: '[I] firmly believe that if the whole materia medica, as now used, could be sunk to the bottom of the sea, it would be all the better for mankind and the worse for the fishes' (see Porter, 1997).

The motivation for understanding what drugs can and cannot do came from clinical practice, but the science could be built only on the basis of secure foundations in physiology, pathology and chemistry. It was not until 1858 that Virchow proposed the cell theory. The first use of a structural formula to describe a chemical compound was in 1868. Bacteria as a cause of disease were discovered by Pasteur in 1878. Previously, pharmacology hardly had the legs to stand on, and we may wonder at the bold vision of Rudolf Buchheim, who created the first pharmacology institute (in his own house) in Estonia in 1847.

In its beginnings, before the advent of synthetic organic chemistry, pharmacology concerned itself exclusively with understanding the effects of natural substances, mainly plant extracts – and a few (mainly toxic) chemicals such as mercury and arsenic. An early development in chemistry was the purification of active compounds from plants. Friedrich Sertürner, a young German apothecary, purified morphine from opium in 1805. Other substances quickly followed, and, even though their structures were unknown, these compounds showed that chemicals, not magic or vital forces, were responsible for the effects that plant extracts produced on living organisms. Early pharmacologists focused most of their attention on such plant-derived drugs as quinine, digitalis, atropine, ephedrine, strychnine and others (many of which are still used today and will have become old friends by the time you have finished reading this book).[4]

PHARMACOLOGY IN THE 20TH AND 21ST CENTURIES

Beginning in the 20th century, the fresh wind of synthetic chemistry began to revolutionise the pharmaceutical industry, and with it the science of pharmacology. New synthetic drugs, such as barbiturates and local anaesthetics, began to appear, and the era of antimicrobial chemotherapy began with the discovery by Paul Ehrlich in 1909 of arsenical compounds for treating syphilis. Around the same time, William Blair-Bell was world renowned for his pioneering work at Liverpool in the treatment of breast cancers with another relatively poisonous agent, lead colloid mixtures. The thinking was that yes, drugs were toxic, but they were slightly more toxic to a microbe or cancer cell. This early chemotherapy has laid the foundations for much of the antimicrobial and anticancer therapies still used today. Further breakthroughs came when the sulfonamides, the first antibacterial drugs, were discovered by Gerhard Domagk in 1935, and with the development of penicillin

by Chain and Florey during the Second World War, based on the earlier work of Fleming.

These few well-known examples show how the growth of synthetic chemistry, and the resurgence of natural product chemistry, caused a dramatic revitalisation of therapeutics in the first half of the 20th century. Each new drug class that emerged gave pharmacologists a new challenge, and it was then that pharmacology really established its identity and its status among the biomedical sciences.

In parallel with the exuberant proliferation of therapeutic molecules – driven mainly by chemistry – which gave pharmacologists so much to think about, physiology was also making rapid progress, particularly in relation to chemical mediators, which are discussed in depth throughout this book. Many hormones, neurotransmitters and inflammatory mediators were discovered in this period, and the realisation that chemical communication plays a central role in almost every regulatory mechanism that our bodies possess immediately established a large area of common ground between physiology and pharmacology, for interactions between chemical substances and living systems were exactly what pharmacologists had been preoccupied with from the outset. Indeed, these fields have developed hand-in-hand as wherever there is either a physiological or pathological mechanism, pharmacology could be there to exploit it with a drug. The concept of 'receptors' for chemical mediators, first proposed by Langley in 1905, was quickly taken up by pharmacologists such as Clark, Gaddum, Schild and others, and is a constant theme in present-day pharmacology (as you will soon discover as you plough through the next two chapters). The receptor concept, and the technologies developed from it, have had a massive impact on drug discovery and therapeutics. Biochemistry also emerged as a distinct science early in the 20th century, and the discovery of enzymes and the delineation of biochemical pathways provided yet another framework for understanding drug effects. The picture of pharmacology that emerges from this brief glance at history (Fig. 1.1) is of a subject evolved from ancient prescientific therapeutics, involved in commerce from the 17th century onwards, and which gained respectability by donning the trappings of science as soon as this became possible in the mid-19th century. Pharmacology grew rapidly in partnership with the evolution of organic chemistry and other biomedical sciences, and was quick to assimilate the dramatic advances in molecular and cell biology in the late 20th century. Signs of its carpetbagger past still cling to pharmacology, for the pharmaceutical industry has become very big business and much pharmacological research nowadays takes place in a commercial environment, a rougher and more pragmatic place than academia.[5] No other biomedical 'ology' is so close to Mammon.

ALTERNATIVE THERAPEUTIC PRINCIPLES

Modern medicine relies heavily on drugs as the main tool of therapeutics. Other therapeutic procedures, such

---

[4]A handful of synthetic substances achieved pharmacological prominence long before the era of synthetic chemistry began. Diethyl ether, first prepared as 'sweet oil of vitriol' in the 16th century, and nitrous oxide, prepared by Humphrey Davy in 1799, were used to liven up parties before being introduced as anaesthetic agents in the mid-19th century (see Ch. 42). Amyl nitrite (see Ch. 21) was made in 1859 and can claim to be the first 'rational' therapeutic drug; its therapeutic effect in angina was predicted on the basis of its physiological effects – a true 'pharmacologist's drug' and the smelly forerunner of the nitrovasodilators that are widely used today. Aspirin (Ch. 27), the most widely used therapeutic drug in history, was first synthesised in 1853, with no therapeutic application in mind. It was rediscovered in 1897 in the laboratories of the German company Bayer, who were seeking a less toxic derivative of salicylic acid. Bayer commercialised aspirin in 1899 and made a fortune.

[5]Some of our most distinguished pharmacological pioneers made their careers in industry: for example, Henry Dale, who laid the foundations of our knowledge of chemical transmission and the autonomic nervous system (Ch. 13); George Hitchings and Gertrude Elion, who described the antimetabolite principle and produced the first effective anticancer drugs (Ch. 57); and James Black, who introduced the first β-adrenoceptor and histamine H_2-receptor antagonists (Chs 15 and 31). It is no accident that in this book, where we focus on the scientific principles of pharmacology, most of our examples are products of industry, not of nature.

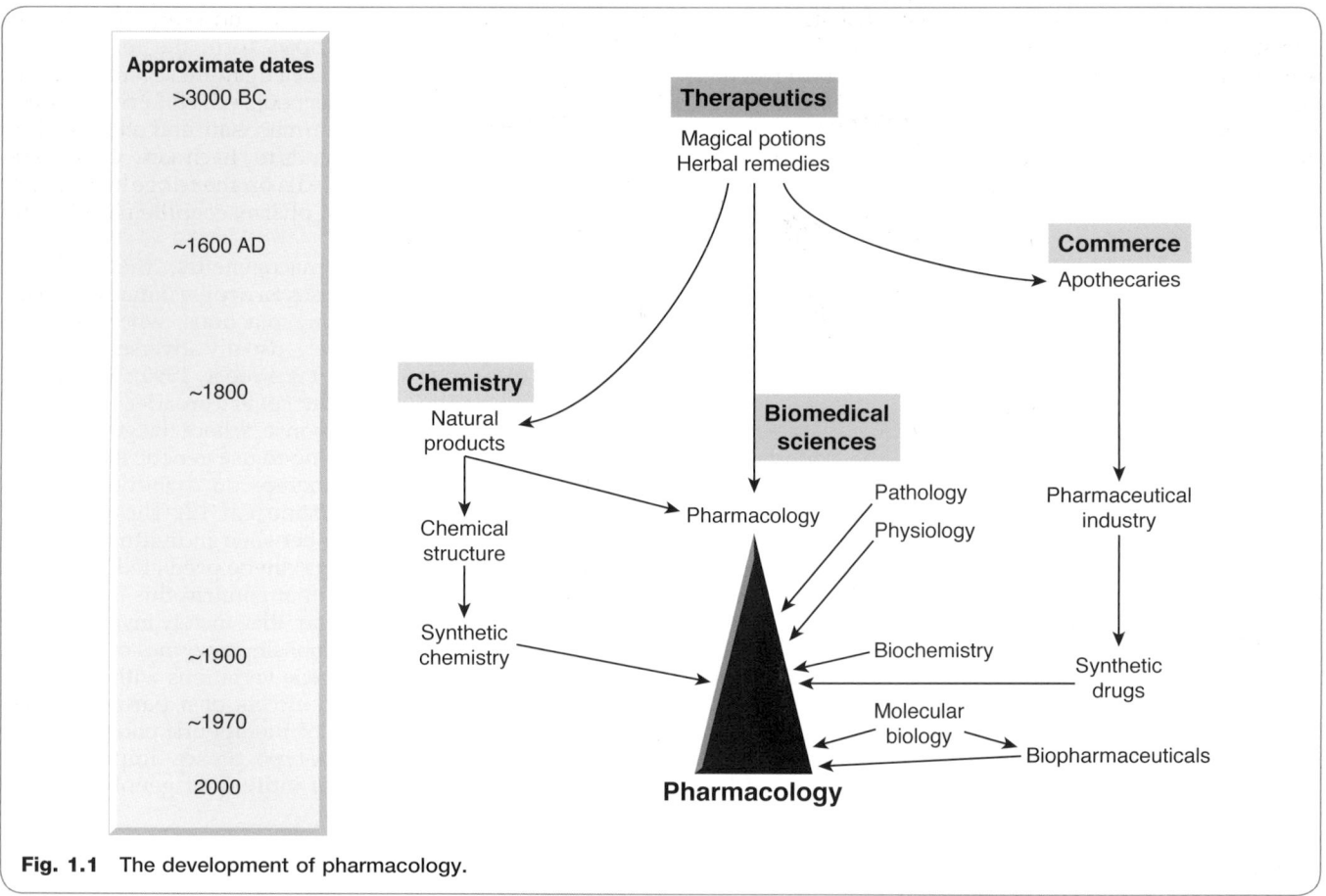

Fig. 1.1 The development of pharmacology.

as surgery, diet, exercise, psychological treatments etc., are also important, of course, as is deliberate non-intervention, but none is so widely applied as drug-based therapeutics.

Before the advent of science-based approaches, repeated attempts were made to construct systems of therapeutics, many of which produced even worse results than pure empiricism. One of these was *allopathy*, espoused by James Gregory (1735–1821). The favoured remedies included bloodletting, emetics and purgatives, which were used until the dominant symptoms of the disease were suppressed. Many patients died from such treatment, and it was in reaction against it that Hahnemann introduced the practice of *homeopathy* in the early 19th century. The implausible guiding principles of homeopathy are:

• like cures like
• activity can be enhanced by dilution

The system rapidly drifted into absurdity: for example, Hahnemann recommended the use of drugs at dilutions of $1:10^{60}$, equivalent to one molecule in a sphere the size of the orbit of Neptune.

Many other systems of therapeutics have come and gone, and the variety of dogmatic principles that they embodied have tended to hinder rather than advance scientific progress. Currently, therapeutic systems that have a basis that lies outside the domain of science remain popular under the general banner of 'alternative' or 'complementary' medicine. Mostly, they reject the 'medical model', which attributes disease to an underlying derangement of normal function that can be defined in physiological or structural terms, detected by objective means, and influenced beneficially by appropriate chemical or physical interventions. They focus instead mainly on subjective malaise, which may be disease-associated or not. Abandoning objectivity in defining and measuring disease goes along with a similar departure from scientific principles in assessing therapeutic efficacy and risk, with the result that principles and practices can gain acceptance without satisfying any of the criteria of validity that would convince a critical scientist, and that are required by law to be satisfied before a new drug can be introduced into therapy. Demand for 'alternative' therapies by the general public, alas, has little to do with demonstrable efficacy.[6]

THE EMERGENCE OF BIOTECHNOLOGY

Since the 1980s, biotechnology has emerged as a major source of new therapeutic agents in the form of antibodies, enzymes and various regulatory proteins, including hormones, growth factors and cytokines (see Clark & Pazdernik, 2015). Although such products (known as *biopharmaceuticals*, *biologicals* or *biologics*) are generally produced by genetic engineering rather than by synthetic chemistry, the pharmacological principles are essentially the same as for conventional drugs, although the details of absorption,

---

[6]The UK Medicines and Healthcare Regulatory Agency (MHRA) requires detailed evidence of therapeutic efficacy based on controlled clinical trials before a new drug is registered, but no clinical trials data for homeopathic products or for the many herbal medicines that were on sale before the Medicines Act of 1968.

distribution and elimination, specificity, harmful effects and clinical effectiveness all differ markedly between high molecular-weight biopharmaceuticals and low molecular-weight drugs – as does their cost! Looking further ahead, gene- and cell-based therapies (Ch. 5), although still in their infancy, are beginning to take therapeutics into a new domain. The principles governing gene suppression, the design, delivery and control of functioning artificial genes introduced into cells, or of engineered cells introduced into the body, are very different from those of drug-based therapeutics and will require a different conceptual framework, which texts such as this will increasingly need to embrace if they are to stay abreast of modern medical treatment.

PHARMACOLOGY TODAY

As with other biomedical disciplines, the boundaries of pharmacology are not sharply defined, nor are they constant. Its exponents are, as befits pragmatists, ever ready to poach on the territory and techniques of other disciplines. If it ever had a conceptual and technical core that it could really call its own, this has now dwindled almost to the point of extinction, and the subject is defined by its purpose – to understand what drugs do to living organisms, and more particularly how their effects can be applied to therapeutics – rather than by its scientific coherence.

Fig. 1.2 shows the structure of pharmacology as it appears today. Within the main subject fall a number of compartments (neuropharmacology, immunopharmacology,

pharmacokinetics, etc.), which are convenient, if not watertight, subdivisions. These topics form the main subject matter of this book. Around the edges are several interface disciplines, not covered in this book, which form important two-way bridges between pharmacology and other fields of biomedicine. Pharmacology tends to have more of these than other disciplines. Recent arrivals on the fringe are subjects such as pharmacogenomics, pharmacoepidemiology and pharmacoeconomics.

Pharmacogenomics. Pharmacogenetics, the study of genetic influences on responses to drugs, initially focused on familial idiosyncratic drug reactions, where affected individuals show an abnormal – usually adverse – response to a class of drug (see Nebert & Weber, 1990). Rebranded as pharmacogenomics, it now covers broader genetically based variations in drug response, where the genetic basis is more complex, the aim being to use genetic information to guide the choice of drug therapy on an individual basis – so-called personalised medicine (Ch. 12). The underlying principle is that differences between individuals in their response to therapeutic drugs can be predicted from their genetic make-up. Examples that confirm this are steadily accumulating (see Ch. 12). So far, they mainly involve genetic polymorphism of drug-metabolising enzymes or receptors. Ultimately, linking specific gene variations with variations in therapeutic or unwanted effects of a particular drug should enable the tailoring of therapeutic choices on the basis of an individual's genotype. Steady improvements in the cost and feasibility of individual genotyping will

Fig. 1.2 Pharmacology today with its various subdivisions. The grey box contains the general areas of pharmacology covered in this book. Interface disciplines *(brown boxes)* link pharmacology to other mainstream biomedical disciplines *(green boxes)*.

increase its applicability, potentially with far-reaching consequences for therapeutics (see Ch. 12).

Pharmacoepidemiology. This is the study of drug effects at the population level (Strom et al., 2013). It is concerned with the variability of drug effects between individuals in a population, and between populations. It is an increasingly important topic in the eyes of the regulatory authorities who decide whether or not new drugs can be licensed for therapeutic use. Variability between individuals or populations detracts from the utility of a drug, even though its overall effect level may be satisfactory. Pharmacoepidemiological studies also take into account patient compliance and other factors that apply when the drug is used under real-life conditions.

Pharmacoeconomics. This branch of health economics aims to quantify in economic terms the cost and benefit of drugs used therapeutically. It arose from the concern of many governments to provide for healthcare from tax revenues, raising questions of what therapeutic procedures represent the best value for money. This, of course, raises fierce controversy, because it ultimately comes down to putting monetary value on health and longevity. As with pharmacoepidemiology, regulatory authorities are increasingly requiring economic analysis, as well as evidence of individual benefit, when making decisions on licensing. For more information on this complex subject, see Rascati (2013).

REFERENCES AND FURTHER READING

Clark, D.P., Pazderink, N.J., 2015. Biotechnology. Elsevier, New York. (*General account of biotechnology and its potential applications*)

Nebert, D.W., Weber, W.W., 1990. Pharmacogenetics. In: Pratt, W.B., Taylor, P. (Eds.), Principles of Drug Action, third ed. Churchill Livingstone, New York. (*A detailed account of genetic factors that affect responses to drugs, with many examples from the pregenomic literature*)

Porter, R., 1997. The Greatest Benefit to Mankind. Harper-Collins, London. (*An excellent and readable account of the history of medicine, with good coverage of the early development of pharmacology and the pharmaceutical industry*)

Rascati, K.L., 2013. Essentials of Pharmacoeconomics, second ed. Lippincott Williams & Wilkins, Philadelphia. (*Introduction to a complex and fraught subject*)

Strom, B.L., Kimmel, S.E., Hennessy, S., 2013. Textbook of Pharmacoepidemiology, second ed. Wiley, Chichester. (*A multiauthor book covering all aspects of a newly emerged discipline, including aspects of pharmacoeconomics*)

2 How drugs act: general principles

OVERVIEW

The emergence of pharmacology as a science came when the emphasis shifted from describing what drugs do to explaining how they work. In this chapter we set out some general principles underlying the interaction of drugs with living systems (Ch. 3 goes into the molecular aspects in more detail). The interaction between drugs and cells is described, followed by a more detailed examination of different types of drug–receptor interaction. The receptor concept has been described as the 'big idea' of pharmacology (Rang, 2006) and will be a recurring theme throughout this book.

INTRODUCTION

To begin with, we should gratefully acknowledge Paul Ehrlich for insisting that drug action must be explicable in terms of conventional chemical interactions between drugs and tissues, and for dispelling the idea that the remarkable potency and specificity of action of some drugs put them somehow out of reach of chemistry and physics and required the intervention of magical 'vital forces'. Although many drugs produce effects in extraordinarily low doses and concentrations, low concentrations still involve very large numbers of molecules. One drop of a solution of a drug at only 10^{-10} mol/L still contains about 3×10^9 drug molecules, so there is no mystery in the fact that it may produce an obvious pharmacological response. Some bacterial toxins (e.g. diphtheria toxin) act with such precision that a single molecule taken up by a target cell is sufficient to kill it.

One of the basic tenets of pharmacology is that drug molecules must exert some chemical influence on one or more cell constituents in order to produce a pharmacological response. In other words, drug molecules must get so close to these constituent cellular molecules that the two interact chemically in such a way that the function of the latter is altered. Of course, the molecules in the organism vastly outnumber the drug molecules, and if the drug molecules were merely distributed at random, the chance of interaction with any particular class of cellular molecule would be negligible. Therefore pharmacological effects require, in general, the non-uniform distribution of the drug molecule within the body or tissue, which is the same as saying that drug molecules must be 'bound' to particular constituents of cells and tissues in order to produce an effect. Ehrlich summed it up thus: 'Corpora non agunt nisi fixata' (in this context, 'A drug will not work unless it is bound').[1]

These critical binding sites are often referred to as 'drug targets' (an obvious allusion to Ehrlich's famous phrase 'magic bullets', describing the potential of antimicrobial drugs). The mechanisms by which the association of a drug molecule with its target leads to a physiological response constitute the major thrust of pharmacological research. Most drug targets are protein molecules. Even general anaesthetics (see Ch. 42), which were long thought to produce their effects by an interaction with membrane lipid, now appear to interact mainly with membrane proteins (see Franks, 2008).

All rules need exceptions, and many antimicrobial and antitumour drugs (Chs 52 and 57), as well as mutagenic and carcinogenic agents (Ch. 58), interact directly with DNA rather than protein; bisphosphonates, used to treat osteoporosis (Ch. 37), bind to calcium salts in the bone matrix, rendering them toxic to osteoclasts, much like rat poison. There are also exceptions among the new generation of *biopharmaceutical drugs* that include nucleic acids, proteins and antibodies (see Ch. 5).

PROTEIN TARGETS FOR DRUG BINDING

Four main kinds of regulatory protein are commonly involved as primary drug targets, namely:

- receptors
- enzymes
- carrier molecules (transporters)
- ion channels

Furthermore, many drugs bind (in addition to their primary targets) to plasma proteins (see Ch. 9) and other tissue proteins, without producing any obvious physiological effect. Nevertheless, the generalisation that most drugs act on one or other of the four types of protein listed above serves as a good starting point.

Further discussion of the mechanisms by which such binding leads to cellular responses is given in Chapters 3–4.

DRUG RECEPTORS

WHAT DO WE MEAN BY RECEPTORS?

▼ As emphasised in Chapter 1, the concept of receptors is central to pharmacology, and the term is most often used to describe the target molecules through which soluble physiological mediators – hormones, neurotransmitters, inflammatory mediators, etc. – produce their effects. Examples such as acetylcholine receptors, cytokine receptors, steroid receptors and growth hormone receptors abound in this book, and generally the term *receptor* indicates a recognition molecule for a chemical mediator through which a response is transduced.

'Receptor' is sometimes used to denote *any* target molecule with which a drug molecule (i.e. a foreign compound rather than an endogenous mediator) has to combine in order to elicit its specific

---

[1]There are, if one looks hard enough, exceptions to Ehrlich's dictum – drugs that act without being bound to any tissue constituent (e.g. osmotic diuretics, osmotic purgatives, antacids and heavy metal chelating agents). Nonetheless, the principle remains true for the great majority.

Targets for drug action

- A drug is a chemical applied to a physiological system that affects its function in a specific way.
- With some exceptions, drugs act on target proteins, namely:
  - receptors
  - enzymes
  - carriers
  - ion channels.
- The term *receptor* is used in different ways. In pharmacology, it describes protein molecules whose function is to recognise and respond to endogenous chemical signals. Other macromolecules with which drugs interact to produce their effects are known as *drug targets*.
- Specificity is reciprocal: individual classes of drug bind only to certain targets, and individual targets recognise only certain classes of drug.
- No drugs are completely specific in their actions. In many cases, increasing the dose of a drug will cause it to affect targets other than the principal one, and this can lead to side effects.

effect. For example, the voltage-sensitive sodium channel is sometimes referred to as the 'receptor' for **local anaesthetics** (see Ch. 44), or the enzyme dihydrofolate reductase as the 'receptor' for **methotrexate** (Ch. 51). The term *drug target*, of which receptors are one type, is preferable in this context.

In the more general context of cell biology, the term receptor is used to describe various cell surface molecules (such as *T-cell receptors*, *integrins*, *Toll receptors*, etc; see Ch. 7) involved in the cell-to-cell interactions that are important in immunology, cell growth, migration and differentiation, some of which are also emerging as drug targets. These receptors differ from conventional pharmacological receptors in that they respond to proteins attached to cell surfaces or extracellular structures, rather than to soluble mediators.

Various carrier proteins are often referred to as receptors, such as the *low-density lipoprotein receptor* that plays a key role in lipid metabolism (Ch. 24) and the *transferrin receptor* involved in iron absorption (Ch. 26). These entities have little in common with pharmacological receptors. Though quite distinct from pharmacological receptors, these proteins play an important role in the action of drugs such as *statins* (Ch. 24).

RECEPTORS IN PHYSIOLOGICAL SYSTEMS

Receptors form a key part of the system of chemical communication that all multicellular organisms use to coordinate the activities of their cells and organs. Without them, we would be unable to function.

Some fundamental properties of receptors are illustrated by the action of **adrenaline** (epinephrine) on the heart. Adrenaline first binds to a receptor protein (the β_1 *adrenoceptor*, see Ch. 15) that serves as a recognition site for adrenaline and other catecholamines. When it binds to the receptor, a train of reactions is initiated (see Ch. 3), leading to an increase in force and rate of the heartbeat. In the absence of adrenaline, the receptor is normally functionally silent. This is true of most receptors for endogenous mediators (hormones, neurotransmitters, cytokines, etc.), although there are examples (see Ch. 3) of receptors that are 'constitutively active' – that is, they exert a controlling

influence even when no chemical mediator is present (see p. 14).

There is an important distinction between *agonists*, which 'activate' the receptors, and *antagonists*, which combine at the same site without causing activation, and block the effect of agonists on that receptor. The distinction between agonists and antagonists only exists for pharmacological receptors; we cannot usefully speak of 'agonists' for the other classes of drug target described above.

The characteristics and accepted nomenclature of pharmacological receptors are described by Neubig et al. (2003). The origins of the receptor concept and its pharmacological significance are discussed by Rang (2006).

DRUG SPECIFICITY

For a drug to be useful as either a therapeutic or a scientific tool, it must act selectively on particular cells and tissues. In other words, it must show a high degree of binding site specificity. Conversely, proteins that function as drug targets generally show a high degree of ligand specificity; they bind only molecules of a certain precise type.

These principles of binding site and ligand specificity can be clearly recognised in the actions of a mediator such as **angiotensin** (Ch. 23). This peptide acts strongly on vascular smooth muscle, and on the kidney tubule, but has very little effect on other kinds of smooth muscle or on the intestinal epithelium. Other mediators affect a quite different spectrum of cells and tissues, the pattern in each case reflecting the specific pattern of expression of the protein receptors for the various mediators. A small chemical change, such as conversion of one of the amino acids in angiotensin from L to D form, or removal of one amino acid from the chain, can inactivate the molecule altogether, because the receptor fails to bind the altered form. The complementary specificity of ligands and binding sites, which gives rise to the very exact molecular recognition properties of proteins, is central to explaining many of the phenomena of pharmacology. It is no exaggeration to say that the ability of proteins to interact in a highly selective way with other molecules – including other proteins – is the basis of living machines. Its relevance to the understanding of drug action will be a recurring theme in this book.

Finally, it must be emphasised that no drug acts with complete specificity. Thus tricyclic antidepressant drugs (Ch. 48) act by blocking monoamine transporters but are notorious for producing side effects (e.g. dry mouth) related to their ability to block various other receptors. In general, the lower the potency of a drug and the higher the dose needed, the more likely it is that sites of action other than the primary one will assume significance. In clinical terms, this is often associated with the appearance of unwanted 'off-target' side effects,[2] of which no drug is free.

Since the 1970s, pharmacological research has succeeded in identifying the protein targets of many different types of drug. Drugs such as opioid analgesics (Ch. 43), cannabinoids (Ch. 20) and benzodiazepine tranquillisers (Ch. 45), whose actions had been described in exhaustive detail for many years, are now known to target well-defined receptors, many of which have been fully characterised by

---

[2]'On-target' side effects are unwanted effects mediated through the same receptor as the clinically desired effect, for example constipation and respiratory depression by opioid analgesic drugs (see Ch. 43), whereas 'off target' side effects are mediated by a different mechanism.

gene-cloning and protein crystallography techniques (see Ch. 3).

RECEPTOR CLASSIFICATION

▼ Where the action of a drug can be associated with a particular receptor, this provides a valuable means for classification and refinement in drug design. For example, pharmacological analysis of the actions of histamine (see Ch. 18) showed that some of its effects (the H_1 effects, such as smooth muscle contraction) were strongly antagonised by the competitive histamine antagonists then known. Black and his colleagues suggested in 1970 that the remaining actions of histamine, which included its stimulant effect on gastric secretion, might represent a second class of histamine receptor (H_2). Testing a number of histamine analogues, they found that some were selective in producing H_2 effects, with little H_1 activity. By analysing which parts of the histamine molecule conferred this type of specificity, they were able to develop selective H_2 antagonists, which proved to be potent in blocking gastric acid secretion, a development of major therapeutic significance (Ch. 31).[3] Two further types of histamine receptor (H_3 and H_4) were recognised later.

Receptor classification based on pharmacological responses continues to be a valuable and widely used approach. Subsequently, newer experimental approaches produced other criteria on which to base receptor classification. The direct measurement of ligand binding to receptors (see later) allowed many new receptor subtypes to be defined that could not easily be distinguished by studies of drug effects. Molecular sequencing of the amino acid structure (see Ch. 3) provided a completely new basis for classification at a much finer level of detail than can be reached through pharmacological analysis. Finally, analysis of the biochemical pathways that are linked to receptor activation (see Ch. 3) provides yet another basis for classification.

The result of this data explosion was that receptor classification suddenly became much more detailed, with a proliferation of receptor subtypes for all the main types of ligand. As alternative molecular and biochemical classifications began to spring up that were incompatible with the accepted pharmacologically defined receptor classes, the International Union of Basic and Clinical Pharmacology (IUPHAR) convened expert working groups to produce agreed receptor classifications for the major types, taking into account the pharmacological, molecular and biochemical information available. These wise people have a hard task; their conclusions will be neither perfect nor final but are essential to ensure a consistent terminology. To the student, this may seem an arcane exercise in taxonomy, generating much detail but little illumination. There is a danger that the tedious lists of drug names, actions and side effects that used to burden the subject will be replaced by exhaustive tables of receptors, ligands and transduction pathways. In this book, we have tried to avoid detail for its own sake and include only such information on receptor classification as seems interesting in its own right or is helpful in explaining the actions of important drugs. A comprehensive database of known receptor classes is available (see <www.guidetopharmacology.org/>), as well as a regularly updated summary (Alexander et al., 2015).

DRUG–RECEPTOR INTERACTIONS

Occupation of a receptor by a drug molecule may or may not result in *activation* of the receptor. By activation, we mean that the receptor is affected by the bound molecule in such a way as to alter the function of the cell and elicit a tissue response. The molecular mechanisms associated with receptor activation are discussed in Chapter 3. Binding and activation represent two distinct steps in the generation of the receptor-mediated response by an agonist (Fig. 2.1). If a drug binds to the receptor without causing activation and thereby prevents the agonist from binding, it is termed a *receptor antagonist*. The tendency of a drug to bind to the

Fig. 2.1 **The distinction between drug binding and receptor activation.** Ligand *A* is an agonist, because when it is bound, the receptor *(R)* tends to become activated, whereas ligand *B* is an antagonist, because binding does not lead to activation. It is important to realise that for most drugs, binding and activation are reversible, dynamic processes. The rate constants k_{+1}, k_{-1}, α and β for the binding, unbinding and activation steps vary between drugs. For an antagonist, which does not activate the receptor, $\beta = 0$.

receptors is governed by its *affinity*, whereas the tendency for it, once bound, to activate the receptor is denoted by its *efficacy*. These terms are defined more precisely later (pp. 9 and 11). Drugs of high potency generally have a high affinity for the receptors and thus occupy a significant proportion of the receptors even at low concentrations. Agonists also possess significant efficacy, whereas antagonists, in the simplest case, have zero efficacy. Drugs with intermediate levels of efficacy, such that even when 100% of the receptors are occupied the tissue response is submaximal, are known as *partial agonists*, to distinguish them from *full agonists*, the efficacy of which is sufficient that they can elicit a maximal tissue response. These concepts, though clearly an oversimplified description of events at the molecular level (see Ch. 3), provide a useful basis for characterising drug effects.

We now discuss certain aspects in more detail, namely drug binding, agonist concentration–effect curves, competitive antagonism, partial agonists and the nature of efficacy. Understanding these concepts at a qualitative level is sufficient for many purposes, but for more detailed analysis a quantitative formulation is needed (see pp. 19–20).

THE BINDING OF DRUGS TO RECEPTORS

▼ The binding of drugs to receptors can often be measured directly by the use of drug molecules (agonists or antagonists) labelled with one or more radioactive atoms (usually ^3H, ^{14}C or ^{125}I). The usual procedure is to incubate samples of the tissue (or membrane fragments) with various concentrations of radioactive drug until equilibrium is reached (i.e. when the rate of association [binding] and dissociation [unbinding] of the radioactive drug are equal). The bound radioactivity is measured after removal of the supernatant.

In such experiments, the radiolabelled drug will exhibit both specific binding (i.e. binding to receptors, which is saturable as there are a finite number of receptors in the tissue) and a certain amount of 'non-specific binding' (i.e. drug taken up by structures other than receptors, which, at the concentrations used in such studies, is normally non-saturable), which obscures the specific component and needs to be kept to a minimum (Fig. 2.2A–B). The amount of non-specific

---

[3]For this work, and the development of β-adrenoceptor antagonists by a similar experimental approach, Sir James Black was awarded the 1984 Nobel Prize in Physiology or Medicine.

Fig. 2.2 **Measurement of receptor binding.** (A) (i) Cartoon depicting radioligand (shown in red) binding to its receptor *(R)* in the membrane as well as to non-specific sites on other proteins and lipid. In (ii) when the concentration of radioligand is increased all the specific sites become saturated but non-specific binding continues to increase. In (iii) addition of a high concentration of a non-radioactive drug *(shown in green)* that also binds to R displaces the radioactive drug from its receptors but not from the non-specific sites. (B–D) Illustrate actual experimental results for radioligand binding to β adrenoceptors in cardiac cell membranes. The ligand was [^{3}H]-cyanopindolol, a derivative of pindolol (see Ch. 15). (B) Measurements of total and non-specific binding at equilibrium. Non-specific binding is measured in the presence of a saturating concentration of a non-radioactive β-adrenoceptor agonist, which prevents the radioactive ligand from binding to β adrenoceptors. The difference between the two lines represents specific binding. (C) Specific binding plotted against concentration. The curve is a rectangular hyperbola (Eq. 2.5). (D) Specific binding as in (C) plotted against the concentration on a log scale. The sigmoid curve is a *logistic curve* representing the logarithmic scaling of the rectangular hyperbola plotted in panel (C) from which the binding parameters K (the equilibrium dissociation constant) and B_{max} (the binding capacity) can be determined.

binding is estimated by measuring the radioactivity taken up in the presence of a saturating concentration of a (non-radioactive) ligand that inhibits completely the binding of the radioactive drug to the receptors, leaving behind the non-specific component. This is then subtracted from the total binding to give an estimate of specific binding (Fig. 2.2C). The *binding curve* (Fig. 2.2C–D) defines the relationship between concentration and the amount of drug bound (B), and in most cases it fits well to the relationship predicted theoretically (see Fig. 2.14), allowing the affinity of the drug for the receptors to be estimated, as well as the *binding capacity* (B_{max}), representing the density of receptors in the tissue. When combined with functional studies, binding measurements have proved very valuable. It has, for example, been confirmed that the *spare receptor hypothesis* (p. 10) for muscarinic receptors in smooth muscle is correct; agonists are found to bind, in general, with rather low affinity, and a maximal biological effect occurs at low receptor occupancy. It has also been shown, in skeletal muscle and other tissues, that denervation leads to an increase in the number of receptors in the target cell, a finding that accounts, at least in part, for the phenomenon of *denervation supersensitivity*. More generally, it appears that receptors tend to increase in number, usually over the course of a few days, if the relevant hormone or transmitter is absent or scarce, and to decrease in number if the receptors are activated for a prolonged period, a process of adaptation to continued administration of drugs or hormones (see p. 18).

Non-invasive imaging techniques, such as *positron emission tomography* (PET), using drugs labelled with an isotope of short half-life (such as ^{11}C or ^{18}Fl), can also be used to investigate the distribution of receptors in structures such as the living human brain. This technique has been used, for example, to measure the degree of dopamine-receptor blockade produced by antipsychotic drugs in the brains of schizophrenic patients (see Ch. 47).

Binding curves with agonists often reveal an apparent heterogeneity among receptors. For example, agonist binding to muscarinic receptors (Ch. 14) and also to β adrenoceptors (Ch. 15) suggests at least two populations of binding sites with different affinities. This may be because the receptors can exist either unattached or coupled within the membrane to another macromolecule, the G protein (see Ch. 3), which constitutes part of the transduction system through which the receptor exerts its regulatory effect. Antagonist binding does not show this complexity, probably because antagonists, by their nature, do not lead to the secondary event of G protein coupling. Because agonist binding results in activation, agonist affinity has proved to be a surprisingly elusive concept, about which aficionados love to argue.

THE RELATION BETWEEN DRUG CONCENTRATION AND EFFECT

Although binding can be measured directly, it is usually a biological response, such as a rise in blood pressure,

Fig. 2.3 Experimentally observed concentration–effect curves. Although the lines, drawn according to the binding Eq. 2.5, fit the points well, such curves do not give correct estimates of the affinity of drugs for receptors. This is because the relationship between receptor occupancy and response is usually non-linear.

contraction or relaxation of a strip of smooth muscle in an organ bath, the activation of an enzyme, or a behavioural response, that we are interested in, and this is often plotted as a *concentration–effect curve* (in vitro) or *dose–response curve* (in vivo), as in Fig. 2.3. This allows us to estimate the *maximal response* that the drug can produce (E_{max}), and the concentration or dose needed to produce a 50% maximal response (EC_{50} or ED_{50}). A logarithmic concentration or dose scale is often used. This transforms the curve from a rectangular hyperbola to a sigmoidal curve in which the mid portion is essentially linear (the importance of the slope of the linear portion will become apparent later in this chapter when we consider antagonism and partial agonists). The E_{max}, EC_{50} and slope parameters are useful for comparing different drugs that produce qualitatively similar effects (see Fig. 2.7 and Ch. 8). Although they look similar to the binding curve in Fig. 2.2D, concentration–effect curves cannot be used to measure the affinity of agonist drugs for their receptors, because the response produced is not, as a rule, directly proportional to receptor occupancy. This often arises because the maximum response of a tissue may be produced by agonists when they occupy less than 100% of the receptors. Under these circumstances the tissue is said to possess spare receptors (see later).

In interpreting concentration–effect curves, it must be remembered that the concentration of the drug at the receptors may differ from the known concentration in the bathing solution. Agonists may be subject to rapid enzymic degradation or uptake by cells as they diffuse from the surface towards their site of action, and a steady state can be reached in which the agonist concentration at the receptors is very much less than the concentration in the bath. In the case of acetylcholine, for example, which is hydrolysed by cholinesterase present in most tissues (see Ch. 14), the concentration reaching the receptors can be less than 1% of that in the bath, and an even bigger difference has been found with noradrenaline (norepinephrine), which is avidly taken up by sympathetic nerve terminals in many tissues (Ch. 15). The problem is reduced but not entirely eradicated

by the use of recombinant receptors expressed in cells in culture. Thus, even if the concentration–effect curve, as in Fig. 2.3, looks just like a facsimile of the binding curve (see Fig. 2.2D), it cannot be used directly to determine the affinity of the agonist for the receptors.

SPARE RECEPTORS

▼ Stephenson (1956), studying the actions of acetylcholine analogues in isolated tissues, found that many full agonists were capable of eliciting maximal responses at very low occupancies, often less than 1%. This means that the mechanism linking the response to receptor occupancy has a substantial reserve capacity. Such systems may be said to possess *spare receptors*, or a receptor reserve. The existence of spare receptors does not imply any functional subdivision of the receptor pool, but merely that the pool is larger than the number needed to evoke a full response. This surplus of receptors over the number actually needed might seem a wasteful biological arrangement. But in fact it is highly efficient in that a given number of agonist–receptor complexes, corresponding to a given level of biological response, can be reached with a lower concentration of hormone or neurotransmitter than would be the case if fewer receptors were provided. Economy of hormone or transmitter secretion is thus achieved at the expense of providing more receptors.

COMPETITIVE ANTAGONISM

Though one drug can inhibit the response to another in several ways (see p. 16), competition at the receptor level is particularly important, both in the laboratory and in the clinic, because of the high potency and specificity that can be achieved.

In the presence of a competitive antagonist, the agonist occupancy (i.e. proportion of receptors to which the agonist is bound) at a given agonist concentration is reduced, because the receptor can accommodate only one molecule at a time. However, because the two are in competition, raising the agonist concentration can restore the agonist occupancy (and hence the tissue response). The antagonism is therefore said to be *surmountable*, in contrast to other types of antagonism (see later) where increasing the agonist concentration fails to overcome the blocking effect. A simple theoretical analysis (see p. 20) predicts that in the presence of a fixed concentration of the antagonist, the log concentration–effect curve for the agonist will be shifted to the right, without any change in slope or maximum – the hallmark of competitive antagonism (Fig. 2.4A). The shift is expressed as a *dose ratio*, r (the ratio by which the agonist concentration has to be increased in the presence of the antagonist in order to restore a given level of response). Theory predicts that the dose ratio increases linearly with the concentration of the antagonist (see p. 20). These predictions are often borne out in practice (Fig. 2.5A), providing a relatively simple method for determining the equilibrium dissociation constant of the antagonist (K_B; Fig. 2.5B). Examples of competitive antagonism are very common in pharmacology. The surmountability of the block by the antagonist may be important in practice, because it allows the functional effect of the agonist to be restored by an increase in concentration. With other types of antagonism (as detailed below), the block is usually insurmountable.

The salient features of competitive antagonism are:

• shift of the agonist log concentration–effect curve to the right, without change of slope or maximum (i.e. antagonism can be overcome by increasing the concentration of the agonist)

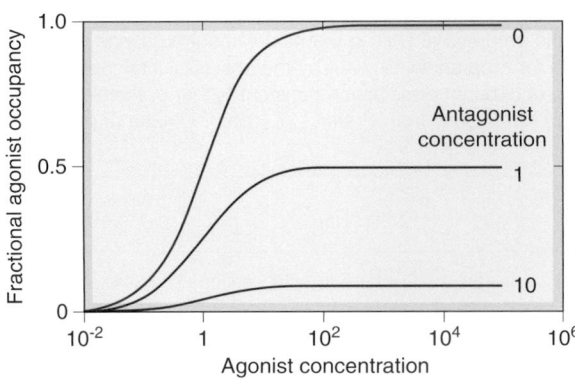

Fig. 2.4 Hypothetical agonist concentration–occupancy curves in the presence of reversible (A) and irreversible (B) competitive antagonists. The concentrations are normalised with respect to the equilibrium dissociation constants, K (i.e. 1.0 corresponds to a concentration equal to K and results in 50% occupancy). Note that in (A) increasing the agonist concentration overcomes the effect of a reversible antagonist (i.e. the block is surmountable), so that the maximal response is unchanged, whereas in (B) the effect of an irreversible antagonist is insurmountable and full agonist occupancy cannot be achieved.

- linear relationship between agonist dose ratio and antagonist concentration
- evidence of competition from binding studies.

Competitive antagonism is the most direct mechanism by which one drug can reduce the effect of another (or of an endogenous mediator).

▼ The characteristics of *reversible competitive antagonism* described above reflect the fact that agonist and competitive antagonist molecules do not stay bound to the receptor but dissociate and rebind continuously. The rate of dissociation of the antagonist molecules is sufficiently high that a new equilibrium is rapidly established on addition of the agonist. In effect, agonist molecules are able to replace the antagonist molecules on the receptors when the antagonist unbinds, although they cannot, of course, evict bound antagonist molecules. Displacement occurs because, by occupying a proportion of the vacant receptors, the agonist effectively reduces the rate of association of the antagonist molecules; consequently, the rate of dissociation temporarily exceeds that of association, and the overall antagonist occupancy falls.

Competitive antagonism

- Reversible competitive antagonism is the commonest and most important type of antagonism; it has two main characteristics.
  - In the presence of the antagonist, the agonist log concentration–effect curve is shifted to the right without change in slope or maximum, the extent of the shift being a measure of the *dose ratio*.
  - The dose ratio increases linearly with antagonist concentration.
- Antagonist affinity, measured in this way, is widely used as a basis for receptor classification.

IRREVERSIBLE COMPETITIVE ANTAGONISM

▼ *Irreversible competitive* (or *non-equilibrium*) *antagonism* occurs when the antagonist binds to the same site on the receptor as the agonist but dissociates very slowly, or not at all, from the receptors, with the result that no change in the antagonist occupancy takes place when the agonist is applied.[4]

The predicted effects of reversible and irreversible antagonists are compared in Fig. 2.4.

In some cases (Fig. 2.6A), the theoretical effect is accurately reproduced with the antagonist reducing the maximum response. However, the distinction between reversible and irreversible competitive antagonism (or even non-competitive antagonism) is not always so clear. This is because of the phenomenon of spare receptors (see p. 10); if the agonist occupancy required to produce a maximal biological response is very small (say 1% of the total receptor pool), then it is possible to block irreversibly nearly 99% of the receptors without reducing the maximal response. The effect of a lesser degree of antagonist occupancy will be to produce a parallel shift of the log concentration–effect curve that is indistinguishable from reversible competitive antagonism (Fig. 2.6B). Only when the antagonist occupancy exceeds 99% will the maximum response will be reduced.

Irreversible competitive antagonism occurs with drugs that possess reactive groups that form covalent bonds with the receptor. These are mainly used as experimental tools for investigating receptor function, and few are used clinically. Irreversible enzyme inhibitors that act similarly are clinically used, however, and include drugs such as **aspirin** (Ch. 27), **omeprazole** (Ch. 31) and monoamine oxidase inhibitors (Ch. 48).

PARTIAL AGONISTS AND THE CONCEPT OF EFFICACY

So far, we have considered drugs either as agonists, which in some way activate the receptor when they occupy it, or as antagonists, which cause no activation. However, the ability of a drug molecule to activate the receptor – namely its efficacy – is actually a graded, rather than an all-or-nothing, property. If a series of chemically related agonist drugs acting on the same receptors is tested on a given biological system, it is often found that the largest response that can be produced differs from one drug to another. Some compounds (known as *full agonists*) can produce a maximal response (the largest response that the tissue is capable of giving), whereas others (*partial agonists*) can produce only a submaximal response. Fig. 2.7A shows concentration–effect curves for several α-adrenoceptor agonists (see Ch. 15), which cause contraction of isolated

---

[4]This type of antagonism is sometimes called non-competitive, but that term is ambiguous and best avoided in this context.

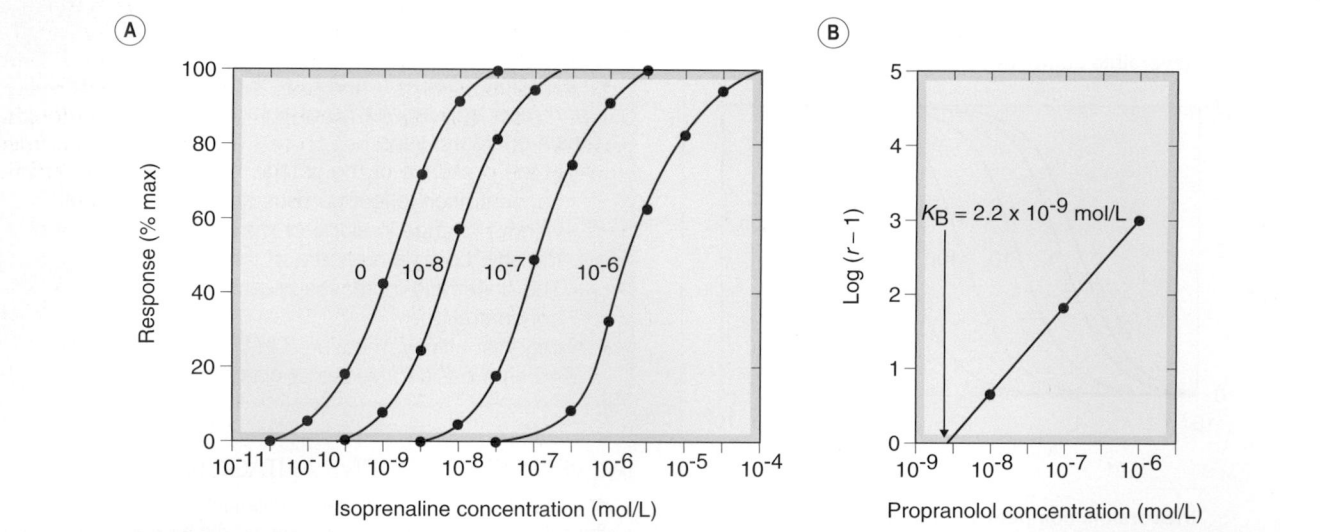

Fig. 2.5 Competitive antagonism of isoprenaline by propranolol measured on isolated guinea pig atria. (A) Concentration–effect curves at various propranolol concentrations (indicated on the curves). Note the progressive shift to the right without a change of slope or maximum. (B) Schild plot (Eq. 2.10). The equilibrium dissociation constant (K_B) for propranolol is given by the abscissal intercept, 2.2×10^{-9} mol/L. Note that the subscript 'B' is now used in 'K_B' to indicate that the equilibrium dissociation constant is that of the antagonist (designated drug B) measured in the presence of the agonist (designated drug A). (Results from Potter, L.T., 1967. Uptake of propranolol by isolated guinea pig atria. J. Pharmacol. Exp. Ther. 55, 91–100.)

Fig. 2.6 Effects of irreversible competitive antagonists on agonist concentration–effect curves. (A) Rat brain neurones responding to the opioid agonist normorphine before and after being exposed to the irreversible competitive antagonist β-funaltrexamine for 30 minutes and then washed to remove the antagonist. Note the depression of the maximum response. (B) Responses of the guinea pig ileum to histamine before and after treatment with increasing concentrations of a receptor alkylating agent (GD121) for 5 minutes and then washed to remove the antagonist. Note the concentration–response curve is initially shifted to the right with no depression of the maximum response. (Panel [A] after Williams, J.T., North, R.A., 1984. Mol. Pharmacol. 26, 489–497; panel [B] after Nickerson, M., 1955. Nature 178, 696–697.)

- ▲ Phenylephrine
- ● Clonidine
- ■ Oxymetazoline
- ▲ Tolazoline
- ■ Naphazoline

Fig. 2.7 Partial agonists. (A) Log concentration–effect curves for a series of α-adrenoceptor agonists causing contraction of an isolated strip of rabbit aorta. Phenylephrine is a full agonist. The others are partial agonists with different efficacies. The lower the efficacy of the drug the lower the maximum response and slope of the log concentration–response curve. (B) The relationship between response and receptor occupancy for the series. Note that the full agonist, phenylephrine, produces a near-maximal response when only about half the receptors are occupied, whereas partial agonists produce submaximal responses even when occupying all of the receptors. The efficacy of tolazoline is so low that it is classified as an α-adrenoceptor antagonist (see Ch. 15). In these experiments, receptor occupancy was not measured directly, but was calculated from pharmacological estimates of the equilibrium constants of the drugs. (Data from Ruffolo, R.R. Jr, et al., 1979. J. Pharmacol. Exp. Ther. 209, 429–436.)

strips of rabbit aorta. The full agonist **phenylephrine** produced the maximal response of which the tissue was capable; the other compounds could only produce submaximal responses and are partial agonists. The difference between full and partial agonists lies in the relationship between receptor occupancy and response. In the experiment shown in Fig. 2.7 it was possible to estimate the affinity of the various drugs for the receptor, and hence (based on the theoretical model described later; p. 19) to calculate the fraction of receptors occupied (known as *occupancy*) as a function of drug concentration. Plots of response as a function of occupancy for the different compounds are shown in Fig. 2.7B, showing that for partial agonists the response at a given level of occupancy is less than for full agonists. The weakest partial agonist, **tolazoline**, produces a barely detectable response even at 100% occupancy, and is usually classified as a *competitive antagonist* (see p. 10 and Ch. 15).

These differences can be expressed quantitatively in terms of *efficacy* (*e*), a parameter originally defined by Stephenson (1956) that describes the 'strength' of the agonist–receptor complex in evoking a response of the tissue. In the simple scheme shown in Fig. 2.1, efficacy describes the tendency of the drug–receptor complex to adopt the active (AR*), rather than the resting (AR), state. A drug with zero efficacy (*e* = 0) has no tendency to cause receptor activation, and causes no tissue response. A full agonist is a drug whose efficacy[5] is sufficient that it produces a maximal response when less than 100% of receptors are occupied. A partial agonist has lower efficacy, such that 100% occupancy elicits only a submaximal response.

▼ Subsequently it was appreciated that efficacy is composed of drug-dependent and tissue-dependent components. The drug-dependent component is referred to as the *intrinsic efficacy*, which is the ability of the agonist drug molecule, once bound, to activate the receptor protein (see Kelly, 2013). The tissue-dependent components of efficacy include the number of receptors that it expresses and the efficiency of coupling of receptor activation to the measured tissue response. The number of receptors expressed is especially relevant to the study of receptors in recombinant expression systems when receptors are often very highly expressed and intermediate efficacy agonists then appear as full agonists. Across different cell types expressing the same receptor but at different densities a given drug of intermediate efficacy may appear as a full agonist in one tissue (high level of receptor expression), a partial agonist in another (lower level of receptor expression), and even as an antagonist in another (very low level of receptor expression). The term 'partial agonist' is therefore only applicable when describing the action of a drug on a specific tissue or cell type.

For G protein–coupled receptors the elucidation of their X-ray crystal structures (described in Ch. 3) and the application of molecular dynamic simulations of drug binding are beginning to tease out the molecular basis of receptor activation and why some ligands are agonists and some are antagonists. For students starting to study pharmacology the simple theoretical two-state model described below provides a useful starting point.

PARTIAL AGONISTS AS ANTAGONISTS

In discussing the efficacy of partial agonists above we considered the situation in which the tissue was exposed

---

[5]In Stephenson's formulation, efficacy is the reciprocal of the occupancy needed to produce a 50% maximal response, thus *e* = 25 implies that a 50% maximal response occurs at 4% occupancy. There is no theoretical upper limit to efficacy.

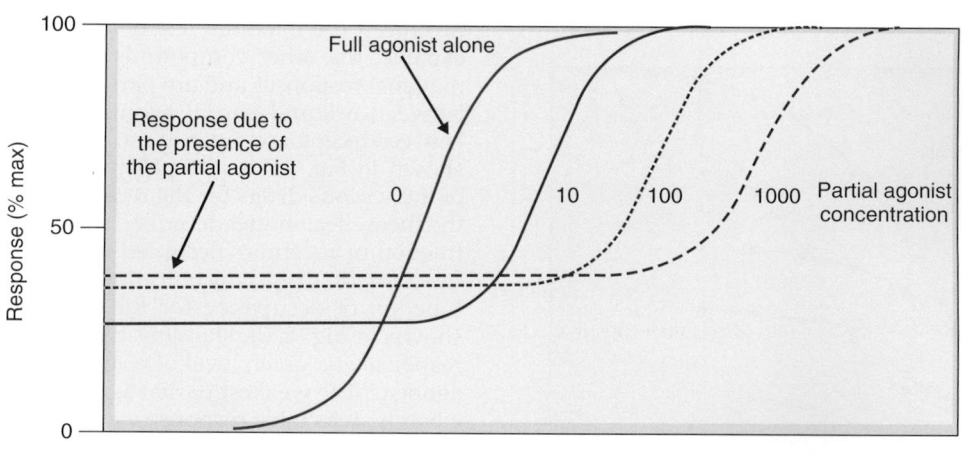

Fig. 2.8 Hypothetical concentration–response curves for a full agonist in the absence and presence of increasing concentrations of a partial agonist. The partial agonist will have agonist action and hence the initial response increases as the partial agonist concentration increases, reaching a maximum equal to the maximum response of the partial agonist. However, when the full agonist is added in the presence of the partial agonist its concentration–response curve is shifted to the right.

to only one drug, the partial agonist. What we should also consider is how the presence of a partial agonist would alter the response of a tissue to a higher efficacy agonist. This is depicted in Fig. 2.8 where it can be seen that the presence of the partial agonist induces some level of response dependent upon the concentration initially applied but in addition because the partial agonist is competing with the full agonist for the receptors it effectively acts as a competitive antagonist, shifting the concentration–response curve of the full agonist to the right. This is not just an obscure theoretical point but something which occurs in clinical practice. In the treatment of heroin users, buprenorphine, a weak partial agonist, not only acts as a weak opioid substitute but also acts as an antagonist and reduces the likelihood of overdose when users relapse and take heroin again (see Ch. 50).

CONSTITUTIVE RECEPTOR ACTIVATION AND INVERSE AGONISTS

▼ Although we are accustomed to thinking that receptors are activated only when an agonist molecule is bound, there are examples (see De Ligt et al., 2000) where an appreciable level of activation (*constitutive activation*) may exist even when no ligand is present. These include receptors for benzodiazepines (see Ch. 45), cannabinoids (Ch. 20), serotonin (Ch. 16) and several other mediators. Furthermore, receptor mutations occur – either spontaneously, in some disease states (see Bond & Ijzerman, 2006), or experimentally created (see Ch. 4) – that result in appreciable constitutive activation. If a ligand reduces the level of constitutive activation; such drugs are known as *inverse agonists* (Fig. 2.9; see De Ligt et al., 2000) to distinguish them from *neutral antagonists*, which do not by themselves affect the level of activation. Inverse agonists can be regarded as drugs with negative efficacy, to distinguish them from agonists (positive efficacy) and neutral antagonists (zero efficacy). Neutral antagonists, by binding to the agonist binding site, will antagonise both agonists and inverse agonists. Inverse agonism was first observed at the benzodiazepine receptor (Ch. 45) but such drugs are proconvulsive and thus not therapeutically useful! New examples of constitutively active receptors and inverse agonists are emerging with increasing frequency (mainly among G protein–coupled receptors). **Pimavanserin**, an inverse agonist at the 5-HT$_{2A}$ receptor, has recently been developed for the treatment of

psychosis associated with Parkinson's disease (see Chs 41 and 47). It turns out that most of the receptor antagonists in clinical use are actually inverse agonists when tested in systems showing constitutive receptor activation. However, most receptors – like cats – show a preference for the inactive state, and for these there is no practical difference between a competitive antagonist and an inverse agonist.

The following section describes a simple model that explains full, partial and inverse agonism in terms of the relative affinity of different ligands for the resting and activated states of the receptor.

The two-state receptor model

▼ As illustrated in Fig. 2.1, agonists and antagonists both bind to receptors, but only agonists activate them. How can we express this difference, and account for constitutive activity, in theoretical terms? The two-state model (Fig. 2.10) provides a simple but useful approach.

As shown in Fig. 2.1, we envisage that the occupied receptor can switch from its 'resting' (R) state to an activated (R*) state, R* being favoured by binding of an agonist but not an antagonist molecule.

As described above, receptors may show constitutive activation (i.e. the R* conformation can exist without any ligand being bound), so the added drug encounters an equilibrium mixture of R and R* (see Fig. 2.10). If it has a higher affinity for R* than for R, the drug will cause a shift of the equilibrium towards R* (i.e. it will promote activation and be classed as an agonist). If its preference for R* is very large, nearly all the occupied receptors will adopt the R* conformation and the drug will be a full agonist; if it shows only a modest degree of selectivity for R* (say 5- to 10-fold), a smaller proportion of occupied receptors will adopt the R* conformation and it will be a partial agonist; if it shows no preference, the prevailing R : R* equilibrium will not be disturbed and the drug will be a neutral antagonist (zero efficacy), whereas if it shows selectivity for R it will shift the equilibrium towards R and be an inverse agonist (negative efficacy). We can therefore think of efficacy as a property determined by the relative affinity of a ligand for R and R*, a formulation known as the *two-state model*, which is useful in that it puts a physical interpretation on the otherwise mysterious meaning of efficacy, as well as accounting for the existence of inverse agonists.

BIASED AGONISM

A major problem with the two-state model is that, as we now know, receptors are not actually restricted to two distinct states but have much greater conformational

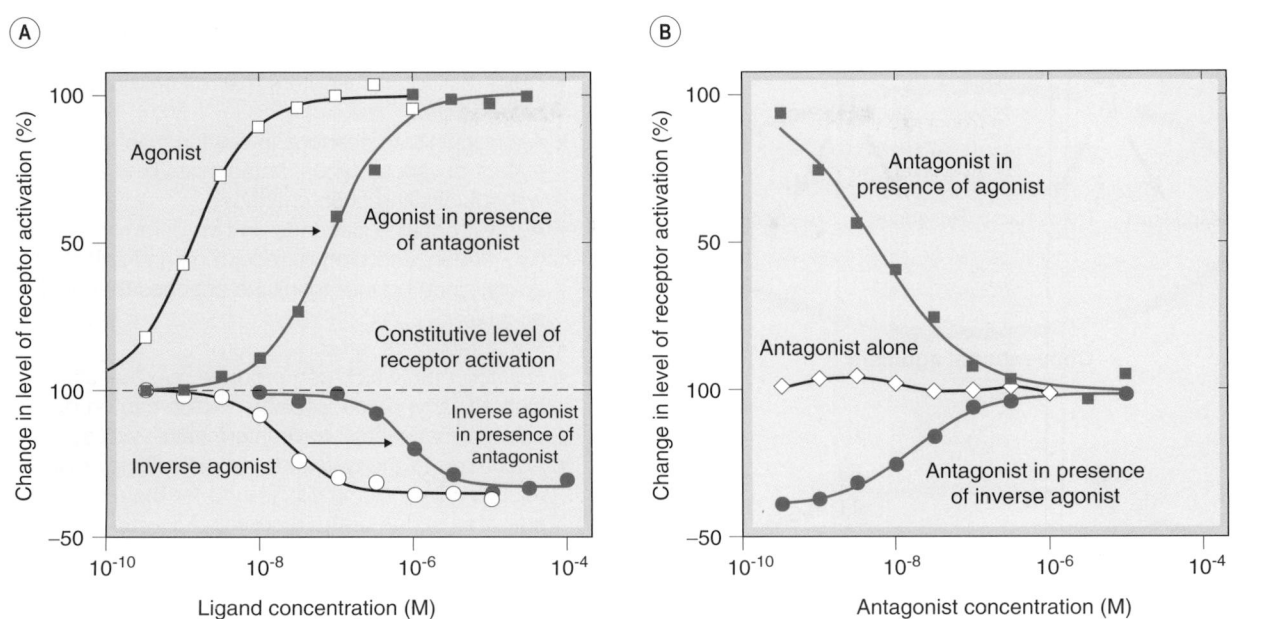

Fig. 2.9 **Inverse agonism.** The interaction of a competitive antagonist with normal and inverse agonists in a system that shows receptor activation in the absence of any added ligands (constitutive activation). (A) The degree of receptor activation (vertical scale) increases in the presence of an agonist *(open squares)* and decreases in the presence of an inverse agonist *(open circles)*. Addition of a competitive antagonist shifts both curves to the right *(closed symbols)*. (B) The antagonist on its own does not alter the level of constitutive activity *(open symbols)*, because it has equal affinity for the active and inactive states of the receptor. In the presence of an agonist *(closed squares)* or an inverse agonist *(closed circles)*, the antagonist restores the system towards the constitutive level of activity. These data (reproduced with permission from Newman-Tancredi, A., et al., 1997. Br. J. Pharmacol. 120, 737–739) were obtained with cloned human 5-hydroxytryptamine (5-HT) receptors expressed in a cell line. (Agonist, 5-carboxamidotryptamine; inverse agonist, spiperone; antagonist, WAY 100635; ligand concentration [M = mol/L]; see Ch. 16 for information on 5-HT receptor pharmacology.)

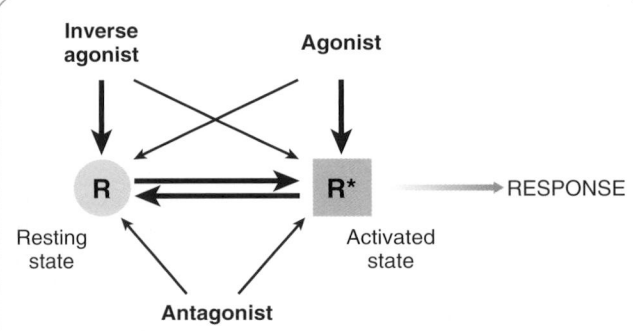

Fig. 2.10 **The two-state model.** The receptor is shown in two conformational states, *resting (R)* and *activated (R*)*, which exist in equilibrium. Normally, when no ligand is present, the equilibrium lies far to the left, and few receptors are found in the R* state. For constitutively active receptors, an appreciable proportion of receptors adopt the R* conformation in the absence of any ligand. Agonists have higher affinity for R* than for R, so shift the equilibrium towards R*. The greater the relative affinity for R* with respect to R, the greater the efficacy of the agonist. An inverse agonist has higher affinity for R than for R* and so shifts the equilibrium to the left. A *neutral* antagonist has equal affinity for R and R* so does not by itself affect the conformational equilibrium but reduces by competition the binding of other ligands.

flexibility, so that there is more than one inactive and active conformation. The different conformations that they can adopt may be preferentially stabilised by different ligands, and may produce different functional effects by activating different signal transduction pathways (see Ch. 3).

Receptors that couple to second messenger systems (see Ch. 3) can couple to more than one intracellular effector pathway, giving rise to two or more simultaneous responses. One might expect that all agonists that activate the same receptor type would evoke the same array of responses (Fig. 2.11A). However, it has become apparent that different agonists can exhibit bias for the generation of one response over another even though they are acting through the same receptor (Fig. 2.11B), probably because they stabilise different activated states of the receptor (see Kelly, 2013). Agonist bias has become an important concept in pharmacology.

Redefining and attempting to measure agonist efficacy for such a multistate model is problematic, however, and requires a more complicated state transition model than the two-state model described above. The errors, pitfalls and a possible way forward have been outlined by Kenakin & Christopoulos (2013).

ALLOSTERIC MODULATION

▼ In addition to the agonist binding site (now referred to as the *orthosteric* binding site), to which competitive antagonists also bind, receptor proteins possess many other *(allosteric)* binding sites (see Ch. 3) through which drugs can influence receptor function in various ways, by increasing or decreasing the affinity of agonists

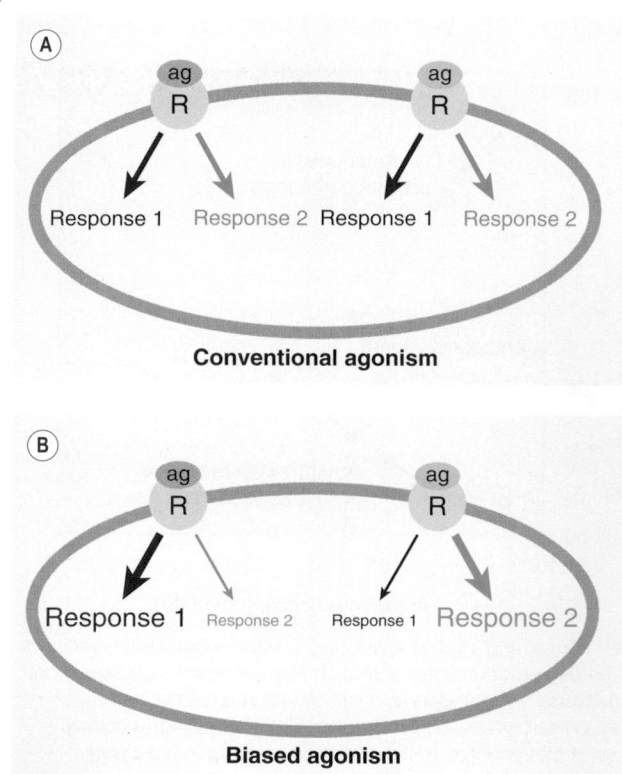

Fig. 2.11 **Biased agonism.** In (A), the receptor *(R)* is coupled to two intracellular responses – *response 1* and *response 2*. When different agonists indicated in *red* and *green* activate the receptor they evoke both responses in a similar manner. This is what we can consider as being conventional agonism. In (B), biased agonism is illustrated in which two agonists bind at the same site on the receptor yet the *red* agonist is better at evoking response 1 and the *green* agonist is better at evoking response 2.

Agonists, antagonists and efficacy

- Drugs acting on receptors may be *agonists* or *antagonists*.
- Agonists initiate changes in cell function, producing effects of various types; antagonists bind to receptors without initiating such changes.
- Agonist potency depends on two parameters: *affinity* (i.e. tendency to bind to receptors) and *efficacy* (i.e. ability, once bound, to initiate changes that lead to effects).
- For antagonists, efficacy is zero.
- *Full agonists* (which can produce maximal effects) have high efficacy; *partial agonists* (which can produce only submaximal effects) have intermediate efficacy.
- According to the two-state model, efficacy reflects the relative affinity of the compound for the resting and activated states of the receptor. Agonists show selectivity for the activated state; antagonists show no selectivity. This model, although helpful, fails to account for the complexity of agonist action.
- *Inverse agonists* show selectivity for the resting state of the receptor, this being of significance only in situations where the receptors show *constitutive activity*.
- *Allosteric modulators* bind to sites on the receptor other than the agonist binding site and can modify agonist activity.

for the agonist binding site, by modifying efficacy or by producing a response themselves (Fig. 2.12). Depending on the direction of the effect, the ligands may be allosteric antagonists or allosteric facilitators of the agonist effect, and the effect may be to alter the slope and maximum of the agonist log concentration–effect curve (see Fig. 2.12). This type of allosteric modulation of receptor function has attracted much attention recently and occurs at different types of receptors (see review by Changeux & Christopoulos, 2016). Well-known examples of allosteric facilitation include glycine at NMDA receptors (Ch. 39), benzodiazepines at $GABA_A$ receptors (Ch. 45) and **cinacalcet** at the Ca^{2+} receptor (Ch. 37). One reason why allosteric modulation may be important to the pharmacologist and future drug development is that across families of receptors such as the muscarinic receptors (see Ch. 14) the orthosteric binding sites are very similar and it has proven difficult to develop selective agonists and antagonists for individual subtypes. The hope is that there will be greater variation in the allosteric sites and that receptor-selective allosteric ligands can be developed. Furthermore, positive allosteric modulators will exert their effects only on receptors that are being activated by endogenous ligands and have no effect on those that are not activated. This might provide a degree of selectivity (e.g. in potentiating spinal inhibition mediated by endogenous opioids, see Ch. 43) and a reduction in side effect profile.

OTHER FORMS OF DRUG ANTAGONISM

Other mechanisms can also account for inhibitory interactions between drugs.

The most important ones are:

- chemical antagonism
- pharmacokinetic antagonism
- block of receptor–response linkage
- physiological antagonism

CHEMICAL ANTAGONISM

Chemical antagonism refers to the uncommon situation where the two substances combine in solution; as a result, the effect of the active drug is lost. Examples include the use of chelating agents (e.g. **dimercaprol**) that bind to heavy metals and thus reduce their toxicity, and the use of the neutralising antibody **infliximab**, which has an anti-inflammatory action due to its ability to sequester the inflammatory cytokine tumour necrosis factor (TNF; see Ch. 19).

PHARMACOKINETIC ANTAGONISM

Pharmacokinetic antagonism describes the situation in which the 'antagonist' effectively reduces the concentration of the active drug at its site of action. This can happen in various ways. The rate of metabolic degradation of the active drug may be increased (e.g. the reduction of the anticoagulant effect of **warfarin** when an agent that accelerates its hepatic metabolism, such as **phenytoin**, is given; see Chs 10 and 58). Alternatively, the rate of absorption of the active drug from the gastrointestinal tract may be reduced, or the rate of renal excretion may be increased. Interactions of this sort, discussed in more detail in Chapter 58, are common and can be important in clinical practice.

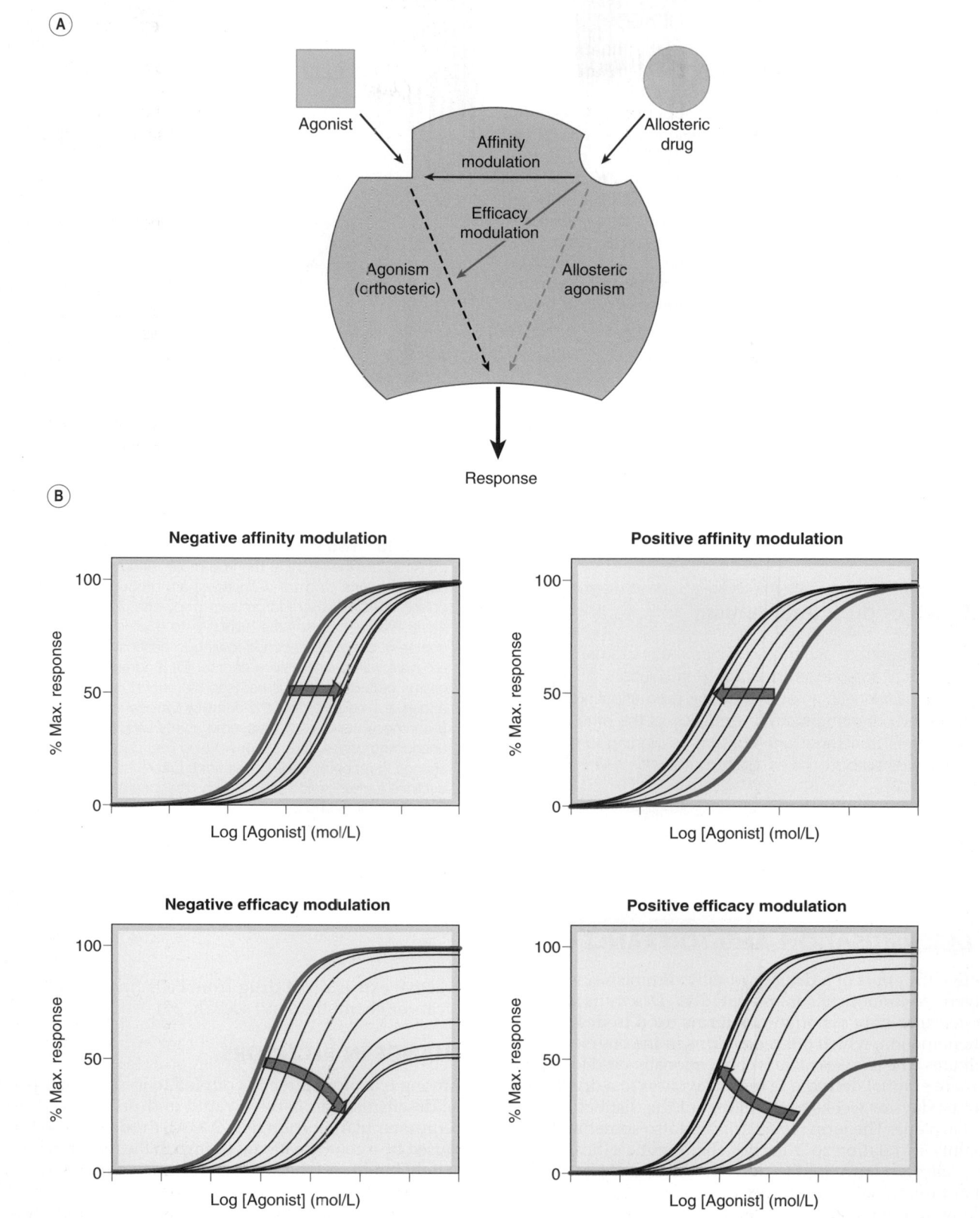

Fig. 2.12   Allosteric modulation. (A) Allosteric drugs bind at a separate site on the receptor to 'traditional' agonists (now often referred to as 'orthosteric' agonists). They can modify the activity of the receptor by (i) altering agonist affinity, (ii) altering agonist efficacy or (iii) directly evoking a response themselves. (B) Effects of affinity- and efficacy-modifying allosteric modulators on the concentration–effect curve of an agonist *(blue line)*. In the presence of the allosteric modulator the agonist concentration–effect curve *(now illustrated in red)* is shifted in a manner determined by the type of allosteric modulator until a maximum effect of the modulator is reached. (Panel [A] adapted with permission from Conn et al., 2009. Nat. Rev. Drug Discov. 8, 41–54; panel [B] courtesy of Christopoulos, A.)

BLOCK OF RECEPTOR–RESPONSE LINKAGE

Non-competitive antagonism describes the situation where the antagonist blocks at some point downstream from the agonist binding site on the receptor, and interrupts the chain of events that leads to the production of a response by the agonist. For example, **ketamine** enters the ion channel pore of the NMDA receptor (see Ch. 39) blocking it, thus preventing ion flux through the channels. Drugs such as **verapamil** and **nifedipine** prevent the influx of Ca^{2+} through the cell membrane (see Ch. 23) and thus non-selectively block the contraction of smooth muscle produced by drugs acting at any receptor that couples to these calcium channels. As a rule, the effect will be to reduce the slope and maximum of the agonist log concentration–response curve, although it is quite possible for some degree of rightward shift to occur as well.

PHYSIOLOGICAL ANTAGONISM

Physiological antagonism is a term used loosely to describe the interaction of two drugs whose opposing actions in the body tend to cancel each other. For example, **histamine** acts on receptors of the parietal cells of the gastric mucosa to stimulate acid secretion, while **omeprazole** blocks this effect by inhibiting the proton pump; the two drugs can be said to act as physiological antagonists.

Types of drug antagonism

Drug antagonism occurs by various mechanisms:
- chemical antagonism (interaction in solution)
- pharmacokinetic antagonism (one drug affecting the absorption, metabolism or excretion of the other)
- competitive antagonism (both drugs binding to the same receptors); the antagonism may be reversible or irreversible
- interruption of receptor–response linkage
- physiological antagonism (two agents producing opposing physiological effects)

DESENSITISATION AND TOLERANCE

Often, the effect of a drug gradually diminishes when it is given continuously or repeatedly. *Desensitisation* and *tachyphylaxis* are synonymous terms used to describe this phenomenon, which often develops in the course of a few minutes. The term *tolerance* is conventionally used to describe a more gradual decrease in responsiveness to a drug, taking hours, days or weeks to develop, but the distinction is not a sharp one. The term *refractoriness* is also sometimes used, mainly in relation to a loss of therapeutic efficacy. *Drug resistance* is a term used to describe the loss of effectiveness of antimicrobial or antitumour drugs (see Chs 51 and 57). Many different mechanisms can give rise to these phenomena. They include:

- change in receptors
- translocation of receptors
- exhaustion of mediators
- increased metabolic degradation of the drug
- physiological adaptation

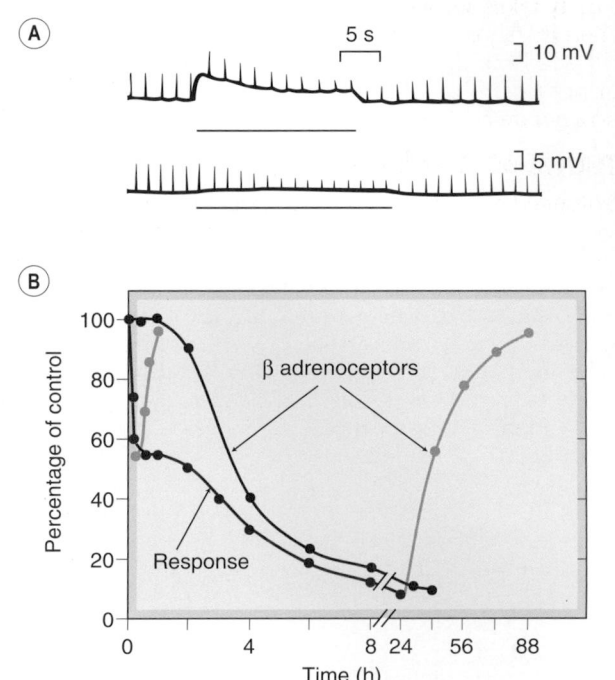

Fig. 2.13 Two kinds of receptor desensitisation.
(A) Acetylcholine (ACh) at the frog motor endplate. Brief depolarisations *(upward deflections)* are produced by short pulses of ACh delivered from a micropipette. A long pulse *(horizontal line)* causes the response to decline with a time course of about 20 seconds, owing to desensitisation, and it recovers with a similar time course. (B) β adrenoceptors of rat glioma cells in tissue culture. Isoproterenol (1 μmol/L) was added at time zero, and the adenylyl cyclase response and β-adrenoceptor density measured at intervals. During the early uncoupling phase, the response *(blue line)* declines with no change in receptor density *(red line)*. Later, the response declines further concomitantly with disappearance of receptors from the membrane by internalisation. The *green* and *orange* lines show the recovery of the response and receptor density after the isoproterenol is washed out during the early or late phase. (Panel [A] from Katz B., Thesleff S., 1957. J. Physiol. 138, 63; panel [B] from Perkins, J.P., 1981. Trends Pharmacol. Sci. 2, 326.)

- active extrusion of drug from cells (mainly relevant in cancer chemotherapy; see Ch. 57)

CHANGE IN RECEPTORS

Among receptors directly coupled to ion channels (see Ch. 3), desensitisation is often rapid and pronounced. At the neuromuscular junction (Fig. 2.13A), the desensitised state is caused by a conformational change in the receptor, resulting in tight binding of the agonist molecule without the opening of the ionic channel. Phosphorylation of intracellular regions of the receptor protein is a second, slower mechanism by which ion channels become desensitised.

Most G protein–coupled receptors (see Ch. 3) also show desensitisation (Fig. 2.13B). Phosphorylation of the receptor interferes with its ability to activate second messenger cascades, although it can still bind the agonist molecule. The molecular mechanisms of this 'uncoupling' are considered further in Chapter 3. This type of desensitisation usually takes seconds to minutes to develop, and recovers when the agonist is removed.

It will be realised that the two-state model in its simple form, discussed earlier, needs to be further elaborated to incorporate additional desensitised states of the receptor.

TRANSLOCATION OF RECEPTORS

Prolonged exposure to agonists often results in a gradual decrease in the number of receptors expressed on the cell surface, as a result of *internalisation* of the receptors. This is shown for β adrenoceptors in Fig. 2.13B and is a slower process than the uncoupling described above. Similar changes have been described for other types of receptor, including those for various peptides. The internalised receptors are taken into the cell by endocytosis of patches of the membrane, a process that normally depends on receptor phosphorylation and the subsequent binding of *arrestin* proteins to the phosphorylated receptor (see Ch. 3, Fig. 3.16). This type of adaptation is common for hormone receptors and has obvious relevance to the effects produced when drugs are given for extended periods. It is generally an unwanted complication when agonist drugs are used clinically.

EXHAUSTION OF MEDIATORS

In some cases, desensitisation is associated with depletion of an essential intermediate substance. Drugs such as **amphetamine**, which acts by releasing amines from nerve terminals (see Chs 15 and 49), show marked tachyphylaxis because the amine stores become depleted.

ALTERED DRUG METABOLISM

Tolerance to some drugs, for example **barbiturates** and **ethanol** (Ch. 49), occurs partly because repeated administration of the same dose produces a progressively lower plasma concentration, as a result of increased metabolic degradation. The degree of tolerance that results is generally modest, and in both of these examples other mechanisms contribute to the substantial tolerance that actually occurs. However, the pronounced tolerance to **nitrovasodilators** (see Chs 21 and 23) results mainly from decreased metabolism, which reduces the release of the active mediator, nitric oxide.

PHYSIOLOGICAL ADAPTATION

Diminution of a drug's effect may occur because it is nullified by a homeostatic response. For example, the blood pressure-lowering effect of **thiazide diuretics** is limited because of a gradual activation of the renin–angiotensin system (see Ch. 23). Such homeostatic mechanisms are very common, and if they occur slowly the result will be a gradually developing tolerance. It is a common experience that many side effects of drugs, such as nausea or sleepiness, tend to subside even though drug administration is continued. We may assume that some kind of physiological adaptation is occurring, presumably associated with altered gene expression resulting in changes in the levels of various regulatory molecules, but little is known about the mechanisms involved.

QUANTITATIVE ASPECTS OF DRUG–RECEPTOR INTERACTIONS

▼ Here we present some aspects of so-called receptor theory, which is based on applying the Law of Mass Action to the drug–receptor interaction and which has served well as a framework for interpreting a large body of quantitative experimental data (see Colquhoun, 2006).

THE BINDING REACTION

▼ The first step in drug action on specific receptors is the formation of a reversible drug–receptor complex, the reactions being governed by the Law of Mass Action. Suppose that a piece of tissue, such as heart muscle or smooth muscle, contains a total number of receptors, N_{tot}, for an agonist such as adrenaline. When the tissue is exposed to adrenaline at concentration x_A and allowed to come to equilibrium, a certain number, N_A, of the receptors will become occupied, and the number of vacant receptors will be reduced to $N_{tot} - N_A$. Normally, the number of adrenaline molecules applied to the tissue in solution greatly exceeds N_{tot}, so that the binding reaction does not appreciably reduce x_A. The magnitude of the response produced by the adrenaline will be related (even if we do not know exactly how) to the number of receptors occupied, so it is useful to consider what quantitative relationship is predicted between N_A and x_A. The reaction can be represented by:

$$\begin{array}{cccc} A & + & R & \xrightleftharpoons[k_{-1}]{k_{+1}} & AR \\ \text{drug} & + & \text{free receptor} & & \text{complex} \\ (x_A) & & (N_{tot} - N_A) & & (N_A) \end{array}$$

The Law of Mass Action (which states that the rate of a chemical reaction is proportional to the product of the concentrations of reactants) can be applied to this reaction.

$$\text{Rate of forward reaction} = k_{+1}x_A(N_{tot} - N_A) \qquad (2.1)$$

$$\text{Rate of backward reaction} = k_{-1}N_A \qquad (2.2)$$

At equilibrium, the two rates are equal:

$$k_{+1}x_A(N_{tot} - N_A) = k_{-1}N_A \qquad (2.3)$$

The *affinity constant* of binding is given by k_{+1}/k_{-1} and from Eq. 2.3 equals $N_A/x_A(N_{tot} - N_A)$. Unfortunately, this has units of reciprocal concentration (L/mol) which for some of us is a little hard to get our heads around. Pharmacologists therefore tend to use the reciprocal of the affinity constant, the *equilibrium dissociation constant (K)*, which has units of concentration (mol/L).

For drug A its equilibrium dissociation constant (K_A)[6] can be represented as

$$K_A = k_{-1}/k_{+1} = x_A(N_{tot} - N_A)/N_A \qquad (2.4)$$

The proportion of receptors occupied, or occupancy (P_A), is N_A/N_{tot}, which is independent of N_{tot}.

$$P_A = \frac{x_A}{x_A + k_{-1}/k_{+1}} = \frac{x_A}{x_A + K_A} \qquad (2.5)$$

Thus if the equilibrium dissociation constant of a drug is known we can calculate the proportion of receptors it will occupy at any concentration.

Eq. 2.5 can be written:

$$P_A = \frac{x_A/K_A}{x_A/K_A + 1} \qquad (2.6)$$

This important result is known as the Hill–Langmuir equation.[7]

---

[6]Here we now use 'K_A' rather than just 'K' because we will in the next section be going on to consider the situation when two drugs, A and B, are present and there we will use 'K_A' and 'K_B' to denote the equilibrium dissociation constants of the two drugs.

[7]A.V. Hill first published it in 1909, when he was still a medical student. Langmuir, a physical chemist working on gas adsorption, derived it independently in 1916. Both subsequently won Nobel Prizes. Until recently, it was known to pharmacologists as the Langmuir equation, even though Hill deserves the credit.

Fig. 2.14 **Theoretical relationship between occupancy and ligand concentration.** The relationship is plotted according to Eq. 2.5. (A) Plotted with a linear concentration scale, this curve is a rectangular hyperbola. (B) Plotted with a log concentration scale, it is a symmetrical sigmoid curve. K_A is defined in the text and footnote 6.

The *equilibrium dissociation constant*, K_A, is a characteristic of the drug and of the receptor; it has the dimensions of concentration and is numerically equal to the concentration of drug required to occupy 50% of the sites at equilibrium. (Verify from Eq. 2.5 that when $x_A = K_A$ then $P_A = 0.5$.) The higher the affinity of the drug for the receptors, the lower will be the value of K_A. Eq. 2.6 describes the relationship between occupancy and drug concentration, and it generates a characteristic curve known as a *rectangular hyperbola*, as shown in Fig. 2.14A. It is common in pharmacological work to use a logarithmic scale of concentration; this converts the hyperbola to a symmetrical sigmoid curve (Fig. 2.14B).

The same approach is used to analyse data from experiments in which drug binding is measured directly (see pp. 8–9, Fig. 2.2). In this case, the relationship between the amount bound (*B*) and ligand concentration (x_A) should be:

$$B = B_{max} x_A / (x_A + K_A) \tag{2.7}$$

where B_{max} is the total number of binding sites in the preparation (often expressed as pmol/mg of protein). To display the results in linear form, Eq. 2.6 may be rearranged to:

$$B/x_A = B_{max}/K_A - B/K_A \tag{2.8}$$

A plot of B/x_A against B (known as a *Scatchard plot*) gives a straight line from which both B_{max} and K_A can be estimated. Statistically, this procedure is not without problems, and it is now usual to estimate these parameters from the untransformed binding values by an iterative non-linear curve-fitting procedure.

To this point, our analysis has considered the binding of one ligand to a homogeneous population of receptors. To get closer to real-life pharmacology, we must consider (a) what happens when more than one ligand is present, and (b) how the tissue response is related to receptor occupancy.

BINDING WHEN MORE THAN ONE DRUG IS PRESENT

▼ Suppose that two drugs, A and B, which bind to the same receptor with equilibrium dissociation constants K_A and K_B, respectively, are present at concentrations x_A and x_B. If the two drugs compete (i.e. the receptor can accommodate only one at a time), then, by application of the same reasoning as for the one-drug situation described above, the occupancy by drug A is given by:

$$P_A = \frac{x_A/K_A}{x_A/K_A + x_B/K_B + 1} \tag{2.9}$$

Comparing this result with Eq. 2.5 shows that adding drug B, as expected, reduces the occupancy by drug A. Fig. 2.4A (p. 11) shows the predicted binding curves for A in the presence of increasing concentrations of B, demonstrating the shift without any change of slope or maximum that characterises the pharmacological effect of a competitive antagonist (see Fig. 2.5). The extent of the rightward shift, on a logarithmic scale, represents the ratio (r_A, given by x_A'/x_A where x_A' is the increased concentration of A) by which the concentration of A must be increased to overcome the competition by B. Rearranging Eq. 2.9 shows that

$$r_A = (x_B/K_B) + 1 \tag{2.10}$$

Thus r_A depends only on the concentration and equilibrium dissociation constant of the competing drug B, not on the concentration or equilibrium dissociation constant of A.

If A is an agonist, and B is a competitive antagonist, and we assume that the response of the tissue will be an unknown function of P_A, then the value of r_A determined from the shift of the agonist concentration–effect curve at different antagonist concentrations can be used to estimate the equilibrium dissociation constant K_B for the antagonist. Such pharmacological estimates of r_A are commonly termed *agonist dose ratios* (more properly concentration ratios, although most pharmacologists use the older term). This simple and very useful Eq. (2.10) is known as the *Schild equation*, after the pharmacologist who first used it to analyse drug antagonism.

Eq. 2.10 can be expressed logarithmically in the form:

$$\log(r_A - 1) = \log x_B - \log K_B \tag{2.11}$$

Thus a plot of log (r_A–1) against log x_B, usually called a *Schild plot* (as in Fig. 2.5, earlier), should give a straight line with unit slope (i.e. its gradient is equal to 1) and an abscissal intercept equal to log K_B. Following the pH and pK notation, antagonist potency can be expressed as a pA_2 value; under conditions of competitive antagonism, $pA_2 = -\log K_B$. Numerically, pA_2 is defined as the negative logarithm of the molar concentration of antagonist required to produce an agonist dose ratio equal to 2. As with pH notation, its principal advantage is that it produces simple numbers, a pA_2 of 6.5 being equivalent to a K_B of 3.2×10^{-7} mol/L.

For competitive antagonism, *r* shows the following characteristics:

- It depends only on the concentration and equilibrium dissociation constant of the antagonist, and not on the size of response that is chosen as a reference point for the measurements (so long as it is submaximal).
- It does not depend on the equilibrium dissociation constant of the agonist.
- It increases linearly with x_B, and the slope of a plot of (r_A–1) against x_B is equal to $1/K_B$; this relationship, being independent of the characteristics of the agonist, should be the same for an antagonist against all agonists that act on the same population of receptors.

These predictions have been verified for many examples of competitive antagonism (see Fig. 2.5).

In this section, we have avoided going into great detail and have oversimplified the theory considerably. As we learn more about the actual molecular details of how receptors work to produce their biological effects (see Ch. 3), the shortcomings of this theoretical treatment become more obvious. The two-state model can be incorporated without difficulty, but complications arise when we include the involvement of G proteins (see Ch. 3) in the reaction scheme (as they shift the equilibrium between R and R*), and when we allow for the fact that receptor activation is not a simple on–off switch, as the two-state model assumes, but may take different forms. Despite strenuous efforts by theoreticians to allow for such possibilities, the molecules always seem to remain one step ahead. Nevertheless, this type of basic theory applied to the two-state model remains a useful basis for developing quantitative models of drug action. The book by Kenakin (1997) is recommended as an introduction, and the later review (Kenakin & Christopoulos, 2011) presents a detailed account of the value of quantification in the study of drug action.

Fig. 2.15 **Early and late responses to drugs.** Many drugs act directly on their targets *(left-hand arrow)* to produce a rapid physiological response. If this is maintained, it is likely to cause changes in gene expression that give rise to delayed effects. Some drugs *(right-hand arrow)* have their primary action on gene expression, producing delayed physiological responses. Drugs can also work by both pathways. Note the bidirectional interaction between gene expression and response.

Binding of drugs to receptors

- Binding of drugs to receptors necessarily obeys the *Law of Mass Action*.
- At equilibrium, receptor occupancy is related to drug concentration by the *Hill–Langmuir equation* (Eq. 2.6).
- The higher the affinity of the drug for the receptor, the lower the concentration at which it produces a given level of occupancy.
- The same principles apply when two or more drugs compete for the same receptors; each has the effect of reducing the apparent affinity for the other.

THE NATURE OF DRUG EFFECTS

In discussing how drugs act in this chapter, we have focused mainly on the rapid consequences of receptor activation. Details of the receptors and their linkage to effects at the cellular level are described in Chapter 3. We now have a fairly good understanding at this level. It is important, however, particularly when considering drugs in a therapeutic context, that their direct effects on cellular function generally lead to secondary, delayed effects, which are often highly relevant in a clinical situation in relation to both therapeutic efficacy and harmful effects (Fig. 2.15). For example, activation of cardiac β adrenoceptors (see Chs 3 and 22) causes rapid changes in the functioning of the heart muscle, but also slower (minutes to hours) changes in the functional state of the receptors (e.g. desensitisation), and even slower (hours to days) changes in gene expression that produce long-term changes (e.g. hypertrophy) in cardiac structure and function. Opioids (see Ch. 43) produce an immediate analgesic effect, but after a time, tolerance and dependence ensue, and in some cases long-term addiction. In these and many other examples, the nature of the intervening mechanism is unclear, although as a general rule any long-term phenotypic change necessarily involves alterations of gene expression. Drugs are often used to treat chronic conditions, and understanding long-term as well

as acute drug effects is becoming increasingly important. Pharmacologists have traditionally tended to focus on short-term physiological responses, which are much easier to study, rather than on delayed effects. The focus is now clearly shifting.

Drug effects

- Drugs act mainly on cellular targets, producing effects at different functional levels (e.g. biochemical, cellular, physiological and structural).
- The direct effect of the drug on its target produces acute responses at the biochemical, cellular or physiological levels.
- Prolonged receptor activation generally leads to *delayed long-term effects*, such as desensitisation or down-regulation of receptors, hypertrophy, atrophy or remodelling of tissues, tolerance, dependence and addiction.
- Long-term delayed responses result from changes in gene expression, although the mechanisms by which the acute effects bring this about are often uncertain.
- Therapeutic effects may be based on acute responses (e.g. the use of bronchodilator drugs to treat asthma; Ch. 29) or delayed responses (e.g. antidepressants; Ch. 48).

REFERENCES AND FURTHER READING

General

Alexander, S.P.H., Kelly, E., Marrion, N., et al., 2015. The Concise Guide to Pharmacology. Br. J. Pharmacol. 172, 5729–6202. (*Summary data on a vast array of receptors, ion channels, transporters and enzymes and of the drugs that interact with them – valuable for reference*)

Colquhoun, D., 2006. The quantitative analysis of drug–receptor interactions: a short history. Trends Pharmacol. Sci. 27, 149–157. (*An illuminating account for those interested in the origins of one of the central ideas in pharmacology*)

Franks, N.P., 2008. General anaesthesia: from molecular targets to neuronal pathways of sleep and arousal. Nat. Rev. Neurosci. 9, 370–386. (*Describes how we now understand that general anaesthetics interact with specific membrane proteins rather than by accumulating in membrane lipids*)

Kenakin, T., 1997. Pharmacologic Analysis of Drug–Receptor Interactions, third ed. Lippincott-Raven, New York. (*Useful and detailed textbook covering most of the material in this chapter in greater depth*)

Kenakin, T., Christopoulos, A., 2013. Signalling bias in new drug discovery: detection, quantification and therapeutic impact. Nat. Rev. Drug Discov. 12, 205–216. (*Detailed discussion of the difficulties in measuring agonist efficacy and bias*)

Neubig, R., Spedding, M., Kenakin, T., Christopoulos, A., 2003. International Union of Pharmacology Committee on receptor nomenclature and drug classification: XXXVIII. Update on terms and symbols in quantitative pharmacology. Pharmacol. Rev. 55, 597–606. (*Summary of IUPHAR-approved terms and symbols relating to pharmacological receptors – useful for reference purposes*)

Rang, H.P., 2006. The receptor concept: pharmacology's big idea. Br. J. Pharmacol. 147 (Suppl. 1), 9–16. (*Short review of the origin and status of the receptor concept*)

Stephenson, R.P., 1956. A modification of receptor theory. Br. J. Pharmacol. 11, 379–393. (*Classic analysis of receptor action introducing the concept of efficacy*)

Receptor mechanisms: agonists and efficacy

Bond, R.A., Ijzerman, A.P., 2006. Recent developments in constitutive receptor activity and inverse agonism, and their potential for GPCR drug discovery. Trends Pharmacol. Sci. 27, 92–96. (*Discussion of pathophysiological consequences of constitutive receptor activation and therapeutic potential of inverse agonists*)

Changeux, J.P., Christopoulos, A., 2016. Allosteric modulation as a unifying mechanism for receptor function and regulation. Cell 166, 1084–1102. (*Extensive review describing allosteric modulation at different types of receptor*)

De Ligt, R.A.F., Kourounakis, A.P., Ijzerman, A.P., 2000. Inverse agonism at G protein-coupled receptors: (patho)physiological relevance and implications for drug discovery. Br. J. Pharmacol. 130, 1–12. (*Useful review article giving many examples of constitutively active receptors and inverse agonists, and discussing the relevance of these concepts for disease mechanisms and drug discovery*)

Kelly, E., 2013. Efficacy and ligand bias at the μ-opioid receptor. Br. J. Pharmacol. 169, 1430–1446. (*A readable account of the problems of measuring efficacy as well as a discussion of agonist bias at an important receptor*)

Kenakin, T., Christopoulos, A., 2011. Analytical pharmacology: the impact of numbers on pharmacology. Trends Pharmacol. Sci. 32, 189–196. (*A theoretical treatment that attempts to take into account recent knowledge of receptor function at the molecular level*)

May, L.T., Leach, K., Sexton, P.M., Christopoulos, A., 2007. Allosteric modulation of G protein-coupled receptors. Annu. Rev. Pharmacol. Toxicol. 47, 1–51. (*Comprehensive review describing the characteristics, mechanisms and pharmacological implications of allosteric interactions at GPCRs*)

How drugs act: molecular aspects

3

OVERVIEW

In this chapter, we move from the general principles of drug action outlined in Chapter 2 to the molecules that are involved in recognising chemical signals and translating them into cellular responses. Molecular pharmacology is advancing rapidly, and the new knowledge is changing our understanding of drug action and opening up many new therapeutic possibilities, further discussed in other chapters.

First, we consider the types of target proteins on which drugs act. Next, we describe the main families of receptors and ion channels. Finally, we discuss the various forms of receptor–effector linkage (signal transduction mechanisms) through which receptors are coupled to the regulation of cell function. The relationship between the molecular structure of a receptor and its functional linkage to a particular type of effector system is a principal theme. In the next two chapters, we see how these molecular events alter important aspects of cell function – a useful basis for understanding the effects of drugs on intact living organisms. We are confident that tomorrow's pharmacology will rest solidly on the advances in cellular and molecular biology that are discussed here.

PROTEIN TARGETS FOR DRUG ACTION

The protein targets for drug action on mammalian cells (Fig. 3.1) that are described in this chapter can be broadly divided into:

- receptors
- ion channels
- enzymes
- transporters (carrier molecules)

The great majority of important drugs act on one or other of these types of protein, but there are exceptions. For example, **colchicine** used to treat arthritic gout attacks (Ch. 27) interacts with the structural protein tubulin, while several immunosuppressive drugs (e.g. **ciclosporin**, Ch. 27) bind to cytosolic proteins known as immunophilins. Therapeutic antibodies that act by sequestering cytokines (protein mediators involved in inflammation; see Chs 5 and 27) are also used. Targets for chemotherapeutic drugs (Chs 51–57), where the aim is to suppress invading microorganisms or cancer cells, include DNA and cell wall constituents as well as other proteins.

RECEPTORS

Receptors (see Fig. 3.1A) are the sensing elements in the system of chemical communications that coordinates the function and responses of all the different cells in the body, the chemical messengers being the various hormones, transmitters and other mediators discussed in Section 2 of this book. Many therapeutically useful drugs act, either as agonists or antagonists, on receptors for known endogenous mediators. In most cases, the endogenous mediator was discovered before – often many years before – the receptor was characterised pharmacologically and biochemically. In some cases, such as the cannabinoid and opioid receptors (see Chs 20 and 43), the endogenous mediators were identified later; in others, known as *orphan receptors* (see later) the mediator, if it exists, still remains unknown. The host defence system also utilises a set of receptors (e.g. the 'Toll' receptors) that are adept at recognising fragments of 'foreign' bacterial and other invading organisms. These are considered separately in Chapter 7.

ION CHANNELS

Ion channels[1] are essentially gateways in cell membranes that selectively allow the passage of particular ions, and that are induced to open or close by a variety of mechanisms. Two important types are *ligand-gated channels* and *voltage-gated channels*. The former open only when one or more agonist molecules are bound, and are properly classified as receptors, since agonist binding is needed to activate them. Voltage-gated channels are gated by changes in the transmembrane potential rather than by agonist binding.

In general, drugs can affect ion channel function in several ways:

1. By binding to the channel protein itself, either to the ligand-binding (*orthosteric*) site of ligand-gated channels, or to other (*allosteric*) sites, or, in the simplest case, exemplified by the action of local anaesthetics on the voltage-gated sodium channel (see Ch. 44), the drug molecule plugs the channel physically (see Fig. 3.1B), blocking ion permeation. Examples of drugs that bind to allosteric sites on the channel protein and thereby affect channel gating include:
   - **benzodiazepine**s (see Ch. 45). These drugs bind to a region of the GABA$_A$ receptor–chloride channel complex (a ligand-gated channel) that is distinct from the GABA binding site and facilitate the opening of the channel by the inhibitory neurotransmitter GABA (see Ch. 39)
   - vasodilator drugs of the **dihydropyridine** type (see Ch. 23), which inhibit the opening of L-type calcium channels (see Ch. 4).

---

[1] 'Ion channels and the electrical properties they confer on cells are involved in every human characteristic that distinguishes us from the stones in a field' (Armstrong, C.M., 2003. Voltage-gated K channels. Sci. STKE 188, re10).

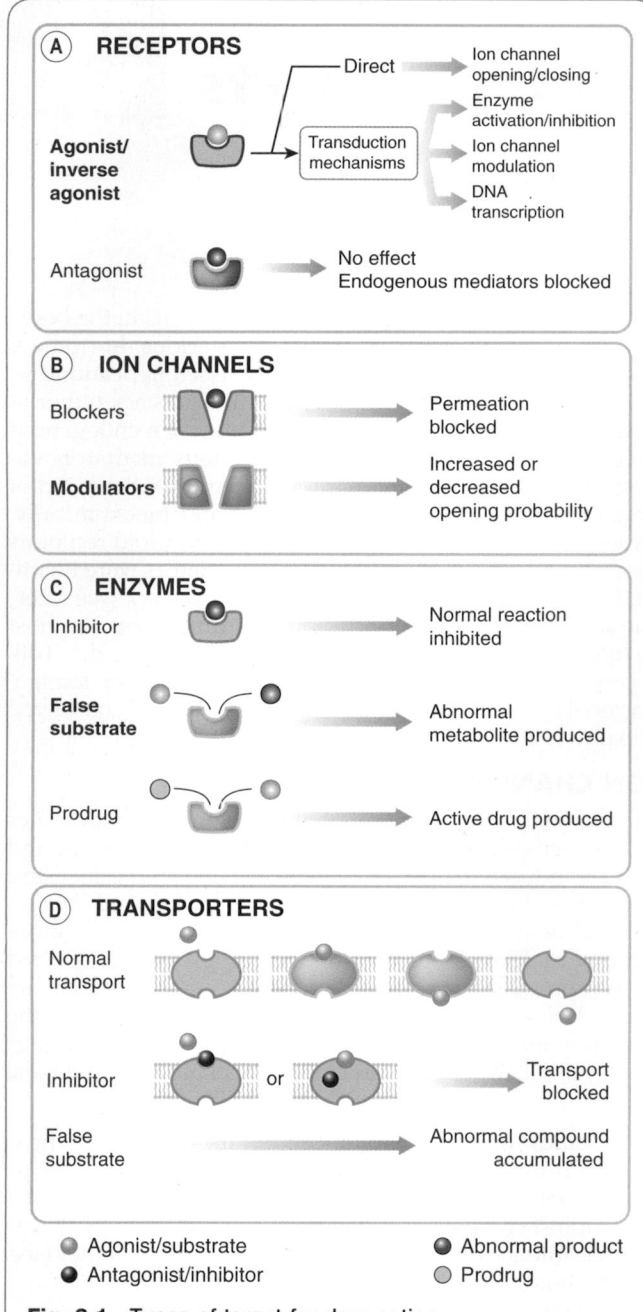

Fig. 3.1 Types of target for drug action.

---

2. By an indirect interaction, involving an activated G protein subunit or other intermediary (see p. 34).
3. By altering the level of expression of ion channels on the cell surface. For example, **gabapentin** reduces the insertion of neuronal calcium channels into the plasma membrane (Ch. 46).

A summary of the different ion channel families and their functions is given later.

ENZYMES

Many drugs target enzymes (see Fig. 3.1C). Often, the drug molecule is a substrate analogue that acts as a competitive inhibitor of the enzyme (e.g. **captopril**, acting on

angiotensin-converting enzyme; Ch. 23); in other cases, the binding is irreversible and non-competitive (e.g. **aspirin**, acting on cyclo-oxygenase; Ch. 27). Drugs may also act as false substrates, where the drug molecule undergoes chemical transformation to form an abnormal product that subverts the normal metabolic pathway. An example is the anticancer drug **fluorouracil**, which replaces uracil as an intermediate in purine biosynthesis but cannot be converted into thymidylate, thus blocking DNA synthesis and preventing cell division (Ch. 57).

It should also be mentioned that drugs may require enzymic degradation to convert them from an inactive form, the prodrug (see Ch. 10), to an active form (e.g. **enalapril** is converted by esterases to enalaprilat, which inhibits angiotensin-converting enzyme). Furthermore, as discussed in Chapter 58, drug toxicity often results from the enzymic conversion of the drug molecule to a reactive metabolite. **Paracetamol** (see Ch. 27) causes liver damage in this way. As far as the primary action of the drug is concerned, this is an unwanted side reaction, but it is of major practical importance.

TRANSPORTERS

The movement of ions and small polar organic molecules across cell membranes generally occurs either through channels, or through the agency of a transport protein (see Fig. 3.1D), because the permeating molecules are often insufficiently lipid-soluble to penetrate lipid membranes on their own. Many such transporters are known; examples of particular pharmacological importance include those responsible for the transport of ions and many organic molecules across the renal tubule, the intestinal epithelium and the blood–brain barrier, the transport of Na^+ and Ca^{2+} out of cells, the uptake of neurotransmitter precursors (such as choline) or of neurotransmitters themselves (such as amines and amino acids) by nerve terminals, and the transport of drug molecules and their metabolites across cell membranes and epithelial barriers. We shall encounter transporters frequently in later chapters.

In many cases, hydrolysis of ATP provides the energy for transport of substances against their electrochemical gradient. Such transport proteins include a distinct ATP-binding site, and are termed ABC (ATP-Binding Cassette) transporters. Important examples include the sodium pump (Na⁺-K⁺-ATPase; see Ch. 4) and *multidrug resistance* (MDR) transporters that eject cytotoxic drugs from cancer and microbial cells, conferring resistance to these therapeutic agents (see Ch. 57). In other cases, including the neurotransmitter transporters, the transport of organic molecules is coupled to the transport of ions (usually Na^+), either in the same direction (*symport*) or in the opposite direction (*antiport*), and therefore relies on the electrochemical gradient for Na^+ generated by the ATP-driven sodium pump. The carrier proteins embody a recognition site that makes them specific for a particular permeating species, and these recognition sites can also be targets for drugs whose effect is to block the transport system (e.g. cocaine blocks monoamine neurotransmitter uptake into nerve terminals; see Ch. 49).

The importance of transporters as a source of individual variation in the pharmacokinetic characteristics of various drugs is increasingly recognised (see Ch. 11).

RECEPTOR PROTEINS

CLONING OF RECEPTORS

In the 1970s, pharmacology entered a new phase when receptors, which had until then been theoretical entities, began to emerge as biochemical realities following the development of receptor-labelling techniques (see Ch. 2), which made it possible to extract and purify the receptor material.

Once receptor proteins were isolated and purified, it was possible to analyse the amino acid sequence of a short stretch, allowing the corresponding base sequence of the mRNA to be deduced and full-length DNA to be isolated by conventional cloning methods, starting from a cDNA library obtained from a tissue source rich in the receptor of interest. The first receptor clones were obtained in this way, but subsequently expression cloning and, with the sequencing of the entire genome of various species, including human, cloning strategies based on sequence homologies, which do not require prior isolation and purification of the receptor protein, were widely used, and now several hundred receptors of all four structural families (see Fig. 3.3) have been cloned. Sequence data so obtained has revealed many molecular variants (subtypes) of known receptors that had not been evident from pharmacological studies (see IUPHAR/BPS, *Guide to Pharmacology*). Much remains to be discovered about the pharmacological, functional and clinical significance of this abundant molecular polymorphism. It is expected, however, that such variations will account for part of the variability between individuals in response to therapeutic agents (see Ch. 12)

Endogenous ligands for many of the novel receptors identified by gene cloning are so far unknown, and they are described as 'orphan receptors'.[2] Identifying ligands for these presumed receptors is often difficult. Increasingly, there are examples (e.g. free fatty acid receptors) where important endogenous ligands have been linked to hitherto orphan receptors. There is optimism that novel therapeutic agents will emerge by targeting this pool of unclaimed receptors.

Much information has been gained by introducing the cloned DNA encoding individual receptors into cell lines, producing cells that express the foreign receptors in a functional form. Such engineered cells allow much more precise control of the expressed receptors than is possible with natural cells or intact tissues, and the technique is widely used to study the binding and pharmacological characteristics of cloned receptors. Expressed human receptors, which often differ in their sequence and pharmacological properties from their animal counterparts, can be studied in this way.

Obtaining crystals of a protein allows its structure to be analysed at very high resolution by X-ray diffraction techniques, but unfortunately, since many receptors are normally embedded in membrane lipid, they have, until relatively recently, proven difficult to crystallise. Much of the information obtained relates to how ligands bind to receptors, but we are now beginning to learn more about

agonist-induced receptor conformational changes and how signalling is initiated.

Now that the genes have been clearly identified, the emphasis has shifted to characterising the receptors pharmacologically and determining their molecular characteristics and physiological functions.

TYPES OF RECEPTOR

Receptors elicit many different types of cellular effect. Some of them are very rapid, such as those involved in fast synaptic transmission, operating within milliseconds, whereas other receptor-mediated effects, such as many of those produced by thyroid hormone or various steroid hormones, occur over hours or days. There are many examples of intermediate timescales – catecholamines, for example, usually act in a matter of seconds, whereas many peptides take rather longer to produce their effects. Not surprisingly, very different types of linkage between receptor occupation and the ensuing response are involved. Based on molecular structure and the nature of this linkage (the transduction mechanism), we can distinguish four receptor types, or superfamilies (Figs 3.2 and 3.3; Table 3.1).

- Type 1: **ligand-gated ion channels** (also known as **ionotropic** receptors[3]). The chain of discoveries culminating in the molecular characterisation of these receptors is described by Halliwell (2007). Typically, these are the receptors on which fast neurotransmitters act (see Table 3.1).
- Type 2: **G protein–coupled receptors** (GPCRs). These are also known as **metabotropic receptors** or **7-transmembrane** (7-TM, serpentine or heptahelical) **receptors**. They are membrane receptors that are coupled to intracellular effector systems primarily via a G protein (see p. 32). They constitute the largest family,[4] and include receptors for many hormones and slow transmitters (Table 3.1).
- Type 3: **kinase-linked and related receptors**. This is a large and heterogeneous group of membrane receptors responding mainly to protein mediators. They comprise an extracellular ligand-binding domain linked to an intracellular domain by a single transmembrane helix. In many cases, the intracellular domain is enzymic in nature (with protein kinase or guanylyl cyclase activity). Some lack enzymic activity themselves but link to intracellular effector enzymes through their binding of adaptor proteins. Examples of these latter receptor types include cytokine receptors (e.g. tumour necrosis factor [TNF] receptors) and pattern recognition receptors (PRRs) that recognise pathogen-associated molecular patterns (PAMPs) or danger-associated molecular patterns (DAMPs) found in pathogens, which stimulate the innate immune system host defence network (see Ch. 7). PRR receptors include the cell surface Toll-like receptors (TLRs), and the cytoplasmic receptors such

---

[2]An oddly Dickensian term that seems inappropriately condescending. Because we can assume that these receptors play defined roles in physiological signalling, their 'orphanhood' reflects our ignorance, not their status. More information on orphan receptors can be found at <www.guidetopharmacology.org/GRAC/FamilyDisplayForward?familyId=115#16>.

[3]Here, focusing on receptors, we include ligand-gated ion channels as an example of a receptor family. Other types of ion channels are described later (p. 46); many are also drug targets, although not receptors in the strict sense.

[4]There are 865 human GPCRs comprising 1.6% of the genome (Fredriksson & Schiöth, 2005). Nearly 500 of these are believed to be odorant receptors involved in smell and taste sensations, the remainder being receptors for known or unknown endogenous mediators – enough to keep pharmacologists busy for some time yet.

Fig. 3.2 Types of receptor–effector linkage. *ACh,* acetylcholine; *E,* enzyme; *G,* G protein; *R,* receptor.

Table 3.1 The four main types of receptor

	Type 1: Ligand-gated ion channels	Type 2: G protein–coupled receptors	Type 3: Receptor kinases	Type 4: Nuclear receptors
Location	Membrane	Membrane	Membrane	Intracellular
Effector	Ion channel	Channel or enzyme	Protein kinases	Gene transcription
Coupling	Direct	G protein or arrestin	Direct	Via DNA
Examples	Nicotinic acetylcholine receptor, $GABA_A$ receptor	Muscarinic acetylcholine receptor, adrenoceptors	Insulin, growth factors, cytokine receptors	Steroid receptors
Structure	Oligomeric assembly of subunits surrounding central pore	Monomeric or oligomeric assembly of subunits comprising seven transmembrane helices with intracellular G protein–coupling domain	Single transmembrane helix linking extracellular receptor domain to intracellular kinase domain	Monomeric structure with receptor- and DNA-binding domains

as RIG-I-like receptors (RLRs) and NOD-like receptors (NLRs). All these immune receptors signal their intracellular effects through adaptor proteins and kinases to alter the cell's transcription to elicit the correct immune response needed to fight against any pathogenic invaders.

- Type 4: **nuclear receptors.** These are receptors that regulate gene transcription.[5] Receptors of this type

also recognise many foreign molecules, inducing the expression of enzymes that metabolise them.

MOLECULAR STRUCTURE OF RECEPTORS

The molecular organisation of typical members of each of these four receptor superfamilies is shown in Fig. 3.3. Although individual receptors show considerable sequence variation in particular regions, and the lengths of the main intracellular and extracellular domains also vary from one to another within the same family, the overall structural patterns and associated signal transduction pathways are

---

[5]The term *nuclear receptor* is something of a misnomer, because some are actually located in the cytosol and migrate to the nuclear compartment when a ligand is present.

Fig. 3.3 General structure of four receptor families. The rectangular segments represent hydrophobic α-helical regions of the protein comprising approximately 20 amino acids, which form the membrane-spanning domains of the receptors. The pink shaded areas illustrate the region of the orthosteric ligand-binding domains. (A) Type 1: ligand-gated ion channels. The example illustrated here shows the subunit structure of the nicotinic acetylcholine receptor. The subunit structure of other ligand-gated ion channels is shown in Fig. 3.5. Many ligand-gated ion channels comprise four or five subunits of the type shown, the whole complex containing 16–20 membrane-spanning segments surrounding a central ion channel. (B) Type 2: G protein–coupled receptors (GPCRs). The two ligand-binding domains shown illustrate the position of the orthosteric ligand-binding domains on different types of GPCRs, there would be only one on each GPCR. (C) Type 3: kinase-linked receptors. Most growth factor receptors incorporate the ligand-binding and enzymatic (kinase) domains in the same molecule, as shown, whereas cytokine receptors lack an intracellular kinase domain but link to cytosolic kinase molecules. Other structural variants also exist. (D) Type 4: nuclear receptors that control gene transcription.

very consistent. The realisation that just four main receptor superfamilies provide a solid framework for interpreting the complex welter of information about the effects of a large proportion of the drugs that have been studied has been one of the most refreshing developments in modern pharmacology.

RECEPTOR HETEROGENEITY AND SUBTYPES

Receptors within a given family generally occur in several molecular varieties, or subtypes, with similar architecture but significant differences in their sequences, and often in their pharmacological properties.[6] Nicotinic acetylcholine receptors are typical in this respect; distinct subtypes occur in different brain regions (see Table 40.2), and these differ from the muscle receptor. Some of the known pharmacological differences (e.g. sensitivity to blocking agents) between muscle and brain acetylcholine receptors correlate with specific sequence differences; however, as far as we know, all nicotinic acetylcholine receptors respond to the same physiological mediator and produce the same kind of synaptic response, so why many variants should have evolved is still a puzzle.

▼ Much of the sequence variation that accounts for receptor diversity arises at the genomic level, that is, different genes give rise to distinct receptor subtypes. Additional variation arises from alternative mRNA splicing, which means that a single gene can give rise to more than one receptor isoform. After translation from genomic DNA, the mRNA normally contains non-coding regions (introns) that are excised by mRNA splicing before the message is translated into protein. Depending on the location of the splice sites, splicing can result in inclusion or deletion of one or more of the mRNA coding regions, giving rise to long or short forms of the protein. This is an important source of variation, particularly for GPCRs, producing receptors with different binding characteristics and different signal transduction mechanisms, although its pharmacological relevance remains to be clarified. Another process that can produce different receptors from the same gene is mRNA editing, which involves the mischievous substitution of one base in the mRNA for another, and hence potentially a small variation in the amino acid sequence of the expressed receptor.

Molecular heterogeneity of this kind is a feature of all kinds of receptors – indeed of functional proteins in general. New receptor subtypes and isoforms continue to be discovered, and regular updates of the catalogue are available (www.guidetopharmacology.org/). The problems of classification, nomenclature and taxonomy resulting from this flood of data have been mentioned earlier.

We will now describe the characteristics of each of the four receptor superfamilies.

TYPE 1: LIGAND-GATED ION CHANNELS

The nicotinic acetylcholine receptor, which we find at the skeletal neuromuscular junction (Ch. 14), in autonomic ganglia (Ch. 14) and in the brain (Ch. 40), is a typical example of a ligand-gated ion channel, known as the cys-loop receptors (so called because they have in their structure a large intracellular domain between transmembrane domains 3 and 4 containing multiple cysteine residues [see Fig. 3.3A]). Others of this type include the GABA_A and glycine receptors (Ch. 39) as well as the 5-hydroxytryptamine type 3 (5-HT_3; Chs 16 and 40) receptor. Other types of ligand-gated ion

[6]Receptors for 5-hydroxytryptamine (see Ch. 16) are currently the champions with respect to diversity, with 13 subtypes of GPCR and 1 ligand-gated ion channel all responding to the same endogenous ligand.

channel exist – namely ionotropic glutamate receptors (Ch. 39) and purinergic P2X receptors (Chs 17 and 40) that differ in several respects from the nicotinic acetylcholine receptor (see Fig. 3.5). In addition to the ligand-gated ion channels found on the cell membrane that mediate fast synaptic transmission, there are also intracellular ligand-gated ion channels – namely the inositol trisphosphate (IP_3) and ryanodine receptors (see Ch. 4) that release Ca^{2+} from intracellular stores.

MOLECULAR STRUCTURE

Ligand-gated ion channels have structural features in common with other ion channels, described on p. 46. The nicotinic acetylcholine receptor cloned from the Torpedo electric ray (Fig. 3.4),[7] consists of a pentameric assembly of different subunits, of which there are four types, termed α, β, γ and δ, each of molecular weight (M_r) 40–58 kDa. The subunits show marked sequence homology, and each contains four membrane-spanning α-helices, inserted into the membrane as shown in Fig. 3.4B. The pentameric structure ($α_2$, β, γ, δ) possesses two acetylcholine binding sites, each lying at the interface between one of the two α subunits and its neighbour. Both must bind acetylcholine molecules for the receptor to be activated. Fig. 3.4B shows the receptor structure. Each subunit spans the membrane four times, so the channel comprises no fewer than 20 membrane-spanning helices surrounding a central pore.

▼ One of the transmembrane helices (M_2) from each of the five subunits forms the lining of the ion channel (see Fig. 3.4). The five M_2 helices that form the pore are sharply kinked inwards halfway through the membrane, forming a constriction. When acetylcholine molecules bind, a conformation change occurs in the extracellular part of the receptor, which twists the α subunits, causing the kinked M_2 segments to swivel out of the way, thus opening the channel. The channel lining contains a series of anionic residues, making the channel selectively permeable to cations (primarily Na^+ and K^+, although some types of nicotinic receptor are permeable to Ca^{2+} as well).

The use of site-directed mutagenesis, which enables short regions, or single residues, of the amino acid sequence to be altered, has shown that a mutation of a critical residue in the M_2 helix changes the channel from being cation permeable (hence excitatory in the context of synaptic function) to being anion permeable (typical of receptors for inhibitory transmitters such as GABA and glycine). Other mutations affect properties such as gating and desensitisation of ligand-gated channels.

Other ligand-gated ion channels, such as glutamate receptors (see Ch. 39) and P2X receptors (see Chs 17 and 40), whose structures are shown in Fig. 3.5, have a different architecture. Ionotropic glutamate receptors are tetrameric and the pore is built from loops rather than transmembrane helices, in common with many other (non-ligand-gated) ion channels (see Fig. 3.20). P2X receptors are trimeric and each subunit has only two transmembrane domains (North, 2002). The nicotinic receptor and other cys-loop receptors are pentamers with two agonist binding sites on each receptor. Binding of one agonist molecule to one site increases the affinity of binding at the other site (positive cooperativity) and both sites need to be occupied for the receptor to be activated and the channel to open. Some ionotropic glutamate receptors have as many as four agonist binding sites and P2X receptors have three, but they appear to open when two agonist molecules are bound. Once again we realise that the simple model of receptor

[7]In early studies the Torpedo electric ray was used to isolate and purify the nicotinic receptor as it expresses a very high density of nicotinic receptors on its electroplaques. We now realise that the subunit compositions of the mammalian neuromuscular (Ch. 14) and neuronal (Chs 14 and 40) nicotinic receptors are different from that of the Torpedo but here we focus on the Torpedo receptor to keep it simple.

Fig. 3.4 **Structure of the nicotinic acetylcholine receptor (a typical ligand-gated ion channel).** (A) Schematic diagram in side view *(upper)* and plan view *(lower)*. The five receptor subunits ($α_2$, β, γ, δ) form a cluster surrounding a central transmembrane pore, the lining of which is formed by the M_2 helical segments of each subunit. These contain a preponderance of negatively charged amino acids, which makes the pore cation selective. There are two acetylcholine binding sites in the extracellular portion of the receptor, at the interface between the α and the adjoining subunits. When acetylcholine binds, the kinked α-helices either straighten out or swing out of the way, thus opening the channel pore. (B) High-resolution image showing revised arrangement of intracellular domains. (Panel [A] based on Unwin, N., 1993. Nicotinic acetylcholine receptor at 9Å resolution. J. Mol. Biol. 229, 1101–1124, and Unwin, N., 1995. Acetylcholine receptor channel imaged in the open state. Nature 373, 37–43; panel [B] reproduced with permission from Unwin, N., 2005. Refined structure of the nicotinic acetylcholine receptor at 4Å resolution. J. Mol. Biol. 346(4), 967–989.)

Fig. 3.5 **Molecular architecture of ligand-gated ion channels.** *Red* and *blue rectangles* represent membrane-spanning α-helices and *blue hairpins* represent the P loop pore-forming regions. *5-HT₃*, 5-hydroxytryptamine type 3 receptor; *GABA_A*, GABA type A receptor; *IP₃R*, inositol trisphosphate receptor; *nAChR*, nicotinic acetylcholine receptor; *NMDA*, N-methyl-D-aspartic acid receptor; *P2XR*, purine P2X receptor; *RyR*, ryanodine receptor.

activation shown in Fig. 2.1 is an oversimplification as it only considered one agonist molecule binding to produce a response. For two or more agonist molecules binding, more complex mathematical models are needed (see Colquhoun, 2006).

THE GATING MECHANISM

Receptors of this type control the fastest synaptic events in the nervous system, in which a neurotransmitter acts on the postsynaptic membrane of a nerve or muscle cell and transiently increases its permeability to particular ions. Most excitatory neurotransmitters, such as acetylcholine at the neuromuscular junction (Ch. 14) or glutamate in the central nervous system (Ch. 39), cause an increase in Na^+ and K^+ permeability and in some instances Ca^{2+} permeability. At negative membrane potentials this results in a net inward current carried mainly by Na^+, which depolarises the cell and increases the probability that it will generate an action potential. The action of the transmitter reaches a peak in a fraction of a millisecond, and usually decays within a few milliseconds. The sheer speed of this response implies that the coupling between the receptor and the ion channel is a direct one, and the molecular structure of the receptor–channel complex (see earlier) agrees with this. In contrast to other receptor families, no intermediate biochemical steps are involved in the transduction process.

▼ The *patch clamp recording technique*, devised by Neher and Sakmann, allows the very small current flowing through a single ion channel to be measured directly (Fig. 3.6). The patch clamp technique provides a view, rare in biology, of the physiological behaviour of individual protein molecules in real time, and has given many new insights into the gating reactions and permeability characteristics of both ligand-gated channels and voltage-gated channels. The magnitude of the single channel conductance confirms that permeation occurs through a physical pore through the membrane, because the ion flow is too large (about 10^7 ions per second) to be compatible with a carrier mechanism. The channel conductance produced by different agonists is the same, whereas the mean channel lifetime varies. The ligand–receptor interaction scheme shown in Chapter 2 is a useful model for ion-channel gating. The conformation R*, representing the open state of the ion channel, is thought to be the same for all agonists, accounting for the finding that the channel conductance does not vary. Kinetically, the mean open time is determined mainly by the closing rate constant, α, and this varies from one drug to another. As explained in Chapter 2 (see Fig. 2.1), an agonist of high efficacy that activates a large proportion of the receptors that it occupies will

be characterised by $\beta/\alpha \gg 1$, whereas for a drug of low efficacy β/α has a lower value.

At some ligand-gated ion channels the situation is more complicated because different agonists may cause individual channels to open to one or more of several distinct conductance levels (see Fig. 3.6B). This implies that there is more than one R* conformation. Furthermore, desensitisation of ligand-gated ion channels (see Ch. 2) also involves one or more additional agonist-induced conformational states. These findings necessitate some elaboration of the simple scheme in which only a single open state, R*, is represented, and are an example of the way in which the actual behaviour of receptors makes our theoretical models look a little threadbare.

Ligand-gated ion channels

- These are sometimes called ionotropic receptors.
- They are involved mainly in fast synaptic transmission.
- There are several structural families, the commonest being heteromeric assemblies of four or five subunits, with transmembrane helices arranged around a central aqueous channel.
- Ligand binding and channel opening occur on a millisecond timescale.
- Examples include the nicotinic acetylcholine, GABA type A (GABA_A), glutamate (e.g. *N*-methyl-D-aspartic acid receptor [NMDA]) and ATP (P2X) receptors.

TYPE 2: G PROTEIN–COUPLED RECEPTORS

GPCRs constitute the commonest single class of targets for therapeutic drugs. The GPCR family comprises many of the receptors that are familiar to pharmacologists, such as muscarinic AChRs, adrenoceptors, dopamine receptors, 5-HT (serotonin) receptors, receptors for many peptides, purine receptors and many others, including the chemo-receptors involved in olfaction and pheromone detection, and also many 'orphans' (see Fredriksson & Schiöth, 2005). For most of these, pharmacological and molecular studies have revealed a variety of subtypes. All have the characteristic heptahelical structure (see Fig. 3.3B).

Many neurotransmitters, apart from peptides, can interact with both GPCRs and ligand-gated channels, allowing the

(A) Nicotinic acetylcholine channel openings

Number of open channels

3 pA

10 ms

(B) NMDA channel openings

Conductance states

18 pS
38 pS

2 pA

20 ms

Fig. 3.6   Single channel openings recorded by the patch clamp technique. (A) Acetylcholine-operated ion channels at the frog motor endplate. The pipette, which was applied tightly to the surface of the membrane, contained 10 μmol/L ACh. The downward deflections show the currents flowing through single ion channels in the small patch of membrane under the pipette tip. Towards the end of the record, two channels can be seen to open with a discrete step from the first to the second. (B) Single-channel *N*-methyl-D-aspartic acid receptor (NMDA) receptor currents recorded from cerebellar neurons in the outside-out patch conformation. NMDA was added to the outside of the patch to activate the channel. The channel opens to multiple conductance levels. In (B) the openings to the higher conductance level and the subsequent closings are smooth, indicating that one channel is opening (two channels would not be expected to open and close simultaneously) whereas in (A) there are discrete steps indicating two channels. (Panel [A] courtesy D. Colquhoun and D.C. Ogden; panel [B] reproduced with permission from Cull-Candy, S.G. & Usowicz, M.M., 1987. Nature 325, 525–528.)

same molecule to produce fast (through ligand-gated ion channels) and relatively slow (through GPCRs) effects. Individual peptide hormones, however, generally act either on GPCRs or on kinase-linked receptors (see later), but rarely on both, and a similar choosiness applies to the many ligands that act on nuclear receptors.[8]

MOLECULAR STRUCTURE

In 1986 the first pharmacologically relevant GPCR, the β_2 adrenoceptor (Ch. 15), was cloned. Thereafter molecular

---

[8]Examples of promiscuity are increasing, however. Steroid hormones, normally faithful to nuclear receptors, make the occasional pass at ion channels and GPCRs, and some eicosanoids act on nuclear receptors as well as GPCRs. Nature is quite open-minded, although such examples are liable to make pharmacologists frown and students despair.

Fig. 3.7   Structure of the M$_2$ muscarinic receptor. High-resolution image showing the conformation of the M$_2$ muscarinic receptor bound with both an agonist (orthosteric) and a positive allosteric modulator. The brown cylinders represent the transmembrane domains. The full extent of the N- and C-terminal domains and the third intracellular loop are not shown. (Courtesy A. Christopoulos.)

biology caught up very rapidly with pharmacology, and with the sequencing of the human genome the amino acid sequence of all the GPCRs hitherto identified by their pharmacological properties was revealed, as was the structure of many novel GPCRs. More recently the difficulties of crystallising GPCRs have been overcome, allowing the use of the powerful technique of X-ray crystallography to study the three-dimensional molecular structure of these receptors in detail (Fig. 3.7) (Zhang et al., 2015). Also, computational molecular docking and nuclear magnetic resonance (NMR) methods have been developed to study ligand binding and subsequent conformational changes associated with activation (see Sounier et al., 2015). This is starting to provide important information on agonist- and antagonist-bound receptor conformations as well as receptor–G protein interactions. From such studies we are gaining a clearer picture of the mechanism of activation of GPCRs and the factors determining agonist efficacy, as well as having a better basis for designing new GPCR ligands.

GPCRs consist of a single polypeptide chain, usually of 350–400 amino acid residues, but in some cases up to 1100 residues. The general anatomy is shown in Fig. 3.3B. Their characteristic structure comprises seven transmembrane α-helices, similar to those of the ion channels discussed previously, with an extracellular N-terminal domain of varying length, and an intracellular C-terminal domain.

GPCRs are divided into three main classes – A, B and C (Table 3.2). There is considerable sequence homology between the members of one class, but little between different classes. They share the same seven transmembrane helix (heptahelical) structure, but differ in other respects, principally in the length of the extracellular N-terminus and the location of the agonist binding domain. Class A is by far the largest, comprising most monoamine, neuropeptide and chemokine receptors. Class B includes receptors for some other peptides, such as calcitonin and glucagon. Class C is the smallest, its main members being the

Table 3.2 Main G protein–coupled receptor classes[a,b]

Class	Receptors[b]	Structural features
A: rhodopsin family	The largest group. Receptors for most amine neurotransmitters, many neuropeptides, purines, prostanoids, cannabinoids, etc.	Short extracellular (N-terminal) tail. Ligand binds to transmembrane helices (amines) or to extracellular loops (peptides)
B: secretin/glucagon receptor family	Receptors for peptide hormones, including secretin, glucagon, calcitonin	Intermediate extracellular tail incorporating ligand-binding domain
C: metabotropic glutamate receptor/calcium sensor family	Small group. Metabotropic glutamate receptors, GABA$_B$ receptors, Ca^{2+}-sensing receptors	Long extracellular tail incorporating ligand-binding domain

[a]Other classes include frizzled G protein–coupled receptors (GPCRs), adhesion GPCRs and receptors for pheromones.
[b]For full lists, see <www.guidetopharmacology.org>.

metabotropic glutamate and GABA receptors, and the Ca^{2+}-sensing receptors.[9]

▼ The understanding of the function of receptors of this type owes much to studies of a closely related protein, *rhodopsin*, which is responsible for transduction in retinal rods. This protein is abundant in the retina, and much easier to study than receptor proteins (which are anything but abundant); it is built on an identical plan to that shown in Fig. 3.3B and also produces a response in the rod (hyperpolarisation, associated with inhibition of Na$^+$ conductance) through a mechanism involving a G protein (see p. 32, Fig. 3.9). The most obvious difference is that a photon, rather than an agonist molecule, produces the response. In effect, rhodopsin can be regarded as incorporating its own inbuilt agonist molecule, namely *retinal*, which isomerises from the *trans* (inactive) to the *cis* (active) form when it absorbs a photon.

For small molecules, such as noradrenaline (norepinephrine) and acetylcholine, the ligand-binding domain of class A receptors is buried in the cleft between the α-helical segments within the membrane (see Figs 3.3B and 3.7), similar to the slot occupied by retinal in the rhodopsin molecule.[10] Peptide ligands, such as substance P (Ch. 19), bind more superficially to the extracellular loops, as shown in Fig. 3.3B. From crystal structures and single-site mutagenesis experiments, it is possible to map the ligand-binding domain of these receptors. Recent advances in computational molecular docking of ligands into the ligand–receptor-binding domain have made it possible to design novel synthetic ligands based primarily on knowledge of the receptor structure (see Manglik et al., 2016) – an important milestone in drug development, which has relied up to now mainly on the structure of endogenous mediators (such as histamine) or plant alkaloids (such as morphine) for its chemical inspiration.[11]

[9]The Ca^{2+}-sensing receptor (see Conigrave et al., 2000) is an unusual GPCR that is activated not by conventional mediators, but by extracellular Ca^{2+} in the range of 1–10 mmol/L – an extremely low affinity in comparison with other GPCR agonists. It is expressed by cells of the parathyroid gland, and serves to regulate the extracellular Ca^{2+} concentration by controlling parathyroid hormone secretion (Ch. 37). This homeostatic mechanism is quite distinct from the mechanisms for regulating intracellular Ca^{2+}, discussed in Chapter 4.
[10]Hydrophilic small molecules access their ligand-binding domain from the extracellular space down the water-filled cleft, however for highly lipophilic molecules such as those activating the cannabinoid CB$_1$ and lysophospholipid S1P$_1$ receptors access appears to be through a membrane-embedded access channel in the side of the receptor.
[11]In the past many lead compounds have come from screening huge chemical libraries (see Ch. 60). No inspiration was required, just robust assays, large computers and efficient robotics. Now with the generation of crystal structures we have moved to a more sophisticated age in drug discovery.

PROTEINASE-ACTIVATED RECEPTORS[12]

▼ Although activation of GPCRs is normally the consequence of a diffusible agonist, it can be the result of proteinase activation. Four types of protease-activated receptors (PARs) have been identified (see review by Ramachandran et al., 2012). Many proteinases, such as thrombin (a proteinase involved in the blood-clotting cascade; see Ch. 25), activate PARs by snipping off the end of the extracellular N-terminal tail of the receptor (Fig. 3.8) to expose five or six N-terminal residues that bind to receptor domains in the extracellular loops, functioning as a 'tethered agonist'. Receptors of this type occur in many tissues and they appear to play a role in inflammation and other responses to tissue damage where tissue proteinases are released. A PAR molecule can be activated only once, because the cleavage cannot be reversed, and thus continuous resynthesis of the receptor protein is necessary. Inactivation occurs by a further proteolytic cleavage that frees the tethered ligand, or by desensitisation, involving phosphorylation (see Fig. 3.8), after which the receptor is internalised and degraded, to be replaced by newly synthesised protein.

G protein–coupled receptors

- These are sometimes called metabotropic or seven-transmembrane-domain (7-TDM) receptors.
- Structures comprise seven membrane-spanning α-helices.
- The G protein is a membrane protein comprising three subunits (α, β, γ), the α subunit possessing GTPase activity.
- The G protein interacts with a binding pocket on the intracellular surface of the receptor.
- When the G protein binds to an agonist-occupied receptor, the α subunit binds GTP, dissociates and is then free to activate an effector (e.g. a membrane enzyme). In some cases, the βγ subunit is the activator species.
- Activation of the effector is terminated when the bound GTP molecule is hydrolysed, which allows the α subunit to recombine with βγ.
- There are several types of G protein, which interact with different receptors and control different effectors.
- Examples include muscarinic acetylcholine receptors, adrenoceptors, neuropeptide and chemokine receptors, and proteinase-activated receptors.

[12]These receptors were formerly called protease-activated receptors.

Fig. 3.8 **Activation of a proteinase-activated receptor by cleavage of the N-terminal extracellular domain.** Inactivation occurs by phosphorylation. Recovery requires resynthesis of the receptor.

Fig. 3.9 **The function of the G protein.** The G protein consists of three subunits (α, β, γ), which are anchored to the membrane through attached lipid residues. Coupling of the α subunit to an agonist-occupied receptor causes the bound GDP to exchange with intracellular GTP; the α–GTP complex then dissociates from the receptor and from the βγ complex, and interacts with a target protein (target 1, which may be an enzyme, such as adenylyl cyclase or phospholipase C). The βγ complex also activates a target protein (target 2, which may be an ion channel or a kinase). The GTPase activity of the α subunit is increased when the target protein is bound, leading to hydrolysis of the bound GTP to GDP, whereupon the α subunit reunites with βγ.

G PROTEINS AND THEIR ROLE

G proteins comprise a family of membrane-resident proteins whose function is to respond to GPCR activation and pass on the message inside the cell to the effector systems that generate a cellular response. They represent the level of middle management in the organisational hierarchy, intervening between the receptors – choosy mandarins, alert to the faintest whiff of their preferred chemical – and the effector enzymes or ion channels – the blue-collar brigade that gets the job done without needing to know which hormone authorised the process. They are the go-between

proteins, but were actually called G proteins because of their interaction with the guanine nucleotides, GTP and GDP. For more detailed information on the structure and functions of G proteins, see reviews by Milligan and Kostenis (2006), and Oldham and Hamm (2008). G proteins consist of three subunits: α, β and γ (Fig. 3.9). Guanine nucleotides bind to the α subunit, which has enzymic (GTPase) activity, catalysing the conversion of GTP to GDP. The β and γ subunits remain together as a βγ complex. The 'γ subunit is anchored to the membrane through a fatty acid chain, coupled to the G protein through a reaction known as *prenylation*. In the 'resting' state (see Fig. 3.9), the G protein

Table 3.3 The main G protein subtypes and their functions[a]

Subtypes	Main effectors	Notes
Gα subunits[b]		
Gα_s	Stimulates adenylyl cyclase, causing increased cAMP formation	Activated by cholera toxin, which blocks GTPase activity, thus preventing inactivation
Gα_i	Inhibits adenylyl cyclase, decreasing cAMP formation	Blocked by pertussis toxin, which prevents dissociation of $\alpha\beta\gamma$ complex
Gα_o	? Limited effects of α subunit (effects mainly due to $\beta\gamma$ subunits)	Blocked by pertussis toxin. Occurs mainly in nervous system
Gα_q	Activates phospholipase C, increasing production of second messengers inositol trisphosphate and diacylglycerol (see pp. 36–38) thus releasing Ca^{2+} from intracellular stores and activating protein kinase C (PKC)	
G$\alpha_{12/13}$	Activates Rho and thus Rho kinase	
G$\beta\gamma$ subunits		
	Activate potassium channels Inhibit voltage-gated calcium channels Activate GPCR kinases (GRKs, pp. 38–39) Activate mitogen-activated protein kinase cascade Interact with some forms of adenylyl cyclase and with phospholipase Cβ	Many $\beta\gamma$ isoforms identified, but specific functions are not yet known

[a]This table lists only those isoforms of major pharmacological significance. Many more have been identified, some of which play roles in olfaction, taste, visual transduction and other physiological functions (see Offermanns, 2003).
[b]Initially the subscripts 's' and 'i' were used to denote <u>s</u>timulatory and <u>i</u>nhibitory actions on adenylyl cyclase but, subsequently, the terms used, 'q' and '12/13', have little logic behind their use.
GPCR, G protein–coupled receptor.

exists as an $\alpha\beta\gamma$ trimer, which may or may not be precoupled to the receptor, with GDP occupying the site on the α subunit. When a GPCR is activated by an agonist this induces small changes in residues around the ligand-binding pocket that translate to larger rearrangements of the intracellular regions of the receptor that open a cavity on the intracellular side of the receptor into which the G protein can bind, resulting in a high-affinity interaction of $\alpha\beta\gamma$ and the receptor. This agonist-induced interaction of $\alpha\beta\gamma$ with the receptor occurs within about 50 ms, causing the bound GDP to dissociate and to be replaced with GTP (GDP–GTP exchange), which in turn causes dissociation of the G protein trimer, releasing α–GTP from the $\beta\gamma$ subunits; these are the 'active' forms of the G protein, which diffuse in the membrane and can associate with various enzymes and ion channels, causing activation of the target (see Fig. 3.9). It was originally thought that only the α subunit had a signalling function, the $\beta\gamma$ complex serving merely as a chaperone to keep the flighty α subunits out of range of the various effector proteins that they might otherwise excite. However, the $\beta\gamma$ complexes actually make assignations of their own, and control effectors in much the same way as the α subunits. Association of α or $\beta\gamma$ subunits with target enzymes or channels can cause either activation or inhibition, depending on which G protein is involved (see Table 3.3). G protein activation results in amplification, because a single agonist–receptor complex can activate several G protein molecules in turn, and each of these can remain associated with their effector enzyme for long enough to produce many molecules of product. The product (see later) is often a 'second messenger', and further amplification occurs before the final cellular response is produced.

Signalling is terminated when the hydrolysis of GTP to GDP occurs through the inherent GTPase activity of the α subunit. The resulting α–GDP then dissociates from the effector, and reunites with $\beta\gamma$, completing the cycle.

▼ Attachment of the α subunit to an effector molecule actually increases its GTPase activity, the magnitude of this increase being different for different types of effector. Because GTP hydrolysis is the step that terminates the ability of the α subunit to produce its effect, regulation of its GTPase activity by the effector protein means that the activation of the effector tends to be self-limiting. In addition, there is a family of about 20 cellular proteins, regulators of G protein signalling (RGS) proteins (see review by Sjögren, 2017), that possess a conserved sequence that binds specifically to α subunits to increase greatly their GTPase activity, so hastening the hydrolysis of GTP and inactivating the complex. RGS proteins thus exert an inhibitory effect on G protein signalling, a mechanism that is thought to have a regulatory function in many situations.

Different GPCRs couple to different G proteins and thus produce distinct cellular responses. For example, M_2 muscarinic acetylcholine receptors (mAChRs) and β_1 adrenoceptors, both of which occur in cardiac muscle cells, produce opposite functional effects (Chs 14 and 15). Four main classes of G protein (G_s, G_i, G_o and G_q) are of pharmacological importance (Table 3.3). These differ primarily in the α subunit they contain.[13] G proteins show selectivity with

---

[13]In humans there are 21 known subtypes of Gα, 6 of Gβ and 12 of Gγ, providing, in theory, about 1500 variants of the trimer. We know little about the role of different α, β and γ subtypes, but it would be rash to assume that the variations are functionally irrelevant. By now, you will be unsurprised (even if somewhat bemused) by such a display of molecular heterogeneity, for it is the way of evolution.

Fig. 3.10 Bidirectional control of a target enzyme, such as adenylyl cyclase by G_s and G_i. Heterogeneity of G proteins allows different receptors to exert opposite effects on a target enzyme.

respect to both the receptors and the effectors with which they couple, having specific recognition domains in their structure complementary to specific G protein-binding domains in the receptor and effector molecules. For example, G_s and G_i produce, respectively, stimulation and inhibition of the enzyme *adenylyl cyclase* (Fig. 3.10).

One functional difference that has been useful as an experimental tool to distinguish which type of G protein is involved in different situations concerns the action of two bacterial toxins, *cholera toxin* and *pertussis toxin* (see Table 3.3). These toxins, which are enzymes, catalyse a conjugation reaction (ADP ribosylation) on the α subunit of G proteins. Cholera toxin acts only on G_s, and it causes persistent activation. Many of the symptoms of cholera, such as the excessive secretion of fluid from the gastro-intestinal epithelium (leading to 'rice-water stools'), are due to the uncontrolled activation of adenylyl cyclase that occurs. Pertussis toxin specifically blocks G_i and G_o by preventing dissociation of the G protein trimer. Pertussis toxin is released from *Bordetella pertussis* bacteria, which cause whooping cough. As with cholera toxin, the symptoms caused by pertussis toxin are related to its effects on G proteins, but in this case by inhibiting G_i and G_o rather than activating G_s and leading to changes in respiratory tract secretion and a distinctive cough rather than the copious diarrhoea of cholera.

TARGETS FOR G PROTEINS

The main targets for G proteins, through which GPCRs control different aspects of cell function (see Table 3.3), are:

- *adenylyl cyclase*, the enzyme responsible for cAMP formation;
- *phospholipase C*, the enzyme responsible for inositol phosphate and diacylglycerol (DAG) formation;
- *ion channels*, particularly calcium and potassium channels;
- *Rho A/Rho kinase*, a system that regulates the activity of many signalling pathways controlling cell growth, proliferation and motility, smooth muscle contraction, etc.;
- *mitogen-activated protein kinase* (MAP kinase), a system that controls many cell functions, including cell division and is also a target of several kinase-linked receptors.

The adenylyl cyclase/cAMP system

The discovery by Sutherland and his colleagues of the role of cAMP (cyclic 3′,5′-adenosine monophosphate) as an intracellular mediator demolished at a stroke the barriers that existed between biochemistry and pharmacology, and

introduced the concept of second messengers in signal transduction. cAMP is a nucleotide synthesised within the cell from ATP by the action of a membrane-bound enzyme, adenylyl cyclase. It is produced continuously and inactivated by hydrolysis to 5′-AMP by the action of a family of enzymes known as phosphodiesterases (PDEs). Many different drugs, hormones and neurotransmitters act on GPCRs and increase or decrease the catalytic activity of adenylyl cyclase (see Fig. 3.10), thus raising or lowering the concentration of cAMP within the cell. In mammalian cells there are 10 different molecular isoforms of the enzyme, some of which respond selectively to $G\alpha_s$ or $G\alpha_i$.

Cyclic AMP regulates many aspects of cellular function including, for example, enzymes involved in energy metabolism, cell division and cell differentiation, ion transport, ion channels and the contractile proteins in smooth muscle. These varied effects are, however, all brought about by a common mechanism, namely the activation of protein kinases by cAMP (known as cyclic AMP-dependent protein kinases) in eukaryotic cells. One important cyclic AMP-dependent protein kinase is *protein kinase A* (PKA). Protein kinases regulate the function of many different cellular proteins by controlling protein phosphorylation. Fig. 3.11 shows how increased cAMP production in response to β-adrenoceptor activation affects enzymes involved in glycogen and fat metabolism in liver, fat and muscle cells. The result is a coordinated response in which stored energy in the form of glycogen and fat is made available as glucose to fuel muscle contraction.

Other examples of regulation by PKA include the increased activity of voltage-gated calcium channels in heart muscle cells (see Ch. 22). Phosphorylation of these channels increases the amount of Ca^{2+} entering the cell during the action potential, and thus increases the force of contraction of the heart.

In smooth muscle, PKA phosphorylates (thereby inactivating) another enzyme, *myosin light-chain kinase*, which is required for contraction. This accounts for the smooth muscle relaxation produced by many drugs that increase cAMP production in smooth muscle (see Ch. 4).

As mentioned earlier, receptors linked to G_i rather than G_s inhibit adenylyl cyclase, and thus reduce cAMP formation to elicit opposing responses to those receptors which activate G_s. Examples include certain types of mAChR (e.g. the M_2 receptor of cardiac muscle; see Ch. 14), α_2 adrenoceptors in smooth muscle (Ch. 15) and opioid receptors (see Ch. 43). Adenylyl cyclase can be activated directly by drugs such as **forskolin**, which is used experimentally to study the role of the cAMP system.

Cyclic AMP is hydrolysed within cells by *PDEs*, an important and ubiquitous family of enzymes. Twenty-four

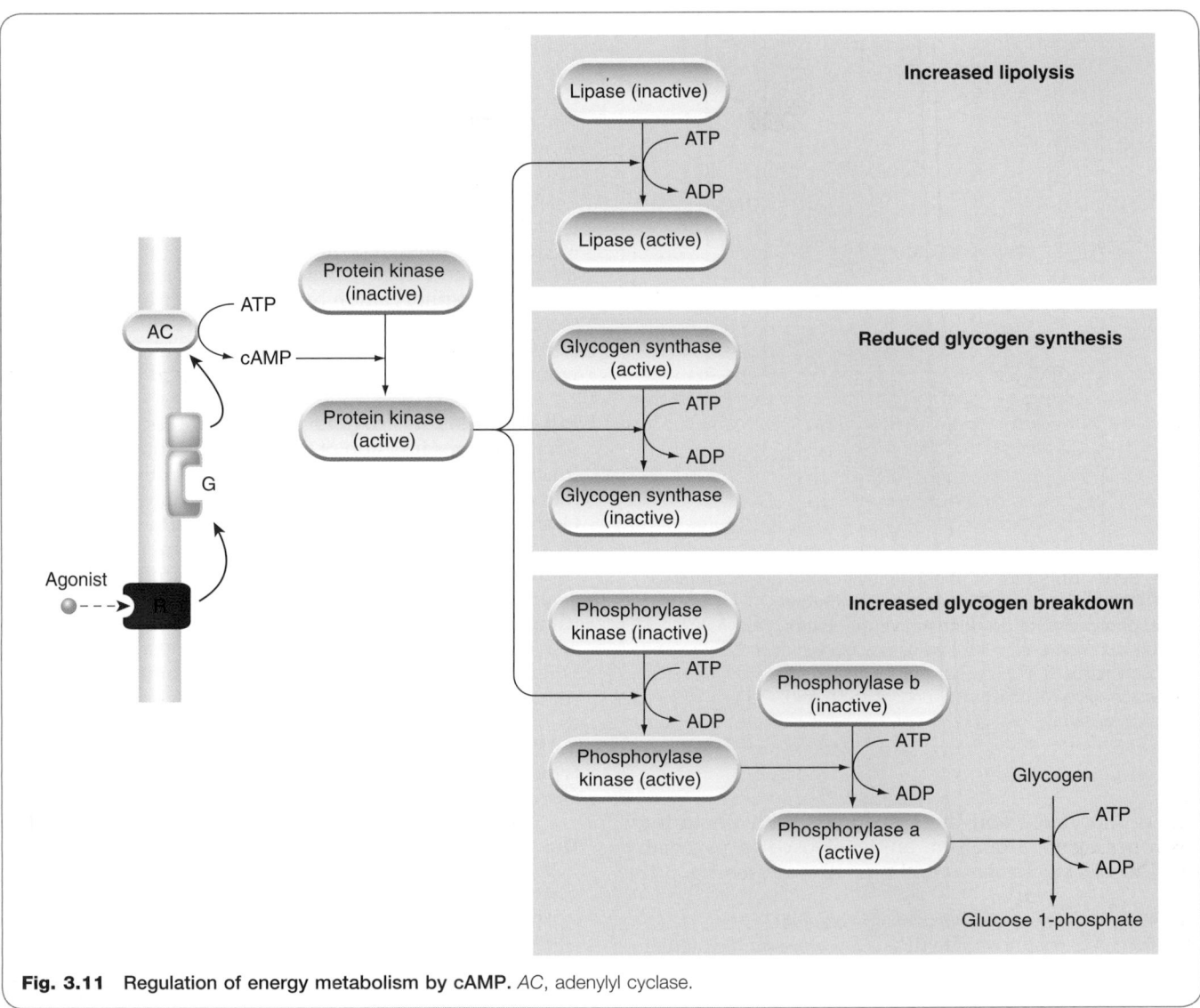

Fig. 3.11 **Regulation of energy metabolism by cAMP.** *AC*, adenylyl cyclase.

PDE subtypes exist, of which some are more selective for cAMP, while others are more selective for cGMP. Most are weakly inhibited by drugs such as methylxanthines (e.g. **theophylline** and **caffeine**; see Chs 29 and 49). **Roflumilast** (used to treat chronic obstructive pulmonary disease [COPD]; Ch. 29) is selective for PDE$_{4B}$, expressed in inflammatory cells; **milrinone** (a positive inotrope that makes the heart beat harder and is sometimes used for symptoms in patients awaiting heart transplantation; Ch. 22) is selective for PDE$_{2A}$, which is expressed in heart muscle; **sildenafil** (better known as Viagra; Ch. 36) is selective for PDE$_{5A}$, and consequently enhances the vasodilator effects of nitric oxide (NO) and drugs that release NO, whose effects are mediated by cGMP (see Ch. 21). The similarity of some of the actions of these drugs to those of sympathomimetic amines (Ch. 15) probably reflects their common property of increasing the intracellular concentration of cAMP.

The phospholipase C/inositol phosphate system
The *phosphoinositide* system, an important intracellular second messenger system, was first discovered in the 1950s by Hokin and Hokin, whose recondite interests centred on the mechanism of salt secretion by the nasal glands of seabirds. They found that secretion was accompanied by increased turnover of a minor class of membrane phospholipids known as phosphoinositides (collectively known as PIs; Fig. 3.12). Subsequently, Michell and Berridge found that many hormones that produce an increase in free intracellular Ca^{2+} concentration (which include, for example, muscarinic agonists and α-adrenoceptor agonists acting on smooth muscle and salivary glands) also increase PI turnover. It was later found that one particular member of the PI family, namely phosphatidylinositol (4,5) bis-phosphate (PIP$_2$), which has additional phosphate groups attached to the inositol ring, plays a key role. PIP$_2$ is the substrate for a membrane-bound enzyme, phospholipase Cβ (PLCβ), which splits it into *DAG* and *inositol (1,4,5) trisphosphate* (IP$_3$; Fig. 3.13), both of which function as second messengers as discussed later (p. 36). The activation of PLCβ by various agonists is mediated through a G protein (G$_q$, see Table 3.3). After cleavage of PIP$_2$, the status quo is restored, as shown in Fig. 3.13, DAG being phosphorylated to form phosphatidic acid (PA), while the IP$_3$ is

Fig. 3.12 Structure of phosphatidylinositol bisphosphate (PIP$_2$), showing sites of cleavage by different phospholipases to produce active mediators. Cleavage by phospholipase A2 (PLA$_2$) yields arachidonic acid. Cleavage by phospholipase C (PLC) yields inositol trisphosphate (I(1,4,5)P$_3$) and diacylglycerol (DAG). *PA*, phosphatidic acid; *PLD*, phospholipase D.

dephosphorylated and then recoupled with PA to form PIP$_2$ once again.[14] Lithium, an agent used in psychiatry (see Ch. 48), blocks this recycling pathway (see Fig. 3.13).

Inositol phosphates and intracellular calcium
Inositol (1,4,5) trisphosphate (IP$_3$) is a water-soluble mediator that is released into the cytosol and acts on a specific receptor – the IP$_3$ receptor – which is a ligand-gated calcium channel present on the membrane of the endoplasmic reticulum (see Fig. 3.5). The main role of IP$_3$, described in more detail in Chapter 4, is to control the release of Ca^{2+} from intracellular stores. Because many drug and hormone effects involve intracellular Ca^{2+}, this pathway is particularly important.

Diacylglycerol and protein kinase C
DAG is produced, as well as IP$_3$, whenever receptor-induced PI hydrolysis occurs. The main effect of DAG is to activate a protein kinase, *protein kinase C* (PKC), which catalyses the phosphorylation of several intracellular proteins. DAG, unlike the inositol phosphates, is highly lipophilic and remains within the membrane. It binds to a specific site on the PKC molecule, causing the enzyme to migrate from the cytosol to the cell membrane, thereby becoming activated. There are at least 10 different mammalian PKC subtypes, which have distinct cellular distributions and phosphorylate different proteins. Several are activated by DAG and raised intracellular Ca^{2+}, both of which are produced by activation of GPCRs.[15] PKCs are also activated

by *phorbol esters* (highly irritant, tumour-promoting compounds produced by certain plants), which have been extremely useful in studying the functions of PKC. One of the subtypes is activated by the lipid mediator *arachidonic acid* (see Ch. 18) generated by the action of phospholipase A$_2$ on membrane phospholipids, so PKC activation can also occur with agonists that activate this enzyme. The various PKC isoforms, like the tyrosine kinases discussed later (p. 40), act on many different functional proteins, such as ion channels, receptors, enzymes (including other kinases), transcription factors and cytoskeletal proteins. Protein phosphorylation by kinases plays a central role in signal transduction, and controls many different aspects of cell function. The DAG–PKC link provides a mechanism whereby GPCRs can mobilise this army of control freaks.

Ion channels as targets for G proteins
Another major function of GPCRs is to control ion channel function directly by mechanisms that do not involve second messengers such as cAMP or inositol phosphates. Direct G protein–channel interaction, through the βγ subunits of G$_i$ and G$_o$ proteins, appears to be a general mechanism for controlling K$^+$ and Ca^{2+} channels. In cardiac muscle, for example, mAChRs enhance K$^+$ permeability in this way (thus hyperpolarising the cells and inhibiting electrical activity; see Ch. 22). Similar mechanisms operate in neurons, where many inhibitory drugs, such as opioid analgesics, reduce excitability by opening certain K$^+$ channels – known as G protein-activated inwardly rectifying K$^+$ channels (GIRK) – or by inhibiting voltage-activated N and P/Q type Ca^{2+} channels, thus reducing neurotransmitter release (see Chs 4 and 43).

The Rho/Rho kinase system
▼ This signal transduction pathway (see Bishop & Hall, 2000) is activated by certain GPCRs (and also by non-GPCR mechanisms), which couple to G proteins of the G$_{12/13}$ type. The free G protein α subunit interacts with a *guanosine nucleotide exchange factor*, which facilitates GDP–GTP exchange at another GTPase, Rho. Rho–GDP, the resting form, is inactive, but when GDP–GTP exchange occurs, Rho is activated, and in turn activates Rho kinase. Rho kinase phosphorylates many substrate proteins and controls a wide variety of cellular functions, including smooth muscle contraction and proliferation, cell movement and migration, angiogenesis and synaptic remodelling. By enhancing hypoxia-induced pulmonary artery vasoconstriction, activation of Rho kinase is thought to be important in the pathogenesis of pulmonary hypertension (see Ch. 23). Specific Rho kinase inhibitors are in development for several clinical indications including glaucoma – an area to watch.

The MAP kinase system
▼ The MAP kinase system involves several signal transduction pathways (Fig. 3.15) that are activated not only by various cytokines and growth factors acting on kinase-linked receptors (see p. 42, Fig. 3.17), but also by ligands activating GPCRs. The coupling of GPCRs to different families of MAP kinases can involve G protein α and βγ subunits as well as *Src* and *arrestins* – proteins also involved in GPCR desensitisation (see p. 38). The MAP kinase system controls many processes involved in gene expression, cell division, apoptosis and tissue regeneration.

---

[14]Alternative abbreviations for these mediators are PtdIns (PI), PtdIns (4,5)-P$_2$ (PIP$_2$), Ins (1,4,5)-P$_3$ (IP$_3$).

[15]PKCs were originally named as Ca^{2+}-dependent protein kinases (PKC), as opposed to cAMP-dependent PKA. Although later subtypes were found not to be Ca^{2+}-dependent, the PKC name has stuck.

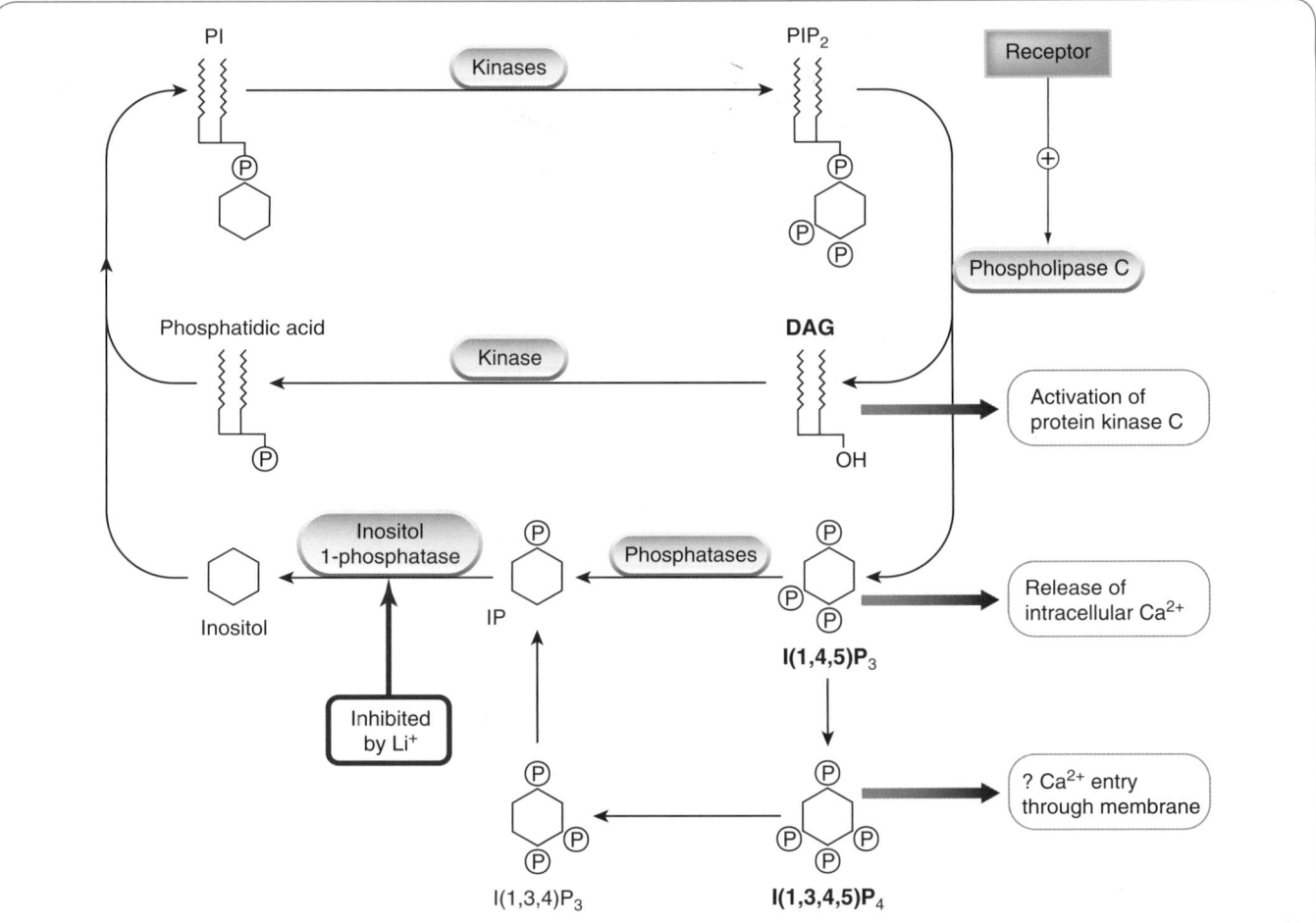

Fig. 3.13 **The phosphatidylinositol (PI) cycle.** Receptor-mediated activation of phospholipase C results in the cleavage of phosphatidylinositol bisphosphate (PIP$_2$), forming diacylglycerol (DAG) (which activates protein kinase C) and inositol trisphosphate (IP$_3$) (which releases intracellular Ca^{2+}). The role of inositol tetraphosphate (IP$_4$), which is formed from IP$_3$ and other inositol phosphates, is unclear, but it may facilitate Ca^{2+} entry through the plasma membrane. IP$_3$ is inactivated by dephosphorylation to inositol. DAG is converted to phosphatidic acid, and these two products are used to regenerate PI and PIP$_2$.

Effectors controlled by G proteins

Two key second messenger pathways are controlled by receptors via G proteins:
- Adenylyl cyclase/cAMP:
  - can be activated or inhibited by pharmacological ligands, depending on the nature of the receptor and G protein;
  - adenylyl cyclase catalyses formation of the intracellular messenger cAMP;
  - cAMP activates protein kinases such as protein kinase A (PKA) that control cell function in many different ways by causing phosphorylation of various enzymes, carriers and other proteins.
- Phospholipase C/inositol trisphosphate (IP$_3$)/diacylglycerol (DAG):
  - catalyses the formation of two intracellular messengers, IP$_3$ and DAG, from membrane phospholipid;
  - IP$_3$ acts to increase free cytosolic Ca^{2+} by releasing Ca^{2+} from intracellular compartments

  - increased free Ca^{2+} initiates many events, including contraction, secretion, enzyme activation and membrane hyperpolarisation;
  - DAG activates various protein kinase C (PKC) isoforms, which control many cellular functions by phosphorylating a variety of proteins.
Receptor-linked G proteins also control:
- Ion channels:
  - opening potassium channels, resulting in membrane hyperpolarisation;
  - inhibiting calcium channels, thus reducing neurotransmitter release.
- Phospholipase A$_2$ (and thus the formation of arachidonic acid and eicosanoids).

The main postulated roles of GPCRs in controlling enzymes and ion channels are summarised in Fig. 3.14.

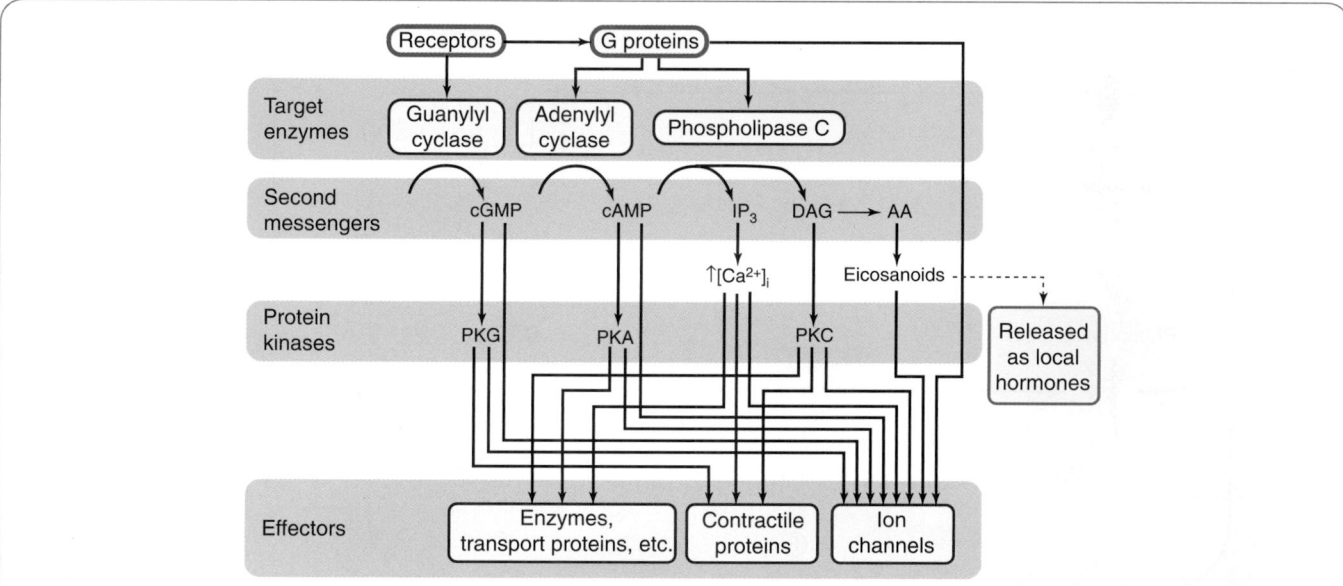

Fig. 3.14 G protein and second messenger control of cellular effector systems. Not shown in this diagram are signalling pathways where arrestins, rather than G proteins, link G protein–coupled receptors to downstream events *(see text and Fig. 3.15)*. *AA*, arachidonic acid; *DAG*, diacylglycerol; *IP₃*, inositol trisphosphate.

Fig. 3.15 G protein–coupled receptor (GPCR) activation of mitogen-activated protein (MAP) kinase cascade. (A) Sequential activation of the multiple components of the MAP kinase cascade. GPCR activation of MAP kinases can involve Gα and βγ subunits (not shown). (B) Activation of ERK and JNK3 through interaction with arrestins (βARR). Activation of ERK can occur either at the plasma membrane involving Src, or by direct activation after internalisation of the receptor/arrestin complex. *ARR*, arrestin; *GRK*, G protein–coupled receptor kinase.

FURTHER DEVELOPMENTS IN GPCR BIOLOGY

▼ By the early 1990s, we thought we had more or less got the measure of GPCR function, as described previously. Since then, the plot has thickened, and further developments have necessitated a substantial overhaul of the basic model.

GPCR desensitisation

▼ As described in Chapter 2, desensitisation is a feature of most GPCRs, and the mechanisms underlying it have been extensively studied. *Homologous desensitisation* is restricted to the receptors activated by the desensitising agonist, while *heterologous desensitisation* affects other GPCRs in addition. Two main processes are involved (see Kelly et al., 2008):

- receptor phosphorylation
- receptor internalisation (endocytosis)

The sequence of GPCRs includes certain residues (serine and threonine), mainly in the C-terminal cytoplasmic tail, which can be phosphorylated by specific GPCR kinases (GRKs) and by kinases such as PKA and PKC.

Fig. 3.16 Desensitisation and trafficking of G protein–coupled receptors (GPCRs). On prolonged agonist activation of the GPCR, selective GPCR kinases (GRKs) are recruited to the plasma membrane and phosphorylate the receptor. Arrestin (ARR) then binds and traffics the GPCR to clathrin-coated pits for subsequent internalisation into endosomes in a dynamin-dependent process. The GPCR is then dephosphorylated by a phosphatase (PP2A) and either recycled back to the plasma membrane or trafficked to lysosomes for degradation. *Dyn*, dynamin; *GRK*, G protein–coupled receptor kinase; *PP2A*, phosphatase 2A.

On receptor activation GRK2 and GRK3 are recruited to the plasma membrane by binding to free G protein βγ subunits. GRKs then phosphorylate the receptors in their activated (i.e. agonist-bound) state. The phosphorylated receptor serves as a binding site for arrestins, intracellular proteins that block the interaction between the receptor and the G proteins producing a selective *homologous desensitisation*. Arrestin binding also targets the receptor for endocytosis in clathrin-coated pits (Fig. 3.16). The internalised receptor can then either be dephosphorylated and reinserted into the plasma membrane (*resensitisation*) or trafficked to lysosomes for degradation (*inactivation*). This type of desensitisation seems to occur with most GPCRs but with subtle differences that fascinate the aficionados.

Phosphorylation by PKA and PKC at residues different from those targeted by GRKs generally leads to impaired coupling between the activated receptor and the G protein, so the agonist effect is reduced. This can give rise to either homologous or heterologous desensitisation, depending on whether or not receptors other than that for the desensitising agonist are simultaneously phosphorylated by the kinases, some of which are not very selective. Receptors phosphorylated by second messenger kinases are probably not internalised and are reactivated by dephosphorylation by phosphatases when the agonist is removed.

GPCR oligomerisation

▼ The earlier view that GPCRs exist and function as monomeric proteins (in contrast to ion channels, which generally comprise multimeric complexes; see p. 28) was first overturned by work on

the GABA_B receptor. Two subtypes of this GPCR exist, encoded by different genes, and the functional receptor consists of a heterodimer of the two (see Ch. 39). A similar situation arises with G protein–coupled glutamate receptors. Oddly, although the GABA_B dimer has two potential agonist binding sites, one on each subunit, only one is functional and signalling is transmitted through the dimer to the other receptor in the dimer which couples to the G protein (see Fig. 39.9).

Other GPCRs are functional as monomers but it now seems likely that most, if not all, GPCRs can exist as either homomeric or heteromeric oligomers (i.e. dimers or larger oligomers) (Ferré et al., 2015). Within the opioid receptor family (see Ch. 43), the μ receptor was crystallised as a dimer and stable and functional heterodimers of κ and δ receptors, whose pharmacological properties differ from those of either parent, have been created in cell lines. More diverse GPCR combinations have also been found, such as that between dopamine (D_2) and somatostatin receptors, on which both ligands act with increased potency. Roaming even further afield in search of functional assignations, the dopamine receptor D_5 can couple directly with a ligand-gated ion channel, the GABA_A receptor, inhibiting the function of the latter without the intervention of any G protein (Liu et al., 2000). These interactions have so far been studied mainly in engineered cell lines, but they also occur in native cells. Functional dimeric complexes between angiotensin (AT_1) and bradykinin (B_2) receptors occur in human platelets and show greater sensitivity to angiotensin than 'pure' AT_1 receptors (AbdAlla et al., 2001). In women suffering from pregnancy-related hypertension (pre-eclamptic toxaemia), the number of these dimers increases due to increased expression of B_2 receptors, resulting – paradoxically – in increased sensitivity to the vasoconstrictor action of angiotensin.

It is too early to say what impact this newly discovered versatility of GPCRs in linking up with other receptors to form functional combinations will have on conventional pharmacology and therapeutics, but it could be considerable.

Constitutively active receptors

▼ GPCRs may be constitutively (i.e. spontaneously) active in the absence of any agonist (see Ch. 2 and review by Costa & Cotecchia, 2005). This was first shown for δ opioid receptors (see Ch. 43). There are now many other examples of native GPCRs that show constitutive activity when studied in vitro. The histamine H_3 receptor also shows constitutive activity in vivo, and this may prove to be a quite general phenomenon. It means that inverse agonists (see Ch. 2), which suppress this basal activity, may exert effects distinct from those of neutral antagonists, which block agonist effects without affecting basal activity.

Agonist specificity

▼ It was thought that the linkage of a particular GPCR to a particular signal transduction pathway depends mainly on the structure of the receptor, which confers specificity for a particular G protein, from which the rest of the signal transduction pathway follows. This would imply, in line with the two-state model discussed in Chapter 2, that all agonists acting on a particular receptor stabilise the same activated (R*) state and should activate the same signal transduction pathway, and produce the same type of cellular response. It is now clear that this is an oversimplification. In many cases, for example, with agonists acting on angiotensin receptors, or with inverse agonists on β adrenoceptors, the cellular effects are qualitatively different with different ligands, implying the existence of more than one – probably many – R* states (sometimes referred to as *biased agonism*; see Ch. 2). Binding of arrestins to GPCRs initiates MAP kinase signalling, such that agonists that induce GRK/arrestin 'desensitisation' will terminate some GPCR signalling but may also activate signalling through arrestins that may continue even after the receptor/arrestin complex has been internalised (see Fig. 3.15).

Biased agonism has profound implications – indeed heretical to many pharmacologists, who are accustomed to thinking of agonists in terms of their affinity and efficacy, and nothing else; it has added a new dimension to the way in which we think about drug efficacy and specificity (see Kenakin and Christopoulos, 2013).

Receptor activity-modifying proteins

▼ Receptor activity-modifying proteins (RAMPs) are a family of membrane proteins that associate with some GPCRs and alter their functional characteristics. They were discovered in 1998 when it was found that the functionally active receptor for the neuropeptide *calcitonin gene-related peptide* (CGRP) (see Chs 16 and 19) consisted of a complex of a GPCR – called calcitonin receptor-like receptor (CRLR) – that by itself lacked activity, with another membrane protein (RAMP1). More surprisingly, CRLR when coupled with another RAMP (RAMP2) showed a quite different pharmacology, being activated by an unrelated peptide, *adrenomedulin*. In other words, the agonist specificity is conferred by the associated RAMP as well as by the GPCR itself. More RAMPs have emerged, and so far nearly all the examples involve Class B peptide receptors (see Table 3.2), the calcium-sensing receptor being an exception. RAMPs are an example of how protein–protein interactions influence the pharmacological behaviour of the receptors in a highly selective way and may be novel targets for drug development (Sexton et al., 2012).

G protein–independent signalling

▼ In using the term *G protein–coupled receptor* to describe the class of receptors characterised by their heptahelical structure, we are following conventional textbook dogma but neglecting the fact that G proteins are not the only link between GPCRs and the various effector systems that they regulate. In this context, signalling mediated through arrestins bound to the receptor (see p. 36), rather than through G proteins, is important (see reviews by Pierce & Lefkowitz, 2001; Delcourt et al., 2007). Arrestins can act as an intermediary for GPCR activation of the MAP kinase cascade (see Fig. 3.15B).

There are many examples where the various 'adapter proteins' that link receptors of the tyrosine kinase type to their effectors (see p. 42) can also interact with GPCRs (see Brzostowski & Kimmel, 2001), allowing the same effector systems to be regulated by receptors of either type.

In summary, the simple dogma that has underpinned much of our understanding of GPCRs, namely, one GPCR gene – one GPCR protein – one functional GPCR – one G protein – one response, is showing distinct signs of wear. In particular:

- one gene, through alternative splicing, RNA editing, etc., can give rise to more than one receptor protein;
- one GPCR protein can associate with others, or with other proteins such as RAMPs, to produce more than one type of functional receptor;
- different agonists may affect a receptor in different ways and elicit qualitatively different responses;
- the signal transduction pathway from 'GPCR' does not invariably require G proteins, and there can be cross-talk with tyrosine kinase-linked receptors.

GPCRs are evidently versatile and adventurous molecules around which much modern pharmacology revolves, and nobody imagines that we have reached the end of the story.

TYPE 3: KINASE-LINKED AND RELATED RECEPTORS

These membrane receptors are quite different in structure and function from ligand-gated channels and GPCRs. They are activated by a wide variety of protein mediators, including growth factors and cytokines (see Ch. 19), and hormones such as insulin (see Ch. 32) and leptin (Ch. 33), whose effects are exerted mainly at the level of gene transcription. Most of these receptors are large proteins consisting of a single chain of up to 1000 residues, with a single membrane-spanning helical region, linking a large extracellular ligand-binding domain to an intracellular domain of variable size and function. The basic structure is shown in Fig. 3.3C, but many variants exist (see later). Over 100 such receptors have been cloned, and many structural variations exist. For more detail, see the review by Hubbard & Miller (2007). These receptors play a major role in controlling cell division, intermediary metabolism, growth, differentiation, inflammation, tissue repair, apoptosis and immune responses, discussed further in Chapters 6 and 19.

The main types are as follows:

Receptor tyrosine kinases (RTKs). These receptors have the basic structure shown in Fig. 3.17A, incorporating a tyrosine kinase moiety in the intracellular region. They include receptors for many growth factors, such as **epidermal growth factor** and **nerve growth factor**, and also the group of *TLRs* that recognise bacterial lipopolysaccharides and play an important role in the body's reaction to infection (see Ch. 7). The insulin receptor (see Ch. 32) also belongs to the RTK class, although it has a more complex dimeric structure, and links indirectly to intracellular tyrosine kinases.

Receptor serine/threonine kinases. This smaller class is similar in structure to RTKs but they phosphorylate serine and/or threonine residues rather than tyrosine. The main example is the receptor for **transforming growth factor** (TGF).

Cytokine receptors. These receptors (Fig. 3.17B) lack intrinsic enzyme activity. When occupied, they activate various tyrosine kinases, such as Jak (the Janus kinase). Ligands for these receptors include cytokines such as **interferons** and **colony-stimulating factors** involved in immunological responses as well as cell growth and differentiation.

Fig. 3.17 **Transduction mechanisms of kinase-linked receptors.** The first step following agonist binding is dimerisation, which leads to autophosphorylation of the intracellular domain of each receptor. SH2-domain proteins then bind to the phosphorylated receptor and are themselves phosphorylated. Two well-characterised pathways are shown: (A) the growth factor (Ras/Raf/mitogen-activated protein [MAP] kinase) pathway (see also Ch. 6). Grb2 can also be phosphorylated but this negatively regulates its signalling. (B) Simplified scheme of the cytokine (Jak/Stat) pathway (see also Ch. 19). Some cytokine receptors may pre-exist as dimers rather than dimerise on cytokine binding. Several other pathways exist, and these phosphorylation cascades interact with components of G protein systems.

Kinase-linked receptors

- Receptors for various growth factors incorporate tyrosine kinase in their intracellular domain.
- Cytokine receptors have an intracellular domain that binds and activates cytosolic kinases when the receptor is occupied.
- The receptors all share a common architecture, with a large extracellular ligand-binding domain connected via a single membrane-spanning helix to the intracellular domain.
- Signal transduction generally involves dimerisation of receptors, followed by autophosphorylation of tyrosine residues. The phosphotyrosine residues act as acceptors for the SH2 domains of a variety of intracellular proteins, thereby allowing control of many cell functions.
- They are involved mainly in events controlling cell growth and differentiation, and act indirectly by regulating gene transcription.
- Two important pathways are:
  - the Ras/Raf/mitogen-activated protein (MAP) kinase pathway, which is important in cell division, growth and differentiation
  - the Jak/Stat pathway activated by many cytokines, which controls the synthesis and release of many inflammatory mediators.

PROTEIN PHOSPHORYLATION AND KINASE CASCADE MECHANISMS

Protein phosphorylation (see Cohen, 2002) is a key mechanism for controlling the function of proteins (e.g. enzymes, ion channels, receptors, transport proteins) involved in regulating cellular processes. Phosphorylation and dephosphorylation are accomplished by *kinases* and *phosphatases*, respectively – enzymes, of which several hundred subtypes are represented in the human genome – which are themselves subject to regulation dependent on their phosphorylation status. Much effort is currently being invested in mapping the complex interactions between signalling molecules that are involved in drug effects and pathophysiological processes such as oncogenesis, neurodegeneration, inflammation and much else. Here we can present only a few pharmacologically relevant aspects of what has become an enormous subject.

In many cases, ligand binding to the receptor leads to dimerisation. The association of the two intracellular kinase domains allows a mutual autophosphorylation of intracellular tyrosine residues to occur. The phosphorylated tyrosine residues then serve as high-affinity docking sites for other intracellular proteins that form the next stage in the signal transduction cascade. One important group of such proteins is known as the *SH2 domain proteins* (standing for *Src* homology, because they were first identified in the *Src* oncogene product).[16] These possess a highly conserved

sequence of about 100 amino acids, forming a recognition site for the phosphotyrosine residues of the receptor. Individual SH2 domain proteins, of which many are now known, bind selectively to particular receptors, so the pattern of events triggered by particular growth factors is highly specific. The mechanism is summarised in Fig. 3.17.

What happens when the SH2 domain protein binds to the phosphorylated receptor varies greatly according to the receptor that is involved; many SH2 domain proteins are enzymes, such as protein kinases or phospholipases. Some growth factors activate a specific subtype of phospholipase C (PLCγ), thereby causing phospholipid breakdown, IP_3 formation and Ca^{2+} release (see p. 35). Other SH2-containing proteins couple phosphotyrosine-containing proteins with a variety of other functional proteins, including many that are involved in the control of cell division and differentiation. The end result is to activate or inhibit, by phosphorylation, a variety of transcription factors that migrate to the nucleus and suppress or induce the expression of particular genes. For more detail, see Jin and Pawson (2012). *Nuclear factor kappa B* (NFκB) is a transcription factor that plays a key role in multiple disorders including inflammation and cancer (see Chs 18 and 57; Karin et al., 2004). It is normally present in the cytosol, complexed with an inhibitor (IκB). Phosphorylation of IκB occurs when a specific kinase (IKK) is activated in response to various inflammatory cytokines and GPCR agonists. This results in dissociation of IκB from NFκB and migration of NFκB to the nucleus, where it switches on various proinflammatory and anti-apoptotic genes.

▼ Two well-defined signal transduction pathways are summarised in Fig. 3.17. The Ras/Raf pathway mediates the effect of many growth factors and mitogens. Ras, which is a proto-oncogene product, functions like a G protein, and conveys the signal (by GDP/GTP exchange) from the SH2-domain protein, Grb. Activation of Ras in turn activates Raf, which is the first of a sequence of three serine/threonine kinases, each of which phosphorylates, and activates, the next in line. The last of these, MAP kinase (which is also activated by GPCRs, see earlier), phosphorylates one or more transcription factors that initiate gene expression, resulting in a variety of cellular responses, including cell division. This three-tiered MAP kinase cascade forms part of many intracellular signalling pathways involved in a wide variety of disease processes, including malignancy, inflammation, neurodegeneration, atherosclerosis and much else. The kinases form a large family, with different subtypes serving specific roles. They are thought to represent an important target for future therapeutic drugs. Many cancers are associated with mutations in the genes coding for proteins involved in this cascade, leading to activation of the cascade in the absence of the growth factor signal (see Chs 6 and 57). For more details, see the review by Avruch (2007).

A second pathway, the Jak/Stat pathway (see Fig. 3.17B), is involved in responses to many cytokines. Dimerisation of these receptors occurs when the cytokine binds, and this attracts a cytosolic tyrosine kinase unit (Jak) to associate with, and phosphorylate, the receptor dimer. Jaks belong to a family of proteins, different members having specificity for different cytokine receptors. Among the targets for phosphorylation by Jak are a family of transcription factors (Stats). These are SH2-domain proteins that bind to the phosphotyrosine groups on the receptor–Jak complex, and are themselves phosphorylated. Thus activated, Stat migrates to the nucleus and activates gene expression.

Other important mechanisms centre on *phosphatidylinositol-3 kinase* (PI₃ kinases, see Vanhaesebroeck et al., 1997), a ubiquitous enzyme family that is activated both by GPCRs and RTKs and attaches a phosphate group to position 3 of PIP_2 to form PIP_3. Other protein

---

[16]*v-Src* is a gene found in Rous sarcoma virus that encodes a tyrosine kinase which causes sarcoma (a malignant tumour) in chickens – it was found to have a closely related sequence to the chicken's own gene termed c-Src (for cellular rather than viral Src). This was the first oncogene to be discovered, in 1979.

---

[17]Protein kinase B was named to fill in the gap between protein kinase A (cAMP-dependent) and protein kinase C (Ca²⁺-dependent). As you can see, nomenclature is highly imaginative!

kinases, particularly protein kinase B (PKB,[17] also known as Akt), have recognition sites for PIP$_3$ and are thus activated, controlling a wide variety of cellular functions, including apoptosis, differentiation, proliferation and trafficking. Akt also causes NO synthase activation in the vascular endothelium (see Ch. 21).

Recent work on signal transduction pathways has produced a bewildering profusion of molecular detail, often couched in a jargon that is apt to deter the faint-hearted. Perseverance will be rewarded, however, for there is no doubt that important new drugs, particularly in the areas of inflammation, immunology and cancer, will come from the targeting of these proteins. A breakthrough in the treatment of chronic myeloid leukaemia was achieved with the introduction of the first explicitly-designed kinase inhibitor, **imatinib**, a drug that inhibits a specific tyrosine kinase involved in the pathogenesis of the disease (see Ch. 57).

Fig. 3.18 illustrates the central role of protein kinases in signal transduction pathways in a highly simplified and schematic way. Many, if not all, of the proteins involved, including the receptors and the kinases themselves, are substrates for kinases, so there are many mechanisms for feedback and cross-talk between the various signalling pathways. Given that there are over 500 protein kinases, and similarly large numbers of receptors and other signalling molecules, the network of interactions can look bewilderingly complex. Dissecting out the details has become a major theme in cell biology. For pharmacologists, the idea of a simple connection between receptor and response, which guided thinking throughout the 20th century, is undoubtedly crumbling, although it will take some time before the complexities of signalling pathways are assimilated into a new way of thinking about drug action.

Protein phosphorylation in signal transduction

- Many receptor-mediated events involve protein phosphorylation, which controls the functional and binding properties of intracellular proteins.
- Receptor-linked tyrosine kinases, cyclic nucleotide-activated tyrosine kinases and intracellular serine/threonine kinases comprise a 'kinase cascade' mechanism that leads to amplification of receptor-mediated events.
- There are many kinases, with differing substrate specificities, allowing specificity in the pathways activated by different hormones.
- Desensitisation of G protein–coupled receptors occurs as a result of phosphorylation by specific receptor kinases, causing the receptor to become non-functional and to be internalised.
- There is a large family of phosphatases that act to dephosphorylate proteins and thus reverse the effects of kinases.

Fig. 3.18 **Central role of kinase cascades in signal transduction.** Kinase cascades (e.g. those shown in Fig. 3.15) are activated by G protein–coupled receptors (GPCRs), either directly or via different second messengers, by receptors that generate cGMP, or by kinase-linked receptors. The kinase cascades regulate various target proteins, which in turn produce a wide variety of short- and long-term effects. *CaM kinase,* Ca^{2+}/calmodulin-dependent kinase; *DAG,* diacylglycerol; *GC,* guanylyl cyclase; *GRK,* GPCR kinase; *IP$_3$,* inositol trisphosphate; *PKA,* cAMP-dependent protein kinase; *PKC,* protein kinase C; *PKG,* cGMP-dependent protein kinase.

TYPE 4: NUCLEAR RECEPTORS

By the 1970s, it was clear that receptors for steroid hormones such as oestrogen and the glucocorticoids (Chs. 36 and 34) were present in the cytoplasm of cells and translocated into the nucleus after binding with their steroid partner. Other hormones, such as the thyroid hormone T_3 (Ch. 35) and the fat-soluble vitamins D and A (retinoic acid), were found to act in a similar fashion. Comparisons of gene and protein sequence data led to the recognition that these receptors were members of a much larger family of related proteins. We now know these as the *nuclear receptor (NR) family*.

As well as NRs such as the glucocorticoid and retinoic acid receptor, whose ligands are well characterised, this family includes a great many (~40%) orphan receptors – receptors with no known well-defined ligands (see earlier). The first of these to be described, in the 1990s, was the *retinoid X receptor* (RXR), a receptor cloned on the basis of its similarity with the vitamin A receptor, and which was subsequently found to bind the vitamin A derivative 9-*cis*-retinoic acid. This event triggered intense interest in the NR field and, during the intervening years, specific binding partners have been characterised for many NRs ('adopted orphans', e.g. RXR) although in the case of many others ('true orphans') these have yet to be identified – or perhaps do not exist as such, as one possible function of these receptors is their 'promiscuous' ability to bind to many related compounds (such as dietary factors) with low affinity.

Unlike the other receptors described in this chapter, NRs can interact with DNA directly, and can be regarded as *ligand-activated transcription factors* that produce their effects by modifying gene transcription. Through this mechanism they can control the transcription and expression of many genes and proteins so, as it might be imagined, they are key players in regulating metabolic, developmental and other critical physiological processes. Another unique property is that NRs are not generally embedded in membranes like GPCRs or ion channels, but are present in other compartments of the cell. Some, such as the steroid receptors, which are predominately located in the cytoplasm, are activated by their ligand and translocate from the cytoplasm to the nucleus, while others, such as the RXR, probably dwell mainly within the nuclear compartment. Having said this, there is increasing evidence for the existence of small pools of some NRs, such as oestrogen and glucocorticoid receptors (ER and GR) at the plasma membrane and in organelles such as the mitochondria (Levin and Hammes, 2016), where they can act directly on other targets such as protein kinases to bring about immediate biological actions.

The NR superfamily probably evolved from a single distant evolutionary ancestral gene by duplication and other events. In man, there are at least 48 members, but more proteins may arise through alternative splicing events. While this represents a rather small proportion of all receptors (less than 10% of the total number of GPCRs), the NRs are very important drug targets (Burris et al., 2013), being responsible for the biological effects of approximately 10%–15% of all prescription drugs. They can recognise an extraordinarily diverse group of substances (mostly small hydrophobic molecules), which may exhibit full or partial agonist, antagonist or inverse agonist activity. Some NRs which bind their ligands with high affinity (e.g. ER and GR) are involved predominantly in endocrine signalling, but many bind their ligands with low affinity and probably act as metabolic (e.g. lipid) sensors. They are thus crucial links between our dietary and metabolic status and the expression of genes that regulate the metabolism and disposition of lipids. NRs also regulate expression of many drug-metabolising enzymes and transporters.

STRUCTURE OF NUCLEAR RECEPTORS

▼ All NRs are monomeric proteins of 50–100 kDa, which share a broadly similar structural design (see Fig. 3.19 and Bourguet et al., 2000, for further details). The *N-terminal domain* displays the most heterogeneity. It harbours the *activation function 1 (AF1)* site that binds to other cell-specific transcription factors in a ligand-independent way and modifies the binding or regulatory capacity of the receptor itself. In the presence of the ligand, it synergises with *AF2* to produce the fully active complex. Alternative splicing of genes may yield several receptor isoforms, each with slightly different N-terminal regions. The *core domain* of the receptor is highly conserved and consists of the structure responsible for DNA recognition and binding. At the molecular level, this comprises two *zinc fingers* – cysteine- (or cystine-/histidine-) rich loops in the amino acid chain that are held in a particular conformation by zinc ions. The main function of this portion of the molecule is to recognise and bind to the *hormone response elements* (HREs) located in the genes that are regulated by this family of receptors, but it also plays a part in regulating receptor dimerisation which is crucial to the function of most NRs.

It is the highly flexible *hinge region* in the molecule that allows it to dimerise with other NRs and regulates the intracellular trafficking of the receptor. This can produce molecular complexes with diverse configurations, able to interact differently with DNA. Finally, the *C-terminal domain* contains the *ligand-binding module* and is specific to each class of receptor, although structurally highly conserved. It is also important in dimerisation and binding co-activator and co-repressor proteins (see later). The AF2 region is important in ligand-dependent activation and is generally highly conserved, although it is absent in *Rev-erbAα* and *Rev-erbAβ*, NRs that regulate metabolism (and also function as part of a circadian molecular clock mechanism). Also located near the C-terminal are motifs that contain *nuclear localisation signals* and others that may, in the case of some receptors, bind *accessory heat shock* and other proteins.

CONTROL OF GENE TRANSCRIPTION

▼ HREs are short (usually 4–6 base pairs) sequences of DNA to which the NRs bind to modify gene transcription. They are generally present symmetrically in pairs or *half-sites*, although these may be arranged together in different ways (e.g. *simple repeats* or *inverted repeats*). Each NR exhibits a preference for a particular *consensus sequence* and the nucleotide spacing between them, but because of the family homology, they share a close similarity. In the nucleus, the AF1 and AF2 domains of the ligand-bound receptor recruit large complexes of other proteins including co-activators or co-repressors to modify gene expression. Some of these co-activators are enzymes involved in chromatin remodelling, such as histone acetylase/deacetylase which, together with other enzymes, regulate the unravelling of the DNA to facilitate access by polymerase enzymes and hence gene transcription. Co-repressor complexes are recruited by some receptors and comprise histone deacetylase and other factors that cause the chromatin to become tightly packed, preventing further transcriptional activation. The case of the *constitutive androstane receptor* (CAR, see later) is particularly interesting: like some G proteins described earlier in this chapter, CAR can form a constitutively active complex that is terminated when it binds its ligand. The mechanisms of negative gene regulation by NRs are particularly complex (see Santos et al., 2011 for a good account of this phenomenon). In addition to agonists, NRs can also be targeted by competitive antagonists, which prevent occupation of the binding site by the endogenous ligand or by inverse agonists (or antagonists), which sterically prevent the binding of co-activator factors, thus reducing the constitutive activity of these

Fig. 3.19 **Schematic diagram of a nuclear receptor.** A greatly simplified diagram of the functional topology of a nuclear receptor (the oestrogen receptor is picked as an example). A schematic diagram shows the various regions of the receptor including the DNA-binding domain (DBD). Below is a diagram illustrating, in the corresponding colours, the configuration of the liganded receptor showing its binding to hormone response elements (HREs) on DNA. In panel A, the ligand (L) is bound in the ligand-binding domain (LBD) and this enables the C-terminal AF2 region to bind to the LBD. In turn, this allows the binding of a co-activator protein at the LBD (only a partial structure shown), which allows gene transcription to proceed. In panel B, an antagonist (A) is bound to the LBD. This sterically inhibits the binding of AF2 and thus the attachment of the co-activator protein. Most nuclear receptors operate as dimers but only a monomer is shown here for clarity. (Based largely upon Shiau et al., 1998.) Cylindrical structures represent regions of α-helical protein structure.

receptors. A very interesting development is the identification of selective receptor modulators (e.g. selective oestrogen receptor modulators - SERMs) which, by altering the binding of co-activator and co-repressor proteins, have agonist activity in some tissues and antagonist activities in others.

CLASSIFICATION OF NUCLEAR RECEPTORS

NRs are usually classified into subfamilies according to their phylogeny. For our purposes, however, it is more useful to classify them on the basis of their molecular action into two main classes (I and II), and two other minor groups of receptors (III, IV).

Class I consists largely of endocrine steroid receptors, including the GRs and mineralocorticoid receptors (MRs), as well as the oestrogen, progesterone and androgen receptors (ER, PR and AR, respectively). The hormones (e.g. glucocorticoids) recognised by these receptors generally act in a negative feedback fashion to control biological events (see Ch. 34 for more details). In the absence of their ligand, these NRs are predominantly located in the cytoplasm, complexed with heat shock and other proteins, and possibly reversibly attached to the cytoskeleton or other intracellular structures. Following diffusion (or possibly transportation) into the cell from the blood, ligands bind their NR partner with high affinity. These liganded receptors generally form homodimers and translocate to the nucleus, where they can *transactivate* or *transrepress* genes by binding to 'positive' or 'negative' HREs. Once bound, the NR recruits other proteins to form complexes that promote transcription of multiple genes. For example, it is estimated that the activated GR itself can regulate

transcription of ~1% of the genome either directly or indirectly.

Class II NRs function in a slightly different way. Their ligands are generally lipids or other metabolites already present to some extent within the cell. This group includes the *peroxisome proliferator-activated receptor* (PPAR) that recognises fatty acids; the *liver oxysterol receptor* (LXR) that recognises and acts as a cholesterol sensor, the *farnesoid (bile acid) receptor* (FXR), a *xenobiotic receptor* (SXR; in rodents the PXR) that recognises a great many foreign substances, including therapeutic drugs, and the *CAR*, which not only recognises the steroid androstane but also some drugs such as **phenobarbital** (see Ch. 46). Indeed, PXR and CAR are akin to airport security guards who alert the bomb disposal squad when suspicious luggage is found. When they sense foreign molecules (xenobiotics), they induce drug-metabolising enzymes such as CYP3A (which is responsible for metabolising about 60% of all prescription drugs; see Ch. 10 and di Masi et al., 2009). They also bind some prostaglandins and non-steroidal drugs, as well as the antidiabetic **thiazolidinediones** (see Ch. 32) and **fibrates** (see Ch. 24).

Unlike the receptors in class I, these NRs almost always operate as heterodimers together with RXR, the retinoid X receptor. Two types of heterodimer may then be formed: a *non-permissive heterodimer*, which can be activated only by the RXR ligand itself, and the *permissive heterodimer*, which can be activated either by retinoic acid itself or by its partner's ligand. Class II NRs are generally bound to co-repressor proteins. These dissociate when the ligand binds and allows recruitment of co-activator proteins

Table 3.4 **Some common pharmacologically significant nuclear receptors**

Receptor name	Abbreviation	Ligand	Drugs	Location	Ligand binding	Mechanism of action
Type I						
Androgen	AR	Testosterone	All natural and synthetic glucocorticoids (Ch. 34), mineralocorticoids (Ch. 30) and sex steroids (Ch. 36) together with their antagonists (e.g. raloxifene, 4-hydroxy-tamoxifen and mifepristone).	Cytosolic	Homodimers	Translocation to nucleus. Binding to HREs with two half-sites with an inverted sequence. Recruitment of co-activators, transcription factors and other proteins.
Oestrogen	ERα, β	17β-oestradiol				
Glucocorticoid	GRα	Cortisol, corticosterone				
Progesterone	PR	Progesterone				
Mineralocorticoid	MR	Aldosterone				
Type II						
Retinoid X	RXR α,β,γ	9-*cis*-retinoic acid	Retinoid drugs (Ch. 28)	Nuclear	Heterodimers often with RXR	Binding to HREs with two half-sites with an inverted or simple repeat sequence. Complexed with co-repressors, which are displaced following ligand binding, allowing the binding of co-activators
Retinoic acid	RAR α,β,γ	Vitamin A				
Thyroid hormone	TR α,β	T3, T4	Thyroid hormone drugs (Ch. 35)			
Peroxisome proliferator	PPAR α,β,γ,δ	Fatty acids, prostaglandins	Rosiglitazone, pioglitazone (Ch. 32)			
Constitutive androstane	CAR	Androstane	Stimulation of CYP synthesis and alteration of drug metabolism (Ch. 10)			
Pregnane X	PXR	Xenobiotics				

Only examples from Classes I and II are included.

and hence changes in gene transcription. They tend to mediate positive feedback effects (e.g. occupation of the receptor amplifies rather than inhibits a particular biological event).

Class III NRs are very similar to Class I in the sense that they form homodimers, but they can bind to HREs, which do not have an inverted repeat sequence. Class IV NRs may function as monomers or dimers but only bind to one HRE half site. Many of the remaining orphan receptors belong to these latter classes.

The discussion here must be taken only as a broad guide to the action of NRs, as many other types of interaction have also been discovered. For example, some of these receptors may bring about non-genomic – or even genomic – actions by directly interacting with factors in the cytosol, or they may be covalently modified by phosphorylation or by protein–protein interactions with other transcription factors such that their function is altered (see Falkenstein et al., 2000).

Table 3.4 summarises the properties of some common NRs of importance to pharmacologists.

ION CHANNELS AS DRUG TARGETS

We have discussed ligand-gated ion channels as one of the four main types of drug receptor. There are many other types of ion channel that represent important drug targets, even though they are not generally classified as 'receptors'

Nuclear receptors

- A family of 48 soluble receptors that sense lipid and hormonal signals and modulate gene transcription.
- Their ligands are many and varied, including steroid drugs and hormone, thyroid hormones, vitamins A and D, various lipids and xenobiotics
- There are two main categories:
  - Class I nuclear receptors (NRs) are present in the cytoplasm, form homodimers in the presence of their ligand, and migrate to the nucleus. Their ligands are mainly endocrine in nature (e.g. steroid hormones);
  - Class II NRs are generally constitutively present in the nucleus and form heterodimers with the retinoid X receptor. Their ligands are usually lipids (e.g. the fatty acids).
- The liganded receptor complexes initiate changes in gene transcription by binding to hormone response elements in gene promoters and recruiting co-activator or co-repressor factors.
- The receptor family is the target of approximately 10% of prescription drugs, and the enzymes that it regulates affect the pharmacokinetics of some 60% of all prescription drugs.

because they are not the immediate targets of fast neuro-transmitters, but drugs can act upon them to alter their ability to open and close.[18]

Here we discuss the structure and function of ion channels at the molecular level; their role as regulators of cell function is described in Chapter 4.

Ions are unable to penetrate the lipid bilayer of the cell membrane, and can get across only with the help of membrane-spanning proteins in the form of channels or transporters. The concept of ion channels was developed in the 1950s on the basis of electrophysiological studies on the mechanism of membrane excitation (see Ch. 4). Electrophysiology, particularly the *voltage clamp technique*, remains an essential tool for studying the physiological and pharmacological properties of ion channels. Since the mid-1980s, when the first ion channels were cloned by Numa in Japan, much has been learned about the structure and function of these complex molecules. The use of patch clamp recording, which allows the behaviour of individual channels to be studied in real time, has been particularly valuable in distinguishing channels on the basis of their conductance and gating characteristics. Accounts by Hille (2001), Ashcroft (2000) and Catterall (2000) give background information.

Ion channels consist of protein molecules designed to form water-filled pores that span the membrane, and can switch between open and closed states. The rate and direction of ion movement through the pore is governed by the electrochemical gradient for the ion in question, which is a function of its concentration on either side of the membrane, and of the membrane potential. Ion channels are characterised by:

- their selectivity for particular ion species, determined by the size of the pore and the nature of its lining;
- their gating properties (i.e. the nature of the stimulus that controls the transition between open and closed states of the channel);
- their molecular architecture.

ION SELECTIVITY

Channels are generally either cation selective or anion selective. The main cation-selective channels are selective for Na^+, Ca^{2+} or K^+, or non-selective and permeable to all three. Anion channels are mainly permeable to Cl^-, although other types also occur. The effect of modulation of ion channels on cell function is discussed in Chapter 4.

GATING

VOLTAGE-GATED CHANNELS

In the main these channels open when the cell membrane is depolarised.[19] They form a very important group because they underlie the mechanism of membrane excitability (see Ch. 4). The most important channels in this group are selective sodium, potassium or calcium channels.

Commonly, the channel opening (activation) induced by membrane depolarisation is short lasting, even if the depolarisation is maintained. This is because, with some channels, the initial activation of the channels is followed by a slower process of inactivation.

The role of voltage-gated channels in the generation of action potentials and in controlling other cell functions is described in Chapter 4.

LIGAND-GATED CHANNELS

These (see Fig. 3.5) are activated by binding of a chemical ligand to a site on the channel molecule. Fast neurotransmitters, such as glutamate, acetylcholine, GABA, 5-HT and ATP (see Chs 14, 16, 17 and 39) act in this way, binding to sites on the outside of the membrane. In addition, there are also ligand-gated ion channels that do not respond to neurotransmitters but to changes in their local environment. For example, the TRPV1 channel on sensory nerves that mediates the pain-producing effect of the chilli pepper ingredient capsaicin responds to extracellular protons when tissue pH falls, as occurs in inflamed tissue, as well as to the physical stimulus, heat (see Ch. 43).

Some ligand-gated channels in the plasma membrane respond to intracellular rather than extracellular signals, the most important being the following:

- Calcium-activated potassium channels, which occur in most cells and open, thus hyperpolarising the cell, when $[Ca^{2+}]_i$ increases.
- Calcium-activated chloride channels, widely expressed in excitable and non-excitable cells where they are involved in diverse functions such as epithelial secretion of electrolytes and water, sensory transduction, regulation of neuronal and cardiac excitability and regulation of vascular tone.
- ATP-sensitive potassium channels, which open when the intracellular ATP concentration falls because the cell is short of energy. These channels, which are quite distinct from those mediating the excitatory effects of extracellular ATP, occur in many nerve and muscle cells, and also in insulin-secreting cells (see Ch. 32), where they are part of the mechanism linking insulin secretion to blood glucose concentration.

Other examples of cell membrane channels that respond to intracellular ligands include arachidonic acid-sensitive potassium channels and DAG-sensitive calcium channels, whose functions are not well understood.

CALCIUM RELEASE CHANNELS

The main ones, IP_3 and **ryanodine** receptors (see Ch. 4), are a special class of ligand-gated calcium channels that are present on the endoplasmic or sarcoplasmic reticulum rather than the plasma membrane and control the release of Ca^{2+} from intracellular stores. Ca^{2+} can also be released from lysosomal stores by nicotinic acid adenine dinucleotide phosphate, which activates two-pore domain calcium channels.

STORE-OPERATED CALCIUM CHANNELS

When the intracellular Ca^{2+} stores are depleted, 'store-operated' channels (SOCs) in the plasma membrane open to allow Ca^{2+} entry. The mechanism by which this linkage

---

[18]In truth, the distinction between ligand-gated channels and other ion channels is an arbitrary one. In grouping ligand-gated channels with other types of receptor in this book, we are respecting the historical tradition established by Langley and others, who first defined receptors in the context of the action of acetylcholine at the neuromuscular junction. The advance of molecular biology may force us to reconsider this semantic issue in the future, but for now we make no apology for upholding the pharmacological tradition.

[19]There is always an exception to the rule! The members of the HCN family of potassium channels found in neurons and cardiac muscle cells are activated by hyperpolarisation.

Fig. 3.20 Molecular architecture of ion channels. *Red and blue rectangles* represent membrane-spanning α-helices. *Blue hairpins* are pore loop (P) domains, present in many channels, *blue rectangles* being the pore-forming regions of the membrane-spanning α-helices. *Cross-shaded rectangles* represent the voltage-sensing regions of voltage-gated channels. The *green symbol* represents the inactivating particle of voltage-gated sodium channels. Further information on ion channels is given in Chapter 4. *ASIC*, acid-sensing ion channel; *ENaC*, epithelial sodium channel; *TRP*, transient receptor potential channel.

occurs involves interaction of a Ca^{2+}-sensor protein in the endoplasmic reticulum membrane with a dedicated Ca^{2+} channel in the plasma membrane (see Stathopulos & Ikura, 2017). In response to GPCRs that elicit Ca^{2+} release, the opening of these channels allows the cytosolic free Ca^{2+} concentration, $[Ca^{2+}]_i$, to remain elevated even when the intracellular stores are running low, and also provides a route through which the stores can be replenished (see Ch. 4).

MOLECULAR ARCHITECTURE OF ION CHANNELS

▼ Ion channels are large and elaborate molecules. Their characteristic structural motifs have been revealed as knowledge of their sequence and structure has accumulated since the mid-1980s, when the first voltage-gated sodium channel was cloned. The main structural subtypes are shown in Fig. 3.20. All consist of several (often four) domains, which are similar or identical to each other, organised either as an oligomeric array of separate subunits, or as one large protein. Each subunit or domain contains a bundle of two to six membrane-spanning helices.

Voltage-gated channels generally include one transmembrane helix that contains an abundance of basic (i.e. positively charged) amino acids. When the membrane is depolarised, so that the interior of the cell becomes less negative, this region – the voltage sensor – moves slightly towards the outer surface of the membrane, which has the effect of opening the channel (see Bezanilla, 2008). Many voltage-activated channels also show *inactivation*, which happens when an intracellular appendage of the channel protein moves to plug the channel from the inside. Voltage-gated sodium and calcium channels

are remarkable in that the whole structure with four six-helix domains consists of a single huge protein molecule, the domains being linked together by intracellular loops of varying length (see Fig. 3.20B). Potassium channels comprise the most numerous and heterogeneous class.[20] Voltage-gated potassium channels resemble sodium channels, except that they are made up of four subunits rather than a single long chain. The class of potassium channels known as 'inward rectifier channels' because of their biophysical properties has the two-helix structure shown in Fig. 3.20A, whereas others are classed as 'two-pore domain' channels, because each subunit contains two P loops.

The various architectural motifs shown in Fig. 3.20 only scrape the surface of the molecular diversity of ion channels. In all cases, the individual subunits come in several molecular varieties, and these can unite in different combinations to form functional channels as *hetero-oligomers* (as distinct from *homo-oligomers* built from identical subunits). Furthermore, the channel-forming structures described are usually associated with other membrane proteins, which significantly affect their functional properties. For example, the ATP-gated potassium channel exists in association with the *sulfonylurea receptor* (SUR), and it is through this linkage that various drugs (including antidiabetic drugs of the sulfonylurea class; see Ch. 32) regulate the channel. Good progress is being made in understanding the relation between molecular structure and ion channel function, but we still have only a fragmentary understanding of the physiological role of many of these channels. Many important drugs exert their effects by influencing channel function, either directly or indirectly.

---

[20]The human genome encodes more than 70 distinct potassium channel subtypes – either a nightmare or a golden opportunity for the pharmacologist, depending on one's perspective.

PHARMACOLOGY OF ION CHANNELS

▼ Many drugs and physiological mediators described in this book exert their effects by altering the behaviour of ion channels.

The gating and permeation of both voltage-gated and ligand-gated ion channels is modulated by many factors, including the following.

- *Ligands that bind directly to various sites on the channel protein.* These include a variety of drugs and toxins that act in different ways, for example by blocking the channel or by affecting the gating process, thereby either facilitating or inhibiting the opening of the channel.
- *Mediators and drugs that act indirectly, mainly by activation of GPCRs.* The latter produce their effects mainly by affecting the state of phosphorylation of individual amino acids located on the intracellular region of the channel protein. As described above, this modulation involves the production of second messengers that activate protein kinases. The opening of the channel may be facilitated or inhibited, depending on which residues are phosphorylated. Drugs such as β-adrenoceptor agonists (Ch. 15) affect calcium and potassium channel function in this way, producing a wide variety of cellular effects.
- *Intracellular signals, particularly Ca^{2+} and nucleotides such as ATP and GTP (see Ch. 4).* Many ion channels possess binding sites for these intracellular mediators. Increased $[Ca^{2+}]_i$ opens certain types of potassium and chloride channels, and inactivates voltage-gated calcium channels. As described in Chapter 4, $[Ca^{2+}]_i$ is itself affected by the function of ion channels and GPCRs. Intracellular ATP binds to and closes a family of potassium channels known as the ATP-gated potassium channels (see Ch. 32) that are also sensitive to sulfonylurea drugs. Intracellular cyclic nucleotides, cAMP and cGMP, activate channels permeable to either calcium and sodium ions or to potassium ions.

Fig. 3.21 summarises the main sites and mechanisms by which drugs affect voltage-gated sodium channels, a typical example of this type of drug target.

CONTROL OF RECEPTOR EXPRESSION

Receptor proteins are synthesised by the cells that express them, and the level of expression is itself controlled, via the pathways discussed previously, by receptor-mediated events. We can no longer think of the receptors as the fixed elements in cellular control systems, responding to changes in the concentration of ligands, and initiating effects through the signal transduction pathway – they are themselves subject to regulation. Short-term regulation of receptor function generally occurs through *desensitisation*, as discussed earlier. Long-term regulation occurs through *an increase or decrease of receptor expression.* Examples of this type of control include the proliferation of various postsynaptic receptors after denervation (see Ch. 13), the up-regulation of various G protein–coupled and cytokine receptors in response to inflammation (see Ch. 18), and the induction of growth factor receptors by certain tumour viruses (see Ch. 6). Long-term drug treatment invariably induces adaptive responses, which, particularly with drugs that act on the central nervous system, can limit their effectiveness as in opioid tolerance (see Ch. 43) or can be the basis for therapeutic efficacy. In the latter instance this may take the form of a very slow onset of the therapeutic effect (e.g. with antidepressant drugs; see Ch. 48). It is likely that changes in receptor expression, secondary to the immediate action of the drug, are involved in delayed effects of this sort – a kind of 'secondary pharmacology', the importance of which is only now becoming clearer. The same principles apply

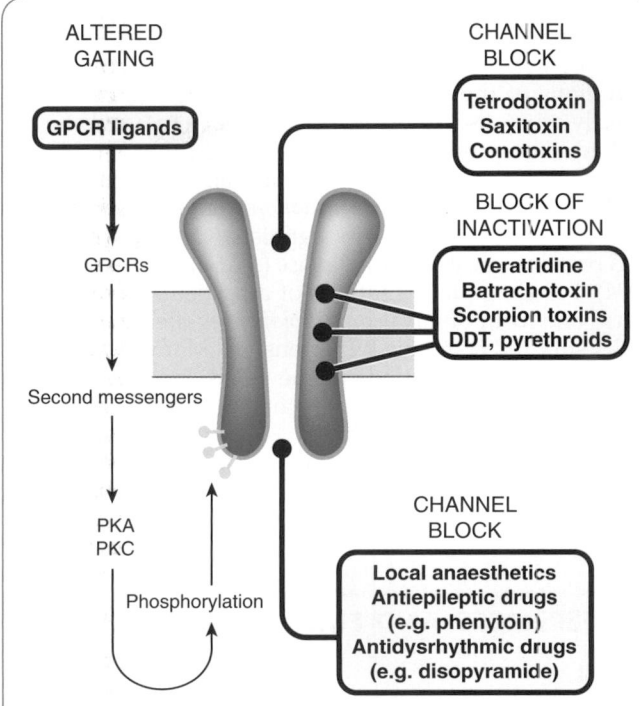

Fig. 3.21 Drug-binding domains of voltage-gated sodium channels (see Ch. 44). The multiplicity of different binding sites and effects appears to be typical of many ion channels. *DDT*, Dichlorodiphenyltrichloroethane (dicophane, a well-known insecticide); *GPCR*, G protein–coupled receptor; *PKA*, protein kinase A; *PKC*, protein kinase C.

to drug targets other than receptors (ion channels, enzymes, transporters, etc.) where adaptive changes in expression and function follow long-term drug administration, resulting, for example, in resistance to certain anticancer drugs (Ch. 57).

RECEPTORS AND DISEASE

Increasing understanding of receptor function in molecular terms has revealed a number of disease states directly linked to receptor malfunction. The principal mechanisms involved are:

- autoantibodies directed against receptor proteins;
- mutations in genes encoding receptors, ion channels and proteins involved in signal transduction.

An example of the former is *myasthenia gravis* (see Ch. 14), a disease of the neuromuscular junction due to autoantibodies that inactivate nicotinic acetylcholine receptors. Autoantibodies can also mimic the effects of agonists, as in many cases of thyroid hypersecretion, caused by activation of **thyrotropin** receptors (Ch. 35).

Inherited mutations of genes encoding GPCRs account for various disease states (see Stoy & Gurevich, 2015). Mutated **vasopressin** and **adrenocorticotrophic hormone** receptors (see Chs 30 and 34) can result in resistance to these hormones. Receptor mutations can result in activation of effector mechanisms in the absence of agonists. One of these involves the receptor for thyrotropin, producing continuous oversecretion of thyroid hormone; another involves the receptor for luteinising hormone and results in precocious puberty. Adrenoceptor polymorphisms are common in humans, and recent studies suggest that certain mutations of the β_2 adrenoceptor, although they do not directly cause disease, are associated with a reduced efficacy of β-adrenoceptor agonists in treating asthma (Ch. 29) and a poor prognosis in patients with cardiac failure, potentially through *constitutively active mutations* that render receptors active in the absence of any agonists (Ch. 22). Mutations in G proteins can also cause disease (see Spiegel & Weinstein, 2004). For example, mutations of a particular Gα subunit cause one form of *hypoparathyroidism*, while mutations of a Gβ subunit result in hypertension. Many cancers are associated with mutations of the genes encoding growth factor receptors, kinases and other proteins involved in signal transduction (see Ch. 6).

Mutations in ligand-gated ion channels (GABA$_A$ and nicotinic) and other ion channels (Na$^+$ and K$^+$) that alter their function give rise to some forms of idiopathic epilepsy (see Ch. 46 and Poduri & Lowenstein, 2011).

Given the fact that the NR family of receptors plays a key part in the regulation and coordination of growth, development and organogenesis, reproduction, the immune system and many other fundamental biological processes, it is not surprising that many illnesses are associated with malfunctioning of the NR system. Such conditions include inflammation, cancer, diabetes, cardiovascular disease, obesity and reproductive disorders (see Kersten et al., 2000; Murphy & Holder, 2000).

Research on genetic polymorphisms affecting receptors, signalling molecules, ion channels and effector enzymes is continuing apace, and it is expected that a clearer understanding of the variability between individuals in their disease susceptibility and response to therapeutic drugs (see Ch. 58) will result, in the foreseeable future.

REFERENCES AND FURTHER READING

General

IUPHAR/BPS. Guide to Pharmacology. www.guidetopharmacology.org/. (*Comprehensive catalogue of molecular and pharmacological properties of known receptor and ion channels – also transporters and some enzymes involved in signal transduction*)

Nelson, N., 1998. The family of Na$^+$/Cl$^-$ neurotransmitter transporters. J. Neurochem. 71, 1785–1803. (*Review article describing the molecular characteristics of the different families of neurotransporters*)

Ion channels

Ashcroft, F.M., 2000. Ion Channels and Disease. Academic Press, London. (*A useful textbook covering all aspects of ion channel physiology and its relevance to disease, with a lot of pharmacological information for good measure*)

Bezanilla, F., 2008. How membrane proteins sense voltage. Nat. Rev. Mol. Cell Biol. 9, 323–332. (*Review of recent studies of how membrane proteins respond to changes in transmembrane potential*)

Catterall, W.A., 2000. From ionic currents to molecular mechanisms: the structure and function of voltage-gated sodium channels. Neuron 26, 13–25. (*General review of sodium channel structure, function and pharmacology*)

Colquhoun, D., 2006. Agonist-activated ion channels. Br. J. Pharmacol. 147, S17–S26. (*Review article discussing the relationship between agonist binding and channel opening*)

Halliwell, R.F., 2007. A short history of the rise of the molecular pharmacology of ionotropic drug receptors. Trends Pharmacol. Sci. 28, 214–219. (*Good account of the main discoveries in this active field*)

Hille, B., 2001. Ionic Channels of Excitable Membranes. Sinauer Associates, Sunderland. (*A clear and detailed account of the basic principles of ion channels, with emphasis on their biophysical properties*)

North, R.A., 2002. Molecular physiology of P2X receptors. Physiol. Rev. 82, 1013–1067. (*Encyclopedic review of P2X receptor structure and function*)

Poduri, A., Lowenstein, D., 2011. Epilepsy genetics—past, present, and future. Curr. Opin. Genet. Dev. 21, 325–332.

Stathopoulos, P.B., Ikura, M., 2017. Store operated calcium entry: From concept to structural mechanisms. Cell Calcium 63, 3–7.

G protein–coupled receptors

AbdAlla, S., Lother, H., El Massiery, A., Quitterer, U., 2001. Increased AT$_1$ receptor heterodimers in preeclampsia mediate enhanced angiotensin II responsiveness. Nat. Med. 7, 1003–1009. (*The first instance of disturbed GPCR heterodimerisation in relation to human disease*)

Adams, M.N., Ramachandran, R., Yau, M.K., et al., 2011. Structure, function and pathophysiology of protease activated receptors. Pharmacol. Ther. 130, 248–282. (*Extensive review of the topic*)

Audet, M., Bouvier, M., 2012. Restructuring G protein-coupled receptor activation. Cell 151, 14–23. (*Review of recent developments related to G protein-coupled receptor crystallisation*)

Conigrave, A.D., Quinn, S.J., Brown, E.M., 2000. Cooperative multi-modal sensing and therapeutic implications of the extracellular Ca^{2+}-sensing receptor. Trends Pharmacol. Sci. 21, 401–407. (*Short account of the Ca^{2+}-sensing receptor, an anomalous type of GPCR*)

Costa, T., Cotecchia, S., 2005. Historical review: negative efficacy and the constitutive activity of G protein-coupled receptors. Trends Pharmacol. Sci. 26, 618–624. (*A clear and thoughtful review of ideas relating to constitutive receptor activation and inverse agonists*)

Ferré, S., Casadó, V., Devi, L.A., et al., 2015. G protein-coupled receptor oligomerization revisited: functional and pharmacological perspectives. Pharmacol. Rev. 66, 413–434. (*Comprehensive review of GPCR olgomerisation and the implications for pharmacology and cellular signalling*)

Fredriksson, R., Schiöth, H.B., 2005. The repertoire of G protein-coupled receptors in fully sequenced genomes. Mol. Pharmacol. 67, 1414–1425. (*Estimation of the number of GPCR genes in different species – nearly 500 more in mouse than in human!*)

Kelly, E., Bailey, C.P., Henderson, G., 2008. Agonist-selective mechanisms of GPCR desensitization. Br. J. Pharmacol. 153 (Suppl. 1), S379–S388. (*Short review of main mechanisms of GPCR desensitisation*)

Kenakin, T., Christopoulos, A., 2013. Signalling bias in new drug discovery: detection, quantification and therapeutic impact. Nat. Rev. Drug Discov. 12, 205–216. (*Detailed discussion of the difficulties in measuring agonist efficacy and bias*)

Liu, F., Wan, Q., Pristupa, Z., et al., 2000. Direct protein–protein coupling enables cross-talk between dopamine D$_5$ and γ-aminobutyric acid A receptors. Nature 403, 274–280. (*The first demonstration of direct coupling of a GPCR with an ion channel. Look, no G protein!*)

Manglik, A., Lin, H., Aryal, D.K., et al., 2016. Structure-based discovery of opioid analgesics with reduced side effects. Nature 537, 185–190. (*Exciting report of the use of computational molecular modelling in the design of a new opioid receptor agonist*)

Milligan, G., Kostenis, E., 2006. Heterotrimeric G proteins: a short history. Br. J. Pharmacol. 147 (Suppl. 1), 46–55.

Offermanns, S., 2003. G proteins as transducers in transmembrane signalling. Prog. Biophys. Mol. Biol. 83, 101–130. (*Detailed review of G protein subtypes and their function in signal transduction*)

Oldham, W.M., Hamm, H.E., 2008. Heterotrimeric G protein activation by G protein-coupled receptors. Nat. Rev. Mol. Cell Biol. 9, 60–71. (*Useful review of the structure and function of G proteins*)

Pierce, K.L., Lefkowitz, R.J., 2001. Classical and new roles of β-arrestins in the regulation of G protein-coupled receptors. Nat. Rev. Neurosci. 2, 727–733. (*Good review of non-G protein-mediated signalling of GPCRs through arrestin*)

Ramachandran, R., Noorbakhsh, F., defea, K., Hollenberg, M.D., 2012. Targeting proteinase-activated receptors: therapeutic potential and challenges. Nat. Rev. Drug Discov. 11, 69–86.

Sexton, P.M., Poyner, D.R., Simms, J., Christopoulos, A., Hay, D.L., 2012. RAMPs as drug targets. Adv. Exp. Med. Biol. 744, 61–74.

Simonds, W.F., 1999. G protein regulation of adenylate cyclase. Trends Pharmacol. Sci. 20, 66–72. (*Review of mechanisms by which G proteins affect adenylyl cyclase at the level of molecular structure*)

Sjögren, B., 2017. The evolution of regulators of G protein signalling proteins as drug targets – 20 years in the making: IUPHAR Review 21. Br. J. Pharmacol. 174, 427–437. (*Useful description of how RGS proteins function and their potential as drug targets*)

Sounier, R., Mas, C., Steyaert, J., et al , 2015. Propagation of conformational changes during μ-opioid receptor activation. Nature 524, 375–378. (*Describes the use of NMR to study conformational changes in a GPCR upon agonist activation*)

Spiegel, A.M., Weinstein, L.S., 2004. Inherited diseases involving G proteins and G protein-coupled receptors. Annu. Rev. Med. 55, 27–39. (*Short review article*)

Stoy, H., Gurevich, V.V., 2015. How genetic errors in GPCRs affect their function: Possible therapeutic strategies. Genes Dis. 2, 108–132. (*Extensive review with many examples of GPCR mutations associated with disease*)

Xie, G.X., Palmer, P.P., 2007. How regulators of G protein signalling achieve selective regulation. J. Mol. Biol. 366, 349–365. (*General review about RGS proteins and how they work*)

Zhang, D., Zhao, Q., Wu, B., 2015. Structural studies of G protein-coupled receptors. Mol. Cells 38, 836–842. (*Informative review of GPCR crystal structures*)

Signal transduction

Avruch, J., 2007. MAP kinase pathways: the first twenty years. Biochim. Biophys. Acta 1773, 1150–1160. (*Short general review. One of a series of articles on MAP kinases in this issue*)

Bishop, A.L., Hall, R.A., 2000. Rho-GTPases and their effector proteins. Biochem. J. 348, 241–255. (*General review article on the Rho/Rho kinase system and the various pathways and functions that it controls*)

Brzostowski, J.A., Kimmel, A.R., 2001. Signaling at zero G: G protein-independent functions for 7TM receptors. Trends Biochem. Sci. 26, 291–297. (*Review of evidence for GPCR signalling that does not involve G proteins, thus conflicting with the orthodox dogma*)

Vanhaesebroeck, B., Leevers, S.J., Panayotou, G., Waterfield, M.D., 1997. Phosphoinositide 3-kinases: a conserved family of signal transducers. Trends Biochem. Sci. 22, 267–272. (*Review by the group that discovered PI-3 kinases, summarising the multiple roles of this signal transduction mechanism – much expanded since 1997*)

Kinase-linked receptors

Cohen, P., 2002. Protein kinases – the major drug targets of the twenty-first century. Nat. Rev. Drug Discov. 1, 309–315. (*General review on pharmacological aspects of protein kinases*)

Cook, D.N., Pisetsky, D.S., Schwartz, D.A., 2004. Toll-like receptors in the pathogenesis of human disease. Nat. Immunol. 5, 975–979. (*Review emphasising the role of this class of receptor tyrosine kinases in many human disease states*)

Delcourt, N., Bockaert, J., Marin, P., 2007. GPCR-jacking: from a new route in RTK signalling to a new concept in GPCR activation. Trends Pharmacol. Sci. 28, 602–607. (*Gives examples of 'cross-talk' between GPCR and RTK signalling pathways*)

Hubbard, S.R., Miller, W.T., 2007. Receptor tyrosine kinases: mechanisms of activation and signaling. Curr. Opin. Cell Biol. 19, 117–123 (*Reviews recent structural results showing mechanism of RTK dimerisation and signalling*)

Ihle, J.N., 1995. Cytokine receptor signalling. Nature 377, 591–594.

Jin, J., Pawson, T., 2012. Modular evolution of phosphorylation-based signalling systems. Philos. Trans. R. Soc. Lond. B. Biol. Sci. 367, 2540–2555. (*Informative review on receptor kinase signalling*)

Karin, M., Yamamoto, Y., Wang, M., 2004. The IKK-NFκB system: a treasure trove for drug development. Nat. Rev. Drug Discov. 3, 17–26. (*Describes the transcription factor NFκB, which plays a key role in inflammation, and its control by kinase cascades*)

Nuclear receptors

Bourguet, W., Germain, P., Gronemeyer, H., 2000. Nuclear receptor ligand-binding domains: three-dimensional structures, molecular interactions and pharmacological implications. Trends Pharmacol. Sci. 21, 381–388. (*Accessible review concentrating on distinction between agonist and antagonist effects at the molecular level*)

Burris, T.P., Solt, L.A., Wang, Y., et al., 2013. Nuclear receptors and their selective pharmacologic modulators. Pharmacol. Rev. 65, 710–778. (*A very comprehensive account of the action of drugs at nuclear receptors. Not light reading, but worthwhile if you really want to dig deeply into this fascinating subject*)

Evans, R.M., Mangelsdorf, D.J., 2014. Nuclear receptors, RXR, and the big bang. Cell 157, 255–266. (*Easy-to-read review of nuclear receptors focusing on the key role that RXR plays in many crucial physiological signalling systems. Contains a lot of useful background material on nuclear receptors and their history*)

Falkenstein, E., Tillmann, H.C., Christ, M., Feuring, M., Wehling, M., 2000. Multiple actions of steroid hormones – a focus on rapid non-genomic effects. Pharm. Rev. 52, 513–553. (*Comprehensive review article describing the 'non-classical' effects of steroids*)

Germain, P., Staels, B., Dacquet, C., Spedding, M., Laudet, V., 2006. Overview of nomenclature of nuclear receptors. Pharmacol. Rev. 58, 685–704. (*Comprehensive and authoritative review that deals with receptor biology as well as nomenclature. Recommended*)

Kersten, S., Desvergne, B., Wahli, W., 2000. Roles of PPARs in health and disease. Nature 405, 421–424. (*General review of an important class of nuclear receptors*)

di Masi, A., De Marinis, E., Ascenzi, P., Marino, M., 2009. Nuclear receptors CAR and PXR: molecular, functional, and biomedical aspects. Mol. Aspects Med. 30, 297–343. (*A very comprehensive account of the role played by these nuclear receptors in xenobiotic metabolism but also contains some useful general background information on the receptor family*)

Levin, E.R., Hammes, S.R., 2016. Nuclear receptors outside the nucleus: extranuclear signalling by steroid receptors. Nat. Rev. Mol. Cell Biol. 17, 783–797. (*This paper reviews the increasing evidence that some of the key effects of steroids are mediated by populations of nuclear receptors outside the nucleus and describes the often rather complex networks through which they bring about these effects*)

Murphy, G.J., Holder, J.C., 2000. PPAR-γ agonists: therapeutic role in diabetes, inflammation and cancer. Trends Pharmacol. Sci. 21, 469–474. (*Account of the emerging importance of nuclear receptors of the PPAR family as therapeutic targets*)

Santos, G.M., Fairall, L., Schwabe, J.W.R., 2011. Negative regulation by nuclear receptors: a plethora of mechanisms. Trends Endocrinol. Metab. 22, 87–93. (*A very accessible and well written introduction to a very complex subject. Highly recommended*)

Shiau, A.K., Barstad, D., Loria, P.M., et al., 1998. The structural basis of estrogen receptor/coactivator recognition and the antagonism of this interaction by tamoxifen. Cell 95, 927–937.

4 How drugs act: cellular aspects – excitation, contraction and secretion

OVERVIEW

The link between a drug interacting with a molecular target and its effect at the pathophysiological level, such as a change in blood glucose concentration or the shrinkage of a tumour, involves events at the cellular level. Whatever their specialised physiological function, cells generally share much the same repertoire of signalling mechanisms. In the next four chapters, we describe the parts of this repertoire that are of particular significance in understanding drug action at the cellular level. In this chapter, we describe mechanisms that operate mainly over a short timescale (milliseconds to hours), particularly excitation, contraction and secretion, which account for many physiological responses; Chapter 5 looks at how biopharmaceuticals and gene therapy may alter the cell's chemical behaviours to have their desired effects; Chapter 6 deals with the slower processes (generally days to months), including cell division, growth, differentiation and cell death, that determine the body's structure and constitution; Chapter 7 describes host defence mechanisms.

The short-term regulation of cell function depends mainly on the following components and mechanisms, which regulate, or are regulated by, the free concentration of Ca^{2+} in the cytosol, $[Ca^{2+}]_i$:

• ion channels and transporters in the plasma membrane
• the storage and release of Ca^{2+} by intracellular organelles
• Ca^{2+}-dependent regulation of a variety of functional proteins, including enzymes, contractile proteins and vesicle proteins

More detailed coverage of the topics presented in this chapter can be found in Berridge (2014) and Kandel et al. (2012).

Because $[Ca^{2+}]_i$ plays such a key role in cell function, a wide variety of drug effects result from interference with one or more of these mechanisms. Knowledge of the molecular and cellular details is extensive, and here we focus on the aspects that help to explain drug effects.

REGULATION OF INTRACELLULAR CALCIUM

Ever since the famous accident in 1882 by Sidney Ringer's technician, which showed that using tap water rather than distilled water to make up the bathing solution for isolated frog hearts would allow them to carry on contracting, the role of Ca^{2+} as a major regulator of cell function has never been in question. Many drugs and physiological mechanisms operate, directly or indirectly, by influencing $[Ca^{2+}]_i$. Here we consider the main ways in which it is regulated, and later we describe some of the ways in which $[Ca^{2+}]_i$ controls cell function. Details of the molecular components and drug targets are presented in Chapter 3, and descriptions of drug effects on integrated physiological function are given in later chapters.

The study of Ca^{2+} regulation took a big step forward in the 1970s with the development of optical techniques based on the Ca^{2+}-sensitive photoprotein *aequorin*, and fluorescent dyes such as *Fura-2*, which, for the first time, allowed free $[Ca^{2+}]_i$ to be continuously monitored in living cells with a high level of temporal and spatial resolution.

Most of the Ca^{2+} in a resting cell is sequestered in organelles, particularly the *endoplasmic* or *sarcoplasmic reticulum* (ER or SR) and the mitochondria, and the free $[Ca^{2+}]_i$ is kept to a low level, about 100 nmol/L. The Ca^{2+} concentration in extracellular fluid, $[Ca^{2+}]_o$, is about 2.4 mmol/L, so there is a large concentration gradient favouring Ca^{2+} entry. $[Ca^{2+}]_i$ is kept low (a) by the operation of active transport mechanisms that eject cytosolic Ca^{2+} through the plasma membrane and pump it into the ER, and (b) by the normally low Ca^{2+} permeability of the plasma and ER membranes. Regulation of $[Ca^{2+}]_i$ involves three main mechanisms:

• control of Ca^{2+} entry
• control of Ca^{2+} extrusion
• exchange of Ca^{2+} between the cytosol and the intracellular stores

These mechanisms are described in more detail later and are summarised in Fig. 4.1.

CALCIUM ENTRY MECHANISMS

There are four main routes by which Ca^{2+} enters cells across the plasma membrane:

• voltage-gated calcium channels
• ligand-gated calcium channels
• store-operated calcium channels (SOCs)
• Na^+–Ca^{2+} exchange (can operate in either direction; see *Calcium extrusion mechanisms*, p. 55)

VOLTAGE-GATED CALCIUM CHANNELS

The pioneering work of Hodgkin and Huxley on the ionic basis of the nerve action potential (see pp. 56–58) identified voltage-dependent Na^+ and K^+ conductances as the main participants. It was later found that some invertebrate nerve and muscle cells could produce action potentials that depended on Ca^{2+} rather than Na^+, and it was then found that vertebrate cells also possess voltage-activated calcium channels capable of allowing substantial amounts

Fig. 4.1 **Regulation of intracellular calcium.** The main routes of transfer of Ca²⁺ into, and out of, the cytosol, endoplasmic reticulum (ER) and lysosomal structures are shown for a typical cell (see text for details). *Black arrows:* routes into the cytosol. *Blue arrows:* routes out of the cytosol. *Red arrows:* regulatory mechanisms. The state of the ER store of Ca²⁺ is monitored by the sensor protein Stim1, which interacts directly with the store-operated calcium channel (SOC) to promote Ca²⁺ entry when the ER store is depleted. Normally, [Ca²⁺]ᵢ is regulated to about 10^{-7} mol/L in a 'resting' cell. Mitochondria (not shown) also function as Ca²⁺ storage organelles but release Ca²⁺ only under pathological conditions, such as ischaemia (see pp. 55–56). There is recent evidence for a lysosomal store of Ca²⁺, activated by the second messenger nicotinic acid adenine dinucleotide phosphate (NAADP) through a two-pore domain calcium channel (TPC). *GPCR*, G protein–coupled receptor; *IP₃*, inositol trisphosphate; *IP₃R*, inositol trisphosphate receptor; *LGC*, ligand-gated cation channel; *NCX*, Na⁺–Ca²⁺ exchange transporter; *PMCA*, plasma membrane Ca²⁺-ATPase; *RyR*, ryanodine receptor; *SERCA*, sarcoplasmic/endoplasmic reticulum ATPase; *VGCC*, voltage-gated calcium channel.

of Ca²⁺ to enter the cell when the membrane is depolarised. These voltage-gated channels are highly selective for Ca²⁺ (although they also conduct Ba²⁺ ions, which are often used as a substitute in electrophysiological experiments), and do not conduct Na⁺ or K⁺; they are ubiquitous in excitable cells and cause Ca²⁺ to enter the cell whenever the membrane is depolarised, for example by a conducted action potential.

A combination of electrophysiological and pharmacological criteria have revealed five distinct subtypes of voltage-gated calcium channels: L, T, N, P/Q and R[1]. The subtypes vary with respect to their activation and inactivation kinetics, their voltage threshold for activation, their conductance and their sensitivity to blocking agents, as summarised in Table 4.1. The molecular basis for this heterogeneity has been worked out in some detail. The main pore-forming subunit (termed

α₁, see Fig. 3.20) occurs in at least 10 molecular subtypes, and associates with other subunits (β, γ and two subunits from the same gene, α₂δ, linked by a disulfide bond) that also exist in different subtypes to form the functional channel. Different combinations of these subunits give rise to the different physiological subtypes[2]. In general, L channels are particularly important in regulating contraction of cardiac and smooth muscle (see p. 64), and N channels (and also P/Q) are involved in neurotransmitter and hormone release, while T channels mediate Ca²⁺ entry into neurons around the resting membrane potential and can control the rate of repolarisation of neurons and cardiac cells as well as various Ca²⁺-dependent functions such as regulation of other channels, enzymes, etc. Clinically used drugs that act directly on some forms of calcium channel include the group of 'Ca²⁺ antagonists' consisting of *dihydropyridines* (e.g. **nifedipine**), **verapamil** and **diltiazem** (used for their

---

[1]P and Q are so similar that they usually get lumped together. The terminology is less than poetic: L stands for *long-lasting*; T stands for *transient*; N stands for *neither long-lasting nor transient*. Although P stands for *Purkinje* – this type of channel was first observed in cerebellar Purkinje cells – it continued the alphabetical sequence (missing out O of course) and so the next discovered were termed Q and R.

[2]Readers interested in knowing more about the subunit composition of different voltage-gated calcium channels should consult the Guide to Pharmacology at <http://www.guidetopharmacology.org/GRAC/FamilyDisplayForward?familyId=80>

Table 4.1 Types and functions of Ca²⁺ channels

Gated by	Main types	Characteristics	Location and function	Drug effects
Voltage	L	High activation threshold Slow inactivation	Plasma membrane of many cells Main Ca²⁺ source for contraction in smooth and cardiac muscle	Blocked by dihydropyridines, verapamil, diltiazem; and calciseptine (peptide from snake venom) Activated by BayK 8644 Phosphorylation by PKA (e.g. following β_1 adrenoceptor activation) increases channel opening
	N	Low activation threshold Slow inactivation	Main Ca²⁺ source for transmitter release by nerve terminals	Blocked by ω-conotoxin GV1A (component of *Conus* snail venom) and ziconotide (marketed preparation of ω-conotoxin used to control pain) (Ch. 43)
	T	Low activation threshold Fast inactivation	Widely distributed Important in cardiac pacemaker and atria (role in dysrhythmias), also neuronal firing patterns	Blocked by mibefradil
	P/Q	Low activation threshold Slow inactivation	Nerve terminals Transmitter release	Blocked by ω-agatoxin-4A (component of funnel-web spider venom)
	R	Low threshold Fast inactivation	Neurons and dendrites Control of firing patterns	Blocked by low concentrations of SNX-482 (a toxin from a member of the tarantula family)
IP₃	IP₃ receptor	Activated by binding of IP₃ and Ca²⁺	Located in endoplasmic/sarcoplasmic reticulum Mediates Ca²⁺ release produced by GPCR activation	Not directly targeted by drugs Some experimental blocking agents known Responds to GPCR agonists and antagonists in many cells
Ca²⁺	Ryanodine receptor	Directly activated in skeletal muscle via dihydropyridine receptor of T-tubules. Activated by Ca²⁺ in cardiac muscle	Located in endoplasmic/sarcoplasmic reticulum. Pathway for Ca²⁺ release in striated muscle	Activated by caffeine and ATP in the presence of Ca²⁺ Ryanodine both activates (low concentrations) and closes (high concentrations) the channel. Also closed by Mg²⁺, K⁺ channel blockers and dantrolene Mutations may lead to drug-induced malignant hyperthermia, sudden cardiac death and central core disease
Store depletion	Store-operated channels	Activated by sensor protein that monitors level of ER Ca²⁺ stores	Located in plasma membrane	Activated indirectly by agents that deplete intracellular stores (e.g. GPCR agonists, thapsigargin) Not directly targeted by drugs

ER, endoplasmic reticulum; *GPCR*, G protein–coupled receptor; *IP₃*, inositol trisphosphate; *PKA*, protein kinase A.

cardiovascular effects; see Chs 22 and 23), and **gabapentin** and **pregabalin** (used to treat epilepsy, pain and anxiety; see Chs 43, 45 and 46). Many drugs affect calcium channels indirectly by acting on G protein–coupled receptors (see Ch. 3). A number of toxins act selectively on one or other type of calcium channel (see Table 4.1), and these are used as experimental tools.

LIGAND-GATED CHANNELS

Most ligand-gated cation channels (see Ch. 3) that are activated by excitatory neurotransmitters are relatively non-selective, and conduct Ca²⁺ ions as well as other cations. Most important in this respect is the glutamate receptor of the NMDA type (Ch. 39), which has a particularly high permeability to Ca²⁺ and is a major contributor to Ca²⁺ uptake by postsynaptic neurons (and also glial cells) in the central nervous system. Activation of this receptor can readily cause so much Ca²⁺ entry that the cell dies, mainly through activation of Ca²⁺-dependent proteases but also by triggering *apoptosis* (see Ch. 6). This mechanism, termed *excitotoxicity*, probably plays a part in various neurodegenerative disorders (see Ch. 41).

For many years, there was dispute about the existence of 'receptor-operated channels' in smooth muscle, responding directly to mediators such as adrenaline (epinephrine), acetylcholine and histamine. Now it seems that the P2X receptor (see Ch. 3), activated by ATP, is the only example of a true ligand-gated channel in smooth muscle, and this constitutes an important route of entry for Ca^{2+}. As mentioned above, many mediators acting on G protein–coupled receptors affect Ca^{2+} entry indirectly, mainly by regulating voltage-gated calcium channels or potassium channels.

STORE-OPERATED CALCIUM CHANNELS (SOCS)

SOCs are very low-conductance channels that occur in the plasma membrane and open to allow entry when the ER stores are depleted, but are not sensitive to cytosolic $[Ca^{2+}]_i$. The linkage between the ER and the plasma membrane involves a Ca^{2+}-sensor protein (*Stim1*) in the ER membrane, which connects directly to the channel protein (*Orai1*) in the plasma membrane. Depletion of ER Ca^{2+} causes Stim1 to accumulate at junctions between the ER and the plasma membrane where it traps and activates Orai1 resulting in Ca^{2+} entry (see Prakriya & Lewis, 2015).

Like the ER and SR channels, these channels can serve to amplify the rise in $[Ca^{2+}]_i$ resulting from Ca^{2+} release from the stores. So far, only experimental compounds are known to block these channels, but efforts are being made to develop specific blocking agents for therapeutic use as relaxants of smooth muscle.

CALCIUM EXTRUSION MECHANISMS

Active transport of Ca^{2+} outwards across the plasma membrane, and inwards across the membranes of the ER or SR, depends on the activity of distinct Ca^{2+}-dependent ATPases,[3] similar to the Na^+/K^+-dependent ATPase that pumps Na^+ out of the cell in exchange for K^+. **Thapsigargin** (derived from a Mediterranean plant, *Thapsia garganica*) specifically blocks the ER pump, causing loss of Ca^{2+} from the ER. It is a useful experimental tool but has no therapeutic significance.

Calcium is also extruded from cells in exchange for Na^+, by Na^+–Ca^{2+} exchange. The exchanger transfers three Na^+ ions for one Ca^{2+}, and therefore produces a net depolarising current when it is extruding Ca^{2+}. The energy for Ca^{2+} extrusion comes from the electrochemical gradient for Na^+, not directly from ATP hydrolysis. This means that a reduction in the Na^+ concentration gradient resulting from Na^+ entry will reduce Ca^{2+} extrusion by the exchanger, causing a secondary rise in $[Ca^{2+}]_i$, a mechanism that is particularly important in cardiac muscle (see Ch. 22). **Digoxin** (derived from the *Digitalis* or 'Foxglove' plant), which inhibits Na^+ extrusion, acts on cardiac muscle in this way (Ch. 22), causing $[Ca^{2+}]_i$ to increase.

CALCIUM RELEASE MECHANISMS

There are two main types of calcium channel in the ER and SR membrane, which play an important part in controlling the release of Ca^{2+} from these stores.

- The *inositol trisphosphate receptor* (IP$_3$R) is activated by inositol trisphosphate (IP$_3$), a second messenger produced by the action of many ligands on G protein–coupled receptors (see Ch. 3). IP$_3$R is a ligand-gated ion channel, although its molecular structure differs from that of ligand-gated channels in the plasma membrane (see Berridge, 2016). This is the main mechanism by which activation of Gq–coupled receptors causes an increase in $[Ca^{2+}]_i$.

- *Ryanodine receptors* (RyR) are so called because they were first identified through the specific blocking action of the plant alkaloid **ryanodine**. There are three isoforms – RyR1–3 (Van Petegem, 2012), which are expressed in many different cell types. RyR1 is highly expressed in skeletal muscle, RyR2 in the heart and RyR3 in brain neurons. In skeletal muscle, RyRs on the SR are physically coupled to *dihydropyridine receptors* on the T-tubules (see Fig. 4.9); this coupling results in rapid Ca^{2+} release following the action potential in the muscle fibre. In other muscle types, RyRs respond to Ca^{2+} that enters the cell through membrane calcium channels by a mechanism known as *calcium-induced calcium release* (CICR).

The functions of IP$_3$Rs and RyRs are modulated by a variety of other intracellular signals (see Berridge, 2016; Van Petegem, 2012), which affect the magnitude and spatiotemporal patterning of Ca^{2+} signals. Fluorescence imaging techniques have revealed a remarkable level of complexity of Ca^{2+} signals, and much remains to be discovered about the importance of this patterning in relation to physiological and pharmacological mechanisms. The Ca^{2+} sensitivity of RyRs is increased by **caffeine**, causing Ca^{2+} release from the SR even at resting levels of $[Ca^{2+}]_i$. This is used experimentally but rarely happens in humans, because the other pharmacological effects of caffeine (see Ch. 49) occur at much lower doses. The blocking effect of **dantrolene**, a compound related to ryanodine, is used therapeutically to relieve muscle spasm in the rare condition of *malignant hyperthermia* (see Ch. 42), which is associated with inherited abnormalities in the RyR protein.

A typical $[Ca^{2+}]_i$ signal resulting from activation of a Gq–coupled receptor is shown in Fig. 4.2A. The response produced in the absence of extracellular Ca^{2+} represents release from intracellular stores. The larger and more prolonged response when extracellular Ca^{2+} is present shows the contribution of SOC-mediated Ca^{2+} entry. The various positive and negative feedback mechanisms that regulate $[Ca^{2+}]_i$ give rise to a variety of temporal and spatial oscillatory patterns (Fig. 4.2B) that are responsible for spontaneous rhythmic activity in smooth muscle and nerve cells (see Berridge, 2008).

OTHER SECOND MESSENGERS

▼ Two intracellular metabolites, cyclic ADP-ribose (cADPR) and nicotinic acid adenine dinucleotide phosphate (NAADP) formed from the ubiquitous coenzymes nicotinamide adenine dinucleotide (NAD) and NAD phosphate, also affect Ca^{2+} signalling (see Morgan et al., 2015; Parrington et al., 2015). cADPR acts by increasing the sensitivity of RyRs to Ca^{2+}, thus increasing the 'gain' of the CICR effect, whereas NAADP has been proposed to release Ca^{2+} from lysosomes by activating two-pore domain calcium channels (Fig. 4.1).

The levels of these messengers in mammalian cells may be regulated mainly in response to changes in the metabolic status of the cell, although the details are not yet clear. Abnormal Ca^{2+} signalling is involved in many pathophysiological conditions, such as ischaemic cell death, endocrine disorders and cardiac dysrhythmias, where the roles of cADPR and NAADP, and their interaction with other mechanisms that regulate $[Ca^{2+}]_i$, are the subject of much current work.

THE ROLE OF MITOCHONDRIA

▼ Under normal conditions, mitochondria accumulate Ca^{2+} passively as a result of the intramitochondrial potential, which is strongly negative with respect to the cytosol. This negativity is maintained

---

[3]These pumps have been likened to Sisyphus, condemned endlessly to push a stone up a hill (also consuming ATP, no doubt), only for it to roll down again.

Fig. 4.2 (A) Increase in intracellular free calcium concentration in response to receptor activation. The records were obtained from a single rat sensory neuron grown in tissue culture. The cells were loaded with the fluorescent Ca^{2+} indicator Fura-2, and the signal from a single cell monitored with a fluorescence microscope. A brief exposure to the peptide bradykinin, which causes excitation of sensory neurons (see Ch. 43), causes a transient increase in $[Ca^{2+}]_i$ from the resting value of about 150 nmol/L. When Ca^{2+} is removed from the extracellular solution, the bradykinin-induced increase in $[Ca^{2+}]_i$ is still present but is smaller and briefer. The response in the absence of extracellular Ca^{2+} represents the release of stored intracellular Ca^{2+} resulting from the intracellular production of inositol trisphosphate. The difference between this and the larger response when Ca^{2+} is present extracellularly is believed to represent Ca^{2+} entry through store-operated ion channels in the cell membrane. (Figure kindly provided by G. M. Burgess and A. Forbes, Novartis Institute for Medical Research.) (B) Spontaneous intracellular calcium oscillations in pacemaker cells from the rabbit urethra that regulate the rhythmic contractions of the smooth muscle. The signals cease when external Ca^{2+} is removed, showing that activation of membrane Ca^{2+} channels is involved in the mechanism. (From McHale, N., et al., 2006. J. Physiol. 570, 23–28.)

by active extrusion of protons, and is lost – thus releasing Ca^{2+} into the cytosol – if the cell runs short of ATP, for example under conditions of hypoxia. This only happens *in extremis*, and the resulting Ca^{2+} release contributes to the cytotoxicity associated with severe metabolic disturbance. Cell death resulting from brain ischaemia or coronary ischaemia (see Chs 22 and 41) involves this mechanism, along with others that contribute to an excessive rise in $[Ca^{2+}]_i$.

CALMODULIN

Calcium exerts its control over cell functions by virtue of its ability to regulate the activity of many different proteins, including enzymes (particularly kinases and phosphatases), channels, transporters, transcription factors, synaptic vesicle proteins and many others either by binding directly to these proteins or through a Ca^{2+}-binding protein that serves as an intermediate between Ca^{2+} and the regulated functional protein, the best known such binding protein being the ubiquitous *calmodulin*. This regulates at least 40 different functional proteins – indeed a powerful fixer. Calmodulin is a dumbbell-shaped protein with a globular domain at either end, each with two Ca^{2+} binding sites. When all are occupied, the protein undergoes a conformational change, exposing a 'sticky' hydrophobic domain that lures many proteins into association, thereby affecting their functional properties.

EXCITATION

Excitability describes the ability of a cell to show a regenerative all-or-nothing electrical response to depolarisation of its membrane, this membrane response being known as

Calcium regulation

Intracellular Ca^{2+} concentration, $[Ca^{2+}]_i$, is critically important as a regulator of cell function.

- Intracellular Ca^{2+} is determined by (a) Ca^{2+} entry; (b) Ca^{2+} extrusion; and (c) Ca^{2+} exchange between the cytosol, endoplasmic or sarcoplasmic reticulum (ER, SR), lysosomes and mitochondria.
- Calcium entry occurs by various routes, including voltage- and ligand-gated calcium channels and Na^+–Ca^{2+} exchange.
- Calcium extrusion depends mainly on an ATP-driven Ca^{2+} pump.
- Calcium ions are actively taken up and stored by the ER/SR, from which they are released in response to various stimuli.
- Calcium ions are released from ER/SR stores by (a) the second messenger inositol trisphosphate (IP_3) acting on IP_3 receptors; or (b) increased $[Ca^{2+}]_i$ itself acting on ryanodine receptors, a mechanism known as Ca^{2+}-induced Ca^{2+} release.
- Other second messengers, cyclic ADP-ribose and nicotinic acid dinucleotide phosphate, also promote the release of Ca^{2+} from Ca^{2+} stores.
- Depletion of ER/SR Ca^{2+} stores promotes Ca^{2+} entry through the plasma membrane, via store-operated channels.
- Calcium ions affect many aspects of cell function by binding to proteins such as calmodulin, which in turn bind other proteins and regulate their function.

an action potential. It is a characteristic of most neurons and muscle cells (including skeletal, cardiac and smooth muscle) and of many endocrine gland cells. In neurons and muscle cells, the ability of the action potential, once initiated, to propagate to all parts of the cell membrane, and often to spread to neighbouring cells, explains the importance of membrane excitation in intra- and intercellular signalling. In the nervous system and in skeletal muscle, action potential propagation is the mechanism responsible for communication over long distances at high speed, indispensable for large, fast-moving creatures. In cardiac and smooth muscle, as well as in some central neurons, spontaneous rhythmic activity occurs. In gland cells, the action potential, where it occurs, serves to amplify the signal that causes the cell to secrete. In each type of tissue, the properties of the excitation process reflect the special characteristics of the ion channels that underlie the process. The molecular nature of ion channels, and their importance as drug targets, is considered in Chapter 3; here we discuss the cellular processes that depend primarily on ion channel function. For more detail, see Hille (2001).

THE 'RESTING' CELL

The resting cell is not resting at all but very busy controlling the state of its interior, and it requires a continuous supply of energy to do so. In relation to the topics discussed in this chapter, the following characteristics are especially important:

- membrane potential
- permeability of the plasma membrane to different ions
- intracellular ion concentrations, especially $[Ca^{2+}]_i$

Under resting conditions, all cells maintain a negative internal potential between about −30 and −80 mV, depending on the cell type. This arises because (a) the membrane is relatively impermeable to Na^+, and (b) Na^+ ions are actively extruded from the cell in exchange for K^+ ions by an energy-dependent transporter, the Na^+ pump (or Na^+-K^+-ATPase). The result is that the intracellular K^+ concentration, $[K^+]_i$, is higher, and $[Na^+]_i$ is lower, than the respective extracellular concentrations. In many cells, other ions, particularly Cl^-, are also actively transported and unequally distributed across the membrane. In many cases (e.g. in neurons), the membrane permeability to K^+ is relatively high, and the membrane potential settles at a value of −60 to −80 mV, close to the equilibrium potential for K^+ (Fig. 4.3). In other cells (e.g. smooth muscle), anions play a larger part, and the membrane potential is generally lower (−30 to −50 mV) and less dependent on K^+.

ELECTRICAL AND IONIC EVENTS UNDERLYING THE ACTION POTENTIAL

Our present understanding of electrical excitability rests firmly on the work of Hodgkin, Huxley and Katz on squid axons, published in 1949–1952. Their experiments (see Katz, 1966) revealed the existence of voltage-gated ion channels (see pp. 60–61) and showed that the action potential is generated by the interplay of two processes:

1. A rapid, transient increase in Na^+ permeability that occurs when the membrane is depolarised beyond about −50 mV.
2. A slower, sustained increase in K^+ permeability.

Because of the inequality of Na^+ and K^+ concentrations on the two sides of the membrane, an increase in Na^+

Fig. 4.3 **Simplified diagram showing the ionic balance of a typical 'resting' cell.** The main transport mechanisms that maintain the ionic gradients across the plasma membrane are the ATP-driven Na^+–K^+ and Ca^{2+} pumps and the Na^+–Ca^{2+} exchange transporter. The membrane is relatively permeable to K^+, because some types of potassium channel are open at rest, but impermeable to other cations. The unequal ion concentrations on either side of the membrane give rise to the 'equilibrium potentials' shown. The resting membrane potential, typically about −60 mV but differing between different cell types, is determined by the equilibrium potentials and the permeabilities of the various ions involved, and by the 'electrogenic' effect of the transporters. For simplicity, anions and other ions, such as protons, are not shown, although these play an important role in many cell types.

permeability causes an inward (depolarising) current of Na^+ ions, whereas an increase in K^+ permeability causes an outward (repolarising) current. The separability of these two currents can be most clearly demonstrated by the use of drugs blocking sodium and potassium channels, as shown in Fig. 4.4. During the physiological initiation or propagation of a nerve impulse, the first event is a small depolarisation of the membrane, produced either by trans-mitter action or by the approach of an action potential passing along the axon. This opens sodium channels, allowing an inward current of Na^+ ions to flow, which depolarises the membrane still further. The process is thus a regenerative one, and the increase in Na^+ permeability is enough to bring the membrane potential towards E_{Na}. The increased Na^+ conductance is transient, because the channels inactivate rapidly and the membrane returns to its resting state.

In many types of cell, including most nerve cells, repolarisation is assisted by the opening of voltage-dependent K^+ channels. These function in much the same way as sodium channels, but their activation kinetics are about 10 times slower and they do not inactivate appreciably. This means that the potassium channels open later than the sodium channels, contributing to the rapid termination of the action potential and to the after-hyperpolarisation that follows the depolarising phase. The behaviour of the sodium and

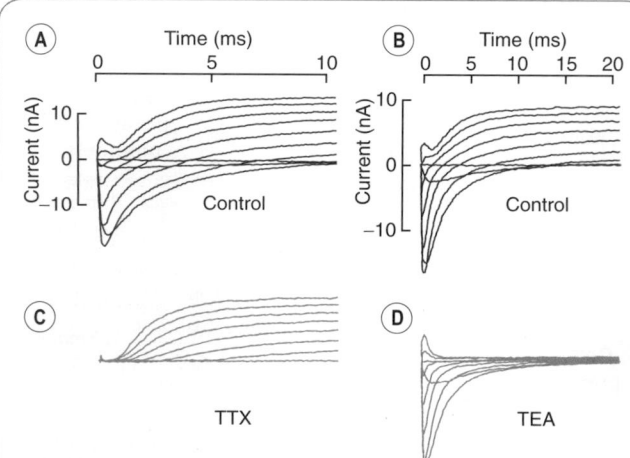

Fig. 4.4 **Separation of sodium and potassium currents in the nerve membrane.** Voltage clamp records from the node of Ranvier of a single frog nerve fibre. At time 0, the membrane potential was stepped to a depolarised level, ranging from −60 mV (lower trace in each series) to +60 mV (upper trace in each series) in 15-mV steps. (A and B) Control records from two fibres. (C) Effect of tetrodotoxin (TTX), which abolishes Na⁺ currents. (D) Effect of tetraethylammonium (TEA), which abolishes K⁺ currents. (From Hille, B., 1970. Ionic channels in nerve membranes. Prog. Biophys. Mol. Biol. 21, 1–32.)

Fig. 4.5 **Behaviour of sodium and potassium channels during a conducted action potential.** Rapid opening of sodium channels occurs during the action potential upstroke. Delayed opening of potassium channels, and inactivation of sodium channels, causes repolarisation. E_m, membrane potential; g_K, membrane conductance to K⁺; g_{Na}, membrane conductance to Na⁺.

potassium channels during an action potential is shown in Fig. 4.5.

The foregoing account, based on Hodgkin and Huxley's work 65 years ago, involves only Na⁺ and K⁺ channels. Subsequently (see Hille, 2001), voltage-gated calcium channels (see Fig. 4.1) were discovered. These function in basically the same way as sodium channels, if on a slightly slower timescale; they contribute to action potential generation in many cells, particularly cardiac and smooth muscle cells, but also in neurons and secretory cells. Ca²⁺ entry

through voltage-gated calcium channels plays a key role in intracellular signalling, as described on pp. 52–56.

CHANNEL FUNCTION

The discharge patterns of excitable cells vary greatly. Skeletal muscle fibres are quiescent unless stimulated by the arrival of a nerve impulse at the neuromuscular junction. Cardiac muscle fibres discharge spontaneously at a regular rate (see Ch. 22). Neurons may be normally silent, or they may discharge spontaneously, either regularly or in bursts; smooth muscle cells show a similar variety of firing patterns. The frequency at which different cells normally discharge action potentials also varies greatly, from 100 Hz or more for fast-conducting neurons, down to about 1 Hz for cardiac muscle cells. These very pronounced functional variations reflect the different characteristics of the ion channels expressed in different cell types. Rhythmic fluctuations of [Ca²⁺]ᵢ underlie the distinct firing patterns that occur in different types of cell (see Berridge, 2016).

Drugs that alter channel characteristics, either by interacting directly with the channel itself or indirectly through second messengers, affect the function of many organ systems, including the nervous, cardiovascular, endocrine, respiratory and reproductive systems, and are a frequent theme in this book. Here we describe some of the key mechanisms involved in the regulation of excitable cells.

In general, action potentials are initiated by membrane currents that cause depolarisation of the cell. These currents may be produced by synaptic activity, by an action potential approaching from another part of the cell, by a sensory stimulus or by spontaneous *pacemaker* activity. The tendency of such currents to initiate an action potential is governed by the *excitability* of the cell, which depends mainly on the state of (a) the voltage-gated sodium and/or calcium channels, and (b) the potassium channels of the resting membrane. Anything that increases the number of available sodium or calcium channels, or reduces their activation threshold, will tend to increase excitability, whereas increasing the resting K⁺ conductance reduces it. Agents that do the reverse, by blocking channels or interfering with their opening, will have the opposite effect. Some examples are shown in Figs 4.6 and 4.7. Inherited mutations of channel proteins are responsible for a wide variety of neurological and other genetic disorders (see Imbrici et al., 2016).

USE DEPENDENCE AND VOLTAGE DEPENDENCE

▼ Voltage-gated channels can exist in three functional states (Fig. 4.8): *resting* (the closed state that prevails at the normal resting potential), *activated* (the open state favoured by brief depolarisation) and *inactivated* (the blocked state resulting from a trapdoor-like occlusion of the open channel by a floppy intracellular appendage of the channel protein). After the action potential has passed, many sodium channels are in the inactivated state; after the membrane potential returns to its resting value, the inactivated channels take time to revert to the resting state and thus become available for activation once more. In the meantime, the membrane is temporarily *refractory*. Each action potential causes the channels to cycle through these states. The duration of the refractory period determines the maximum frequency at which action potentials can occur. Drugs that block sodium channels, such as local anaesthetics (Ch. 44), antidysrhythmic drugs (Ch. 22) and antiepileptic drugs (Ch. 46), commonly show a selective affinity for one or other of these functional states of the channel, and in their presence the proportion of channels in the high-affinity state is increased. Of particular importance are drugs that bind most strongly to the inactivated state of the channel and thus favour the adoption of this state, prolonging the refractory period and reducing the maximum frequency at which action potentials can

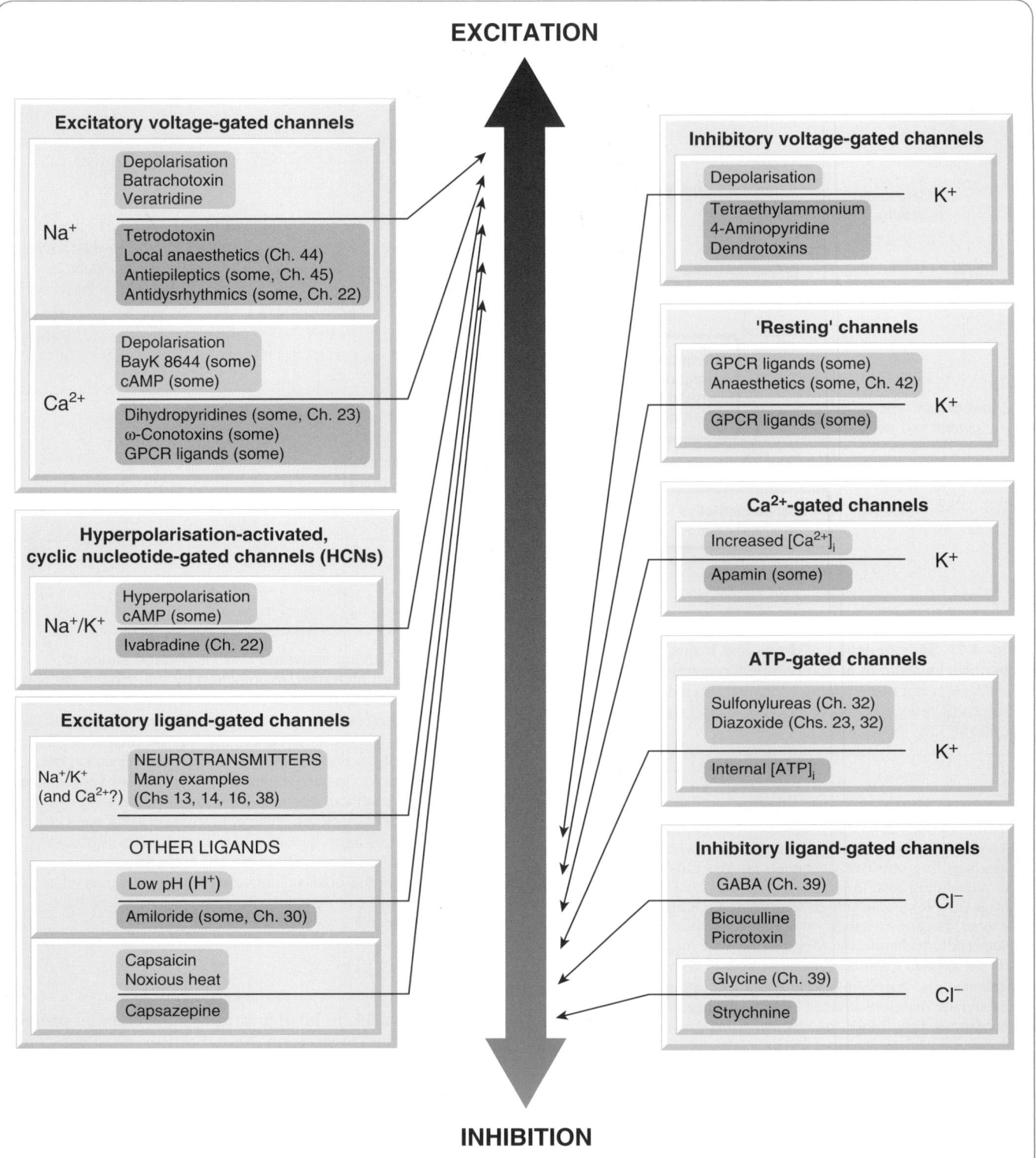

Fig. 4.6 Ion channels associated with excitatory and inhibitory membrane effects, and some of the drugs and other ligands that affect them. Channel openers are shown in green boxes, blocking agents and inhibitors in pink boxes. Hyperpolarisation-activated Na⁺/K⁺ channels are known as hyperpolarisation-activated, cyclic nucleotide-gated channels (HCNs); H⁺ activated channels are known as acid-sensing ion channels (ASICs). *GPCR,* G protein–coupled receptor.

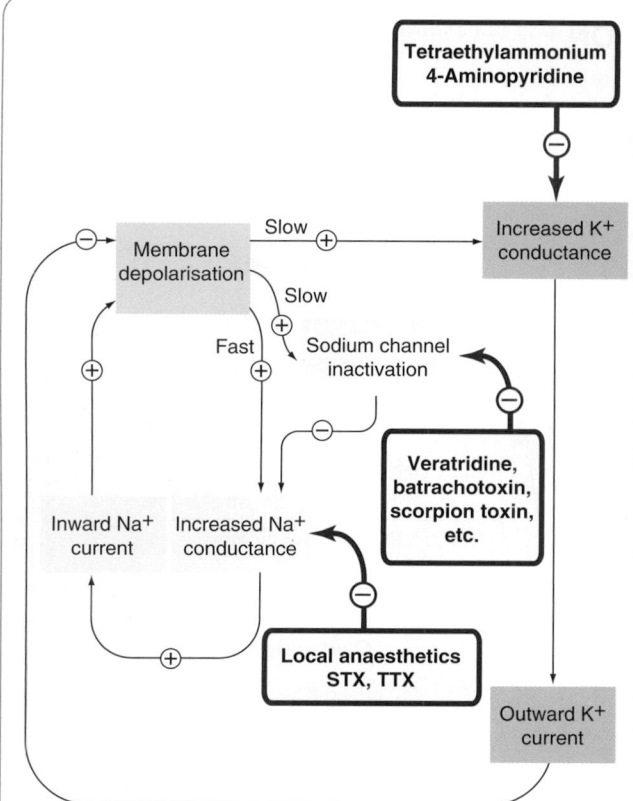

Fig. 4.7 Sites of action of drugs and toxins that affect channels involved in action potential generation. Many other mediators affect these channels indirectly via membrane receptors, through phosphorylation or altered expression. *STX*, saxitoxin; *TTX*, tetrodotoxin.

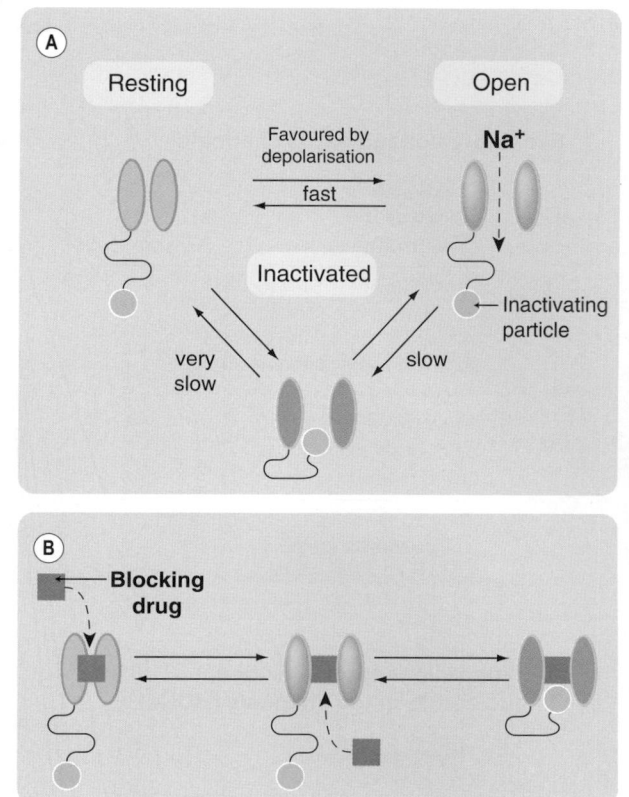

Fig. 4.8 Resting, activated and inactivated states of voltage-gated channels, exemplified by the sodium channel. (A) Membrane depolarisation causes a rapid transition from the resting (closed) state to the open state. The inactivating particle (part of the intracellular domain of the channel protein) is then able to block the channel. With prolonged depolarisation below the threshold for opening, channels can go directly from resting to inactivated without opening. (B) Some blocking drugs (such as tetrodotoxin) block the channel from the outside like a plug, whereas others (such as local anaesthetics and antiepileptic drugs) enter from the inside of the cell and often show preference for the open or inactivated states, and thus affect the kinetic behaviour of the channels, with implications for their clinical application.

be generated. This type of block is called *use dependent*, because the binding of such drugs increases as a function of the rate of action potential discharge, which governs the rate at which inactivated – and therefore drug-sensitive – channels are generated. This is important for some antidysrhythmic drugs (see Ch. 22) and for antiepileptic drugs (Ch. 46), because high-frequency discharges can be inhibited without affecting excitability at normal frequencies. Drugs that readily block sodium channels in their resting state (e.g. local anaesthetics, Ch. 44) prevent excitation at low as well as high frequencies.

Most sodium channel-blocking drugs are cationic at physiological pH and are therefore affected by the voltage gradient across the cell membrane. They block the channel from the inside, so that their blocking action is favoured by depolarisation. This phenomenon, known as *voltage dependence*, is also of relevance to the action of antidysrhythmic and antiepileptic drugs, because the cells that are the seat of dysrhythmias or seizure activity are generally somewhat depolarised and therefore more strongly blocked than healthy cells. Similar considerations apply also to drugs that block potassium or calcium channels, but we know less about the importance of use and voltage dependence for these than we do for sodium channels.

SODIUM CHANNELS

In most excitable cells, the regenerative inward current that initiates the action potential results from activation of voltage-gated sodium channels. The early voltage clamp studies by Hodgkin and Huxley on the squid giant axon, described on p. 57, revealed the essential functional properties of these channels. Later, advantage was taken of the potent and highly selective blocking action of **tetrodotoxin**

(TTX, see Ch. 44) to label and purify the channel proteins, and subsequently to clone them. Sodium channels consist of a central, pore-forming α subunit (shown in Fig. 3.20) and two auxiliary β subunits. Nine α-subunits (Na$_v$1.1 through Na$_v$1.9) and four β subunits have been identified in mammals. The α subunits contain four similar domains, each comprising six membrane-spanning helices (see Catterall & Swanson, 2015). One of these helices, S4, which contains several basic amino acids and forms the voltage sensor, moves outwards, thus opening the channel, when the membrane is depolarised. One of the intracellular loops is designed to swing across and block the channel when S4 is displaced, thus inactivating the channel.

It was known from physiological studies that the sodium channels of heart and skeletal muscle differ in various ways from those of neurons. In particular, cardiac sodium channels (and those of some sensory neurons) are relatively insensitive to TTX and slower in their kinetics, compared with most neuronal sodium channels. This is explained by the relative insensitivity of some α subunits ($Na_v1.5$, $Na_v1.8$ and $Na_v1.9$) to tetrodotoxin. Changes in the level of expression of some sodium channel subunits is thought to underlie the hyperexcitability of sensory neurons in different types of neuropathic pain (see Ch. 43).

In addition to channel-blocking compounds such as tetrodotoxin, other compounds affect sodium channel gating. For example, the plant alkaloid **veratridine** and the frog skin poison **batrachotoxin** cause persistent activation, while various scorpion toxins prevent inactivation, mechanisms resulting in enhanced neuronal excitability.

POTASSIUM CHANNELS

In a typical resting cell (see p. 57, Fig. 4.3), the membrane is selectively permeable to K^+ and the membrane potential (about −60 mV) is somewhat positive to the K^+ equilibrium (about −90 mV). This resting permeability comes about because some potassium channels are open. If more potassium channels open, the membrane hyperpolarises and the cell is inhibited, whereas the opposite happens if potassium channels close. As well as affecting excitability in this way, potassium channels also play an important role in regulating the duration of the action potential and the temporal patterning of action potential discharges; altogether, these channels play a central role in regulating cell function. As mentioned in Chapter 3, the number and variety of potassium channel subtypes is extraordinary, implying that evolution has been driven by the scope for biological advantage to be gained from subtle variations in the functional properties of these channels. A recent résumé lists over 60 different pore-forming subunits, plus another 20 or so auxiliary subunits. An impressive evolutionary display, maybe, but hard going for most of us.

▼ Potassium channels fall into three main classes (Table 4.2),[4] of which the structures are shown in Fig. 3.20.

- *Voltage-gated potassium channels*, which possess six membrane-spanning helices, one of which serves as the voltage sensor, causing the channel to open when the membrane is depolarised. Included in this group are channels of the shaker family, accounting for most of the voltage-gated K^+ currents familiar to electrophysiologists, and others such as Ca^{2+}-activated potassium channels and two subtypes that are important in the heart, HERG and LQT channels. Many of these channels are blocked by drugs such as **tetraethylammonium** and **4-aminopyridine**.
- *Inwardly rectifying potassium channels*, so called because they allow K^+ to pass inwards much more readily than outwards. These have two membrane-spanning helices and a single pore-forming loop (P loop). These channels are regulated by interaction with G proteins (see Ch. 3) and mediate the inhibitory effects of many agonists acting on G protein–coupled receptors. Certain types are important in the heart, particularly in regulating the duration of the cardiac action potential (Ch. 22); others are the target for the action of **sulfonylureas** (antidiabetic drugs that stimulate insulin secretion by blocking

them; see Ch. 32) and smooth muscle relaxant drugs, such as **minoxidil** and **diazoxide**, which open them (see Ch. 23).
- *Two-pore domain potassium channels*, with four helices and two P loops. These show outward rectification and therefore exert a strong repolarising influence, opposing any tendency to excitation. They may contribute to the resting K^+ conductance in many cells and are susceptible to regulation via G proteins; certain subtypes have been implicated in the action of volatile anaesthetics such as **isoflurane** (Ch. 42).

For more details, and information on potassium channels and the various drugs and toxins that affect them, see Jenkinson (2006) and Alexander et al. (2015).

Inherited abnormalities of potassium channels (channelopathies) contribute to a rapidly growing number of cardiac, neurological and other diseases. These include the *long QT syndrome* associated with mutations in cardiac voltage-gated potassium channels, causing episodes of ventricular arrest that can result in sudden death. Drug-induced prolongation of the *QT* interval is an unwanted side effect of several drugs (see Ch 22), including **methadone** and various antipsychotic agents. Nowadays, new drugs are screened for this property at an early stage in the development process (see Ch. 60). Certain familial types of deafness and epilepsy are associated with mutations in voltage-gated potassium channels (Imbrici et al., 2016).

Ion channels and electrical excitability

- Excitable cells generate an all-or-nothing action potential in response to membrane depolarisation. This occurs in most neurons and muscle cells, and in some gland cells. The ionic basis and time course of the response varies between tissues.
- The regenerative response results from the depolarising current associated with opening of voltage-gated cation channels (mainly Na^+ and Ca^{2+}). It is terminated by inactivation of these channels accompanied by opening of K^+ channels.
- These voltage-gated channels exist in many molecular varieties, with specific functions in different types of cell.
- The membrane of the 'resting' cell is relatively permeable to K^+ but impermeable to Na^+ and Ca^{2+}. Drugs or mediators that open K^+ channels reduce membrane excitability, as do inhibitors of Na^+ or Ca^{2+} channel function. Blocking K^+ channels or activating Na^+ or Ca^{2+} channels increases excitability.
- Cardiac muscle cells, some neurons and some smooth muscle cells generate spontaneous action potentials whose amplitude, rate and rhythm are affected by drugs that affect ion channel function.

MUSCLE CONTRACTION

Effects of drugs on the contractile machinery of smooth muscle are the basis of many therapeutic applications, for smooth muscle is an important component of most physiological systems, including blood vessels and the gastrointestinal, respiratory and urinary tracts. For many decades, smooth muscle pharmacology with its trademark

---

[4]Potassium channel terminology is confusing, to put it mildly. Electrophysiologists have named K^+ currents prosaically on the basis of their functional properties (I_{KV}, I_{KCa}, I_{KATP}, I_{KIR}, etc.); geneticists have named genes somewhat fancifully according to the phenotypes associated with mutations ('shaker', 'ether-a-go-go', etc.), while molecular biologists have introduced a rational but unmemorable nomenclature on the basis of sequence data (KCNK, KCNQ, etc., with numerical suffixes). The rest of us must make what we can of the unlovely jargon of labels such as HERG (which – don't blink – stands for 'Human Ether-a-go-go Related Gene'), TWIK, TREK and TASK.

Table 4.2 Types and functions of K⁺ channels

Structural class[a]	Functional subtypes[b]	Functions	Drug effects	Notes
Voltage-gated (6T, 1P)	Voltage-gated K⁺ channels	Action potential repolarisation Limits maximum firing frequency	Blocked by tetraethylammonium, 4-aminopyridine Certain subtypes blocked by dendrotoxins (from mamba snake venom)	Subtypes in the heart include HERG and LQT channels, which are involved in congenital and drug-induced dysrhythmias Other subtypes may be involved in inherited forms of epilepsy
	Ca²⁺-activated K⁺ channels	Inhibition following stimuli which increase [Ca²⁺]ᵢ	Certain subtypes blocked by apamin (from bee venom), and charybdotoxin (from scorpion venom)	Important in many excitable tissues to limit repetitive discharges, also in secretory cells
Inward rectifying (2T, 1P)	G protein-activated	Mediate effects of Gi/Go-coupled GPCRs which cause inhibition by increasing K⁺ conductance	GPCR agonists and antagonists Some are blocked by tertiapin (from honey bee venom)	Other inward rectifying K⁺ channels important in kidney
	ATP-sensitive	Found in many cells Channels open when [ATP] is low, causing inhibition Important in control of insulin secretion in the pancreas	Association of one subtype with the sulfonylurea receptor (SUR) results in modulation by sulfonylureas (e.g. glibenclamide) which close channel, and by K⁺ channel openers (e.g. diazoxide, minoxidil) which relax smooth muscle	
Two-pore domain (4T, 2P)	Several subtypes identified (TWIK, TRAAK, TREK, TASK, etc.)	Most are voltage-insensitive; some are normally open and contribute to the 'resting' K⁺ conductance Modulated by GPCRs	Certain subtypes are activated by volatile anaesthetics (e.g. isoflurane) No selective blocking agents	The nomenclature is misleading, especially when they are incorrectly referred to as two-pore channels

[a]K⁺ channel structures (see Fig. 3.20) are defined according to the number of transmembrane helices (T) and the number of pore-forming loops (P) in each α subunit. Functional channels contain several subunits (often four) which may be identical or different, and they are often associated with accessory (β) subunits.
[b]Within each functional subtype, several molecular variants have been identified, often restricted to particular cells and tissues. The physiological and pharmacological significance of this heterogeneity is not yet understood.
GPCR, G protein–coupled receptor.

technology – the isolated organ bath – held the centre of the pharmacological stage, and neither the subject nor the technology shows any sign of flagging, even though the stage has become much more crowded. Cardiac and skeletal muscle contractility are also the targets of important drug effects.

Although in each case the basic molecular basis of contraction is similar, namely an interaction between actin and myosin, fuelled by ATP and initiated by an increase in [Ca²⁺]ᵢ, there are differences between these three kinds of muscle that account for their different responsiveness to drugs and chemical mediators.

These differences (Fig. 4.9) involve (a) the linkage between membrane events and increase in [Ca²⁺]ᵢ, and (b) the mechanism by which [Ca²⁺]ᵢ regulates contraction.

SKELETAL MUSCLE

Skeletal muscle possesses an array of transverse T-tubules extending into the cell from the plasma membrane. The action potential of the plasma membrane depends on voltage-gated sodium channels, as in most nerve cells, and propagates rapidly from its site of origin, the motor endplate (see Ch. 14), to the rest of the fibre. The T-tubule membrane contains voltage-gated calcium channels termed dihydropyridine receptors (DHPRs),[5] that respond to membrane depolarisation conducted passively along the T-tubule when the plasma membrane is invaded by an action potential. DHPRs are located extremely close to *RyRs* (see Ch. 3) in the adjacent SR membrane and activation of these RyRs causes release of Ca²⁺ from the SR. Direct coupling between the DHPRs of the T-tubule and the RyRs of the SR (as

[5]Although these are, to all intents and purposes, just a form of L-type calcium channel the term dihydropyridine receptor (DHPR) is used to reflect that they are not identical to the L-type channels in neurons and cardiac muscle.

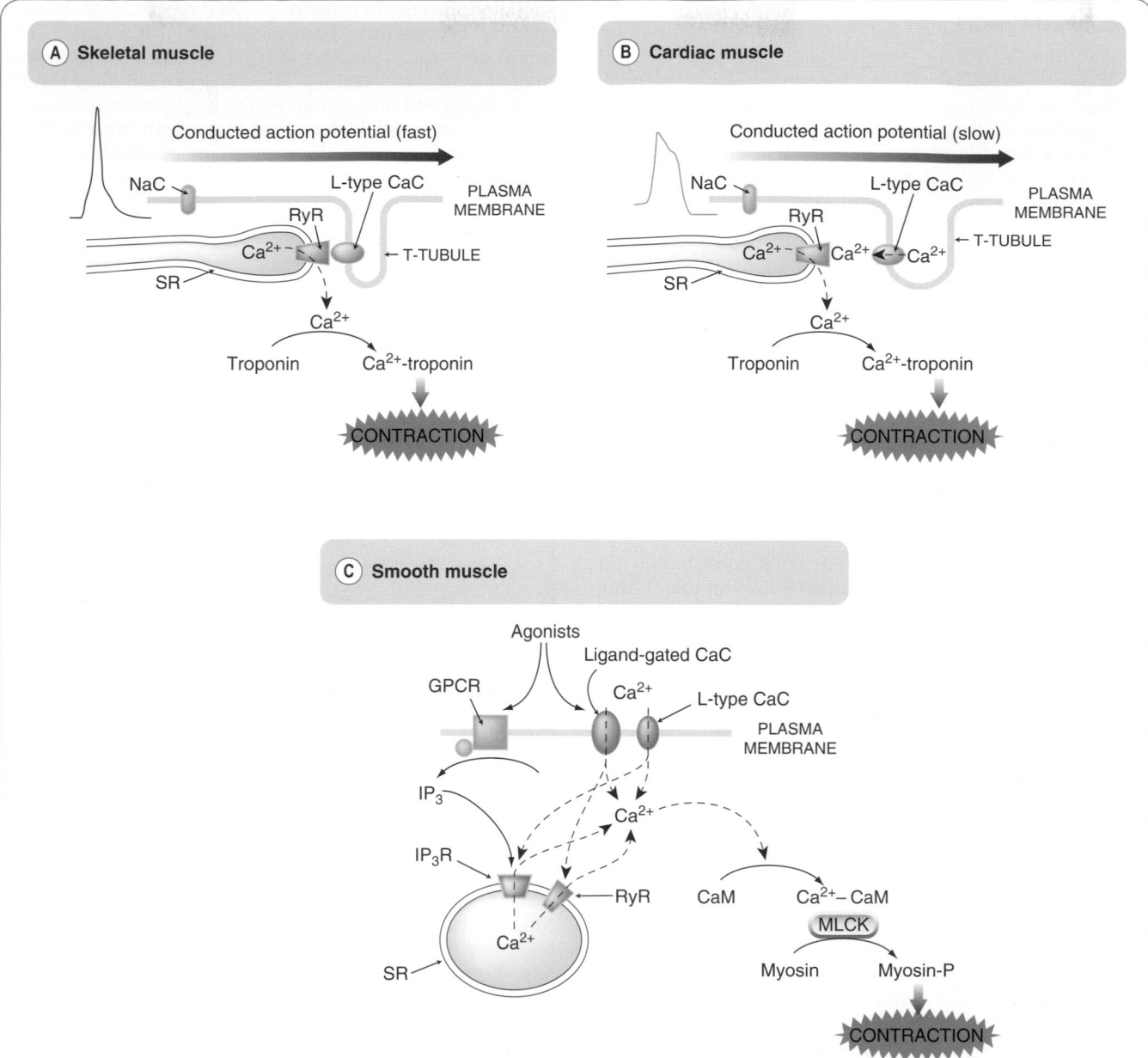

Fig. 4.9 Comparison of excitation–contraction coupling in (A) skeletal muscle, (B) cardiac muscle and (C) smooth muscle. Skeletal and cardiac muscle differ mainly in the mechanism by which membrane depolarisation is coupled to Ca^{2+} release. The calcium channel (CaC) and ryanodine receptor (RyR) are very closely positioned in both types of muscle. In cardiac muscle, Ca^{2+} entry via voltage-gated calcium channels initiates Ca^{2+} release through activation of the Ca^{2+}-sensitive RyRs, whereas in skeletal muscle the sarcolemmal calcium channels activate the RyRs through a voltage-dependent physical interaction. The control of intracellular Ca^{2+} in smooth muscle cells may vary depending upon the type of smooth muscle. In general terms, smooth muscle contraction is largely dependent upon inositol trisphosphate (IP_3)-induced Ca^{2+} release from SR stores through IP_3 receptors (IP_3R). Smooth muscle contraction can also be produced either by Ca^{2+} entry through voltage- or ligand-gated calcium channels. The mechanism by which Ca^{2+} activates contraction is different, and operates more slowly, in smooth muscle compared with in skeletal or cardiac muscle. *CaC*, calcium channel; *CaM*, calmodulin; *GPCR*, G protein–coupled receptor; *MLCK*, myosin light-chain kinase; *NaC*, voltage-gated sodium channel; *RyR*, ryanodine receptor; *SR*, sarcoplasmic reticulum.

shown in Fig. 4.9) causes the opening of the RyRs on membrane depolarisation. Through this link, depolarisation rapidly activates the RyRs, releasing a short puff of Ca^{2+} from the SR into the sarcoplasm. The Ca^{2+} binds to troponin, a protein that normally blocks the interaction between actin and myosin. When Ca^{2+} binds, troponin moves out of the way and allows the contractile machinery to operate. Ca^{2+} release is rapid and brief, and the muscle responds with a short-lasting 'twitch' response. This is a relatively fast and direct mechanism compared with the arrangement in cardiac and smooth muscle (see later), and consequently less susceptible to pharmacological modulation.

CARDIAC MUSCLE

Cardiac muscle differs from skeletal muscle in several important respects. The nature of the cardiac action potential, the ionic mechanisms underlying its inherent rhythmicity and the effects of drugs on the rate and rhythm of the heart are described in Chapter 22. The cardiac action potential varies in its configuration in different parts of the heart, but commonly shows a plateau lasting several hundred milliseconds following the initial rapid depolarisation. T-tubules in cardiac muscle contain L-type calcium channels, which open during this plateau and allow Ca^{2+} to enter. This Ca^{2+} entry acts on RyRs (a different molecular type from those of skeletal muscle) to release Ca^{2+} from the SR (see Fig. 4.9). With minor differences, the subsequent mechanism by which Ca^{2+} activates the contractile machinery is the same as in skeletal muscle. Ca^{2+}-induced Ca^{2+} release via RyRs may play a role in some forms of cardiac arrhythmia. Mutations of RyRs are implicated in various disorders of skeletal and cardiac muscle function (see Priori & Napolitano, 2005).

SMOOTH MUSCLE

The properties of smooth muscle vary considerably in different organs, and the mechanisms linking membrane events and contraction are correspondingly variable and more complex than in other kinds of muscle. Spontaneous rhythmic activity occurs in many organs, by mechanisms producing oscillations of $[Ca^{2+}]_i$ (see Fig. 4.2B). The action potential of smooth muscle is generally a rather lazy and vague affair compared with the more military behaviour of skeletal and cardiac muscle, and it propagates through the tissue much more slowly and uncertainly. The action potential is, in most cases, generated by L-type calcium channels rather than by voltage-gated sodium channels, and this is one important route of Ca^{2+} entry. In addition, many smooth muscle cells possess P2X receptors, ligand-gated cation channels, which allow Ca^{2+} entry when activated by ATP released from autonomic nerves (see Ch. 13). Smooth muscle cells also store Ca^{2+} in the ER, from which it can be released when the IP3R is activated (see Ch. 3). IP3 is generated by activation of many types of G protein–coupled receptor. Thus in contrast to skeletal and cardiac muscle, Ca^{2+} release and contraction can occur in smooth muscle when such receptors are activated without necessarily involving depolarisation and Ca^{2+} entry through the plasma membrane. RyRs are also present in many smooth muscle cells and calcium-induced Ca^{2+} release via these channels may play a role in generating muscle contraction (see Fig. 4.9) or couple to plasma membrane calcium-activated K^+ channels resulting in cell hyperpolarisation, thereby reducing Ca^{2+} entry through voltage-gated calcium channels (Fig. 4.10).

The contractile machinery of smooth muscle is activated when the *myosin light chain* undergoes phosphorylation, causing it to become detached from the actin filaments. This phosphorylation is catalysed by a kinase, *myosin light-chain kinase* (MLCK), which is activated when it binds to Ca^{2+}–calmodulin (see p. 56, Fig. 4.9). A second enzyme, *myosin phosphatase*, reverses the phosphorylation and causes relaxation. The activity of MLCK and myosin phosphatase thus exerts a balanced effect, promoting contraction and relaxation, respectively. Both enzymes are regulated by cyclic nucleotides (cAMP and cGMP; see Ch. 3), and many drugs that cause smooth muscle contraction or relaxation

mediated through G protein–coupled receptors or through guanylyl cyclase-linked receptors act in this way. Fig. 4.10 summarises the main mechanisms by which drugs control smooth muscle contraction. The complexity of these control mechanisms and interactions explains why pharmacologists have been entranced for so long by smooth muscle. Many therapeutic drugs work by contracting or relaxing smooth muscle, particularly those affecting the cardiovascular, respiratory and gastrointestinal systems, as discussed in later chapters, where details of specific drugs and their physiological effects are given.

Muscle contraction

- Muscle contraction occurs in response to a rise in $[Ca^{2+}]_i$.
- In skeletal muscle, depolarisation causes rapid Ca^{2+} release from the sarcoplasmic reticulum (SR); in cardiac muscle, Ca^{2+} enters through voltage-gated channels, and this initial entry triggers further release from the SR; in smooth muscle, the Ca^{2+} signal is due partly to Ca^{2+} entry and partly to inositol trisphosphate (IP3)-mediated release from the SR.
- In smooth muscle, contraction can occur without action potentials, for example, when agonists at G protein–coupled receptors lead to IP3 formation.
- Activation of the contractile machinery in smooth muscle involves phosphorylation of the myosin light chain, a mechanism that is regulated by a variety of second messenger systems.

RELEASE OF CHEMICAL MEDIATORS

Much of pharmacology is based on interference with the body's own chemical mediators, particularly neurotransmitters, hormones and inflammatory mediators. Here we discuss some of the common mechanisms involved in the release of such mediators, and it will come as no surprise that Ca^{2+} plays a central role. Drugs and other agents that affect the various control mechanisms that regulate $[Ca^{2+}]_i$ will therefore also affect mediator release, and this accounts for many of the physiological effects that they produce.

Chemical mediators that are released from cells fall into two main groups (Fig. 4.11):

- Mediators that are preformed and packaged in storage vesicles – sometimes called storage granules – from which they are released by *exocytosis*. This large group comprises all the conventional neurotransmitters and neuromodulators (see Chs 13 and 38), and many hormones. It also includes secreted proteins such as cytokines and various growth factors (Ch. 19).
- Mediators that are produced on demand and are released by diffusion or by membrane carriers.[6] This group includes nitric oxide (Ch. 21) and many lipid mediators (e.g. prostanoids, Ch. 18) and

---

[6]Carrier-mediated release can also occur with neurotransmitters that are stored in vesicles but is quantitatively less significant than exocytosis.

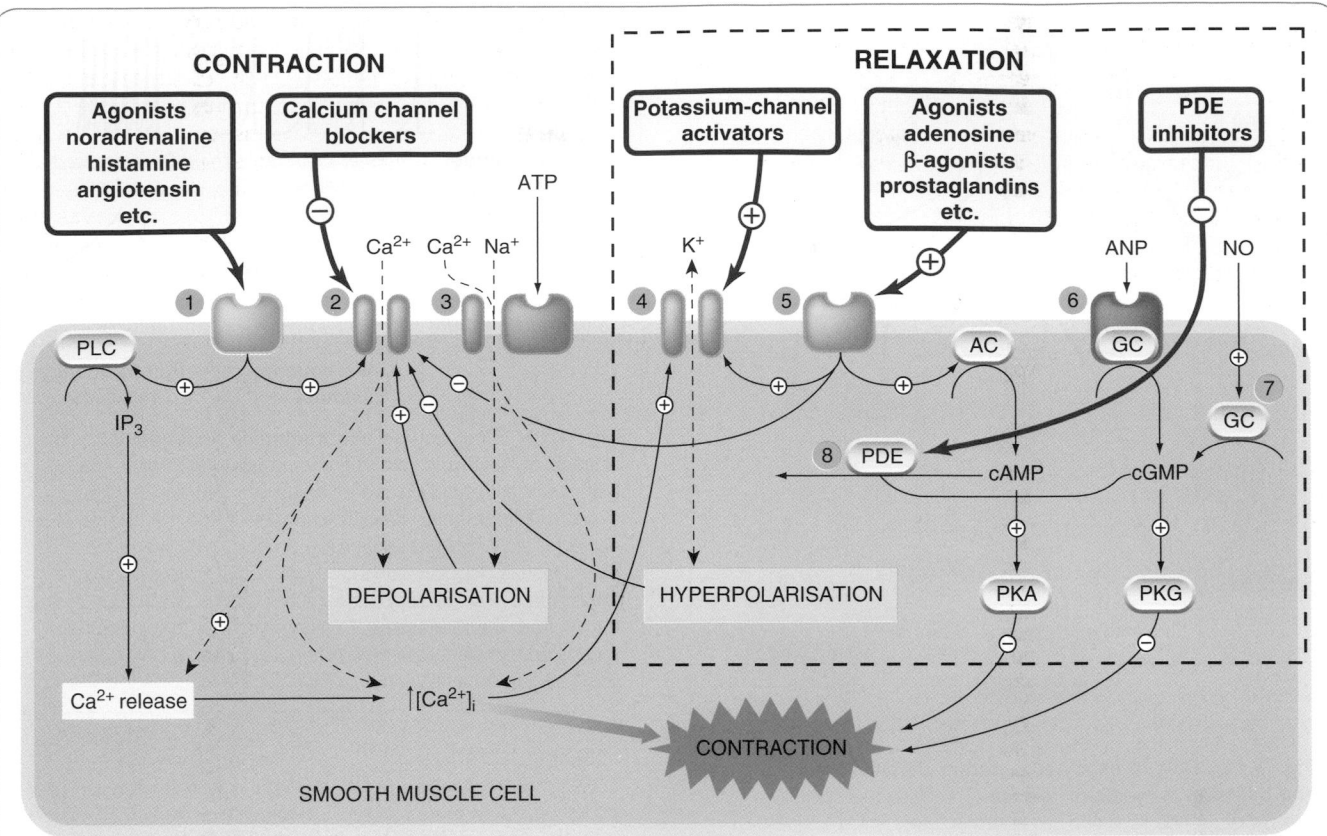

Fig. 4.10 Mechanisms controlling smooth muscle contraction and relaxation. *1.* G protein–coupled receptors for excitatory agonists, mainly regulating inositol trisphosphate formation and calcium channel function. *2.* Voltage-gated calcium channels. *3.* P2X receptor for ATP (ligand-gated cation channel). *4.* Potassium channels. *5.* G protein–coupled receptors for inhibitory agonists, mainly regulating cAMP formation and potassium and calcium channel function. *6.* Receptor for atrial natriuretic peptide (ANP), coupled directly to guanylyl cyclase (GC). *7.* Soluble GC, activated by nitric oxide (NO). *8.* Phosphodiesterase (PDE), the main route of inactivation of cAMP and cGMP. *AC*, adenylyl cyclase; *PKA*, protein kinase A; *PKG*, protein kinase G; *PLC*, phospholipase C.

endocannabinoids (Ch. 20), which are released from the postsynaptic cell to act retrogradely on nerve terminals.

Calcium ions play a key role in both cases, because a rise in $[Ca^{2+}]_i$ initiates exocytosis and is also the main activator of the enzymes responsible for the synthesis of diffusible mediators.

In addition to mediators that are released from cells, some are formed from precursors in the plasma, two important examples being *kinins* (Ch. 19) and *angiotensin* (Ch. 23), which are peptides produced by protease-mediated cleavage of circulating proteins.

EXOCYTOSIS

Exocytosis, occurring in response to an increase of $[Ca^{2+}]_i$, is the principal mechanism of transmitter release (see Fig. 4.11) in the peripheral and central nervous systems, as well as in endocrine cells and mast cells. The secretion of enzymes and other proteins by gastrointestinal and exocrine glands and by vascular endothelial cells is also basically similar. Exocytosis (see Thorn et al., 2016) involves fusion between the membrane of synaptic vesicles and the inner surface of the plasma membrane. The vesicles are preloaded with stored transmitter, and release occurs in discrete packets, or quanta, each representing the contents of a single vesicle. The first evidence for this came from the work of Katz and his colleagues in the 1950s, who recorded spontaneous 'miniature endplate potentials' at the frog neuromuscular junction, and showed that each resulted from the spontaneous release of a packet of the transmitter, acetylcholine. They also showed that release evoked by nerve stimulation occurred by the synchronous release of several hundred such quanta and was highly dependent on the presence of Ca^{2+} in the bathing solution. Unequivocal evidence that the quanta represented vesicles releasing their contents by exocytosis came from electron microscopic studies, in which the tissue was rapidly frozen in mid-release, revealing vesicles in the process of extrusion, and from elegant electrophysiological measurements showing that membrane capacitance (reflecting the area of the presynaptic membrane) increased in a stepwise manner as each vesicle fused and then gradually returned to the surface as the vesicle membrane was recovered from the surface. There is also biochemical evidence showing that, in addition to the transmitter, other constituents of the vesicles are released at the same time.

▼ In nerve terminals specialised for fast synaptic transmission, Ca^{2+} enters through voltage-gated calcium channels, mainly of the N and P/Q type (see p. 52 and Table 4.1), and the synaptic vesicles are 'docked' at active zones – specialised regions of the presynaptic

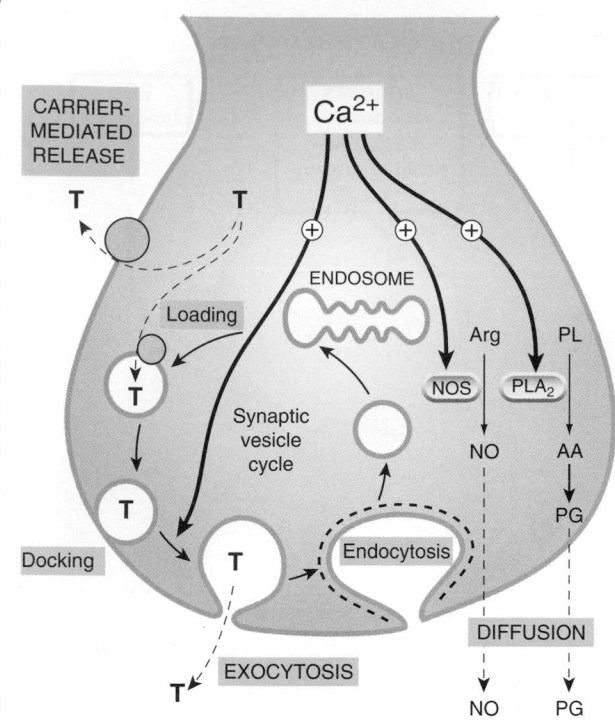

Fig. 4.11 Role of exocytosis, carrier-mediated transport and diffusion in mediator release. The main mechanism of release of monoamine and peptide mediators is Ca²⁺-mediated exocytosis, but carrier-mediated release from the cytosol also occurs. T represents a typical amine transmitter, such as noradrenaline (norepinephrine) or 5-hydroxytryptamine. Nitric oxide (NO) and prostaglandins (PGs) are released by diffusion as soon as they are formed, from arginine (Arg) and arachidonic acid (AA), respectively, through the action of Ca²⁺-activated enzymes, nitric oxide synthase (NOS) and phospholipase A₂ (PLA₂) (see Chs 18 and 21 for more details).

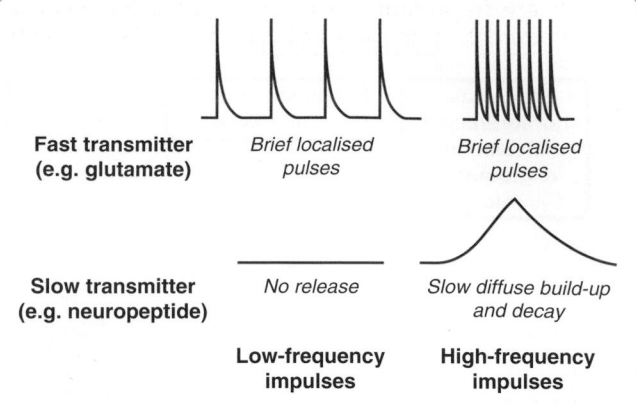

Fig. 4.12 Time course and frequency dependence of the release of 'fast' and 'slow' transmitters. Fast transmitters (e.g. glutamate) are stored in synaptic vesicles that are 'docked' close to voltage-gated calcium channels in the membrane of the nerve terminal and are released in a short burst when the membrane is depolarised (e.g. by an action potential). Slow transmitters (e.g. neuropeptides) are stored in separate vesicles further from the membrane. Release is slower, because they must first migrate to the membrane, and occurs only when [Ca²⁺]ᵢ builds up sufficiently.

membrane from which exocytosis occurs, situated close to the relevant calcium channels and opposite receptor-rich zones of the postsynaptic membrane. Elsewhere, where speed is less critical, Ca²⁺ may come from intracellular stores and the spatial organisation of active zones is less clear. It is common for secretory cells, including neurons, to release more than one mediator (for example, a 'fast' transmitter such as glutamate and a 'slow' transmitter such as a neuropeptide) from different vesicle pools (see Ch. 13). The fast transmitter vesicles are located close to active zones, while the slow transmitter vesicles are further away. Release of the fast transmitter, because of the tight spatial organisation, occurs as soon as the neighbouring calcium channels open, before the Ca²⁺ has a chance to diffuse throughout the terminal, whereas release of the slow transmitter requires the Ca²⁺ to diffuse more widely. As a result, release of fast transmitters occurs impulse by impulse, even at low stimulation frequencies, whereas release of slow transmitters builds up only at higher stimulation frequencies. The release rates of the two therefore depend critically on the frequency and patterning of firing of the presynaptic neuron (Fig. 4.12). In non-excitable cells (e.g. most exocrine and endocrine glands), the slow mechanism predominates and is activated mainly by Ca²⁺ release from intracellular stores.

Calcium causes exocytosis by binding to the vesicle-bound protein *synaptotagmin*, and this favours association between a second vesicle-bound protein, *synaptobrevin*, and a related protein, *synaptotaxin*, on the inner surface of the plasma membrane. This association brings the vesicle membrane into close apposition with the plasma membrane, causing membrane fusion. This group of proteins, known collectively as SNAREs, plays a key role in exocytosis.

Having undergone exocytosis, the empty vesicle[7] is recaptured by endocytosis and returns to the interior of the terminal, where it fuses with the larger endosomal membrane. The endosome buds off new vesicles, which take up transmitter from the cytosol by means of specific transport proteins and are again docked on the presynaptic membrane. This sequence, which typically takes several minutes, is controlled by various trafficking proteins associated with the plasma membrane and the vesicles, as well as cytosolic proteins. So far, there are few examples of drugs that affect transmitter release by interacting with synaptic proteins, although the botulinum neurotoxins (see Ch. 14) produce their effects by proteolytic cleavage of SNARE proteins.

NON-VESICULAR RELEASE MECHANISMS

If this neat and tidy picture of transmitter packets ready and waiting to pop obediently out of the cell in response to a puff of Ca²⁺ seems a little too good to be true, rest assured that the picture is not quite so simple. Acetylcholine, noradrenaline (norepinephrine) and other mediators can leak out of nerve endings from the cytosolic compartment, independently of vesicle fusion, by utilising carriers in the plasma membrane (see Fig. 4.11). Drugs such as **amphetamines**, which release amines from central and peripheral nerve terminals (see Chs 15 and 40), do so by displacing the endogenous amine from storage vesicles into the cytosol, whence it escapes via the monoamine transporter in the plasma membrane, a mechanism that does not depend on Ca²⁺.[8]

Nitric oxide (see Ch. 21), arachidonic acid metabolites (e.g. prostaglandins; Ch. 18) and endocannabinoids (see

---

[7]The vesicle contents may not always discharge completely. Instead, vesicles may fuse transiently with the cell membrane and release only part of their contents before becoming disconnected (termed *kiss-and-run exocytosis*).
[8]Some cheeses may have high levels of the trace amino acid tyramine, which can act akin to amphetamines and release noradrenaline (particularly in those being treated with monoamine oxidase (MAO) inhibitors, see Ch. 48) giving a dramatic sympathetic episode known as a 'cheese effect'.

Ch. 20) are important examples of mediators that are released from the cytosol by diffusion across the membrane or by carrier-mediated extrusion, rather than by exocytosis. The mediators are not stored but escape from the cell as soon as they are synthesised. In each case, the synthetic enzyme(s) is activated by Ca^{2+}, and the moment-to-moment control of the rate of synthesis depends on $[Ca^{2+}]_i$. This kind of release is necessarily slower than the classic exocytotic mechanism, but in the case of nitric oxide is fast enough for it to function as a true transmitter (see Fig. 13.5 and Ch. 21).

Mediator release

- Most chemical mediators are packaged into storage vesicles and released by exocytosis. Some are not stored but synthesised on demand and released by diffusion or the operation of membrane carriers.
- Exocytosis occurs in response to increased $[Ca^{2+}]_i$ as a result of a Ca^{2+}-mediated interaction between proteins of the synaptic vesicle and the plasma membrane, causing the membranes to fuse.
- After releasing their contents, vesicles are recycled and reloaded with transmitter.
- Many secretory cells contain more than one type of vesicle, loaded with different mediators and secreted independently.
- Stored mediators (e.g. neurotransmitters) may be released directly from the cytosol independently of Ca^{2+} and exocytosis, by drugs that interact with membrane transport mechanisms.
- Non-stored mediators, such as prostanoids, nitric oxide and endocannabinoids are released by increased $[Ca^{2+}]_i$, which activates the enzymes responsible for their synthesis.

EPITHELIAL ION TRANSPORT

Fluid-secreting epithelia include the renal tubule, salivary glands, gastrointestinal tract and airways epithelia. In each case, epithelial cells are arranged in sheets separating the interior (blood-perfused) compartment from the exterior lumen compartment, into which, or from which, secretion takes place. Fluid secretion involves two main mechanisms, which often co-exist in the same cell and indeed interact with each other. The two mechanisms (Fig. 4.13) are concerned, respectively, with Na^+ transport and Cl^- transport.

In the case of Na^+ transport, secretion occurs because Na^+ enters the cell passively at one end and is pumped out actively at the other, with water following passively. Critical to this mechanism is a class of highly regulated epithelial sodium channels (ENaCs) that allow Na^+ entry.

ENaCs (see Hanukoglu & Hanukoglu, 2016) are widely expressed, not only in epithelial cells but also in neurons and other excitable cells, where their function is largely unknown. They are regulated mainly by aldosterone, a hormone produced by the adrenal cortex that enhances Na^+ reabsorption by the kidney (see Ch. 30). Aldosterone, like other steroid hormones, exerts its effects by regulating

Fig. 4.13 Generalised mechanisms of epithelial ion transport. Such mechanisms are important in renal tubules (see Ch. 30 for more details) and in many other situations, such as the gastrointestinal and respiratory tracts. The exact mechanism may vary from tissue to tissue depending upon channel and pump expression and location. (A) Sodium transport. A special type of epithelial sodium channel (ENaC) controls entry of Na^+ into the cell from the lumenal surface, the Na^+ being actively pumped out at the apical surface by the Na^+–K^+ exchange pump. K^+ moves passively via potassium channels. (B) Chloride transport. Cl^- leaves the cell via a special membrane channel, the cystic fibrosis transmembrane conductance regulator (CFTR), after entering the cell either from the apical surface via the Na^+/Cl^- co-transporter, or at the lumenal surface via the Cl^-/HCO_3^- co-transporter.

gene expression (see Ch. 3), and causes an increase in ENaC expression, thereby increasing the rate of Na^+ and fluid transport. ENaCs are selectively blocked by certain diuretic drugs, notably **amiloride** (see Ch. 30), a compound that is widely used to study the functioning of ENaCs in other situations.

Chloride transport is particularly important in the airways and gastrointestinal tract. In the airways it is essential for fluid secretion, whereas in the colon it mediates fluid reabsorption, the difference being due to the different arrangement of various transporters and channels with respect to the polarity of the cells. The simplified diagram in Fig. 4.13B represents the situation in the pancreas, where secretion depends on Cl⁻ transport. The key molecule in Cl⁻ transport is the *cystic fibrosis transmembrane conductance regulator* (CFTR), so named because early studies on the inherited disorder cystic fibrosis showed it to be associated with impaired Cl⁻ conductance in the membrane of secretory epithelial cells, and the CFTR gene, identified through painstaking genetic linkage studies and isolated in 1989, was found to encode a Cl⁻-conducting ion channel. Severe physiological consequences follow from CFTR mutations and the resulting impairment of secretion, particularly in the airways but also in many other systems, such as sweat glands and pancreas. Studies on the disease-associated mutations of the CFTR gene have revealed much about the molecular mechanisms involved in Cl⁻ transport (Wang et al., 2014).

Both Na⁺ and Cl⁻ transport are regulated by intracellular messengers, notably by Ca^{2+} and cAMP, the latter exerting its effects by activating protein kinases and thereby causing phosphorylation of channels and transporters. CFTR itself is activated by cAMP. In the gastrointestinal tract, increased cAMP formation causes a large increase in the rate of fluid secretion, an effect that leads to the copious diarrhoea produced by cholera infection (see Ch. 3) and by inflammatory conditions in which prostaglandin formation is increased (see Ch. 18). Activation of G protein–coupled receptors, which cause release of Ca^{2+}, also stimulates secretion, possibly also by activating CFTR. Many examples of therapeutic drugs that affect epithelial secretion by activating or blocking G protein–coupled receptors appear in later chapters.

Epithelial ion transport

- Many epithelia (e.g. renal tubules, exocrine glands and airways) are specialised to transport specific ions.
- This type of transport depends on a special class of epithelial sodium channels (ENaCs) which allow Na⁺ entry into the cell at one surface, coupled to active extrusion of Na⁺, or exchange for another ion, from the opposite surface.
- Anion transport depends on a specific chloride channel (the cystic fibrosis transmembrane conductance regulator [CFTR]), mutations of which result in cystic fibrosis.
- The activity of channels, pumps and exchange transporters is regulated by various second messengers and nuclear receptors, which control the transport of ions in specific ways.

REFERENCES AND FURTHER READING

General references

Alexander, S.P., Catterall, W.A., Kelly, E., et al., 2015. The concise guide to pharmacology 2015/16: Voltage-gated ion channels. Br. J. Pharmacol. 172, 5904–5941. (*Contains a brief description of a range of ion channels and the drugs that interact with them*)

Berridge, M.J., 2014. Cell Signalling Biology. Portland Press. doi:10.1042/csb0001002. (*Free ebook available online at www.cellsignallingbiology.org; a regularly updated resource that covers various aspects of cell signalling in a highly readable format*)

Kandel, E.R., Schwartz, J.H., Jessell, T.M., Siegelbaum, S.A., Hudspeth, A.J., 2012. Principles of Neural Science. McGraw-Hill, New York. (*Excellent, well-written textbook of neuroscience*)

Katz, B., 1966. Nerve, Muscle and Synapse. McGraw–Hill, New York. (*A classic account of the ground-breaking electrophysiological experiments that established the basis of nerve and muscle function*)

Berridge, M.J., 2016. The inositol trisphosphate/calcium signaling pathway in health and disease. Physiol. Rev. 96, 1261–1296. (*Clear and readable up-to-date account of the mechanisms and versatility of calcium signaling and how it may be altered in disease states*)

Morgan, A.J., Davis, L.C., Ruas, M., Galione, A., 2015. TPC: the NAADP discovery channel? Biochem. Soc. Trans. 43, 384–389. (*Interesting discussion of this controversial topic from the laboratory of one of the main protagonists*)

Parrington, J., Lear, P., Hachem, A., 2015. Calcium signals regulated by NAADP and two-pore channels–their role in development, differentiation and cancer. Int. J. Dev. Biol. 59, 341–355. (*Review of the potential pathophysiological importance*)

Prakriya, M., Lewis, R.S., 2015. Store-operated calcium channels. Physiol. Rev. 95, 1383–1436. (*Comprehensive review of this topic*)

Excitation and ion channels

Catterall, W.A., Swanson, T.M., 2015. Structural basis for pharmacology of voltage-gated sodium and calcium channels. Mol. Pharmacol. 88, 141–150. (*Useful, authoritative review article*)

Hille, B., 2001. Ionic Channels of Excitable Membranes. Sinauer Associates, Sunderland. (*Still probably the best, clear and detailed account of the basic principles of ion channels, with emphasis on their biophysical properties*)

Imbrici, P., Liantonio, A., Camerino, G.M., et al., 2016. Therapeutic approaches to genetic ion channelopathies and perspectives in drug discovery. Front. Pharmacol. 7, 121. (*Detailed review of the importance of channelopathies in multiple disorders*)

Jenkinson, D.H., 2006. Potassium channels – multiplicity and challenges. Br. J. Pharmacol. 147 (Suppl. 1), 63–71. (*Useful short article on the many types of K⁺ channel*)

Muscle contraction

Berridge, M.J., 2008. Smooth muscle cell calcium activation mechanisms. J. Physiol. 586, 5047–5061. (*Excellent review article describing the various mechanisms by which calcium signals control activity in different types of smooth muscle – complicated but clear*)

Priori, S.G., Napolitano, C., 2005. Cardiac and skeletal muscle disorders caused by mutations in the intracellular Ca^{2+} release channels. J. Clin. Invest. 115, 2033–2038. (*Focuses on RyR mutations in various inherited diseases*)

Van Petegem, F., 2012. Ryanodine receptors: structure and function. J. Biol. Chem. 287 (31), 31624–31632.

Secretion and exocytosis

Hanukoglu, I., Hanukoglu, A., 2016. Epithelial sodium channel (ENaC) family: phylogeny, structure-function, tissue distribution, and associated inherited diseases. Gene 579, 95–132. (*Extensive review of the function and importance of these channels in health and disease*)

Thorn, P., Zorec, R., Rettig, J., Keating, D.J., 2016. Exocytosis in non-neuronal cells. J. Neurochem. 137, 849–859.

Wang, Y., Wrennall, J.A., Cai, Z., Li, H., Sheppard, D.N., 2014. Understanding how cystic fibrosis mutations disrupt CFTR function: from single molecules to animal models. Int. J. Biochem. Cell Biol. 52, 47–57.

How drugs act: biopharmaceuticals and gene therapy

5

OVERVIEW

In this chapter, we discuss the properties of a group of therapeutic agents known collectively as *biopharmaceuticals*. These are relatively recent additions to our therapeutic armoury, but they have already made a major impact on treatment of diseases such as rheumatoid arthritis and cancer. The number of biopharmaceuticals approved for clinical use is growing and the sector will assume more significance in the future. In this chapter, we first introduce protein- and oligonucleotide-based biopharmaceuticals, highlight the major differences with 'conventional' small molecule drugs and explain how they are manufactured, how they work and how they are metabolised. We then introduce the central concepts of *gene therapy*, discuss the promise and problems associated with this therapeutic modality and highlight some limited successes.

INTRODUCTION

This chapter deals with the general pharmacological characteristics of protein and nucleic acid-based pharmaceuticals produced using genetic engineering techniques (i.e. biotechnology, as distinct from synthetic chemistry). Such agents currently account for 20%–25% of new registrations, and are increasingly important therapeutically. Individual agents are discussed in later chapters.

▼ Annoyingly for authors of textbooks and their readers, there is no consensus on what actually constitutes a 'biopharmaceutical' as opposed to a conventional drug. An apparently obvious distinguishing feature is whether it is predominantly 'chemical' in nature (like almost all the small molecule drugs in this book) or of 'biological' origin (like insulin or growth hormone, for example). Unfortunately, this simplistic distinction breaks down rather quickly when we consider that some 'small molecule' drugs (such as **morphine** or **penicillin**) are plant or fungal products whilst other 'biological molecules' such as short peptides or antisense oligonucleotides are produced by synthetic organic chemistry techniques.

A further problem is the stance adopted by the main drug regulatory agencies. The FDA and their European counterparts use slightly different definitions when classifying 'biopharmaceuticals' and this has profound effects on the companies that manufacture them, affecting their regulatory obligations, their business models, patent filings, investment funding and even public relations. As one commentator (Rader, 2008) put it, 'The result is a Babel-like situation with terminological chaos and anarchy confounding communication, comparative and industry analyses, understanding and regulation'.

To simplify the situation, we will adopt a largely pragmatic definition in this chapter; there is no doubt that biopharmaceuticals[1] are different in many respects from conventional small molecule drugs

(including their pharmacology) and we will use these as our criteria for distinguishing between them. We will begin with a discussion of protein and oligonucleotide biopharmaceuticals.

PROTEIN AND OLIGONUCLEOTIDE BIOPHARMACEUTICALS

The use of proteins as therapeutic agents is not a novel idea; insulin, extracted from animal pancreas tissue (Ch. 32), and human growth hormone, extracted at one time from human cadaver pituitary glands (Ch. 34), were among the first therapeutic proteins to be used and, for many years, such purified extracts provided the only option for treating protein hormone deficiency disorders. However, there were problems. Technical difficulties in extraction of the hormone from tissue often led to disappointing yields. Administration of animal hormones (e.g. pig insulin) to humans could evoke an immune response and there was another insidious danger – transmission of infectious agents across species or between people. This was highlighted in the 1970s, when cases of *Creutzfeldt–Jakob disease* (see Ch. 41) were seen in patients treated with human growth hormone obtained from cadavers. This serious problem was later traced to contamination of the donor pituitary glands with infectious *prions* (Ch. 41). The advent of 'genetic engineering' techniques offered a new way to deal with these perennial problems.

Biopharmaceuticals and gene therapy: definition and potential uses

- *Biopharmaceuticals* include proteins and antibodies (and oligonucleotides) used as drugs:
  - *First-generation* biopharmaceuticals are mainly copies of endogenous proteins or antibodies, produced by recombinant DNA technology.
  - *Second-generation* biopharmaceuticals have been 'engineered' to improve the performance of the protein, antibody or antisense agent.
- Applications:
  - therapeutic monoclonal antibodies
  - recombinant hormones
  - controlling gene expression (oligonucleotides)
- *Gene therapy* is the addition of genetic material to cells to prevent, alleviate or cure disease.
- Potential applications:
  - radical cure of monogenic diseases (e.g. cystic fibrosis, haemoglobinopathies);
  - amelioration of diseases with or without a genetic component, including many malignant, neurodegenerative and infectious diseases.

---

[1]There is a tiresome terminological issue here too: such drugs are often known simply as 'biologics', but this term is also used to refer to *any* biological reagents (e.g. antibody-based laboratory tests, plasma expanders and so on).

PROTEINS AND POLYPEPTIDES

The biopharmaceuticals in use today are generally classified as first- or second-generation agents. *First-generation* biopharmaceuticals are usually straightforward copies of human hormones or other proteins, prepared by *transfecting* the human gene into a suitable *expression system* (a cell line that produces the protein in good yield), harvesting and purifying the *recombinant protein* for use as a drug. The first agent to be produced in this way was recombinant human insulin in 1982.

Second-generation biopharmaceuticals are those that have been *engineered*; that is to say, either the gene has been deliberately altered prior to transfection such that the structure of the recombinant protein is changed, or some alteration is made to the purified end product. Such changes are generally made to improve some aspect of the protein's activity profile. Human recombinant insulins designed to act faster or last longer were among the first in this class to be marketed; Table 5.1 contains other examples.

Production methods

▼ There are several problems associated with the manufacture of any type of recombinant protein, and one of the most pressing is the choice of expression system. Many recombinant proteins are expressed in bacterial systems (*Escherichia coli*, for example), which is useful because cultures grow quickly and are generally easy to manipulate. Disadvantages include the fact that the product may contain bacterial endotoxins, which must be removed before administration to patients, and also that bacterial cells differ from mammalian cells in patterns of *post-translational processing* (e.g. glycosylation) of proteins, which may affect the protein's biological action. To circumvent these problems, mammalian (e.g. Chinese hamster ovary [CHO]) cells can also be used as expression systems, although such cells require more careful culture, grow more slowly than bacteria and produce less product, all of which contributes to the cost of the final medicine.

A number of emergent technologies are set to transform the production process. The use of plants to produce recombinant proteins has attracted considerable interest (see Melnik & Stoger, 2013). Several species have shown promise, including the tobacco plant. Human genes of interest can readily be transfected into the plant using tobacco mosaic virus as a vector; the crop grows rapidly (yields a high *biomass*) and offers a number of other advantages. Edible plants

Table 5.1 Some examples of biopharmaceuticals

Class	Type	Biopharmaceutical	Change	Target	Indication	Reason for change
First generation	Protein	Human insulin	None	Insulin receptor	Diabetes	N/A
	Protein	Human growth hormone	None	Growth hormone receptor (agonist)	Pituitary dwarfism, Turner's syndrome	N/A
Second generation	Protein	Insulin	AA sequence	Insulin receptor	Diabetes	Faster acting hormone
	Protein	Interferon analogue	AA sequence	Viral replication	Viral infection	Superior antiviral activity
	Protein	Glucocerebrosidase enzyme	Carbohydrate residue	Glucocerebrosides	Gaucher's disease	Promotes phagocytic uptake
	Protein	Erythropoietin analogue	Carbohydrate residue	Erythropoietin receptor	Anaemia	Prolongs half-life
	Protein	Human growth hormone	AA sequence, prosthetic group	Growth hormone receptor (antagonist)	Acromegaly	Converts agonist into antagonist with long duration of action
	Protein	Adalimumab[a]	Humanised mAb	Tumour necrosis factor	Rheumatoid disease	Persists in circulation
	Protein	Omalizumab	Humanised mAb	IgE	IgE-mediated asthma	Persists in circulation
	Antisense oligonucleotide	Mipomersin	Modified nucleotides	Apolipoprotein B gene	Familial hypercholesteraemia	Stability
	Antisense oligonucleotide	Eteplirsen	Modified nucleotides	Dystrophin gene	Duchenne muscular dystrophy	Stability
	Antisense oligonucleotide	Nusinersen	Modified nucleotides	Survival motor neuron protein (SMN 1)	Spinal muscular atrophy	Stability

[a]Therapeutic monoclonal antibody names all end in '-mab', prefixed by an indication of their species nature: -umab (human), -omab (mouse), -ximab (chimera), -zumab (humanised).
AA, amino acids; *IgE*, immunoglobulin E; *mAb*, monoclonal antibody.
(Source: Walsh, 2004; The British National Formulary; and others.)

such as lettuce and bananas could be used to produce some orally active proteins, such as vaccines, which could then be consumed directly without the need for prior purification. Several such proteins have already been produced in plants, and have entered clinical trials (Kwon et al., 2013).

Another technology that could dramatically increase the yield of human recombinant proteins is the use of transgenic cattle. A dairy cow can produce some 10,000 litres of milk per year, and recombinant proteins introduced into the genome and under the control of promoters that regulate production of other milk proteins, can generate yields as high as 1 g/L (see Brink et al., 2000).

Engineered proteins

There are several ways in which proteins can be altered prior to expression. Alteration of the nucleotide sequence of the coding gene can be used to change single amino acids or, indeed, whole regions of the polypeptide chain. There are good reasons why it may be an advantage to engineer proteins in this way. These include:

- modification of pharmacokinetic properties
- creation of novel *fusion* or other proteins
- reducing immunogenicity, for example, by *humanising* the protein

It is often useful to modify the pharmacokinetic properties of recombinant proteins. Changes in the structure of human insulin, for example, provided a form of the hormone that did not self-associate during storage and was thus faster acting and easier to manage. The half-life of proteins in the blood can often be extended by *PEGylation* (see Ch. 11), the addition of polyethylene glycol to the molecule. This *post-translational engineering* approach has been applied to some human hormones, such as recombinant growth hormone, interferons and others. This is not merely a convenience to patients; it also reduces the overall cost of the treatment, an important factor in the adoption of this type of therapy.

Fusion proteins comprise two or more proteins engineered to be expressed as one single polypeptide chain, sometimes joined by a short linker. An example is **etanercept**, an anti-inflammatory drug used in the treatment of rheumatoid arthritis and other conditions (see Ch. 27). Etanercept consists of the ligand-binding domain taken from the tumour necrosis factor (TNF) receptor, joined to the Fc domain of a human immunoglobulin G antibody. The receptor moiety sequesters endogenous TNF ligand in a complexed inactive form, while the immunoglobulin increases persistence of the drug in the blood. Reduction of immunogenicity through bioengineering is discussed later.

MONOCLONAL ANTIBODIES

Although antisera preparations can be used to confer *passive immunity*, there are a number of inherent disadvantages that limit their utility. Conventionally, antisera are produced from the blood of immunised humans or animals. Antiserum containing high levels of specific antibodies (e.g. to tetanus toxin or snake venom) is prepared from the plasma and this can then be used therapeutically to neutralise pathogens or other dangerous substances in the blood of the patient.

Such preparations are comprised of *polyclonal antibodies* – that is, a *polyvalent* mixture of antibodies from all the plasma cell clones that reacted to that particular antigen. The actual composition and efficacy of these varies over time, and obviously there is a limit to how much plasma can be collected on any one occasion. However, in 1975,

Milstein and Köhler[2] discovered a method of producing from immunised mice an immortalised *hybridoma*, a fusion of one particular lymphocytic clone with an immortalised tumour cell. This furnished a method of producing *monoclonal antibodies (mAbs)* – a single species of monovalent antibody – at high abundance in vitro. The hybridoma cell line could be retained and expanded indefinitely while preserving the integrity of its product.

mAbs can be classified into first- or second-generation reagents along similar lines to the other therapeutic proteins discussed above. First-generation mAbs were simply murine monoclonals (or fragments thereof) but had several drawbacks. As mouse proteins, they provoked an immune response in 50%–75% of all human recipients, had a short half-life in the human circulation and were unable to activate human complement.

Most of these problems can now be surmounted by using either *chimeric* or *humanised* mAbs. These two terms refer to the degree to which they have been engineered. Fig. 5.1 shows how this is done; the antibody molecule consists of a *constant* domain (Fc) and the antibody-binding domain (Fab), with *hypervariable* regions that recognise and bind to the antigen in question. The genes for chimeric mAbs are engineered to contain the cDNA of the *murine* Fab domain coupled with the *human* Fc domain sequences. This

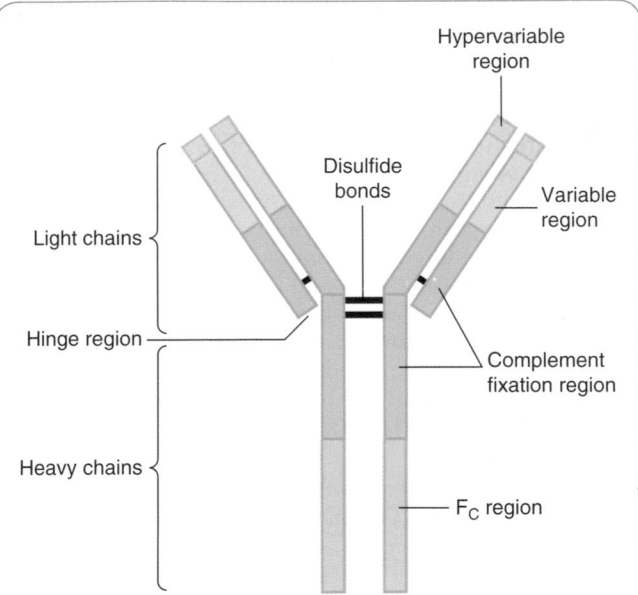

Fig. 5.1 Production of engineered 'chimeric' and 'humanised' monoclonal antibodies. The Y-shaped antibody molecule consists of two main domains: the Fc (constant) domain and the Fab (antigen-binding) domain. At the tip of the Fab regions (on the arms of the 'Y') are the hypervariable regions that actually bind the antigen. Chimeric antibodies are produced by replacing the murine Fc region with its human equivalent by altering and splicing the gene. For humanised antibodies, only the murine hypervariable regions are retained, the remainder of the molecule being human in origin. (After Walsh, 2004.)

[2]They won the 1984 Nobel Prize for Physiology or Medicine for this work.

Fig. 5.2 Using antisense oligonucleotides to correct mild-moderate hyperlipidaemia. The antisense oligonucleotide mipomersen was administered to 50 patients for 13 weeks. The data shows the mean reduction in low-density lipoprotein (LDL) cholesterol expressed in percentage terms from the baseline readings at day 1 with doses of 200 mg/week *(red)* and 400 mg/week *(blue)* compared with a placebo *(black)*. The reduction in expression of apolipoprotein B caused by the drug exactly paralleled the LDL cholesterol data. After discontinuation of the treatment (indicated by dotted line) the blood levels showed signs of returning to baseline values, but were still depressed by 20%–30% at the conclusion of the study at these doses (Redrawn from Geary et al., 2015).

greatly (around five-fold) extends the plasma half-life because whilst most plasma proteins turn over quite rapidly immunoglobulins are an exception (it is easy to see why this provides a selective advantage to the host). Incorporation of human Fc sequences also improves the functionality of the antibody in human medicine. A further development (and now the preferred approach) is to replace the entire Fc and Fab region with the human equivalent with the exception of the hypervariable regions, giving a molecule which, while essentially human in nature, contains just the minimal murine antibody-binding sites. The anticancer monoclonal **Herceptin (trastuzumab**; see Ch. 57) is an example of such an antibody, and some others (together with an explanation of the tongue-twisting nomenclature system) are given in Table 5.1.

OLIGONUCLEOTIDES

We turn next to another type of biopharmaceutical, this time based upon oligonucleotide structures. These offer an alternative way of modifying genetic material that is far less problematic than delivering entire genes (see later). Amongst the most useful approaches is the use of *antisense oligonucleotides*. These are short oligonucleotides that are complementary to part of a gene or gene product that one wishes to modify or suppress. The oligomer needs to be at least 15 bases long to confer specificity and tight binding to its target sequence (most antisense oligos are 15–25 mers). These snippets of genetic material can be designed to suppress the expression of a harmful gene either by forming a triplex (three-stranded helix) with a regulatory component of chromosomal DNA, or by complexing a region of mRNA as a duplex. Unlike entire gene constructs, oligonucleotides can cross plasma and nuclear membranes by endocytosis as well as by direct diffusion, despite their molecular size and charge. To avoid destruction by nucleotidases which

are ubiquitous in biological fluids, enzyme-resistant *methylphosphorate*, *phosphothiorate* or other analogues have been developed.

Following parenteral administration, such oligomers distribute widely throughout the body (although not to the CNS) and work in part by interfering with the transcription of mRNA and in part by stimulating its breakdown by ribonuclease H. **Mipomersen**, the first ever licensed antisense therapeutic (2013), is a phosphothiorate analogue that suppresses the expression of apolipoprotein B, acts through this mechanism. It can be used to treat a rare form of hypercholesterolaemia (Fig. 5.2). Another oligonucleotide drug recently (2016) approved by the FDA, **etiplersen**, targets a specific region of the *dystrophin* gene that is mutated in Duchenne muscular dystrophy, changing the reading frame and causing the faulty exon to be removed, with the result that the final translated product is a partially functional version of the protein.

After a slow start with only two agents actually reaching the market prior to 2017, at the time of writing, several candidate drugs are being tested for use in the treatment of viral diseases including HIV, cytomegalovirus and haemorrhagic virus infections as well as cancer, spinal muscular atrophy and other disorders.

A related approach (see Castanatto & Rossi, 2009), which provides more efficient gene silencing than antisense oligonucleotides, is the use of *short interfering RNA* (siRNA),[3] whereby short lengths of double-stranded RNA recruit an enzyme complex, known as RISC (**R**NA-**I**nduced **S**ilencing **C**omplex), which selectively degrades the corresponding

---

[3]Discovered when plant scientists found, to their surprise, that introducing RNA which encoded the colour-producing enzyme in petunias made the flowers *less* colourful, not more so. Subsequently siRNA has emerged as an important physiological mechanism for controlling gene expression and was recognised by the award in 2006 of the Nobel Prize to Craig Mello and Andrew Fire.

Table 5.2 Differences between biopharmaceuticals and conventional small molecule drugs

Property	Conventional drug	Biopharmaceutical
Size	Generally <500 kDa (10^2)	Generally >5000 kDa (10^3), e.g. oligonucleotides, 10^3; small proteins 10^3–10^4; mAbs 10^5; genes >10^6.
Synthesis	Easy to synthesise identical batches	Most biopharmaceuticals are unique (except small peptides and short oligonucleotides which can be synthesised chemically)
Relationship between dose and effect	Usually a predictable relationship between dose and effect	Complex mechanisms of action, usually high-affinity binding, slow on- and off-rates, unusual shaped D/R curves
Pharmacokinetics	Often oral administration, variable absorption and bioavailability, phase 1 and phase 2 metabolism, excretion of drug in urine or faeces	Usually parenteral administration, bioavailability high, long half-life, atypical biodistribution and removal mechanisms
Toxicology and adverse effects	Variable, possible drug interactions	Immunogenicity, few drug interactions, generally fewer adverse effects

mRNA produced by the cell, thereby blocking expression. These silencing RNA sequences can also be efficiently produced in a cell infected with a virus that is engineered to express the right sequence. Clinical trials of siRNA therapeutics are in progress.

PHARMACOLOGY OF PROTEIN AND OLIGONUCLEOTIDE PHARMACEUTICALS

There are important differences between the pharmacological properties of protein and oligonucleotide biopharmaceuticals and those of conventional small molecule drugs (Table 5.2), attributable in part to their difference in molecular mass. Most conventional drugs have molecular masses of less than 1000 and are usually less than 500 – in fact, it is thought that this factor is important in achieving optimal distribution in the body and for the biological activity of the drug. In contrast, even the smallest protein biopharmaceutical, insulin, has a molecular mass of almost 6000. Antibodies usually weigh in at about 150,000 and oligonucleotides about 2000–3000. Their size obviously affects the absorption and bioavailability of biopharmaceuticals.

Another distinguishing factor is a consequence of their production. Conventional drugs and short oligonucleotides are produced by total (occasionally partial) chemical synthesis, with identical characteristics wherever the compound is made. However, this is not the case with many protein-based biopharmaceuticals. The gene expression system used to produce therapeutically active proteins differs from one company to another – deliberately so in most cases because, unlike genes themselves, proprietary gene constructs and expression systems can be patented, enabling pharma to protect its intellectual property. Each expression system produces a slightly different product in terms of its purity, post-translational modifications and protein 'fingerprint'[4]. This has important consequences for drug regulation, because unlike synthetic small molecule drugs, each biopharmaceutical is unique and a common saying in the biotech industry is that 'the product is the process'. Compared to the first-in-the-field drug, *subsequent*

entry biologics (SEBs) or *follow-on biologics* (FOBs), may be *bioequivalents* (i.e. drugs that are interchangeable with, and therapeutically equivalent to, the original preparation); more often, while still therapeutically effective, they have different clinical properties.[5] However, each requires separate regulatory approval.

Another manufacturing issue concerns the number of steps required to prepare biopharmaceuticals. With chemical synthesis, one can assess the exact purity of the final product, but preparations of biopharmaceuticals may not be homogenous and could contain mixtures of different glycoforms of the protein or possibly bacterial proteins or endotoxins. This means that there is a requirement for greatly enhanced quality control and this obviously has profound implications for ease of manufacture and final cost (Revers & Furzcon, 2010).

Some actions of biopharmaceuticals resemble those of conventional drugs: for example, insulin or growth hormone have identical actions to the native hormone. But there are differences too. Some mAbs immunoneutralise unwanted substances: for example, **infliximab** directly neutralises the cytokine TNF to produce its therapeutic effect. However, another mAb, **rituximab**, binds to CD20 on lymphocytes and causes actual destruction of the cells to diminish an unwanted immune response. **Ibritumomab tiuxetan** also binds CD20, but delivers ^{90}Y to kill the cells.

Because of these different modes of action, the relationship between dose and effect, so beloved of pharmacologists, is much less clear cut. Agoram (2009) highlights some of the problems. In the case of mAbs, high-affinity binding is usual (sometimes a mixture of specific and non-specific binding), slow on- and off-rates are common and the mAb may be internalised, thus modifying its target cell. Dose–response relationships are sometimes bell-shaped or U-shaped. Human recombinant erythropoietin has a bell-shaped dose–response and, in the case of many mAbs, there is a single optimal dose at which effective immunoneutralisation

---

[4]This 'biological variation' using cells to produce a drug is obviously not inherent in more exact medicinal chemistry processes.

[5]More bewildering terminology: *biosimilars* are generic drugs with a similar function to the original but with different pharmacology or toxicology; *biobetters* are generic drugs with a similar function to the original but with superior pharmacology or toxicology.

Table 5.3 A comparison of pharmacokinetics between two conventional small molecule drugs and some biopharmaceuticals

Type	Drug	Route[a]	Dosing frequency	T_{max}	$T_{1/2}$	Bioavailability	V
Conventional drug	20 mg simvastatin	p.o.	1 per day	0.7 h	1.5 h	<5%	215 L/kg
	75 mg indometacin	p.o.	1–2 per day	2–3 h	2–3 h	>90%	1.0 L/kg
Biopharmaceutical	25 mg etanercept	i.m.	1–2 per week	69 h	102 h	58%	6–11 L/kg
	40 mg adalimumab	i.m.	1 per 2 weeks	131 h	10–20 days	64%	4.7–6.0 L/kg
	75 mg omalizumab	i.m.	1 per month	7–8 days	26 days	62%	5.5 L/kg

[a]Route of administration: *i.m.*, intramuscular; *p.o.*, by mouth. All data approximated from information from manufacturers. T_{max}, time to maximum plasma concentration; $t_{1/2}$, half-life; V, volume of distribution.

occurs, instead of the proportional effects that we are more accustomed to when dealing with small molecule drugs. In the case of oligonucleotides, there are also several different mechanisms of action, as we saw previously.

The differences in the nature and size of most biopharmaceuticals when compared with conventional drugs also have implications for their pharmacokinetic properties. Because proteins do not usually survive oral administration, most are administered subcutaneously, intramuscularly or intravenously and so bioavailability is typically high compared with many small molecule drugs, often in the region of 80%–100%. But, except in the case of intravenous administration, absorption from the injection site is usually slow and the time taken to achieve attain the T_{max} reflects this. Once in the circulation however, the half-life is typically long. Because antibodies bind to their target with high affinity, the volume of distribution is often small, but transcellular and unusual trafficking may redistribute the drug to other tissues (Zhao et al., 2012). A comparison of the pharmacokinetics of conventional small molecule drugs with several biopharmaceuticals is shown in Table 5.3.

Biopharmaceuticals are not removed from the body following metabolic transformation and excretion of the type described in Chapter 10 and indeed, some antibodies can persist in the circulation for weeks. Instead, uptake of large biopharmaceuticals by the lymphatic system is the usual first step, followed by lysosomal degradation. However, some 'small' (<69 kDa) mAbs may be eliminated directly by the kidney. Immunogenicity is an issue that plagued early development of proteins as drugs and whilst this has been largely overcome by 'humanisation' of antibodies and proteins, it is still important because it alters the pharmacokinetic properties of the drug (Richter et al., 1999) by increasing its clearance from the circulation.

Drug interactions are less of an issue with biopharmaceuticals, as are general toxicity problems and adverse side effects, an advantage that is reflected in their relatively rapid approval by regulatory agencies. In part, this is due to their extraordinary specificity. In fact, few drugs come closer to the idea of a 'magic bullet'[6] than biopharmaceuticals which, because of the specificity of the immune system,

can inactivate single targets with an extraordinary degree of precision. Ironically, this can cause major problems when testing these drugs.

▼ In 2006, for example, a UK clinical trial of a new mAb (TGN 1412) designed to activate T cells (see Ch. 7) and thus treat B-cell lymphocytic leukaemia went badly wrong. All six participants became severely ill following a 'cytokine storm' and suffered lasting damage. The incident provoked wide media publicity[7] and, while the subsequent investigation blamed an 'unpredictable' biological reaction, it caused many to think hard about how such trials should be conducted in the future (see Muller & Brennan, 2009). Highly specific reagents, such as monoclonals intended for human use, pose particular problems as they may not cross-react with the corresponding proteins of other species, thus evading detection in the usual preclinical animal safety screens. It may be the case that 'surrogate' mAbs which are species-specific will have to be developed to test in animal models of the disease.

GENE THERAPY

Astonishingly, the first study to demonstrate the theoretical feasibility of gene transfer took place in 1944 when Avery and his colleagues showed that a virulence factor could be transferred between two strains of pneumococcus and identified the factor as (what we now call) DNA, which was not even recognised at that time as the genetic material. Following the molecular biology revolution in the 1980s however, the significance of this experiment became clear and the notion that one could replace faulty or missing genes became a thrilling – if distant – prospect. Despite the high hopes and intensive research efforts in the intervening years, the full potential of gene therapy is still unrealised. However, the idea commands such appeal that vast resources (both public and private) have been committed to its development. There are several reasons why it is so attractive. First, it is a (deceptively) simple approach to a radical cure of single-gene diseases such as *cystic fibrosis* and the *haemoglobinopathies*, which are collectively responsible for much misery throughout the world. Second, many other more common conditions, including malignant, neurodegenerative and infectious diseases, have a large genetic component. Conventional treatment of such disorders is (as readers of later chapters will appreciate) far from ideal, so the promise of a completely new approach has enormous allure.

[6]It was Weber's opera, *Der Freischütz* (The Sharpshooter, 1821), that introduced the idea of a 'magic bullet' which, once fired, always found its mark. Ehrlich liked the idea and thought that it was a good description of a highly specific drug. The term, and the concept, has haunted our discipline ever since.

[7]One tabloid headline read: 'We saw human guinea pigs explode' (quoted by Stobbart et al., 2007).

Table 5.4 Characteristics of some delivery systems for gene therapy

Vector	Advantages	Disadvantages	Utilisation of system[a]
Liposomes	Virus-free, cheap to produce	Low efficiency, sometimes cytotoxic	6%
DNA cassettes	Virus-free	Low efficiency, expression temporary	18%
Herpes simplex virus type I	Highly infective, persistent expression	No integration with host DNA, cytotoxic, difficult to handle	3%
Adenovirus	Highly infective in epithelia	Immunogenic and transient, requires repeated administration	23%
Adeno-associated virus	Stable	Low capacity	5%
Retrovirus	Efficient, permanent	Low capacity, unstable, must integrate into host DNA, requires dividing cells	22%

[a]The approximate percentage of trials employing this type of delivery system. (After Wolf & Jenkins, 2002; and with data from Wirth et al., 2013.)

The gurus are emphatic that 'the conceptual part of the gene therapy revolution has indeed occurred …' – so where are the therapies? The devil, of course, is in the detail: in this case, the details of:

- *pharmacokinetics*: delivery of the gene to the interior of appropriate target cells (especially those in the CNS);
- *pharmacodynamics*: the controlled expression of the gene in question;
- *safety*;
- *clinical efficacy* and *long-term practicability*.

There is a broad consensus that the *Weismann barrier*[8] should not be breached and so a moratorium has been agreed on making alterations to the DNA of germ cells (which could influence future generations) and gene therapy trials have focused on somatic cells only.

Here we focus first on the main problems and approaches being used to transform gene therapy into useful medicines, and conclude with a final section on the limited success achieved so far.

GENE DELIVERY

The transfer of large sections of recombinant nucleic acid into target cells is critical to the success of gene therapy. In the words of one commentator (Galun, quoted in Bender, 2016), 'Gene therapy is actually three things: delivery, delivery and delivery'. To overcome this first and most fundamental hurdle, techniques borrowed from viruses, which are masters of the sort of molecular hijacking that is required to introduce functional genes into mammalian cells, are often used in gene therapy research. The constructs must pass from the extracellular space across the plasma and nuclear membranes, and be incorporated into the chromosomes. Because DNA is negatively charged and single genes have molecular weights around 10^4 times greater than conventional drugs, the problem is of a different order from the equivalent stage of routine drug development.

There are several important considerations in choosing a gene delivery system; these include:

- the *capacity* of the system (e.g. how much DNA it can carry);
- the *transfection efficiency* (its ability to enter and become utilised by cells);
- the *lifetime* of the transfected material (determined by the lifetime of the targeted cells);
- the *safety issue*, especially important in the case of viral delivery systems.

Various approaches have been developed (Table 5.4) in an attempt to produce the optimal system.

There are two main gene therapy strategies. Using the in vivo technique, the vector containing the therapeutic gene is injected into the patient, either intravenously (in which case some form of organ or tissue targeting is required) or directly into the target tissue (e.g. the retina). When using the ex vivo strategy, cells are removed from the patient (e.g. stem cells from bone marrow or circulating blood, or myoblasts from a biopsy of striated muscle), and treated with the vector in the laboratory. The genetically altered cells are injected back into the patient they came from, thus avoiding any immune rejection (autologous rather than allogenic).

An ideal vector should be *safe*, highly *efficient* (i.e. insert the therapeutic gene into a high proportion of target cells and under control of the appropriate promoter) and *selective* in that it should lead to expression of the therapeutic protein in the target cells but *not* to the expression of other viral proteins. Ideally, and provided that the cell into which it is inserted is itself long-lived, the vector should cause persistent expression, avoiding the need for repeated treatment. The latter consideration can be a problem in some tissues. In the autosomal recessive disorder *cystic fibrosis*, for example, the airway epithelium malfunctions because it lacks a membrane Cl^- transporter known as the *cystic fibrosis transport regulator* (CFTR). Epithelial cells in the airways are continuously dying and being replaced, so even if the unmutated CFTR gene could be stably transfected into the epithelium, there would still be a periodic need for further treatment unless the gene could be inserted into the progenitor (stem) cells. Similar problems are anticipated in other cells that turn over continuously, such as gastrointestinal epithelium and skin.

[8]Named after August Weismann (1834–1914), who formulated the concept that inheritance utilises only germ, and not somatic, cells.

VIRAL VECTORS

Many contemporary gene delivery strategies aim to capitalise on the capacity of viruses to subvert the transcriptional machinery of the cells they infect and their ability (in some cases) to fuse with the host genome. While seemingly simple, there remain substantial practical problems with this *viral vector* approach. As viruses have evolved the means to invade human cells, so humans have evolved immune responses and other protective countermeasures. Although limiting in some respects, this is not all bad news from the point of view of safety. As many of the viruses used for vectors are pathogenic, they are usually modified such that they are 'replication defective' to avoid toxicity.

Retroviruses

▼ If introduced into stem cells, *retroviral vectors* have long-lasting effects because they are incorporated into, and replicate along with, host DNA, and so the 'therapeutic' gene is passed down to each daughter cell during division. Against this, the *retroviral integrase* inserts the construct into chromosomes randomly, so it may cause damage. Also, retroviruses could infect germ or non-target cells and produce undesired effects if administered in vivo. For this reason, retroviruses have been used mainly for ex vivo gene therapy. The life cycle of naturally occurring retroviruses may be exploited to create useful vectors for gene therapy (Fig. 5.3).

Many viruses are equipped to infect specific cell types, though not necessarily the target cell of interest. It is possible to alter the retroviral envelope to alter specificity, such that the vector could be administered systemically but would target only the desired cell population. An example of this approach with a *lentivirus* (a type of retrovirus) is the substitution of the envelope protein of a non-pathogenic vector (e.g. mouse leukaemia virus) with the envelope protein of human vesicular stomatitis virus, to specifically target human epithelial cells.

Most retrovirus vectors are unable to penetrate the nuclear envelope, and because this dissolves during cell division, they only infect dividing cells rather than non-dividing cells (such as adult neurons).

Adenovirus

▼ *Adenovirus vectors* are popular because of the high transgene expression that can be achieved. They transfer genes to the nucleus of the host cell, but (unlike retroviruses) these are not inserted into the host genome and so do not produce effects that outlast the lifetime of the transfected cell. This property also obviates the risk of disturbing the function of other cellular genes and the theoretical risks of carcinogenicity and germ cell transfection. Because of these favourable properties, adenovirus vectors have been used for in vivo gene therapy. Engineered deletions in the viral genome render it unable to replicate or cause widespread infection in the host while at the same time creating space in the viral genome for the therapeutic transgene to be inserted.

One of the first adenoviral vectors lacked part of a growth-controlling region called E_1, while incorporating the desired transgene. This vector gave excellent results, demonstrating gene transfer to cell lines and animal models of disease, but it proved disappointing as a treatment for cystic fibrosis in human trials. Low doses (administered by aerosol to patients with this disease) produced only a very low-efficiency transfer, whereas higher doses caused inflammation, a host immune response and short-lived gene expression. Furthermore, treatment

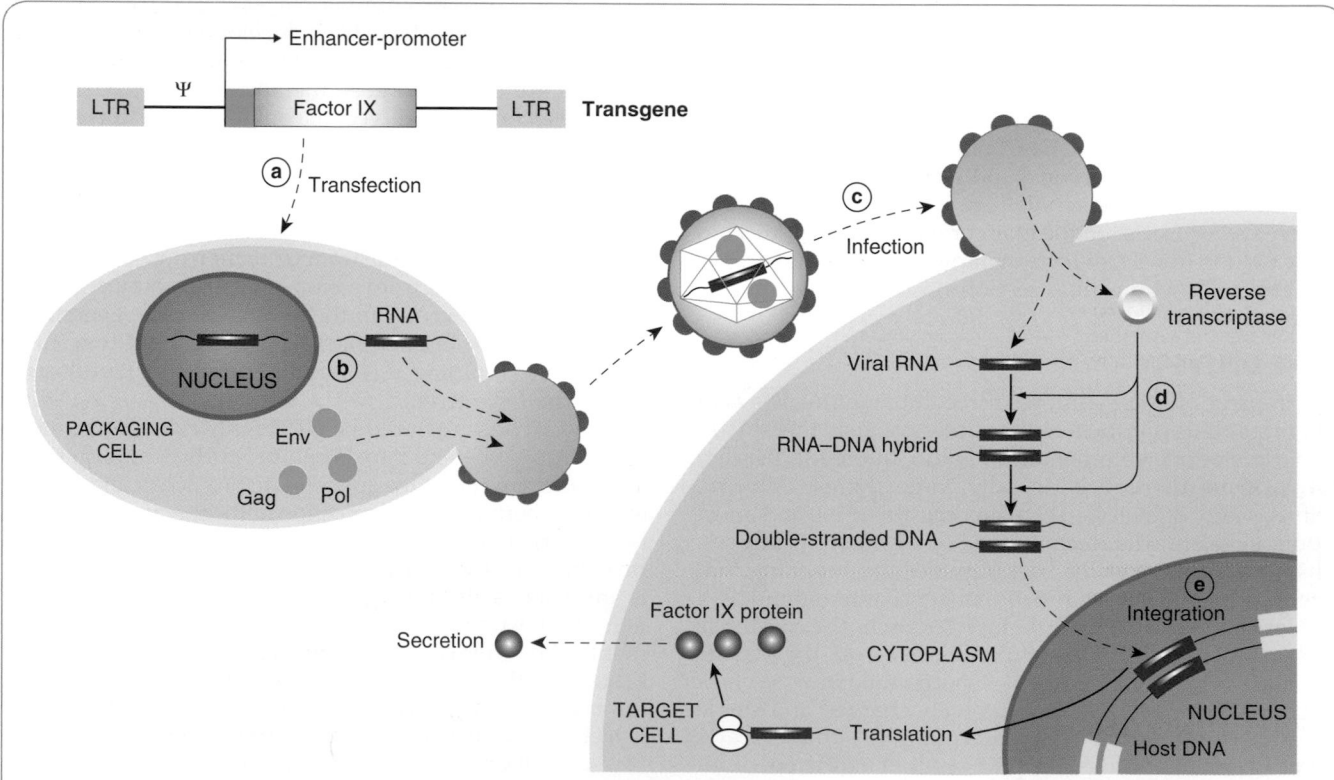

Fig. 5.3 Strategy for making retroviral vectors. The transgene (the example shows the gene for factor IX) in a vector backbone is introduced *(a)* into a packaging cell, where it is integrated into a chromosome in the nucleus, and *(b)* transcribed to make vector mRNA, which is packaged into the retroviral vector and shed from the packaging cell. It then infects the target cell *(c)*. Virally encoded reverse transcriptase *(d)* converts vector RNA into an RNA–DNA hybrid, and then into double-stranded DNA, which is integrated *(e)* into the genome of the target cell. It can then be transcribed and translated to make (in this case) factor IX protein. 'Env', Gag' and 'Pol' represent components of the retroviral vector. *LTR*, long terminal repeat. (Redrawn from Verma & Somia, 1997.)

could not be repeated because of the appearance, in the circulation, of neutralising antibodies. This has led to attempts to manipulate adenoviral vectors to mutate or remove the genes that are most strongly immunogenic.

Other viral vectors

▼ Other potential viral vectors under investigation include *adeno-associated virus*, *herpes virus* and disabled versions of *human immuno-deficiency virus* (HIV). Adeno-associated virus associates with host DNA but is not activated unless the cell is infected with an adenovirus. It is less immunogenic than other vectors but is difficult to mass produce and cannot be used to carry large transgenes. Herpes virus does not associate with host DNA but is very long lived in nervous tissue (so could have a specific application in treating neurological disease). HIV, unlike most other retroviruses, can infect non-dividing cells such as neurons. It is possible to remove the genes from HIV that control replication and substitute other genes. Alternatively, it may prove possible to transfer to other non-pathogenic retroviruses those genes that permit HIV to penetrate the nuclear envelope.

NON-VIRAL VECTORS

To reduce the problems associated with viral vectors, a variety of other substances have been used to deliver genes and other material. These are often collectively known as *nanocarriers*. The list includes the following (but see also Xu et al., 2014):

Liposomes

▼ Non-viral vectors include a variant of liposomes (Ch. 9). Plasmids (diameter up to approximately 2 μm) are too big to package in regular liposomes (diameter 0.025–0.1 μm), but larger particles can be made from positively charged lipids ('lipoplexes'), which interact with both negatively charged cell membranes and DNA, improving delivery into the cell nucleus and incorporation into the host chromosome. Such particles have been used to deliver the genes for HLA-B7, interleukin-2 and CFTR. They are much less efficient than viruses, and attempts are currently under way to improve this by incorporating various viral signal proteins (membrane fusion proteins, for example) in their outer coat. Direct injection of these complexes into solid tumours (e.g. melanoma, breast, kidney and colon cancers) can, however, achieve high local concentrations within the tumour.

Microspheres

▼ Biodegradable microspheres made from polyanhydride co-polymers of fumaric and sebacic acids (see Ch. 9) can be loaded with plasmid DNA. A plasmid with bacterial β-galactosidase activity formulated in this way and given by mouth to rats has resulted in systemic absorption and expression of the bacterial enzyme in the rat liver, raising the possibility of oral gene therapy.

Plasmid DNA

▼ Surprisingly, plasmid DNA itself ('naked DNA') enters the nucleus of some cells and is expressed, albeit much less efficiently than when it is packaged in a vector. Such DNA carries no risk of viral replication and is not usually immunogenic, but it cannot be targeted precisely. There is considerable interest in the possibility of using naked DNA for vaccines, which has several theoretical advantages and numerous trials are using the technique (Liu, 2011).

CONTROLLING GENE EXPRESSION

To realise the full potential of gene therapy, it is not enough to transfer the gene selectively to the desired target cells and maintain acceptable expression of its product – difficult though these goals are. It is also essential that the activity of the gene is controlled. Historically, it was the realisation of the magnitude of this task that diverted attention from the haemoglobinopathies (which were the first projected targets of gene therapy). Correction of these disorders demands an appropriate balance of normal α- and β-globin chain synthesis to be effective, and for this, and many other potential applications, precisely controlled gene expression is essential.

▼ It has not yet proved possible to control transgenes precisely in human recipients, but there are techniques that may eventually enable us to achieve this goal. One hinges on the use of an inducible expression system. This is a fairly standard laboratory technique whereby the inserted gene also includes a **doxycycline**-inducible promoter such that expression of the gene can be switched on or off by treatment with, or withdrawal of, doxycycline.

The control of transfected genes is important in gene targeting as well. By splicing the gene of interest with a tissue-specific promoter, it should be possible to restrict expression of the gene to the target tissue. Such an approach has been used in the design of gene therapy constructs for use in ovarian cancer, the cells of which express several proteins at high abundance, including the proteinase inhibitor SLP1. In combination with the SLP1 promoter, plasmids carrying various genes were successfully and selectively expressed in ovarian cancer cell lines (Wolf & Jenkins, 2002).

SAFETY AND SOCIETAL ISSUES

Experiments or protocols involving the transfer of genetic material tend to provoke deep unease in some sectors of society – witness the genetically modified (GM) crop debate (and see Freier et al., 2014). Partly, this may be traced to ignorance or prejudice but it is nevertheless a problem that can hinder the introduction of new agents. Societal issues aside, the technique does raise a number of specific concerns that generally relate to the use of viral vectors. These are usually selected because they are non-pathogenic, or modified to render them innocuous, but there is a concern that such agents might still acquire virulence during use. Retroviruses, which insert randomly into host DNA, could damage the genome and interfere with the protective mechanisms that normally regulate the cell cycle (see Ch. 6), and if they happen to disrupt essential cellular functions, this could increase the risk of malignancy.[9]

Another problem is that immunogenic viral proteins may elicit an inflammatory response, and this could be harmful in some situations (e.g. in the airways of patients with cystic fibrosis). Initial clinical experience was reassuring, but the death of Jesse Gelsinger, an 18-year-old volunteer in a gene therapy trial for the non-fatal disease *ornithine decarboxylase deficiency* (which can be controlled, albeit tediously, by diet and drugs anyway), led to the appreciation that safety concerns related to immune-mediated responses to vectors are very real (see Marshall, 1999).

THERAPEUTIC APPLICATIONS

Despite the plethora of technical problems and safety concerns, there have been some encouraging successes and interest – and confidence – in the area is still very strong with some 3000 new publications appearing each year.

---

[9]This risk is more than a theoretical possibility; several children treated for *severe combined immunodeficiency* (SCID) with a retrovirus vector developed a leukaemia-like illness (Woods et al., 2006). The retroviral vector was shown to have inserted itself into a gene called *LMO-2*, mutations of which are associated with childhood cancers.

Gene delivery and expression

- Gene delivery is the main hurdle to practical gene therapy.
- Recombinant genes are transferred using a *vector*, often a suitably modified virus.
- There are two main strategies for delivering genes into patients:
  - *in vivo* injection of the vector directly into the patient (e.g. into a malignant tumour);
  - *ex vivo* treatment of cells from the patient (e.g. stem cells from marrow or circulating blood), which are then returned to the patient.
- An ideal vector should be safe, efficient, selective and produce long-lasting expression of the therapeutic gene.
- Viral vectors include retroviruses, adenoviruses, adeno-associated virus, herpesvirus and disabled HIV:
  - *Retroviruses* infect many different types of dividing cells and become incorporated randomly into host DNA.
  - *Adenoviruses* are genetically modified to prevent replication and accommodate the therapeutic transgene. They transfer genes to the nucleus but not to the genome of the host cell. Problems include a strong host immune response, inflammation and short-lived expression. Treatment can be compromised by neutralising antibodies.
  - *Adeno-associated virus* associates with host DNA and is non-immunogenic but is hard to mass produce and has a small capacity.
  - Herpesvirus does not associate with host DNA but persists in nervous tissue and may be useful in treating neurological disease.
  - Disabled versions of HIV differ from most other retroviruses in that they infect non-dividing cells, including neurons.
- Non-viral vectors include:
  - a variant of liposomes, made using positively charged lipids and called 'lipoplexes';
  - biodegradable microspheres, which may offer orally active gene therapy;
  - plasmid DNA ('naked DNA'), which can be used as a vaccine.
- A *tetracycline-inducible expression system* or similar technique can control the activity of the therapeutic gene.

According to a recent reviewer (Tani, 2016) 2210 gene therapy trials had been approved by regulatory agencies around the world by 2015, with six gene therapies already approved by a limited number of countries. The first was **Gendicine**, a treatment for replacing the faulty p53 protein causing head and neck cancer, which was licensed in China in 2003. The European Medicines Agency granted its first license for a gene therapy product, **Glybera,** in 2012[10]. This is an adeno-associated virus construct that delivers a correct copy of lipoprotein lipase to patients lacking this enzyme (a very rare disorder that causes severe pancreatitis) and in 2016, **Strimvelis** was also approved in Europe. This is an ex vivo gene therapy approach to replace adenosine deaminase which is absent in children with a rare (~15 patients per year in Europe) type of SCID. At the time of writing, no gene therapy-based therapeutics had been approved in the United States although intense interest continues.

Recently, a system of gene editing originally discovered in bacteria is promising to transform gene therapy (garnering nearly 7000 publications over the last few years). This bears the rather complex name of *Clustered Regulatory Interspersed Short Palindromic Repeats (CRISPR)* and can target nucleases (notably *Cas9*) to precisely edit genes of interest. Viruses can deliver the CRISPR-Cas9 components, thereby acting as delivery vehicles for the biochemical machinery required to repair faulty genes in humans (see for example, Gori et al., 2015; Gee et al., 2017). To date, no successful gene therapy using CRISPR-Cas9 has been approved for therapeutic use, but several human trials are underway[11], and are very close to getting this therapy into the clinic.

▼ Target diseases eliciting interest from companies specialising in gene therapy applications include:

Single-Gene Defects

Single-gene (*monogenic*), often rare, disorders, were the obvious starting point for gene therapy trials and haemoglobinopathies were the first projected targets, but early attempts (in the 1980s) were put 'on hold' because of the problem (mentioned previously) of controlling precisely the expression of the genes encoding the different polypeptide chains of the haemoglobin molecule. Recent trials have proved encouraging in the treatment of thalassaemia (the commonest monogenic disease) and sickle cell disease (see Rai & Malik, 2016) although no products have yet been approved.

Another early target was cystic fibrosis, but progress here has been disappointing (see Kim et al., 2016 for details) largely because of the biological barriers that must be penetrated. There have been other successes though. For example, *X-linked chronic granulomatous disease* has been successfully treated using a retroviral technique to deliver a functional version of the mutated NADPH oxidase protein (Ott et al., 2006 and Fig. 5.4) and a form of inherited blindness, *Leber's congenital amaurosis*, associated with a mutation in a gene that produces retinal pigment, has been rectified using an adeno-associated virus vector bearing a cDNA coding for the intact gene (Maguire et al., 2009). Several other ocular conditions also seem to be promising candidates for gene therapy approaches (see Borras, 2017; Boye et al., 2013). Williams and Thrasher (2014) have reviewed the general

---

[10]With an annual cost of at least US$1 million per treatment, Glybera has been called the most expensive medicine in the world. No wonder that only one patient has been treated so far! (see Regolado, 2016)

[11]Allogenic transplants in childhood leukaemias, autologous immune cell PD-1 knock-out in lung cancer patients, and OCT4's role in human embryo development are all recent examples of breakthroughs using CRISPR-Cas9 in human cells.

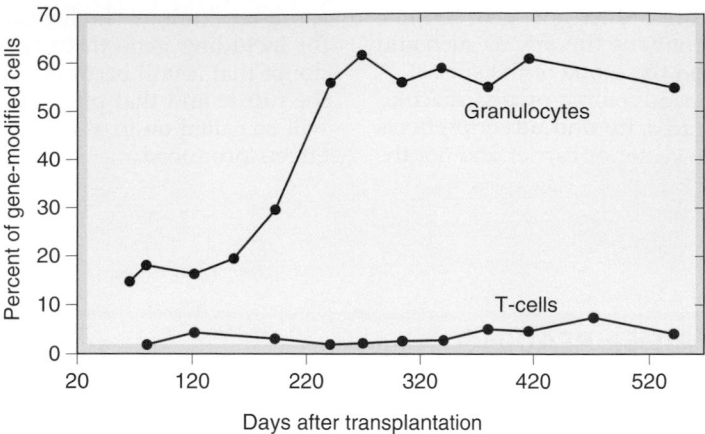

Fig. 5.4 Correcting an inherited defect using gene therapy. In this clinical trial, two patients with X-linked chronic granulomatous disease were transfused with GM–CSF (Granulocyte-Macrophage Colony Stimulating Factor)-treated peripheral blood cells that had been genetically modified with a retroviral vector bearing the intact *gp91phox* gene ('in vitro protocol' – see text). The graph shows that the number of gene-modified peripheral blood leukocytes remained high for well over a year and this was accompanied by good levels of superoxide production in these cells – a clinical 'cure'. (Data redrawn from Ott et al., 2006.)

Safety issues for gene therapy

- There are those safety concerns that are specific to any particular therapy (e.g. polycythaemia from overexpression of **erythropoietin**) and also additional general concerns relating, for example, to the nature of the vectors used.
- Viral vectors:
  - might acquire virulence during use
  - contain viral proteins, which may be immunogenic
  - can elicit an inflammatory response
  - could damage the host genome and interfere with the cell cycle, provoking malignancy.
- The limited clinical experience to date has not so far provided evidence of insurmountable problems.

problems associated with gene therapy in the treatment of monogenic immunodeficiency diseases.

Cancer

Gene therapy for cancer and related diseases currently comprise almost 70% of gene therapy trials. Several therapeutic approaches (see Barar & Omidi, 2012) are under investigation, including:

- restoring 'protective' proteins, such as the tumour suppressor gene (see Ch. 6);
- inactivating oncogene expression (e.g. by using a retroviral vector bearing an antisense transcript RNA to the K-Ras oncogene);
- delivering a gene to malignant cells that renders them sensitive to cytotoxic drugs (e.g. thymidylate kinase, which activates **ganciclovir**) – the so-called 'suicide gene' approach;
- delivery of proteins to healthy host cells, which, for example, renders them resistant to chemotherapy (e.g. addition of the multidrug resistance channel to bone marrow cells ex vivo);

- tagging cancer cells with genes expressing proteins that render malignant cells more visible to the immune system (e.g. for antigens such as HLA-B7 or cytokines such as granulocyte-macrophage colony-stimulating factor and interleukin-2).
- Recent progress in research in some of these areas has been reviewed by Gilham et al. (2015).

Gene Therapy and Infectious Disease

In addition to DNA vaccines mentioned previously, there is considerable interest in the potential of gene therapy for HIV and other viral infections. The aim is to render stem cells (which differentiate into immune cells) resistant to HIV before they mature. For an account of the strategies under investigation, see Chung et al. (2013).

Gene Therapy and Cardiovascular Disease

Gene therapy trials for treating cardiovascular diseases are reviewed by Bradshaw and Baker (2013). Vascular gene transfer is attractive not least because cardiologists and vascular surgeons routinely perform invasive studies that offer the opportunity to administer gene therapy vectors ex vivo (e.g. to a blood vessel that has been removed to use as an autograft) or locally in vivo (e.g. by injection through a catheter directly into a diseased coronary or femoral artery). The nature of many vascular disorders, such as restenosis following angioplasty (stretching a narrowed artery using a balloon that can be inflated via a catheter), is such that transient gene expression might be all that is required therapeutically. Extension of vein graft patency by gene therapy approaches has been reviewed by Chandiwal et al. (2005). This seems to be a promising area (see Hammond & McKirnan, 2001; Ghosh et al., 2008) although Hammer and Steiner (2013) concluded that most trials had proved disappointing.

CONCLUDING REMARKS

Whilst protein and oligonucleotide biopharmaceuticals share some of the characteristics of other drugs described in this book, the same cannot be said for gene therapy. Is a gene a drug? Is a virus a drug? You could argue that it satisfies the broad definition that we posited in on page 1 of this book in that 'administration to a living organism produces a biological effect', but it does not seem sensible to discuss the pharmacology of gene therapy as such and most would consider it beyond the scope of the subject. A gene has no inherent pharmacodynamic or pharmacokinetic properties, most of the toxicity and adverse effects mentioned here are due to the vector or carrier and not the gene itself. And how do you assess the dose of a 'drug' that is self-replicating? Having said that, we make no apologies for including gene therapy in this section. There is little doubt that it will become a major therapeutic modality in the future and that physicians and pharmacologists alike will be called on to assess and comment on the biological effects produced.

REFERENCES AND FURTHER READING

General reviews on biopharmaceuticals, gene therapy and utilities

Agoram, B.M., 2009. Use of pharmacokinetic/ pharmacodynamic modelling for starting dose selection in first-in-human trials of high-risk biologics. Br. J. Clin. Pharmacol. 67, 153–160. (*Interesting review of the PK problems of biopharmaceuticals*)

Bender, E., 2016. Gene therapy: Industrial strength. Nature 537, S57–S59. (*Short commentary on recent progress*)

Brink, M.F., Bishop, M.D., Pieper, F.R., 2000. Developing efficient strategies for the generation of transgenic cattle which produce biopharmaceuticals in milk. Theriogenology 53, 139–148. (*A bit specialised, as it focuses mainly on the husbandry of transgenic cattle, but interesting nonetheless*)

Castanatto, D., Rossi, J.J., 2009. The promises and pitfalls of RNA-interference-based therapeutics. Nature 457, 426–433. (*Useful review of the mechanism, current status and potential applications of RNAi as a means of controlling gene expression*)

Guttmacher, A.E., Collins, F.S., 2002. Genomic medicine: a primer. N. Engl. J. Med. 347, 1512–1520. (*First in a series on genomic medicine*)

Kwon, K.C., Verma, D., Singh, N.D., Herzog, R., Daniell, H., 2013. Oral delivery of human biopharmaceuticals, autoantigens and vaccine antigens bioencapsulated in plant cells. Adv. Drug Deliv. Rev. 65, 782–799. (*The title is self-explanatory*)

Liu, M.A., 2011. DNA vaccines: an historical perspective and view to the future. Immunol. Rev. 239, 62–84.

Melnik, S., Stoger, E., 2013. Green factories for biopharmaceuticals. Curr. Med. Chem. 20, 1038–1046. (*Another paper on the use of plants to produce biologics*)

Rader, R.A., 2008. (Re)defining biopharmaceutical. Nat. Biotechnol. 26, 743–751. (*Short commentary dealing with the vexed problem of defining what biopharmaceuticals are*)

Regolado, A., 2016. The world's most expensive medicine is a bust. MIT Technology Review. May issue.

Revers, L., Furczon, E., 2010. An introduction to biologics and biosimilars. Part II: Subsequent entry biologics: biosame or biodifferent? Can. Pharm. J. 143, 184–191. (*Useful review on regulatory issues surrounding the introduction of follow-on biopharmaceuticals*)

Tani, K., 2016. Current status of ex vivo gene therapy for hematological disorders: a review of clinical trials in Japan around the world. Int. J. Hematol. 104, 42–72.

Verma, I.M., Somia, N., 1997. Gene therapy – promises, problems and prospects. Nature 389, 239–242. (*The authors, from the Salk Institute, describe the principle of inserting corrective genetic material into cells to alleviate disease, the practical obstacles to this and the hopes that better delivery systems will overcome them*)

Walsh, G., 2004. Second-generation biopharmaceuticals. Eur. J. Pharm. Biopharm. 58, 185–196. (*Excellent overview of therapeutic proteins and antibodies; some good tables and figures*)

Wirth, T., Parker, N., Yla-Herttuala, S., 2013. History of gene therapy. Gene 525, 162–169. (*An excellent review of the area from its very beginnings. Highly recommended*)

Xu, H., Li, Z., Si, J., 2014. Nanocarriers in gene therapy: a review. J. Biomed. Nanotechnol. 10, 3483–3507.

Zhao, L., Ren, T.H., Wang, D.D., 2012. Clinical pharmacology considerations in biologics development. Acta Pharmacol. Sin. 33, 1339–1347. (*Review article stressing the differences between conventional drugs and biopharmaceuticals. Good place to start reading*)

Problems

Check, E., 2002. A tragic setback. Nature 420, 116–118. (*News feature describing efforts to explain the mechanism underlying a leukaemia-like illness in a child previously cured of SCID by gene therapy*)

Freire, J.E., Medeiros, S.C., Lopes Neto, A.V., et al., 2014. Bioethical conflicts of gene therapy: a brief critical review. Rev. Assoc. Med. Bras. (1992) 60, 520–524. (*The title is self-explanatory. Easy to read*)

Kim, N., Duncan, G.A., Hanes, J., Suk, J.S., 2016. Barriers to inhaled gene therapy of obstructive lung diseases: A review. J. Control. Release 240, 465–488. (*Describes the rather disappointing results obtained in the cystic fibrosis trials. See also Pickett et al., 2013 below*)

Hammer, A., Steiner, S., 2013. Gene therapy for therapeutic angiogenesis in peripheral arterial disease - a systematic review and meta-analysis of randomized, controlled trials. Vasa 42, 331–339.

Marshall, E., 1999. Gene therapy death prompts review of adenovirus vector. Science 286, 2244–2245. (*Deals with the tragic 'Gelsinger affair'*)

Muller, P.Y., Brennan, F.R., 2009. Safety assessment and dose selection for first-in-human clinical trials with immunomodulatory monoclonal antibodies. Clin. Pharmacol. Ther. 85, 247–258. (*A sober and, at times, rather technical assessment of the safety procedures required for the 'first-in-man' testing of therapeutic monoclonals. Written in the wake of the TGN 1412 affair*)

Richter, W.F., Gallati, H., Schiller, C.D., 1999. Animal pharmacokinetics of the tumor necrosis factor receptor-immunoglobulin fusion protein lenercept and their extrapolation to humans. Drug Metab. Dispos. 27, 21–25.

Stobbart, L., Murtagh, M.J., Rapley, T., et al., 2007. We saw human guinea pigs explode. BMJ 334, 566–567. (*Analysis of the, often grotesque, press coverage of the above clinical trial*)

Woods, N.B., Bottero, V., Schmidt, M., von Kalle, C., Verma, I.M., 2006. Gene therapy: therapeutic gene causing lymphoma. Nature 440, 1123.

Williams, D.A., Thrasher, A.J., 2014. Concise review: lessons learned from clinical trials of gene therapy in monogenic immunodeficiency diseases. Stem Cells Transl. Med. 3, 636–642.

Therapeutic uses

Barar, J., Omidi, Y., 2012. Translational approaches towards cancer gene therapy: hurdles and hopes. Bioimpacts 2, 127–143.

Borras, T., 2017. The pathway from genes to gene therapy in glaucoma: a review of possibilities for using genes as glaucoma drugs. Asia Pac. J. Ophthalmol. (Phila.) 6, 80–93.

Boye, S.E., Boye, S.L., Lewin, A.S., Hauswirth, W.W., 2013. A comprehensive review of retinal gene therapy. Mol. Ther. 21, 509–519.

Bradshaw, A.C., Baker, A.H., 2013. Gene therapy for cardiovascular disease: perspectives and potential. Vasc. Pharm. 58, 174–181.

Chandiwal, A., Balasubramanian, V., Baldwin, Z.K., Conte, M.S., Schwartz, L.B., 2005. Gene therapy for the extension of vein graft patency: a review. Vasc. Endovasc. Surg. 39, 1–14.

Chung, J., DiGiusto, D.L., Rossi, J.J., 2013. Combinatorial RNA-based gene therapy for the treatment of HIV/AIDS. Expert Opin. Biol. Ther. 13 (3), 437–445. (*Review on prophylactic gene therapy approaches for HIV*)

Gee, P., Xu, H., Hotta, A., 2017. Cellular reprogramming, genome editing, and alternative CRISPR Cas9 technologies for precise gene therapy of Duchenne muscular dystrophy. Stem Cells Int. 2017, 8765154. (*A rather technical paper but gives a good idea of the power of the technique*)

Geary, R.S., Baker, B.F., Crooke, S.T., 2015. Clinical and preclinical pharmacokinetics and pharmacodynamics of mipomersen (Kynamro®): a second-generation antisense oligonucleotide inhibitor of apolipoprotein B. Clin. Pharmacokinet. 54, 133 146.

Ghosh, R., Walsh, S.R., Tang, T.Y., Noorani, A., Hayes, P.D., 2008. Gene therapy as a novel therapeutic option in the treatment of peripheral vascular disease: systematic review and meta-analysis. Int. J. Clin. Pract. 62, 1383–1390.

Gori, J.L., Hsu, P.D., Maeder, M.L., Shen, S., Welstead, G.G., Bumcrot, D., 2015. Delivery and specificity of CRISPR-Cas9 genome editing technologies for human gene therapy. Hum. Gene Ther. 26, 443–451.

Hammond, H.K., McKirnan, M.D., 2001. Angiogenic gene therapy for heart disease: a review of animal studies and clinical trials. Cardiovasc. Res. 49, 561–567. (*Comprehensive review spanning animal and human trials of gene therapy for myocardial ischaemia*)

Maguire, A.M., High, K.A., Auricchio, A., et al., 2009. Age-dependent effects of RPE65 gene therapy for Leber's congenital amaurosis: a phase 1 dose-escalation trial. Lancet 374, 1597–1605.

Nathwani, A.C., Davidoff, A.M., Linch, D.C., 2005. A review of gene therapy for haematological disorders. Br. J. Haematol. 128, 3–17. (*The title is self-explanantory; easy to read and comprehensive in scope*)

Ott, M.G., Schmidt, M., Schwarzwaelder, K., et al., 2006. Correction of X-linked chronic granulomatous disease by gene therapy, augmented by insertional activation of MDS1-EVI1, PRDM16 or SETBP1. Nat. Med. 12, 401–409. (*Clinical trial of gene therapy to correct hereditary neutrophil dysfunction*)

Rai, P., Malik, P., 2016. Gene therapy for hemoglobin disorders - a mini-review. J. Rare Dis. Res. Treat. 1, 25–31.

Prickett, M., Jain, M., 2013. Gene therapy in cystic fibrosis. Transl. Res. 161, 255–264. (*Cystic fibrosis was one of the first monogenic disorders identified as a candidate for gene therapy. This review explains how and why things haven't quite worked out the way it was hoped. See also Kim et al., 2016, above*)

Wolf, J.K., Jenkins, A.D., 2002. Gene therapy for ovarian cancer (review). Int. J. Oncol. 21, 461–468. (*Excellent review and broad introduction to gene therapy in general*)

6 Cell proliferation, apoptosis, repair and regeneration

OVERVIEW

About 10 billion new cells are created daily in US through cell division and this must be counterbalanced by the elimination of a similar number from the body in an ordered manner. This chapter explains how this homeostasis is managed. We deal with the life and death of the cell – the processes of replication, proliferation, apoptosis, repair and regeneration and how these relate to the actions of drugs. We begin with cell replication. We explain how stimulation by growth factors causes cells to divide and then consider the interaction of these cells with the extracellular matrix (ECM) which regulates further cell proliferation. We describe the crucial phenomenon of apoptosis (the programmed series of events that lead to cell death), outlining the changes that occur in a cell that is preparing to die and the intracellular pathways that culminate in its demise. We explain how these processes relate to the repair of damaged tissue, to the possibility of its regeneration and whether there is scope for modulating this with novel drugs.

CELL PROLIFERATION

Cell proliferation is, of course, a fundamental biological event. It is integral to many physiological and pathological processes including growth, healing, repair, hypertrophy, hyperplasia and the development of tumours. Because cells need oxygen and nutrients to survive, *angiogenesis* (the development of new blood vessels) necessarily accompanies many of these processes.

Proliferating cells go through what is termed *the cell cycle*, during which they replicate all their components and then divide into two identical daughter cells.[1] The process is tightly regulated by signalling pathways, including receptor tyrosine kinases or receptor-linked kinases and the mitogen-activated protein kinase (MAP kinase) cascade (see Ch. 3). In all cases, the pathways eventually lead to transcription of the genes that control the cell cycle.

THE CELL CYCLE

In the adult, few cells divide repeatedly and most remain in a quiescent phase outside the cycle in the phase termed G_0 (Fig. 6.1). Some cells such as neurons and skeletal muscle cells spend all their lifetime in G_0 whereas others being more stem cell–like in phenotype, including bone marrow

cells and the epithelium of the gastrointestinal tract, divide daily.

The cell cycle is an ordered sequential series of phases (see Fig. 6.1). These are known as S (Synthesis), M (Mitosis) and G (Gap between S or M phases), and they always occur in this order:

- G_1: (Gap1) preparation for DNA synthesis
- S: (Synthesis) DNA synthesis and chromosome duplication of the parental cell
- G_2: (Gap2) preparation for division
- M: (Mitosis) division into two identical daughter cells.

In cells that are dividing continuously, G_1, S and G_2 comprise *interphase* – the phase between one mitosis and the next.

Cell division requires the controlled timing of the critical S phase and M phases. Entry into each of these phases is tightly regulated at *check points* (restriction points) at the start of the S and M phases. Any DNA damage stops the cycle at one or other of these check points to allow repair and thus maintain the integrity of our DNA sequence in each cell. This process is critical for the maintenance of genetic stability. Failure of the check points to stop the cycle when it is appropriate to do so leads to genetic instability, which is a hallmark of cancer.[2]

Quiescent (G_0) cells enter G_1 after exposure to chemical mediators, some of which are associated with damage. For example, a wound can stimulate a quiescent skin cell to divide, thus repairing the lesion. The impetus for a cell to enter the cycle (i.e. to move from G_0 into G_1) may be *growth factors* acting on *growth factor receptors*, though the action of other types of ligands on G protein–coupled receptors (see Ch. 3) can also initiate the process.

Growth factors stimulate the synthesis of both positive regulators of the cell cycle that control the changes necessary for cell division and negative regulators that counterbalance the positive regulators. The maintenance of normal cell numbers in tissues and organs requires a balance between the positive and the negative regulatory signals. *Apoptosis*[3] also controls cell numbers.

POSITIVE REGULATORS OF THE CELL CYCLE

The cycle begins when a growth factor acts on a quiescent cell, provoking it to divide. Growth factors stimulate

---

[1]Not strictly identical in the case of stem cells, as one differentiates and the other remains stem.

[2]The main daily job of our immune system is to detect and destroy cells which have genetic instability, which may become cancerous if missed. This immuno-surveillance gets rid of thousands of incorrectly divided or dangerously damaged cells each day. Occasionally, our immune system will encounter a foreign body such as a virus or bacteria, and will then 'moonlight' on that job for a while too.

[3]The term is originally a Greek word that describes the falling of leaves or petals from plants. Termed in 1972 by Professor James Cormack of Aberdeen University's Greek Department, the second 'p' is silent – APE oh TOE sis.

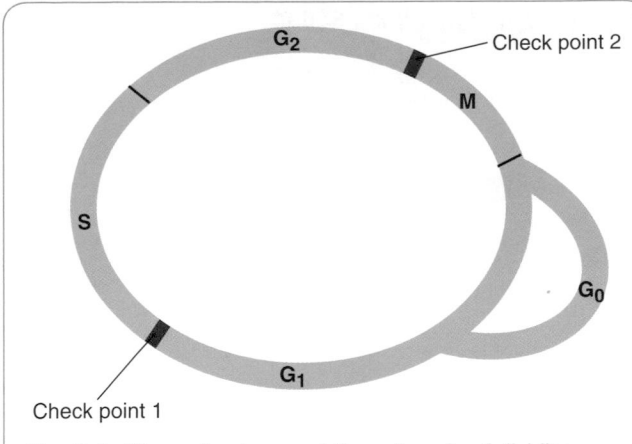

Fig. 6.1 The main phases of the cell cycle of dividing cells.

Fig. 6.2 Schematic representation of the activation of a cyclin-dependent kinase (cdk). (A) An inactive cdk. (B) The inactive cdk binds to a cyclin and is activated; it can now phosphorylate a specific protein substrate (e.g. an enzyme). (C) After the phosphorylating event, the cyclin is degraded.

production of two families of proteins, namely *cyclins* and serine/threonine protein kinases called *cyclin-dependent kinases* (cdks), coded for by the *delayed response* genes. The cdks sequentially phosphorylate various enzymes – activating some and inhibiting others – to coordinate the progression of the cell through the cycle.

Each cdk is inactive and must bind to a cyclin partner, before it can phosphorylate its target protein(s). After the phosphorylation event the cyclin is degraded (Fig. 6.2) by the *ubiquitin/protease system*. Here, several enzymes sequentially add small molecules of ubiquitin to the cyclin. The resulting ubiquitin polymer acts as an 'address label' that directs the cyclin to the *proteasome* where it is degraded.

There are eight main groups of cyclins. According to the 'classical model' of the cell cycle (see Satyanarayana & Kaldis, 2009), those of principal importance in the control of the cycle are cyclins A, B, D and E. Each cyclin is associated with, and activates, a particular cdk. Cyclin A activates cdks 1 and 2; cyclin B, cdk 1; cyclin D, cdks 4 and 6; and cyclin E, cdk 2. Precise timing of each step is essential and many cycle proteins are degraded after they have carried out their functions.[4]

The actions of the cyclin/cdk complexes throughout the cell cycle are depicted in Fig. 6.3.

The activity of these cyclin/cdk complexes is negatively modulated at one or other of the two check points. In quiescent G_0 cells, cyclin D is present in low concentration, and an important regulatory protein – the *Rb protein*[5] is hypophosphorylated. This restrains the cell cycle at check point 1 by inhibiting the expression of several proteins critical for further cycle progression. The Rb protein accomplishes this restraint by binding to transcription factors and preventing them from promoting expression of the genes that code for proteins needed for DNA replication during S phase (such as cyclins E and A, DNA polymerase, thymidine kinase and dihydrofolate reductase). This configuration is maintained until a cell is instructed to divide.

- Growth factor action on a cell in G_0 propels it into G_1, which prepares the cell for S phase. The concentration of cyclin D increases and the cyclin D/cdk complex phosphorylates and activates the proteins required for DNA replication.
- In mid-G_1, the cyclin D/cdk complex phosphorylates the Rb protein, releasing a transcription factor that activates the genes for the components essential for the next phase – DNA synthesis. The action of the cyclin E/cdk complex is necessary for transition from G_1, past check point 1, into S phase.
- Once into S phase, the processes that have been set in motion cannot be reversed and the cell is committed to DNA replication and mitosis. Cyclin E/cdk and cyclin A/cdk regulate progress through S phase, phosphorylating and thus activating the proteins/enzymes involved in DNA synthesis.
- In G_2 phase, the cell, which now has double the number of chromosomes, produces the messenger RNAs and proteins needed to duplicate all other cellular components for allocation to the two daughter cells.
- Cyclin A/cdk and cyclin B/cdk complexes are active during G_2 phase and are necessary for entry into M phase, i.e. for passing check point 2. The presence of cyclin B/cdk complexes in the nucleus is required for mitosis to commence.

Mitosis occurs in four stages:

- *Prophase*. The duplicated chromosomes (which are at this point a tangled mass in the nucleus) condense, each now consisting of two *daughter chromatids* (the original chromosome and an identical copy). These are released into the cytoplasm as the nuclear membrane disintegrates.
- *Metaphase*. The chromosomes are aligned at the equator of the cell (see Fig. 6.3).
- *Anaphase*. A specialised cytoskeletal device, the mitotic apparatus, captures the chromosomes and draws them to opposite poles of the dividing cell (see Fig. 6.3).
- *Telophase*. A nuclear membrane forms round each set of chromosomes. Finally, the cytoplasm divides between the two forming daughter cells. The last step in mitosis is *cytokinesis*, where the plasma membrane between each daughter cell is pinched-off and split.[6]

---

[4]This sequencing ensures that cells cycle in one direction only, i.e. there's no point dividing before you made two identical copies of your chromosome set. That would be asking for trouble, and disease.

[5]So named because mutations of the *Rb* gene are associated with retinoblastoma tumours.
[6]IPMATC – the whole cell cycle processes and order are summed up in this acronym for Interphase, Prophase, Metaphase, Anaphase, Telophase and Cytokinesis.

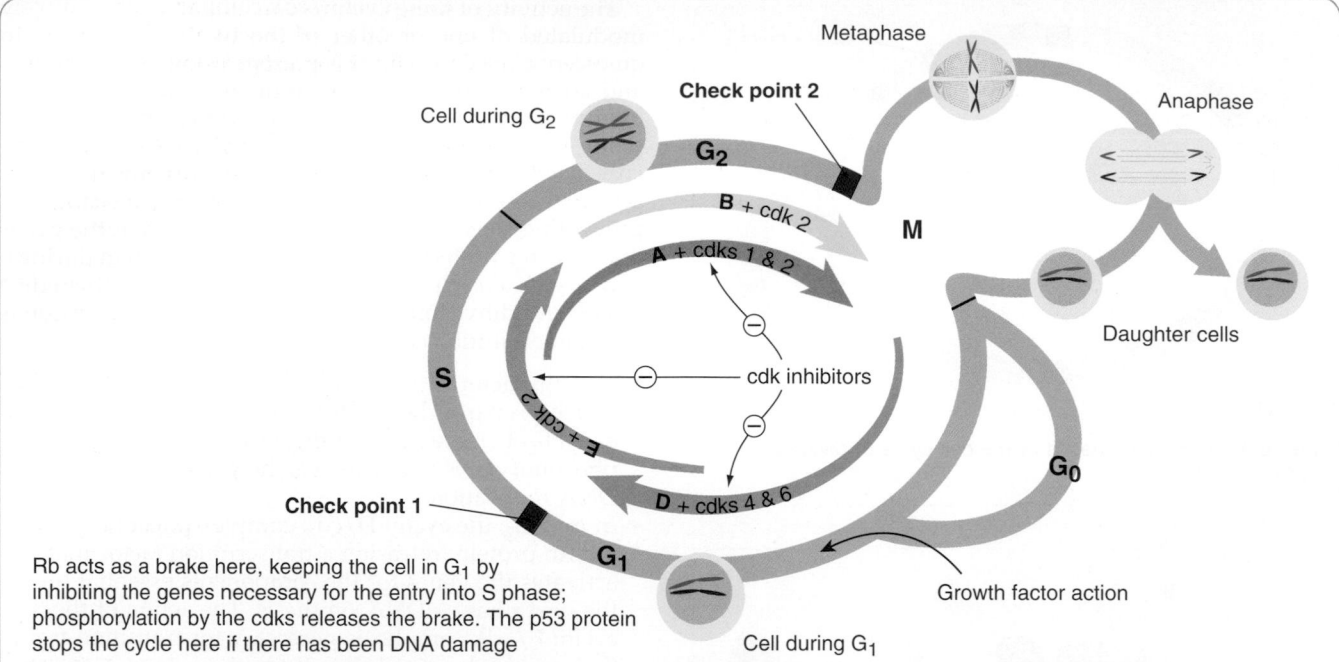

Fig. 6.3 Schematic diagram of the cell cycle, showing the role of the cyclin/cyclin-dependent kinase (cdk) complexes. The processes outlined in the cycle occur inside a cell such as the one shown in Fig. 6.4. A quiescent cell (in G_0 phase), when stimulated to divide by growth factors, is propelled into G_1 phase and prepares for DNA synthesis. Progress through the cycle is determined by sequential action of the cyclin/cdk complexes – depicted here by *coloured arrows*, the arrows being given the names of the relevant cyclins: D, E, A and B. The cdks are given next to the relevant cyclins. The thickness of each arrow represents the intensity of the cdk action at that point in the cycle. The activity of the cdks is regulated by cdk inhibitors. If there is DNA damage, the products of the tumour suppressor gene *p53* arrest the cycle at check point 1, allowing for repair. If repair fails, apoptosis (see Fig. 6.5) is initiated. The state of the chromosomes is shown schematically in each G phase – as a single pair in G_1, and each duplicated and forming two daughter chromatids in G_2. Some changes that occur during mitosis (metaphase, anaphase) are shown in a subsidiary circle. After the mitotic division, the daughter cells may enter G_1 or G_0 phase. *Rb*, retinoblastoma gene.

Each daughter cell will be in G_0 phase and will remain there unless stimulated into G_1 phase once more, as described earlier.

During metaphase, the cyclin A and B complexes phosphorylate cytoskeletal proteins, nuclear histones and possibly components of the spindle (the microtubules along which the chromatids are pulled during metaphase).

NEGATIVE REGULATORS OF THE CELL CYCLE

One of the main negative regulators is the Rb protein, which restrains the cell cycle while it is hypophosphorylated.

Inhibitors of the cdks also serve as negative regulators, their main action being at check points. There are two known families of inhibitors: the *CIP family* (cdk inhibitory proteins, also termed KIP or kinase inhibitory proteins) – proteins p21, p27 and p57; and the *Ink family* (inhibitors of kinases) – proteins p16, p19 and p15.

Protein p21 is a good example of the role of a cyclin/cdk inhibitor. It is under the control of the *p53* gene – a particularly important negative regulator which is relevant in carcinogenesis – that operates at check point 1.

Inhibition of the cycle at check point 1

The *p53* gene has been called the 'guardian of the genome'. It codes for the p53 protein, a transcription factor found in only low concentrations in normal healthy cells. However,

following DNA damage, the protein accumulates and activates the transcription of several genes, one of which codes for p21. Protein p21 inactivates cyclin/cdk complexes, thus Rb phosphorylation is prevented, and it becomes hypophosphorylated (below normal phosphorylation levels). This causes arrest of the cycle at check point 1, allowing DNA repair to take place. If the repair is successful, the cycle proceeds past check point 1 into S phase. If the repair is unsuccessful, the *p53* gene triggers apoptosis or cell suicide.[7]

Inhibition of the cycle at check point 2

DNA damage can arrest the cycle at check point 2, but the mechanisms involved are poorly understood. Inhibition of the accumulation of cyclin B/cdk complex in the nucleus seems to be a factor. For more detail on the control of the cell cycle, see section on microRNAs (p. 88) and Swanton (2004).

---

[7]Thus p53 is the guardian of the genome by preventing any unrepairable errors or genomic instability that occur in a cell from passing on to daughter cells. Another healthy cell will have to step in and replace the p53-destroyed cell. It is better for an organism to kill off less than perfect cells than to have any error whatsoever kept for future generations – 'the needs of the many outweigh the needs of the few' as Spock would say.

The cell cycle

- The term *cell cycle* refers to the sequence of events that take place within a cell as it prepares for division. The quiescent or resting state is called G_0.
- Growth factor action stimulates a cell in G_0 to enter the cycle.
- The phases of the cell cycle are:
  - G_1: preparation for DNA synthesis
  - S: DNA synthesis
  - G_2: preparation for division
  - M, mitosis: division into two daughter cells
- In G_0 phase, a hypophosphorylated protein, coded for by the *Rb* gene, arrests the cycle by inhibiting expression of critical factors necessary for DNA replication.
- Progress through the cycle is controlled by specific kinases (cyclin-dependent kinases; cdks) that are activated by binding to specific proteins termed cyclins.
- Four main cyclins D, E, A and B, together with their cdk complexes drive the cycle; cyclin D/cdk also releases the Rb protein-mediated inhibition.
  There are protein inhibitors of cdks in the cell. Protein p21 is particularly important; it is expressed when DNA damage triggers transcription of gene *p53* and arrests the cycle at check point 1.

INTERACTIONS BETWEEN CELLS, GROWTH FACTORS AND THE EXTRACELLULAR MATRIX

Cell proliferation is regulated by the integrated interplay between growth factors, cells, the ECM and the matrix metalloproteinases (MMPs). The ECM is secreted by the cells and provides a supportive framework. It also profoundly influences cell behaviour by signalling through the cell's integrins (proteins on a cell's extracellular surface that sense the ECM and signal to the cell what environment it is in or the neighbours it has). Matrix expression by cells is regulated by growth factors and cytokines (see Verrecchia & Mauviel, 2007; Järveläinen et al., 2009). The activity of some growth factors is, in turn, determined by the matrix, because they are sequestered by matrix components and released by proteinases (e.g. MMPs) secreted by the cells.

The action of growth factors acting through receptor tyrosine kinases or receptor-coupled kinases (see Ch. 3) is a fundamental part of these processes. Important examples include *fibroblast growth factor* (FGF), *epidermal growth factor* (EGF), *platelet-dependent growth factor* (PDGF), *vascular endothelial growth factor* (VEGF) and *transforming growth factor* (TGF)-β.

The main components of the ECM are:

- Fibre-forming elements, e.g. *collagen species* (the main proteins of the matrix) and *elastin*.
- Non-fibre-forming elements, e.g. proteoglycans, glycoproteins and adhesive proteins such as *fibronectin*. Proteoglycans have a growth-regulating role, in part by functioning as a reservoir of sequestered growth factors. Other elements are associated with the cell surface, where they bind cells to the matrix. Adhesive proteins link the various elements of the matrix together and also form links between the cells and the matrix through cell surface integrins.

Other proteins in the ECM are *thrombospondin* and *osteopontin*, which are not structural elements but modulate cell–matrix interactions and repair processes. The production of the ECM components is regulated by growth factors, particularly TGF-β.

▼ The ECM is a target for drug action. Both beneficial and adverse effects have been reported. Thus glucocorticoids decrease collagen synthesis in chronic inflammation and cyclo-oxygenase (COX)-2 inhibitors can modify fibrotic processes through a proposed action on TGF-β. Statins can decrease fibrosis by inhibiting angiotensin-induced connective tissue growth factor production (Rupérez et al., 2007) and reducing MMP expression. This may contribute to their effects in cardiovascular diseases (Tousoulis et al., 2010). The adverse actions of some drugs attributable to an effect on the ECM include the osteoporosis and skin thinning caused by glucocorticoids (discussed in Järveläinen et al., 2009). The ECM is also an important target in the search for new drugs that regulate tissue repair.

THE ROLE OF INTEGRINS

▼ Integrins are transmembrane kinase-linked receptors (see Ch. 3) comprising α and β subunits. Interaction with the ECM elements (e.g. fibronectin) triggers various cell responses, such as cytoskeletal rearrangement (not considered here) and co-regulation of growth factor function.

Intracellular signalling by both growth factor receptors and integrins is important for optimal cell proliferation (Fig. 6.4). Following integrin stimulation an adapter protein and an enzyme (*focal adhesion kinase*), activate the kinase cascade that comprises the growth factor signalling pathway. There is extensive cross-talk between the integrin and growth factor pathways (Streuli & Akhtar, 2009). Autophosphorylation of growth factor receptors (Ch. 3) is enhanced by integrin activation and integrin-mediated adhesion to the ECM (see Fig. 6.4) not only suppresses the concentrations of cdk inhibitors, but is required for the expression of cyclins A and D, and therefore for the progression of the cell cycle. Furthermore, integrin activation inhibits apoptosis (see later), further facilitating growth factor action (see reviews by Gahmberg et al., 2009 and Barczyk et al., 2010).

Several monoclonal antibodies are targeted at integrins, including **natalizumab**, used to treat multiple sclerosis and **abciximab**, an antithrombotic (Ch. 25).

THE ROLE OF MATRIX METALLOPROTEINASES

▼ Degradation of the ECM by metalloproteinases is necessary for tissue growth, repair and remodelling. When growth factors stimulate a cell to enter the cell cycle, they also stimulate the secretion of metalloproteinases (as inactive precursors), which then sculpt the matrix, producing the local changes necessary to accommodate the increased cell numbers. Metalloproteinases in turn release growth factors from the ECM and, in some cases (e.g. interleukin [IL]-1β), process them from precursor to their active form. The action of these enzymes is regulated by tissue inhibitors of metalloproteinases (TIMPS), which are also secreted by local cells.

In addition to their physiological function, metalloproteinases are involved in the tissue destruction that accompanies various diseases, such as rheumatoid arthritis, osteoarthritis, periodontitis, macular degeneration and myocardial restenosis. They also have a critical role in the growth, invasion and metastasis of tumours (Clark et al., 2008; Marastoni et al., 2008; Jackson et al., 2017). Because of this, much effort has gone into developing synthetic MMP inhibitors for treating cancers and inflammatory disorders, although clinical trials so far have shown limited efficacy and significant adverse effects (see Gialeli et al., 2011). **Doxycycline**, an antibiotic, also inhibits MMPs, and is used experimentally for this purpose.

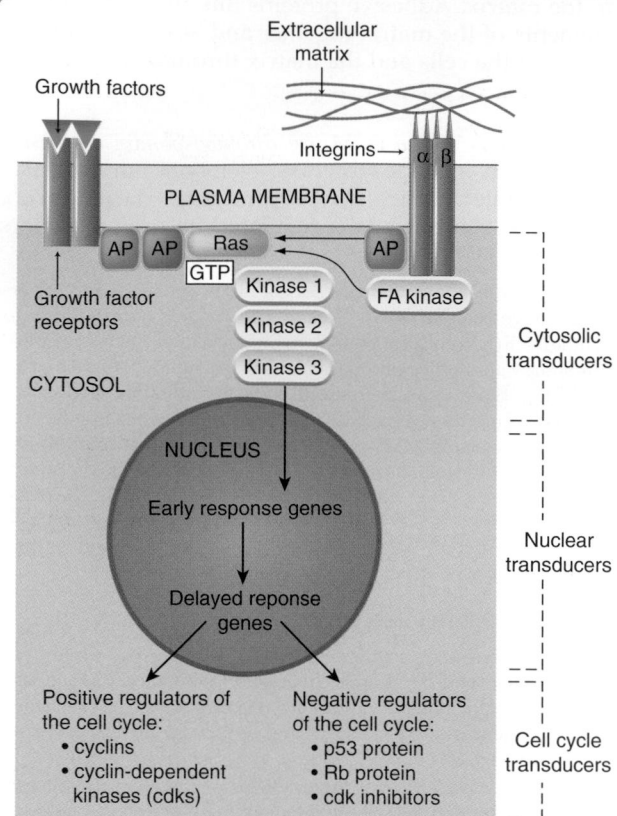

Fig. 6.4 Simplified diagram of the effect of growth factors on a cell in G_0. The overall effect of growth factor action is the generation of the cell cycle transducers. A cell such as the one depicted will then embark on G_1 phase of the cell cycle. Most growth factor receptors have integral tyrosine kinase (see Fig. 3.17). These receptors dimerise, then cross-phosphorylate their tyrosine residues. The early cytosolic transducers include proteins that bind to the phosphorylated tyrosine residues. Optimum effect requires cooperation with integrin action. Integrins (which have α and β subunits) connect the extracellular matrix with intracellular signalling pathways and also with the cell cytoskeleton (not shown here). G protein–coupled receptors can also stimulate cell proliferation, because their intracellular pathways can connect with the Ras/kinase cascade (not shown). *AP*, adapter protein; *FA kinase*, focal adhesion kinase; *Rb*, retinoblastoma protein.

ANGIOGENESIS

Angiogenesis, which normally accompanies cell proliferation, is the formation of new capillaries from existing small blood vessels. Without this, new tissues (including tumours) cannot feed and grow. Angiogenic stimuli include cytokines and various growth factors, in particular *VEGF*. The sequence of events in angiogenesis is as follows:

1. The basement membrane is degraded locally by proteinases.
2. Endothelial cells migrate out, forming a 'sprout'.
3. Following these leading cells, other endothelial cells proliferate under the influence of VEGF.
4. Matrix material is laid down around the new capillary.

Interactions between cells, growth factors and the matrix

- Cells secrete the components of the extracellular matrix (ECM) and become embedded in this tissue.
- The ECM influences the growth and behaviour of the cells. It also acts as a reservoir of growth factors.
- Integrins are transmembrane cellular receptors that can interact with elements of the ECM. They modulate growth factor signalling pathways and also mediate cytoskeletal adjustments within the cell.
- Growth factors cause cells to release metalloproteinases that degrade the local matrix so that it can accommodate the increase in cell numbers.
- Metalloproteinases release growth factors from the ECM and can activate some that are present in precursor form.

A monoclonal antibody, **bevacizumab**, which neutralises VEGF, is used as adjunct treatment for various cancers (see Ch. 57), and following injection into the eye, to treat age-related macular degeneration, a condition in which retinal blood vessels over-proliferate, causing blindness.

APOPTOSIS AND CELL REMOVAL

Apoptosis is cell suicide. It is regulated by a built-in genetically programmed self-destruct mechanism consisting of a specific sequence of biochemical events. It is thus unlike *necrosis*, which is a wholly disorganised disintegration of a damaged cells that releases substances which trigger the inflammatory response.[8]

Apoptosis plays an essential role in embryogenesis, shaping organs during development by eliminating cells that have become redundant. It is the mechanism that each day unobtrusively removes some 10 billion cells from the human body. It is involved in numerous physiological events, including the shedding of the intestinal lining, the death of time-expired neutrophils and the turnover of tissues as the newborn infant grows to maturity. It is the basis for the development of self-tolerance in the immune system (Ch. 7) and acts as a first-line defence against carcinogenic mutations by purging cells that could become malignant.

Disorders of apoptosis are also implicated in the pathophysiology of many conditions, including:

- chronic neurodegenerative diseases such as Alzheimer's and Parkinson's disease and multiple sclerosis (Ch. 41);
- conditions with acute tissue damage or cell loss, such as myocardial infarction (Ch. 22), stroke and spinal cord injury (Ch. 41);
- depletion of T cells in HIV infection (Ch. 53);
- osteoarthritis (Ch. 37);
- haematological disease, such as aplastic anaemia (Ch. 26);

[8]There are other forms of programmed cell death (PCD) including *autophagy* and (confusingly) *programmed necrosis or necroptosis*. Here we will focus on apoptosis, also known as 'Type I PCD'.

- evasion of the immune response by cancer cells and resistance to cancer chemotherapy (Ch. 57);
- autoimmune/inflammatory diseases such as myasthenia gravis (Ch. 14), rheumatoid arthritis (Ch. 27), and bronchial asthma (Ch. 29);
- viral infections with ineffective eradication of virus-infected cells (Ch. 53).

▼ Apoptosis is particularly important in the regulation of the immune response and in the many conditions in which it is an underlying component. There is evidence that T cells have a negative regulatory pathway controlled by surface *programmed cell death receptors* (e.g. the PD-1 receptor), and that there is normally a balance between the stimulatory pathways triggered by antigens and this negative regulatory apoptosis-inducing pathway. The balance is important in the maintenance of peripheral tolerance. A disturbance of this balance is seen in autoimmune disease, in the 'exhaustion' of T cells in chronic viral diseases such as HIV, and possibly in tumour escape from immune destruction (Zha et al., 2004). Indeed PD-1 generally acts to inhibit T-cell receptor signalling, and PD-1 inhibitors (checkpoint inhibitors) cause activation of T cells, allowing them to once more recognise and attack the tumour (see also Ch. 57).

Apoptosis is a *default response*, i.e. continuous active signalling by tissue-specific trophic factors, cytokines and hormones, and cell-to-cell contact factors (adhesion molecules, integrins, etc.) are required for cell survival and viability. The self-destruct mechanism is automatically triggered unless it is actively and continuously inhibited by these antiapoptotic factors. Different cell types require differing sets of survival factors, which function only locally. If a cell strays or is dislodged from the area protected by its paracrine survival signals, it will die.

Withdrawal of these survival factors – which has been termed 'death by neglect' – is not the only pathway to apoptosis (Fig. 6.5). The death machinery can be activated by ligands that stimulate *death receptors* and by DNA damage. But it is generally accepted that cell proliferation processes and apoptosis are tightly integrated.

MORPHOLOGICAL CHANGES IN APOPTOSIS

As the cell dies it 'rounds up', the chromatin condenses into dense masses, nucleases chop up the genome into unusable different sized fragments (seen on a gel as DNA 'laddering'), the cytoplasm shrinks and there is blebbing of the plasma membrane. Finally, mediated by a family of proteolytic enzymes known as caspases, the cell is transformed into a cluster of membrane-bound entities. This cellular 'corpse' displays 'eat me' signals, such as phosphatidylserine on its surface, which are recognised by macrophages, which then phagocytose the remains. It is important that these cellular fragments are enclosed by a membrane because otherwise the release of cell constituents could trigger an inflammatory reaction. An additional safeguard against this is that phagocytosing macrophages release anti-inflammatory mediators such as TGF-β, annexin-1 and IL-10.

THE MAJOR PLAYERS IN APOPTOSIS

The repertoire of reactions in apoptosis is extremely complex and varies between species and cell types. Yet it could be that the pivotal reaction(s) that lead to either cell survival or cell death are controlled by a single gene or combination of genes. If so, these genes could be desirable targets for drugs used to treat many proliferative diseases.

Only a simple outline of apoptosis can be given here. Portt et al. (2011) have reviewed the whole area in detail.

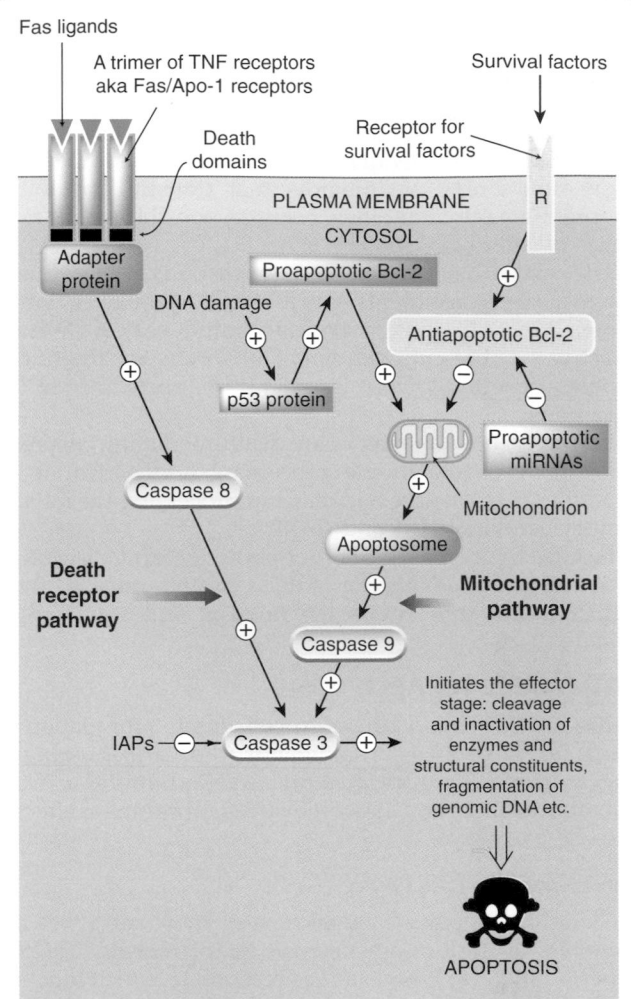

Fig. 6.5 A simplified diagram of the two main signalling pathways in apoptosis. The 'death receptor' pathway is activated when death receptors such as members of the tumour necrosis factor (TNF) family are stimulated by specific death ligands. This recruits adapter proteins that activate initiator caspases (e.g. caspase 8), which in turn activate effector caspases such as caspase 3. The mitochondrial pathway is activated by diverse signals, one being DNA damage. In the presence of DNA damage that cannot be repaired, the p53 protein (see text and Figs 6.3 and 6.4) activates a subpathway that releases cytochrome C from the mitochondrion, with subsequent involvement of the *apoptosome* and activation of an initiator caspase, caspase 9. The apoptosome is a complex of procaspase 9, cytochrome C and apoptotic-activating protease factor-1 (Apaf-1). Both these pathways converge on the effector caspase (e.g. caspase 3), which brings about the demise of the cell. The survival factor subpathway normally restrains apoptosis by inhibiting the mitochondrial pathway through activation of the antiapoptotic factor Bcl-2. The receptor labelled 'R' represents the respective receptors for trophic factors, growth factors, cell-to-cell contact factors (adhesion molecules, integrins), etc. Continuous stimulation of these receptors is necessary for cell survival/proliferation. If this pathway is non-functional (*shown in grey*), this antiapoptotic drive is withdrawn. *IAP*, inhibitor of apoptosis.

The major players are a family of cysteine aspartate-directed proteinases (*caspases*) present in the cell in inactive form. These undertake delicate protein surgery, selectively cleaving a specific set of target proteins (enzymes, structural components, all of which contain a characteristic motif recognised by the caspases), inactivating some and activating others. A cascade of about nine different caspases is required, some functioning as initiators that transmit the initial apoptotic signals, and others being responsible for the final phase of cell death (see Fig. 6.5).

The 'executioner' caspases (e.g. caspase 3) cleave and inactivate cell constituents such as the DNA repair enzymes, protein kinase C, and cytoskeletal components. A DNAase is activated that cuts genomic DNA between the nucleosomes, generating DNA fragments of approximately 180 base pairs.

However, not all caspases are death-mediating enzymes; some have a role in the processing and activating of cytokines (e.g. caspase 8 is active in processing the inflammatory cytokines IL-1 and IL-18).

Besides the caspases, another pathway can be triggered by *apoptotic initiating factor* (AIF), a protein released from mitochondria that enters the nucleus and triggers cell suicide.

PATHWAYS TO APOPTOSIS

There are two main routes to cell death: stimulation of death receptors by external ligands (the *extrinsic pathway*) and an internal *mitochondrial pathway*. Both routes activate initiator caspases and converge on a final common effector caspase pathway.

THE EXTRINSIC PATHWAY

Lurking in the plasma membrane of most cell types are members of the tumour necrosis factor receptor (TNFR) superfamily (also known as Fas receptors), which function as 'death receptors' (see Fig. 6.5). Important family members include TNFR-1 and CD95 (also known as Fas ligands or Apo-1), but there are many others (e.g. PD-1, a death receptor that can be induced on activated T cells, as discussed previously).

Each receptor has a 'death domain' in its cytoplasmic tail. Stimulation of the receptors by a ligand such as tumour necrosis factor (TNF[9]) itself or TRAIL[10] causes them to trimerise and recruit an adapter protein that binds to their death domains. The resulting complex activates caspase 8 (and probably caspase 10), which in turn activate the effector caspases (see Fig. 6.5).

The mitochondrial pathway

This pathway can be triggered by DNA damage or by withdrawal of cell survival factors or other factors. In some way, the cell can 'audit' such damage and decide whether to initiate the apoptotic pathway. It is possible that

promyelocytic leukaemia bodies, large complexes of proteins in the nucleus, participate in this task (Wyllie, 2010), although how they do so is not clear.

Regulating the apoptotic event are the members of the Bcl-2 protein family, a group of proteins with homologous domains allowing interactions between individual members. If the cell selects the apoptotic route, the p53 protein activates p21 and proapoptotic members of the Bcl-2 family – Bid, Bax and Bak. In addition to these proapoptotic individuals, this family has antiapoptotic members (e.g. Bcl-2 itself[11]). These factors compete with each other on the surface of the mitochondria and the outcome depends upon the relative competing concentrations of these molecular players. In the case of a proapoptotic signal, oligomers of Bax and or Bak form pores in the mitochondrial membrane through which proteins such as cytochrome C can leak.

When released, cytochrome C complexes with a protein termed Apaf-1 (apoptotic protease-activating factor-1); the pair then combining with procaspase 9 to activate it. This latter enzyme orchestrates the effector caspase pathway. The triumvirate of cytochrome C, Apaf-1 and procaspase 9 is termed the *apoptosome* (see Fig. 6.5 and see Riedl & Salvesen, 2007). Nitric oxide (see Ch. 21) is another mediator that can have proapoptotic and antiapoptotic actions.

In normal cells, survival factors (specified earlier) continuously activate antiapoptotic mechanisms. The withdrawal of survival factors can cause death in several different ways depending on the cell type. A common mechanism is tipping the balance between Bcl-2 family members leading to loss of the antiapoptotic protein action, with the resultant unopposed action of the proapoptotic members of the Bcl-2 family of proteins (see Fig. 6.5).

The two main cell death pathways are connected to each other, in that caspase 8 in the death receptor pathway can activate the proapoptotic Bcl-2 family proteins and thus activate the mitochondrial pathway.

MicroRNAs, the cell cycle and apoptosis

MicroRNAs (miRNAs), discovered only around the turn of the millennium, are a family of small 'non-coding' RNAs present within plants and animals. Coded by sections of the genome found outside the normal coding sequences of genes, miRNAs negatively regulate the ribosomal translation processes of many other genes. They are now known to inhibit the expression of genes coding for cell cycle regulation, apoptosis (see Fig. 6.5), cell differentiation and development (Carleton et al., 2007; Lynam-Lennon et al., 2009). About 3% of human genes encode for miRNA and some 30% of human genes coding for proteins are regulated by miRNAs.

Altered miRNA expression is now believed to be linked to a variety of diseases, including diabetes, obesity, Alzheimer's disease, cardiovascular system diseases, inflammatory conditions and neurodegenerative diseases (Barbato et al., 2009), as well as carcinogenesis, metastasis and resistance to cancer therapies (Wurdinger & Costa, 2007; Garzon et al., 2009). miRNAs are also believed to function as oncogenes and/or tumour suppressor genes and to regulate T cells (Zhou et al., 2009). Not surprisingly, miRNAs are being heralded as targets for new drug development for a variety of disease states (Christopher et al., 2016; Cho 2010).

[9]Tumour necrosis factor was first thought to be secreted by bacteria, since it was known that infected tumours would sometimes recede and be cured. This 'bacterial-secreted' *tumour killing factor* was discovered to be TNF, released instead from our macrophages responding to the bacterial infection. A side effect of the TNF was to kill the tumour, hence its name. TNF is also known as *cachexin*, the agent responsible for muscle apoptosis and wastage in cancer patients.
[10]TRAIL is **t**umour necrosis factor-α–**r**elated **a**poptosis-**i**nducing **l**igand, of course; what else? See Janssen et al. (2005) for discussion of a role of TRAIL. PD-L1, a ligand for the PD-1 receptor, is found on all haemopoietic cells and many other tissues.

[11]Another brake on cell death is a family of caspase-inhibiting proteins called IAPs (inhibitors of apoptosis proteins).

Apoptosis

- Apoptosis is programmed cell death. It is an essential biological process and critical, for example, embryogenesis and tissue homeostasis.
- Apoptosis depends upon a cascade of proteinases called caspases. Two sets of initiator caspases converge on a set of effector caspases, which bring about the apoptotic event.
- Two main pathways activate the effector caspases: the death receptor pathway and the mitochondrial pathway.
  - Stimulation of the tumour necrosis factor receptor family initiates the death receptor pathway. The main initiator is caspase 8.
  - The mitochondrial pathway is activated by internal factors such as DNA damage, which results in transcription of gene *p53*. The p53 protein activates a subpathway that releases cytochrome C from the mitochondrion. This, in turn, complexes with protein Apaf-1 and together they activate initiator caspase 9.
- In undamaged cells, survival factors (cytokines, hormones, cell-to-cell contact factors) continuously activate antiapoptotic mechanisms. Withdrawal of survival factors causes cell death through the mitochondrial pathway.
- The effector caspases (e.g. caspase 3) initiate a cascade of proteases that cleave cell constituents, DNA, cytoskeletal components, enzymes, etc. This reduces the cell to a cluster of membrane-bound entities that are eventually phagocytosed by macrophages.

REPAIR AND HEALING

Repair occurs when tissues are damaged or lost. It is also implicated in the resolution of the local inflammatory reaction to a pathogen or chemical irritant. In some instances, damage or tissue loss can lead to *regeneration*, which is different from repair and is considered below.

There is considerable overlap between the mechanisms activated in inflammation and repair. Both entail an ordered series of events including cell migration, angiogenesis, proliferation of connective tissue cells, synthesis of ECM and finally remodelling – all coordinated by the growth factors and cytokines that are appropriate for the particular tissue involved. TGF-β is a key regulator of several of these processes.[12]

Repair, healing and regeneration

- Repair and healing occurs when tissues are damaged. It is a common sequel to inflammation. Connective tissue cells, white blood cells and blood vessels are commonly involved.
- Regeneration is the replacement of the tissue or organ that has been damaged or lost. It depends upon the presence of a pool of primitive stem cells that have the potential to develop into any cell in the body. Complete regeneration of a tissue or organ is rare in mammals. The more rapid repair processes – often accompanied by scarring – usually make good the damage. This may be an evolutionary trade-off in mammals for the lost power of regeneration.
- However, it might be possible to activate regenerative pathways in mammals – at least to some extent and in some organs.

PATHOPHYSIOLOGICAL IMPLICATIONS

As mentioned before, cell proliferation and apoptosis are involved in many physiological and pathological processes. These are:

- the growth of tissues and organs in the embryo and later during development;
- the replenishment of lost or time-expired cells such as leukocytes, gut epithelium and uterine endometrium;
- immunological responses, including development of immunological tolerance to host proteins;
- repair and healing after injury or inflammation;
- the hyperplasia (increase in cell number and in connective tissue) associated with chronic inflammatory, hypersensitivity and autoimmune diseases (Ch. 7);
- the growth, invasion and metastasis of tumours (Ch. 57);
- regeneration of tissues.

The role of cell proliferation and apoptosis in the first two processes listed is self-evident and needs no further comment. Their involvement in immune tolerance is discussed briefly above but the other processes require further discussion.

HYPERPLASIA

Hyperplasia (cell proliferation and matrix expansion) is a hallmark of chronic inflammatory and autoimmune diseases such as rheumatoid arthritis (Chs 7 and 27), psoriasis, chronic ulcers and chronic obstructive lung disease. It also underlies the bronchial hyper-reactivity of chronic asthma (Ch. 29) and glomerular nephritis.

Cell proliferation and apoptotic events are also implicated in atherosclerosis (Ch. 24), restenosis and myocardial repair after infarction (Ch. 22).

THE GROWTH, INVASION AND METASTASIS OF TUMOURS

Growth factor signalling systems, antiapoptotic pathways and cell cycle controllers are of increasing interest as targets for novel approaches to the treatment of cancer. See Chapter 57.

---

[12]Next time you cut yourself, have a look at the scar exactly a week later. It may be that almost all signs of the scar have nearly vanished. This impressive biological process (bleeding, scabbing, scarring, wound healing) in a week is thanks to growth factors from the scab stimulating epithelial and endothelial stem cells into action to remodel and match what was damaged – even down to replicating a fingerprint.

STEM CELLS AND REGENERATION

Regeneration of tissue replaces that lost following damage or disease and allows restoration of function. Many animals (e.g. amphibians) have impressive regenerative powers and can even regrow an entire organ such as a limb or a tail. The essential process is the activation of *stem cells* – a pool of undifferentiated cells that have the potential to develop into any of the more specialised cells in the body – 'totipotent' or 'pluripotent' cells (Slack, 2014; Burgess, 2016). Not only do amphibians have a plentiful supply of these primitive cells but many of their more specialised cells can de-differentiate, becoming stem cells again. These can then multiply and retrace the fetal developmental pathways that generated the organ, by differentiating into the various cell types needed to replace the missing structure.

However, during evolution, mammals have lost this ability in all but a few tissues. Blood cells, intestinal epithelium and the outer layers of the skin are replaced continuously throughout life but there is a low turnover and replacement of cells in organs such as liver, kidney and bone. This 'physiological renewal' is effected by local tissue-specific stem cells.

Almost alone among mammalian organs, the liver has significant ability to replace itself. It can regenerate to its original size in a remarkably short time, provided that at least 25% has been left intact.[13] The mature parenchymal liver cells participate in this process as well as all the other cellular components of the liver.

It is necessary to distinguish *embryonic stem cells* (ES cells) from *adult stem cells* (AS cells) and *progenitor cells*. ES cells are the true pluripotent cells of the embryo that can differentiate into any other cell type. AS cells have a more restricted capability, whereas progenitor cells are able to differentiate only into a single cell type. ES cells are absent in the adult mammal, but AS cells are present, although they are few in number. In mammals, tissue or organ damage (with the exception of the liver, mentioned previously) normally leads to repair, rather than regeneration.

Until recently, it was assumed that this was (with a few exceptions) an unalterable situation, but recent work has suggested that it might be possible to activate the regenerative pathways in mammals – at least to some extent and in some organs. For this to happen, it is necessary to encourage some stem cells to proliferate, develop and differentiate at the relevant sites; or – and this is a rather more remote prospect in humans – to persuade some local specialised cells to de-differentiate. This can occur in some mammals under special circumstances. However, it may be that repair is the Janus face of regeneration, being an evolutionary trade-off in mammals for the lost power of regeneration.[14]

▼ Where are the relevant stem cells that could be coaxed into regenerative service? Various possibilities are being vigorously investigated and in some cases tested clinically. These include:
- ES cells (limited availability and serious ethical issues)
- bone marrow-derived mesenchymal stem cells (Zhang et al., 2017)
- muscle-derived stem cells (Kelc et al., 2013)
- human-induced pluripotent stem cells (Nishikawa et al., 2008)
- tissue-resident progenitor cells.

For a tissue such as the liver to regenerate, local tissue-specific stem cells must be stimulated by growth factors to enter the cell cycle and to proliferate. Other essential processes include those already discussed such as angiogenesis, activation of MMPs and interaction between the matrix and fibronectin to link all the new elements together. The concomitant replacement of components of the lost connective tissue (fibroblasts, macrophages, etc.) would also be necessary.

Because most tissues do not regenerate spontaneously, mechanisms that could restore regenerative ability could be of immense therapeutic value. Stem cell therapy has become an attractive prospect for treating all manner of diseases, ranging from erectile dysfunction and urinary incontinence to heart disease and neurodegeneration. Animal studies have confirmed that this is a potentially rewarding area although routine stem cell therapy in humans is still a distant prospect. The literature is daunting but the following examples provide an insight into the obstacles and aspirations of the field: repair of damaged heart muscle (Ch. 22; see Lovell & Mathur, 2011), repair of retinal degeneration (Ong & da Cruz, 2012), stroke (Banerjee et al., 2011) and replacement of insulin-secreting cells to treat type 1 diabetes mellitus (Ch. 32; Voltarelli et al., 2007).

THERAPEUTIC PROSPECTS

Theoretically, all the processes described in this chapter could constitute useful targets for new drug development. Below, we list those approaches that are proving or are likely to prove fruitful.

APOPTOTIC MECHANISMS

Compounds that could modify apoptosis are being intensively investigated (Melnikova & Golden, 2004; MacFarlane, 2009). Here we can only outline some of the more important approaches.

Drugs that promote apoptosis by various mechanisms were heralded as a potential new approach to cancer treatment, and are actively being studied, though none has yet been approved for clinical use. Potential proapoptotic therapeutic approaches need to be targeted precisely to the diseased tissue to avoid the obvious risks of damaging other tissues. Examples include the following:

- An antisense compound against Bcl-2 (**oblimersen**) is being tested for chronic lymphocytic leukaemia.
- **Obatoclax**, and **Navitoclax** are small molecule inhibitors of Bcl-2 action, being tested for treating haematological malignancies. For details see MacFarlane (2009).
- MicroRNA technology could also be used to promote apoptosis (see Fig. 6.5).
- Monoclonal agonist antibodies to the death receptor ligand TRAIL (e.g. **lexatumumab**) are undergoing

[13]There is an account of liver regeneration in Greek mythology. Prometheus stole the secret of fire from Zeus and gave it to mankind. To punish him, Zeus had him shackled to a crag in the Caucasus and every day an eagle tore at his flesh and devoured much of his liver. During the night, however, it regenerated and in the morning was whole again. The legend doesn't say whether the requisite 25% was left after the eagle had had its fill, and the regeneration described seems unrealistically fast – rat liver takes 2 weeks or more to get back to the original size after 66% hepatectomy.
[14]Bovine myosatellite stem cells have been used to grow burgers in the lab (a slightly vegetarian alternative). The fact that one burger can cost up to £250,000 to make may mean that only professional footballers can afford them for now.

clinical trials for treatment of solid tumours and lymphomas (MacFarlane, 2009).

- **Bortezomib**, which inhibits the proteasome, is available for the treatment of selected cancers. It causes the build-up of Bax, an apoptotic promoter protein of the Bcl-2 family that acts by inhibiting antiapoptotic Bcl-2. Bortezomib acts partly by inhibiting NF-κB action (see Ch. 3).
- One of the most cancer-specific genes codes for an endogenous caspase inhibitor, *survivin*. This occurs in high concentrations in certain tumours and a small molecule suppressor of survivin is in clinical trial (Giaccone & Rajan, 2009), the objective being to induce cancer cell suicide.

Inhibiting apoptosis might prevent or treat a wide range of common degenerative disorders. Unfortunately, success in developing such inhibitors for clinical use has so far proved elusive and a number have been found to lack efficacy in clinical trials. Current areas of interest include the following:

- Blocking the PD-1 death receptor with a targeted antibody (such as **Nivolumab**) is a potentially fruitful new avenue to explore for the treatment of HIV, hepatitis B and hepatitis C infections, as well as other chronic infections and some cancers that express the ligand for PD-1 (Trivedi et al., 2015).
- Several caspase inhibitors are under investigation for treating myocardial infarction, stroke, liver disease, organ transplantation and sepsis. **Emricasan** is one such candidate undergoing trials in patients requiring liver transplants.

ANGIOGENESIS AND METALLOPROTEINASES

The search for clinically useful anti-angiogenic drugs and MMP inhibitors is continuing, but has not so far been successful. At present, only one new drug has been approved for use in cancer treatment: **bevacizumab**, a monoclonal antibody that neutralises VEGF, which is also used to treat age-related macular degeneration, a disease also associated with excessive proliferation of retinal blood vessels.

CELL CYCLE REGULATION

The main endogenous positive regulators of the cell cycle are the cdks. Several small molecules that inhibit cdks by targeting the ATP-binding sites of these kinases have been developed; an example is **flavopiridol**, currently in clinical trials, which inhibits all the cdks, causing arrest of the cell cycle; it also promotes apoptosis, has anti-angiogenic properties and can induce differentiation (Dickson & Schwartz, 2009).

Some compounds affect upstream pathways for cdk activation and may find a use in cancer treatment. Examples are **perifosine** (although its future is uncertain at the moment) and **lovastatin** (a cholesterol-lowering drug, see Ch. 24, which may also have anticancer properties).

Bortezomib, a boronate compound, covalently binds the proteasome, inhibiting the degradation of proapoptotic proteins. It is used in treating multiple myeloma (see Ch. 57).

Of the various components of the growth factor signalling pathway, receptor tyrosine kinases, the Ras protein and cytoplasmic kinases have been the subjects of most interest. Kinase inhibitors recently introduced for cancer treatment include **imatinib**, **gefitinib lapatinib**, **sunitinib** and **erlotinib** (see Ch. 57).

REFERENCES AND FURTHER READING

Cell cycle and apoptosis (general)

Ashkenasi, A., 2002. Targeting death and decoy receptors of the tumour necrosis receptor superfamily. Nat. Rev. Cancer 2, 420–429. (*Exemplary review, comprehensive; good diagrams*)

Aslan, J.E., Thomas, G., 2009. Death by committee: organellar trafficking and communication in apoptosis. Traffic 10, 1390–1404.

Barbato, C., Ruberti, F., Cogoni, C., 2009. Searching for MIND: microRNAs in neurodegenerative diseases. J. Biomed. Biotechnol. 2009, 871313.

Carleton, M., Cleary, M.C., Linsley, P.S., 2007. MicroRNAs and cell cycle regulation. Cell Cycle 6, 2127–2132. (*Describes how specific microRNAs act to control cell cycle check points*)

Cho, W.C., 2010. MicroRNAs: potential biomarkers for cancer diagnosis, prognosis and targets for therapy. Int. J. Biochem. Cell Biol. 42, 1273–1281.

Christopher, A.F., Kaur, R.P., Kaur, G., Kaur, A., Gupta, V., Bansal, P., 2016. MicroRNA therapeutics: Discovering novel targets and developing specific therapy. Perspectives Clin. Res. 7, 68–74.

Cummings, J., Ward, T., Ranson, M., Dive, C., 2004. Apoptosis pathway-targeted drugs – from the bench to the clinic. Biochim. Biophys. Acta 1705, 53–66. (*Good review discussing – in the context of anticancer drug development – Bcl-2 proteins, IAPs, growth factors, tyrosine kinase inhibitors and assays for apoptosis-inducing drugs*)

Danial, N.N., Korsmeyer, S.J., 2004. Cell death: critical control points. Cell 116, 205–219. (*Definitive review of the biology and control of apoptosis; includes evidence from C. elegans, Drosophila and mammals*)

Dickson, M.A., Schwartz, G.K., 2009. Development of cell-cycle inhibitors for cancer therapy. Curr. Oncol. 16, 36–43. (*Discusses drugs that target the cell cycle that have entered clinical trials*)

Elmore, S., 2007. Apoptosis: a review of programmed cell death. Toxicol. Pathol. 35, 495–516. (*A general overview of apoptosis, including structural changes, biochemistry and the role of apoptosis in health and disease*)

Garzon, R., Calin, G.A., Croce, C.M., 2009. MicroRNAs in cancer. Annu. Rev. Med. 60, 167–179.

Giaccone, G., Rajan, A., 2009. Met amplification and HSP90 inhibitors. Cell Cycle 8, 2682.

Janssen, E.M., Droin, N.M., Lemmens, E.E., 2005. CD4+ T-cell-help controls CD4+ T cell memory via TRAIL-mediated activation-induced cell death. Nature 434, 88–92. (*Control of TRAIL expression could explain the role of CD4+ T cells in CD8+ T-cell function*)

Lynam-Lennon, N., Maher, S.M., Reynolds, J.V., 2009. The roles of microRNAs in cancer and apoptosis. Biol. Rev. 84, 55–71. (*Detailed review of the role of microRNAs in cell proliferation and cell death and their potential roles as oncogenes and tumour suppressor genes*)

MacFarlane, M., 2009. Cell death pathways – potential therapeutic targets. Xenobiotica 39, 616–624. (*Excellent up-to-date review with table of agents in early clinical trial*)

Melnikova, A., Golden, J., 2004. Apoptosis-targeting therapies. Nat. Rev. Drug Discov. 3, 905–906. (*Crisp overview*)

Ouyang, L., Shi, Z., Zhao, S., et al., 2012. Programmed cell death pathways in cancer: a review of apoptosis, autophagy and programmed necrosis. Cell Prolif. 45, 487–498. (*A wide-ranging review dealing with all types of programmed cell death in cancer cells*)

Portt, L., Norman, G., Clapp, C., Greenwood, M., Greenwood, M.T., 2011. Anti-apoptosis and cell survival: a review. Biochim. Biophys. Acta 1813, 238–259. (*A very detailed review which deals with both pro- and antiapoptotic mechanisms as well as other types of programmed cell death*)

Riedl, S.J., Salvesen, G.S., 2007. The apoptosome: signalling platform of cell death. Nat. Rev. Mol. Cell Biol. 8, 405–413. (*Discusses the formation of the apoptosome and the activation of its effector, caspase 9*)

Riedl, S.J., Shi, Y., 2004. Molecular mechanisms of caspase regulation during apoptosis. Nat. Rev. Mol. Cell Biol. 5, 897–905. (*Systematic review*)

Satyanarayana, A., Kaldis, P., 2009. Mammalian cell-cycle regulation: several Cdks, numerous cyclins and diverse compensatory mechanisms. Oncogene 28, 2925–2939. (*Summarises the results of gene knockout experiments which point to the ability of the cell to compensate for the loss of most cyclins. Interesting review for those who want to delve deeper into the subject*)

Swanton, C., 2004. Cell-cycle targeted therapies. Lancet 5, 27–36. (*Definitive review of the protein families controlling the cell cycle, their alterations in malignancy and their potential as targets for new drugs*)

Tousoulis, D., Andreou, I., Tentolouris, C., et al., 2010. Comparative effects of rosuvastatin and allopurinol on circulating levels of matrix metalloproteinases in patients with chronic heart failure. Int. J. Cardiol. 145, 438–443.

Trivedi, M.S., Hoffner, B., Winkelmann, J.L., Abbott, M.E., Hamid, O., Carvajal, R.D., 2015. Programmed death 1 immune checkpoint inhibitors. Clin. Adv. Hematol. Oncol. 13, 858–868. (*Review that appraises the recent work on reversing T cell exhaustion*)

Wurdinger, T., Costa, F.F., 2007. Molecular therapy in the microRNA era. Pharmacogenomics J. 7, 297–304.

Wyllie, A.H., 2010. 'Where, O death, is thy sting?' A brief review of apoptosis biology. Mol. Neurobiol. 42, 4–9. (*A short and very accessible review by one of the founders of the field. Highly recommended*)

Yang, B.F., Lu, Y.J., Wang, Z.G., 2009. MicroRNAs and apoptosis: implications in molecular therapy of human disease. Clin. Exp. Pharmacol. Physiol. 36, 951–960. (*Comprehensive review of the apotosis-regulating miRNAs and apoptotic cell death*)

Zha, Y., Blank, C., Gajewski, T.F., 2004. Negative regulation of T-cell function by PD-1. Crit. Rev. Immunol. 24, 229–237. (*Article on the balance between stimulatory and inhibitory signalling and its relevance to self-tolerance and the pathogenesis of autoimmune diseases*)

Zhou, L., Seo, K.H., Wong, H.K., Mi, Q.S., 2009. MicroRNAs and immune regulatory T cells. Int. Immunopharmacol. 9, 524–527.

Integrins, extracellular matrix, metalloproteinases and angiogenesis

Barczyk, M., Carracedo, S., Gullberg, D., 2010. Integrins. Cell Tissue Res. 339, 269–280.

Clark, I.M., Swingler, T.E., Sampieri, C.L., Edwards, D.R., 2008. The regulation of matrix metalloproteinases and their inhibitors. Int. J. Biochem. Cell Biol. 40, 1362–1378.

Gialeli, C., Theocharis, A.D., Karamanos, N.K., 2011. Roles of matrix metalloproteinases in cancer progression and their pharmacological targeting. FEBS J. 278, 16–27. (*Somewhat discouraging review of clinical trials data with MMP inhibitors*)

Gahmberg, C.G., Fagerholm, S.C., Nurmi, S.M., et al., 2009. Regulation of integrin activity and signalling. Biochim. Biophys. Acta 1790, 431–444. (*Crisp review of the control of cell signalling by integrins*)

Jackson, H.W., Defamie, V., Waterhouse, P., Khokha, R., 2017. TIMPs: versatile extracellular regulators in cancer. Nat. Rev. Cancer 17, 38–53. (*Thorough review of the roles of TIMPs, ADAMs and MMPs in cancer*)

Järveläinen, H., Sainio, A., Koulu, M., Wight, T.N., Penttinen, R., 2009. Extracellular matrix molecules: potential targets in pharmacotherapy. Pharmacol. Rev. 61, 198–223. (*Comprehensive review of the role of the extracellular matrix [ECM] in the cellular events involved in proliferation and differentiation with discussion of the ECM as a potential target for new drug development*)

Marastoni, S., Ligresti, G., Lorenzon, E., Colombatti, A., Mongiat, M., 2008. Extracellular matrix: a matter of life and death. Connect. Tissue Res. 49, 203–206. (*Crisp analysis of the ECM and its role in cell survival, growth and proliferation*)

Rupérez, M., Rodrigues-Diez, R., Blanco-Colio, L.M., et al., 2007. HMG-CoA reductase inhibitors decrease angiotensin II-induced vascular fibrosis: role of RhoA/ROCK and MAPK pathways. Hypertension 50, 377–383.

Streuli, C.H., Akhtar, N., 2009. Signal co-operation between integrins and other receptor systems. Biochem. J. 418, 491–506. (*Deals with integrin interaction with growth factors to regulate angiogenesis, their interplay with tyrosine kinases and with cytokine receptors*)

Verrecchia, F., Mauviel, A., 2007. Transforming growth factor-beta and fibrosis. World J. Gastroenterol. 13, 3056–3062.

Stem cells, regeneration and repair

Aldhous, P., 2008. How stem cell advances will transform medicine. New Scientist 2654, 40–43. (*Clear, simple article*)

Banerjee, S., Williamson, D., Habib, N., Gordon, M., Chataway, J., 2011. Human stem cell therapy in ischaemic stroke: a review. Age. Ageing 40, 7–13.

Burgess, R., 2016. Stem Cells: A Short Course. Wiley-Blackwell. ISBN: 978-1-118-43919-7.

Gaetani, R., Barile, L., Forte, E., et al., 2009. New perspectives to repair a broken heart. Cardiovasc. Hematol. Agents Med. Chem. 7, 91–107. (*Discusses sources of cardiomyogenic cells and their potential for diseased or injured myocardium*)

Kelc, R., Trapecar, M., Vogrin, M., Cencic, A., 2013. Skeletal muscle-derived cell cultures as potent models in regenerative medicine research. Muscle Nerve 47, 477–482.

Lovell, M.J., Mathur, A., 2011. Republished review: cardiac stem cell therapy: progress from the bench to bedside. Postgrad. Med. J. 87, 558–564. (*Useful review on the state of cardiac stem cell therapy highlighting the problems as well as the potential. Easy to read*)

Nature Reviews Drug Discovery, 2006. Vol. 5 (August) has a series of articles on nerve regeneration. (*The articles 'highlight recent progress in knowledge of the molecular, cellular and circuitry level responses to injuries to the adult mammalian CNS, with a view to understanding the underlying mechanism that will enable the development of appropriate therapeutic strategies'*)

Nishikawa, S., Goldstein, R.A., Nierras, C.R., 2008. The promise of human induced pluripotent stem cells for research and therapy. Nat. Rev. Mol. Cell Biol. 9, 725–729. (*Induced pluripotent stem cells [iPS] are human somatic cells that have reprogrammed to be pluripotent*)

Ong, J.M., da Cruz, L., 2012. A review and update on the current status of stem cell therapy and the retina. Br. Med. Bull. 102, 133–146. (*Easy to read review*)

Rosenthal, N., 2003. Prometheus's vulture and the stem-cell promise. N. Engl. J. Med. 349, 267–286. (*Excellent article on the problem of regeneration of tissues and organs*)

Slack, J.M.W., 2014. Genes. A Very Short Introduction. Oxford University Press. ISBN: 9780199603381.

Voltarelli, J.C., Couri, C.E., Stracieri, A.B., et al., 2007. Autologous nonmyeloablative hematopoietic stem cell transplantation in newly diagnosed type 1 diabetes mellitus. JAMA 297, 1568–1576. (*Successful early trial of stem cell transplantation*)

Zhang, X., Bendeck, M.P., Simmons, C.A., Santerre, J.P., 2017. Deriving vascular smooth muscle cells from mesenchymal stromal cells: evolving differentiation strategies and current understanding of their mechanisms. Biomaterials 145, 9–22.

Wilson, C., 2003. The regeneration game. New Scientist 179, 2414–2427. (*Very readable article on the possibility of regeneration of mammalian tissues and organs*)

Cellular mechanisms: host defence

OVERVIEW

Everyone has experienced an inflammatory episode at some time or other, and will be familiar with the characteristic symptoms such as redness, swelling, heat, pain and loss of function at the site of injury sometimes accompanied by fever and malaise. Inflammatory mediators are considered separately in Chapters 18 and 19; here we focus on the cellular players involved in the host defence response and explain the bare bones of this crucial and sophisticated mechanism. Understanding these cellular responses and their functions provides an essential basis for understanding the actions of anti-inflammatory and immunosuppressant drugs – a major class of therapeutic agents with multiple clinical applications (see Ch. 27).

INTRODUCTION

All living creatures are born into a world that poses a constant challenge to their physical well-being and survival. Evolution, which has equipped us with homeostatic systems that maintain a stable internal environment in the face of changing external temperatures and fluctuating supplies of food and water, has also provided us with mechanisms for combating the ever-present threat of infection and for promoting healing and restoration of normal function in the event of injury. In mammals, this function is subserved by the *innate* and *acquired* (or *adaptive*) immune systems, working together with a variety of mediators and mechanisms which, when deployed collectively, give rise to what we term the *inflammatory response*. Generally, this acts to protect us, but occasionally it goes awry, leading to a spectrum of autoimmune and inflammatory diseases which require drug therapy to restore order.

The main functions of this host inflammatory response then, are *defence* and *repair* – in other words, nothing less than the on-going biosecurity and survival of the organism. Immunodeficiency due, for example, to genetic causes (e.g. *leukocyte adhesion deficiency*), infection with organisms such as HIV, radiation overexposure or immunosuppressant drugs, is usually a life-threatening condition.

Like airport security systems in the mundane world, the body has the cellular and molecular equivalents of guards, identity checks, alarm systems and a communication network with which to summon back-up when required. It also has access to an astonishing data bank that stores precise molecular details of previous illegal intruders and prevents them from returning. This host response has two main components, which work hand-in-hand. These are:

- The *innate*, 'non-adaptive' response. This developed early in evolution and is present in virtually all

organisms. In fact, some of the key mammalian gene families and other components were first identified in plants and insects. This is the first line of defence.
- The *adaptive* immune response. This appeared much later in evolutionary terms and is found only in vertebrates. It provides the physical basis for our immunological 'memory' and is the second, and supremely effective, line of defence.

The inflammatory response

- The inflammatory response occurs in tissues following injury or exposure to a pathogen or other noxious substance.
- It usually has two components: an *innate* non-adaptive response and an *adaptive* (acquired or specific) immunological response.
- These reactions are generally protective, but if inappropriately deployed they are deleterious.
- The normal outcome of the response is healing with or without scarring; alternatively, if the underlying cause persists, chronic inflammation results.
- Many of the diseases that require drug treatment involve inflammation. Understanding the action and use of anti-inflammatory and immunosuppressive drugs necessitates understanding the inflammatory reaction.

THE INNATE IMMUNE RESPONSE

Mucosal epithelial tissues, which are exposed to the external environment, constantly secrete antibacterial proteins such as *defensins* together with a type of 'all purpose' immunoglobulin (Ig)A as a sort of pre-emptive defensive strategy, but elsewhere the innate response is activated immediately following infection or injury.[1]

PATTERN RECOGNITION

One of the most important functions of any security system is the ability to establish identity. How does an organism decide whether a cell or stray molecule is a *bona fide* citizen or an unwanted and potentially dangerous intruder? In the case of the innate response this is achieved through a network of *pattern recognition receptors* (PRRs). They recognise

---

[1]One immunologist described the innate immune response as the organism's 'knee jerk' response to infection; it is an excellent description.

The innate immune response

- The innate response occurs immediately on injury or infection. It comprises vascular and cellular elements. Mediators generated by cells or from plasma modify and regulate the magnitude of the response.
- Utilising Toll and other recognition receptors, sentinel cells in body tissues, such as macrophages, mast and dendritic cells detect specific pathogen-associated molecular patterns. This triggers the release of cytokines, particularly interleukin (IL)-1 and tumour necrosis factor (TNF)-α, as well as various chemokines.
- IL-1 and TNF-α act on local postcapillary venular endothelial cells, causing:
  - vasodilatation and fluid exudation
  - expression of adhesion molecules on the cell surfaces
- Exudate contains enzyme cascades that generate bradykinin (from kininogen), and C5a and C3a (from complement). Complement activation lyses bacteria.
- C5a and C3a stimulate mast cells to release histamine, which dilates local arterioles.
- Tissue damage and cytokines release prostaglandins PGI_2 and PGE_2 (vasodilators) and leukotriene $(LT)B_4$ (a chemotaxin).
- Cytokines stimulate synthesis of vasodilator nitric oxide, which increases vascular permeability.
- Using adhesion molecules, leukocytes roll on, adhere to and finally migrate through activated vascular endothelium towards the pathogen (attracted by chemokines, IL-8, C5a, and LTB_4), where phagocytosis and bacterial killing takes place.

pathogen-associated molecular patterns (PAMPs) – common products produced by bacteria, fungi, parasites and viruses, which they cannot readily change to evade detection. PRRs include G protein–coupled receptors such as the FPR (formyl peptide receptor) family that recognises N-formylated peptides characteristic of bacterial protein synthesis (and liberated from damaged mitochondria too), and cytoplasmic receptors such as the *NOD-like receptors* (**N**ucleotide-binding **O**ligomerization **D**omain-like receptors) – a large family of intracellular proteins that can recognise fragments of bacterial proteoglycan, as well as several other families of molecules.

Among the best-studied of these PRRs are the *Toll-like receptors* (TLRs: see Jimenez et al., 2016, for a recent review). The Toll[2] gene was first identified in *Drosophila* in the mid-1990s. Analogous genes were soon found in vertebrates and it was quickly established that as a family, their main job was to detect highly conserved components in pathogens and to signal their presence to both arms of the immune system.

---

[2]The name, which loosely translates from German as 'Great!' or 'Eureka!', has remained firmly attached to the family. Discovered in fruit fly experiments, Christiane Nüsslein-Volhard exclaimed 'Das ist ja toll!' The name has stuck since then.

Humans have a repertoire of 10 TLRs but some other animals have more. Structurally, they are transmembrane glycoproteins belonging to the *receptor tyrosine kinase* family (see Ch. 3). Phylogenetically they are highly conserved. Unlike the antigen receptors on T and B cells that develop and change through life, endowing each lymphocyte clone with a structurally unique receptor (see later), TLRs are encoded for by discrete genes in the host DNA. Table 7.1 lists these receptors and the chief pathogenic products they recognise, where these are known. There are two main types of TLR, located respectively on the cell surface and in endosomes. The latter type generally recognises pathogen RNA/DNA (presumably because they appear in phagosomes), while the former recognises other pathogen components such as cell wall material, endotoxin, etc. Some TLRs also recognise *damage associated molecular patterns* (DAMPs), substances released when host cells are damaged (e.g. heat shock proteins) thus providing an additional way of monitoring internal damage.

How a single family of receptors can recognise such a wide spectrum of different chemicals is a molecular mystery. Some act together (e.g. TLR 1, 2 and 6), in other cases they solve the problem by recruiting additional 'accessory' proteins that modulate their binding properties (e.g. TLR 4). When activated, Toll receptors dimerise and initiate complex signalling pathways that activate genes coding for proteins and factors crucial to the deployment or modulation of the inflammatory response, many of which we will discuss further. Interestingly from the pharmacological viewpoint, TLR 7 also recognises some synthetic antiviral compounds such as *imidazoquinolones*. The ability of these drugs to provoke TLR activation probably underlies their clinical effectiveness (see Ch. 53).

TLRs are strategically located on 'sentinel' cells – those likely to come into early contact with invaders. These include *macrophages* as well as *mast cells* and (crucially) *dendritic cells*, which are especially abundant in skin and other inside–outside interfaces, as well as some *intestinal epithelial cells* that are exposed to pathogens in the food that we eat. Genetic defects in the TLR system have been observed. These can lead to an inability to mount an effective host defence response or sometimes to a constitutively active inflammatory response.

Having outlined how 'non-self' pathogens are detected by the innate immune system, we can now describe the events that follow the 'raising of the alarm'.

RESPONSES TO PATTERN RECOGNITION

Vascular events

Interaction of a PAMP with TLRs triggers the sentinel cells to respond by producing a range of pro-inflammatory polypeptides called *cytokines*, including *tumour necrosis factor (TNF)-α* and *interleukin (IL)-1*. The maturation and processing of IL-1 (and some other cytokines) is managed by *inflammasomes*, intracellular multiprotein complexes that vary according to the type of inflammatory stimulus. The inflammasome thus initiates a precisely tailored inflammatory response appropriate to the situation (see Yang et al., 2015, for a recent overview).

Also released, either as a direct consequence of tissue damage or following cytokine stimulation, are lower molecular-weight inflammatory mediators (such as prostaglandins and histamine). These act on the vascular endothelial cells of the postcapillary venules, causing expression of *adhesion molecules* on the intimal surface and an

Table 7.1 The human toll-like receptor (TLR) family of pattern recognition receptors (PRRs)

PRR	Pathogen or endogenous product recognised	Ligand	Sites of expression	Location
TLR 2 (usually acting together with **TLR 1**, **TLR 6** and possibly **TLR 10**)	Bacteria (Gm pos) *Mycoplasma* Parasites Yeast Damaged host cells	Lipoproteins Lipoteichoic acid GPI anchors Cell wall carbohydrates Heat shock proteins	Monocyte/macrophages Some dendritic cells B lymphocytes Mast cells	Surface
TLR 4[a]	Bacteria (Gm neg) Virus Damaged host cells	Lipopolysaccharide Some viral proteins Heat shock proteins Fibrinogen Hyaluronic acid	Monocyte/macrophages Some dendritic cells Mast cells Intestinal epithelium	
TLR 5	Bacteria	Flagellin	Monocyte/macrophages Some dendritic cells Intestinal epithelium	
TLR 3	Virus	Viral dsRNA	Dendritic cells B lymphocytes	Intracellular (endosomal)
TLR 7	Virus	Viral ssRNA Some synthetic drugs	Monocyte/macrophages	
TLR 8	Virus	Viral ssRNA	Mast cells	
TLR 9	Bacteria	Bacterial CpG containing Bacterial DNA Self DNA	B lymphocytes	

[a]Operates in conjunction with MD-2 (lymphocyte antigen 96, a lipopolysaccharide binding protein).
CpG DNA, unmethylated CG dinucleotide; *Gm neg/pos*, Gram-negative/positive (bacteria); *GPI*, glycosylphosphatidylinositol anchoring proteins; *ssRNA*, single-stranded RNA; *dsRNA*, double-stranded RNA.

increase in vascular permeability (which allows immune cells to pass from the blood to the affected tissue).

Leukocytes adhere to the endothelial cells through interactions between their cell surface *integrins* and adhesion molecules on endothelial cells, and this halts their flow through the microcirculation. They are then able to migrate out of the vessels, attracted by *chemotaxins* generated by the microorganisms themselves or as a result of their interaction with the tissues. Polypeptide *chemokines* released during TLR activation play an important part in this. (Cytokines and chemokines are considered separately in Ch. 19.)

The initial vascular events also include dilatation of the small arterioles, resulting in increased blood flow. This is followed by a slowing (and sometimes a cessation) of blood flow and an increase in the permeability of the postcapillary venules allowing exudation of fluid. This vasodilatation is brought about by mediators, including histamine, prostaglandin (PG)E$_2$ and PGI$_2$ (prostacyclin) released from injured cells, some of which act together with cytokines to increase vascular permeability.

The resulting fluid exudate contains the components for four proteolytic enzyme cascades: the *complement system*, the *coagulation system*, the *fibrinolytic system* and the *kinin system* (Fig. 7.1). The components of these cascades are inactive proteases that are activated by cleavage, each activated component then activating the next.

▼ The *complement system* comprises nine major components, designated C1 to C9. Activation of the cascade is initiated by substances derived from microorganisms, such as yeast cell walls or endotoxins. This pathway of activation is termed the *alternative pathway* (see Fig. 7.1) as opposed to the *classic pathway*, which is dealt with later. One of the main events is the enzymatic splitting of C3, giving rise to various peptides, one of which, *C3a* (termed an *anaphylatoxin*), stimulates mast cells to secrete further chemical mediators and can also directly stimulate smooth muscle, while *C3b* (termed an *opsonin*) attaches to the surface of a microorganism, facilitating ingestion by phagocytes. *C5a*, generated enzymatically from C5, also releases mediators from mast cells and is a powerful chemotactic attractant and activator of leukocytes.

The final components in the sequence, complement-derived mediators (C5 to C9), coalesce to form a *membrane attack complex* that can attach to certain bacterial membranes, leading to lysis. Complement can therefore mediate the destruction of invading bacteria or damage multicellular parasites; however, it may sometimes cause injury to the host. The principal enzymes of the coagulation and fibrinolytic cascades, thrombin and plasmin, can also activate the cascade by hydrolysing C3, as can enzymes released from leukocytes.

The *coagulation system* and the *fibrinolytic system* are described in Chapter 25. Factor XII is activated to XIIa (e.g. by collagen), and the end product, fibrin, laid down during a host–pathogen interaction, may also serve to limit the extent of the infection. Thrombin is additionally involved in the activation of the kinin (see Fig. 7.1) and, indirectly, the fibrinolytic systems (see Ch. 25).

The *kinin system* is another enzyme cascade relevant to inflammation. It yields several pro-inflammatory and pain-producing mediators, in particular bradykinin (see Fig. 7.1).

Eventually, the exudate drains through the lymphatics to local lymph nodes or lymphoid tissue, where the products of the invading microorganism trigger the adaptive phase of the response.

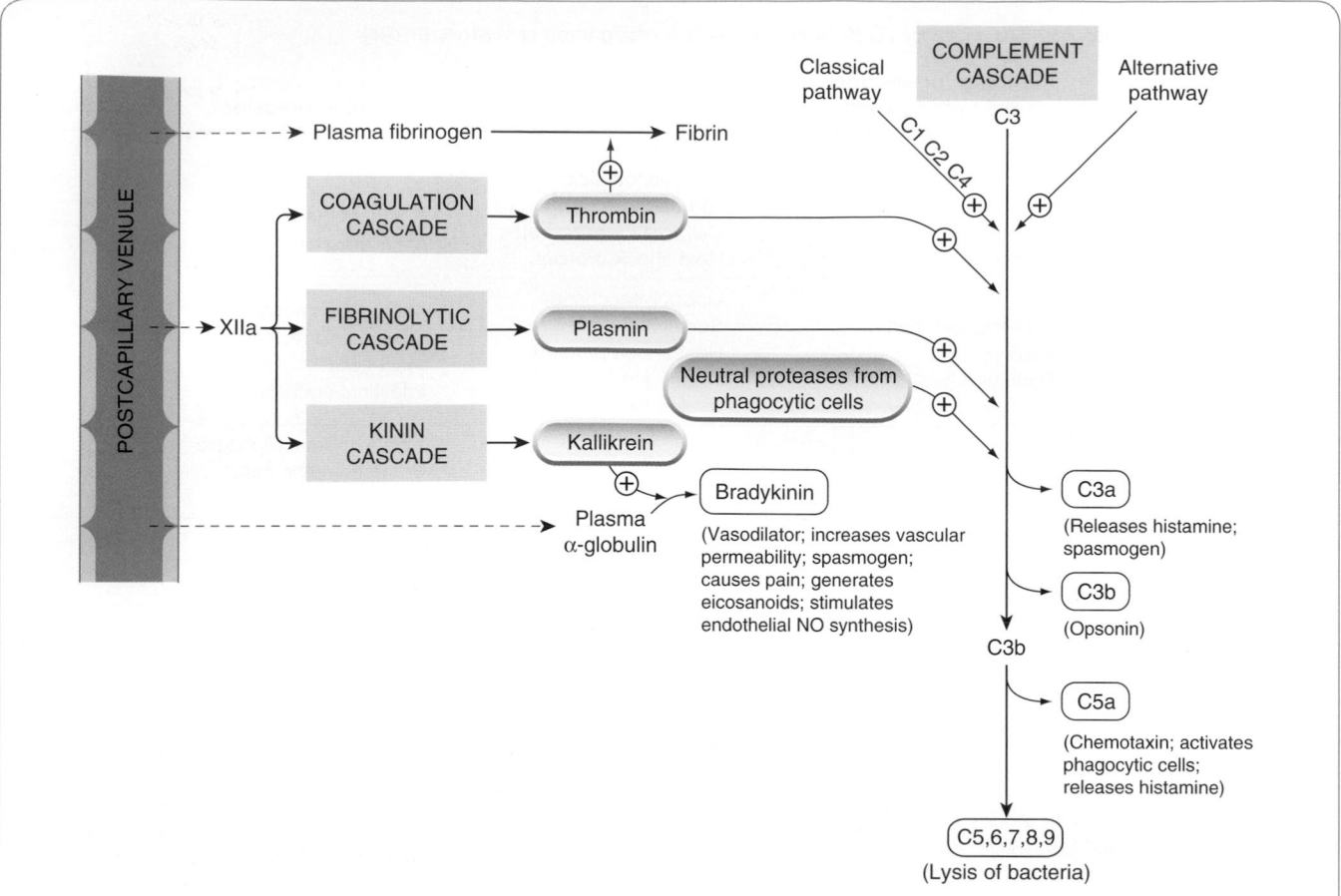

Fig. 7.1 Four enzyme cascades are activated when plasma leaks out into the tissues as a result of the increased vascular permeability of inflammation. Factors causing exudation are depicted in Fig. 7.2. Mediators generated are shown in *red-bordered boxes*. Complement components are indicated by C1, C2, etc. When plasmin is formed, it tends to increase kinin formation and decrease the coagulation cascade. XIIa, Factor XIIa, see text. (Adapted from Dale, M.M., Foreman, J.C., Fan, T-P. (eds), 1994. Textbook of Immunopharmacology. 3rd ed. Blackwell Scientific, Oxford.)

Cellular events

Of the cells involved in inflammation, some (e.g. vascular endothelial cells, mast cells, dendritic cells and tissue macrophages) are normally present in tissues, while other actively motile cells (e.g. leukocytes) gain access from the circulating blood.

Polymorphonuclear leukocytes

Neutrophil polymorphs – the 'shock troops' of inflammation – are the first blood leukocytes to enter an infected or damaged tissue (Fig. 7.2). The whole process is cleverly choreographed: under direct observation, the neutrophils may be seen first to *roll* along the activated endothelium, then to *adhere* and finally to *migrate* out of the blood vessel and into the extravascular space. This process is regulated by the successive activation of different families of adhesion molecules (*selectins, intercellular adhesion molecule* [ICAM] and *integrins*) on the inflamed endothelium that engage corresponding *counter-ligands* on the neutrophil, capturing it as it rolls along the surface, stabilising its interaction with the endothelial cells and enabling it to migrate out of the vessel (using a further adhesion molecule termed *PECAM*, **P**latelet **E**ndothelial **C**ell **A**dhesion **M**olecule). The neutrophil is attracted to the invading pathogen by chemicals termed *chemotaxins*, some of which (such as the tripeptide formyl-Met-Leu-Phe) are released by the microorganism,

whereas others, such as C5a, are produced locally or in some cases released (e.g. chemokines such as IL-8), from nearby cells such as macrophages.

Neutrophils can engulf, kill and digest microorganisms. Together with eosinophils, they have surface receptors for C3b, which acts as an *opsonin* that forms a link between neutrophil and invading bacterium (an even more effective link may be made by antibodies.) Neutrophils kill microorganisms by internalising them into internal vacuoles. An NADPH oxidase enzyme on the leukocyte surface regulates ion transport such that the pH of the normally acidic vacuole is raised and optimal enzymatic digestion of the organism by neutral proteases can occur. Toxic oxygen radicals are also produced by this enzyme but it is now believed that these are less important in microbial killing (see Segal, 2016). However, if the neutrophil is inappropriately activated, these biochemical weapons may be turned inadvertently on the host's tissues, causing damage. When neutrophils have exhausted their potential, they undergo apoptosis and are cleared by phagocytic macrophages. It is this mass of live and apoptotic neutrophils that constitutes 'pus'.

Mast cells

Important 'sentinel' cells that express TLRs, mast cells also have surface receptors both for IgE and for the complement-derived *anaphylatoxins* C3a and C5a. Ligands acting at these

Fig. 7.2 Simplified diagram of the events leading up to polymorphonuclear leukocyte (PMN) migration in a local acute inflammatory reaction. In response to activation of pattern recognition receptors, tissue macrophages release the pro-inflammatory cytokines interleukin (IL)-1 and tumour necrosis factor (TNF)-α. These act on the endothelial cells of postcapillary venules, causing exudation of fluid and expression of adhesion factors that recognise counter-ligands on blood-borne neutrophils. Free flowing neutrophils in the blood are first 'captured' by *selectins* on activated endothelial cells. These cells then roll along the endothelium before their progress is arrested by the action of *integrins* and they adhere to the vessel wall. The activated cells then 'crawl' along the endothelium until they find a suitable site for transmigration. In a minority of cases, neutrophils can actually move through endothelial cells (*transcellular transmigration*) but they mainly migrate through the junction between endothelial cells (*paracellular transmigration*). Further adhesion molecules then guide the cell through the gaps. The migrating cells must also migrate through gaps in the layer of pericytes (contractile cells) that surround the venules as well as the basement membrane (comprised of connective tissue). Chemotactic gradients formed by the release of substances released by or from the pathogen guide the cell to its target where it can kill and/or phagocytose the invader. Neutrophils characteristically die after this event, in which case they enter apoptosis and are phagocytosed by macrophages, resolving the inflammatory event. *Photo inset:* Photomicrograph of a normal, un-inflamed microcirculation in the mesenteric bed of mouse *(left-hand panel)* and following a period of inflammation *(right-hand panel).* The arrows indicate neutrophils adhering to the endothelium as well as some that have already transmigrated. (Diagram modified from Nourshargh et al., 2010. Picture courtesy Drs S. Yazid, G. Leoni and D. Cooper.)

receptors trigger mediator release, as does direct physical damage. One of the main substances released is *histamine*; others include *heparin, leukotrienes, PGD₂, platelet-activating factor (PAF), nerve growth factor* and some *interleukins* and proteases. Unusually, mast cells have preformed packets of cytokines that they can release instantaneously (by Ca^{2+}-mediated exocytosis, Ch. 4) when stimulated. This makes them extremely effective triggers of the inflammatory response.

Monocytes/macrophages
Monocytes follow polymorphs into inflammatory lesions after a delay (sometimes several hours). Adhesion to endothelium and migration into the tissue follow a similar pattern of adhesive molecule binding to that seen with neutrophils, although monocyte chemotaxis utilises additional chemokines, such as MCP-1[3] (which, reasonably

enough, stands for **M**onocyte **C**hemoattractant **P**rotein-1) and RANTES (which very *unreasonably* stands for **R**egulated on **A**ctivation **N**ormal **T** cell **E**xpressed and **S**ecreted; immunological nomenclature has excelled itself here!).

Once in tissues, blood monocytes differentiate into *macrophages.*[4] The newly differentiated cell may acquire an *M1* or an *M2 phenotype*, depending upon the types of cytokines it secretes. The former is generally regarded as a pro-inflammatory cell, whereas the latter is probably more involved in tissue repair and healing (although this simplistic distinction is currently a subject of debate: see Martinez & Gordon, 2014). Macrophages therefore have a remarkable range of abilities, being not only a jack-of-all-trades but also a master of many.

Activation of monocyte/macrophage TLRs stimulates the generation and release of chemokines and other cytokines that act on vascular endothelial cells, attract other leukocytes to the area and give rise to systemic manifestations of the

[3]Human immunodeficiency virus-1 binds to the surface CD4 glycoprotein on monocytes/macrophages but is able to penetrate the cell only after binding also to MCP-1 and RANTES receptors. This is a case where the innate immune system inadvertently aids the enemy.

[4]Literally 'big eaters', compared with neutrophils, originally called *microphages* or 'little eaters'.

inflammatory response such as fever (many of these inflammatory mediators have pyrogenic properties). Macrophages engulf tissue debris and dead cells, as well as phagocytosing and killing most (but unfortunately not all) microorganisms. They also play an important part in *antigen presentation*. When stimulated by glucocorticoids, macrophages also secrete *annexin 1* (a potent anti-inflammatory polypeptide; see Ch. 34), which controls the development of the local inflammatory reaction helping to limit any collateral damage.

Dendritic cells

These are present in many tissues, especially those that subserve a barrier function (e.g. the skin, where they are sometimes referred to as *Langerhans cells* after their discoverer). As a key 'sentinel cell' they can detect the presence of pathogens and when thus activated they can migrate into lymphoid tissue, where they play an crucial part in antigen presentation.

Eosinophils

These cells have similar capacities to neutrophils but, like mast cells, are also 'armed' with a battery of substances stored in their granules, which, when released, kill multicellular parasites (e.g. helminths). These include *eosinophil cationic protein*, a *peroxidase* enzyme, the *eosinophil major basic protein* and a *neurotoxin*. The eosinophil is considered by many to be of primary importance in the pathogenesis of the late phase of asthma where, it is suggested, secreted granule proteins cause damage to bronchiolar epithelium (see Fig. 29.4).

Basophils

Basophils are very similar in many respects to mast cells. Except in certain inflammatory diseases, such as viral infections and myeloproliferative disorders, the basophil content of the tissues is generally tiny and in health they form only <0.1% of circulating white blood cells.

Vascular endothelial cells

Vascular endothelial cells (see also Chs 23 and 24), originally considered as passive lining cells, are now known to play an active part in inflammation. Small arteriole endothelial cells secrete nitric oxide (NO), causing relaxation of the underlying smooth muscle (see Ch. 21), vasodilatation and increased delivery of plasma and blood cells to the inflamed area. The endothelial cells of the postcapillary venules regulate plasma exudation and thus the delivery of plasma-derived mediators (see Fig. 7.1). Vascular endothelial cells express several adhesion molecules (the ICAM and selectin families; see Fig. 7.2), as well as a variety of receptors, including those for histamine, acetylcholine and IL-1. In addition to NO, the cells can synthesise and release the vasodilator agents PGI_2 and PGE_2, the vasoconstrictor agent endothelin, plasminogen activator, PAF and several cytokines. Endothelial cells also participate in the angiogenesis that occurs during inflammatory resolution, chronic inflammation and cancer (see Chs 6, 7 and 57).

Platelets

Platelets are involved primarily in coagulation and thrombotic phenomena (see Ch. 25) but also play a part in inflammation. They have low-affinity receptors for IgE, and may contribute to the first phase of allergic asthma (Fig. 29.1). In addition to generating thromboxane (TX)A_2

and PAF, they can generate free radicals and pro-inflammatory cationic proteins. Platelet-derived growth factor contributes to the repair processes that follow inflammatory responses or damage to blood vessels.

Natural killer cells

Natural killer (NK) cells are a specialised type of lymphocyte. In an unusual twist to the receptor concept, NK cells kill targets (e.g. virus-infected or tumour cells) that lack ligands for inhibitory receptors on the NK cells themselves. These ligands are known as *major histocompatibility complex* (MHC) molecules, and any cells lacking these become a target for NK-cell attack, a strategy sometimes called the 'mother turkey strategy'.[5] MHC proteins are expressed on the surface of most host cells and, in simple terms, are specific for that individual, enabling the NK cells to avoid damaging their host's cells. NK cells have other functions: they are equipped with Fc receptors and, in the presence of antibodies directed against a target cell, they can kill the cell by antibody-dependent cellular cytotoxicity.

THE ADAPTIVE IMMUNE RESPONSE

The adaptive response provides the cellular basis for an 'immunological memory'. It provides a more powerful defence than the innate response, as well as being highly specific for the invading pathogen. Here we will provide only a simplified outline, stressing those aspects relevant for an understanding of drug action; for more detailed coverage, see textbooks in the References and Further Reading section at the end of this chapter.

The key cells are the *lymphocytes*[6]. These are long-lived cells derived from precursor stem cells within the bone marrow. Following release into the blood and maturation, they dwell in the lymphoid tissues such as the lymph nodes and spleen. Here, they are poised to detect, intercept and identify foreign proteins presented to them by *antigen-presenting cells* (APCs) such as the macrophage or the dendritic cells. The three main groups of lymphocytes are:

- *B cells*, which mature in the bone marrow. They are responsible for antibody production, i.e. the *humoral* immune response.
- *T cells*, which mature in the thymus. They are important in the induction phase of the immune response and in *cell-mediated* immune reactions.
- *NK cells*. These are really part of the innate system. They are activated by *interferons* and release cytotoxic granules that destroy target cells identified as 'foreign' or abnormal.

▼ Fig. 7.3 shows how these cells arise. APCs ingest and process antigen (*A–D*) and present fragments to naive, uncommitted CD4 T cells in conjunction with MHC class II molecules, or to naive CD8 T

[5]Richard Dawkins in *River Out of Eden*, citing the zoologist Schliedt, explains that the 'rule of thumb a mother turkey uses to recognise nest robbers is a dismayingly brusque one; in the vicinity of the nest, attack anything that moves unless it makes a noise like a baby turkey'.
[6]White blood cells (WBC) or leukocytes in blood are mostly neutrophils (50%–60%) or lymphocytes (20%–40%), with the rest being monocytes (3%–7%), eosinophils (1%–5%) and less than 1% basophils. The WBC count in a healthy adult is in the range 3.5–11 million per mL of blood – higher values may indicate chronic bacterial or viral infection; lower levels occur in anaemia or in immunosuppressed individuals (e.g. when undergoing treatment with chemotherapeutic drugs [see Ch. 57]).

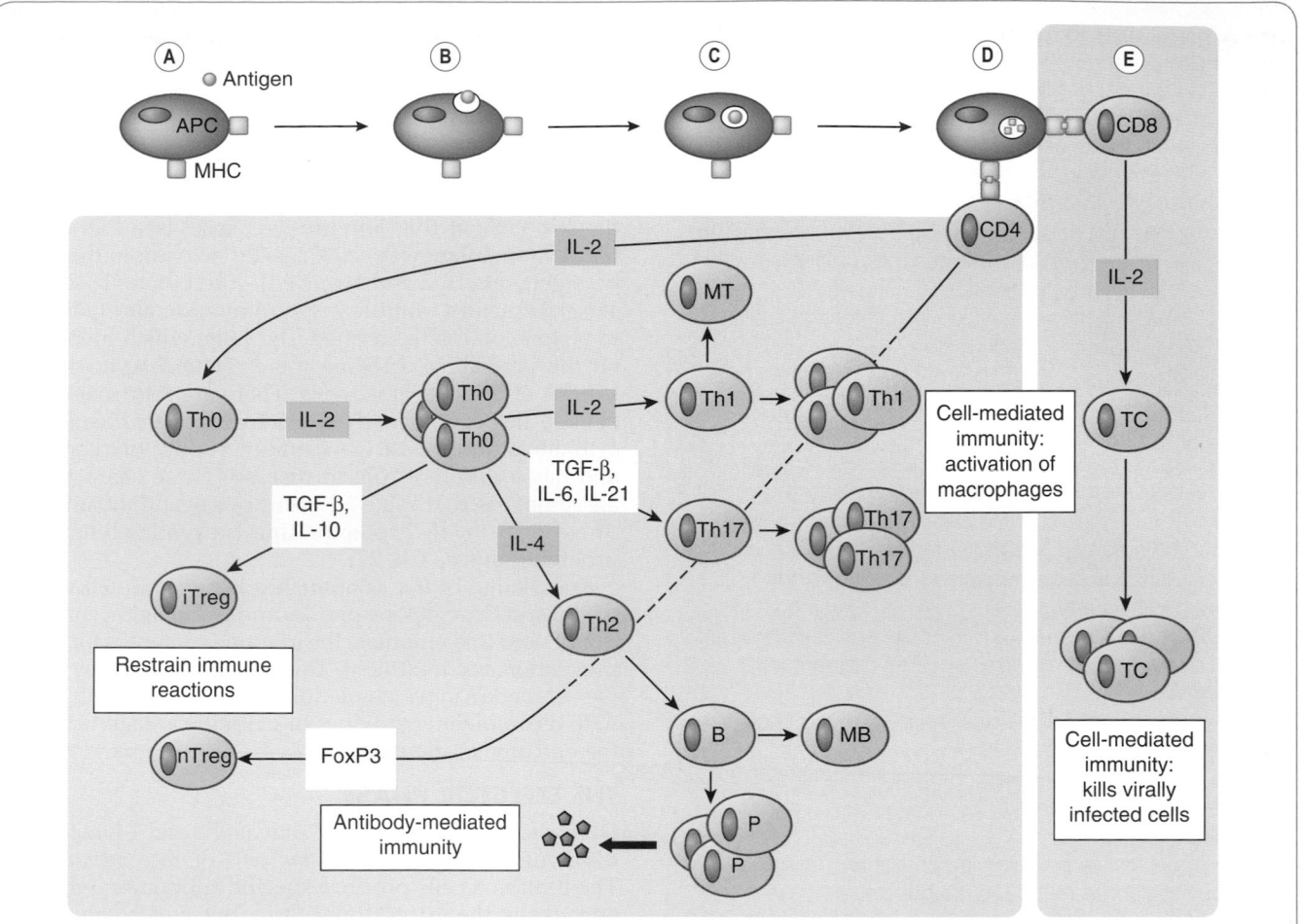

Fig. 7.3 Simplified diagram of the induction and effector phases of lymphocyte activation. See text for details. *MT*, memory T cell; *MB*, memory B cell; *TC*, cytotoxic T cell; *P*, plasma cell; *Treg*, regulatory T cell.

cells in conjunction with MHC class I molecules, thus 'arming' them. The armed CD4+ T cells synthesise and express IL-2 receptors and release this cytokine, which stimulates the cells by autocrine action, causing generation and proliferation of T-helper zero (Th0) cells. Autocrine cytokines (e.g. IL-4) cause differentiation of some Th0 cells to give Th2 cells, which are responsible for the development of antibody-mediated immune responses. These Th2 (and sometimes Th1) cells cooperate with and activate B cells to proliferate and give rise eventually to memory B cells (MB) and plasma cells (P), which secrete antibodies. The T cells that aid B cells in this way are referred to as T_{FH} (follicular homing) cells. Further stimulation by autocrine cytokines (e.g. IL-2,6) cause proliferation of Th0 cells to give Th1, Th17 or iTreg cells. Th1 and Th17 cells secrete cytokines that activate macrophages (responsible for some cell-mediated immune reactions). iTreg (inducible Treg derived from Th0 precursors) and nTreg (naturally occurring Treg matured in the thymus) cells restrain and inhibit the development of the immune response, thus preventing autoimmunity and excessive immune activation. The armed CD8+ T cells (E) also synthesise and express IL-2 receptors and release IL-2, which stimulates the cells by autocrine action to proliferate and give rise to cytotoxic T cells (TC). These can kill virally infected cells. IL-2 secreted by CD4+ cells also plays a part in stimulating CD8+ cells to proliferate. Note that the 'effector phase' depicted above relates to the 'protective' action of the immune response. When the response is inappropriately deployed – as in chronic inflammatory conditions such as rheumatoid arthritis – the Th1/Th17 component of the immune response is dominant and the activated macrophages release IL-1 and TNF-α, which in turn trigger the release of the chemokines and inflammatory cytokines that play a major role in the pathology of the disease.

T and B lymphocytes express antigen-specific receptors that recognise and react with virtually all foreign proteins and polysaccharides that we are likely to encounter during our lifetime. This receptor repertoire is generated randomly and so could recognise 'self' proteins as well as foreign antigens, with devastating results. However, *tolerance* to self-antigens is acquired during fetal life by apoptotic deletion of T-cell clones in the thymus that recognise the host's own tissues. Dendritic cells and macrophages involved in the innate response also have a role in preventing harmful immune reactions against the host's own cells.

The adaptive immune response occurs in two phases, termed the *induction phase* and the *effector phase*.

THE INDUCTION PHASE

During the induction phase, antigen is 'presented' to T cells in the lymph nodes by macrophages or large dendritic cells. This antigen may constitute part of an invading pathogen (e.g. the coat of a bacterium) or be released by such an organism (e.g. a bacterial toxin), or it may be a vaccine, an environmental agent such as pollen, an insect bite, a foodstuff or a substance introduced experimentally to study the immune response (e.g. the injection of egg albumin into the guinea pig). APCs ingest and proteolytically 'process' the antigen and once they reach local lymph nodes, they 'present' the fragments on their surface to lymphocytes

The adaptive response

- The adaptive (specific, acquired) immunological response boosts the effectiveness of the innate responses. It has two phases, the induction phase and the effector phase, the latter consisting of (i) antibody-mediated and (ii) cell-mediated components.
- During the *induction phase*, naive T cells bearing either the CD4 or the CD8 co-receptors are presented with antigen, triggering proliferation:
  - CD8-bearing T cells develop into cytotoxic T cells that can kill virally infected cells
  - CD4-bearing T-helper (Th) cells are stimulated by different cytokines to develop into Th1, Th2, Th17 or Treg cells
  - *Th1* cells develop into cells that release cytokines that activate macrophages; these cells, along with cytotoxic T cells, control cell-mediated responses
  - *Th2* cells control antibody-mediated responses by stimulating B cells to proliferate, giving rise to antibody-secreting plasma cells and memory cells
  - *Th17* cells are similar to Th1 cells and are important in some human diseases such as rheumatoid arthritis
  - *Treg* cells restrain the development of the immune response.
- The effector phase utilises both antibody- and cell-mediated responses.
- Antibodies provide:
  - more selective complement activation
  - more effective pathogen phagocytosis
  - more effective attachment to multicellular parasites, facilitating their destruction
  - direct neutralisation of some viruses and of some bacterial toxins.
- Cell-mediated reactions provide:
  - CD8$^+$ cytotoxic T cells that kill virus-infected cells
  - cytokine-releasing CD4$^+$ T cells that enable macrophages to kill intracellular pathogens such as the tubercle bacillus
  - memory cells primed to react rapidly to a known antigen
  - help for B-cell activation.
- Inappropriately deployed immune reactions are termed *hypersensitivity reactions*.
- Anti-inflammatory and immunosuppressive drugs are used when the normally protective inflammatory and/or immune responses escape control.

in combination with various *MHC* molecules. This is followed by complex interactions of those T cells with B cells and other T cells (Fig. 7.4). Two types of lymphocytes 'attend' APCs. They are generally distinguished by the presence, on their surface, of *CD4* or *CD8* receptors. These are *co-receptors* that cooperate with the main antigen-specific receptors in antigen recognition. Macrophages also carry surface CD4 proteins.

The two types of lymphocyte involved in the adaptive response are:

- Uncommitted (naive) CD4$^+$ T-helper (Th) lymphocytes, or T-helper precursor (Thp) cells, in association with class II MHC molecules (see Fig. 7.4).
- Naive CD8$^+$ T lymphocytes in association with class I MHC molecules.[7]

Activation of a T cell by an APC requires that several 'identification' and 'authentication' signals pass between the two cells at this 'immune synapse' (see Fig. 7.4; see Medzhitov & Janeway, 2000). After activation, the T cells both generate IL-2 and acquire IL-2 receptors. IL-2 has an *autocrine*[8] action, stimulating proliferation and giving rise to a clone of T cells, termed *Th0* cells, which, depending on the prevailing cytokine milieu, give rise to different subsets of armed helper cells. There are four major types of these 'helper cells', each of which generates a characteristic cytokine profile, possesses a unique surface marker profile and has a different role in disease. These characteristics are summarised in Table 7.2. Some potent anti-inflammatory drugs block the IL-2 receptor, thus preventing lymphocyte proliferation (see Ch. 27).

Knowledge of the relationship between T-cell subsets, their respective cytokine profiles and pathological conditions can be used to manipulate the immune responses for disease prevention and treatment. There are already many experimental models in which modulation of the Th1/Th2 balance with recombinant cytokines or cytokine antagonists alters the outcome of the disease.

THE EFFECTOR PHASE

During the effector phase, the activated B and T lymphocytes differentiate either into *plasma cells* or into *memory cells*. The B plasma cells produce specific antibodies, which are effective in the extracellular fluid, but which cannot neutralise pathogens within cells. T-cell-mediated immune mechanisms overcome this problem by activating macrophages or directly killing virus-infected host cells. Antigen-sensitive *memory cells* are formed when the clone of lymphocytes that are programmed to respond to an antigen is greatly expanded after the first contact with the organism. They allow a greatly accelerated and more effective response to subsequent antigen exposure. In some cases, the response is so rapid and efficient that, after one exposure, the pathogen can never gain a foothold again. Vaccination and immunisation procedures make use of this invaluable phenomenon.

THE ANTIBODY-MEDIATED (HUMORAL) RESPONSE

There are five main classes of antibody – IgG, IgM, IgE, IgA and IgD – which differ from each other in certain structural respects. All are *γ-globulins* (immunoglobulins), which both recognise and interact specifically with antigens (i.e. proteins or polysaccharides foreign to the host), as well as activating one or more further components of the host's defence systems.

---

[7]The main reason that it is difficult to transplant organs such as kidneys from one person to another is that their respective MHC molecules are different. Lymphocytes in the recipient will react to non-self (*allogenic*) MHC molecules in the donor tissue, which is then likely to be rejected by a rapid and powerful immunological reaction.

[8]In 'autocrine' signalling the mediator acts on the cell that released it. In 'paracrine' signalling, the mediator acts on neighbouring cells, whilst in 'juxtacrine' signalling, it acts on cells in direct contact.

Fig. 7.4 **The activation of a T cell by an antigen-presenting cell (APC).** (A) The APC encounters a foreign protein and this is proteolytically processed into peptide fragments. The activation process then involves three stages: (i) Interaction between the complex of pathogen-derived antigen peptide fragments with major histocompatibility complex (MHC) class II and the antigen-specific receptor on the T cell; (B) (ii) Interaction between the CD4 co-receptor on the T cell and an MHC molecule on the APC; (iii) The B7 protein on the APC cell surface binds to CD28 on the T cell providing a co-stimulatory signal. The CD4 co-receptor, together with a T-cell chemokine receptor, constitute the main binding sites for the HIV virus (see Fig. 53.3).

Table 7.2 **Lymphocyte subsets, their role in host defence and relationship to inflammatory disease**

Subset	Cytokine trigger	Main role in adaptive response	Main cytokines produced	Role in disease
Th0	IL-2	Precursor cells for further differentiation	—	—
Th1	IL-2	'Cell-mediated immunity' • Cytokines released from these cells: activate macrophages to phagocytose and kill microorganisms and kill tumour cells; drive proliferation and maturation of the clone into *cytotoxic T cells* that kill virally infected host cells; reciprocally inhibit Th2 cell maturation	IFN-γ, IL-2 and TNF-α	Insulin-dependent diabetes mellitus (Ch. 32), multiple sclerosis, *Helicobacter pylori*-induced peptic ulcer (Ch. 31), aplastic anaemia (Ch. 26) and rheumatoid arthritis (Ch. 27). Allograft rejection
Th2	IL-4	'Humoral immunity' • Cytokines released from these cells: stimulate B cells to proliferate and mature into plasma cells producing antibodies; enhance differentiation and activation of eosinophils and reciprocally inhibit Th1/Th17-cell functions. For this reason, they are often thought of as having a predominately anti-inflammatory action.	IL-4, IL-5, TGF-β, IL-10 and IL-13	Asthma (Ch. 29) and allergy. AIDS progression is associated with loss of Th1 cells and is facilitated by Th2 responses
Th17	TGF-β, IL-6 and IL-21	A specialised type of Th1 cell	IL-17	The response to infection, organ-specific immune responses and in the pathogenesis of diseases such as rheumatoid arthritis and multiple sclerosis
Treg[a]	IL-10 and TGF-β or FOX P3 Matured in the thymus	Restraining the immune response, preventing autoimmunity and curtailing potentially damaging inflammatory responses	IL-10 and TGF-β	Failure of this mechanism can provoke excessive inflammation

[a]Two populations are commonly encountered: inducible (iTreg) and naturally occurring Treg cells (nTreg).
IFN, interferon; *IL*, interleukin; *TGF*, transforming growth factor; *TNF*, tumour necrosis factor.

▼ An antibody is a Y-shaped protein molecule (see Ch. 5) in which the arms of the Y (the **A**ntigen **B**inding **F**ragment - *Fab* portion) include a variable recognition site for specific antigens, and the invariable stem of the Y (the '**C**onstant' *Fc* portion) activates host defences. The B cells that are responsible for antibody production recognise foreign molecules by means of surface receptors that are similar to the immunoglobulin that the B-cell clone will eventually produce. Mammals harbour a vast number of B-cell clones that produce different antibodies with recognition sites for different antigens.

The induction of antibody-mediated responses varies with the type of antigen. With most antigens, a cooperative process between Th2 cells and B cells is generally necessary to produce a response. B cells can also present antigen to T cells which then release cytokines that act further on the B cell. The anti-inflammatory glucocorticoids (see Chs 27 and 34) and the immunosuppressive drug **ciclosporin** (see Ch. 27) affect the molecular events crucial to induction. The cytotoxic immunosuppressive drugs (see Ch. 27) inhibit the proliferation of both B and T cells. Eicosanoids may play a part in controlling these processes as prostaglandins of the E series can inhibit lymphocyte proliferation, probably by inhibiting the release of IL-2.

As you might guess, the ability to make antibodies has huge survival value; children born without this ability[9] suffer repeated infections such as pneumonia, skin infections and tonsillitis. Before the days of antibiotics, they died in early childhood, and even today they require regular replacement therapy with immunoglobulin. Apart from their ability to neutralise pathogens, antibodies can boost the effectiveness and specificity of the host's defence reaction in several ways.

Antibodies and complement
Formation of the antigen–antibody complex exposes a binding site for complement on the Fc domain. This activates the complement sequence and sets in train its attendant biological effects (see Fig. 7.1). This route to C3 activation (the *classic pathway*) provides an especially selective way of activating complement in response to a particular pathogen, because the antigen–antibody reaction that initiates it is not only a highly specific recognition event, but also occurs in close association with the pathogen. The lytic property of complement can be used therapeutically: monoclonal antibodies (mAbs) and complement together can be used to rid bone marrow of cancer cells as an adjunct to chemotherapy or radiotherapy (see Ch. 57).

Antibodies and the phagocytosis of bacteria
When antibodies are attached to their antigens on microorganisms by their Fab portions, the Fc domain is exposed. Phagocytic cells (neutrophils and macrophages) express surface receptors for these projecting Fc portions, which serve as a very specific link between microorganism and phagocyte.

Antibodies and cellular toxicity
In some cases, for example, with parasitic worms, the invader may be too large to be ingested by phagocytes. Antibody molecules can form a link between parasite and the host's white cells (in this case, eosinophils), which are then able to damage or kill the parasite. NK cells in conjunction with Fc receptors can also kill antibody-coated target cells (an example of *antibody-dependent cell-mediated cytotoxicity*; ADCC).

Antibodies and mast cells or basophils
Mast cells and basophils have receptors for IgE, a particular form of antibody that can attach ('fix') to their cell membranes. When this cell-fixed antibody reacts with an antigen, an entire panoply of pharmacologically active mediators is secreted. This very complex reaction is found widely throughout the animal kingdom and presumably confers clear survival value to the host. Having said that, its precise biological significance is not always entirely clear, although it may be of importance in association with eosinophil activity as a defence against parasitic worms. When inappropriately triggered by substances not inherently damaging to the host, it is implicated in certain types of allergic reaction and seemingly contributes more to illness than to survival in the modern world.

THE CELL-MEDIATED IMMUNE RESPONSE
Cytotoxic T cells (derived from CD8[+] cells) and inflammatory (cytokine-releasing) Th1 cells are attracted to inflammatory sites in a similar manner to neutrophils and macrophages, and are involved in cell-mediated responses (see Fig. 7.3).

Cytotoxic T cells
Armed cytotoxic T cells kill intracellular microorganisms such as viruses. When a virus infects a mammalian cell, there are two aspects to the resulting defensive response. The first step is the expression on the cell surface of peptides derived from the pathogen in association with MHC molecules. The second step is the recognition of the peptide–MHC complex by specific receptors on cytotoxic (CD8[+]) T cells (Fig. 7.4 shows a similar process for a CD4[+] T cell). The cytotoxic T cells then destroy virus-infected cells by programming them to undergo apoptosis. Cooperation with macrophages may be required for killing to occur.

Macrophage activating CD4[+] Th1 cells
Some pathogens (e.g. *Mycobacteria*, *Listeria*) survive and actually multiply within macrophages after ingestion. Armed CD4[+] Th1 cells release cytokines that activate macrophages to kill these intracellular pathogens. Th1 cells also recruit macrophages by releasing cytokines that act on vascular endothelial cells (e.g. TNF-α) and chemokines (e.g. *macrophage chemotactic factor-1; MCP-1*) that attract the macrophages to the sites of infection.

A complex of microorganism-derived peptides plus MHC molecules is expressed on the macrophage surface and is recognised by cytokine-releasing Th1 cells, which then generate cytokines that enable the macrophage to deploy its killing mechanisms. Activated macrophages (with or without intracellular pathogens) are veritable factories for the production of chemical mediators: they can generate and secrete not only many cytokines but also toxic oxygen metabolites and neutral proteases that kill extracellular organisms (e.g. *Pneumocystis jiroveci* and helminths), complement components, eicosanoids, NO, a fibroblast-stimulating factor, pyrogens and the 'tissue factor' that initiates the extrinsic pathway of the coagulation cascade (Ch. 25), as well as various other coagulation factors. It is primarily

---

[9]Mainly boys: 'Bruton's agammaglobulinaemia' is caused by a defect in a tyrosine kinase (BTK) coded on the X chromosome (Col. Bruton was chief of paediatrics at the Walter Reid army hospital). BTKs promote leukocyte survival and proliferation and BTK inhibitors are proving useful in treating certain leukaemias (see Ch. 57).

the cell-mediated reaction that is ultimately responsible for allograft rejection. Macrophages are also important in coordinating the repair processes that must occur for inflammation to resolve.

The specific cell-mediated or humoral immunological response is superimposed on the innate non-specific vascular and cellular reactions described previously, making them not only markedly more effective but much more selective for particular pathogens.

The general events of the inflammatory and hypersensitivity reactions specified above vary in some tissues. For example, in the airway inflammation of asthma, eosinophils and neuropeptides play a particularly significant role (see Ch. 29). In central nervous system (CNS) inflammation, there is less neutrophil infiltration and monocyte influx is delayed, possibly because of lack of adhesion molecule expression on CNS vascular endothelium and deficient generation of chemokines. It has long been known that some tissues – the CNS parenchyma, the anterior chamber of the eye and the testis – are *immunologically privileged* sites, in that a foreign antigen introduced directly does not provoke an immune reaction (which could be very disadvantageous to the host)[10]. However, introduction elsewhere of an antigen already in the CNS parenchyma will trigger the development of immune/inflammatory responses in the CNS.

SYSTEMIC RESPONSES IN INFLAMMATION

In addition to the local changes in an inflammatory site, there are commonly more general systemic manifestations of inflammatory disease. Typically, these could include fever, an increase in blood leukocytes and the release from the liver of *acute-phase proteins*. These include C-reactive protein, α_2-macroglobulin, fibrinogen, α_1-antitrypsin, serum amyloid A and some complement components. While the function of many of these components is still a matter of conjecture, many seem to have some antimicrobial actions. C-reactive protein, for example, binds to some microorganisms, and the resulting complex activates complement. Other proteins scavenge iron (an essential nutrient for invading organisms) or block proteases, perhaps protecting the host against the worst excesses of the inflammatory response.

THE ROLE OF THE NERVOUS SYSTEM IN INFLAMMATION

It has become clear in recent years that the central, autonomic and peripheral nervous systems all play an important part in the regulation of the inflammatory response. This occurs at various levels:

- *The neuroendocrine system.* Adrenocorticotrophic hormone (ACTH), released from the anterior pituitary gland in response to endogenous circadian rhythm or

to stress, releases cortisol from the adrenal glands. This hormone plays a crucial role in regulating immune function at all levels, hence the use of glucocorticoid drugs in the treatment of inflammatory disease. This topic is explored fully in Chapters 27 and 34.
- *The CNS.* Surprisingly, cytokines such as IL-1 can signal the development of an inflammatory response directly to the brain through receptors on the vagus nerve. This may elicit an 'inflammatory reflex' and trigger activation of a cholinergic anti-inflammatory pathway. See Tracey (2002) and Sternberg (2006) for interesting discussions of this topic.
- *The autonomic nervous system.* Both the sympathetic and parasympathetic systems can modulate the development of the inflammatory response. Generally speaking, their influence is anti-inflammatory. Receptors for noradrenaline and acetylcholine are found on macrophages and many other cells involved in the immune response although the origins of these ligands are unclear. Opioid receptors are also found on inflammatory cells and they also have multiple effects on many aspects of the inflammatory response (Liang et al., 2016).
- *Peripheral sensory neurons.* Some sensory neurons release inflammatory neuropeptides when appropriately stimulated. These neurons are fine afferents (capsaicin-sensitive C and Aδ fibres; see Ch. 43) with specific receptors at their peripheral terminals. Kinins, 5-hydroxytryptamine (5-HT) and other chemical mediators generated during inflammation act on these receptors, stimulating the release of neuropeptides such as the tachykinins (neurokinin A, substance P) and calcitonin gene-related peptide (CGRP), which have pro-inflammatory or algesic actions. The neuropeptides are considered further in Chapter 19.

UNWANTED INFLAMMATORY AND IMMUNE RESPONSES

The immune response has to strike a delicate balance. According to one school of thought, an infection-proof immune system would be a possibility but would come at a serious cost to the host. With many millions of potential antigenic sites in the host, such a 'super-immune' system would be some 1000 times more likely to attack the host itself, triggering *autoimmune disease*. It is not uncommon to encounter patients in whom exposure to ordinarily innocuous substances such as pollen or peanuts inadvertently activates the immune system. When this happens, the ensuing inflammation itself inflicts self-harm – either acutely as in (for example) anaphylaxis, or chronically in (for example) asthma or rheumatoid arthritis. In either case, anti-inflammatory or immunosuppressive therapy may be required.

▼ Unwanted immune responses, termed *allergic* or *hypersensitivity* reactions, are generally classified into four types.

Type I hypersensitivity

▼ Also called *immediate* or *anaphylactic hypersensitivity* (often known simply as 'allergy'), type I hypersensitivity occurs in individuals who predominantly exhibit a Th2 rather than a Th1 response to antigen. In these individuals, substances that are not inherently noxious (such as grass pollen, house dust mites, certain foodstuffs or drugs, animal

---

[10]Cold sore sufferers can blame this phenomenon for their misery – herpes simplex virus resides in the facial nervous tissue and becomes activated following stress or environmental stimuli, for example, exposure to the sun. The virus can reside in the CNS tissue for a whole lifetime from infancy, stubbornly resistant to the attempts of our immune cells to remove it. It can be transmitted to the baby from a carrier via a kiss, before the infant's immune system can eliminate the virus (usually by 6 months old). Bonnie babies are destined to suffer forever more.

fur and so on) provoke the production of antibodies of the IgE type.[11] These fix on mast cells, in the lung, and also to eosinophils. Subsequent contact with the problematic substance causes the release of histamine, PAF, eicosanoids and cytokines. The effects may be localised to the nose (hay fever), the bronchial tree (the initial phase of asthma), the skin (urticaria) or the gastrointestinal tract. In some cases, the reaction is more generalised and produces *anaphylactic shock*, which can be severe and life-threatening. Some important unwanted effects of drugs include anaphylactic hypersensitivity responses (see Ch. 58).

Type II hypersensitivity

▼ Also called *antibody-dependent cytotoxic hypersensitivity*, type II hypersensitivity occurs when the mechanisms outlined above are directed against cells within the host that are (or appear to be) foreign. For example, host cells or proteins altered by drugs are sometimes mistaken by the immune system for foreign organisms and evoke antibody formation. The antigen–antibody reaction triggers complement activation (and its sequelae) and may promote attack by NK cells. Examples include alteration by drugs of neutrophils, leading to *agranulocytosis* (see Ch. 57), or of platelets, leading to *thrombocytopenic purpura* (Ch. 25). These type II reactions are also implicated in some types of *autoimmune thyroiditis* (e.g. *Hashimoto's disease*; see Ch. 35).

Type III hypersensitivity

▼ Also called *complex-mediated hypersensitivity*, type III hypersensitivity occurs when antibodies react with *soluble* antigens. The antigen–antibody complexes can activate complement or attach to mast cells and stimulate the release of inflammatory mediators.

An experimental example of this is the *Arthus reaction* that occurs if a foreign protein is injected subcutaneously into a rabbit or guinea pig with high pre-existing circulating concentrations of antibody. Within 3–8 hours the area becomes red and swollen because the antigen–antibody complexes precipitate in small blood vessels and activate complement. Neutrophils are attracted and activated (by C5a) to generate toxic oxygen species and to secrete enzymes.

Mast cells are also stimulated by C3a to release mediators. Damage caused by this process is involved in *serum sickness*, which occurs when antigen persists in the blood after sensitisation, causing a severe reaction, as in the response to mouldy hay (known as *farmer's lung*), and in certain types of autoimmune kidney and arterial disease. Type III hypersensitivity is also implicated in *lupus erythematosus* (a chronic, autoimmune inflammatory disease).

Type IV hypersensitivity

▼ The prototype of type IV hypersensitivity (also known as *cell-mediated* or *delayed hypersensitivity*) is the *tuberculin reaction*, a local inflammatory response seen when proteins derived from cultures of the tubercle bacillus are injected into the skin of a person who has been sensitised by a previous infection or immunisation. An 'inappropriate' cell-mediated immune response is stimulated, accompanied by infiltration of mononuclear cells and the release of various cytokines. Cell-mediated hypersensitivity is also the basis of the reaction seen in some other infections (e.g. mumps and measles), as well as with mosquito and tick bites. It is also important in the skin reactions to

drugs or industrial chemicals (see Ch. 58), where the chemical (termed a *hapten*) combines with proteins in the skin to form the 'foreign' substance that evokes the cell-mediated immune response (see Fig. 7.3).

In essence, inappropriately deployed T-cell activity underlies all types of hypersensitivity, initiating types I, II and III, and being involved in both the initiation and the effector phase in type IV. These reactions are the basis of the clinically important group of autoimmune diseases.[12] Immunosuppressive drugs (Ch. 27) and/or glucocorticoids (Ch. 34) are routinely employed to treat such disorders.

THE OUTCOME OF THE INFLAMMATORY RESPONSE

It is important not to lose sight of the fact that the inflammatory response is a defence mechanism and not a disease *per se*. Its role is to restore normal structure and function to the infected or damaged tissue and, in the vast majority of cases, this is what occurs. The healing and resolution phase of the inflammatory response is an active process and does not simply 'happen' in the absence of further inflammation. It is now clear that resolution involves its own unique palette of mediators and cytokines (including various growth factors, annexin A1, lipoxins, resolvins and IL-10; see Ch. 19) to terminate residual inflammation and to promote remodelling and repair of damaged tissue.

In some cases, healing will be complete, but if there has been marked damage, repair is usually necessary and this may result in scarring. If the pathogen persists, it is enclosed by the host in a fibrous capsule 'prison' to prevent any further damage. Alternatively, the acute inflammatory response may transform into a chronic inflammatory response. This is a slow, smouldering reaction that can continue indefinitely, destroying tissue and promoting local proliferation of cells and connective tissue. The principal cell types found in areas of chronic inflammation are mononuclear cells and abnormal macrophage-derived cells. During healing or chronic inflammation, growth factors trigger angiogenesis and cause fibroblasts to lay down fibrous tissue. Infection by some microorganisms, such as syphilis, tuberculosis and leprosy, bear the characteristic hallmarks of chronic inflammation from the start. The cellular and mediator components of this type of inflammation are also seen in many, if not most, chronic autoimmune and hypersensitivity diseases, and are important targets for drug action.

---

[11]Such individuals are said to be 'atopic', from a Greek word meaning 'out of place'.

[12]Leukaemias are more likely in individuals who haven't been regularly exposed to infectious agents throughout their lives. Our immune systems have evolved to fight invaders – if our world is too sterile and our immune system unchallenged, then it is more likely to turn on itself predisposing us to cancerous pre-leukaemic cells (Cornwall, 2015). Dairy farmers who drink unpasteurized milk and breath farm air, suffer less from asthma and other autoimmune disorders (Kaiser, 2015).

REFERENCES AND FURTHER READING

The innate and adaptive responses

Abbas, A.K., Murphy, K.M., Sher, A., 1996. Functional diversity of helper lymphocytes. Nature 383, 787–793. (*Excellent review, helpful diagrams; commendable coverage of Th1 and Th2 cells and their respective cytokine subsets*)

Adams, D.H., Lloyd, A.R., 1997. Chemokines: leukocyte recruitment and activation cytokines. Lancet 349, 490–495. (*Commendable review*)

Cornwall, W., 2015. Study may explain mysterious cancer–day care connection. Science doi:10.1126/science.aac4614. http://www.sciencemag.org/news/2015/05/study-may-explain-mysterious-cancer-day-care-connection.

Delves, P.J., Roitt, I.M., 2000. The immune system. N. Engl. J. Med. 343, 37–49, 108–117. (*A good overview of the immune system – a mini-textbook of major areas in immunology; colourful three-dimensional figures*)

Gabay, C., Kushner, I., 1999. Acute phase proteins and other systemic responses to inflammation. N. Engl. J. Med. 340, 448–454. (*Lists the acute-phase proteins and outlines the mechanisms controlling their synthesis and release*)

Jimenez-Dalmaroni, M.J., Gerswhin, M.E., Adamopoulos, I.E., 2016. The critical role of toll-like receptors–From microbial recognition to autoimmunity: a comprehensive review. Autoimmun. Rev. 15, 1–8. (*Whilst it focusses on bone destruction, this has a good overview of the TLR family*)

Kaiser, J., 2015. Dirty farm air may ward off asthma in children. Science doi:10.1126/science.aad1700. http://www.sciencemag.org/news/2015/09/dirty-farm-air-may-ward-off-asthma-children.

Kennedy, M.A., 2010. A brief review of the basics of immunology: the innate and adaptive response. Vet. Clin. North Am. Small Anim. Pract. 40, 369–379. (*Actually written for vets, this little review is an easy-to-read introduction to the subject*)

Kay, A.B., 2001. Allergic diseases and their treatment. N. Engl. J. Med. 344, 30–37, 109–113. (*Covers atopy and Th2 cells, the role of Th2 cytokines in allergies, IgE, the main types of allergy and new therapeutic approaches*)

Liang, X., Liu, R., Chen, C., Ji, F., Li, T., 2016. Opioid system modulates the immune function: a review. Transl. Perioper. Pain Med. 1, 5–13.

Mackay, C.R., Lanzavecchia, A., Sallusto, F., 1999. Chemoattractant receptors and immune responses. Immunologist 7, 112–118. (*Masterly short review covering the role of chemoattractants in orchestrating immune responses – both the innate reaction and the Th1 and Th2 responses*)

Martinez, F.O., Gordon, S., 2014. The M1 and M2 paradigm of macrophage activation: time for reassessment. F1000Prime Rep. 6, 13. (*For those who want to dig a bit deeper into macrophage biology. Some very good diagrams*)

Medzhitov, R., 2001. Toll-like receptors and innate immunity. Nat. Rev. Immunol. 1, 135–145. (*Excellent review of the role of Toll-like receptors in (a) the detection of microbial infection, and (b) the activation of innate non-adaptive responses, which in turn lead to antigen-specific adaptive responses*)

Medzhitov, R., Janeway, C., 2000. Innate immunity. N. Engl. J. Med. 343, 338–344. (*Outstandingly clear coverage of the mechanisms involved in innate immunity and its significance for the adaptive immune response*)

Mills, K.H., 2008. Induction, function and regulation of IL-17-producing T cells. Eur. J. Immunol. 38, 2636–2649. (*This paper covers the biology of Th17 cells – a relatively recent addition to our understanding of Th biology. Accessible and has good diagrams*)

Murphy, P.M., 2001. Viral exploitation and subversion of the immune system through chemokine mimicry. Nat. Immunol. 2, 116–122. (*Excellent description of viral/immune system interaction*)

Nourshargh, S., Hordijk, P.L., Sixt, M., 2010. Breaching multiple barriers: leukocyte motility through venular walls and the interstitium. Nature Rev. Mol. Cell Biol. 11, 366–378. (*Excellent review of leukocyte mechanisms of transmigration through blood vessels. Contains excellent diagrams. Recommended*)

Parkin, J., Cohen, B., 2001. An overview of the immune system. Lancet 357, 1777–1789. (*A competent, straightforward review covering the role of the immune system in recognising, repelling and eradicating pathogens and in reacting against molecules foreign to the body*)

Segal, A.W., 2016. NADPH oxidases as electrochemical generators to produce ion fluxes and turgor in fungi, plants and humans. Open Biol. 6, 1–15. (*Very good review of the role of neutrophil killing mechanisms which suggests a new paradigm for understanding their microbiocidal actions. Very good diagrams*)

Sternberg, E.M., 2006. Neural regulation of innate immunity: a coordinated nonspecific host response to pathogens. Nat. Rev. Immunol. 6, 318–328. (*This paper and the paper by Tracey (below) are both excellent and easy-to-read reviews covering the role of the CNS in inflammation. Some good diagrams*)

Strowig, T., Henao-Mejia, J., Elinav, E., Flavell, R., 2012. Inflammasomes in health and disease. Nature 481, 278–286. (*Excellent, comprehensive review if you want to keep up to date in this area*)

Tracey, K.J., 2002. The inflammatory reflex. Nature 420, 853–859.

Wills-Karp, M., Santeliz, J., Karp, C.L., 2001. The germless theory of allergic diseases. Nat. Rev. Immunol. 1, 69–75. (*Discusses the hypothesis that early childhood infections inhibit the tendency to develop allergic disease*)

Yang, C.A., Chiang, B.L., 2015. Inflammasomes and human autoimmunity: a comprehensive review. J. Autoimmun. 61, 1–8.

Books

Dawkins, R., 1995. River out of Eden, first ed. Weidenfeld & Nicholson, London.

Murphy, K.M., Travers, P., Walport, M., 2011. Janeway's Immunobiology, eighth ed. Taylor & Francis, London. (*A classic textbook, updated and available as an e-book also. Excellent diagrams*)

Nijkamp, F.P., Parnham, M. (Eds.), 2011. Principles of Immunopharmacology, third ed. Birkhauser, Basle. (*A popular textbook that covers most of the topics in more depth than is possible in this book. Well written and illustrated. Recommended*)

Serhan, C., Ward, P.A., Gilroy, D.W. (Eds.), 2010. Fundamentals of Inflammation. Cambridge University Press, New York. (*A different type of textbook. Individual topics are written by appropriate experts and combined into a single volume. An authoritative and comprehensive volume that provides access to cutting-edge thinking in the field. Recommended*)

8 Method and measurement in pharmacology

OVERVIEW

We emphasised in Chapters 2 to 5 that drugs, being molecules, produce their effects by interacting with other molecules. This interaction can lead to effects at all levels of biological organisation, from molecules to human populations.[1]

Gaddum, a pioneering pharmacologist, commented in 1942: 'A branch of science comes of age when it becomes quantitative.' In this chapter, we cover the principles of metrication at the various organisational levels, ranging from laboratory methods to clinical trials. Assessment of drug action at the population level is the concern of pharmacoepidemiology and pharmacoeconomics (see Ch. 1), disciplines that are beyond the scope of this book.

We consider first the general principles of bioassay and its extension to studies in human beings; we describe the development of animal models to bridge the predictive gap between animal physiology and human disease; we next discuss aspects of clinical trials used to evaluate therapeutic efficacy in a clinical setting; finally, we consider the principles of balancing benefit and risk. Experimental design and statistical analysis are central to the interpretation of all types of pharmacological data. Kirkwood and Sterne (2003) provide an excellent introduction.

BIOASSAY

Bioassay, defined as the estimation of the concentration or potency of a substance by measurement of the biological response that it produces, has played a key role in the development of pharmacology. Quantitation of drug effects by bioassay is necessary to compare the properties of different substances, or the same substance under different circumstances. It is used:

- to measure the pharmacological activity of new or chemically undefined substances;
- to investigate the function of endogenous mediators;
- to measure drug toxicity and unwanted effects.

▼ Bioassay plays a key role in the development of new drugs, discussed in Chapter 60.

The use of bioassay to measure the *concentration* of drugs and other active substances in the blood or other body fluids – once an important technology – has now been largely replaced by analytical chemistry techniques.

Many hormones and chemical mediators have been discovered by the biological effects that they produce. For example, the ability of extracts of the posterior lobe of the pituitary to produce a rise in blood pressure and a contraction of the uterus was observed at the beginning of the 20th century. Quantitative assay procedures based on these actions enabled a standard preparation of the extract to be established by international agreement in 1935. By use of these assays, it was shown that two distinct peptides – vasopressin and oxytocin – were responsible, and they were eventually identified and synthesised in 1953. Biological assay had already revealed much about the synthesis, storage and release of the hormones, and was essential for their purification and identification. Nowadays, it does not take 50 years of laborious bioassays to identify new hormones before they are chemically characterised,[2] but bioassay still plays a key role. The recent growth of *biopharmaceuticals* (see Ch. 5) as registered therapeutic agents has relied on bioassay techniques and the establishment of standard preparations. Biopharmaceuticals, whether derived from natural sources (e.g. monoclonal antibodies, vaccines) or by recombinant DNA technology (e.g. erythropoietin), tend to vary from batch to batch, and need to be standardised with respect to their biological activity. Varying glycosylation patterns, for example, which are not detected by immunoassay techniques, may affect biological activity.

BIOLOGICAL TEST SYSTEMS

Nowadays, an important use of bioassay is to provide information that will predict the effect of the drug in the clinical situation (where the aim is to improve function in patients suffering from the effects of disease). The choice of laboratory test systems (in vitro and in vivo 'models') that provide this predictive link is an important aspect of quantitative pharmacology.

By the 1960s, pharmacologists had become adept at using isolated organs and laboratory animals (usually under anaesthesia) for quantitative experiments, and had developed the principles of bioassay to allow reliable measurements to be made with these sometimes difficult and unpredictable test systems.

Bioassays on different test systems may be run in parallel to reveal the profile of activity of an unknown mediator. Vane and his colleagues studied the generation and destruction of endogenous active substances such as prostanoids (see Ch. 18) in blood by the technique of *cascade superfusion*, measuring contraction or relaxation of a series of different smooth muscle test preparations chosen to differentiate between different active constituents of the sample. This technique has been invaluable in studying the production and fate of short-lived mediators such as thromboxane, prostacyclin and nitric oxide (Chs 18 and 21).

These 'traditional' assay systems address drug action at the physiological level – roughly, the mid-range of the organisational hierarchy shown in Fig. 8.1. Extension of

---

[1]Consider the effect of cocaine on organised crime, of organophosphate 'nerve gases' on the stability of dictatorships or of anaesthetics on the feasibility of surgical procedures for examples of molecular interactions that affect the behaviour of populations and societies.

[2]In 1988, a Japanese group (Yanagisawa et al., 1988) described in a single remarkable paper the bioassay, purification, chemical analysis, synthesis and DNA cloning of a new vascular peptide, *endothelin* (Ch. 23).

Level of biological organisation	Test system (examples)	Response measures (example relating to analgesia)	Methods	
Population & society	Socioeconomic group	Impact on healthcare costs, social costs, disability costs, disease prevalence	Pharmaco-economics, pharmaco-epidemiology	Socioeconomic
Family	Patients' family members	Impact on relationships, job prospects, suicide risk	Social medicine	Socioeconomic
Patient	Patients undergoing medical treatment	Pain relief, improvement of disability, etc.	Clinical trials	Clinical
Individual — Human volunteer	Normal healthy subjects	Subjective pain intensity and threshold	Clinical pharmacology	Clinical
Experimental animal	Rat, mouse, primate, etc.	Behavioural responses to noxious and non-noxious stimuli		Laboratory methods
Physiological system	CNS	Reflex responses to noxious stimuli	Physiological	Laboratory methods
Tissue & organ	Spinal cord	Synaptic responses in dorsal horn	Physiological	Laboratory methods
Cell	Spinal cord neurons	Membrane responses	Cellular	Laboratory methods
DRUG ACTION	Transfected cell lines	Second messenger responses	Cellular / Molecular	Laboratory methods
Molecule	Substance P (NK-1) receptor	Binding studies on cloned receptor expressed in cell lines	Molecular	Laboratory methods

Fig. 8.1 Levels of biological organisation and types of pharmacological measurement. *CNS,* central nervous system; *NK-1,* neurokinin-1.

the range in both directions, towards the molecular and towards the clinical, has taken place since. Binding assays (Ch. 3) and the use of engineered cell lines expressing normal and mutated receptors and signalling molecules are now widely used. Techniques based on X-ray crystallography, nuclear magnetic resonance spectroscopy and fluorescence signals have thrown much new light on drug action at the molecular level (see reviews by Lohse et al., 2012; Nygaard et al., 2013), and allow, for the first time, measurement as well as detection of the initial molecular events. Indeed, the range of techniques for analysing drug effects at the molecular and cellular levels is now very impressive and expanding rapidly. An example (Fig. 8.2) is the use of fluorescence-activated cell sorting (FACS) to measure the effect of a corticosteroid on the expression of a cell surface marker protein by human blood monocytes. Quantitative cellular assays of this kind are now widely used in pharmacology.

These approaches have important implications for basic understanding of drug action, and for drug design, but the need remains for measurement of drug effects at the physiological and clinical level – the focus of this chapter.

Bridging the gap between events at the molecular level and at the physiological and therapeutic levels presents difficulties, because human illness cannot, in many cases, be accurately reproduced in experimental animals. The use of transgenic animals to model human disease is discussed in more detail later.

GENERAL PRINCIPLES OF BIOASSAY
THE USE OF STANDARDS

J.H. Burn wrote in 1950: 'Pharmacologists today strain at the king's arm, but they swallow the frog, rat and mouse, not to mention the guinea pig and the pigeon.' He was referring to the fact that the 'king's arm' had been long

Fig. 8.2 **Measuring the effect of glucocorticoid drugs on cell surface receptor expression using FACS (fluorescence-activated cell sorting).** FACS technology enables the detection and measurement of fluorescent-tagged antibodies attached to structures on individual cells. In this experiment the effect of three glucocorticoids is tested on the expression of a cell surface haemoglobin scavenger receptor (CD 163). *(A)* Human monocytes were isolated from human venous blood and *(B)* incubated for 8 h alone or with various concentrations of the glucocorticoids dexamethasone, prednisone or hydrocortisone (see Chs 27 and 34). *(C)* The cells were then placed on ice and incubated with fluorescent-tagged antibodies to the receptor. *(D)* The cells were then fixed, washed and *(E)* subjected to FACS analysis. In this technique, cells flow through a small tube and are individually scanned by a laser. The reflected light is analysed using a series of filters (so that different coloured fluorescent tags can be used) and the data collected as *fluorescence intensity units*, compared with a standard (FITC) and expressed as 'FITC equivalents' to produce the final results *(F)*, which can be plotted as a conventional log-concentration curve. (Data courtesy N. Goulding.)

since abandoned as a standard measure of length, whereas drug activity continued to be defined in terms of dose needed to cause, say, vomiting of a pigeon or cardiac arrest in a mouse. A plethora of 'pigeon units', 'mouse units' and the like, which no two laboratories could agree on, contaminated the literature.[3] Even if two laboratories cannot agree – because their pigeons differ – on the activity in pigeon units of the same sample of an active substance, they should nonetheless be able to agree that preparation X is, say, 3.5 times as active as standard preparation Y on

the pigeon test. Biological assays are therefore designed to measure the *relative potency* of two preparations, usually a standard and an unknown. Maintaining stable preparations of various hormones, antisera and other biological materials as reference standards is the task of the UK National Board for Biological Standards Control.

THE DESIGN OF BIOASSAYS

▼ Given the aim of comparing the activity of two preparations, a standard (S) and an unknown (U), on a particular preparation, a bioassay must provide an estimate of the dose or concentration of U that will produce the same biological effect as that of a known dose or concentration of S. As Fig. 8.3 shows, provided that the log dose–effect curves for S and U are parallel, the ratio, *M*, of equiactive doses will not depend on the magnitude of response chosen. Thus *M* provides an estimate of the potency ratio of the two preparations. A comparison of the magnitude of the effects produced by equal doses of S and U does not provide an estimate of *M* (see Fig. 8.3).

---

[3]More picturesque examples of absolute units of the kind that Burn would have frowned on are the PHI and the mHelen. PHI, cited by Colquhoun (1971), stands for 'purity in heart index' and measures the ability of a virgin pure-in-heart to transform, under appropriate conditions, a he-goat into a youth of surpassing beauty. The mHelen is a unit of beauty, 1 mHelen being sufficient to launch one ship.

Fig. 8.3 Comparison of the potency of unknown and standard by bioassay. Note that comparing the magnitude of responses produced by the same dose (i.e. volume) of standard and unknown gives no quantitative estimate of their relative potency. (The differences, A_1 and A_2, depend on the dose chosen.) Comparison of equieffective doses of standard and unknown gives a valid measure of their relative potencies. Because the lines are parallel, the magnitude of the effect chosen for the comparison is immaterial; i.e. log M is the same at all points on the curves.

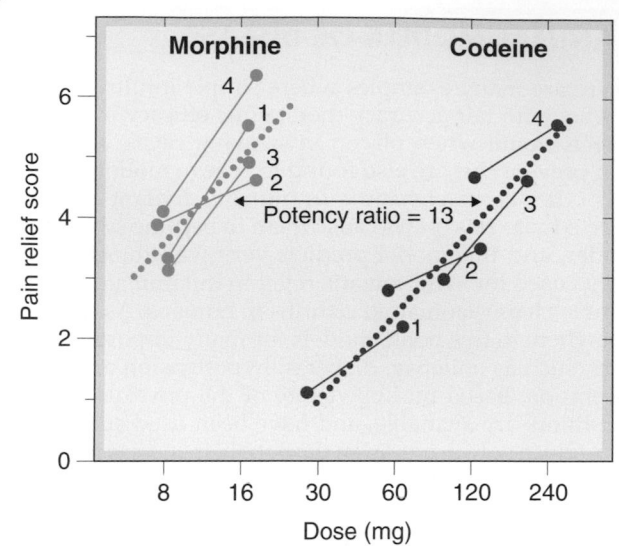

Fig. 8.4 Assay of morphine and codeine as analgesics in humans. Each of four patients (numbered 1–4) was given, on successive occasions in random order, four different treatments (high and low morphine, and high and low codeine) by intramuscular injection, and the subjective pain relief score calculated for each. The calculated regression lines gave a potency ratio estimate of 13 for the two drugs. (After Houde, R.W. et al., 1965. In: Analgetics. Academic Press, New York.)

The main problem with all types of bioassay is that of biological variation, and the design of bioassays is aimed at:

• minimising variation
• avoiding systematic errors resulting from variation
• estimation of the limits of error of the assay result.

Commonly, comparisons are based on analysis of *dose–response curves*, from which the matching doses of S and U are calculated. The use of a logarithmic dose scale means that the curves for S and U will normally be parallel, and the potency ratio (M) is estimated from the horizontal distance between the two curves (see Fig. 8.3). Assays of this type are known as *parallel line* assays, the minimal design being the 2 + 2 assay, in which two doses of standard (S_1 and S_2) and two of unknown (U_1 and U_2) are used. The doses are chosen to give responses lying on the linear part of the log dose–response curve, and are given repeatedly in randomised order, providing an inherent measure of the variability of the test system, which can be used, by means of straightforward statistical analysis, to estimate the confidence limits of the final result.

A simple example of an experiment to compare two analgesic drugs, **morphine** and **codeine** (see Ch. 43) in humans, based on a modified 2 + 2 design is shown in Fig. 8.4. Each of the four doses was given on different occasions to each of the four subjects, the order being randomised and both subject and observer being unaware of the dose given. Subjective pain relief was assessed by a trained observer, and the results showed morphine to be 13 times as potent as codeine. This, of course, does not prove its superiority, but merely shows that a smaller dose is needed to produce the same effect. Such a measurement is, however, an essential preliminary to assessing the relative therapeutic merits of the two drugs, for any comparison of other factors, such as side effects, duration of action, tolerance or dependence, needs to be done on the basis of doses that are equiactive as analgesics.

Problems arise if the two log dose–response curves are not parallel, or if the maximal responses differ, which can happen if the mechanism of action of the two drugs differs, or if one is a partial agonist (see Ch. 2). In this case it is not possible to define the relative potencies of S and U unambiguously in terms of a simple ratio and the experimenter must then face up to the fact that the comparison requires measurement of more than a single dimension of potency.

Bioassay

• Bioassay is the measurement of potency of a drug or unknown mediator from the magnitude of the biological effect that it produces.

• Bioassay normally involves comparison of the unknown preparation with a standard. Estimates that are not based on comparison with standards are liable to vary from laboratory to laboratory.

• Comparisons are best made on the basis of dose–response curves, which allow estimates of the equiactive concentrations of unknown and standard to be used as a basis for the potency comparison. Parallel line assays follow this principle.

• The biological response may be *quantal* (the proportion of tests in which a given all-or-nothing effect is produced) or *graded*. Different statistical procedures are appropriate in each case.

• Different approaches to metrication apply according to the level of biological organisation at which the drug effect needs to be measured. Approaches range through molecular and chemical techniques, in vitro and in vivo animal studies and clinical studies on volunteers and patients, to measurement of effects at the socioeconomic level.

ANIMAL MODELS OF DISEASE

There are many examples where simple intuitive models predict with fair accuracy therapeutic efficacy in humans. Ferrets vomit when placed in swaying cages, and drugs that prevent this are also found to relieve motion sickness and other types of nausea in humans. Irritant chemicals injected into rats' paws cause them to become swollen and tender, and this model predicts very well the efficacy of drugs used for symptomatic relief in inflammatory conditions such as rheumatoid arthritis in humans. As discussed elsewhere in this book, models for many important disorders, such as epilepsy, diabetes, hypertension and gastric ulceration, based on knowledge of the physiology of the condition, are available, and have been used successfully to produce new drugs, even though their success in predicting therapeutic efficacy is far from perfect.[4]

Ideally, an animal model should resemble the human disease in the following ways:

1. similar pathophysiological phenotype (*face validity*)
2. similar causation (*construct validity*)
3. similar response to treatment (*predictive validity*)

In practice, there are many difficulties, and the shortcomings of animal models are one of the main roadblocks on the route from basic medical science to improvements in therapy. The difficulties include the following.

- Many diseases, particularly in psychiatry, are defined by phenomena in humans that are difficult or impossible to observe in animals, which rules out face validity. As far as we know, mania or delusions have no counterpart in rats, nor does anything resembling a migraine attack or autism. Pathophysiological similarity is also inapplicable to conditions such as depression or anxiety disorders, where no clear brain pathology has been defined.
- The 'cause' of many human diseases is complex or unknown. To achieve construct validity for many degenerative diseases (e.g. Alzheimer's disease, osteoarthritis, Parkinson's disease), we need to model the upstream (causative) factors rather than the downstream (symptomatic) features of the disease, although the latter are the basis of most of the simple physiological models used hitherto. The inflammatory pain model mentioned earlier lacks construct validity for rheumatoid arthritis, which is an autoimmune disease.
- Relying on response to treatment as a test of predictive validity carries the risk that drugs acting by novel mechanisms could be missed, because the model will have been selected on the basis of its responsiveness to known drugs. With schizophrenia (Ch. 47), for example, it is clear that dopamine antagonists are effective, and many of the models used are designed to assess dopamine antagonism in

the brain, rather than other potential mechanisms that need to be targeted if drug discovery is to move on to address new targets.

GENETIC AND TRANSGENIC ANIMAL MODELS

Nowadays, genetic approaches are increasingly used as an adjunct to conventional physiological and pharmacological approaches to disease modelling.

Animal models

- Animal models of disease are important for investigating pathogenesis and for the discovery of new therapeutic agents. Animal models generally reproduce imperfectly only certain aspects of human disease states. Models of psychiatric illness are particularly problematic.
- Transgenic animals are produced by introducing mutations into the germ cells of animals (usually mice), which allow new genes to be introduced ('knock-ins') or existing genes to be inactivated ('knockouts') or mutated in a stable strain of animals.
- Transgenic animals are widely used to develop disease models for drug testing. Many such models are now available.
- The induced mutation operates throughout the development and lifetime of the animal, and may be lethal. Techniques of conditional mutagenesis allow the abnormal gene to be switched on or off at a chosen time.

By selective breeding, it is possible to obtain pure animal strains with characteristics closely resembling certain human diseases. Genetic models of this kind include spontaneously hypertensive rats, genetically obese mice, epilepsy-prone dogs and mice, rats with deficient vasopressin secretion, and many other examples. In many cases, the genes responsible have not been identified.

▼ The obese mouse, which arose from a spontaneous mutation in a mouse-breeding facility, is one of the most widely used models for the study of obesity and type 2 diabetes (see Ch. 32). The phenotype results from inactivation of the *leptin* gene, and shows good face validity (high food intake, gross obesity, impaired blood glucose regulation, vascular complications – features characteristic of human obesity) and good predictive validity (responding to pharmacological intervention similarly to humans), but poor construct validity, since most obese humans are not leptin deficient.

Genetic manipulation of the germline to generate *transgenic animals* (see Rudolph & Moehler, 1999; Offermanns & Hein, 2004) is important as a means of generating animal models that replicate human disease and are expected to be predictive of therapeutic drug effects in humans. This versatile technology, first reported in 1980, can be used in many different ways, for example:

- to inactivate individual genes, or mutate them to pathological forms
- to introduce new (e.g. human) genes

---

[4]There have been many examples of drugs that were highly effective in experimental animals (e.g. in reducing brain damage following cerebral ischaemia) but ineffective in humans (stroke victims). Similarly, substance P antagonists (Ch. 19) are effective in animal tests for analgesia, but they proved inactive when tested in humans. How many errors in the opposite direction may have occurred we shall never know, because such drugs will never have been tested in humans.

- to overexpress genes by inserting additional copies
- to allow gene expression to be controlled by the experimenter[5]

Currently, most transgenic technologies are applicable in mice but much more difficult in other mammals. Other vertebrates (e.g. zebrafish) and invertebrates (*Drosophila, Caenorhabditis elegans*) are increasingly used for drug screening purposes.

Examples of such models include transgenic mice that overexpress mutated forms of the *amyloid precursor protein* or *presenilins*, which are important in the pathogenesis of Alzheimer's disease (see Ch. 41). When they are a few months old, these mice develop pathological lesions and cognitive changes resembling Alzheimer's disease, and provide very useful models with which to test possible new therapeutic approaches. Another neurodegenerative condition, Parkinson's disease (Ch. 41), has been modelled in transgenic mice that overexpress *synuclein*, a protein found in the brain inclusions that are characteristic of the disease. Transgenic mice with mutations in tumour suppressor genes and oncogenes (see Ch. 6) are widely used as models for human cancers. Mice in which the gene for a particular adenosine receptor subtype has been inactivated show distinct behavioural and cardiovascular abnormalities, such as increased aggression, reduced response to noxious stimuli and raised blood pressure. These findings serve to pinpoint the physiological role of this receptor, whose function was hitherto unknown, and to suggest new ways in which agonists or antagonists for these receptors might be developed for therapeutic use (e.g. to reduce aggressive behaviour or to treat hypertension). Transgenic mice can, however, be misleading in relation to human disease. For example, the gene defect responsible for causing cystic fibrosis (a disease affecting mainly the lungs in humans), when reproduced in mice, causes a disorder that mainly affects the intestine.

PHARMACOLOGICAL STUDIES IN HUMANS

Studies involving human subjects range from experimental pharmacodynamic or pharmacokinetic investigations to formal clinical trials. Non-invasive recording methods, such as *functional magnetic resonance imaging* (FMRI) to measure regional blood flow in the brain (a surrogate for neuronal activity) and *ultrasonography* to measure cardiac performance, have greatly extended the range of what is possible. The scientific principles underlying experimental work in humans designed (for example) to check whether mechanisms that operate in other species also apply to humans, or to take advantage of the much broader response capabilities of a person compared with a rat, are the same as for animals, but the ethical and safety issues are paramount.

Ethics committees associated with all medical research centres tightly control the type of experiment that can be done, weighing up not only safety and ethical issues, but also the scientific importance of the proposed study. At the other end of the spectrum of experimentation on humans are formal *clinical trials*, often involving thousands of patients, aimed at answering specific questions regarding the efficacy and safety of new drugs.

CLINICAL TRIALS

Clinical trials are an important and highly specialised form of biological assay, designed specifically to measure therapeutic efficacy and detect adverse effects. The need to use patients undergoing treatment for experimental purposes raises serious ethical considerations, and imposes many restrictions. Here, we discuss some of the basic principles involved in clinical trials; the role of such trials in the course of drug development is described in Chapter 60.

A clinical trial is a method for comparing objectively, by a prospective study, the results of two or more therapeutic procedures. For new drugs, this is carried out during phases II and III of clinical development (Ch. 60). It is important to realise that, until about 60 years ago, methods of treatment were chosen on the basis of clinical impression and personal experience rather than objective testing.[6] Although many drugs, with undoubted effectiveness, remain in use without ever having been subjected to a controlled clinical trial, any new drug is now required to have been tested in this way before being licensed for clinical use.[7]

On the other hand, **digitalis** (see Ch. 22) was used for 200 years to treat cardiac failure before a controlled trial showed it to be of very limited value except in a particular type of patient.

An introduction to the principles and organisation of clinical trials is given by Hackshaw (2009). A clinical trial aims to compare the response of a test group of patients receiving a new treatment (A) with that of a control group receiving an existing 'standard' treatment (B). Treatment A might be a new drug or a new combination of existing drugs, or any other kind of therapeutic intervention, such as a surgical operation, a diet, physiotherapy and so on. The standard against which it is judged (treatment B) might be a drug or non-drug treatment that is in current clinical practice, or (if there is no currently available effective treatment), a placebo or no treatment at all.

The use of controls is crucial in clinical trials. Claims of therapeutic efficacy based on reports that, for example, 16

---

[5]With conventional transgenic technology, the genetic abnormality is expressed throughout development, sometimes proving lethal or causing major developmental abnormalities. *Conditional transgenesis* (see Ristevski, 2005), allows the modified gene to remain unexpressed until triggered by the administration of a chemical promoter (e.g. the tetracycline analogue, **doxycycline**, in the most widely used *Cre-Lox* conditional system). This avoids the complications of developmental effects and long-term adaptations, and may allow adult disease to be modelled more accurately.

[6]Not exclusively. James Lind conducted a controlled trial in 1753 on 12 mariners, which showed that oranges and lemons offered protection against scurvy. However, 40 years passed before the British Navy acted on his advice, and a further century before the US Navy did.
[7]It is fashionable in some quarters to argue that to require evidence of efficacy of therapeutic procedures in the form of a controlled trial runs counter to the doctrines of 'holistic' medicine. This is a fundamentally antiscientific view, for science advances only by generating predictions from hypotheses and by subjecting the predictions to experimental test. 'Alternative' medical procedures, such as homeopathy, aromatherapy, acupuncture or 'detox', have rarely been so tested, and where they have, they generally lack efficacy. Standing up for the scientific approach is the *evidence-based medicine* movement (see Sackett et al., 1996), which sets out strict criteria for assessing therapeutic efficacy, based on randomised controlled clinical trials, and urges scepticism about therapeutic doctrines whose efficacy has not been so demonstrated.

out of 20 patients receiving drug X got better within 2 weeks are of no value (particularly so with minor illnesses that are self-resolving), without a knowledge of how 20 patients receiving a different treatment, or none at all, would have fared. In a *parallel-group design*, the controls are provided by a separate group of patients from those receiving the test treatment, but sometimes a *crossover design* is possible in which the same patients are switched from test to control treatment or vice versa, and the results compared. Randomisation is essential to avoid bias in assigning individual patients to test or control groups. Hence, the *randomised controlled clinical trial* is now regarded as *the* essential tool for assessing clinical efficacy of new drugs.

Concern inevitably arises over the ethics of assigning patients at random to particular treatment groups (or to no treatment). However, the reason for setting up a trial is that doubt exists whether the test treatment offers greater benefit than the control treatment, and there is genuine clinical equipoise in treatment selection. All would agree on the principle of informed consent,[8] whereby each patient must be told the nature and risks of the trial, and agree to participate on the basis that he or she will be randomly and unknowingly assigned to either the test or the control group. The regularly updated 'Declaration of Helsinki' sets out the widely accepted ground rules governing research on human subjects.

Unlike the kind of bioassay discussed earlier, the clinical trial does not normally give any information about potency or the form of the dose–response curve, but merely compares the response produced by two or more stipulated therapeutic regimens. Survival curves provide one commonly used measure. Fig. 8.5 shows rates of disease-free survival in two groups of breast cancer patients treated with conventional chemotherapy with and without the addition of paclitaxel (see Ch. 57). The divergence of the curves shows that paclitaxel significantly improved the clinical response. Additional questions may be posed, such as the incidence and severity of side effects, or whether the treatment works better or worse in particular classes of patient, but only at the expense of added complexity and numbers of patients. The investigator must decide in advance, using a protocolised approach, what dose to use and how often to give it, and the trial will reveal only whether the chosen regimen performed better or worse than the control treatment. Unless different doses are compared, it will not say whether increasing or decreasing the dose would have improved the response.

A considerable amount of preliminary or fundamental work has to be completed prior to designing and embarking on a clinical trial that measures patient outcomes with a new drug. The basic question or hypothesis posed by a clinical trial is thus simpler than that addressed by most conventional bioassays. However, the organisation of clinical trials, with controls against bias, is immeasurably more

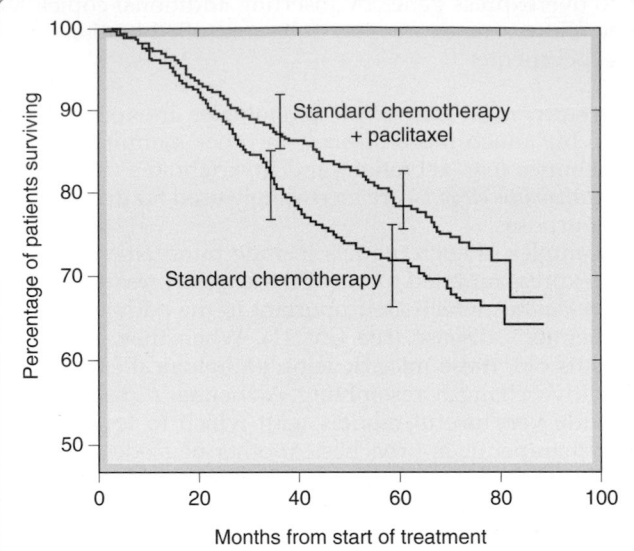

Fig. 8.5 Disease-free survival curves followed for 8 years in matched groups of breast cancer patients treated with a standard chemotherapy regime alone (629 patients), or with addition of paclitaxel (613 patients), showing a highly significant ($p = 0.006$) improvement with paclitaxel. Error bars represent 95% confidence intervals. (Redrawn from Martin et al., 2008. J. Natl. Cancer Inst. 100, 805–814.)

complicated, time-consuming and expensive than that of any laboratory-based assay. Observational studies may therefore be more practical or appropriate for assessing rare adverse effects where large sample sizes and long-term follow-up are needed.

AVOIDANCE OF BIAS

There are three main strategies that aim to minimise bias in clinical trials, namely:

1. randomisation
2. the double-blind technique
3. rigorous follow-up and ascertainment of outcomes

If two treatments, A and B, are being compared on a series of selected patients, the simplest form of randomisation is to allocate each patient to A or B by reference to a series of random numbers, toss of a coin, or even drawing lots. In a properly randomised trial, neither the patient nor the investigator should have any influence on which treatment the patient will end up receiving. One difficulty, particularly if the groups are small, is that the two groups may turn out to be ill-matched with respect to characteristics such as age, sex or disease severity. *Stratified randomisation* avoids the difficulty by dividing the subjects into age, sex, severity, or other categories, random allocation to A or B being used within each category. It is possible to treat two or more characteristics of the trial population in this way, but the number of strata can quickly become large, and the process is self-defeating when the number of subjects in each becomes too small. As well as avoiding error resulting from imbalance of groups assigned to A and B, stratification can also allow more sophisticated conclusions to be reached. B might, for example, prove to be better than A in a particular group of patients even if it is not significantly better overall.

---

[8]Even this can be contentious, because patients who are unconscious, demented or mentally ill are unable to give such consent, yet no one would want to preclude trials that might offer improved therapies to these needy patients. Clinical trials in children are particularly problematic but are necessary if the treatment of childhood diseases is to be placed on the same evidence base as is judged appropriate for adults. There are many examples where experience has shown that children respond differently from adults, and there is now increasing pressure on pharmaceutical companies to perform trials in children, despite the difficulties of carrying out such studies. The same concerns apply to trials in elderly patients.

The double-blind technique, whereby neither subject nor investigator is aware at the time of the assessment which treatment is being used, is intended to minimise subjective bias. It has been repeatedly shown that, with the best will in the world, subjects and investigators both contribute to bias if they know which treatment is which. Awareness of the specific trial intervention may lead to changes in clinical management, or to biased reporting and measurement of outcomes Although the use of a double-blind technique is an important safeguard this is not always possible. A dietary regimen, for example, can seldom be disguised; with drugs, pharmacological effects may reveal to patients what they are taking and predispose them to report accordingly.[9] In general, however, the double-blind procedure, with precautions if necessary to disguise such clues as the taste or appearance of the two drugs, is used whenever possible.[10] If full-blinding of participants and investigators is not possible, one option is to have a follow-up of outcomes conducted by assessors who are unaware of the treatments being used.

High-quality clinical trials have pre-specified follow-up time points where outcomes are measured in a defined manner. Study results may be incomplete and potentially biased if patients drop out of the study or fail to attend follow-up because the intervention did not improve their symptoms. Inadequate follow-up or missing data means that important outcomes (such as serious adverse events) may not have been detected.

THE SIZE OF THE SAMPLE

Both ethical and financial considerations dictate that the trial should involve the minimum number of subjects, and much statistical thought has gone into the problem of deciding in advance how many subjects will be required to produce a useful – and statistically meaningful – result (a *power* calculation). The results of a trial cannot be absolutely conclusive, because it is based on a sample of patients (selected on the basis of specific eligibility criteria), and there is always a chance that the sample was atypical of the population from which it came. Thus, the trial findings may not be generalisable to the routine clinical practice.

Judgements on the appropriate sample size should be based on whether the aim is to demonstrate that two treatments are equivalent (e.g. new treatment is non-inferior to the one that is currently in use), or whether the aim is to demonstrate a significant difference between interventions. Two types of erroneous conclusion are possible, referred to as *type I* and *type II errors*. A type I error occurs if the results show a difference between A and B when none actually exists (false positive). A type II error occurs if no

difference is found although A and B do actually differ (false negative). A major factor that determines the size of sample needed is the degree of certainty the investigator seeks in avoiding either type of error. The probability of incurring a type I error is expressed as the *significance* of the result. To say that A and B are different at the $p < 0.05$ level of significance means that the probability of obtaining a false positive result (i.e. incurring a type I error) is less than 1 in 20. For most purposes, this level of significance is considered acceptable as a basis for drawing conclusions.

The probability of detecting a genuine difference that exists between interventions, and avoiding a type II error is termed the *power* of the trial. We tend to regard type II errors more leniently than type I errors, and it is often acceptable to design trials with a power of 0.8–0.9, which means that there is an 80%–90% chance of detecting a real effect. A larger sample size will confer greater power or ability to detect any difference that exists.

The second factor that determines the sample size required is the magnitude of difference between A and B that is regarded as clinically important. For example, to detect that a given treatment reduces the mortality in a certain condition by at least 10 percentage points, say from 50% (in the control group) to 40% (in the treated group), would require 850 subjects, assuming that we wanted to achieve a $p < 0.05$ level of significance and a power of 0.9. If we were content only to detect a larger treatment effect of a 20-percentage point reduction in mortality (and very likely miss a reduction by 10 points), only 210 subjects would be needed. In this example, missing a real 10-point reduction in mortality could result in abandonment of a treatment that would save 100 lives for every 1000 patients treated – an extremely serious mistake from society's point of view. This simple example emphasises the need to assess clinical benefit (which is often difficult to quantify) in parallel with statistical considerations (which are fairly straightforward) in planning trials.

▼ A trial may give a significant result (of benefit or harm) before the planned number of patients have been enrolled, so it is common for interim analyses to be carried out at intervals (by an independent *data monitoring* team so that the trial team remains unaware of the results). If this analysis gives a conclusive result, or if it shows that continuation is unlikely to give a conclusive result (i.e. futility), the trial can be terminated, thus reducing the number of subjects tested. In one such large-scale trial (Beta-blocker Heart Attack Trial Research Group, 1982) of the value of long-term treatment with the β-adrenoceptor-blocking drug **propranolol** (Ch. 15) following heart attacks, the interim results showed a significant reduction in mortality, which led to the early termination of the trial. Another trial, the Cardiac Arrhythmia Suppression Trial (CAST, Echt et al., 1991), was stopped because the treatment group, contrary to expectation, showed increased mortality compared with placebo.

Recently, the tendency has been to perform very large-scale trials, to allow several different treatment protocols in various different patient groups to be compared. An example is the ALLHAT trial of various antihypertensive and lipid-lowering drugs to improve the outcome in cardiovascular disease (see Ch. 23). This ran from 1994 to 2002, cost US$130 million, and involved more than 42,000 patients in 623 treatment centres, with an army of coordinators and managers to keep it on track. One of its several far-reaching conclusions was that a cheap and familiar diuretic drug in use for more than 50 years was more effective than more recent and expensive antihypertensive drugs.[11]

---

[9]The distinction between a true pharmacological response and a beneficial clinical effect produced by the knowledge (based on the pharmacological effects that the drug produces) that an active drug is being administered is not easy to draw, and we should not expect a mere clinical trial to resolve such a tricky semantic issue.

[10]Maintaining the blind can be problematic. In an attempt to determine whether **melatonin** is effective in countering jet lag, a pharmacologist investigator recruited a group of fellow pharmacologists attending a congress in Australia, providing them with unlabelled capsules of melatonin or placebo, with a jet lag questionnaire to fill in when they arrived. Some of them (one of the authors included), with analytical resources easily to hand, opened the capsules and consigned them to the bin on finding that they contained placebo. Pharmacologists are only human.

---

[11]Though without much impact so far on prescribing habits, owing to the marketing muscle of pharmaceutical companies.

CLINICAL OUTCOME MEASURES

The measurement of clinical outcome can be a complicated business, and is becoming increasingly so as society becomes more preoccupied with assessing the efficacy of therapeutic procedures in terms of improved length and quality of life, and societal and economic benefit. Various scales for assessing 'health-related quality of life' have been devised and tested (see Walley & Haycocks, 1997); these may be combined with measures of life expectancy to arrive at the measure 'quality-adjusted life years' (QALYs) as an overall measure of therapeutic efficacy, which attempts to combine both survival time and relief from suffering in assessing overall benefit.[12] In planning clinical trials, it is necessary to decide the purpose of the trial in advance, and to define the outcome measures accordingly, particularly in light of the modern-day emphasis on outcomes that are important to patients.

Measuring long-term patient benefit may take years, so objective clinical effects, such as lowering of blood pressure, improved airways conductance or change in white cell count are often used as trial outcome measures. These *surrogate markers* reflect pathophysiological changes of which the patient is most likely unaware. In many cases such changes correlate well with clinical outcome as it affects the patient; not always, though. In the CAST trial (see previously), anti-arrhythmic drugs were found to suppress certain ventricular arrhythmias (the surrogate marker), but to *increase* sudden cardiac deaths. Regulatory authorities are therefore rightly cautious about accepting surrogate end points as a measure of actual patient benefit.

PLACEBOS

▼ A placebo is a dummy medicine containing no active ingredient (or alternatively, a dummy surgical procedure, diet or other kind of therapeutic intervention), which the patient believes is (or could be, in the context of a controlled trial) the real thing. The 'placebo response' (see review by Enck et al., 2013) is widely believed to be a powerful therapeutic effect,[13] producing a significant beneficial effect in about one-third of patients. While many clinical trials include a placebo group that shows improvement, few have compared this group directly with untreated controls, particularly where the natural history of the disease is symptom resolution without any intervention. The role of placebo is a topic of major debate, with some arguing that placebo has limited effect, except perhaps in trials involving pain or nausea (Hróbjartsson & Gøtzsche, 2010), whilst others have reported clinically meaningful effects with placebo (Howick et al, 2013). There are also growing numbers of pragmatic trials where the new treatment is compared against 'standard or usual' care, rather than the rather artificial construct of a placebo dummy pill that does not represent what the patient would actually receive in clinical practice.

The risks of placebo therapies should not be underestimated. The use of active medicines may be delayed. The necessary element of deception[14] risks undermining the confidence of patients in the integrity of doctors. A state of 'therapy dependence' may be produced in people who are not ill, because there is no way of assessing whether a patient still 'needs' the placebo.

META-ANALYSIS

▼ It is possible, using statistical techniques, to combine the data obtained in several individual trials (provided each has been conducted according to a randomised design) in order to gain greater power and significance. This procedure, known as *meta-analysis* or *overview analysis*, can be very useful in arriving at a conclusion on the basis of several published trials, of which some claimed superiority of the test treatment over the control while others did not. As an objective procedure with defined study selection and quality assessment criteria, it is certainly preferable to the 'take your pick' approach to conclusion-forming adopted by most human beings when confronted with contradictory data. It has several drawbacks, however (see Naylor, 1997), the main ones being susceptibility to selective reporting of results and 'publication bias', because negative studies (or unfavourable findings) are less likely to be published than positive studies, partly because they are considered less interesting or, more seriously, because publication would harm the business of the pharmaceutical company that performed the trial.[15] Double counting, caused by the same data being incorporated into more than one trial report, is another problem.

The published clinical trials literature contains reports of many trials that are poorly designed and unreliable. The Cochrane Collaboration (<www.cochrane.org>) sifts carefully through the literature and produces *systematic reviews* that collate and combine data only from trials (of drugs and other therapeutic interventions) that meet strict quality criteria. About 7000 such 'gold-standard' summaries are available, and provide the most reliable evaluation of trials data on a wide range of therapeutic drugs.

BALANCING BENEFIT AND RISK
THERAPEUTIC INDEX

▼ The concept of therapeutic index aims to provide a measure of the margin of safety of a drug, by drawing attention to the relationship between the effective and toxic doses:

$$\text{Therapeutic index} = LD_{50}/ED_{50}$$

where LD_{50} is the dose that is lethal in 50% of the population, and ED_{50} is the dose that is 'effective' in 50%. Obviously, it can only be measured in animals, and it is not a useful guide to the safety of a drug in clinical use for several reasons:

- LD_{50} does not reflect the incidence of adverse effects in the therapeutic setting.[16]
- ED_{50} depends on what measure of effectiveness is used. For example, the ED_{50} for **aspirin** used for a mild headache is much lower than for aspirin as an antirheumatic drug.
- Both efficacy and toxicity are subject to individual variation. Individual differences in the effective dose or the toxic dose of a drug makes it inherently less predictable, and therefore less safe, although this is not reflected in the therapeutic index.

---

[12]As may be imagined, trading off duration and quality of life raises issues about which many of us feel decidedly squeamish. Not so economists, however. They approach the problem by asking such questions as: 'How many years of life would you be prepared to sacrifice in order to live the rest of your life free of the disability you are currently experiencing?' Or, even more disturbingly: 'If, given your present condition, you could gamble on surviving free of disability for your normal lifespan, or (if you lose the gamble) dying immediately, what odds would you accept?' Imagine being asked this by your doctor. 'But I only wanted something for my sore throat,' you protest weakly.
[13]Its opposite, the *nocebo effect*, describes the adverse effects reported with dummy medicines.

[14]Surprisingly, deception may not even be necessary. Kaptchuk et al. (2010) found that symptoms of irritable bowel syndrome were improved slightly more in patients given inert sugar pills, described as such by the physician, than in patients given no pills. The effect was, however, small, and the patients were encouraged to think that the pills might engage 'mind-body healing processes'.
[15]To reduce this bias, measures are now in place to ensure that most clinical trials are registered and the results publicly disclosed.
[16]Ironically, **thalidomide** – probably the most harmful drug ever marketed – was promoted specifically on the basis of its exceptionally high therapeutic index (i.e. it killed rats only when given in extremely large doses).

Clinical trials

- A clinical trial is a special type of bioassay done to compare the clinical efficacy of a new drug or procedure with that of a known drug or procedure (or a placebo).
- At its simplest, the aim is a straight comparison of unknown (A) with standard (B) at a single-dose level. The result may be: 'B better than A', 'B worse than A', or 'No difference detected'. Efficacy, not potency, is compared.
- To avoid bias, clinical trials should be:
  - *controlled* (comparison of A with B, rather than study of A alone);
  - *randomised* (assignment of subjects to A or B on a random basis);
  - *double-blind* (neither subject nor assessor knows whether A or B is being used).
- Type I errors (concluding that A is better than B when the difference is actually due to chance) and type II errors (concluding that A is not different from B because a real difference has escaped detection) can occur; the likelihood of either kind of error decreases as the methodological quality, sample size and number of end-point events is increased.
- Interim analysis of data, carried out by an independent group, may be used as a basis for terminating a trial prematurely if the data are already conclusive, or if a clear result is unlikely to be reached.
- All experiments on human subjects require approval by an independent ethics committee.
- Clinical trials require very careful planning and execution, and are inevitably expensive.
- Clinical outcome measures may comprise:
  - physiological measures (e.g. blood pressure, liver function tests, airways function);
  - subjective assessments (e.g. pain relief, mood);
  - long-term outcome (e.g. survival or freedom from recurrence);
  - overall '*quality of life*' measures;
  - '*quality-adjusted life years*' (QALYs), which combine survival with quality of life.
- Meta-analysis is a statistical technique used to pool the data from several independent trials.

OTHER MEASURES OF BENEFIT AND RISK

▼ Alternative ways of quantifying the benefits and risks of drugs in clinical use have received much attention. One useful approach is to estimate from clinical trial data the proportion of test and control patients who will experience (A) a defined level of clinical benefit (e.g. survival beyond 2 years, pain relief to a certain predetermined level, slowing of cognitive decline by a given amount) and (B) adverse effects of defined degree. These estimates of proportions of patients showing beneficial or harmful reactions can be expressed as *number needed to treat* (NNT; i.e. the number of patients who need to be treated in order for one to show the given effect, whether beneficial or adverse). For example, in a recent study of pain relief by antidepressant drugs compared with placebo, the findings were: for benefit (a defined level of pain relief), NNT = 3; for minor unwanted effects, NNT = 3; for major adverse effects, NNT = 22. Thus of 100 patients treated with the drug, on average 33 will experience pain relief, 33 will experience minor unwanted effects, and 4 or 5 will experience major adverse effects, information that is helpful in guiding therapeutic choices. One advantage of this type of analysis is that it can take into account the underlying disease severity in quantifying benefit. Thus if drug A halves the mortality of an often fatal disease (reducing it from 50% to 25%, say), the NNT to save one life is 4; if drug B halves the mortality of a rarely fatal disease (reducing it from 5% to 2.5%, say), the NNT to save one life is 40. Notwithstanding other considerations, drug A is judged to be more valuable than drug B, even though both reduce mortality by one-half. Furthermore, the clinician must realise that to save one life with drug B, 40 patients must be exposed to a risk of adverse effects, whereas only four are exposed for each life saved with drug A.

Determination of risk and benefit

- *Therapeutic index* (lethal dose for 50% of the population divided by effective dose for 50%) is unsatisfactory as a measure of drug safety because:
  - it is based on animal toxicity data, which may not reflect forms of toxicity or adverse reactions that are important clinically;
  - it takes no account of idiosyncratic toxic reactions.
- More sophisticated measures of risk–benefit analysis for drugs in clinical use are available, and include the *number needed to treat* (NNT) principle.

REFERENCES AND FURTHER READING

General references

Colquhoun, D., 1971. Lectures on Biostatistics. Oxford University Press, Oxford. (*Standard textbook*)

Kirkwood, B.R., Sterne, J.A.C., 2003. Medical Statistics, second ed. Blackwell, Malden. (*Clear introductory textbook covering statistical principles and methods*)

Walley, T., Haycocks, A., 1997. Pharmacoeconomics: basic concepts and terminology. Br. J. Clin. Pharmacol. 43, 343–348. (*Useful introduction to analytical principles that are becoming increasingly important for therapeutic policy makers*)

Yanagisawa, M., Kurihara, H., Kimura, S., et al., 1988. A novel potent vasoconstrictor peptide produced by vascular endothelial cells. Nature 332, 411–415. (*The first paper describing endothelin – a remarkably full characterisation of an important new mediator*)

Molecular methods

Lohse, M.J., Nuber, S., Hoffmann, C., 2012. Fluorescence/ bioluminescence resonance energy transfer techniques to study G protein-coupled receptor activation and signaling. Pharmacol. Rev. 64, 299–336. (*Review of modern fluorescence-based methods for studying GPCR function*)

Nygaard, R., Zou, Y., Dror, R.O., et al., 2013. The dynamic process of β(2)-adrenergic receptor activation. Cell 152 (3), 532–542. (*Review demonstrating the use of modern spectroscopic techniques to measure the effects of ligands on receptor conformation*)

Animal models

Offermanns, S., Hein, L. (Eds.), 2004. Transgenic models in pharmacology. Handb. Exp. Pharmacol. 159. (*A comprehensive series of review articles describing transgenic mouse models used to study different pharmacological mechanisms and disease states)*

Ristevski, S., 2005. Making better transgenic models: conditional, temporal, and spatial approaches. Mol. Biotechnol. 29, 153–164. *(Description of methods for controlling transgene expression)*

Rudolph, U., Moehler, H., 1999. Genetically modified animals in pharmacological research: future trends. Eur. J. Pharmacol. 375, 327–337. *(Good review of uses of transgenic animals in pharmacological research, including application to disease models)*

Clinical trials

Beta-blocker Heart Attack Trial Research Group, 1982. A randomised trial of propranolol in patients with acute myocardial infarction. 1. Mortality results. JAMA 247, 1707–1714. *(A trial that was terminated early when clear evidence of benefit emerged)*

Echt, D.S., Liebson, P.R., Mitchell, L.B., et al., 1991. Mortality and morbidity in patients receiving encainide, flecainide, or placebo. The Cardiac Arrhythmia Suppression Trial. N. Engl. J. Med. 324, 781–788. *(Important trial showing that antiarrhythmic drugs, which were expected to reduce sudden deaths after a heart attack, have the opposite effect)*

Enck, P., Bigel, U., Schedlowski, M., Rief, W., 2013. The placebo response in medicine: minimize, maximize or personalize? Nat. Rev. Drug Discov. 12, 191–204. *(Comprehensive review of a slippery phenomenon)*

Hackshaw, A., 2009. A Concise Guide to Clinical Trials. Wiley Blackwell. *(Short introductory textbook)*

Howick, J., Friedemann, C., Tsakok, M., et al., 2013. Are treatments more effective than placebos? A systematic review and meta-analysis. PLoS ONE 8, e62599.

Hrobjartsson, A., Gotzsche, P.C., 2010. Placebo interventions for all clinical conditions. Cochrane Database Syst. Rev. CD003974.

Kaptchuk, T.J., Friedlander, E., Kelley, J.M., et al., 2010. Placebos without deception: a randomized controlled trial in irritable bowel syndrome. PLoS ONE 5 (12), e15591. *(Study showing that placebo pills have a significant effect even if the patient knows that they contain no active ingredient)*

Naylor, C.D., 1997. Meta-analysis and the meta-epidemiology of clinical research. Br. Med. J. 315, 617–619. *(Thoughtful review on the strengths and weaknesses of meta-analysis)*

Sackett, D.L., Rosenburg, W.M.C., Muir-Gray, J.A., et al., 1996. Evidence-based medicine: what it is and what it isn't. Br. Med. J. 312, 71–72. *(Balanced account of the value of evidence-based medicine – an important recent trend in medical thinking)*

Absorption and distribution of drugs

9

OVERVIEW

The physical processes of diffusion, penetration of membranes, binding to plasma protein and partition into fat and other tissues underlie the absorption and distribution of drugs. These processes are described, followed by more specific coverage of the process of drug absorption and related practical issue of routes of drug administration, and of the distribution of drugs into different bodily compartments. Drug interactions caused by one drug altering the absorption or distribution of another are described. There is a short final section on special drug delivery systems designed to deliver drugs efficiently and selectively to their sites of action.

INTRODUCTION

Drug disposition is divided into four stages designated by the acronym 'ADME':

- **A**bsorption from the site of administration
- **D**istribution within the body
- **M**etabolism
- **E**xcretion

General aspects of drug absorption and distribution are considered here, together with routes of administration. Absorption and distribution of inhaled general anaesthetics (a special case) are described in Chapter 42. Metabolism and excretion are covered in Chapter 10. We begin with a description of the physical processes that underlie drug disposition.

PHYSICAL PROCESSES UNDERLYING DRUG DISPOSITION

Drug molecules move around the body in two ways:

- bulk flow (i.e. in the bloodstream, lymphatics or cerebrospinal fluid)
- diffusion (i.e. molecule by molecule, over short distances).

The chemical nature of a drug makes no difference to its transfer by bulk flow. The cardiovascular system provides a rapid long-distance distribution system. In contrast, diffusional characteristics differ markedly between different drugs. In particular, ability to cross hydrophobic diffusion barriers is strongly influenced by lipid solubility. Aqueous diffusion is part of the overall mechanism of drug transport, because it is this process that delivers drug molecules to and from the non-aqueous barriers. The rate of diffusion

of a substance depends mainly on its molecular size, the *diffusion coefficient* being inversely proportional to the square root of molecular weight. Consequently, while large molecules diffuse more slowly than small ones, the variation with molecular weight is modest. Classical 'small molecule' drugs mainly fall within the molecular weight range 200–1000 Da, and variations in aqueous diffusion rate have only a small effect on their overall pharmacokinetic behaviour, whereas biopharmaceuticals are typically much larger molecules (Ch. 5). Thus the molecular weight of a monoclonal antibody drug is approximately 150 kDa and of a small interfering RNA 7.5 kDa, so diffusion can be an important limitation to the rate of onset of action of biopharmaceutical drugs.

For small molecule drugs, we can treat the body as a series of interconnected, well-stirred compartments, within each of which the drug concentration is uniform. It is movement *between* compartments, generally involving penetration of non-aqueous diffusion barriers, that determines where, and for how long, a drug will be present in the body after it has been administered. The analysis of drug movements with the help of a simple compartmental model is discussed in Chapter 11.

THE MOVEMENT OF DRUG MOLECULES ACROSS CELL BARRIERS

Cell membranes form the barriers between aqueous compartments in the body. A single layer of membrane separates the intracellular from the extracellular compartments. An epithelial barrier, such as the gastrointestinal mucosa or renal tubule, consists of a layer of cells tightly connected to each other so that molecules must traverse at least two cell membranes (inner and outer) to pass from one side to the other. The anatomical disposition and permeability of vascular endothelium (the cell layer that separates intravascular from extravascular compartments) varies from one tissue to another. Gaps between endothelial cells are packed with a loose matrix of proteins that act as filters, retaining large molecules and letting smaller ones through. The cut-off of molecular size is not exact: water permeates rapidly whereas molecules of 80,000–100,000 Da permeate very slowly. In some regions, especially the *blood–brain barrier* (see p. 129) of the CNS, and the placenta, there are tight junctions between the cells, and the endothelium is encased in an impermeable layer of periendothelial cells (*pericytes*). These features prevent potentially harmful molecules from penetrating to brain or fetus and have major consequences for drug distribution and activity.

In other organs (e.g. the liver and spleen), endothelium is discontinuous, allowing free passage between cells. In the liver, hepatocytes form the barrier between intra- and extravascular compartments and take on several endothelial cell functions. Fenestrated endothelium occurs in endocrine glands, facilitating transfer to the bloodstream of hormones or other molecules through pores in the endothelium. Formation of fenestrated endothelium is controlled by a specific endocrine gland-derived vascular endothelial growth factor (dubbed EG-VEGF). Endothelial cells lining postcapillary venules have specialised functions relating to leukocyte migration and inflammation, and the sophistication of the intercellular junction can be appreciated from the observation that leukocyte migration can occur without any detectable leak of water or small ions (see Ch. 7).

There are four main ways by which small molecules cross cell membranes (Fig. 9.1):

- by diffusing directly through the lipid;
- by combination with a *solute carrier* (SLC) or other membrane transporter;
- by diffusing through aqueous pores formed by special membrane glycoproteins (*aquaporins*) that traverse the lipid;
- by *pinocytosis*.

Of these routes, diffusion through lipid and carrier-mediated transport are particularly important in relation to pharmacokinetic mechanisms.

▼ Diffusion through aquaporins is probably important in the transfer of gases such as carbon dioxide, but the pores are too small in diameter (about 0.4 nm) to allow most drug molecules (which usually exceed 1 nm in diameter) to pass through. Consequently, drug distribution is not notably abnormal in patients with genetic diseases affecting aquaporins. Pinocytosis involves invagination of part of the cell membrane and the trapping within the cell of a small vesicle containing extracellular constituents. The vesicle contents can then be released within the cell, or extruded from its other side. This mechanism is important for the transport of some macromolecules (e.g. **insulin**, which crosses the blood–brain barrier by this process), but not for small molecules.

DIFFUSION THROUGH LIPID

Non-polar molecules (in which electrons are uniformly distributed) dissolve freely in membrane lipids, and consequently diffuse readily across cell membranes. The number of molecules crossing the membrane per unit area in unit time is determined by the *permeability coefficient*, P, and the concentration difference across the membrane. Permeant molecules must be present within the membrane in sufficient numbers and must be mobile within the membrane if rapid permeation is to occur. Thus, two physicochemical factors contribute to P, namely *solubility* in the membrane (which can be expressed as a partition coefficient for the substance distributed between the membrane phase and the aqueous environment) and *diffusivity*, which is a measure of the mobility of molecules within the lipid and is expressed as a diffusion coefficient. The diffusion coefficient varies only modestly between conventional drugs, as noted above, so the most important determinant of membrane permeability for conventional low molecular-weight drugs is the partition coefficient (Fig. 9.2). Many pharmacokinetic characteristics of a drug – such as rate of absorption from the gut, penetration into different tissues and the extent of renal elimination – can be predicted from knowledge of its lipid solubility.

ION TRAPPING

Ionisation and membrane permeability affect not only the rate at which drugs permeate membranes but also the steady-state distribution of drug molecules between aqueous compartments. Lipid-soluble molecules diffuse into cells where they can be metabolised (e.g. by esterases); this may

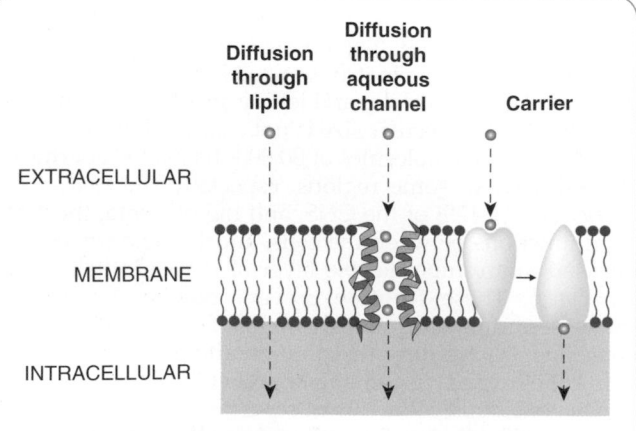

Fig. 9.1 **Routes by which solutes can traverse cell membranes.** (Molecules can also cross cellular barriers by pinocytosis.)

Fig. 9.2 **The importance of lipid solubility in membrane permeation.** (A) and (B) show the concentration profile in a lipid membrane separating two aqueous compartments. A lipid-soluble drug (A) is subject to a much larger transmembrane concentration gradient (ΔC_m) than a lipid-insoluble drug (B). It therefore diffuses more rapidly, even though the aqueous concentration gradient ($C_1 - C_2$) is the same in both cases.

liberate a functionally important charged (and hence impermeant) metabolite, which is consequently trapped within the cell. This has been extensively exploited, notably in probing the function of intracellular mediators such as Ca^{2+} using fluorescent indicators such as fura-2, which is loaded into cells as an uncharged ester and trapped intracellularly as the charged form (see, for example, Fig. 4.2). The same approach has been used recently by pharmaceutical chemists seeking to target drugs (several of which are in development) to intracellular sites of action within monocytes and macrophages using esterase-sensitive chemical motifs conjugated to a drug such as a histone deacetylase inhibitor (Ch. 29). This forms a prodrug (see later, p. 131) that delivers the drug to cells of the monocyte macrophage lineage which selectively express human carboxylesterase-1, the charged active drug product being trapped in the monocyte cytoplasm, which is its site of action (Needham et al., 2011).

pH and ionisation
One important complicating factor in relation to membrane permeation is that many drugs are weak acids or bases, and therefore exist in both un-ionised and ionised form, the ratio of the two forms varying with pH. For a weak base, B, the ionisation reaction is:

$$BH^+ \xrightleftharpoons{K_a} B + H^+$$

and the dissociation constant pK_a is given by the Henderson–Hasselbalch equation

$$pK_a = pH + \log_{10}\frac{[BH^+]}{[B]}$$

For a weak acid, AH:

$$AH \xrightleftharpoons{K_a} A^- + H^+$$

$$pK_a = pH + \log_{10}\frac{[AH]}{[A^-]}$$

In either case, the ionised species, BH^+ or A^-, has very low lipid solubility and is virtually unable to permeate membranes except where a specific transport mechanism exists. The lipid solubility of the uncharged species, B or AH, depends on the chemical nature of the drug; for many drugs, the uncharged species is sufficiently lipid-soluble to permit rapid membrane permeation, although there are exceptions (e.g. aminoglycoside antibiotics; see Ch. 52) where even the uncharged molecule is insufficiently lipid-soluble to cross membranes appreciably. This is usually because of hydrogen-bonding groups (such as hydroxyl in sugar moieties in aminoglycosides) that render the uncharged molecule hydrophilic.

pH partition and ion trapping
If a pH difference exists between body compartments, this can alter the steady-state distribution of drugs that are weak acids or weak bases via its influence on their ionisation. Fig. 9.3 shows how a weak acid (e.g. **aspirin**, pK_a 3.5) and a weak base (e.g. **pethidine**, pK_a 8.6) would be distributed at equilibrium between three body compartments, namely plasma (pH 7.4), alkaline urine (pH 8) and gastric juice (pH 3). Within each compartment, the ratio of ionised to un-ionised drug is governed by the pK_a of the drug and

the pH of that compartment. It is assumed that the un-ionised species can cross the membrane, and therefore reaches an equal concentration in each compartment. The ionised species is assumed not to cross at all. The result is that, at equilibrium, the total (ionised + un-ionised) concentration of the drug will be different in each compartment, with an acidic drug being concentrated in the compartment with high pH ('ion trapping'), and vice versa. The concentration gradients produced by ion trapping can theoretically be very large if there is a large pH difference between compartments. Thus, aspirin would be concentrated more than four-fold with respect to plasma in an alkaline renal tubule, and about 6000-fold in plasma with respect to the acidic gastric contents. Such large gradients are not achieved in reality for two main reasons. First, assuming total impermeability of the charged species is not realistic, and even a small permeability will attenuate considerably the concentration difference that can be reached. Second, body compartments rarely approach equilibrium. Neither the gastric contents nor the renal tubular fluid stands still, and the resulting bulk flow of drug molecules reduces the concentration gradients well below the theoretical equilibrium conditions. The pH partition mechanism nonetheless correctly explains some of the qualitative effects of pH changes in different body compartments on the pharmacokinetics of weakly acidic or basic drugs, particularly in relation to renal excretion and to penetration of the blood–brain barrier.

pH partition is not the main determinant of the site of absorption of drugs from the gastrointestinal tract. This is because the enormous absorptive surface area of the villi and microvilli in the ileum compared with the much smaller absorptive surface area in the stomach is of overriding importance. Thus absorption of an acidic drug such as aspirin is promoted by drugs that accelerate gastric emptying (e.g. **metoclopramide**) and retarded by drugs that slow gastric emptying (e.g. **propantheline**), even though the acidic pH of the stomach contents favours absorption of weak acids. Values of pK_a for some common drugs are shown in Fig. 9.4.

There are several important consequences of pH partition:

- Free-base trapping of some antimalarial drugs (e.g. **chloroquine**, see Ch. 55) in the acidic environment in the food vacuole of the malaria parasite contributes to the disruption of the haemoglobin digestion pathway that underlies their toxic effect on the parasite.
- Urinary acidification accelerates excretion of weak bases and retards that of weak acids (see Ch. 10).
- Urinary alkalinisation has the opposite effects: it reduces excretion of weak bases and increases excretion of weak acids.
- Increasing plasma pH (e.g. by administration of sodium bicarbonate) causes weakly acidic drugs to be extracted from the CNS into the plasma. Conversely, reducing plasma pH (e.g. by administration of a carbonic anhydrase inhibitor such as **acetazolamide**, see Ch. 30) causes weakly acidic drugs to become concentrated in the CNS, potentially increasing their neurotoxicity. This has practical consequences in choosing a means to alkalinise urine in treating aspirin overdose: bicarbonate and acetazolamide each increase urine pH and hence increase salicylate elimination, but bicarbonate reduces whereas acetazolamide increases distribution of salicylate to the CNS.

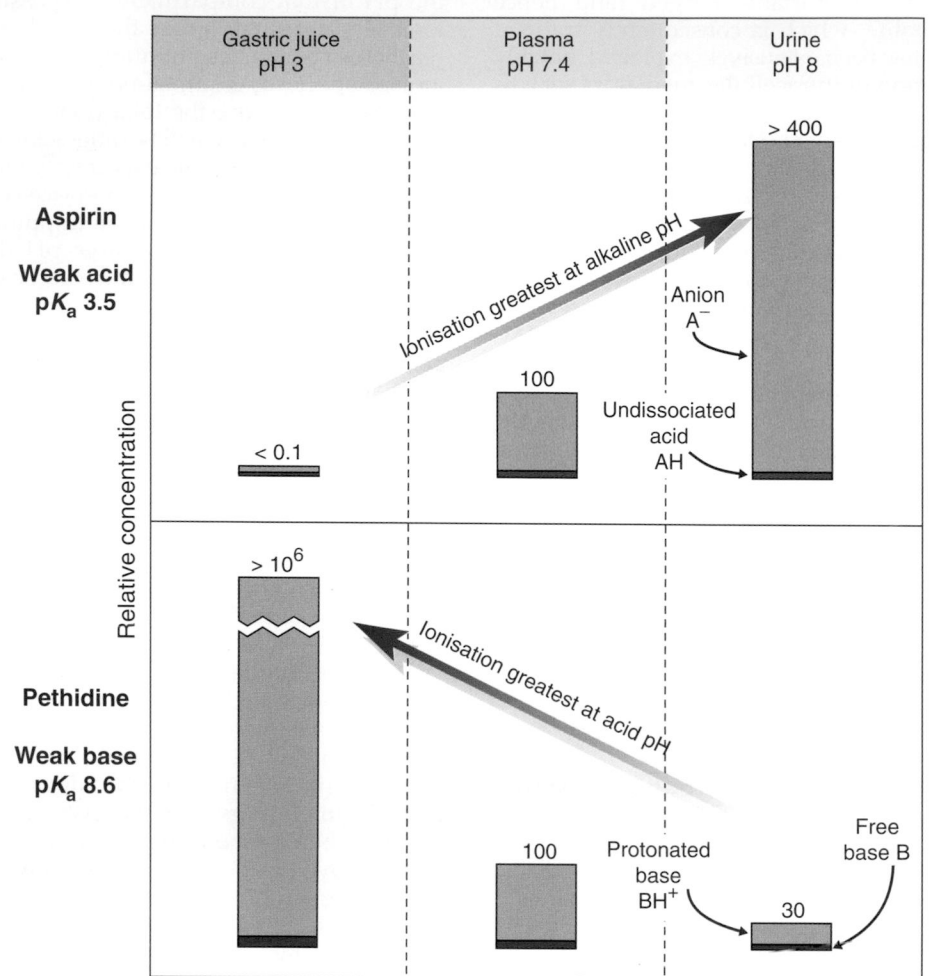

Fig. 9.3 Theoretical partition of a weak acid (aspirin) and a weak base (pethidine) between aqueous compartments (urine, plasma and gastric juice) according to the pH difference between them. Numbers represent relative concentrations (total plasma concentration = 100). It is assumed that the uncharged species in each case can permeate the cellular barrier separating the compartments, and therefore reaches the same concentration in all three. Variations in the fractional ionisation as a function of pH give rise to the large total concentration differences with respect to plasma.

CARRIER-MEDIATED TRANSPORT

Many cell membranes possess specialised transport mechanisms that regulate entry and exit of physiologically important molecules, such as sugars, amino acids, neurotransmitters and metal ions. They are broadly divided into *SLC transporters* and *ATP-binding cassette (ABC) transporters*. The former facilitate passive movement of solutes down their electrochemical gradient, while the latter are active pumps fuelled by ATP. Over 300 human genes are believed to code these transporters, most of which act mainly on endogenous substrates, but some also transport foreign chemicals ('xenobiotics') including drugs. The role of such transporters in neurotransmitter function is discussed in Chapters 14, 15 and 38.

Organic cation transporters and organic anion transporters

Two structurally related SLCs of importance in drug distribution are the organic cation transporters (OCTs) and organic anion transporters (OATs). The carrier molecule consists of a transmembrane protein that binds one or more molecules or ions, changes conformation and releases its cargo on the other side of the membrane. Such systems may operate purely passively, without any energy source; in this case, they merely facilitate the process of transmembrane equilibration of a single transported species in the direction of its electrochemical gradient. The OCTs translocate dopamine, choline and various drugs including **vecuronium**, **quinine** and **procainamide**. They are 'uniporters' (i.e. each protein transporter molecule binds one solute molecule at a time and transports it down its gradient). OCT2 (present in proximal renal tubules) concentrates drugs such as **cisplatin** (an important anticancer drug, see Ch. 57) in these cells, resulting in its selective nephrotoxicity; related drugs (e.g. **carboplatin**, **oxaliplatin**) are not transported by OCT2 and are less nephrotoxic; competition with **cimetidine** for OCT2 offers possible protection against cisplatin nephrotoxicity (Fig. 9.5). Other SLCs are coupled to the electrochemical gradient of Na^+ or other ions across the membrane, generated by ATP-dependent ion pumps (see Ch. 4); in this case, transport can occur against an electrochemical gradient. It may involve exchange of one molecule for another ('antiport') or transport of two

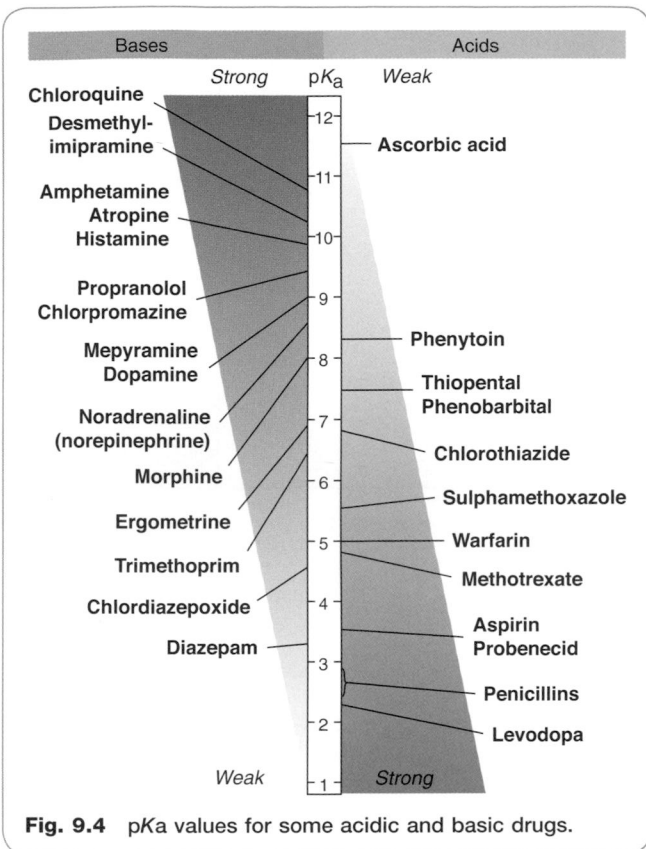

Bases		Acids
Strong	pK_a	*Weak*

Chloroquine
Desmethyl-
imipramine

Amphetamine
Atropine
Histamine

Propranolol
Chlorpromazine

Mepyramine
Dopamine

Noradrenaline
(norepinephrine)

Morphine

Ergometrine

Trimethoprim

Chlordiazepoxide

Diazepam

Weak

—12—
—11—
—10—
—9—
—8—
—7—
—6—
—5—
—4—
—3—
—2—
—1

Ascorbic acid

Phenytoin

Thiopental
Phenobarbital

Chlorothiazide

Sulphamethoxazole

Warfarin

Methotrexate

Aspirin
Probenecid

Penicillins

Levodopa

Strong

Fig. 9.4 pK_a values for some acidic and basic drugs.

molecules together in the same direction ('symport'). The OATs are responsible for the renal secretion of urate, prostaglandins, several vitamins and *p*-amino hippurate, and for drugs such as **probenecid**, many antibiotics, antiviral, non-steroidal anti-inflammatory and antineoplastic drugs. Uptake is driven by exchange with intracellular dicarboxylic acids (mainly α-ketoglutarate, partly derived from cellular metabolism and partly by co-transport with Na^+ entering cells down its concentration gradient). Metabolic energy is provided by ATP for Na^+/K^+ exchange. Carrier-mediated transport, because it involves a binding step, shows the characteristic of saturation.

Carriers of this type are ubiquitous, and many pharmacological effects are the result of interference with them. Thus, some nerve terminals have transport mechanisms that accumulate specific neurotransmitters or their precursors, and there are many examples of drugs that act by inhibiting these transport mechanisms (see Chs 14, 15, 38, 48 and 49). From a general pharmacokinetic point of view, however, the main sites where SLCs, including OCTs and OATs, are expressed and carrier-mediated drug transport is important are:

- the blood–brain barrier
- the gastrointestinal tract
- the renal tubule
- the biliary tract
- the placenta

P-glycoprotein transporters

P-glycoproteins (P-gp; P for 'permeability'), which belong to the ABC transporter superfamily, are the second important

class of transporters, and are responsible for multidrug resistance in cancer cells, many of which express an ATP-dependent pump with broad specificity called multidrug resistance protein 1 (mdr1) – see Chapter 57. This is expressed in animals, fungi and bacteria and may have evolved as a defence mechanism against toxins. P-gps are present in renal tubular brush border membranes, in bile canaliculi, in astrocyte foot processes in brain microvessels[1], and in the gastrointestinal tract. They play an important part in absorption, distribution and elimination of many drugs, and are often co-located with SLC drug carriers, so that a drug that has been concentrated by, for example, an OAT transporter in the basolateral membrane of a renal tubular cell may then be pumped out of the cell by a P-gp in the lumenal membrane (see Ch. 30).

Polymorphic variation in the genes coding SLCs and P-gp contributes to individual genetic variation in responsiveness to different drugs, and competition between drugs for the same transporter cause drug–drug interactions (see Yoshida et al., 2013 for a review). OCT1 transports several drugs, including **metformin** (used to treat diabetes; see Ch. 32), into hepatocytes (in contrast to OCT2 which is active in renal proximal tubular cells, see previously). Metformin acts partly through effects within hepatocytes. Single nucleotide polymorphisms (SNPs) that impair the function of OCT1 influence the effectiveness of metformin (Fig. 9.6). This is but one example of many genetic influences on drug effectiveness or toxicity via altered activity of carriers that influence drug disposition. Furthermore, induction or competitive inhibition of transporter molecules can occur in the presence of a second ligand that binds the carrier, so there is a potential for drug interaction (see Fig. 9.5 and Ch. 12).

Plasma protein and tissue partition of drugs

In addition to the processes so far described, which govern the transport of drug molecules across the barriers between different aqueous compartments, two additional factors have a major influence on drug distribution and elimination. These are:

- binding to plasma proteins
- partition into body fat and other tissues

BINDING OF DRUGS TO PLASMA PROTEINS

At therapeutic concentrations in plasma, many drugs exist mainly in bound form. The fraction of drug that is unbound and pharmacologically active in plasma can be less than 1%, the remainder being associated with plasma protein. Seemingly small differences in protein binding (e.g. 99.5% vs 99.0%) can have large effects on free drug concentration and drug effect. Such differences are common between human plasma and plasma from species used in preclinical drug testing, and must be taken into account when estimating a suitable dose for 'first time in human' studies during drug development. The most important plasma protein in relation to drug binding is albumin, which binds many acidic drugs (e.g. warfarin, non-steroidal anti-inflammatory

---

[1]This is illustrated by strain and species differences. For example, Collie dogs lack the multidrug resistance gene (*mdr1*), that encodes a P-glycoprotein which extrudes toxins from the cerebrospinal fluid across the blood–brain barrier. This has consequences for veterinary medicine because **ivermectin** (an anthelminthic drug, Ch. 56) is severely neurotoxic in the many breeds with Collie ancestry.

Fig. 9.5 **Human organic cation transporter 2 (OCT2) mediates cisplatin nephrotoxicity.** OCT2 is expressed in kidney whereas OCT1 is expressed in liver. Cisplatin (100 μmol/L) influences the activity of OCT2 but not of OCT1, each expressed in a cultured cell line (A), whereas the less nephrotoxic drugs carboplatin and oxaliplatin do not. Cisplatin similarly influences OCT2 activity in fresh human kidney tubule cells but not in fresh hepatocytes or kidney cells from diabetic patients who are less susceptible to cisplatin nephrotoxicity (B). Cisplatin accumulates in cells that express OCT2 (C) and causes cell death (D). Cimetidine competes with cisplatin for OCT2 and concentration dependently protects against cisplatin-induced apoptosis (D) – cimetidine concentrations are in μmol/L. (Data redrawn from Ciarimboli, G et al., 2005. Am. J. Pathol. 167, 1477–1484.)

drugs, sulfonamides) and a smaller number of basic drugs (e.g. tricyclic antidepressants and chlorpromazine). Other plasma proteins, including β-globulin and an acid glyco-protein that increases in inflammatory disease, have also been implicated in the binding of certain basic drugs such as quinine.

The amount of a drug that is bound to protein depends on three factors:

• the concentration of free drug
• its affinity for the binding sites
• the concentration of protein

As a first approximation, the binding reaction can be regarded as a simple association of the drug molecules with a finite population of binding sites, exactly analogous to drug–receptor binding (see Ch. 2):

$$\underset{\substack{\text{free}\\\text{drug}}}{D} + \underset{\substack{\text{binding}\\\text{site}}}{S} \rightleftharpoons \underset{\text{complex}}{DS}$$

The usual concentration of albumin in plasma is approximately 0.6 mmol/L (4 g/100 mL). With two sites per albumin molecule, the drug-binding capacity of plasma albumin would therefore be about 1.2 mmol/L. For most drugs, the total plasma concentration required for a clinical effect is much less than 1.2 mmol/L, so with usual therapeutic doses the binding sites are far from saturated, and the concentration bound [DS] varies nearly in direct proportion to the free concentration [D]. Under these conditions, the fraction bound, [DS]/([D] + [DS]), is independent of the drug concentration. However, some drugs, for example, **tolbutamide** (see Ch. 32), act at plasma concentrations at which its binding to plasma albumin approaches saturation (i.e. on the flat part of the binding curve). This means that increasing the dose increases the free (pharmacologically active) concentration disproportionately. This is illustrated in Fig. 9.7.

Plasma albumin binds many different drugs, so competition can occur between them. If two drugs (A and B) compete

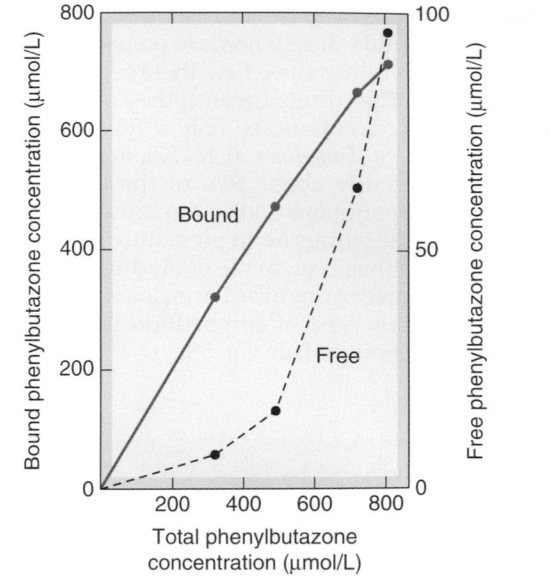

Fig. 9.7 **Binding of phenylbutazone to plasma albumin.** The graph shows the disproportionate increase in free concentration as the total concentration increases, owing to the binding sites approaching saturation. (Data from Brodie, B., Hogben, C.A.M., 1957. J. Pharm. Pharmacol. 9, 345.)

Fig. 9.6 **Genetic variants of organic cation transporter 1 (OCT1) are associated with different responses to metformin in healthy humans.** (A) An oral glucose tolerance test (OGTT) gave similar plasma glucose responses in control subjects with only reference *OCT1* alleles versus subjects with at least one reduced function *OCT1* allele. (B) In contrast, after metformin treatment, the OGTT response was less in the same reference subjects than in those with reduced function *OCT1* alleles – i.e. the effect of metformin was blunted in the variant-allele group. (C) Glucose exposure estimated by area under the glucose time curves (AUC) was significantly lower in subjects with only reference *OCT1* alleles, $p = 0.004$. (Data redrawn from Yan Shu, et al., 2007. J. Clin. Invest. 117, 1422–1431.)

Movement of drugs across cellular barriers

- To traverse cellular barriers (e.g. gastrointestinal mucosa, renal tubule, blood–brain barrier, placenta), drugs have to cross lipid membranes.
- Drugs cross lipid membranes mainly (a) by passive diffusional transfer and (b) by carrier-mediated transfer.
- The main factor that determines the rate of passive diffusional transfer across membranes is a drug's lipid solubility.
- Many drugs are weak acids or weak bases; their state of ionisation varies with pH according to the Henderson–Hasselbalch equation.
- With weak acids or bases, only the uncharged species (the protonated form for a weak acid, the unprotonated form for a weak base) can diffuse across lipid membranes; this gives rise to pH partition.
- pH partition means that weak acids tend to accumulate in compartments of relatively high pH, whereas weak bases do the reverse.
- Carrier-mediated transport is mediated by solute carriers (SLCs), which include organic cation transporters (OCTs) and organic anion transporters (OATs), and P-glycoproteins (P-gps) (ATP-binding cassette [ABC] transporters) in the renal tubule, blood–brain barrier and gastrointestinal epithelium. These are important in determining the distribution of many drugs, are prone to genetic variation and are targets for drug interactions.

in this way, administration of drug B can reduce the protein binding, and hence increase the free plasma concentration, of drug A. To do this, drug B needs to occupy an appreciable fraction of the binding sites. Few therapeutic drugs affect the binding of other drugs because they occupy, at therapeutic plasma concentrations, only a tiny fraction of the available sites. *Sulfonamides* (Ch. 52) are an exception, because they occupy about 50% of the binding sites at therapeutic concentrations and so can cause harmful effects by displacing other drugs or, in premature babies, bilirubin (see later). Much has been made of binding interactions of this kind as a source of untoward drug interactions in clinical medicine, but this type of competition is less important than was once thought (see Ch. 58).

Binding of drugs to plasma proteins

- Plasma albumin binds mainly acidic drugs (approximately two molecules per albumin molecule).
- Saturable binding can lead to a non-linear relation between dose and free (active) drug concentration, but the effective concentration range of most therapeutic drugs is below that at which this would be important.
- Binding to plasma protein is a source of species variation, important in interpreting preclinical pharmacology studies and estimating the first-in-human dose.
- β-Globulin and acid glycoprotein also bind some drugs.
- Extensive protein binding slows drug elimination (metabolism and/or glomerular filtration).
- Competition between drugs for protein binding can lead to clinically significant drug interactions, but this is uncommon.

PARTITION INTO BODY FAT AND OTHER TISSUES

Fat represents a large, non-polar compartment. In practice, this is important for only a few drugs, mainly because the effective fat:water partition coefficient is relatively low for most drugs. Morphine, for example, although lipid-soluble enough to cross the blood–brain barrier, has a lipid:water partition coefficient of only 0.4, so sequestration of the drug by body fat is of little importance. Thiopental, by comparison (fat:water partition coefficient approximately 10), accumulates substantially in body fat. This has important consequences that limit its usefulness as an intravenous anaesthetic to short-term initiation ('induction') of anaesthesia, and it has been replaced by propofol even for this indication in many countries (Ch. 42).

The second factor that limits the accumulation of drugs in body fat is its low blood supply – less than 2% of the cardiac output. Consequently, drugs are delivered slowly to body fat, and the theoretical equilibrium distribution between fat and body water is delayed. For practical purposes, therefore, partition into body fat when drugs are given acutely is important only for a few highly lipid-soluble drugs (e.g. general anaesthetics; Ch. 42). When

lipid-soluble drugs are given chronically, however, accumulation in body fat is often significant (e.g. benzodiazepines; Ch. 45). Some drugs and environmental contaminants (such as insecticides), if ingested intermittently, accumulate slowly but progressively in body fat.

Fat is not the only tissue in which drugs can accumulate. **Chloroquine** – an antimalarial drug (Ch. 55) – has a high affinity for melanin and is taken up by the retina, which is rich in melanin granules, accounting for chloroquine's ocular toxicity. Tetracyclines (Ch. 52) accumulate slowly in bones and teeth, because they have a high affinity for calcium, and should not be used in children for this reason. Very high concentrations of **amiodarone** (an antidysrhythmic drug; Ch. 22) accumulate in liver and lung during chronic use, causing hepatitis and interstitial pulmonary fibrosis.

DRUG ABSORPTION AND ROUTES OF ADMINISTRATION

The main routes of drug administration and elimination are shown schematically in Fig. 9.8. Absorption is defined as the passage of a drug from its site of administration into the plasma. It is important for all routes of administration except intravenous injection, where it is complete by definition. There are instances, such as topical administration of a steroid cream to skin or inhalation of a bronchodilator aerosol to treat asthma (Ch. 29), where absorption as just defined is not required for the drug to act, but in most cases the drug must enter plasma before reaching its site of action.

The main routes of administration are:

- oral (drug is swallowed)
- sublingual or buccal (drug is kept in contact with the oral mucosa)
- rectal
- application to other epithelial surfaces (e.g. skin, cornea, vagina and nasal mucosa)
- inhalation
- injection
  - subcutaneous
  - intramuscular
  - intravenous
  - intrathecal
  - intravitreal

ORAL ADMINISTRATION

Most small molecule drugs are taken by mouth and swallowed. Little absorption occurs until the drug enters the small intestine, although non-polar drugs applied to the buccal mucosa or under the tongue are absorbed directly from the mouth (e.g. organic nitrates, Ch. 21, and buprenorphine, Ch. 43). Peptides and proteins are subject to digestion as well as epithelial barriers, so the oral route is not generally suitable to biopharmaceuticals and despite ingenious pharmaceutical approaches to circumvent these problems, success has been limited (Renukuntla et al., 2013).

DRUG ABSORPTION FROM THE INTESTINE

For most drugs, the mechanism of absorption is the same as for other epithelial barriers, namely, passive transfer at a rate determined by the ionisation and lipid solubility of the drug molecules. Fig. 9.9 shows the absorption of various

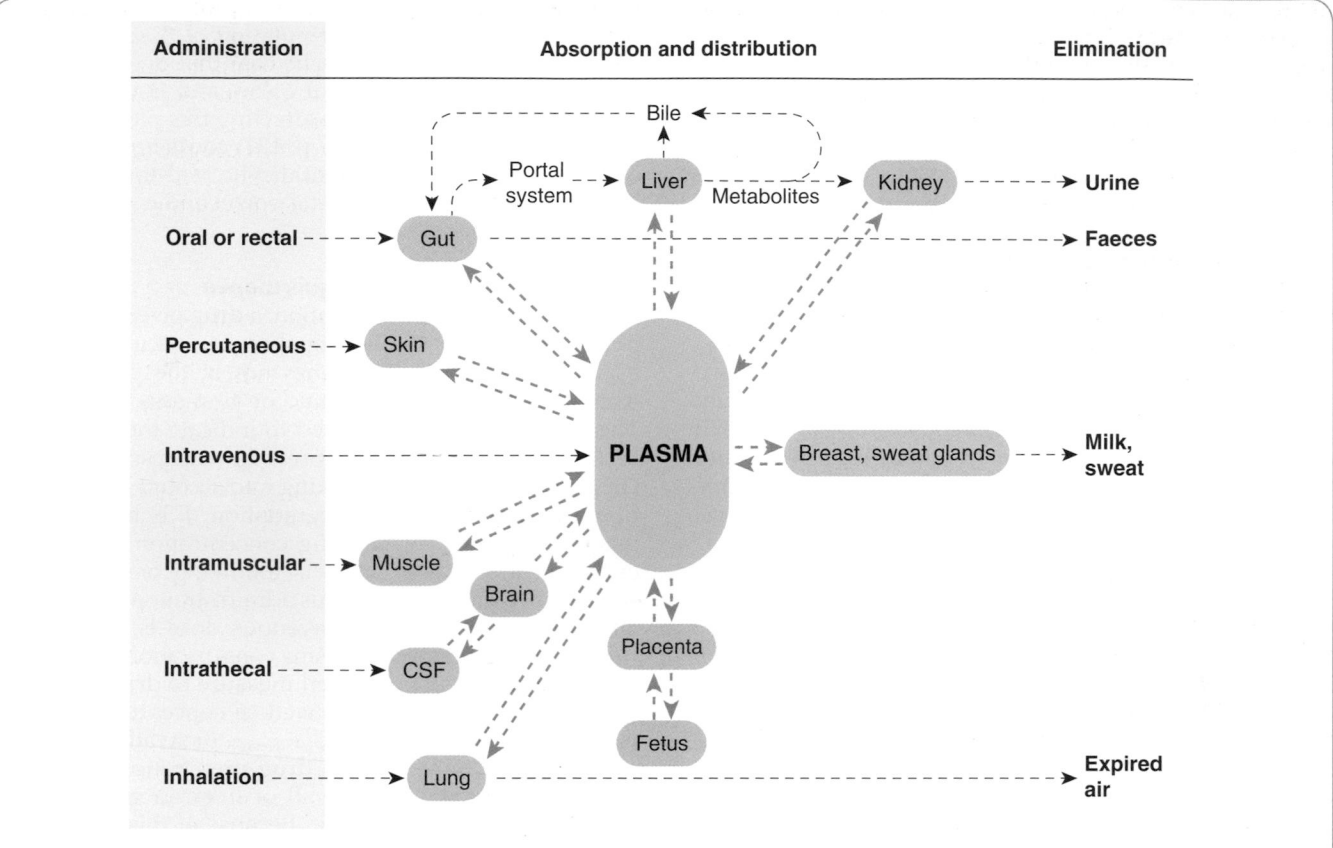

Fig. 9.8 The main routes of drug administration and elimination. *CSF*, cerebrospinal fluid.

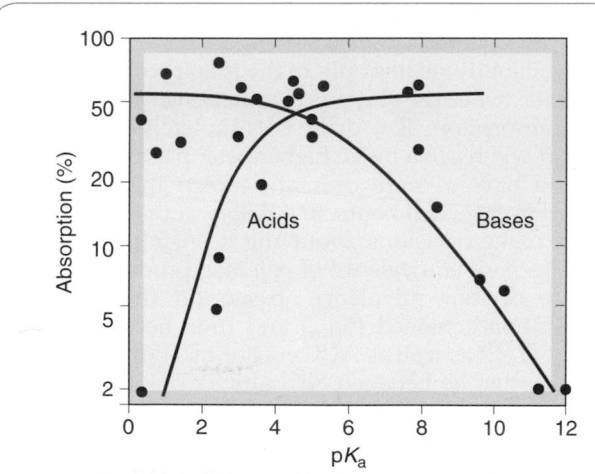

Fig. 9.9 Absorption of drugs from the intestine, as a function of pKa, for acids and bases. Weak acids and bases are well absorbed; strong acids and bases are poorly absorbed. (Redrawn from Schanker, L.S. et al., 1957. J. Pharmacol. 120, 528.)

weak acids and bases as a function of pK_a. As expected, strong bases of pK_a 10 or higher are poorly absorbed, as are strong acids of pK_a less than 3, because they are fully ionised. The arrow poison curare used by South American Indians contains quaternary ammonium compounds that block neuromuscular transmission (Ch. 14). These strong bases are poorly absorbed from the gastrointestinal tract, so the meat from animals killed in this way was safe to eat.

In some instances, intestinal drug absorption depends on carrier-mediated transport rather than simple lipid diffusion. Examples include **levodopa**, used in treating Parkinson's disease (see Ch. 41), which is taken up by the carrier that normally transports phenylalanine, and **fluorouracil** (Ch. 57), a cytotoxic drug that is transported by the carrier for pyrimidines (thymine and uracil). Iron is absorbed via specific carriers in the epithelial cell membranes of jejunal mucosa, and calcium is absorbed by a vitamin D–dependent carrier.

FACTORS AFFECTING GASTROINTESTINAL ABSORPTION

Typically, about 75% of a drug given orally is absorbed in 1–3 h, but numerous factors alter this, some physiological and some to do with the formulation of the drug. The main factors are:

- gut content (e.g. fed vs fasted)
- gastrointestinal motility
- splanchnic blood flow
- particle size and formulation
- physicochemical factors, including some drug interactions
- genetic polymorphisms in, and drug–drug competition for, transporters

The influence of feeding, which influences both gut content and splanchnic blood flow, is routinely examined in early phase clinical trials and prescribing advice tailored accordingly. Gastrointestinal motility has a large effect.

Many disorders (e.g. migraine, diabetic neuropathy) cause gastric stasis and slow drug absorption. Drug treatment can also affect motility, either reducing (e.g. drugs that block muscarinic receptors; see Ch. 14) or increasing it (e.g. **metoclopramide**, an antiemetic used in migraine to facilitate absorption of analgesic). Excessively rapid movement of gut contents (e.g. in some forms of diarrhoea) can impair absorption. Several drugs (e.g. **propranolol**) reach a higher plasma concentration if they are taken after a meal, probably because food increases splanchnic blood flow. Conversely, splanchnic blood flow is greatly reduced by hypovolaemia or heart failure, with a resultant reduction of drug absorption.

Particle size and formulation have major effects on absorption. In 1971, patients in a New York hospital were found to require unusually large maintenance doses of **digoxin** (Ch. 22). In a study on normal volunteers, it was found that standard digoxin tablets from different manufacturers resulted in different plasma concentrations (Fig. 9.10), even though the digoxin content of the tablets was the same, probably in part because of differences in particle size.

Therapeutic drugs are formulated to produce desired absorption characteristics. Capsules may be designed to remain intact for some hours after ingestion in order to delay absorption, or tablets may have a resistant coating to give the same effect. In some cases, a mixture of slow- and fast-release particles is included in a capsule to produce rapid but sustained absorption. More elaborate pharmaceutical systems include modified-release preparations that permit less frequent dosing. Such preparations not only permit an increased dose interval but also reduce adverse effects related to high peak plasma concentrations following administration of a conventional formulation.

When drugs are swallowed, the intention is usually that they should be absorbed and cause a systemic effect, but there are exceptions. **Vancomycin** is very poorly absorbed, and is administered orally to eradicate toxin-forming *Clostridium difficile* from the gut lumen in patients with pseudomembranous colitis (an adverse effect of broad-spectrum

antibiotics caused by appearance of this organism in the bowel). **Mesalazine** is a formulation of 5-aminosalicylic acid in a pH-dependent acrylic coat that degrades in the terminal ileum and proximal colon, and is used to treat inflammatory bowel disease affecting this part of the gut. **Olsalazine** is a prodrug (see p. 131) consisting of a dimer of two molecules of 5-aminosalicylic acid that is cleaved by colonic bacteria in the distal bowel and is used to treat patients with distal colitis.

Bioavailability and bioequivalence

To access the systemic circulation, a drug given orally must not only penetrate the intestinal mucosa, it must also run a gauntlet of inactivating enzymes in the gut wall and liver, referred to as 'presystemic' or 'first-pass' metabolism. The term *bioavailability* is used to indicate the fraction (F) of an orally administered dose that reaches the systemic circulation as intact drug, taking into account both absorption and local metabolic degradation. F is measured by determining the plasma drug concentration versus time curves in a group of subjects following oral and (on a separate occasion) intravenous administration (the fraction absorbed following an intravenous dose is 1 by definition). The area under the plasma concentration time curves (AUC) provides an integrated measure of drug exposure, taking into account time as well as concentration, and F is estimated as $AUC_{oral} / AUC_{intravenous}$. Bioavailability is not a characteristic solely of the drug preparation: variations in enzyme activity of gut wall or liver, in gastric pH or intestinal motility all affect it. Because of this, one cannot speak strictly of the bioavailability of a particular preparation, but only of that preparation in a given individual on a particular occasion, and F determined in a group of healthy volunteer subjects may differ substantially from the value determined in patients with diseases of gastrointestinal or circulatory systems.

Bioavailability relates only to the total proportion of the drug that reaches the systemic circulation and neglects the rate of absorption. If a drug is completely absorbed in 30 min, it will reach a much higher peak plasma concentration (and have a more dramatic effect) than if it were absorbed over several hours. Regulatory authorities – which have to make decisions about the licensing of products that are 'generic equivalents' of patented products – require evidence of 'bioequivalence' based on the maximum concentration achieved (C_{max}) and time between dosing and C_{max} (T_{max}) as well as $AUC_{(0-t)}$. For most drugs, $AUC_{(0-t)}$ and C_{max} must lie between 80% and 125% of a marketed preparation for the new generic product to be accepted as bioequivalent (EMEA, 2010).

OROMUCOSAL (SUBLINGUAL OR BUCCAL) ADMINISTRATION

Absorption directly from the oral cavity is sometimes useful when a rapid response is required, particularly when the drug is either unstable at gastric pH or rapidly metabolised by the liver. **Glyceryl trinitrate** and **buprenorphine** are examples of drugs that are often given sublingually (Chs 22 and 43, respectively). Buccal midazolam is as effective and safe as intravenous or rectal diazepam in terminating early *status epilepticus* (Ch. 46) in children (Brigo et al., 2015). Times from arrival in the emergency department to drug administration and to seizure cessation are shortened and the drug is easier to administer. Drugs absorbed from the mouth pass directly into the systemic circulation without

Fig. 9.10 Variation in oral absorption among different formulations of digoxin. The four curves show the mean plasma concentrations attained for the four preparations, each of which was given on separate occasions to four subjects. The large variation has caused the formulation of digoxin tablets to be standardised since this study was published. (From Lindenbaum, J. et al., 1971. N Engl J Med 285, 1344.)

entering the portal system, and so escape first-pass metabolism by enzymes in the gut wall and liver.

RECTAL ADMINISTRATION

Rectal administration is used for drugs that are required either to produce a local effect (e.g. anti-inflammatory drugs such as **mesalazine** suppositories or enemas for use in ulcerative colitis, see Ch. 31) or to produce systemic effects. Absorption following rectal administration may be unreliable, but can be rapid and more complete than following oral administration, since only a fraction of the capillary drainage returns to the systemic circulation via the portal vein. This route can be useful in patients who are vomiting or are unable to take medication by mouth (e.g. postoperatively or during palliative care), but rectal administration has not been widely adopted even when there is a seemingly good rationale and suppositories commercially available, for example, ergotamine-containing suppositories for treating migraine attacks – a condition where gastric stasis and vomiting can limit the effectiveness of oral tablets (Ch. 16).

APPLICATION TO EPITHELIAL SURFACES

CUTANEOUS ADMINISTRATION

Cutaneous administration is used when a local effect on the skin is required (e.g. topically applied steroids, Ch. 28). Appreciable absorption may nonetheless occur and lead to systemic effects; absorption is sometimes exploited therapeutically, for example, in local application of rub-on gels of non-steroidal anti-inflammatory agents such as **ibuprofen** (Ch. 27).

Most drugs are absorbed very poorly through unbroken skin. However, a number of organophosphate insecticides (see Ch. 14), which need to penetrate an insect's cuticle to work, are absorbed through skin, and accidental poisoning occurs in farm workers.

▼ A case is recounted of a 35-year-old florist in 1932. 'While engaged in doing a light electrical repair job at a work bench he sat down in a chair on the seat of which some "Nico-Fume liquid" (a 40% solution of free nicotine) had been spilled. He felt the solution wet through his clothes to the skin over the left buttock, an area about the size of the palm of his hand. He thought nothing further of it and continued at his work for about 15 minutes, when he was suddenly seized with nausea and faintness … and found himself in a drenching sweat. On the way to hospital he lost consciousness.' He survived, just, and then 4 days later: 'On discharge from the hospital he was given the same clothes that he had worn when he was brought in. The clothes had been kept in a paper bag and were still damp where they had been wet with the nicotine solution.' The sequel was predictable. He survived again but felt thereafter 'unable to enter a greenhouse where nicotine was being sprayed'. Transdermal dosage forms of nicotine are now used to reduce the withdrawal symptoms that accompany stopping smoking (Ch. 50).

Transdermal dosage forms, in which the drug is incorporated in a stick-on patch applied to the skin, are used increasingly, and several drugs – for example **oestrogen** and **testosterone** for hormone replacement (Ch. 36) are available in this form. Such patches produce a steady rate of drug delivery and avoid presystemic metabolism. **Fentanyl** is available in a patch to treat intermittent breakthrough pain (Ch. 43). However, the method is suitable only for lipid-soluble drugs and is relatively expensive.

NASAL SPRAYS

Some peptide hormone analogues, for example, **antidiuretic hormone** (Ch. 34) and **gonadotrophin-releasing hormone** (see Ch. 36), are given as nasal sprays, as is **calcitonin** (Ch.

37). Absorption is believed to take place through mucosa overlying nasal-associated lymphoid tissue. This is similar to the mucosa overlying Peyer's patches in the small intestine, which is also unusually permeable.

EYE DROPS

Many drugs are applied as eye drops, relying on absorption through the epithelium of the conjunctival sac to produce their effects. Desirable local effects within the eye can be achieved without causing systemic side effects; for example, **dorzolamide** is a carbonic anhydrase inhibitor that is given as eye drops to lower ocular pressure in patients with glaucoma. It achieves this without affecting the kidney (see Ch. 30), thus avoiding the acidosis that is caused by oral administration of acetazolamide. Some systemic absorption from the eye occurs, however, and can result in unwanted effects (e.g. bronchospasm in asthmatic patients using **timolol** eye drops for glaucoma).

ADMINISTRATION BY INHALATION

Inhalation is the route used for volatile and gaseous anaesthetics, the lung serving as the route of both administration and elimination. The rapid exchange resulting from the large surface area and blood flow makes it possible to achieve rapid adjustments of plasma concentration. The pharmacokinetic behaviour of inhalation anaesthetics is discussed in Chapter 42.

Drugs used for their effects on the lung are also given by inhalation, usually as an aerosol. Glucocorticoids (e.g. **beclometasone dipropionate**) and bronchodilators (e.g. **salbutamol**; Ch. 29) are given in this way to achieve high local concentrations in the lung while minimising systemic effects. However, drugs given by inhalation in this way are usually partly absorbed into the circulation, and systemic side effects (e.g. tremor following salbutamol) can occur. Chemical modification of a drug may minimise such absorption. For example, **ipratropium**, a muscarinic-receptor antagonist (Chs 14 and 29), is a quaternary ammonium ion analogue of atropine. It is used as an inhaled bronchodilator because its poor absorption reduces the likelihood of systemic adverse effects.

ADMINISTRATION BY INJECTION

Intravenous injection is the fastest and most certain route of drug administration. Bolus injection rapidly produces a high concentration of drug, first in the right heart and pulmonary vessels and then in the systemic circulation. The peak concentration reaching the tissues depends critically on the rate of injection. Administration by intravenous infusion using a mechanical pump avoids the uncertainties of absorption from other sites, while avoiding high peak plasma concentrations caused by bolus injection.

Subcutaneous or intramuscular injection of drugs usually produces a faster effect than oral administration, but the rate of absorption depends greatly on the site of injection and on local blood flow. The rate-limiting factors in absorption from the injection site are:

- diffusion through the tissue
- removal by local blood flow

Absorption from a site of injection (sometimes but not always desirable, see later) is increased by increased blood flow. *Hyaluronidase* (an enzyme that breaks down the intercellular matrix, thereby increasing diffusion) also increases drug absorption from the site of injection. Conversely, absorption is reduced in patients with circulatory failure (shock) in whom tissue perfusion is reduced (Ch. 23).

METHODS FOR DELAYING ABSORPTION

It may be desirable to delay absorption, either to produce a local effect or to prolong systemic action. For example, addition of adrenaline (epinephrine) to a local anaesthetic reduces absorption of the anaesthetic into the general circulation, usefully prolonging the anaesthetic effect (Ch. 44). Formulation of insulin with protamine and zinc produces a long-acting form (see Ch. 32). Procaine penicillin (Ch. 52) is a poorly soluble salt of **penicillin**; when injected as an aqueous suspension, it is slowly absorbed and exerts a prolonged action. Esterification of steroid hormones (e.g. medroxyprogesterone acetate, testosterone propionate; Ch. 36) and antipsychotic drugs (e.g. fluphenazine decanoate; Ch. 47) increases their solubility in oil and slows their absorption when they are injected in an oily solution.

Another method used to achieve slow and continuous absorption of certain steroid hormones (e.g. **oestradiol**; Ch. 36) is the subcutaneous implantation of drug substance, for example, formulated as a solid pellet. The rate of absorption is proportional to the surface area of the implant.

INTRATHECAL INJECTION

Injection of a drug into the subarachnoid space via a lumbar puncture needle is used for some specialised purposes. **Methotrexate** (Ch. 57) is administered in this way in the treatment of certain childhood leukaemias to prevent relapse in the CNS. Regional anaesthesia can be produced by intrathecal administration of a local anaesthetic such as **bupivacaine** (see Ch. 44); opioid analgesics can also be used in this way (Ch. 43). **Baclofen** (a GABA analogue; Ch. 39) is used to treat disabling muscle spasms. It has been administered intrathecally to minimise its adverse effects. Some antibiotics (e.g. aminoglycosides) cross the blood–brain barrier very slowly, and in rare clinical situations where they are essential (e.g. nervous system infections with bacteria resistant to other antibiotics) can be given intrathecally or directly into the cerebral ventricles via a reservoir. **Nusinersen**, an antisense oligonucleotide used to treat spinal muscular atrophy (Ch. 41) is administered intrathecally and this route may become increasingly important in view of the therapeutic potential of biopharmaceuticals in neurological disorders and the access problem posed to these agents by the blood–brain barrier (see p. 129).

INTRAVITREAL INJECTION

Ranibizumab (monoclonal antibody fragment that binds to vascular endothelial growth factor; Ch. 23) or a fusion protein, **aflibercept**, are given by intravitreal injection by ophthalmologists treating patients with wet age-related macular degeneration, macular oedema and choroidal neovascularisation. Intravitreal implants that slowly release corticosteroids (such as **fluocinolone** or **dexamethasone**) over a period of months are used in macular oedema.

DISTRIBUTION OF DRUGS IN THE BODY

BODY FLUID COMPARTMENTS

Body water is distributed into four main compartments (Fig. 9.11). Water constitutes 50% to 70% of body weight, being rather less in women than in men.

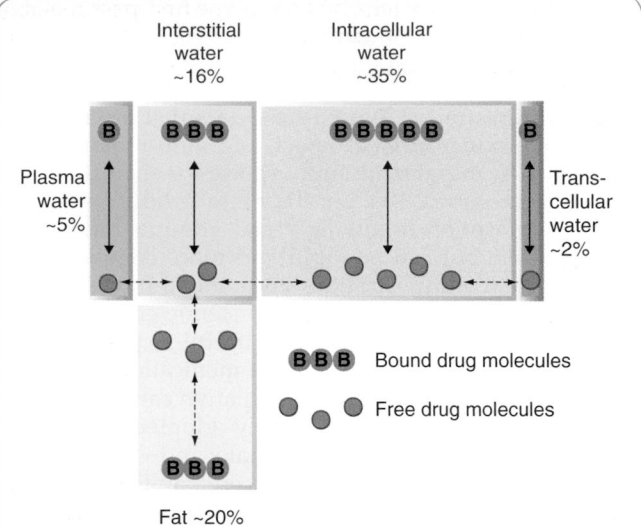

Fig. 9.11 The main body fluid compartments, expressed as a percentage of body weight. Drug molecules exist in bound or free form in each compartment, but only the free drug is able to move between the compartments.

Drug absorption and bioavailability

- Drugs of very low lipid solubility, including those that are strong acids or bases, are generally poorly absorbed from the gut.
- Some drugs (e.g. **levodopa**) are absorbed by carrier-mediated transfer.
- Absorption from the gut depends on many factors, including:
  - gastrointestinal motility
  - gastrointestinal pH
  - particle size
  - physicochemical interaction with gut contents (e.g. chemical interaction between calcium and tetracycline antibiotics)
  - genetic polymorphisms in drug transporters and competition for transporters.
- Bioavailability is the fraction of an ingested dose of a drug that gains access to the systemic circulation. It may be low because absorption is incomplete, or because the drug is metabolised in the gut wall or liver before reaching the systemic circulation.
- Bioequivalence implies that if one formulation of a drug is substituted for another, no clinically untoward consequences will ensue.

Extracellular fluid comprises the blood plasma (about 4.5% of body weight), interstitial fluid (16%) and lymph (1.2%). Intracellular fluid (30%–40%) is the sum of the fluid contents of all cells in the body. Transcellular fluid (2.5%) includes the cerebrospinal, intraocular, peritoneal, pleural and synovial fluids, and digestive secretions. The fetus may also be regarded as a special type of transcellular compartment. Within each of these aqueous compartments, drug molecules usually exist both in free solution and in bound form; furthermore, drugs that are weak acids or bases will exist as an equilibrium mixture of the charged and uncharged forms, the position of the equilibrium depending on the pH.

The equilibrium pattern of distribution between the various compartments will therefore depend on:

- permeability across tissue barriers
- binding within compartments
- pH partition
- fat:water partition

To enter the transcellular compartments from the extracellular compartment, a drug must cross a cellular barrier, a particularly important example being the blood–brain barrier.

THE BLOOD–BRAIN BARRIER

The concept of the blood–brain barrier was introduced by Paul Ehrlich to explain his observation that intravenously injected dye stained most tissues but not the brain. The barrier consists of a continuous layer of endothelial cells joined by tight junctions and surrounded by pericytes. The brain is consequently inaccessible to many drugs of low lipid solubility. However, inflammation can disrupt the integrity of the blood–brain barrier, allowing normally impermeant substances to enter the brain (Fig. 9.12) and

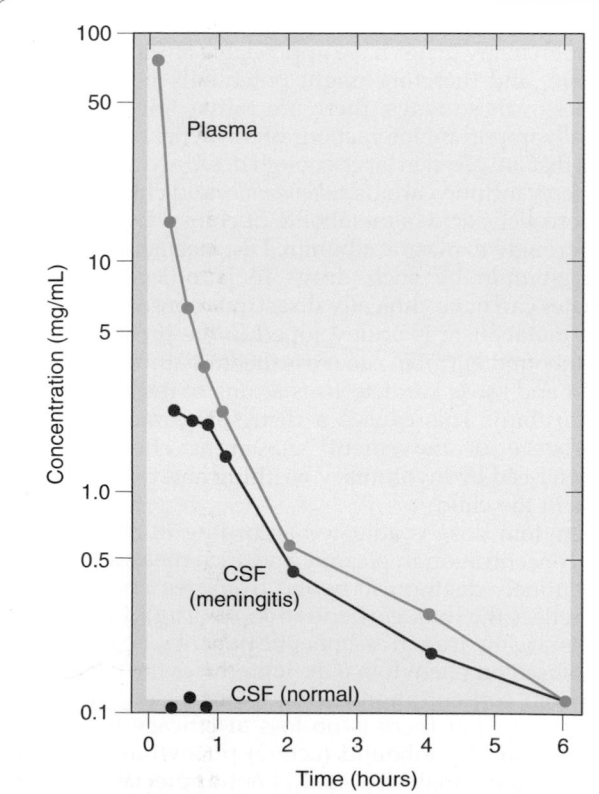

Fig. 9.12 Plasma and cerebrospinal fluid concentrations of an antibiotic (thienamycin) following an intravenous dose (25 mg/kg). In normal rabbits, no drug reaches the cerebrospinal fluid (CSF), but in animals with experimental *Escherichia coli* meningitis the concentration of drug in CSF approaches that in the plasma. (From Patamasucon, P., McCracken Jr, G.H., 1973. Antimicrob. Agents Chemother. 3, 270.)

can also disrupt drug efflux mechanisms; consequently, penicillin (Ch. 52) can be given intravenously (rather than intrathecally) to treat bacterial meningitis, which is accompanied by intense inflammation.

Furthermore, in some parts of the CNS, including the *chemoreceptor trigger zone*, the barrier is leaky. This enables **domperidone**, an antiemetic dopamine–receptor antagonist (Chs 31 and 41) that does not penetrate the blood–brain barrier but does access the chemoreceptor trigger zone, to be used to prevent the nausea caused by dopamine agonists such as **apomorphine** when these are used to treat advanced Parkinson's disease. This is achieved without loss of efficacy, because dopamine receptors in the basal ganglia are accessible only to drugs that have traversed the blood–brain barrier.

Methylnaltrexone bromide is a peripherally acting μ-opioid–receptor antagonist used in treating opioid-induced constipation in patients requiring opioids as part of palliative care (Ch. 43). It has limited gastrointestinal absorption and does not cross the blood–brain barrier, so does not block the desired CNS opioid effects. Several peptides, including bradykinin, increase blood–brain barrier permeability. There is interest in exploiting this to improve penetration of anticancer drugs during treatment of brain tumours.

VOLUME OF DISTRIBUTION

The apparent volume of distribution, V_d, (see Ch. 11) is defined as the volume that would contain the total body content of the drug (Q) at a concentration equal to that present in the plasma (C_P):

$$V_d = \frac{Q}{C_P}$$

It is important to avoid identifying a given range of V_d too closely with a particular anatomical compartment. Drugs may act at very low concentrations in the key compartment that provides access to their receptors. For example, insulin has a measured V_d similar to the volume of plasma water but exerts its effects on muscle, fat and liver via receptors that are exposed to interstitial fluid but not to plasma (Ch. 32).

DRUGS LARGELY CONFINED TO THE PLASMA COMPARTMENT

The plasma volume is about 0.05 L/kg body weight. A few drugs, such as **heparin** (Ch. 25), are confined to plasma because the molecule is too large to cross the capillary wall easily. More often, retention of a drug in the plasma following a single dose reflects strong binding to plasma protein. It is, nevertheless, the free drug in the interstitial fluid that exerts a pharmacological effect. Following repeated dosing, equilibration occurs and measured V_d increases. Some dyes bind exceptionally strongly to plasma albumin, as with Evans blue, such that its V_d is used experimentally to measure plasma volume.

DRUGS DISTRIBUTED IN THE EXTRACELLULAR COMPARTMENT

The total extracellular volume is about 0.2 L/kg, and this is the approximate V_d for many polar compounds, such as vecuronium (Ch. 14), **gentamicin** and **carbenicillin** (Ch. 52). These drugs cannot easily enter cells because of their low lipid solubility, and they do not traverse the blood–brain or placental barriers freely. Many macromolecular biopharmaceuticals, notably monoclonal antibodies (Ch. 5), distribute in the extracellular space and access receptors on cell surfaces but do not readily enter cells. Nucleic acid-based biopharmaceuticals which work on intracellular DNA or RNA are often packaged in special delivery systems (see p. 131) that facilitate access to the cell interior.

DISTRIBUTION THROUGHOUT THE BODY WATER

Total body water represents about 0.55 L/kg. This approximates the distribution of many drugs that readily cross cell membranes, such as **phenytoin** (Ch. 46) and **ethanol** (Ch. 50). The binding of drugs outside the plasma compartment, or partitioning into body fat, increases V_d beyond total body water. Consequently, there are also many drugs with V_d greater than the total body volume, such as morphine (Ch. 43), tricyclic antidepressants (Ch. 48) and **haloperidol** (Ch. 47). Such drugs are not efficiently removed from the body by haemodialysis, which is therefore unhelpful in managing overdose with such agents.

Drug distribution

- The major compartments are:
  - plasma (5% of body weight)
  - interstitial fluid (16%)
  - intracellular fluid (35%)
  - transcellular fluid (2%)
  - fat (20%).
- Volume of distribution (V_d) is defined as the volume of solvent that would contain the total body content of the drug (Q) at a concentration equal to the measured plasma concentration (C_p), $V_d = Q/C_p$.
- Lipid-insoluble drugs are mainly confined to plasma and interstitial fluids; most do not enter the brain following acute dosing.
- Lipid-soluble drugs reach all compartments and may accumulate in fat.
- For drugs that accumulate outside the plasma compartment (e.g. in fat or by being bound to tissues), V_d may exceed total body volume.

DRUG INTERACTIONS CAUSED BY ALTERED ABSORPTION (SEE CH. 12 FOR A GENERAL APPROACH TO DRUG INTERACTIONS)

Gastrointestinal absorption is slowed by drugs that inhibit gastric emptying, such as atropine or opiates, or accelerated by drugs that hasten gastric emptying (e.g. metoclopramide; see Ch. 31). Alternatively, drug A may interact physically or chemically with drug B in the gut in such a way as to inhibit absorption of B. For example, Ca^{2+} and Fe^{2+} each form insoluble complexes with **tetracycline** that retard their absorption; **colestyramine**, a bile acid-binding resin, binds several drugs (e.g. warfarin, digoxin), preventing their absorption if administered simultaneously. Another example is the addition of **adrenaline** (**epinephrine**) to local anaesthetic injections; the resulting vasoconstriction slows the absorption of the anaesthetic, thus prolonging its local effect (Ch. 44). Physiologically based modelling is now beginning to be used to predict quantitatively the effects of genetic polymorphisms of drug transporters in intestine and hepatocytes and of drug–drug interactions due to competition for these transporters (Yoshida et al., 2013).

DRUG INTERACTIONS CAUSED BY ALTERED DISTRIBUTION (SEE CH. 12 FOR A GENERAL APPROACH TO DRUG INTERACTIONS)

One drug may alter the distribution of another, by competing for a common binding site on plasma albumin or tissue protein, but such interactions are seldom clinically important unless accompanied by a separate effect on drug elimination (see Chs 10, 12). Displacement of a drug from binding sites in plasma or tissues transiently increases the concentration of free (unbound) drug, but this is followed by increased elimination, so a new steady state results in which total drug concentration in plasma is reduced but the free drug concentration is similar to that before introduction of the second 'displacing' drug. Consequences of potential clinical importance include:

- Harm from the transient increase in concentration of free drug before the new steady state is reached.
- If dose is being adjusted according to measurements of total plasma concentration, it must be appreciated that the target therapeutic concentration range will be altered by co-administration of a displacing drug.
- When the displacing drug additionally reduces elimination of the first, so that the free concentration is increased not only acutely but also chronically at the new steady state, severe toxicity may ensue.

Although many drugs have appreciable affinity for plasma albumin, and therefore might potentially be expected to interact in these ways, there are rather few instances of clinically important interactions of this type. Protein-bound drugs that are given in large enough dosage to act as displacing agents include various *sulfonamides* and **chloral hydrate**; trichloroacetic acid, a metabolite of chloral hydrate, binds very strongly to plasma albumin. Displacement of bilirubin from albumin by such drugs in jaundiced premature neonates can have clinically disastrous consequences: bilirubin metabolism is undeveloped in the premature liver, and unbound bilirubin can cross the immature blood–brain barrier and cause kernicterus (staining of the basal ganglia by bilirubin). This causes a distressing and permanent disturbance of movement known as choreoathetosis, characterised by involuntary writhing and twisting movements in the child.

Phenytoin dose is adjusted according to measurement of its concentration in plasma, and such measurements do not routinely distinguish bound from free phenytoin (i.e. they reflect the total concentration of drug). Introduction of a displacing drug in an epileptic patient whose condition is stabilised on phenytoin (Ch. 46) reduces the total plasma phenytoin concentration owing to increased elimination of free drug, but there is no loss of efficacy because the concentration of unbound (active) phenytoin at the new steady state is unaltered. If it is not appreciated that the therapeutic range of plasma concentrations has been reduced in this way, an increased dose may be prescribed, causing harm.

Drugs that alter protein binding sometimes additionally reduce elimination of the displaced drug, causing clinically important interactions. *Salicylates* displace **methotrexate** from binding sites on albumin and reduce its secretion into the nephron by competition with the OAT (Ch. 10).

Quinidine and several other antidysrhythmic drugs including **verapamil** and **amiodarone** (Ch. 22) displace digoxin from tissue-binding sites while simultaneously reducing its renal excretion; they consequently can cause severe dysrhythmias through digoxin toxicity.

SPECIAL DRUG DELIVERY SYSTEMS

Several approaches are used or in development to improve drug delivery and localise the drug to the target tissue. They include:

- prodrugs
- antibody–drug conjugates
- packaging in liposomes
- coated implantable devices

PRODRUGS

Prodrugs are inactive precursors that are metabolised to active metabolites; they are described in Chapter 10. Some of the examples in clinical use confer no obvious benefits and have been found to be prodrugs only retrospectively, not having been designed with this in mind. However, some do have advantages. For example, the cytotoxic drug **cyclophosphamide** (see Ch. 57) becomes active only after it has been metabolised in the liver; it can therefore be taken orally without causing serious damage to the gastrointestinal epithelium. Levodopa is absorbed from the gastrointestinal tract and crosses the blood–brain barrier via an amino acid transport mechanism before conversion to active dopamine in nerve terminals in the basal ganglia (Ch. 41). **Zidovudine** is phosphorylated to its active triphosphate metabolite only in cells containing the appropriate reverse transcriptase, hence conferring selective toxicity towards cells infected with HIV (Ch. 53). **Valaciclovir** and **famciclovir** are each ester prodrugs, respectively of **aciclovir** and of **penciclovir**. Their bioavailability is greater than that of aciclovir and penciclovir, which are themselves prodrugs that are converted into active metabolites in virally infected cells (Ch. 53). **Diacetyl morphine** (heroin) is a prodrug that penetrates the blood–brain barrier even faster than its active metabolites morphine and 6-monoacetyl morphine (Ch. 43), accounting for increased 'buzz' and hence abuse potential.

Delivering nucleic acid-based drugs (antisense oligonucleotides and small interfering RNA drugs) to their intracellular sites of action is a major issue with this class of biopharmaceutical (Ch. 5). Modifying these agents with chemical groups that bind specific surface transporters permits drug delivery to specific cells. The asialoglycoprotein receptor (ASGR) is a lectin that is abundantly expressed on the cell surface of hepatocytes and binds terminal galactose and *N*-acetyl galactosamine (GalNAc) residues, leading to selective hepatocyte uptake (Prakash et al., 2016).

Other problems could theoretically be overcome by using suitable prodrugs; for example, instability of drugs at gastric pH, direct gastric irritation (aspirin was synthesised in the 19th century in a deliberate attempt to produce a prodrug of salicylic acid that would be tolerable when taken by mouth), failure of drug to cross the blood–brain barrier and so on. While the optimistic prodrug designer 'will have to bear in mind that an organism's normal reaction to a foreign substance is to burn it up for food', the successes mentioned above in delivering nucleic acid drugs to hepatocytes is a notable encouragement, with early human studies that have provided proof of concept in patients with dyslipidaemia, haemophilia and one form of amyloidosis, for example.

ANTIBODY–DRUG CONJUGATES

▼ One of the aims of cancer chemotherapy is to improve the selectivity of cytotoxic drugs (see Ch. 57). One approach is to attach the drug or toxin to an antibody directed against a tumour-specific antigen, which will bind selectively to tumour cells (Thomas et al., 2016). **Ado-trastuzumab emtansine** and **brentuximab vedotin** have been approved by the FDA for treatment of selected cases of, respectively, metastatic breast cancer and Hodgkin's lymphoma.

PACKAGING IN LIPOSOMES

▼ Liposomes are vesicles 0.1–1 µm in diameter produced by sonication of an aqueous suspension of phospholipids. They can be filled with non lipid-soluble drugs, which are retained until the liposome is disrupted. Liposomes are taken up by reticuloendothelial cells, especially in the liver. They are also concentrated in malignant tumours, and several liposomal chemotherapeutic formulations are commercially available (see Yingchoncharoeu et al., 2016). **Amphotericin**, an antifungal drug used to treat systemic mycoses (Ch. 54), is available in a liposomal formulation that is less nephrotoxic and better tolerated than the conventional form, albeit considerably more expensive. A long-acting form of **doxorubicin** encapsulated in liposomes is available for the treatment of malignancies (including ovarian cancer and myeloma), and **paclitaxel** is available in an albumin nanoparticle used to treat breast cancer (Ch. 57). A liposomal preparation of **cytarabine** is available for intrathecal treatment of lymphomatous meningitis, and a liposomal formulation of **vincristine** is available for selected patients with acute lymphoblastic leukaemia.

COATED IMPLANTABLE DEVICES

▼ Impregnated coatings have been developed that permit localised drug delivery from implants. Examples include hormonal delivery to the endometrium from intrauterine devices, and delivery of antithrombotic and antiproliferative agents (drugs or radiopharmaceuticals) to the coronary arteries from *stents* (tubular devices inserted via a catheter after a diseased coronary artery has been dilated with a balloon). Stents reduce the occurrence of re-stenosis, but this can still occur at the margin of the device. Coating stents with drugs such as **sirolimus** (a potent immunosuppressant; see Ch. 27) embedded in a surface polymer prevents this important clinical problem.

REFERENCES AND FURTHER READING

Drug absorption and bioequivalence
EMEA, 2010. Guideline on the investigation of bioequivalence. http://www.ema.europa.eu/docs/en_GB/document_library/Scientific_guideline/2010/01/WC500070039.pdf. (Accessed 19 March 2017).
Yoshida, K., Maeda, K., Sugiyama, Y., 2013. Hepatic and intestinal drug transporters: prediction of pharmacokinetic effects caused by drug-drug interactions and genetic polymorphisms. Ann. Rev. Pharmacol. Toxicol. 53, 581–612. (*Reviews the status of predicting pharmacokinetic behaviour on the basis of transporter-mediated drug interactions and pharmacogenetics*)

Drug distribution (including blood–brain barrier)
Ciarimboli, G., 2008. Organic cation transporters. Xenobiotica 38, 936–971. (*Discusses species- and tissue-specific distribution of different OCT isoforms and polymorphisms in OCTs as a source of variation in drug response*)

Miller, D.S., Bauer, B., Hartz, A.M.S., 2008. Modulation of P-glycoprotein at the blood–brain barrier: opportunities to improve central nervous system pharmacotherapy. Pharmacol. Rev. 60, 196–209.

Drug delivery and routes of administration

Brigo, F., Nardone, R., Tezzon, F., Trinka, E., 2015. Nonintravenous midazolam versus intravenous or rectal diazepam for the treatment of early status epilepticus: a systematic review with meta-analysis. Epilepsy Behav. 49, 325–336. (*"Non-intravenous midazolam is as effective and safe as intravenous or rectal diazepam in terminating early status epilepticus in children and probably also in adults."* Buccal midazolam was socially more acceptable and easier to administer, and might also have a higher efficacy than rectal diazepam in seizure control)

Huttunen, K.M., Raunio, H., Rautio, J., 2011. Prodrugs – from serendipity to rational design. Pharmacol. Rev. 63, 750–771. (*Reviews prodrug strategy*)

Needham, L.A., Davidson, A.H., Bawden, L.J., Belfield, A., 2011. Drug targeting to monocytes and macrophages using esterase-sensitive chemical motifs. J. Pharmacol. Exp. Ther. 339, 132–142. (*Ingenious method of targeting drugs to this cell lineage which selectively expresses an esterase that releases the charged form of drug intracellularly where it is trapped and where its target resides*)

Prakash, T.P., Yu, J., Migawa, M.T., et al., 2016. Comprehensive structure activity relationship of triantennary N-acetylgalactosamine conjugated antisense oligonucleotides for targeted delivery to hepatocytes. J. Med. Chem. 59, 2718–2733. (*Enabling technology: potential gateway to a flood of nucleic acid based therapeutics*)

Renukuntla, J., Vadlapudi, A.D., Patel, A., Boddu, S.H.S., Mitra, A.K., 2013. Approaches for enhancing oral bioavailability of peptides and proteins. Int. J. Pharm. 447, 75–93. (*Limited success only*)

Thomas, A., Teichner, B.A., Hassan, R., 2016. Antibody-drug conjugates for cancer therapy. Lancet Oncol. 17 (6), e254–e262. (*Attractive approach, two FDA-licensed products*)

Yingchoncharoeu, P., Kanilowski, D.S., Richardson, D.R., 2016. Lipid-based drug delivery systems in cancer therapy: what is available and what is yet to come. Pharmacol. Rev. 63, 701–787. (*Potential of lipid nanoparticles – several have already been licensed*)

Drug metabolism and elimination

OVERVIEW

We describe phases 1 and 2 of drug metabolism, emphasising the importance of the cytochrome P450 monooxygenase system. We then cover the processes of biliary excretion and enterohepatic recirculation of drugs, and of drug interactions caused by induction or inhibition of metabolism. Drug and drug metabolite elimination by the kidney are described and drug interactions due to effects on renal elimination considered.

INTRODUCTION

Drug elimination is the irreversible loss of drug from the body. It occurs by two processes: *metabolism* and *excretion*. Metabolism consists of anabolism and catabolism, that is, respectively, the build-up and breakdown of substances by enzymic conversion of one chemical entity to another within the body, whereas excretion consists of elimination from the body of drug or drug metabolites. The main excretory routes are:

- the kidneys
- the hepatobiliary system
- the lungs (important for volatile/gaseous anaesthetics)

Most drugs leave the body in the urine, either unchanged or as polar metabolites. Some drugs are secreted into bile via the liver, but most of these are then reabsorbed from the intestine. There are, however, instances (e.g. **rifampicin**; Ch. 52) where faecal loss accounts for the elimination of a substantial fraction of unchanged drug in healthy individuals, and faecal elimination of drugs such as **digoxin** that are normally excreted in urine (Ch. 22) becomes progressively more important in patients with advancing renal impairment. Excretion via the lungs occurs only with highly volatile or gaseous agents (e.g. general anaesthetics; Ch. 42). Small amounts of some drugs are also excreted in secretions such as milk or sweat. Elimination by these routes is quantitatively negligible compared with renal excretion, although excretion into milk can sometimes be important because of effects on the baby (<www.fpnotebook.com/ob/Pharm/MdctnsInLctn.htm>).

Lipophilic substances are not eliminated efficiently by the kidney (see later, p. 140). Consequently, most lipophilic drugs are metabolised to more polar products, which are then excreted in urine. Drugs are metabolised predominantly in the liver, especially by the cytochrome P450 (CYP) system. Some P450 enzymes are extrahepatic and play an important part in the biosynthesis of steroid hormones (Ch. 34) and eicosanoids (Ch. 18), but here we are concerned with catabolism of drugs by the hepatic P450 system.

DRUG METABOLISM

Animals have evolved complex systems that detoxify foreign chemicals ('xenobiotics'), including carcinogens and toxins present in poisonous plants. Drugs are a special case of such xenobiotics and, like plant alkaloids, they often exhibit *chirality* (i.e. there is more than one stereoisomer), which affects their overall metabolism. Drug metabolism involves two kinds of reaction, known as phase 1 and phase 2, which often occur sequentially. Both phases decrease lipid solubility, thus increasing renal elimination.

PHASE 1 REACTIONS

Phase 1 reactions (e.g. oxidation, reduction or hydrolysis) are catabolic, and the products are often more chemically reactive and hence, paradoxically, sometimes more toxic or carcinogenic than the parent drug. Phase 1 reactions often introduce a reactive group, such as hydroxyl, into the molecule, a process known as 'functionalisation'. This group then serves as the point of attack for the conjugating system to attach a substituent such as glucuronide (Fig. 10.1), explaining why phase 1 reactions so often precede phase 2 reactions. The liver is especially important in phase 1 reactions. Many hepatic drug-metabolising enzymes, including CYP enzymes, are embedded in the smooth endoplasmic reticulum. They are often called 'microsomal' enzymes because, on homogenisation and differential centrifugation, the endoplasmic reticulum is broken into very small fragments that sediment only after prolonged high-speed centrifugation in the microsomal fraction. To reach these metabolising enzymes in life, a drug must cross the plasma membrane. Polar molecules do this less readily than non-polar molecules except where there are specific transport mechanisms (Ch. 9), so intracellular metabolism is important for lipid-soluble drugs, while polar drugs are, at least partly, excreted unchanged in the urine.

THE P450 MONOOXYGENASE SYSTEM

Nature, classification and mechanism of P450 enzymes

Cytochrome P450 enzymes are haem proteins, comprising a large family ('superfamily') of related but distinct enzymes, each referred to as CYP followed by a defining set of numbers and a letter. P450 enzymes (reviewed by Guengerich et al., 2016 and Nair et al., 2016) differ from one another in amino acid sequence, in sensitivity to inhibitors and inducing agents (see later), and in the specificity of the reactions that they catalyse. Different members of the family have distinct, but often overlapping, substrate specificities. Purification and cloning of P450 enzymes form the basis of the current classification, which is based on amino acid sequence similarities. Not all 57 human CYPs are involved in drug metabolism, but it has been estimated that CYP enzymes in families 1–3 mediate 70%–80% of all

133

Fig. 10.1 The two phases of drug metabolism.

Table 10.1 Examples of drugs that are substrates of P450 isoenzymes

Isoenzyme P450	Drug(s)
CYP1A2	Caffeine, paracetamol (→NAPQI), tacrine, theophylline
CYP2B6	Cyclophosphamide, methadone
CYP2C8	Paclitaxel, repaglinide
CYP2C19	Omeprazole, phenytoin
CYP2C9	Ibuprofen, tolbutamide, warfarin
CYP2D6	Codeine, debrisoquine, S-metoprolol
CYP2E1	Alcohol, paracetamol
CYP3A4, 5, 7	Ciclosporin, nifedipine, indinavir, simvastatin

NAPQI, N-acetyl-*p*-benzoquinone imine – the metabolite responsible for paracetamol toxicity in overdose.
(Adapted from http://medicine.iupui.edu/flockhart/table.htm)

phase 1-dependent metabolism of clinically used small-molecule drugs (Ingelman-Sundberg, 2004). Twelve CYPs accounted for 93.0% of drug metabolism of 1839 known drug-metabolising reactions in a large international database (Preissner et al., 2013). CYPs 1A2, 3A4, 2D6, 2C9 and 2C19 were responsible for approximately 60% of drug metabolism. Examples of therapeutic drugs that are substrates for some important P450 isoenzymes are shown in Table 10.1, and a useful table of drug substrates, inhibitors and inducers of CYP subtypes is provided by the Indiana University Department of Medicine/Clinical Pharmacology (<http://medicine.iupui.edu/clinpharm/ddis/main-table/ - accessed August 2018>).

Drug oxidation by the monooxygenase P450 system requires drug (substrate, 'DH'), P450 enzyme, molecular oxygen, NADPH and NADPH–P450 reductase (a flavoprotein). The mechanism involves a complex cycle (Fig. 10.2), but the outcome of the reaction is quite simple, namely the addition of one atom of oxygen (from molecular oxygen) to the drug to form a hydroxylated product (DOH), the other atom of oxygen being converted to water.

▼ P450 enzymes have unique spectral properties, and the reduced forms combine with carbon monoxide to form a pink compound (hence 'P') with absorption peaks near 450 nm (range 447–452 nm). The first clue that there is more than one form of CYP came from the observation that treatment of rats with 3-methylcholanthrene (3-MC), an inducing agent (see later), causes a shift in the absorption maximum from 450 to 448 nm – the 3-MC-induced isoform of the enzyme absorbs light maximally at a slightly shorter wavelength than the un-induced enzyme.

P450 and biological variation

There are important variations in the expression and regulation of P450 enzymes between species. For instance, the pathways by which certain dietary heterocyclic amines (formed when meat is cooked) generate genotoxic products involves one member of the P450 superfamily (CYP1A2) that is constitutively present in humans and rats (which develop colon tumours after treatment with such amines) but not in cynomolgus monkeys (which do not). Such species differences have crucial implications for the choice of species to be used for toxicity and carcinogenicity testing during the development of new drugs for use in humans.

Within human populations, there are major sources of inter-individual variation in P450 enzymes that are of great importance in therapeutics. These include genetic polymorphisms (alternative sequences at a locus within the DNA strand – alleles – that persist in a population through several generations; Ch. 12). Environmental factors are also important, since enzyme inhibitors and inducers are present in the diet and environment. For example, a component of grapefruit juice inhibits drug metabolism (leading to potentially disastrous consequences, including cardiac

Fig. 10.2 The monooxygenase P450 cycle. Each of the *pink* or *blue* rectangles represents one single molecule of cytochrome P450 (P450) undergoing a catalytic cycle. Iron in P450 is in either the ferric *(pink rectangles)* or ferrous *(blue rectangles)* state. P450 containing ferric iron (Fe^{3+}) combines with a molecule of drug ('DH'), and receives an electron from NADPH–P450 reductase, which reduces the iron to Fe^{2+}. This combines with molecular oxygen, a proton and a second electron (either from NADPH–P450 reductase or from cytochrome b_5) to form an $Fe^{2+}OOH$–DH complex. This combines with another proton to yield water and a ferric oxene $(FeO)^{3+}$–DH complex. $(FeO)^{3+}$ extracts a hydrogen atom from DH, with the formation of a pair of short-lived free radicals (see text), liberation from the complex of oxidised drug ('DOH'), and regeneration of P450 enzyme.

Fig. 10.3 The glucuronide conjugation reaction. A glucuronyl group is transferred from uridine diphosphate glucuronic acid (UDPGA) to a drug molecule.

dysrhythmias), whereas Brussels sprouts and cigarette smoke induce P450 enzymes. Components of the herbal medicine St John's wort (Ch. 48) induce CYP450 isoenzymes as well as P-glycoprotein (P-gp) (see Ch. 9). Drug interactions based on one drug altering the metabolism of another are common and clinically important (see Ch. 12).

Not all drug oxidation reactions involve the P450 system. Some drugs are metabolised in plasma (e.g. hydrolysis of **suxamethonium** by plasma cholinesterase; Ch. 14), lung (e.g. various prostanoids; Ch. 18) or gut (e.g. **tyramine**, **salbutamol**; Chs 15 and 29). **Ethanol** (Ch. 50) is metabolised by a soluble cytoplasmic enzyme, alcohol dehydrogenase, in addition to CYP2E1. Other P450-independent enzymes involved in drug oxidation include xanthine oxidase, which inactivates **6-mercaptopurine** (Ch. 57), and mono-amine oxidase, which inactivates many biologically active amines (e.g. **noradrenaline** [norepinephrine], tyramine, 5-hydroxytryptamine; Chs 15 and 16).

HYDROLYTIC REACTIONS

Hydrolysis (e.g. of **aspirin**; see Fig. 10.1) occurs in plasma and in many tissues. Both ester and (less readily) amide bonds are susceptible to hydrolytic cleavage. Reduction is less common in phase 1 metabolism than oxidation, but

warfarin (Ch. 25) is inactivated by reduction of a ketone to a hydroxyl group by CYP2A6.

PHASE 2 REACTIONS

Phase 2 reactions are synthetic ('anabolic') and involve conjugation (i.e. attachment of a substituent group), which usually results in inactive products, although there are exceptions (e.g. the active sulphate metabolite of **minoxidil**, a potassium channel activator used to treat severe hypertension (Ch. 23) and (as a cream) to promote hair growth. Phase 2 reactions take place mainly in the liver. If a drug molecule or phase 1 product has a suitable 'handle' (e.g. a hydroxyl, thiol or amino group), it is susceptible to conjugation. The chemical group inserted may be glucuronyl (Fig. 10.3), sulphate, methyl or acetyl. The tripeptide glutathione conjugates drugs or their phase 1 metabolites via its sulfhydryl group, as in the detoxification of **paracetamol** (see Fig. 58.1). Glucuronidation involves the formation of a high-energy phosphate ('donor') compound, uridine diphosphate glucuronic acid (UDPGA), from which glucuronic acid is transferred to an electron-rich atom (N, O or S) on the substrate, forming an amide, ester or thiol bond. UDP-glucuronyl transferase, which catalyses these reactions, has very broad substrate specificity embracing many drugs and other foreign molecules. Several important endogenous substances, including bilirubin and adrenal corticosteroids, are conjugated by the same pathway.

Acetylation and methylation reactions occur with acetyl-CoA and S-adenosyl methionine, respectively, acting as the donor groups. Many conjugation reactions occur in the liver, but other tissues, such as lung and kidney, are also involved.

STEREOSELECTIVITY

Many clinically important drugs, such as **sotalol** (Ch. 22), **warfarin** (Ch. 25) and **cyclophosphamide** (Ch. 57), are mixtures of stereoisomers, the components of which differ not only in their pharmacological effects but also in their metabolism, which may follow completely distinct pathways (Campo et al., 2009). Several clinically important drug interactions involve stereospecific inhibition of metabolism of one drug by another (see Table 10.6). In some cases, drug toxicity is mainly linked to one of the stereoisomers, not necessarily the pharmacologically active one. Where practicable, regulatory authorities urge that new drugs should consist of single isomers to lessen these complications.[1]

INHIBITION OF P450

Inhibitors of P450 differ in their selectivity towards different isoforms of the enzyme, and are classified by their mechanism of action. Some drugs compete for the active site but are not themselves substrates (e.g. **quinidine** is a potent competitive inhibitor of CYP2D6 but is not a substrate for it). Non-competitive inhibitors include drugs such as **ketoconazole**, which forms a tight complex with the Fe^{3+} form of the haem iron of CYP3A4, causing reversible non-competitive inhibition. So-called mechanism-based inhibitors require oxidation by a P450 enzyme. Examples include the oral contraceptive **gestodene** (CYP3A4) and the anthelmintic drug **diethylcarbamazine** (CYP2E1). An oxidation product (e.g. a postulated epoxide intermediate of gestodene) binds covalently to the enzyme, which then destroys itself ('suicide inhibition'; see Pelkonen et al., 2008).

INDUCTION OF MICROSOMAL ENZYMES

A number of drugs, such as **rifampicin** (Ch. 52), **ethanol** (Ch. 50) and **carbamazepine** (Ch. 46), increase the activity of microsomal oxidase and conjugating systems when administered repeatedly. Many carcinogenic chemicals (e.g. benzpyrene, 3-MC) also have this effect, which can be substantial; Fig. 10.4 shows a nearly 10-fold increase in the rate of benzpyrene metabolism 2 days after a single dose. The effect is referred to as *induction*, and is the result of increased synthesis and/or reduced breakdown of microsomal enzymes (Pelkonen et al., 2008).

Enzyme induction can increase drug toxicity and carcinogenicity, because several phase 1 metabolites are toxic or carcinogenic: paracetamol is an important example of a drug with a highly toxic metabolite (see Ch. 58). Enzyme induction is exploited therapeutically by administering **phenobarbital** to premature babies to induce glucuronyl-transferase, thereby increasing bilirubin conjugation and reducing the risk of kernicterus (staining and neurological damage of the basal ganglia by bilirubin, Ch. 9).

▼ The mechanism of induction is incompletely understood but is similar to that involved in the action of steroid and other hormones that bind to nuclear receptors (see Ch. 3). The most thoroughly studied inducing agents are polycyclic aromatic hydrocarbons (e.g. 3-MC). These bind to the ligand-binding domain of a soluble protein, termed the aromatic hydrocarbon (Ah) receptor. This complex is transported to the nucleus by an Ah receptor nuclear translocator and binds Ah receptor response elements in the DNA, thereby promoting transcription of the gene *CYP1A1*. In addition to enhanced transcription, some inducing agents (e.g. ethanol, which induces CYP2E1 in humans) also stabilise mRNA or P450 protein.

PRESYSTEMIC ('FIRST-PASS') METABOLISM

Some drugs are extracted so efficiently by the liver or gut wall that the amount reaching the systemic circulation is considerably less than the amount absorbed. This is known as presystemic (or first-pass) metabolism and reduces bioavailability (Ch. 9), even when a drug is well absorbed. Presystemic metabolism is important for many therapeutic drugs (Table 10.2 shows some examples), and is a problem because:

- A much larger dose of the drug is needed when it is taken by mouth than when it is given parenterally.
- Marked individual variations occur in the extent of first-pass metabolism, both in the activities of drug-metabolising enzymes and also as a result of variations in hepatic or intestinal blood flow. Hepatic blood flow can be reduced in disease (e.g. heart failure) or by drugs, such as β-adrenoceptor antagonists, which impair the clearance of unrelated drugs, such as lidocaine, that are subject to presystemic metabolism due to a high hepatic extraction ratio. Intestinal blood flow is strongly influenced by eating and studies on the pharmacokinetic effects of food are routine in the development of orally administered drugs.

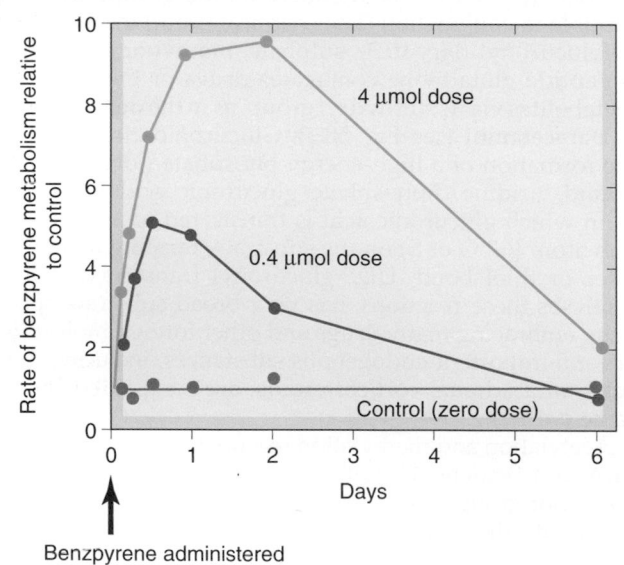

Fig. 10.4 Stimulation of hepatic metabolism of benzpyrene. Young rats were given benzpyrene (intraperitoneally) in the doses shown, and the benzpyrene-metabolising activity of liver homogenates was measured at times up to 6 days. (From Conney, A.H. et al., 1957. J. Biol. Chem. 228, 753.)

---

[1]Well-intentioned – though the usefulness of expensive 'novel' entities that are actually just the pure active isomer of well-established and safe racemates has been questioned, and enzymic interconversion of stereoisomers may subvert such chemical sophistication.

Table 10.2 Examples of drugs that undergo substantial pre-systemic ("first-pass") elimination

Aspirin	Metoprolol
Glyceryl trinitrate	Morphine
Isosorbide dinitrate	Propranolol
Levodopa	Salbutamol
Lidocaine	Verapamil

PHARMACOLOGICALLY ACTIVE DRUG METABOLITES

In some cases (Table 10.3) a drug becomes pharmacologically active only after it has been metabolised. For example, **azathioprine**, an immunosuppressant drug (Ch. 27), is metabolised to **mercaptopurine**; and **enalapril**, an angiotensin-converting enzyme inhibitor (Ch. 23), is hydrolysed to its active form **enalaprilat**. Such drugs, in which the parent compound lacks activity of its own, are known as *prodrugs*. These are sometimes designed deliberately to overcome problems of drug delivery (Ch. 9). Metabolism can alter the pharmacological actions of a drug qualitatively. **Aspirin** inhibits platelet function and has anti-inflammatory activity (Chs 25 and 27). It is hydrolysed to salicylic acid (see Fig. 10.1), which has anti-inflammatory but not antiplatelet activity. In other instances, metabolites have pharmacological actions similar to those of the parent compound (e.g. benzodiazepines, many of which form long-lived active metabolites that cause sedation to persist after the parent drug has disappeared; Ch. 45). There are also cases in which metabolites are responsible for toxicity. Bladder toxicity of **cyclophosphamide**, which is caused by its toxic metabolite acrolein (Ch. 57), is an example. Methanol and ethylene glycol both exert their toxic effects via metabolites formed by alcohol dehydrogenase. Poisoning with these agents is treated with ethanol (or with a more potent inhibitor), which competes for the active site of the enzyme.

DRUG INTERACTIONS DUE TO ENZYME INDUCTION OR INHIBITION

INTERACTIONS CAUSED BY ENZYME INDUCTION

Enzyme induction is an important cause of drug interaction. The slow onset of induction and slow recovery after withdrawal of the inducing agent, together with the potential for selective induction of one or more CYP isoenzymes,

Drug metabolism

- Phase 1 reactions involve oxidation, reduction and hydrolysis. They:
  - usually form more chemically reactive products, which can be pharmacologically active, toxic or carcinogenic.
  - often involve a monooxygenase system in which cytochrome P450 plays a key role.
- Phase 2 reactions involve conjugation (e.g. glucuronidation) of a reactive group (often inserted during phase 1 reaction) and usually lead to inactive and polar products that are readily excreted in urine.
- Some conjugated products are excreted via bile, are reactivated in the intestine and then reabsorbed ('enterohepatic circulation').
- Induction of P450 enzymes can greatly accelerate hepatic drug metabolism. It can increase the toxicity of drugs with toxic metabolites, and is an important cause of drug–drug interaction, as is enzyme inhibition.
- Presystemic metabolism in liver or gut wall reduces the bioavailability of several drugs when they are administered by mouth.

contribute to the insidious nature of the clinical problems that induction presents. Adverse clinical outcomes from such interactions are very diverse, including graft rejection as a result of loss of effectiveness of immunosuppressive treatment, seizures due to loss of anticonvulsant effectiveness, unwanted pregnancy from loss of oral contraceptive action and thrombosis (from loss of effectiveness of warfarin) or bleeding (from failure to recognise the need to reduce warfarin dose when induction wanes after an inducing agent is discontinued). Over 200 drugs cause enzyme induction and thereby decrease the pharmacological activity

Table 10.3 Some drugs that produce active or toxic metabolites

Inactive (prodrugs)	Active drug	Active metabolite	Toxic metabolite	See Chapter
Azathioprine ⟶		Mercaptopurine		27
Cortisone ⟶		Hydrocortisone		34
Prednisone ⟶		Prednisolone		34
Enalapril ⟶		Enalaprilat		23
Zidovudine ⟶		Zidovudine trisphosphate		53
Cyclophosphamide ⟶		Phosphoramide mustard ⟶	Acrolein	57
	Diazepam ⤏	Oxazepam		45
	Morphine ⟶	Morphine 6-glucuronide		43
	Halothane ⟶		Trifluoroacetic acid	42
	Methoxyflurane ⟶		Fluoride	42
	Paracetamol ⟶		*N*-Acetyl-*p*-benzoquinone imine	27, 58

of a range of other drugs. Some examples are given in Table 10.4, and further examples are given at the Indiana University Department of Medicine website cited previously (p. 134). Because the inducing agent is often itself a substrate for the induced enzymes, the process can result in slowly developing tolerance. This pharmacokinetic kind of tolerance is generally less marked than pharmacodynamic tolerance, for example, to opioids (Ch. 43), but it is clinically important when starting treatment with the antiepileptic drug **carbamazepine** (Ch. 46). Treatment starts at a low dose to avoid toxicity (because liver enzymes are not induced initially) and is gradually increased over a period of a few weeks, during which it induces its own metabolism.

Fig. 10.5 shows how the antibiotic **rifampicin**, given for 3 days, reduces the effectiveness of **warfarin** as an anticoagulant. Conversely, enzyme induction can increase toxicity of a second drug if the toxic effects are mediated via an active metabolite. **Paracetamol (acetaminophen)** toxicity is a case in point (see Fig. 58.1): this is caused by its CYP metabolite *N*-acetyl-*p*-benzoquinone imine (NAPQI). Consequently, the risk of serious hepatic injury following paracetamol overdose is increased in patients in whom CYP has been induced, for example, by chronic alcohol consumption.

INTERACTIONS CAUSED BY ENZYME INHIBITION

As with induction, interactions caused by enzyme inhibition are hard to anticipate from first principles. If in doubt about the possibility of an interaction, it is best to look it up (e.g. in the *British National Formulary*, which has an invaluable appendix on drug interactions indicating which are of known clinical importance) or at the Indiana University Department of Medicine website cited previously (p. 134).

Enzyme inhibition, particularly of CYP enzymes, slows the metabolism and hence increases the action of other drugs inactivated by the enzyme. Such effects can be clinically important and are major considerations in the treatment of patients with HIV infection with combination therapy, because several protease inhibitors are potent CYP inhibitors (Ch. 53). Other examples of drugs that are enzyme inhibitors are shown in Table 10.5. To make life even more difficult, several inhibitors of drug metabolism influence the metabolism of different stereoisomers selectively. Examples of drugs that inhibit the metabolism of the active (*S*) and less active (*R*) isomers of warfarin in this way are shown in Table 10.6.

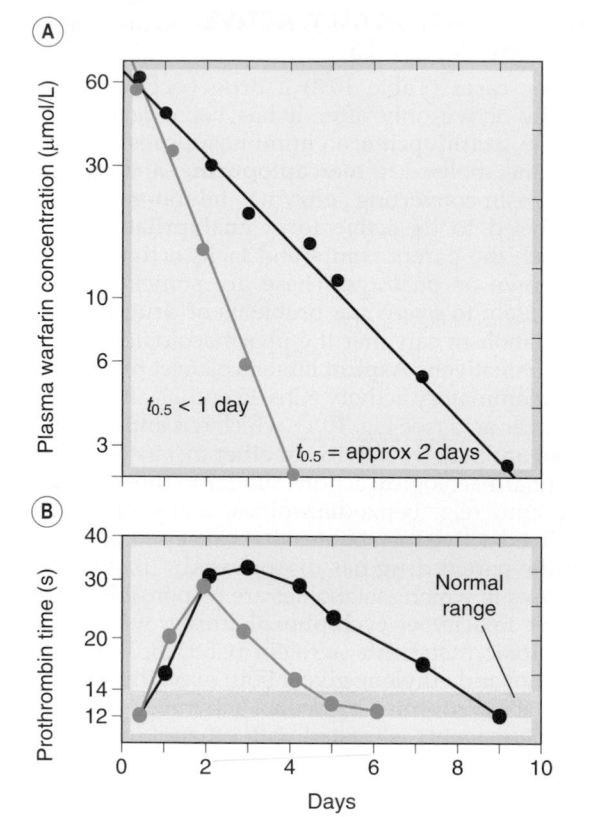

Fig. 10.5 Effect of rifampicin on the metabolism and anticoagulant action of warfarin. (A) Plasma concentration of warfarin (log scale) as a function of time following a single oral dose of 5 µmol/kg body weight. After the subject was given rifampicin (600 mg daily for a few days), the plasma half-life of warfarin decreased from approximately 2 days to <1 day. (B) The effect of a single dose of warfarin on prothrombin time under normal conditions (*red curve*) and after rifampicin administration (*green curve*). (Redrawn from O' Reilly, R.A. 1974. Ann. Intern. Med. 81, 337.)

Table 10.4 Examples of drugs that induce drug-metabolising enzymes

Drugs inducing enzyme action	Examples of drugs with metabolism affected
Phenobarbital	Warfarin
Rifampicin	Oral contraceptives
Griseofulvin	Corticosteroids
Phenytoin	Ciclosporin
Ethanol Carbamazepine	Drugs listed in left-hand column will also be affected

Table 10.5 Examples of drugs that inhibit drug-metabolising enzymes

Drugs inhibiting enzyme action	Drugs with metabolism affected
Allopurinol	Mercaptopurine, azathioprine
Chloramphenicol	Phenytoin
Cimetidine	Amiodarone, phenytoin, pethidine
Ciprofloxacin	Theophylline
Corticosteroids	Tricyclic antidepressants, cyclophosphamide
Disulfiram	Warfarin
Erythromycin	Ciclosporin, theophylline
Monoamine oxidase inhibitors	Pethidine
Ritonavir	Saquinavir

Table 10.6 Stereoselective and non-stereoselective inhibition of warfarin metabolism

Inhibition of metabolism	Drug(s)
Stereoselective for (S) isomer	Phenylbutazone
	Metronidazole
	Sulfinpyrazone
	Trimethoprim–sulfamethoxazole
	Disulfiram
Stereoselective for (R) isomer	Cimetidine[a]
	Omeprazole[a]
Non-stereoselective effect on both isomers	Amiodarone

[a]Minor effect only on prothrombin time.
(From Hirsh, J., 1991. N. Engl. J. Med. 324, 1865–1875.)

The therapeutic effects of some drugs are a direct consequence of enzyme inhibition (e.g. the xanthine oxidase inhibitor **allopurinol**, used to prevent gout; Ch. 27). Xanthine oxidase metabolises several cytotoxic and immunosuppressant drugs, including **mercaptopurine** (the active metabolite of **azathioprine**), the action of which is thus potentiated and prolonged by allopurinol. **Disulfiram**, an inhibitor of aldehyde dehydrogenase that is used to produce an aversive reaction to ethanol (see Ch. 50), also inhibits metabolism of other drugs, including **warfarin**, which it potentiates. **Metronidazole**, an antimicrobial used to treat anaerobic bacterial infections and several protozoal diseases (Chs 52 and 55), also inhibits this enzyme, and patients prescribed it are advised to avoid alcohol for this reason.

There are also examples of drugs that inhibit the metabolism of other drugs, even though enzyme inhibition is not the main mechanism of action of the offending agents. Thus, glucocorticosteroids and **cimetidine** potentiate a range of drugs, including some antidepressant and cytotoxic drugs.

Inhibition of the conversion of a prodrug to its active metabolite can result in *loss* of activity. Proton pump inhibitors (such as **omeprazole**, Ch. 31) and the antiplatelet drug **clopidogrel** (Ch. 25) have been widely co-prescribed, because clopidogrel is often used with other antithrombotic drugs predisposing to bleeding from the stomach – omeprazole reduces gastric acid secretion and the risk of gastric haemorrhage (Ch. 31). Clopidogrel works through an active metabolite formed by CYP2C19 which is inhibited by omeprazole, possibly thereby reducing the antiplatelet effect. It is unclear how clinically important this may be, but the FDA continues to warn against concomitant use of these drugs for this reason.

DRUG AND METABOLITE EXCRETION

BILIARY EXCRETION AND ENTEROHEPATIC CIRCULATION

Liver cells transfer various substances, including drugs, from plasma to bile by transport systems similar to those of the renal tubule; these include organic cation transporters (OCTs), organic anion transporters (OATs) and P-glycoproteins (P-gps) (see Ch. 9). Various hydrophilic drug conjugates (particularly glucuronides) are concentrated in bile and delivered to the intestine, where the glucuronide can be hydrolysed, regenerating active drug; free drug can

then be reabsorbed and the cycle repeated, a process referred to as *enterohepatic circulation*. The result is a 'reservoir' of recirculating drug that can amount to about 20% of total drug in the body, prolonging drug action. Examples where this is important include **morphine** (Ch. 43) and **ethinylestradiol** (Ch. 36). Several drugs are excreted to an appreciable extent in bile. **Vecuronium** (a non-depolarising muscle relaxant; Ch. 14) is an example of a drug that is excreted mainly unchanged in bile. **Rifampicin** (Ch. 52) is absorbed from the gut and slowly deacetylated, retaining its biological activity. Both forms are secreted in the bile, but the deacetylated form is not reabsorbed, so eventually most of the drug leaves the body in this form in the faeces.

RENAL EXCRETION OF DRUGS AND METABOLITES

RENAL CLEARANCE

Elimination of drugs by the kidneys is best quantified by the renal clearance (CL_{ren}, see Chs 11, 30). This is defined as the volume of plasma containing the amount of substance that is removed from the body by the kidneys in unit time. It is calculated from the plasma concentration, C_p, the urinary concentration, C_u, and the rate of flow of urine, V_u, by the equation:

$$CL_{ren} = (C_u \times V_u)/C_p.$$

CL_{ren} varies greatly for different drugs, from less than 1 mL/min to the theoretical maximum set by the renal plasma flow, which is approximately 700 mL/min, measured by *p*-aminohippuric acid (PAH) clearance (renal extraction of PAH approaches 100%).

Drugs differ greatly in the rate at which they are excreted by the kidney, ranging from **penicillin** (Ch. 52), which is (like PAH) cleared from the blood almost completely on a single transit through the kidney, to **amiodarone** (Ch. 22) and **risedronate** (Ch. 37), which are cleared extremely slowly. Most drugs fall between these extremes. Three fundamental processes account for renal drug excretion:

1. glomerular filtration
2. active tubular secretion
3. passive reabsorption (diffusion from the concentrated tubular fluid back across tubular epithelium)

GLOMERULAR FILTRATION

Glomerular capillaries allow drug molecules of molecular weight below about 20 kDa to pass into the glomerular filtrate. Plasma albumin (molecular weight approximately 68 kDa) is almost completely impermeant, but most drugs – with the exception of macromolecules such as **heparin** (Ch. 25) or biopharmaceuticals (Ch. 5) – cross the barrier freely. If a drug binds to plasma albumin, only free drug is filtered. If, like **warfarin** (Ch. 25), a drug is approximately 98% bound to albumin, the concentration in the filtrate is only 2% of that in plasma, and clearance by filtration is correspondingly reduced.

TUBULAR SECRETION

Up to 20% of renal plasma flow is filtered through the glomerulus, leaving at least 80% of delivered drug to pass on to the peritubular capillaries of the proximal tubule. Here, drug molecules are transferred to the tubular lumen by two independent and relatively non-selective carrier

Table 10.7 Important drugs and related substances secreted into the proximal renal tubule by OAT or OCT transporters

OAT	OCT
p-Aminohippuric acid	Amiloride
Furosemide	Dopamine
Glucuronic acid conjugates	Histamine
Glycine conjugates	Mepacrine
Indometacin	Morphine
Methotrexate	Pethidine
Penicillin	Quaternary ammonium
Probenecid	compounds
Sulfate conjugates	Quinine
Thiazide diuretics	5-Hydroxytryptamine
Uric acid	(serotonin)
	Triamterene

Table 10.8 Examples of drugs that are excreted largely unchanged in the urine

Percentage	Drugs excreted
100–75	Furosemide, gentamicin, methotrexate, atenolol, digoxin
75–50	Benzylpenicillin, cimetidine, oxytetracycline, neostigmine
~50	Propantheline, tubocurarine

systems (see Ch. 9). One of these, the OAT, transports acidic drugs in their negatively charged anionic form (as well as various endogenous acids, such as uric acid), while an OCT handles organic bases in their protonated cationic form. Some important drugs that are transported by these two carrier systems are shown in Table 10.7. The OAT carrier can transport drug molecules against an electrochemical gradient, and can therefore reduce the plasma concentration nearly to zero, whereas OCT facilitates transport down an electrochemical gradient. Because at least 80% of the drug delivered to the kidney is presented to the carrier, tubular secretion is potentially the most effective mechanism of renal drug elimination. Unlike glomerular filtration, carrier-mediated transport can achieve maximal drug clearance even when most of the drug is bound to plasma protein.[2] **Penicillin** (Ch. 52), for example, although about 80% protein-bound and therefore cleared only slowly by filtration, is almost completely removed by proximal tubular secretion, and is therefore rapidly eliminated.

Many drugs compete for the same transport systems (Table 10.7), leading to drug interactions. For example, **probenecid** was developed originally to potentiate penicillin by retarding its tubular secretion (see later).

DIFFUSION ACROSS THE RENAL TUBULE

Water is reabsorbed as fluid traverses the tubule, the volume of urine emerging being only about 1% of that of the glomerular filtrate. Consequently, if the tubule is freely permeable to drug molecules, some 99% of the filtered drug will be reabsorbed passively down the resulting concentration gradient. Lipid-soluble drugs are therefore excreted poorly, whereas polar drugs of low tubular

permeability remain in the lumen and become progressively concentrated as water is reabsorbed. Polar drugs handled in this way include **digoxin** and aminoglycoside antibiotics. These exemplify a relatively small but important group of drugs (Table 10.8) that are not inactivated by metabolism, the rate of renal elimination being the main factor that determines their duration of action. These drugs have to be used with special care in individuals whose renal function may be impaired, including the elderly and patients with renal disease or any severe acute illness.

The degree of ionisation of many drugs – weak acids or weak bases – is pH-dependent, and this markedly influences their renal excretion. The ion-trapping effect (see Ch. 9) means that a basic drug is more rapidly excreted in an acid urine that favours the charged form and thus inhibits reabsorption. Conversely, acidic drugs are most rapidly excreted if the urine is alkaline (Fig. 10.6).

DRUG INTERACTIONS DUE TO ALTERED DRUG EXCRETION

The main mechanisms by which one drug can affect the rate of renal excretion of another are by:

- altering protein binding, and hence filtration
- inhibiting tubular secretion
- altering urine flow and/or urine pH

INHIBITION OF TUBULAR SECRETION

Probenecid (Ch. 27) was developed to inhibit secretion of **penicillin** and thus prolong its action. It also inhibits the excretion of other drugs, including **zidovudine** (see Ch. 53). Other drugs have an incidental probenecid-like effect and can enhance the actions of substances that rely on tubular secretion for their elimination. Table 10.9 gives some examples. Because diuretics, such as furosemide, act from within the tubular lumen, drugs that inhibit their secretion into the tubular fluid, such as non-steroidal anti-inflammatory drugs, reduce their effect.

ALTERATION OF URINE FLOW AND PH

Diuretics tend to increase the urinary excretion of other drugs and their metabolites, but this is seldom immediately clinically important. Conversely, loop and thiazide diuretics indirectly *decrease* the excretion of **lithium**; they cause Na⁺ depletion, to which the kidney responds by increased proximal tubular reabsorption of Na⁺, and Li⁺, which is handled in a similar way to Na⁺, and this can cause lithium toxicity in patients treated with lithium carbonate for mood disorders (Ch. 48). The effect of urinary pH on the excretion of weak acids and bases is put to use in the treatment of poisoning with *salicylate* (see Ch. 27), but is not a cause of accidental interactions.

---

[2]Because filtration involves isosmotic movement of both water and solutes, it does not affect the free concentration of drug in the plasma. Thus the equilibrium between free and bound drug is not disturbed, and there is no tendency for bound drug to dissociate as blood traverses the glomerular capillary. The rate of clearance of a drug by filtration is therefore reduced directly in proportion to the fraction that is bound. In the case of active tubular secretion, this is not so because the carrier transports drug molecules unaccompanied by water. As free drug molecules are taken from the plasma, therefore, the free plasma concentration falls, causing dissociation of bound drug from plasma albumin. Secretion is only retarded slightly, even though the drug is mostly bound, because effectively 100% of the drug, both bound and free, is available to the carrier.

Fig. 10.6 **The effect of urinary pH on drug excretion.** (A) Phenobarbital clearance in the dog as a function of urine flow. Because phenobarbital is acidic, alkalinising the urine increases clearance about five-fold. (B) Amphetamine excretion in humans. Acidifying the urine increases the rate of renal elimination of amphetamine, reducing its plasma concentration and its effect on the subject's mental state. (Data from Gunne & Anggard, 1974. In: Torrell, T. et al. (eds) Pharmacology and Pharmacokinetics. Plenum, New York.)

Table 10.9 Examples of drugs that inhibit renal tubular secretion

Drug(s) causing inhibition	Drug(s) affected
Probenecid Sulfinpyrazone Phenylbutazone Sulfonamides Aspirin Thiazide diuretics Indometacin	Penicillin Azidothymidine Indometacin
Verapamil Amiodarone Quinidine	Digoxin
Indometacin	Furosemide (frusemide)
Aspirin Non-steroidal anti-inflammatory drugs	Methotrexate

Elimination of drugs by the kidney

- Most drugs, unless highly bound to plasma protein, cross the glomerular filter freely.
- Many drugs, especially weak acids and weak bases, are actively secreted into the renal tubule and rapidly excreted.
- Lipid-soluble drugs are passively reabsorbed along with water by diffusion across the tubular barrier, so are not efficiently excreted in the urine.
- Because of pH partition, weak acids are more rapidly excreted in alkaline urine, and vice versa.
- Several important drugs are removed predominantly by renal excretion, and are liable to cause toxicity in elderly persons and patients with renal disease.
- There are instances of clinically important drug–drug interactions due to one drug reducing the renal clearance of another (examples include diuretics/lithium and indometacin/methotrexate), but these are less common than interactions due to altered drug metabolism.

REFERENCES AND FURTHER READING

General further reading

Coon, M.J., 2005. Cytochrome P450: nature's most versatile biological catalyst. Annu. Rev. Pharmacol. Toxicol. 45, 1–25. (*Summarises the individual steps in the P450 and reductase reaction cycles*)

Nassar, A.F., 2009. Drug Metabolism Handbook: Concepts and Applications. Wiley-Blackwell, Hoboken, NJ. (*Multi-authored handbook aimed at bench scientists; will be invaluable for pharmaceutical industry scientists*)

Testa, B., Krämer, S.D., 2009. The Biochemistry of Drug Metabolism. Wiley-VCH, Weinheim. (*Two-volume reference work*)

Drug metabolism

Campo, V.L., Bernardes, L.S.C., Carvalho, I., 2009. Stereoselectivity in drug metabolism: molecular mechanisms and analytical methods. Curr. Drug Metab. 10, 188–205.

Guengerich, F.P., Waterman, M.R., Egli, M., 2016. Recent structural insights into cytochrome P450 function. Trends Pharmacol. Sci. 37, 625–640. (*Review*)

Ingelman-Sundberg, M., 2004. Pharmacogenetics of cytochrome P450 and its applications in drug therapy: the past, present and future. Trends Pharmacol. Sci. 25, 193–200. (*Estimates that personalized P450 gene-based treatment would be relevant for 10%–20% of all small molecule drug therapy*)

Nair, P.C., McKinnon, R.A., Miners, J.O., 2016. Cytochrome P450 structure-function: insights from molecular dynamics simulations. Drug Metab. Rev. 48, 434–452. (*Structure-function relations in P450*)

Preissner, S.C., Hoffmann, M.F., Preissner, R., Dunkel, M., Gewiess, A., Preissner, S., 2013. Polymorphic Cytochrome P450 Enzymes (CYPs) and their role in personalized therapy. PLoS ONE 8 (12), e82562. (*Use of a text mining approach to identify the most relevant polymorphisms in human CYPs. The most important polymorphic CYPs were 1A2, 2D6, 2C9 and 2C19. Thirty-four common allele variants in caucasians led to altered enzyme activity*)

P450 enzyme induction and inhibition

Henderson, L., Yue, Q.Y., Bergquist, C., et al., 2002. St John's wort (*Hypericum perforatum*): drug interactions and clinical outcomes. Br. J. Clin. Pharmacol. 54, 349–356. (*Reviews the induction of CYP450 isoenzymes and of P-glycoprotein by constituents in this herbal remedy*)

Pelkonen, O., Turpeinen, M., Hakkola, J., et al., 2008. Inhibition and induction of human cytochrome P450 enzymes: current status. Arch. Toxicol. 82, 667–715. (*Review*)

Drug elimination

Kusuhara, H., Sugiyama, Y., 2009. In vitro–in vivo extrapolation of transporter-mediated clearance in the liver and kidney. Drug Metab. Pharmacokinet. 24, 37–52. (*Review*)

Pharmacokinetics

OVERVIEW

We explain the importance of pharmacokinetic analysis and present a simple approach to this topic. We explain how drug clearance determines the steady-state plasma concentration during constant-rate drug administration and how the characteristics of absorption and distribution (considered in Ch. 9) plus metabolism and excretion (considered in Ch. 10) determine the time course of drug concentration in blood plasma during and following drug administration. The effect of different dosing regimens on the time course of drug concentration in plasma is explained. Population pharmacokinetics is mentioned briefly, and a final section considers limitations to the pharmacokinetic approach.

INTRODUCTION: DEFINITION AND USES OF PHARMACOKINETICS

Pharmacokinetics is the branch of pharmacology dedicated to determining the fate of chemical substances administered to a living organism – 'what the body does to the drug'. In practice this involves the measurement and formal interpretation of changes with time of drug and drug metabolite concentrations in plasma, urine and sometimes other accessible regions of the body, in relation to dosing. It provides a framework for understanding what happens to a drug when given to an animal or human, where it goes in the body, and how quickly, that enables one to understand the effects that it produces. In contrast, pharmacodynamics ('what the drug does to the body'), describes events consequent on interaction of the drug with its receptor or other primary site of action. The distinction is useful, although the words cause dismay to etymological purists.

'Pharmacodynamic' received an entry in a dictionary of 1890 ('relating to the powers or effects of drugs') whereas pharmacokinetic studies only became possible in the latter part of the 20th century with the development of sensitive, specific and accurate physicochemical analytical techniques, especially high-performance chromatography and mass spectrometry, for measuring drug concentrations in biological fluids. The time course of drug concentration following dosing depends on the processes of absorption, distribution, metabolism and excretion (ADME) that we have considered qualitatively in Chapters 9 and 10.

In practice, pharmacokinetics usually focuses on concentrations of drug in *blood plasma*, which is easily sampled via venepuncture, since plasma concentrations are assumed usually to bear a clear relation to the concentration of drug in extracellular fluid surrounding cells that express the receptors or other targets with which drug molecules combine. This underpins what is termed the *target concentration strategy*. Individual variation in *response* to a given dose of a drug is often greater than variability in the *plasma concentration* at that dose. Plasma concentrations (C_p) are therefore useful in the early stages of drug development (see later), and in the case of a few drugs plasma drug concentrations are also used in routine clinical practice to individualise dosage, to achieve the desired therapeutic effect while minimising adverse effects in each individual patient – an approach known as *therapeutic drug monitoring*, often abbreviated TDM. Table 11.1 shows examples of some drugs where a therapeutic range of plasma concentrations has been established, enabling TDM. Concentrations of drug in other body fluids (e.g. urine,[1] saliva, cerebrospinal fluid, milk) may add useful information.

Formal interpretation of pharmacokinetic data consists of fitting concentration-versus-time data to a model (whether abstract or, more usefully, physiologically based) and determining parameters that describe the observed behaviour. The parameters can then be used to adjust the dose regimen to achieve a desired target plasma concentration, The pharmacologically active concentration range is estimated from experiments on cells, tissues or laboratory animals, and modified as data emerge from early human pharmacology trials, which often test single doses of the new drug administered to successive groups of volunteers in progressively increasing doses - single ascending dose (SAD) studies (Ch. 8). Some descriptive pharmacokinetic characteristics can be estimated directly by inspecting the time course of drug concentration in plasma following dosing – important examples,[2] illustrated more fully later, are the *maximum plasma concentration* following a given dose of a drug administered in a defined dosing form (C_{max}) and the *time* (T_{max}) between drug administration and achieving C_{max}. Other pharmacokinetic parameters are estimated mathematically from experimental data; examples include *volume of distribution* (V_d) and *clearance* (CL), concepts that have been introduced in Chapters 9 and 10, respectively, and to which we return below. This approach applies both to classical low molecular-weight drugs and to macromolecular biopharmaceuticals (Ch. 5), although qualitative aspects of absorption, distribution and elimination are, of course, very different and pharmacokinetic parameters differ markedly – for example, antibodies have evolved to persist for long periods after exposure to antigen, and therapeutic antibodies commonly have low rates of clearance and long elimination half-lives in consequence.

---

[1]*Clinical* pharmacology became at one time so associated with the measurement of drugs in urine that the canard had it that clinical pharmacologists were the new alchemists – they turned urine into airline tickets.

[2]Important because dose-related adverse effects often occur around C_{max}.

Table 11.1 Examples of drugs where therapeutic drug monitoring (TDM) of plasma concentrations is used clinically

Category	Example(s)	See chapter
Immunosuppressants	Ciclosporin, tacrolimus	27
Cardiovascular	Digoxin	22
Respiratory	Theophylline	17, 29
CNS	Lithium, phenytoin	48, 46
Antibacterials	Aminoglycosides	52
Anticancer drugs	Methotrexate	57

USES OF PHARMACOKINETICS

Knowledge of the pharmacokinetic behaviour of drugs in animals and man is crucial in drug development, both to make sense of preclinical toxicological and pharmacological data[3] and to decide on an appropriate dose and dosing regimen for clinical trials (see Ch. 60). Drug regulators have developed concepts such as *bioavailability* and *bioequivalence* (Ch. 9) to support the licensing of generic versions of drugs produced when originator products lose patent protection. Understanding the general principles of pharmacokinetics is also important in clinical practice, to understand the rationale of recommended dosing regimens, to interpret drug concentrations for TDM and to adjust dose regimens rationally, and to identify and evaluate possible drug interactions (see Chs 9 and 10). In particular, intensive-care specialists and anaesthetists dealing with a severely ill patient often need to individualise the dose regimen depending on the urgency of achieving a therapeutic plasma concentration, and whether the pharmacokinetic behaviour of the drug is likely to be affected by illness such as renal impairment or liver disease.

SCOPE OF THIS CHAPTER

We describe:

- how total drug clearance determines steady-state plasma concentration during continuous administration;
- how drug concentration versus time can be described by a simple model in which the body is represented as a single well-stirred compartment, of volume V_d. This describes the situation before steady state (or after drug is discontinued) in terms of elimination half-life ($t_{1/2}$);

- situations where this model is inadequate, and introduce a two-compartment model;
- situations where clearance varies with drug concentration ('non-linear kinetics');
- situations (such as paediatric pharmacokinetics) where only a few samples are available and population kinetics may be used.

Finally, we consider some of the limitations inherent in the pharmacokinetic approach. More detailed accounts are provided by Atkinson et al. (2012), Birkett (2010) and Rowland and Tozer (2010).

DRUG ELIMINATION EXPRESSED AS CLEARANCE

The overall clearance of a drug by all routes (CL_{tot}) is the fundamental pharmacokinetic parameter describing drug elimination. It is defined as the volume of plasma which contains the total amount of drug that is removed from the body in unit time. It is thus expressed as volume per unit time, e.g. mL/min or L/h. Renal clearance (CL_{ren}), an important component of CL_{tot}, was described in Chapter 10.

The overall clearance of a drug (CL_{tot}) is the sum of clearance rates for each mechanism involved in eliminating the drug, usually renal clearance (CL_{ren}) and metabolic clearance (CL_{met}) plus any additional appreciable routes of elimination (faeces, breath, etc.). It relates the rate of elimination of a drug (in units of mass/unit time) to the plasma concentration, C_p:

$$\text{Rate of drug elimination} = C_p \times CL_{tot} \qquad (11.1)$$

Drug clearance can be determined in an individual subject by measuring the plasma concentration of the drug (in units of, say, mg/L) at intervals during a constant-rate intravenous infusion (delivering, say, X mg of drug per h), until a steady state is approximated (Fig. 11.1A). At steady state, the rate of input to the body is equal to the rate of elimination, so:

$$X = C_{ss} \times CL_{tot} \qquad (11.2)$$

Rearranging this,

$$CL_{tot} = \frac{X}{C_{ss}} \qquad (11.3)$$

where C_{ss} is the plasma concentration at steady state, and CL_{tot} is in units of volume/time (L/h in the example given).

For many drugs, clearance in an individual subject is independent of dose (at least within the range of doses used therapeutically – but see the section on saturation kinetics later for exceptions), so knowing the clearance enables one to calculate the dose rate needed to achieve a desired steady-state ('target') plasma concentration from Eq. 11.2.

CL_{tot} can also be estimated by measuring plasma concentrations at intervals following a single intravenous bolus dose of, say, Q mg (Fig. 11.1B):

$$CL_{tot} = \frac{Q}{AUC_{0-\infty}} \qquad (11.4)$$

---

[3]For example, doses used in experimental animals often need to be much greater than those in humans (on a 'per unit body weight' basis), because drug metabolism is commonly much more rapid in rodents – **methadone** (Ch. 43) is one of many such examples. When using animal data to estimate a 'human equivalent dose' in planning the first-in-human study, doses of low molecular-weight drugs are normalised (so-called 'allometric scaling') to estimated body surface area rather than to body weight. Paediatricians commonly use the same approach, estimating appropriate doses for babies and young children from adult human doses in terms of dose/unit of estimated body surface area rather than dose/kg body weight.

Fig. 11.1 Plasma drug concentration–time curves.
(A) During a constant intravenous infusion at rate X mg/h, indicated by the horizontal bar, the plasma concentration (C) increases from zero to a steady-state value (C_{SS}); when the infusion is stopped, C declines to zero. (B) Following an intravenous bolus dose (Q mg), the plasma concentration rises abruptly and then declines towards zero. (C) Data from panel (B) plotted with plasma concentrations on a logarithmic scale. The straight line shows that concentration declines exponentially. Extrapolation back to the ordinate at zero time gives an estimate of C_0, the concentration at zero time, and hence of V_d, the volume of distribution.

Fig. 11.2 Single-compartment pharmacokinetic model. This model is applicable if the plasma concentration falls exponentially after drug administration (as in Fig. 11.1).

effects in patients with disordered kidney or liver function may differ from those observed in healthy volunteer subjects. In early phase clinical trials these measures of drug exposure are determined at each dose level and the protocol includes 'stopping rules' to avoid dose increments that caused toxicity during animal experiments. See Chapter 9, and Birkett, 2010 for a fuller account.

Note that these estimates of CL_{tot}, unlike estimates based on the rate constant or half-life (see later), do not depend on any particular compartmental model.

SINGLE-COMPARTMENT MODEL

Consider a highly-simplified model of a human being, which consists of a single well-stirred compartment, of volume V_d (distribution volume), into which a quantity of drug Q is introduced rapidly by intravenous injection, and from which it is removed either by being metabolised or by being excreted (Fig. 11.2). For most drugs, V_d is an apparent volume rather than the volume of an anatomical compartment. It links the total amount of drug in the body to its concentration in plasma (see Ch. 9). The quantity of drug in the body immediately after it is administered as a single bolus is equal to the administered dose Q. The initial concentration, C_0, will therefore be given by:

$$C_0 = \frac{Q}{V_d} \quad (11.5)$$

In practice, C_0 is estimated by extrapolating the linear portion of a semilogarithmic plot of C_p against time back to its intercept at time 0 (Fig. 11.1C). C_p at any time depends on the rate of elimination of the drug (i.e. on its total clearance, CL_{tot}) as well as on the dose and V_d. Many drugs exhibit *first-order kinetics*, where the rate of elimination is directly proportional to drug concentration. (An analogy is letting your bath drain down the plug hole where the water, analogous to drug, initially rushes out whereas the last bit always takes an age to drain away. Contrast this with so-called *zero-order kinetics* where the water is pumped out of the bath at a constant rate.) With first-order kinetics

where $AUC_{0-\infty}$ is the area under the full curve[4] relating C_p to time following a bolus dose given at time $t = 0$. $AUC_{0-\infty}$ provides an integrated measure of tissue exposure to the drug in units of time multiplied by drug concentration. Together with C_{max} it informs as to drug effects, both desired and toxic, and so is important in anticipating possible effects in humans from those observed during animal pharmacology and toxicology experiments, and in anticipating how

---

[4]The area is obtained by integrating from time = 0 to time = ∞, and is designated $AUC_{0-\infty}$. The area under the curve has units of time – on the abscissa – multiplied by concentration (mass/volume) – on the ordinate; so $CL = Q/AUC_{0-\infty}$ has units of volume/time as it should.

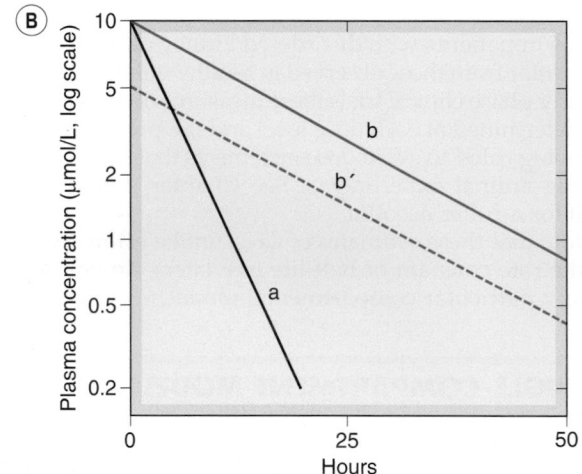

Fig. 11.3 Predicted behaviour of single-compartment model following intravenous drug administration at time 0. Drugs *a* and *b* differ only in their elimination rate constant, k_{el}. Curve *b'* shows the plasma concentration time course for a smaller dose of *b*. Note that the half-life ($t_{1/2}$) (indicated by *broken lines*) does not depend on the dose. (A) Linear concentration scale. (B) Logarithmic concentration scale.

drug concentration decays exponentially (Fig. 11.3), being described by the equation:

$$C_t = C_0 \exp\frac{-CL_{tot}}{V_d}t \qquad (11.6)$$

(Note that exp is another way of writing 'e to the power of', so this has the same form as $C_t = C_0.e^{-kt}$.)

Taking logarithms to the base e (written as ln):

$$\ln C_t - \ln C_0 - \frac{-CL_{tot}}{V_d}t \qquad (11.7)$$

Plotting C_t on a logarithmic scale against *t* (on a linear scale) yields a straight line with slope $-CL_{tot}/V_d$. The constant CL_{tot}/V_d is the *elimination rate constant* k_{el}, which has units

of 1/time. It represents the *fraction* of drug in the body eliminated per unit of time. For example, if the rate constant is 0.1/h this implies that one-tenth of the drug remaining in the body is eliminated each hour.

The *elimination half-life*, $t_{1/2}$, is the time taken for C_p to decrease by half, and is equal to $\ln2/k_{el}$ (=$0.693/k_{el}$). The plasma half-life is therefore determined by V_d as well as by CL_{tot}. It enables one to predict the time course of C_p after a bolus of drug is given or after the start or end of an infusion, when C_p is rising to its steady-state level or declining to zero.

When a single-compartment model is applicable, the drug concentration in plasma approaches the steady-state value approximately exponentially during a constant infusion (see Fig. 11.1A). When the infusion is discontinued, the concentration falls exponentially towards zero with the same half-life: after one half-life, the concentration will have fallen to half the initial concentration; after two half-lives, it will have fallen to one-quarter the initial concentration; after three half-lives, to one-eighth; and so on. It is intuitively obvious that the longer the half-life, the longer the drug will persist in the body after dosing is discontinued. It is less obvious, but nonetheless true, that during chronic drug administration, the longer the half-life, the longer it will take for the drug to accumulate to its steady-state level: one half-life to reach 50% of the steady-state value, two to reach 75%, three to reach 87.5% and so on. This is extremely helpful to a clinician deciding how to start treatment. If the drug in question has a half-life of approximately 24 h, for example, it will take 3–5 days to approximate the steady-state concentration during a constant-rate infusion. If this is too slow in the face of the prevailing clinical situation, a *loading dose* may be used in order to achieve a therapeutic concentration of drug in the plasma more rapidly (see later). The size of such a dose is determined by the volume of distribution (Eq. 11.5).

EFFECT OF REPEATED DOSING

Drugs are usually given therapeutically as repeated doses rather than single injections or a constant infusion. Repeated injections (each of dose *Q*) give a more complicated pattern than the smooth exponential rise during intravenous infusion, but the principle is the same (Fig. 11.4). The concentration will rise to a mean steady-state concentration with an approximately exponential time course, but will oscillate (through a range Q/V_d). The smaller and more frequent the doses, the more closely the situation approaches that of a continuous infusion, and the smaller the swings in concentration. The exact dosage schedule, however, does not affect the mean steady-state concentration, or the rate at which it is approached. In practice, a steady state is effectively achieved after three to five half-lives. Speedier attainment of the steady state can be achieved by starting with a larger dose, as mentioned earlier. Such a loading dose is sometimes used when starting treatment with a drug with a half-life that is long in the context of the urgency of the clinical situation, as may be the case when treating cardiac dysrhythmias with drugs such as **amiodarone** or **digoxin** (Ch. 22) or initiating anticoagulation with **heparin** (Ch. 25).

EFFECT OF VARIATION IN RATE OF ABSORPTION

If a drug is absorbed slowly from the gut or from an injection site into the plasma, it is (in terms of a compartmental

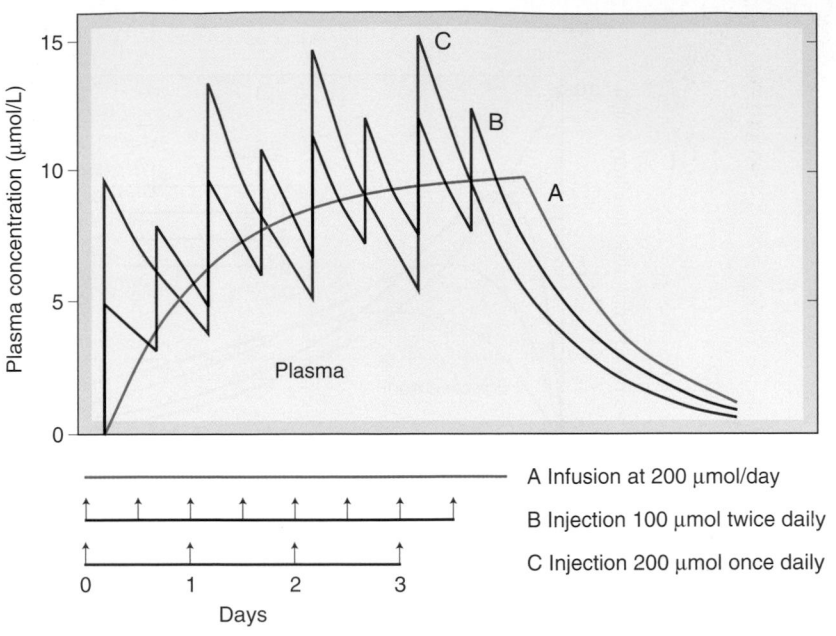

Fig. 11.4 **Predicted behaviour of single-compartment model with continuous or intermittent drug administration.** Smooth *curve A* shows the effect of continuous infusion for 4 days; *curve B* the same total amount of drug given in eight equal doses; and *curve C* the same total amount of drug given in four equal doses. The drug has a half-life of 17 h and a volume of distribution of 20 L. Note that in each case a steady state is effectively reached after about 2 days (about three half-lives), and that the mean concentration reached in the steady state is the same for all three schedules.

A Infusion at 200 μmol/day

B Injection 100 μmol twice daily

C Injection 200 μmol once daily

Pharmacokinetics

- Total clearance (CL_{tot}) of a drug is the fundamental parameter describing its elimination: the rate of elimination equals CL_{tot} multiplied by plasma concentration.
- CL_{tot} determines steady-state plasma concentration (C_{SS}): C_{SS} = rate of drug administration/CL_{tot}.
- For many drugs, disappearance from the plasma follows an approximately exponential time course. Such drugs can be described by a model where the body is treated as a single well-stirred compartment of volume V_d. V_d is an apparent volume linking the amount of drug in the body at any time to the plasma concentration.
- Elimination half-life ($t_{1/2}$) is directly proportional to V_d and inversely proportional to CL_{tot}.
- With repeated dosage or sustained delivery of a drug, the plasma concentration approaches a steady value within three to five plasma half-lives.
- In urgent situations, a loading dose may be needed to achieve therapeutic concentration rapidly.
- The loading dose (L) needed to achieve a desired initial plasma concentration C_{target} is determined by V_d: $L = C_{target} \times V_d$.
- A two-compartment model is often needed. In this case, the kinetics are biexponential. The two components roughly represent the processes of transfer between plasma and tissues (α phase) and elimination from the body (β phase).
- Some drugs show non-exponential 'saturation' kinetics, with important clinical consequences, especially a disproportionate increase in steady-state plasma concentration when daily dose is increased.

model) as though it were being slowly infused at a variable rate into the bloodstream. For the purpose of kinetic modelling, the transfer of drug from the site of administration to the central compartment can be represented approximately by a rate constant, k_{abs} (see Fig. 11.2). This assumes that the rate of absorption is directly proportional, at any moment, to the amount of drug still unabsorbed, which is at best a rough approximation to reality. The effect of slow absorption on the time course of the rise and fall of the plasma concentration is shown in Fig. 11.5. The curves show the effect of spreading out the absorption of the same total amount of drug over different times. In each case, the drug is absorbed completely, but the peak concentration appears later and is lower and less sharp if absorption is slow. In the limiting case, a dosage form that releases drug at a constant rate as it traverses the ileum (Ch. 9) approximates a constant-rate infusion. Once absorption is complete, the plasma concentration declines with the same half-time, irrespective of the rate of absorption.

▼ For the kind of pharmacokinetic model discussed here, the area under the plasma concentration–time curve (*AUC*) is directly proportional to the total amount of drug introduced into the plasma compartment, irrespective of the rate at which it enters. Incomplete absorption, or destruction by first-pass metabolism before the drug reaches the plasma compartment, reduces *AUC* after oral administration (see Ch. 9). Changes in the rate of absorption, however, do not affect *AUC*. Again, it is worth noting that provided absorption is complete, the relation between the rate of administration and the steady-state plasma concentration (Eq. 11.3) is unaffected by k_{abs}, although the size of the oscillation of plasma concentration with each dose is reduced if absorption is slowed.

MORE COMPLICATED KINETIC MODELS

So far, we have considered a single-compartment pharmacokinetic model in which the rates of absorption, metabolism

Fig. 11.5 **The effect of slow drug absorption on plasma drug concentration.** (A) Predicted behaviour of single-compartment model with drug absorbed at different rates from the gut or an injection site. The elimination half-time is 6 h. The absorption half-times ($t_{1/2}$ abs) are marked on the diagram. (Zero indicates instantaneous absorption, corresponding to intravenous administration.) Note that the peak plasma concentration is reduced and delayed by slow absorption, and the duration of action is somewhat increased. (B) Measurements of plasma aminophylline concentration in humans following equal oral and intravenous doses. (Data from Swintowsky, J.V., 1956. J. Am. Pharm. Assoc. 49, 395.)

and excretion are all assumed to be directly proportional to the concentration of drug in the compartment from which transfer is occurring. This is a useful way to illustrate some basic principles but is clearly a physiological oversimplification. The characteristics of different parts of the body, such as brain, body fat and muscle, are quite different in terms of their blood supply, partition coefficient for drugs and the permeability of their capillaries to drugs. These differences, which the single-compartment model ignores, can markedly affect the time courses of drug distribution and action, and much theoretical work has gone into the mathematical analysis of more complex models (see Atkinson et al., 2012; Rowland & Tozer, 2010). They are beyond the scope of this book, and perhaps also beyond the limit of what is actually useful, for the experimental data on pharmacokinetic properties of drugs are seldom accurate or reproducible enough to enable complex models to be tested critically.

The two-compartment model, which introduces a separate 'peripheral' compartment to represent the tissues, in communication with the 'central' plasma compartment, more closely resembles the real situation without involving excessive complications.

TWO-COMPARTMENT MODEL

The two-compartment model is a widely used approximation in which the tissues are lumped together as a peripheral compartment. Drug molecules can enter and leave the peripheral compartment only via the central compartment (Fig. 11.6), which usually represents the plasma (or plasma plus some extravascular space in the case of a few drugs that distribute especially rapidly). The effect of adding a second compartment to the model is to introduce a second exponential component into the predicted time course of the plasma concentration, so that it comprises a fast and a slow phase. This pattern is often found experimentally, and is most clearly revealed when the concentration data

Fig. 11.6 Two-compartment pharmacokinetic model.

are plotted semilogarithmically (Fig. 11.7). If, as is often the case, the transfer of drug between the central and peripheral compartments is relatively fast compared with the rate of elimination, then the fast phase (often called the α *phase*) can be taken to represent the redistribution of the drug (i.e. drug molecules passing from plasma to tissues, thereby rapidly lowering the plasma concentration). The plasma concentration reached when the fast phase is complete, but before appreciable elimination has occurred, allows a measure of the combined distribution volumes of the two compartments; the half-time for the slow phase (the β *phase*) provides an estimate of k_{el}. If a drug is rapidly metabolised or excreted, the α and β phases are not well separated, and the calculation of separate V_d and k_{el} values for each phase is not straightforward. Problems also arise with drugs (e.g. very fat-soluble drugs)

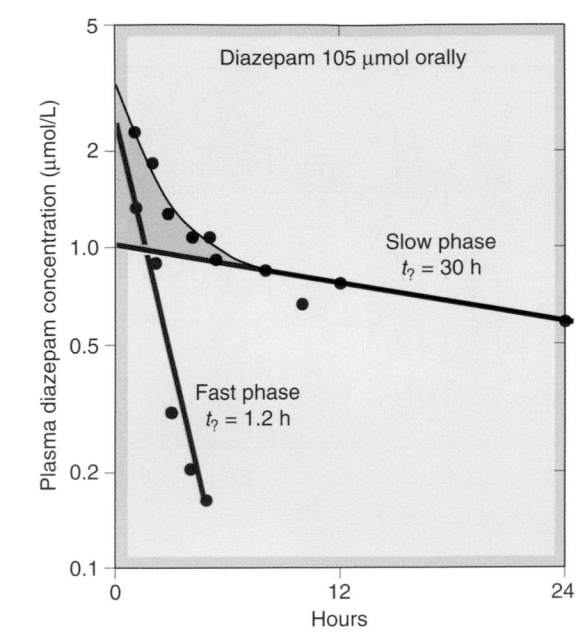

Fig. 11.7 Kinetics of diazepam elimination in humans following a single oral dose. The graph shows a semilogarithmic plot of plasma concentration versus time. The experimental data *(black symbols)* follow a curve that becomes linear after about 8 h (slow phase). Plotting the deviation of the early points *(pink shaded area)* from this line on the same coordinates *(red symbols)* reveals the fast phase. This type of two-component decay is consistent with the two-compartment model (see Fig. 11.6) and is obtained with many drugs. (Data from Curry, S.H., 1980. Drug Disposition and Pharmacokinetics. Blackwell, Oxford.)

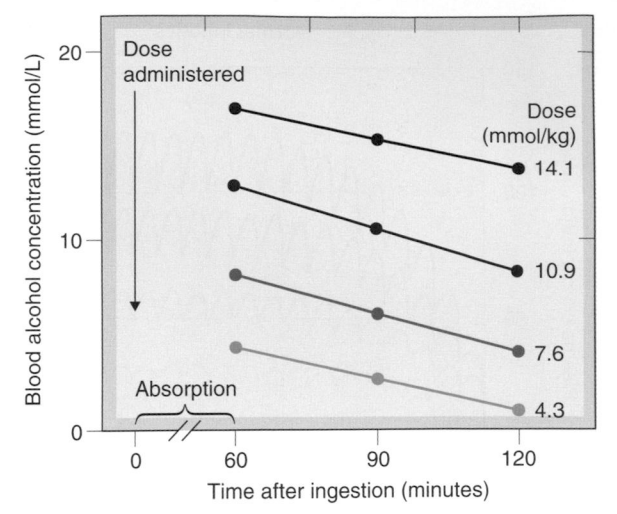

Fig. 11.8 Saturating kinetics of alcohol elimination in humans. The blood alcohol concentration falls linearly rather than exponentially, and the rate of fall does not vary with dose. (From Drew, G.C. et al., 1958. Br. Med. J. 2, 5103.)

for which it is unrealistic to lump all the peripheral tissues together.

SATURATION KINETICS

In the case of some drugs, including **ethanol**, **phenytoin** and **salicylate**, the time course of disappearance of drug from the plasma does not follow the exponential or biexponential patterns shown in Figs 11.3 and 11.7 but is initially linear (i.e. drug is removed at a constant rate that is independent of plasma concentration). This is often called *zero-order kinetics* to distinguish it from the usual first-order kinetics that we have considered so far (these terms have their origin in chemical kinetic theory). *Saturation kinetics* is a better term, because it conveys the underlying mechanism, namely that a carrier or enzyme saturates and so as the concentration of drug substrate increases, the rate of elimination approaches a constant value. Fig. 11.8 shows the example of ethanol. It can be seen that the rate of disappearance of ethanol from the plasma is constant at approximately 4 mmol/L per h, irrespective of dose or of the plasma concentration of ethanol. The explanation for this is that the rate of oxidation by the enzyme alcohol dehydrogenase reaches a maximum at low ethanol concentrations, because of limited availability of the cofactor NAD^+ (see Ch. 49, Fig. 49.6).

Saturation kinetics has several important consequences (Fig. 11.9). One is that the duration of action is more strongly dependent on dose than is the case with drugs that do not show metabolic saturation. Another consequence is that the relationship between dose and steady-state plasma concentration is steep and unpredictable, and it does not obey the proportionality rule implicit in Eq. 11.3 for non-saturating drugs (see Fig. 49.6 for another example related to ethanol). The maximum rate of metabolism sets a limit to the rate at which the drug can be administered; if this rate is exceeded, the amount of drug in the body will, in principle, increase indefinitely and never reach a steady state (see Fig. 11.9). This does not actually happen, because there is always some dependence of the rate of elimination on the plasma concentration (usually because other, non-saturating metabolic pathways or renal excretion contribute significantly at high concentrations). Nevertheless, steady-state plasma concentrations of drugs of this kind vary widely and unpredictably with dose. Similarly, variations in the rate of metabolism (e.g. through enzyme induction) cause disproportionately large changes in the plasma concentration. These problems are well recognised for drugs such as phenytoin, an anticonvulsant for which plasma concentration needs to be closely controlled to achieve an optimal clinical effect (see Ch. 46, Fig. 46.4). Drugs showing saturation kinetics are less predictable in clinical use than ones with first-order kinetics, so may be rejected during drug development if a pharmacologically similar candidate with first-order kinetics is available (Ch. 60).

Clinical applications of pharmacokinetics are summarised in the clinical box.

POPULATION PHARMACOKINETICS

▼ In some situations, for example when a drug is intended for use in chronically ill children, it is desirable to obtain pharmacokinetic data in a patient population rather than in healthy adult volunteers. Such studies in children are inevitably limited and samples for drug analysis are often obtained opportunistically during clinical care, with limitations as to quality of the data and on the number

Fig. 11.9 **Comparison of non-saturating and saturating kinetics for drugs given orally every 12 h.** (A) The curves showing an imaginary drug, similar to the antiepileptic drug phenytoin at the lowest dose, but with linear kinetics. The steady-state plasma concentration is reached within a few days, and is directly proportional to dose. (B) Curves for saturating kinetics calculated from the known pharmacokinetic parameters of phenytoin (see Ch. 45). Note that no steady state is reached with higher doses of phenytoin, and that a small increment in dose results after a time in a disproportionately large effect on plasma concentration. (Curves were calculated with the Sympak pharmacokinetic modelling program written by Dr J.G. Blackman, University of Otago.)

Uses of pharmacokinetics

- Pharmacokinetic studies performed during drug development underpin the standard dose regimens approved by regulatory agencies.
- Clinicians sometimes need to individualise dose regimens to account for individual variation in a particular patient (e.g. a neonate, a patient with impaired and changing renal function, or a patient taking drugs that interfere with drug metabolism; see Ch. 10).
- Drug effect (pharmacodynamics) is often used for such individualisation, but there are drugs (including some anticonvulsants, immunosuppressants and antineoplastics) where a therapeutic range of plasma concentrations has been defined, and for which it is useful to adjust the dose to achieve a concentration in this range.
- Knowledge of kinetics enables rational dose adjustment. For example:
  - the frequency of dosing of a drug such as **gentamicin** eliminated by renal excretion may need to be markedly reduced in a patient with renal impairment (Ch. 52);
  - the dose increment needed to achieve a target plasma concentration range of a drug such as **phenytoin** with saturation kinetics (Ch. 46, Fig. 46.4) is much less than for a drug with linear kinetics.
- Knowing the approximate $t_{1/2}$ of a drug can be very useful, even if a therapeutic concentration is not known:
  - in correctly interpreting adverse events that occur some considerable time after starting regular treatment (e.g. benzodiazepines; see Ch. 45);
  - in deciding on the need or otherwise for an initial loading dose when starting treatment with drugs such as **digoxin** and **amiodarone** (Ch. 22).
- The volume of distribution (V_d) of a drug determines the size of loading dose needed. If V_d is large (as for many tricyclic antidepressants), haemodialysis will not be an effective way of increasing the rate of elimination in treating overdose.

of samples collected from each patient. Population pharmacokinetics addresses how best to analyse such data. Fitting data from all subjects as if there were no kinetic differences between individuals, and fitting each individual's data separately and then combining the individual parameter estimates, each have obvious shortcomings. A better method is to use non-linear mixed effects modelling (NONMEM). The statistical technicalities are considerable and beyond the scope of this chapter: the interested reader is referred to Sheiner et al. (1997).

LIMITATIONS OF PHARMACOKINETICS

Some limitations of the pharmacokinetic approach will be obvious from the above account, such as the proliferation of parameters in even quite conceptually simple models. There are also limitations in the usefulness of monitoring drug concentrations in plasma as an approach to reducing individual variability in drug response (see Ch. 12). Two main assumptions underpin the expectation that by relating response to a drug to its plasma concentration we can reduce variability of response by accounting for pharmacokinetic variation – that is, variation in ADME. They are:

1. That plasma concentration of a drug bears a precise relation to the concentration of drug in the immediate environment of its target (receptor, enzyme, etc.).
2. That drug response depends only on the concentration of the drug in the immediate environment of its target.

While the first of these assumptions is very plausible for those few drugs that work through a target in the circulating blood (e.g. a fibrinolytic drug working on fibrinogen) and reasonably plausible for a drug working on an enzyme, ion channel or G protein–coupled or kinase-linked receptor located in the cell membrane, it is less likely in the case of a nuclear receptor or when an active metabolite is involved. Because of the blood–brain barrier, plasma concentrations rarely reflect local drug concentrations in the brain, so, with exception of lithium (Ch. 48) and some antiepileptic drugs (Ch. 46), monitoring of plasma concentrations is not clinically useful.,

The second assumption is untrue in the case of drugs that form a stable covalent attachment with their target, and so produce an effect that outlives their presence in solution. Examples include the antiplatelet effects of **aspirin** and **clopidogrel** (Ch. 25) and the effect of some monoamine oxidase inhibitors (Ch. 48). In other cases, drugs in therapeutic use act only after delay (e.g. antidepressants, Ch. 48), or gradually induce tolerance (e.g. opioids, Ch. 43) or physiological adaptations (e.g. corticosteroids, Ch. 34) that alter the relation between concentration and drug effect in a time-dependent manner.

REFERENCES AND FURTHER READING

Atkinson, A., Huang, S.M., Lertora, J., Markey, S. (Eds.), 2012. Principles of Clinical Pharmacology, third ed. Academic Press, London. (*Includes detailed section on pharmacokinetics*)

Birkett, D.J., 2010. Pocket Guide: Pharmacokinetics Made Easy. McGraw–Hill Australia, Sydney. (*Excellent slim volume that lives up to the promise of its title*)

Rowland, M., Tozer, T.N., 2010. Clinical Pharmacokinetics and Pharmacodynamics. Concepts and Applications. Wolters Kluwer/ Lippincott Williams & Wilkins, Baltimore. Online simulations by H. Derendorf and G. Hochhaus. (*Excellent text; emphasises clinical applications*)

Population pharmacokinetics

Sheiner, L.B., Rosenberg, B., Marethe, V.V., 1997. Estimation of population characteristics of pharmacokinetic parameters from routine clinical data. J. Pharmacokinet. Biopharm. 5, 445–479.

12 Individual variation, pharmacogenomics and personalised medicine

OVERVIEW

This chapter addresses sources of variation between individuals (inter-individual variation) in their responses to drugs. Important factors, including ethnicity, age, pregnancy, disease and drug interaction (i.e. modification of the action of one drug by another), are described. The concept of individualising drug therapy in light of genomic information ('personalised medicine') – a rapidly developing area of clinical pharmacology – is introduced. We explain relevant elementary genetic concepts and describe briefly several single-gene pharmacogenetic disorders that affect drug responses. We then cover pharmacogenomic tests, including tests for variations in human leukocyte antigen (HLA) genes, in genes influencing drug metabolism, and encoding drug targets.

INTRODUCTION

Therapeutics would be a great deal easier if the same dose of drug always produced the same response. In reality, inter- and even intra-individual variation is often substantial and this can lead to important differences in the balance between benefit and harm of treatment. Physicians need to be aware of the sources of such variation to prescribe drugs safely and effectively. Variation can be caused by different concentrations at sites of drug action or by different responses to the same drug concentration. The first kind is called *pharmacokinetic variation* and can occur because of differences in absorption, distribution, metabolism or excretion (ADME; Chs 9 and 10). The second kind is called *pharmacodynamic variation*. Responses to some therapeutic agents, for example, most vaccines and oral contraceptives (Ch. 36), are sufficiently predictable to permit a standard dose regimen, whereas treatment with **lithium** (Ch. 48), antihypertensive drugs (Ch. 23), anticoagulants (Ch. 25) and many other drugs is individualised, doses being adjusted on the basis of monitoring the drug concentration in the plasma or a response such as change in blood pressure, together with any adverse effects.

Inter-individual variation in response to some drugs is a serious problem; if not taken into account, it can result in lack of efficacy or unexpected adverse effects. Whilst large-scale clinical trials may be able to predict the 'average' effect of a drug, clinicians also recognise that there are subgroups of individuals who have a greater potential for beneficial response than others. Variation is partly caused by environmental factors, but studies comparing identical with non-identical twins suggest that much of the variation in response to some drugs is genetically determined; for example, elimination half-lives of antipyrine, a probe of hepatic drug oxidation, and of **warfarin**, an oral anticoagulant (Ch. 25), differ much less between identical than between fraternal twins. However, even for drugs with a known genetic component such as **warfarin** (see p. 161 and Ch. 25), addition of pharmacogenetic information to a dosing algorithm incorporating other clinical sources of variation (age, sex and so on) does not improve outcome significantly, although when compared with a standardised (i.e. trial and error) loading dose strategy, a genetically guided dose-initiation strategy does result in a greater fraction of time in the therapeutic range during the first weeks of treatment (see Zineh et al., 2013 and Stergiopoulos et al., 2014 for a discussion of randomised controlled trials of pharmacogenetics and warfarin dosing).

Genes influence pharmacokinetics by altering the expression of proteins involved in drug ADME; pharmacodynamic variation reflects differences in drug targets, G proteins or other downstream pathways; and individual susceptibility to uncommon qualitatively distinct adverse reactions (Ch. 58) can result from genetically determined differences in enzymes or immune mechanisms. It is hoped that as our understanding of the human genome improves, together with the introduction of simpler methods to identify genetic differences between individuals, it will become possible to use genetic information specific to an individual patient to preselect a drug that will be effective and not cause toxicity, rather than relying on trial and error supported by physiological clues as at present – an aspiration referred to as *personalised medicine*. Thus far, this approach, which was initially over-hyped, has yielded relatively little in the way of clinical benefit. Research continues at a breakneck pace however, and the US FDA has approved over 200 pharmacogenomic biomarkers for inclusion in drug labelling information – a doubling since the last edition of this book. The Genetic Testing Registry in the United States accepts submissions from laboratories worldwide regarding the genetic tests that are made available for the purposes of screening, diagnosis, drug/disease monitoring and treatment response. As of April 2017, the registry has recorded information on 49,500 tests covering 16,233 genes that are associated with 10,733 diseases (Khoury, 2017). However, the use of pharmacogenomic tests is not consistently supported by evidence of improved outcomes from clinical trials (Zineh et al., 2013; Phillips, 2017) and indeed the FDA approach to pharmacogenetic labelling has been criticised (Shah & Shah, 2012). Nevertheless, pharmacogenetic testing seems likely ultimately to make an important contribution to therapeutics, though at a cost.

In this chapter we first describe the most important epidemiological sources of variation in drug responsiveness, before revisiting some elementary genetics as a basis for understanding genetic disorders characterised by abnormal responses to drugs. We conclude with a brief account of currently available pharmacogenomic tests and how these are beginning to be applied to individualise drug therapy (*pharmacogenomics*).

Variation is usually quantitative in the sense that the drug produces a larger or smaller effect, or acts for a longer or shorter time, while still exerting qualitatively the same effect. But, importantly, the effect may be qualitatively different in susceptible individuals, often because of genetic or immunological differences. Examples include **primaquine**-induced haemolysis in individuals with glucose 6-phosphate dehydrogenase deficiency whose red blood cells are thereby more susceptible to the effect of oxidative stress (Ch. 55), and immune-mediated haemolytic anaemia caused by **methyldopa** – a drug that commonly causes antidrug antibodies – whereas only a few individuals expressing such antibodies develop haemolysis (Ch. 15).

Individual variation

- Variability is a serious problem; if not taken into account, it can result in:
  - lack of efficacy
  - unexpected harmful effects
- Types of variability may be classified as:
  - pharmacokinetic
  - pharmacodynamic
- The main causes of variability are:
  - age
  - genetic factors
  - immunological factors (Ch. 58)
  - disease (especially when this influences drug elimination or metabolism, e.g. kidney or liver disease)
  - drug interactions

EPIDEMIOLOGICAL FACTORS AND INTER-INDIVIDUAL VARIATION OF DRUG RESPONSE

ETHNICITY

Ethnic means 'pertaining to race', and many anthropologists are sceptical as to the value of this concept (see, for example, Cooper et al., 2003). Members of racial groups share some characteristics on the basis of common genetic and cultural heritage, but there is enormous diversity within each group.

Despite the crudeness of such categorisation, it can give some pointers to drug responsiveness (Wood, 2001). One example is the evidence discussed in Chapter 23 that the life expectancy of African-Americans with heart failure is increased by treatment with a combination of **hydralazine** plus a nitrate, whereas that of white Americans may not be.

Some adverse effects may also be predicted on the basis of race; for example, many Chinese subjects differ from Europeans in the way that they metabolise ethanol (Ch. 49), producing a higher plasma concentration of acetaldehyde, which can cause flushing and palpitations. Chinese subjects are considerably more sensitive to the cardiovascular effects of **propranolol** (Ch. 15) than white Europeans, whereas Afro-Caribbean individuals are less sensitive. Despite their increased sensitivity to β-adrenoceptor antagonists, Chinese subjects metabolise propranolol faster than white people, implying that the difference relates to pharmacodynamic differences at or beyond the β adrenoceptors.

Overall effectiveness of **gefitinib** (Ch. 57) in treating patients with advanced lung tumours has been disappointing, but in about 10% of patients, lung tumours shrink rapidly in response to this drug. Japanese patients are three times as likely as whites to respond in this way. The underlying difference is that patients who respond well have specific mutations in the receptor for epidermal growth factor (see Wadman, 2005). It is probable that many such ethnic differences are genetic in origin, but environmental factors, for example, relating to distinctive dietary habits, may also contribute. It is important not to abandon the much more sophisticated search for ways to individualise medicine on the basis of pharmacogenomics just because the much simpler and cheaper process of asking patients to define their ethnic group has had some success: this should rather act as a spur. If such a crude and imperfect approach has had some success, we ought surely to be able to do better with genomic testing!

AGE

The main reason that age affects drug action is that drug elimination is less efficient in newborn babies and in older people, so that drugs commonly produce greater and more prolonged effects at the extremes of life. Other age-related factors, such as variations in pharmacodynamic sensitivity, are also important with some drugs. Body composition changes with age, fat contributing a greater proportion to body mass in the elderly, with consequent changes in distribution volume of drugs. Elderly people typically consume more drugs than do younger adults, so the potential for drug interactions is also increased. For fuller accounts of drug therapy in paediatrics and in the elderly, see the chapters on renal and hepatic disease in Atkinson et al. (2012).

EFFECT OF AGE ON RENAL EXCRETION OF DRUGS

Glomerular filtration rate (GFR) in the newborn, normalised to body surface area, is only about 20% of the adult value. Accordingly, plasma elimination half-lives of renally eliminated drugs are longer in neonates than in adults (Table 12.1). In babies born at term, renal function increases to values similar to those in young adults in less than a week, and continues to increase to a maximum of approximately twice the adult value at 6 months of age. Improvement in renal function occurs more slowly in premature infants. Renal immaturity in premature infants can have a substantial effect on drug elimination. For example, in premature newborn babies, the antibiotic **gentamicin** (see Ch. 52) has a plasma half-life of ≥18 h, compared with 1–4 h for adults and approximately 10 h for babies born at term. It is therefore necessary to reduce and/or space out doses to avoid toxicity in premature babies.

GFR declines slowly from about 20 years of age, falling by about 25% at 50 years and by 50% at 75 years. Fig. 12.1 shows that the renal clearance of **digoxin** in young and elderly subjects is closely correlated with creatinine clearance, a measure of GFR. Consequently, chronic administration over the years of the same daily dose of digoxin to an individual as he or she ages leads to a progressive increase in plasma concentration, and this is a common cause of glycoside toxicity in elderly people (see Ch. 22).

Table 12.1 Effect of age on plasma elimination half-lives of various drugs

Drug	Mean or range of half-life (h)		
	Term neonate[a]	Adult	Elderly person
Drugs that are mainly excreted unchanged in the urine			
Gentamicin	10	2	4
Lithium	120	24	48
Digoxin	200	40	80
Drugs that are mainly metabolised			
Diazepam	25–100	15–25	50–150
Phenytoin	10–30	10–30	10–30
Sulfamethoxypyridazine	140	60	100

[a]Even greater differences from mean adult values occur in premature babies.

(Data from Reidenberg, M.M., 1971. Renal Function and Drug Action. Saunders, Philadelphia; and Dollery, C.T., 1991. Therapeutic Drugs. Churchill Livingstone, Edinburgh.)

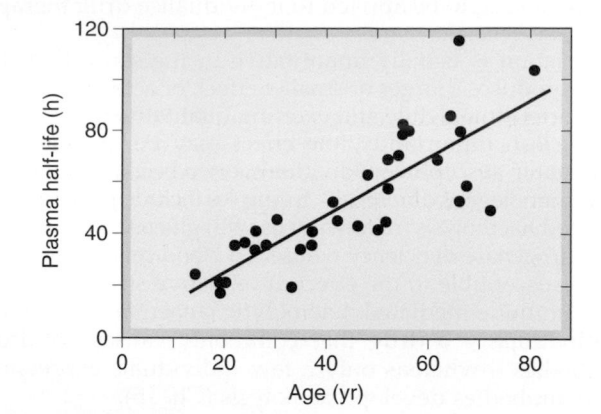

Fig. 12.2 Increasing plasma half-life for diazepam with age in 33 normal subjects. Note the increased variability as well as increased half-life with ageing. (From Klotz, U. et al., 1975. J. Clin. Invest. 55, 347.)

Fig. 12.1 Relationship between renal function (measured as creatinine clearance) and digoxin clearance in young and older subjects. (From Ewy, G.A. et al., 1969. Circulation 34, 452.)

EFFECT OF AGE ON DRUG METABOLISM

Several important enzymes, including hepatic microsomal oxidase, glucuronyltransferase, acetyltransferase and plasma esterases, have low activity in neonates, especially if premature. These enzymes take 8 weeks or longer to reach the adult level of activity. The relative lack of conjugating activity in the newborn can have serious consequences, as in *kernicterus* caused by drug displacement of bilirubin from its binding sites on albumin (Ch. 9) and in the 'grey baby' syndrome caused by the antibiotic **chloramphenicol** (see Ch. 52). This sometimes-fatal condition, at first thought to be a specific biochemical sensitivity to the drug in young babies, actually results simply from accumulation of very high tissue concentrations of chloramphenicol because of slow hepatic conjugation. Chloramphenicol is no more toxic to babies than to adults, provided the dose is reduced to make allowance for this. Slow conjugation is also one reason why **morphine** (which is excreted mainly as the glucuronide, see Ch. 43) is not used as an analgesic in labour, because drug transferred via the placenta has a long half-life in the newborn baby and can cause prolonged respiratory depression.

The activity of hepatic microsomal enzymes declines slowly (and very variably) with age, and the distribution volume of lipid-soluble drugs increases, because the proportion of the body that is fat increases with advancing age. The increasing half-life of the anxiolytic drug **diazepam** with advancing age (Fig. 12.2) is one consequence of this. Some other benzodiazepines and their active metabolites show even greater age-related increases in half-life. Because half-life determines the time course of drug accumulation during repeated dosing (Ch. 11), insidious effects, developing over days or weeks, can occur in elderly people and may be misattributed to age-related memory impairment rather than to drug accumulation. Even if the mean half-life of a drug is little affected, there is often a striking increase in the *variability* of half-life between individuals with increasing age (as in Fig. 12.2). This is important, because a population of older people will contain some individuals with grossly reduced rates of drug metabolism, whereas such extremes do not occur so commonly in young adult populations. Drug regulatory authorities therefore usually

▼ The age-related decline in GFR is not reflected by an increase in plasma creatinine *concentration*, as distinct from creatinine *clearance*. Plasma creatinine typically remains within the normal adult range in elderly persons despite substantially diminished GFR. This is because creatinine synthesis is reduced in elderly persons because of their reduced muscle mass. Consequently, a 'normal' plasma creatinine in an elderly person does not indicate that they have a normal GFR. Failure to recognise this and reduce the dose of drugs that are eliminated by renal excretion can lead to drug toxicity.

require studies in elderly persons as part of the evaluation of drugs likely to be used in older people.

AGE-RELATED VARIATION IN SENSITIVITY TO DRUGS

The same plasma concentration of a drug can cause different effects in young and old subjects. Benzodiazepines (Ch. 45) exemplify this, producing more confusion and less sedation in elderly than in young subjects; similarly, hypotensive drugs (Ch. 23) cause postural hypotension more commonly in elderly than in younger adult patients.

PREGNANCY

Pregnancy causes physiological changes that influence drug disposition in mother and fetus. Maternal plasma albumin concentration is reduced, influencing drug protein binding. Cardiac output is increased, leading to increased renal blood flow and GFR, and increased renal elimination of drugs. Lipophilic molecules rapidly traverse the placental barrier, whereas transfer of hydrophobic drugs is slow, limiting fetal drug exposure following a single maternal dose. The placental barrier excludes some drugs (e.g. low molecular-weight heparins; Ch. 25) so effectively that they can be administered chronically to the mother without causing effects in the fetus. However, drugs that are transferred to the fetus are eliminated more slowly than from the mother. The activity of most drug-metabolising enzymes in fetal liver is much less than in the adult. Furthermore, the fetal kidney is not an efficient route of elimination because excreted drug enters the amniotic fluid, which is swallowed by the fetus. For a fuller account, see Atkinson et al. (2012).

DISEASE

Therapeutic drugs are prescribed to patients, so effects of disease on drug response are very important, especially disease of the major organs responsible for drug metabolism and drug (and drug metabolite) excretion. Detailed consideration is beyond the scope of this book, and interested readers should refer to a clinical text such as the chapters on renal and hepatic disease in Atkinson et al. (2012). Disease can cause pharmacokinetic or pharmacodynamic variation. Common disorders such as impaired renal or hepatic function predispose to toxicity by causing unexpectedly intense or prolonged drug effects as a result of increased drug concentration following a 'standard' dose. Drug absorption is slowed in conditions causing gastric stasis (e.g. migraine, diabetic neuropathy) and may be incomplete in patients with malabsorption owing to ileal or pancreatic disease or to oedema of the ileal mucosa caused by heart failure or nephrotic syndrome. *Nephrotic syndrome* (characterised by heavy proteinuria, oedema and a reduced concentration of albumin in plasma) alters drug absorption because of oedema of intestinal mucosa; alters drug disposition through changes in binding to plasma albumin; and causes insensitivity to diuretics such as **furosemide** that act on ion transport mechanisms in the lumenal surface of tubular epithelium (Ch. 30), through drug binding to albumin in tubular fluid. *Hypothyroidism* is associated with increased sensitivity to several drugs (e.g. **pethidine**), for reasons that are poorly understood. *Hypothermia* (to which elderly persons, in particular, are predisposed) markedly reduces the clearance of many drugs.

Other disorders affect drug sensitivity by altering receptor or signal-transduction mechanisms (see Ch. 3). Examples include the following:

- Diseases that influence receptors:
  - *myasthenia gravis*, an autoimmune disease characterised by antibodies to nicotinic acetylcholine receptors (Ch. 14) and increased sensitivity to neuromuscular-blocking agents (e.g. **vecuronium**) and other drugs that may influence neuromuscular transmission (e.g. *aminoglycoside antibiotics*, Ch. 52);
  - *X-linked nephrogenic diabetes insipidus*, characterised by abnormal antidiuretic hormone (ADH, vasopressin) receptors (Ch. 30) and insensitivity to ADH;
  - *familial hypercholesterolaemia*, an inherited disease of low-density lipoprotein receptors (Ch. 24); the homozygous form is relatively resistant to treatment with statins (which act partly by causing increased hepatic expression of these receptors), whereas the much commoner heterozygous form responds well to statins.
- Diseases that influence signal-transduction mechanisms:
  - *pseudohypoparathyroidism*, which stems from impaired coupling of G protein–coupled receptors with adenylyl cyclase;
  - *familial precocious puberty* and *hyperthyroidism* caused by functioning thyroid adenomas, which are each caused by mutations in G protein–coupled receptors that result in the receptors remaining 'turned on' even in the absence of the hormones that are their natural agonists.

DRUG INTERACTIONS

Many patients, especially elderly ones, are treated continuously with one or more drugs for chronic diseases such as hypertension, heart failure, osteoarthritis and so on. Acute events (e.g. infections, myocardial infarction) are treated with additional drugs. The potential for drug interactions is therefore substantial, and drug interactions account for 5%–20% of adverse drug reactions. These may be serious (approximately 30% of fatal adverse drug reactions are estimated to be the consequence of drug interaction). Drugs can also interact with chemical entities in other dietary constituents (e.g. grapefruit juice, which down-regulates expression of CYP3A4 in the gut) and herbal remedies (such as St John's wort; Ch. 48). The administration of one chemical entity (A) can alter the action of another (B) by one of two general mechanisms[1]:

1. Modifying the pharmacological effect of B without altering its concentration in the tissue fluid (pharmacodynamic interaction).
2. Altering the concentration of B at its site of action (pharmacokinetic interaction), as described in Chapters 9 and 10.

---

[1]A third category of pharmaceutical interactions should be mentioned, in which drugs interact in vitro so that one or both are inactivated. No pharmacological principles are involved, just chemistry. An example is the formation of a complex between **thiopental** and **suxamethonium**, which must not be mixed in the same syringe. **Heparin** is highly charged and interacts in this way with many basic drugs; it is sometimes used to keep intravenous lines or cannulae open and can inactivate basic drugs if they are injected without first clearing the line with saline.

PHARMACODYNAMIC INTERACTION

Pharmacodynamic interaction can occur in many different ways (including those discussed under *Drug antagonism* in Ch. 2). There are many mechanisms, and some examples of practical importance are probably more useful than attempts at classification.

- β-Adrenoceptor antagonists diminish the effectiveness of β-adrenoceptor agonists such as **salbutamol** (Ch. 15).
- Many diuretics lower plasma K⁺ concentration (see Ch. 30), and thereby predispose to **digoxin** toxicity and to toxicity with *class III antidysrhythmic drugs* (Ch. 22).
- **Sildenafil** inhibits the isoform of phosphodiesterase (type V) that inactivates cGMP (Chs 21 and 36); consequently, it potentiates organic nitrates, which activate guanylyl cyclase, and can cause severe hypotension in patients taking these drugs.
- *Monoamine oxidase inhibitors* increase the amount of noradrenaline stored in noradrenergic nerve terminals and interact dangerously with drugs, such as **ephedrine** or **tyramine**, that release stored noradrenaline. This can also occur with tyramine-rich foods – particularly fermented cheeses such as Camembert (see Ch. 48).
- **Warfarin** competes with vitamin K, preventing hepatic synthesis of various coagulation factors (see Ch. 25). If vitamin K production in the intestine is inhibited (e.g. by antibiotics), the anticoagulant action of warfarin is increased.
- The risk of bleeding, especially from the stomach, caused by warfarin is increased by drugs that cause bleeding by different mechanisms (e.g. **aspirin**, which inhibits platelet thromboxane A₂ biosynthesis and which can damage the stomach; Ch. 27).
- *Sulfonamides* prevent the synthesis of folic acid by bacteria and other microorganisms; **trimethoprim** inhibits its reduction to its active tetrahydrofolate form. Given together, the drugs have a synergistic action of value in treating *Pneumocystis* infection (Chs 54 and 55).
- *Non-steroidal anti-inflammatory drugs* (NSAIDs; Ch. 27), such as **ibuprofen** or **indometacin**, inhibit biosynthesis of prostaglandins, including renal vasodilator/natriuretic prostaglandins (prostaglandin E₂, prostaglandin I₂). If administered to patients receiving treatment for hypertension, they increase the blood pressure. If given to patients being treated with diuretics for chronic heart failure, they cause salt and water retention and hence cardiac decompensation.[2]
- Histamine H₁-receptor antagonists, such as **promethazine**, commonly cause drowsiness as an unwanted effect. This is more troublesome if such drugs are taken with alcohol, leading to accidents at work or on the road.

Pharmacokinetic interaction

All the four major processes that determine pharmacokinetics – absorption, distribution, metabolism and excretion (ADME) – can be affected by drugs. Such interactions are covered in Chapters 9 and 10.

> ### Drug interactions
>
> - These are many and varied: if in doubt, look it up.
> - Interactions may be pharmacodynamic or pharmacokinetic.
> - Pharmacodynamic interactions are often predictable from the actions of the interacting drugs.
> - Pharmacokinetic interactions can involve effects on:
>   - absorption (Ch. 9)
>   - distribution (e.g. competition for protein binding, Ch. 9)
>   - hepatic metabolism (induction or inhibition, Ch. 10)
>   - renal excretion (Ch. 10)

GENETIC VARIATION IN DRUG RESPONSIVENESS

A patient's response to a particular drug may be influenced by a rare genetic trait, or a complex multifactorial trait involving effects of several genetic and environmental factors. Complex traits may not adhere to typical Mendelian or familial inheritance because they involve the additive or synergistic influence of multiple gene variants that can interact with environmental factors to result in a wide spectrum of inter-individual drug response. Potential pharmacogenetic markers of variation may include measurable differences in gene expression or functional deficiencies related to genetic factors, i.e. somatic or germline mutations and chromosomal abnormalities.

Mutations are heritable changes in the base sequence of DNA. These may, or may not,[3] result in a change in the amino acid sequence of the protein for which the gene codes. *Germline* or *hereditary* mutations are those that affect the body's reproductive cells (egg or sperm) and can be passed to the next generation where they are present in all cells. In practice, tests for such germline mutations in individuals are usually made on venous blood samples that contain chromosomal and mitochondrial DNA in white blood cells. Germline genetic variations that contribute to differences in drug response and adverse effects in specific populations can be assessed in large cohort or case–control studies that use microarrays or whole genome/exome sequencing strategies to analyse several million genetic variants. The recent emergence of high-throughput genotyping technology has enabled genome wide association studies to identify loci that are potentially linked to drug effect.

Somatic or *acquired* mutations are not present at birth, but can occur in any of the body cells (except the ova and

---

[2]The interaction with diuretics may involve a pharmacokinetic interaction in addition to the pharmacodynamic effect described here, because NSAIDs compete with weak acids, including diuretics, for renal tubular secretion; see Ch. 9.

[3]The genetic code is said to be 'degenerate' because of presence of redundancy, where more than one set of nucleotide base triplets code for each amino acid. A 'silent' mutation with no change in the protein and consequently no change in function can stem from a base change involving a triplet that codes for the same amino acid as the original. Such mutations are neither advantageous nor disadvantageous, so they will neither be eliminated by natural selection nor accumulate in the population at the expense of the wild-type gene.

sperm) during a lifetime, and are not passed on to the offspring. Whilst the vast majority of somatic mutations are thought to have no clinical consequence, those that affect key signalling pathways involved in cell growth, division and differentiation can predispose to carcinogenesis, as well as late-onset mitochondrial and neurogenerative disorders. Somatic cell mutations underlie the pathogenesis of some tumours (Ch. 6), and the presence or absence of such somatic cell mutations guides drug selection. The genomic tests are performed on DNA from samples of the tumour obtained surgically. The tests themselves involve amplification of the relevant sequence(s) and molecular biological methods, often utilising chip technology, to identify the various polymorphisms.

Genetic variation or mutations are not always deleterious and they may confer an advantage under some environmental circumstances. A pharmacogenetically relevant example is the X-linked gene for *glucose 6-phosphate dehydrogenase* (G6PD); deficiency of this enzyme confers partial resistance to malaria (a considerable selective advantage in parts of the world where this disease is common) at the expense of susceptibility to haemolysis in response to oxidative stress in the form of exposure to various dietary constituents, including several drugs (e.g. the antimalarial drug **primaquine**; see Ch. 55). This ambiguity gives rise to the abnormal gene being preserved in future generations, at a frequency that depends on the balance of selective pressures in the environment. Thus the distribution of G6PD deficiency is similar to the geographical distribution of malaria. The situation where functionally distinct forms of a gene are common in a population is called a 'balanced' polymorphism (balanced because a disadvantage, for example in a homozygote, is balanced by an advantage, for example in a heterozygote).

Polymorphisms are relatively common variants (alternative sequences at a locus within the DNA strand) that are found in >1% of individuals within a given population. They arise initially because of a mutation, and are stable if they are non-functional, or die out during subsequent generations if (as is usually the case) they are disadvantageous. However, if the prevailing selective pressures in the environment are favourable, leading to a selective advantage, a polymorphism may increase in frequency over successive generations. Now that genes can be sequenced readily, it has become apparent that *single nucleotide polymorphisms* ([SNPs] – DNA sequence variations that occur when a single nucleotide in the genome sequence is altered) are very common. They may entail substitution of one nucleotide for another (substitution of C for T in two-thirds of SNPs), or deletion or insertion of a nucleotide. Insertions and deletions of one or more nucleotides (other than when the change in number of nucleotides is a multiple of three) result in a 'frame shift' in translation. For example, after an insertion of one nucleotide, the first element of the next triplet in the code becomes the second and all subsequent bases are shifted one 'to the right'. Changes to the coding region of a gene may result in loss of protein synthesis, abnormal protein synthesis or an abnormal rate of protein synthesis.

On average, SNPs occur once in every 300 bases along the 3-billion base human genome, thus resulting in the presence of about 10 million SNPs. They can occur in coding (gene) and non-coding regions of the genome, and they may have a greater role in physiological function if located within a gene or in a regulatory sequence close to the gene. Whilst many SNPs do not have a clear association with

health conditions, some SNPs have a demonstrable relationship with susceptibility to harmful chemicals, magnitude of drug response, and likelihood of developing a disease. For example, SNPs affecting the *F5* gene can cause factor V Leiden blood-clotting disorder, which is the commonest form of inherited thrombophilia (Ch. 25). The abnormality in the factor V clotting factor confers an increased risk of venous thrombosis in response to environmental factors such as prolonged immobility, but might perhaps have been an advantage to ancestors more at risk of haemorrhage than of thrombosis.

SINGLE-GENE PHARMACOKINETIC DISORDERS

The classical Mendelian model contrasts with the complex disease paradigm because it applies to single-gene or monogenic disorders where a mutation in a gene is the primary or sole cause of profound disruption. These are typically rare disorders where the underlying genetic variants have very high penetrance with inheritance patterns that are readily predicted in a Mendelian fashion. This was recognised for albinism (albinos lack an enzyme that is needed to synthesise the brown pigment melanin) and other 'inborn errors of metabolism' in the early part of the 20th century by Archibald Garrod, a British physician who initiated the study of biochemical genetics. Investigation of this large group of individually rare diseases has contributed to our understanding of this particular aspect of molecular pathology – familial hypercholesterolaemia and the mechanism of action of statins (Ch. 24) is one example; further examples of single-gene disorders are given below.

PLASMA CHOLINESTERASE DEFICIENCY

In the 1950s Walter Kalow discovered that **suxamethonium** sensitivity is due to genetic variation in the rate of drug metabolism as a result of a Mendelian autosomal recessive trait. This short-acting neuromuscular-blocking drug is widely used in anaesthesia and is normally rapidly hydrolysed by plasma cholinesterase (Ch. 14). About 1 in 3000 individuals fail to inactivate suxamethonium rapidly and experience prolonged neuromuscular block if treated with it; this is because a recessive gene gives rise to an abnormal type of plasma cholinesterase. The abnormal enzyme has a modified pattern of substrate and inhibitor specificity. It is detected by a blood test that measures the effect of **dibucaine**, which inhibits the abnormal enzyme less than the normal enzyme. Heterozygotes can hydrolyse suxamethonium at a more or less normal rate, but their plasma cholinesterase has reduced sensitivity to dibucaine, intermediate between normal subjects and homozygotes. Only homozygotes express the disease: they appear completely healthy unless exposed to suxamethonium or **mivacurium** (which is also inactivated by plasma cholinesterase) but experience prolonged paralysis if exposed to a dose that would cause neuromuscular block for only a few minutes in a healthy person.[4] There are other reasons why responses

[4]An apparently healthy middle-aged man saw one of the authors over several months because of hypertension; he also saw a psychiatrist because of depression. This failed to improve with other treatment and he underwent electroconvulsive therapy (ECT). Suxamethonium was used to prevent injury caused by convulsions; this usually results in short-lived paralysis but this poor man recovered consciousness some 2 days later to find himself being weaned from artificial ventilation in an intensive care unit. Subsequent analysis showed him to be homozygous for an ineffective form of plasma cholinesterase.

Fig. 12.3 **Distribution of individual plasma concentrations for two drugs in humans.** (A) Plasma salicylate concentration 3 h after oral dosage with sodium salicylate. (B) Plasma isoniazid concentration 6 h after oral dosage. Note the normally distributed values for salicylate, compared with the bimodal distribution of isoniazid. (Panel [A] from Evans, D.A., Clarke, C.A., 1961. Br. Med. Bull. 17, 234–280; panel [B] from Price-Evans, D.A., 1963. Am. J. Med. 3, 639.)

to suxamethonium may be abnormal in an individual patient, notably *malignant hyperpyrexia* (Ch. 14), a genetically determined idiosyncratic adverse drug reaction involving the ryanodine receptor (Ch. 4). It is important to check the family history and test family members who may be affected, but the disorder is so rare that it is currently impractical to screen for it routinely before therapeutic use of suxamethonium.

ACUTE INTERMITTENT PORPHYRIA

The hepatic *porphyrias* are prototypic pharmacogenetic disorders in which patients may be symptomatic even if they are not exposed to a drug, but where many drugs can provoke very severe worsening of the course of the disease. They are inherited disorders involving the biochemical pathway of porphyrin haem biosynthesis. *Acute intermittent porphyria* is the most common acute and severe form. It is inherited as an autosomal dominant trait and is due to one of many different mutations in the gene coding *porphobilinogen deaminase* (PBGD), a key enzyme in haem biosynthesis in red cell precursors, hepatocytes and other cells. All of these mutations reduce the activity of this enzyme, and clinical features are caused by the resulting build-up of haem precursors, including porphyrins. There is a strong interplay with the environment through exposure to drugs, hormones and other chemicals. The use of sedative, anticonvulsant or other drugs in patients with undiagnosed porphyria can be lethal, though with appropriate supportive management most patients recover completely.[5] Many drugs, especially but not exclusively those that induce CYP

enzymes (e.g. barbiturates, **griseofulvin**, **carbamazepine**, oestrogens – see Ch. 10), can precipitate acute attacks in susceptible individuals. Porphyrins are synthesised from δ-amino laevulinic acid (ALA) which is formed by ALA synthase in the liver. This enzyme is induced by drugs such as barbiturates, resulting in increased ALA production and, hence, increased porphyrin accumulation. As mentioned previously, the genetic trait is inherited as an autosomal dominant trait, but frank disease is approximately five times more common in women than in men, because hormonal fluctuations precipitate acute attacks.

DRUG ACETYLATION DEFICIENCY

Both examples considered so far are uncommon diseases. However, in the 1960s Price-Evans demonstrated that the rate of drug acetylation varied in different populations as a result of balanced polymorphism. Fig. 12.3 contrasts the approximately Gaussian distribution of plasma concentrations achieved 3 h after administration of a dose of **salicylate** with the bimodal distribution of plasma concentrations after a dose of **isoniazid**. The isoniazid concentration was <20 μmol/L in about half the population, and in this group the mode was approximately 9 μmol/L. In the other half of the population (plasma concentration >20 μmol/L), the mode was approximately 30 μmol/L. Elimination of isoniazid depends mainly on acetylation, catalysed by an acetyltransferase enzyme, and some studies have reported that slow acetylators are at higher risk of isoniazid-associated hepatotoxicity. However, ongoing research has suggested that adverse effects can arise through several different mechanisms, and that no single pathway or genetic variant is fully responsible for liver toxicity with isoniazid.

Acetyltransferase is also important in the metabolism of other drugs, including **hydralazine** (Ch. 22), **procainamide** (Ch. 22), **dapsone** and various other sulfonamides (Ch. 52) and acetylator status influences drug-induced *lupus* (an autoimmune disorder affecting many organs including skin,

[5]Life expectancy, obtained from parish records, of patients with porphyria diagnosed retrospectively within large kindreds in Scandinavia was normal until the advent and widespread use of barbiturates and other sedative and anticonvulsant drugs in the 20th century, when it plummeted. There is a long and useful list of drugs to avoid in the *British National Formulary*, together with the warning that drugs not on the list may not necessarily be safe in such patients!

joints and kidneys) caused by several of these agents. However, neither phenotyping (by measuring kinetics of drug transformation) nor genotyping for acetyltransferase has found a way into routine clinical practice, probably because these drugs are relatively little used and there are several alternative treatments available that are usually preferred.

AMINOGLYCOSIDE OTOTOXICITY

In the examples above, variations in chromosomal genes cause variations in drug response. Increased susceptibility to hearing loss caused by aminoglycoside antibiotics (see Ch. 52) is, in some families, inherited quite differently, namely exclusively through the mother to all her children. This is the pattern expected of a mitochondrial gene, and indeed the most common predisposing mutation is a single nucleotide (A to G) substitution at position 1555 of the mitochondrial genome which is referred to as *m.1555A>G*. This mutation accounts for 30%–60% of aminoglycoside ototoxicity in China, where aminoglycoside use is common. Aminoglycosides work by binding to bacterial ribosomes (Ch. 52), which share properties with human mitochondrial ribosomes (mitochondria are believed to have evolved from symbiotic bacteria); aminoglycosides cause ototoxicity in all individuals exposed to too high a dose. The *m.1555A>G* mutation makes mitochondrial ribosomes even more similar to their bacterial counterpart, increasing the affinity of the drug which remains bound to ribosomes in the hair cells in the ear for several months following a single dose in susceptible individuals. Although the clinical utility has yet to be proven, some experts have suggested that screening for this variant may be appropriate in children who are likely to require treatment with aminoglycosides (Linden Phillips, 2013).

THERAPEUTIC DRUGS AND CLINICALLY AVAILABLE PHARMACOGENOMIC TESTS

Clinical tests to predict drug responsiveness were anticipated to be one of the first applications of sequencing the human genome. Although a profusion of new pharmacogenetic tests are now marketed to healthcare professionals as well as direct to consumer, the adoption and implementation in routine clinical practice has been slowed by various scientific, commercial, political and educational barriers. Reimbursement for expensive tests and drugs, whether provided by the state or by insurance schemes, depends increasingly on evidence of cost-effectiveness. Here, new pharmacogenetic tests are required to have a positive or meaningful influence on prescribing practice, such as the use of an alternative drug or a different dosing regimen that leads to measurable improvements in patient outcomes (Khoury & Galea, 2016; Manrai et al., 2016). So far the evidence in support of any pharmacogenetic test is less convincing and falls short of the ideal of a randomised controlled trial of a pharmacogenomics-informed prescribing strategy versus current best practice.

Moreover, evaluation of drug response in complex multifactorial traits is a major challenge because multiple genes and genetic variants interact with environmental factors, and the genetic component may only have a modest influence on treatment effect. Much of the earlier research has been focused on striking single pathogenic variants that have readily apparent or clear-cut 'all or none' treatment

effect. In reality, however, the probability of drug benefit and harm is often a continuum with a wide range of variation across individuals in a population (Manrai et al., 2016), and reliance on a single predictive biomarker may not be sufficiently precise or reliable to guide treatment of serious disease.

The key steps in evaluating pharmacogenetic markers in clinical care should be confirmation of analytic validity (accuracy and reliability of the test) and determination of a robust, replicable relationship between the marker and drug response in the population (clinical validity). Clinical utility must then be demonstrated through improved efficacy or safety in patients receiving the biomarker-guided therapeutic regimens. There are also health economic considerations as to whether the genetic markers are of sufficiently high frequency in their patient population to justify the costs of screening. Policy makers and funding agencies will then have to look at feasibility of using the biomarker testing strategy in a way that does not delay patient treatment. Here, the historical approach of single-gene as needed, or 'one at a time' testing can seem slow, inefficient and costly when compared with the recent availability of pre-emptive testing for multiple genetic markers. The growing availability of rapid testing using multi-gene panels means that the individual's genetic data from a single sample can be used to inform many different treatment decisions that subsequently arise in their lifetime.

At present, pharmacogenetic evaluation can include tests for (a) variants of different HLAs that have been strongly linked to susceptibilities to several severe harmful drug reactions that are likely to have arisen from an immunological interaction between the drug molecule and the major histocompatibility molecules in the patient (Chan et al., 2015); (b) genes controlling aspects of drug metabolism; and (c) genes encoding drug targets, where the concept of 'companion diagnostics' (defined by the FDA as: 'a diagnostic test used as a companion to a therapeutic drug to determine its applicability to a specific person') involves detection of a pharmacogenetic marker so that rational drug selection can be made based on the pathway related to the underlying mutation. For one drug (**warfarin**), a test combines genetic information about metabolism with information about its target.

HLA GENE TESTS
ABACAVIR AND *HLAB*5701*

▼ **Abacavir** (Ch. 53) is a reverse transcriptase inhibitor that is highly effective in treating HIV infection. Its use has been limited by severe rashes. Susceptibility to this adverse effect is closely linked to the HLA variant *HLAB*5701*, and testing for this variant is now considered a standard of care supported by prospective randomised trials (Fig. 12.4; Martin, 2013).

ANTICONVULSANTS AND *HLAB*1502*

▼ **Carbamazepine** (Ch. 46) can also cause severe (life-threatening) rashes including *Stevens–Johnson syndrome* and *toxic epidermal necrolysis* (multiform rashes with painful blistering lesions and skin detachment sometimes extending into the gastrointestinal tract) and now considered to be a disease continuum distinguished chiefly by severity, based upon the percentage of body surface involved with skin detachment. These are associated with a particular HLA allele, *HLAB*1502*, which occurs more commonly in ethnic groups in Thailand, Malaysia and Taiwan (Barbarino, 2015), but with far lower frequencies in Korean, Japanese and Caucasian populations. Screening for this allele before starting treatment is potentially worthwhile in ethnic populations where the allele frequency is high. People who develop such a reaction

159

Pharmacogenetics and pharmacogenomics

- Several inherited disorders influence responses to drugs, including:
  - *glucose 6-phosphatase deficiency*, a sex-linked disorder in which affected men (or rare homozygous women) experience haemolysis if exposed to various chemicals including the antimalarial drug **primaquine**;
  - *plasma cholinesterase deficiency*, an autosomal recessive disorder that confers sensitivity to the neuromuscular blocker suxamethonium;
  - *acute intermittent porphyria*, an autosomal dominant disease more severe in women and in which severe attacks are precipitated by drugs or endogenous sex hormones that induce CYP enzymes;
  - *drug acetylator deficiency*, a balanced polymorphism;
  - *increased susceptibility to ototoxicity from aminoglycosides*, which is conferred by a mutation in mitochondrial DNA.
- These pharmacogenetic disorders prove that drug responses can be genetically determined in individuals.
- Single nucleotide polymorphisms (SNPs) and combinations of SNPs (haplotypes) in genes coding for proteins involved in drug disposition or drug action are common and may predict drug response. Pharmacogenomic tests in blood or tissue removed surgically have established associations between several such variants and individual drug response, and several such tests are available for clinical use although their status in individualising drug treatment is still being established.
- Such tests are available for:
  - several human leukocyte antigen (HLA) variants that predict toxicity of **abacavir**, **carbamazepine** and **clozapine**;
  - genes for several enzymes in drug metabolism including CYP2D6 and CYP2C9, and thiopurine-*S*-methyltransferase (TPMT);
  - germline and somatic mutations in growth factor receptors that predict responsiveness to cancer treatments including **imatinib** and **trastuzumab**.

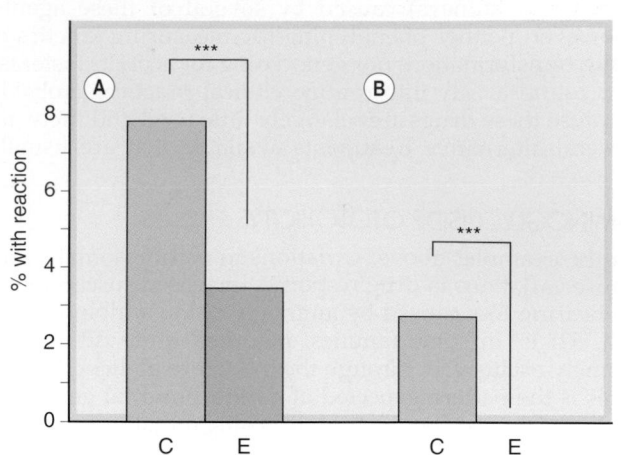

Fig. 12.4 Incidence of abacavir hypersensitivity is reduced by pharmacogenetic screening. In the PREDICT-1 study (Mallal et al., 2008), patients were randomised to standard care (*C*, control group) or prospective pharmacogenetic screening (*E*, experimental group). All the control subjects were treated with abacavir, but only those experimental subjects who were *HLA-B*5701* negative were treated with abacavir. There were two prespecified end points: clinically suspected hypersensitivity reactions (A) and clinically suspected reactions that were immunologically confirmed by a positive patch test (B). Both end points favoured the experimental group ($p < 0.0001$). (Figure redrawn from Hughes, A.R. et al., 2008. Pharmacogenet. J. 8, 365–374.)

to carbamazepine may develop a similar problem if treated with **phenytoin**, and the same allele has been associated with hypersensitivity reactions to this drug too.

DRUG METABOLISM-RELATED GENE TESTS
THIOPURINES AND TPMT

▼ Thiopurine drugs (**tioguanine**, **mercaptopurine** and its prodrug **azathioprine**; Ch. 57) have been used for the past 50 years to treat leukaemias, including acute lymphoblastic leukaemia (ALL, which accounts for approximately one-fifth of all childhood malignancies), and more recently to cause immunosuppression, for example, in treating inflammatory bowel disease. All of these drugs cause bone marrow and liver toxicity, and are detoxified by thiopurine-*S*-methyltransferase (TPMT), which is present in blood cells, as well as by xanthine oxidase. There are large inherited variations in TPMT activity with a trimodal frequency distribution (Weinshilboum &

Sladek, 1980); low TPMT activity in blood is associated with high concentrations of active 6-thioguanine nucleotides (TGN) in blood and with bone marrow toxicity, whereas high TPMT activity is associated with lower concentrations of TGN and reduced efficacy. Before starting treatment, phenotyping (by a blood test for TPMT activity) or genotyping of *TMPT* alleles *TPMT*3A*, *TPMT*3C*, *TPMT*2* is recommended. Even with such testing, careful monitoring of the white blood cell count is needed because of environmental susceptibility factors (e.g. drug interaction with **allopurinol** via inhibition of xanthine oxidase).

5-FLUOROURACIL (5-FU) AND DPYD

▼ **5-FU** (see Ch. 57, Fig. 57.6) and related compounds such as capecitabine and tegafur are used extensively to treat solid tumours, but have variable efficacy and unpredictable mucocutaneous toxicity. It is detoxified by dihydropyrimidine dehydrogenase (DPYD), which has multiple clinically identifiable functional genetic variants. Deficiency of DPYD occurs in 4%–5% of the population and is associated with serious toxicity from 5-FU. Currently available genetic information is not completely sensitive nor specific, and recent proposals have focused on dosage adjustments that are guided by gene activity scores that take several polymorphisms into account.

TAMOXIFEN, OPIOID ANALGESICS AND CYP2D6

▼ **Tamoxifen** (Chs 36 and 57) is metabolised to an oestrogen antagonist endoxifen by CYP2D6, an enzyme that is subject to marked polymorphic variation; several small association studies have suggested a link between *CYP2D6* genotype and efficacy. Genotyping tests for *CYP2D6* are available, but results from larger comparative trials of tamoxifen have yielded less consistent findings.

Opioid analgesics such as codeine and tramadol are metabolised by CYP2D6 into active opioid compounds that have analgesic properties, but also carry serious adverse effects such as sedation and respiratory depression. Slow metabolisers may only obtain limited pain relief from codeine or tramadol, whereas rapid metabolisers may suffer excess toxicity.

DRUG TARGET-RELATED GENE TESTS ('COMPANION DIAGNOSTICS')

TRASTUZUMAB AND HER2

▼ **Trastuzumab** ('Herceptin'; Ch. 57) is a monoclonal antibody that antagonises epidermal growth factor (EGF) by binding to one of its receptors (human EGF receptor 2 – HER2) which can occur in tumour tissue as a result of somatic mutation. It is used in patients with breast cancer whose tumour tissue overexpresses this receptor. Other patients do not benefit from it.

DASATINIB, IMATINIB AND BCR-ABL1

▼ **Dasatinib** and imatinib are first-line tyrosine kinase inhibitors used in haematological malignancies characterised by the presence of a Philadelphia chromosome, namely chronic myeloid leukaemia (CML) and in some adults with ALL. The Philadelphia chromosome results from a translocation defect when parts of two chromosomes (9 and 22) swap places; part of a 'breakpoint cluster region' (BCR) in chromosome 22 links to the 'Abelson-1' (ABL) region of chromosome 9. A mutation (T315I) in BCR/ABL confers resistance to the inhibitory effect of dasatinib and patients with this variant do not benefit from this drug. Ponatinib is licensed in the United States for treatment of patients who have this BCR-ABL T315I mutation.

COMBINED (METABOLISM AND TARGET) GENE TESTS

WARFARIN AND CYP2C9 + VKORC1 GENOTYPING

▼ **Warfarin** is a *par excellence* example of a drug with a narrow benefit:harm balance where dosing must be individualised. This is done by measuring the *international normalised ratio* (INR), a measure of its effect on blood coagulability (Ch. 25), but thrombotic events despite treatment (lack of efficacy) and serious adverse effects (usually bleeding) remain all too common. Warfarin is the most widely used drug for which pharmacogenetic testing has been proposed, based on a study showing that polymorphisms in its key target, vitamin K epoxide reductase (VKOR; see Fig. 25.5) and in CYP2C9, involved in its metabolism, are associated with outcomes. Fig. 12.5 shows the effects of VKOR haplotype and of CYP2C9 genotype on the mean dose of warfarin needed to achieve therapeutic INR. Dosing algorithms have been proposed based on the results of testing for polymorphisms of these genes. A randomised trial favoured this strategy for initiating treatment versus a standard loading dose approach, but genetic testing did not improve on an individualised algorithm for dose initiation based on other clinical variables (Zineh et al., 2013).

CONCLUSIONS

Twin studies as well as several well-documented single-gene disorders (including Mendelian chromosomal – autosomal recessive, autosomal dominant and X-linked – and

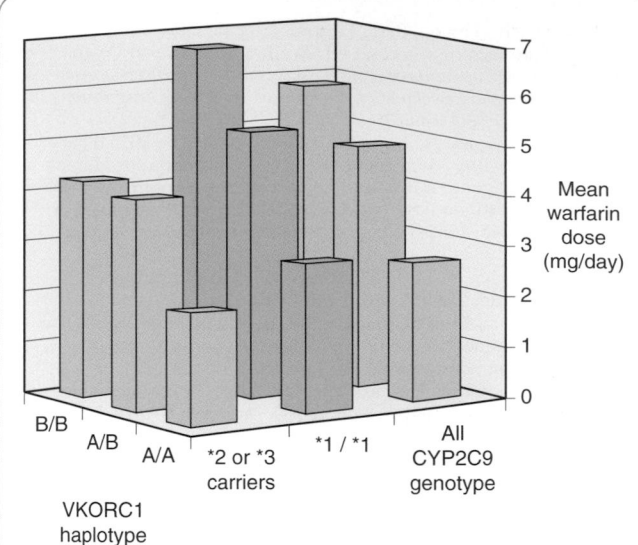

Fig. 12.5 Effect of *VKOR* haplotype and *CYP2C9* genotype on warfarin dose. A series of 186 patients on long-term warfarin treatment who had already been studied for *CYP2C9* were studied retrospectively for genetic variants of *VKOR* (Rieder et al., 2005). *VKOR* haplotype as well as *CYP2C9* genotype influenced the mean warfarin dose (which had been adjusted to achieve therapeutic INR). *A*, Haplotypes 1 and 2; *B*, haplotypes 7, 8 and 9. *A/A*, *A/B* and *B/B* represent haplotype combinations. **1/*1* represents CYP2C9 wild-type homozygotes; **2* and **3* represent CYP2C9 variants. (Figure redrawn from Beitelshees, A.L., McLeod, H.L., 2006. Applying pharmacogenomics to enhance the use of biomarkers for drug effect and drug safety. TIPS 27, 498–502.)

maternally inherited mitochondrial disorders) prove the concept that susceptibility to adverse drug effects can be genetically determined. Pharmacogenomic testing offers the possibility of more precise 'personalised' therapeutics for several drugs and disorders, but high-quality trial evidence of clinical utility in a large population is lacking, particularly in instances where drug response is influenced by complex multifactorial traits. This is a field of intense research activity, rapid progress and high expectations, but proving that these tests add to present best practice and improve outcomes remains a challenge.

REFERENCES AND FURTHER READING

Further reading

Doogue, M.P., Polasek, T.M., 2011. Drug dosing in renal disease. Clin. Biochem. Rev. 32, 69–73. (*Principles and practice of dose adjustment in patients with renal failure*)

Chan, S.L., Jin, S., Loh, M., Brunham, L.R., 2015. Progress in understanding the genomic basis for adverse drug reactions: a comprehensive review and focus on the role of ethnicity. Pharmacogenomics 16, 1161–1178. (*Describes how genetic testing has progressed in assessing susceptibility for adverse drug reactions*)

Khoury, M.J., 2017. No shortcuts on the long road to evidence-based genomic medicine. JAMA 318 (1), 27–28.

Pavlos, R., Mallal, S., Phillips, E., 2012. HLA and pharmacogenetics of drug hypersensitivity. Pharmacogenomics 13, 1285–1306.

Phillips, E.J., Mallal, S.A., 2011. HLA-B*1502 screening and toxic effects of carbamazepine. N. Engl. J. Med. 365, 672.

Phillips, K.A., Deverka, P.A., Sox, H.C., et al., 2017. Making genomic medicine evidence-based and patient-centered: a structured review and landscape analysis of comparative effectiveness research. Genet. Med. 19 (10), 1081–1091. (*Comprehensive review that reports lack of evidence of clinical utility and patient benefit*)

Relling, M.V., Evans, W.E., 2015. Pharmacogenomics in the clinic. Nature 526, 343–350. (*Excellent review article about pharmacogenetic tests that are clinically important, and the barriers to widespread adoption*)

Weng, L.M., Zhang, L., Peng, Y., Huang, R.S., 2013. Pharmacogenetics and pharmacogenomics: a bridge to individualized cancer therapy. Pharmacogenomics 14, 315–324.

References

Atkinson, A.J., Jr., Huang, S.M., Lertora, J., et al., 2012. Principles of Clinical Pharmacology, second ed. Academic Press, San Diego. (*Includes detailed accounts of clinical aspects including effects of renal and liver disease on pharmacokinetics, of effects of age and on drug therapy in pregnant and nursing women*)

Barbarino, J.M., Kroetz, D.L., Klein, T.E., Altman, R.B., 2015. PharmGKB summary: very important pharmacogene information for Human Leukocyte Antigen B (HLA-B). Pharmacogenet. Genomics 25, 205–221.

Cooper, R.S., Kaufman, J.S., Ward, R., 2003. Race and genomics. N. Engl. J. Med. 348, 1166–1170. (*Scholarly and appropriately sceptical analysis*)

Khoury, M.J., Galea, S., 2016. Will precision medicine improve population health? JAMA 316, 1357–1358.

Linden Phillips, L., Bitner-Glindzicz, M., Lench, N., et al., 2013. The future role of genetic screening to detect newborns at risk of childhood-onset hearing loss. Int. J. Audiol. 52, 124–133.

Manrai, A.K., Ioannidis, J.A., Kohane, I.S., 2016. Clinical genomics: from pathogenicity claims to quantitative risk estimates. JAMA 315, 1233–1234. (*Argues that clinically useful impact on patient care has yet to be consistently demonstrated with pharmacogenetic testing*)

Mallal, S., Phillips, E., Carosi, G., et al., 2008. HLA-B*5701 screening for hypersensitivity to abacavir. N. Engl. J. Med. 358, 568–579.

Martin, M.A., Kroetz, D.L., 2013. Abacavir pharmacogenetics – from initial reports to standard of care. Pharmacotherapy 33, 765–775.

Rieder, M.J., Reiner, A.P., Gage, B.F., et al., 2005. Effect of VKORC1 haplotype on transcriptional regulation and warfarin dose. N. Engl. J. Med. 352, 2285–2293.

Shah, R.R., Shah, D.R., 2012. Personalized medicine: is it a pharmacogenetic mirage? Br. J. Clin. Pharmacol. 74, SI 698–SI 721.

Stergiopoulos, K., Brown, D.L., 2014. Genotype-guided vs clinical dosing of warfarin and its analogues: meta-analysis of randomized clinical trials. JAMA Intern. Med. 174, 1330–1338. (*Meta-analysis of randomised controlled trials of genotype guided warfarin regimens*)

Teml, A., Schaeffeler, E., Schwab, M., 2009. Pretreatment determination of TPMT – state of the art in clinical practice. Eur. J. Clin. Pharmacol. 65, 219–221, and related articles. (*Introduces an issue devoted to the impact of TPMT polymorphisms on thiopurine use in clinical practice*)

Wadman, M., 2005. Drug targeting: is race enough? Nature 435, 1008–1009. (*No!*)

Weinshilboum, R.M., Sladek, S.L., 1980. Mercaptopurine pharmacogenetics: monogenic inheritance of erythrocyte thiopurine methyltransferase activity. Am. J. Hum. Genet. 32, 651–662.

Wood, A.J.J., 2001. Racial differences in response to drugs – pointers to genetic differences. N. Engl. J. Med. 344, 1393–1396.

Zineh, I., Pacanowski, M., Woodcock, J., 2013. Pharmacogenetics and coumarins dosing – recalibrating expectations. N. Engl. J. Med. 369, 2273–2275.

Chemical mediators and the autonomic nervous system

13

OVERVIEW

The network of chemical signals and associated receptors by which cells in the body communicate with one another provides many targets for drug action, and has always been a focus of attention for pharmacologists. Chemical transmission in the peripheral autonomic nervous system, and the various ways in which the process can be pharmacologically subverted, is the main focus of this chapter, but the mechanisms described operate also in the central nervous system (CNS). In addition to neurotransmission, we also consider briefly the less clearly defined processes, collectively termed neuromodulation, by which many mediators and drugs exert control over the function of the nervous system. The relative anatomical and physiological simplicity of the peripheral nervous system has made it the proving ground for many important discoveries about chemical transmission, and the same general principles apply to the CNS (see Ch. 38). For more detail than is given here, see Robertson et al. (2012) and Iversen et al. (2009).

HISTORICAL ASPECTS

▼ Studies initiated on the peripheral nervous system have been central to the understanding and classification of many major types of drug action, so it is worth recounting a little history. Excellent accounts are given by Bacq (1975), Valenstein (2005) and Burnstock (2009).

Experimental physiology became established as an approach to the understanding of the function of living organisms in the middle of the 19th century. The peripheral nervous system, and particularly the autonomic nervous system, received a great deal of attention. The fact that electrical stimulation of nerves could elicit a whole variety of physiological effects – from blanching of the skin to arrest of the heart – presented a real challenge to comprehension, particularly of the way in which the signal was passed from the nerve to the effector tissue. In 1877, Du Bois-Reymond was the first to put the alternatives clearly: 'Of known natural processes that might pass on excitation, only two are, in my opinion, worth talking about – either there exists at the boundary of the contractile substance a stimulatory secretion … or the phenomenon is electrical in nature.' The latter view was generally favoured. In 1869, it had been shown that an exogenous substance, **muscarine**, could mimic the effects of stimulating the vagus nerve, and that **atropine** could inhibit the actions both of muscarine and of nerve stimulation. In 1905, Langley showed the same for **nicotine** and **curare** acting at the neuromuscular junction. Most physiologists interpreted these phenomena as stimulation and inhibition of the nerve endings, respectively, rather than as evidence for chemical transmission. Hence the suggestion of T.R. Elliott, in 1904, that **adrenaline (epinephrine)** might act as a chemical transmitter mediating the actions of the sympathetic nervous system was coolly received, until Langley, the Professor of Physiology at Cambridge and a powerful figure at that time, suggested, a year later, that transmission

to skeletal muscle involved the secretion by the nerve terminals of a substance related to nicotine.

One of the key observations for Elliott was that degeneration of sympathetic nerve terminals did not abolish the sensitivity of smooth muscle preparations to adrenaline (which the electrical theory predicted) but actually enhanced it. The hypothesis of chemical transmission was put to direct test in 1907 by Dixon, who tried to show that vagus nerve stimulation released from a dog's heart into the blood a substance capable of inhibiting another heart. The experiment failed, and the atmosphere of scepticism prevailed.

It was not until 1921, in Germany, that Loewi showed that stimulation of the vagosympathetic trunk connected to an isolated and cannulated frog's heart could cause the release into the cannula of a substance ('*Vagusstoff*') that, if the cannula fluid was transferred from the first heart to a second, would inhibit the second heart. This is a classic and much-quoted experiment that proved extremely difficult for even Loewi to perform reproducibly. In an autobiographical sketch, Loewi tells us that the idea of chemical transmission arose in a discussion that he had in 1903, but no way of testing it experimentally occurred to him until he dreamt of the appropriate experiment one night in 1920. He wrote some notes of this very important dream in the middle of the night, but in the morning could not read them. The dream obligingly returned the next night and, taking no chances, he went to the laboratory at 3 a.m. and carried out the experiment successfully. Loewi's experiment may be, and was, criticised on numerous grounds (it could, for example, have been potassium rather than a neurotransmitter that was acting on the recipient heart), but a series of further experiments proved him to be right. His findings can be summarised as follows:

- Stimulation of the vagus caused the appearance in the perfusate of the frog heart of a substance capable of producing, in a second heart, an inhibitory effect resembling vagus stimulation.
- Stimulation of the sympathetic nervous system caused the appearance of a substance capable of accelerating a second heart. By fluorescence measurements, Loewi concluded later that this substance was adrenaline.
- Atropine prevented the inhibitory action of the vagus on the heart but did not prevent release of Vagusstoff. Atropine thus prevented the effects, rather than the release, of the transmitter.
- When Vagusstoff was incubated with ground-up heart muscle, it became inactivated. This effect is now known to be due to enzymatic destruction of acetylcholine by cholinesterase.
- **Physostigmine**, which potentiated the effect of vagus stimulation on the heart, prevented destruction of Vagusstoff by heart muscle, providing evidence that the potentiation is due to inhibition of cholinesterase, which normally destroys the transmitter substance acetylcholine.

A few years later, in the early 1930s, Dale showed convincingly that acetylcholine was also the transmitter substance at the neuromuscular junction of striated muscle and at autonomic ganglia. One of the keys to Dale's success lay in the use of highly sensitive bioassays, especially the leech dorsal muscle, for measuring acetylcholine release. Chemical transmission at sympathetic nerve terminals was demonstrated at about the same time as cholinergic transmission and by very similar methods. Cannon and his colleagues at Harvard first showed unequivocally the phenomenon of chemical transmission at

163

sympathetic nerve endings, by experiments in vivo in which tissues made supersensitive to adrenaline by prior sympathetic denervation were shown to respond, after a delay, to the transmitter released by stimulation of the sympathetic nerves to other parts of the body. The chemical identity of the transmitter, tantalisingly like adrenaline but not identical to it, caused confusion for many years, until, in 1946, von Euler showed it to be the non-methylated derivative **noradrenaline** (**norepinephrine**).

THE AUTONOMIC NERVOUS SYSTEM

The autonomic nervous system for a long time occupied centre stage in the pharmacology of chemical transmission.

BASIC ANATOMY AND PHYSIOLOGY

The autonomic nervous system (see Robertson et al., 2012) consists of three main anatomical divisions: *sympathetic*, *parasympathetic* and *enteric* nervous systems. The sympathetic and parasympathetic systems (Fig. 13.1) provide a link between the CNS and peripheral organs. The enteric nervous system comprises the intrinsic nerve plexuses of the gastrointestinal tract, which are closely interconnected with the sympathetic and parasympathetic systems.

The autonomic nervous system conveys all the outputs from the CNS to the rest of the body, except for the motor innervation of skeletal muscle. The enteric nervous

system has sufficient integrative capabilities to allow it to function independently of the CNS, but the sympathetic and parasympathetic systems are agents of the CNS and cannot function without it. The autonomic nervous system is largely outside the influence of voluntary control. The main processes that it regulates, to a greater or lesser extent, are:

- contraction and relaxation of vascular and visceral smooth muscle
- all exocrine and certain endocrine secretions
- the heartbeat
- energy metabolism, particularly in liver and skeletal muscle

A degree of autonomic control also affects many other systems, including the kidney, immune system and somatosensory system. The autonomic efferent pathway consists of two neurons arranged in series, whereas in the somatic motor system a single motor neuron connects the CNS to the skeletal muscle fibre (Fig. 13.2). The two neurons in the autonomic pathway are known, respectively, as *preganglionic* and *postganglionic*. In the sympathetic nervous system, the intervening synapses lie in *autonomic* ganglia, which are outside the CNS, and contain the nerve endings of preganglionic fibres and the cell bodies of postganglionic neurons. In parasympathetic pathways, the postganglionic cells are mainly found in the target organs, discrete parasympathetic

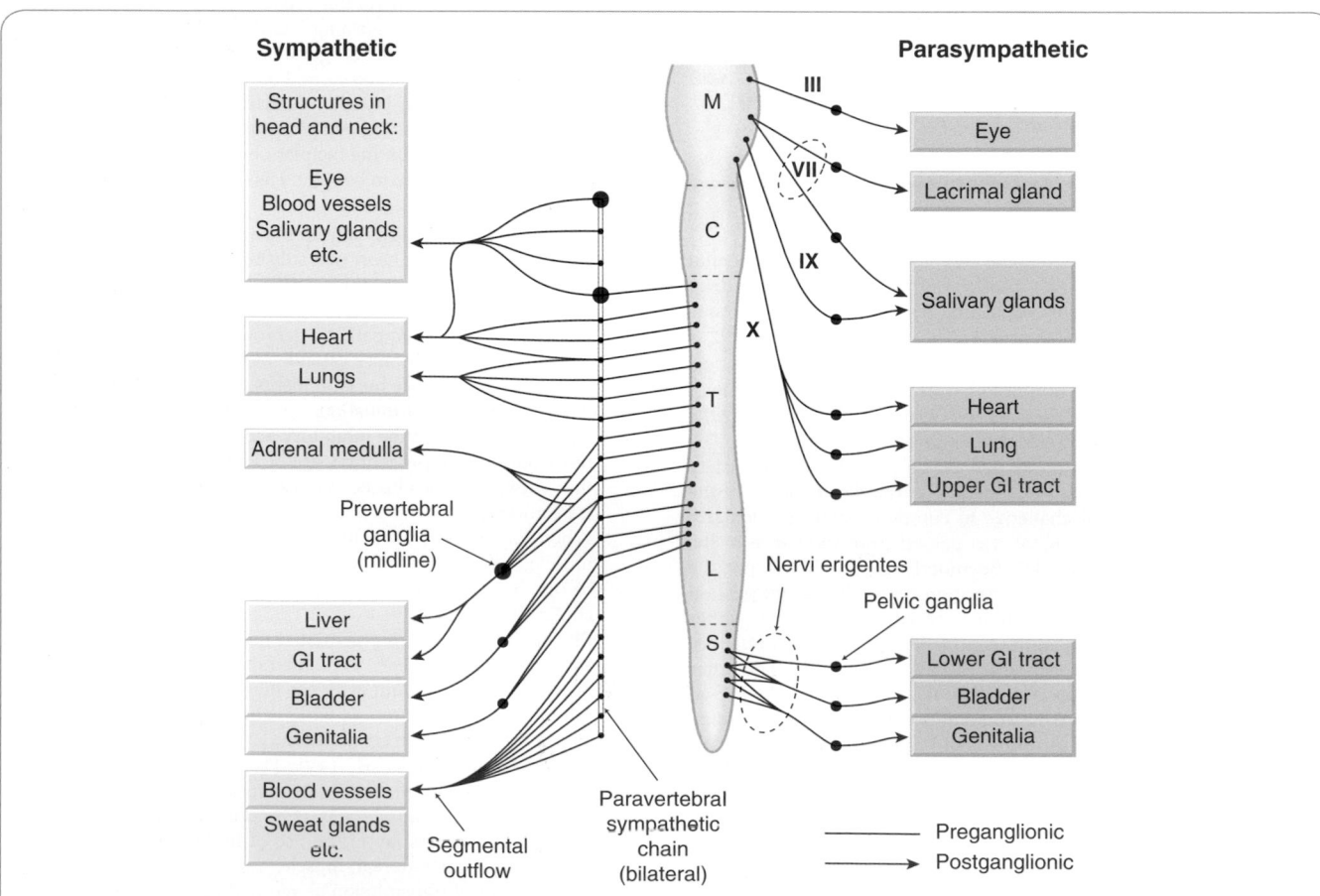

Fig. 13.1 Basic plan of the mammalian autonomic nervous system. *C*, cervical; *GI*, gastrointestinal; *L*, lumbar; *M*, medullary; *S*, sacral; *T*, thoracic.

Fig. 13.2 **Acetylcholine and noradrenaline as transmitters in the peripheral nervous system.** The two main types of acetylcholine (ACh) receptor, nicotinic (nic) and muscarinic (mus) (see Ch. 14) and two types of adrenoceptor, α and β (Ch. 15), are indicated. NA, noradrenaline (norepinephrine).

ganglia (e.g. the ciliary ganglion) being found only in the head and neck.

The cell bodies of the sympathetic preganglionic neurons lie in the *lateral horn* of the grey matter of the thoracic and lumbar segments of the spinal cord, and the fibres leave the spinal cord in the spinal nerves as the *thoracolumbar sympathetic outflow*. The preganglionic fibres synapse in the *paravertebral chains* of sympathetic ganglia, lying on either side of the spinal column. These ganglia contain the cell bodies of the postganglionic sympathetic neurons, the axons of which rejoin the spinal nerve. Many of the postganglionic sympathetic fibres reach their peripheral destinations via the branches of the spinal nerves. Others, destined for abdominal and pelvic viscera, have their cell bodies in a group of unpaired *prevertebral ganglia* in the abdominal cavity. The only exception to the two-neuron arrangement is the innervation of the adrenal medulla. The catecholamine-secreting cells of the adrenal medulla are, in effect, modified postganglionic sympathetic neurons, and the nerves supplying the gland are equivalent to preganglionic fibres.

The parasympathetic nerves emerge from two separate regions of the CNS. The *cranial outflow* consists of preganglionic fibres in certain cranial nerves, namely the *oculomotor nerve* (carrying parasympathetic fibres destined for the eye), the *facial* and *glossopharyngeal nerves* (carrying fibres to the salivary glands and the nasopharynx), and the *vagus nerve* (carrying fibres to the thoracic and abdominal viscera). The ganglia lie scattered in close relation to the target organs; the postganglionic axons are very short compared with those of the sympathetic system. Parasympathetic fibres destined for the pelvic and abdominal viscera emerge as the *sacral outflow* from the spinal cord in a bundle of nerves known as the *nervi erigentes* (because stimulation of these nerves evokes genital erection – a fact of some importance to those responsible for artificial insemination of livestock). These fibres synapse in a group of scattered *pelvic ganglia*, whence the short postganglionic fibres run to target tissues

such as the bladder, rectum and genitalia. The pelvic ganglia carry both sympathetic and parasympathetic fibres, and the two divisions are not anatomically distinct in this region.

The enteric nervous system (reviewed by Furness et al., 2014) consists of the neurons whose cell bodies lie in the intramural plexuses in the wall of the intestine. It is estimated that there are more cells in this system than in the spinal cord, and functionally they do not fit simply into the sympathetic/parasympathetic classification. Incoming nerves from both the sympathetic and the parasympathetic systems terminate on enteric neurons, as well as running directly to smooth muscle, glands and blood vessels. Some enteric neurons function as mechanoreceptors or chemoreceptors, providing local reflex pathways that can control gastrointestinal function without external inputs. The enteric nervous system is pharmacologically more complex than the sympathetic or parasympathetic systems, involving many neuropeptide and other transmitters (such as 5-hydroxytryptamine, nitric oxide and ATP; see Ch. 31).

In some places (e.g. in the visceral smooth muscle of the gut and bladder, and in the heart), the sympathetic and the parasympathetic systems produce opposite effects, but there are others where only one division of the autonomic system operates. The *sweat glands* and most *blood vessels*, for example, have only a sympathetic innervation, whereas the *ciliary muscle* of the eye has only a parasympathetic innervation. *Bronchial smooth muscle* has only a parasympathetic (constrictor) innervation (although its tone is highly sensitive to circulating adrenaline). *Resistance arteries* (see Ch. 23) have a sympathetic vasoconstrictor innervation but no parasympathetic innervation; instead, the constrictor tone is opposed by a background release of nitric oxide from the endothelial cells (see Ch. 21). There are other examples, such as the *salivary glands*, where the two systems produce similar, rather than opposing, effects.

It is therefore a mistake to think of the sympathetic and parasympathetic systems simply as physiological opponents. Each serves its own physiological function and can be more or less active in a particular organ or tissue according to the need of the moment. Cannon rightly emphasised the general role of the sympathetic system in evoking 'fight or flight' reactions in an emergency, but emergencies are rare for most animals. In everyday life, the autonomic nervous system functions continuously to control specific local functions, such as adjustments to postural changes, exercise or ambient temperature. The popular concept of a continuum from the extreme 'rest and digest' state (parasympathetic active, sympathetic quiescent) to the extreme emergency fight or flight state (sympathetic active, parasympathetic quiescent) is an oversimplification, albeit one that provides the student with a generally reliable *aide memoire*.

Table 13.1 lists some of the more important autonomic responses in humans.

TRANSMITTERS IN THE AUTONOMIC NERVOUS SYSTEM

The two main neurotransmitters that operate in the autonomic system are **acetylcholine** and **noradrenaline**, whose sites of action are shown diagrammatically in Fig. 13.2. This diagram also shows the type of postsynaptic receptor with which the transmitters interact at the different sites (discussed more fully in Chs 14 and 15). Some general rules apply:

Table 13.1 **The main effects of the autonomic nervous system**

Organ	Sympathetic effect	Adrenoceptor type[a]	Parasympathetic effect	Cholinoceptor type[a]
Heart				
Sinoatrial node	Rate ↑	β_1	Rate ↓	M_2
Atrial muscle	Force ↑	β_1	Force ↓	M_2
Atrioventricular node	Automaticity ↑	β_1	Conduction velocity ↓	M_2
			Atrioventricular block	M_2
Ventricular muscle	Automaticity ↑ Force ↑	β_1	No effect	M_2
Blood vessels				
ARTERIOLES				
Large coronary	Constriction	α_1, α_2	No effect	—
Small coronary	Dilatation	β_2	No effect	—
Muscle	Dilatation	β_2	No effect	—
Viscera, skin, brain	Constriction	α_1	No effect	—
Erectile tissue	Constriction	α_1	Dilatation	M_3[b]
VEINS	Constriction	α_1, α_2	No effect	—
	Dilatation	β_2	No effect	—
Viscera				
BRONCHI				
Smooth muscle	No sympathetic innervation, but dilated by circulating adrenaline (epinephrine)	β_2	Constriction	M_3
Glands	No effect	—	Secretion	M_3
GASTROINTESTINAL TRACT				
Smooth muscle	Motility ↓	$\alpha_1, \alpha_2, \beta_2$	Motility ↑	M_3
Sphincters	Constriction	$\alpha_1, \alpha_2, \beta_2$	Dilatation	M_3
Glands	No effect	—	Secretion	M_3
		—	Gastric acid secretion	M_1
BLADDER	Relaxation	β_2	Contraction	M_3
	Sphincter contraction	α_1	Sphincter relaxation	M_3
UTERUS				
Pregnant	Contraction	α_1	Variable	—
Non-pregnant	Relaxation	β_2		
MALE SEX ORGANS	Ejaculation	α_1	Erection	M_3[b]
Eye				
Pupil	Dilatation	α_1	Constriction	M_3
Ciliary muscle	Relaxation (slight)	β_2	Contraction	M_3
Skin				
Sweat glands	Secretion (mainly cholinergic via M_3 receptors)	—	No effect	—
Pilomotor	Piloerection	α_1	No effect	—
Salivary glands	Secretion	$\alpha_1, \beta_1, \beta_2$	Secretion	M_3
Lacrimal glands	No effect	—	Secretion	M_3
Kidney	Renin secretion	β_1	No effect	—
Liver	Glycogenolysis Gluconeogenesis	α_1, β_2	No effect	—
Adipose tissue[c]	Lipolysis Thermogenesis	β_3	No effect	—
Pancreatic islets[c]	Insulin secretion ↓	α_2	No effect	—

[a]The adrenoceptor and cholinoceptor types shown are described more fully in Chapters 14 and 15. Transmitters other than acetylcholine and noradrenaline contribute to many of these responses (see Table 13.2).
[b]Vasodilator effects of M_3 receptors are due to nitric oxide release from endothelial cells (see Ch. 21).
[c]No direct innervation. Effect mediated by circulating adrenaline released from the adrenal medulla.

Basic anatomy and physiology of the autonomic nervous system

Anatomy
- The autonomic nervous system comprises three divisions: *sympathetic*, *parasympathetic* and *enteric*.
- The basic (two-neuron) pattern of the sympathetic and parasympathetic systems consists of a *preganglionic* neuron with a cell body in the central nervous system (CNS) and a *postganglionic* neuron with a cell body in an autonomic ganglion.
- The parasympathetic system is connected to the CNS via:
  - cranial nerve outflow (III, VII, IX, X)
  - sacral outflow.
- Parasympathetic ganglia usually lie close to or within the target organ.
- Sympathetic outflow leaves the CNS in thoracic and lumbar spinal roots. Sympathetic ganglia form two paravertebral chains, plus some midline ganglia.
- The enteric nervous system consists of neurons lying in the intramural plexuses of the gastrointestinal tract. It receives inputs from sympathetic and parasympathetic systems, but can act on its own to control the motor and secretory functions of the intestine.

Physiology
- The autonomic system controls smooth muscle (visceral and vascular), exocrine (and some endocrine) secretions, rate and force of contraction of the heart, and certain metabolic processes (e.g. glucose utilisation).
- Sympathetic and parasympathetic systems have opposing actions in some situations (e.g. control of heart rate, gastrointestinal smooth muscle), but not in others (e.g. salivary glands, ciliary muscle).
- Sympathetic activity increases in stress ('fight or flight' response), whereas parasympathetic activity predominates during satiation and repose. Both systems exert a continuous physiological control of specific organs under normal conditions, when the body is at neither extreme.

- All autonomic nerve fibres leaving the CNS release acetylcholine, which acts on *nicotinic receptors* (although in autonomic ganglia a minor component of excitation is due to activation of *muscarinic receptors*; see Ch. 14).
- All postganglionic parasympathetic fibres release acetylcholine, which acts on *muscarinic receptors*.
- All postganglionic sympathetic fibres (with one important exception) release noradrenaline, which may act on either α or β adrenoceptors (see Ch. 15). The exception is the sympathetic innervation of sweat glands, where transmission is due to acetylcholine acting on muscarinic receptors. In some species, but not humans, vasodilatation in skeletal muscle is produced by cholinergic sympathetic nerve fibres.

Acetylcholine and noradrenaline are the grandees among autonomic transmitters, and are central to understanding autonomic pharmacology. However, many other chemical mediators are also released by autonomic neurons (see pp. 170–173), and their functional significance is gradually becoming clearer.

SOME GENERAL PRINCIPLES OF CHEMICAL TRANSMISSION

The essential processes in chemical transmission – the release of mediators, and their interaction with receptors on target cells – are described in Chapters 4 and 3, respectively. Here we consider some general characteristics of chemical transmission of particular relevance to pharmacology. Many of these principles apply also to the CNS and are taken up again in Chapter 38.

PRESYNAPTIC MODULATION

The presynaptic terminals that synthesise and release transmitter in response to electrical activity in the nerve fibre

Transmitters of the autonomic nervous system

- The principal transmitters are **acetylcholine** (ACh) and **noradrenaline**.
- Preganglionic neurons are cholinergic, and ganglionic transmission occurs via nicotinic ACh receptors (although excitatory muscarinic ACh receptors are also present on postganglionic cells).
- Postganglionic parasympathetic neurons are cholinergic, acting on muscarinic receptors in target organs.
- Postganglionic sympathetic neurons are mainly noradrenergic, although a few are cholinergic (e.g. sweat glands).
- Transmitters other than noradrenaline and acetylcholine (NANC transmitters) are also abundant in the autonomic nervous system. The main ones are nitric oxide and vasoactive intestinal peptide (parasympathetic), ATP and neuropeptide Y (sympathetic). Others, such as 5-hydroxytryptamine, GABA and dopamine, also play a role.
- Co-transmission is a general phenomenon.

are often themselves sensitive to transmitter substances and to other substances that may be produced locally in tissues (for review see Boehm & Kubista, 2002). Such presynaptic effects most commonly act to inhibit transmitter release, but may enhance it. Fig. 13.3A shows the inhibitory effect of adrenaline on the release of acetylcholine (evoked by electrical stimulation) from the postganglionic parasympathetic nerve terminals of the intestine. The release of noradrenaline from nearby sympathetic nerve terminals can also inhibit release of acetylcholine. Noradrenergic and cholinergic nerve

Fig. 13.3 **Examples of presynaptic inhibition.** (A) Inhibitory effect of adrenaline on acetylcholine (ACh) release from postganglionic parasympathetic nerves in the guinea pig ileum. The intramural nerves were stimulated electrically where indicated, and the ACh released into the bathing fluid determined by bioassay. Adrenaline strongly inhibits ACh release. (B) Noradrenaline release from mouse hippocampal slices in response to trains of electrical stimuli. *Blue bars* show normal (wild-type) mice. *Red bars* show α_2-adrenoceptor knockout mice. The lack of presynaptic autoinhibition in the knockout mice results in a large increase in release with a long stimulus train, but does not affect release by fewer than four stimuli, because the autoinhibition takes a few seconds to develop. This example is taken from a study of brain noradrenergic nerves, but similar findings have been made on sympathetic nerves. (Panel [A] from Vizi, E.S., 1979. Prog. Neurobiol. 12, 181; panel [B] redrawn from Trendelenburg, et al., 2001. Naunyn Schmiedeberg's Arch Pharmacol 364, 117–130.)

terminals often lie close together in the myenteric plexus, so the opposing effects of the sympathetic and parasympathetic systems result not only from the opposite effects of the two transmitters on the smooth muscle cells, but also from the inhibition of acetylcholine release by noradrenaline acting on the parasympathetic nerve terminals. A similar situation of mutual presynaptic inhibition exists in the heart, where noradrenaline inhibits acetylcholine release and acetylcholine also inhibits noradrenaline release. These are examples of *heterotropic interactions*, where one neurotransmitter affects the release of another. *Homotropic interactions* also occur, where the transmitter, by binding to presynaptic autoreceptors, affects the nerve terminals from which it is being released. This type of *autoinhibitory feedback* acts powerfully at noradrenergic nerve terminals (see Starke et al., 1989). Fig. 13.3B shows that in normal mice, noradrenaline release increases only slightly as the number of stimuli increases from 1 to 64. In transgenic mice lacking a specific type of presynaptic α_2 adrenoceptor (see Ch. 15), the amount released by the longer stimulus train is greatly increased, though the amount released by a single stimulus is unaffected. This is because with one or a few stimuli, there is no opportunity for autoinhibitory feedback to develop, whereas with longer trains the inhibition operates powerfully. A similar autoinhibitory feedback occurs with many transmitters, including acetylcholine and 5-hydroxytryptamine.

In both the noradrenergic and cholinergic systems, the presynaptic autoreceptors are pharmacologically distinct from the postsynaptic receptors (see Fig. 13.4 and Chs 14 and 15), and there are drugs that act selectively, as agonists or antagonists, on the pre- or postsynaptic receptors.

Cholinergic and noradrenergic nerve terminals respond not only to acetylcholine and noradrenaline, as described above, but also to other substances that are released as co-transmitters, such as ATP and neuropeptide Y (NPY), or derived from other sources, including nitric oxide, prostaglandins, adenosine, dopamine, 5-hydroxytryptamine, γ-aminobutyric acid (GABA), opioid peptides, endocannabinoids and many other substances. The description of the autonomic nervous system represented in Fig. 13.2 is undoubtedly oversimplified. Fig. 13.4 shows some of the main presynaptic interactions between autonomic neurons, and summarises the many chemical influences that regulate transmitter release from noradrenergic neurons.

Presynaptic receptors regulate transmitter release mainly by affecting Ca^{2+} entry into the nerve terminal (see Ch. 4), but also by other mechanisms (see Kubista & Boehm, 2006). Most presynaptic receptors are of the G protein–coupled type (see Ch. 3), which control the function of calcium channels and potassium channels either through a direct interaction of G proteins with the channels or by second messengers that regulate the state of phosphorylation of the channel proteins. Transmitter release is inhibited when calcium channel opening is inhibited, or when potassium channel opening is increased (see Ch. 4); in many cases, both mechanisms operate simultaneously. Presynaptic regulation by receptors linked directly to ion channels (ionotropic receptors; see Ch. 3) rather than to G proteins also occurs (see Dorostkar & Boehm, 2008). Nicotinic acetylcholine receptors (nAChRs) are particularly important in this respect. They can either facilitate or inhibit the release of other transmitters, such as glutamate (see Ch. 39), and most of the nAChRs expressed in the CNS are located presynaptically. Another example is the $GABA_A$ receptor,

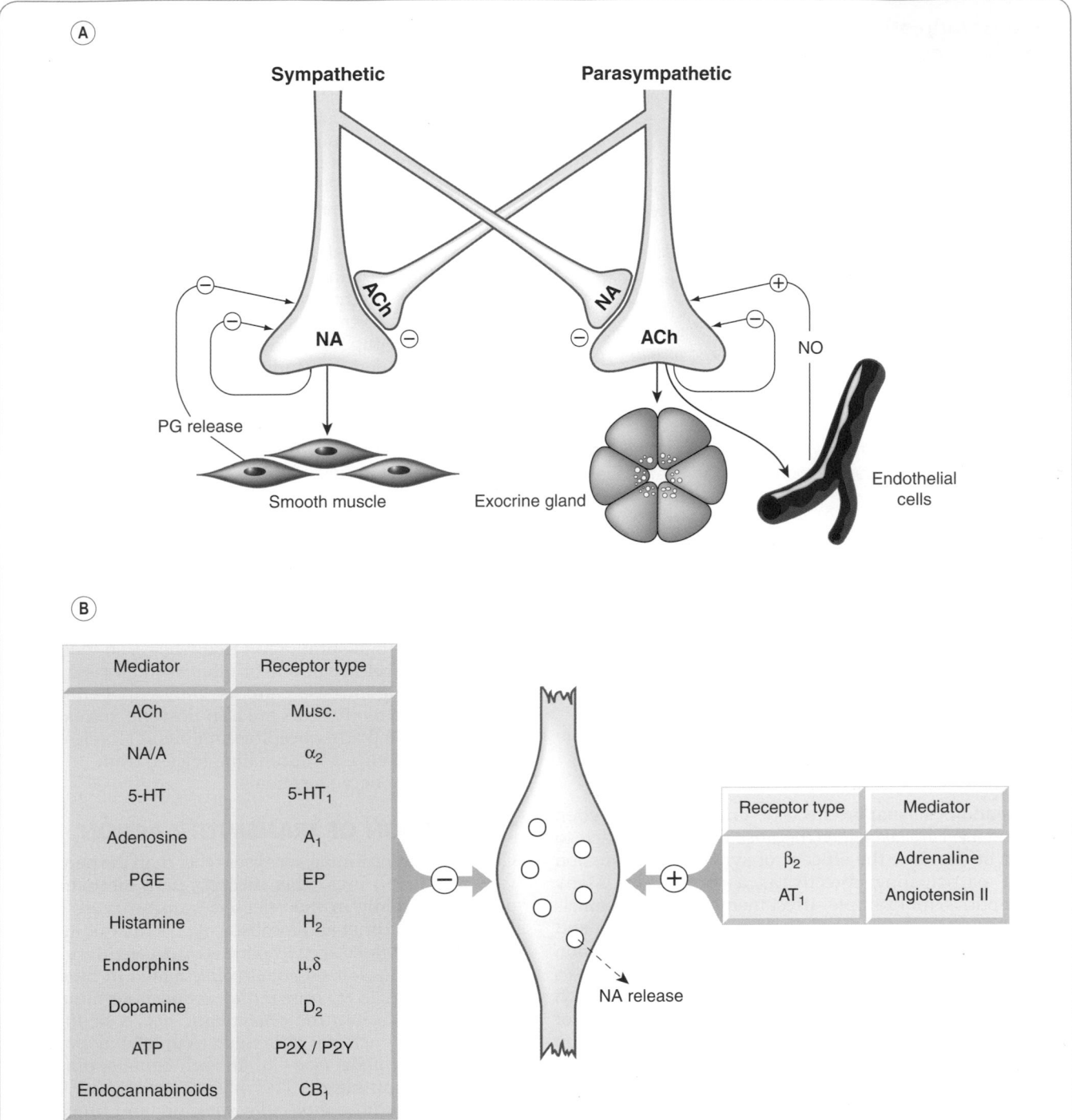

Fig. 13.4 **Presynaptic regulation of transmitter release from noradrenergic and cholinergic nerve terminals.** (A) Postulated homotropic and heterotropic interactions between sympathetic and parasympathetic nerves. (B) Some of the known inhibitory and facilitatory influences on noradrenaline release from sympathetic nerve endings. *5-HT*, 5-hydroxytryptamine; *ACh*, acetylcholine; *NA*, noradrenaline; *NO*, nitric oxide; *PG*, prostaglandin; *PGE*, prostaglandin E.

whose action is to inhibit transmitter release (see Chs 4 and 38). Other ionotropic receptors, such as those activated by ATP and 5-hydroxytryptamine (Chs 16, 17 and 40), have similar effects on transmitter release.

POSTSYNAPTIC MODULATION

Chemical mediators often act on postsynaptic structures, including neurons, smooth muscle cells, cardiac muscle cells, and so on, in such a way that their excitability or spontaneous firing pattern is altered. In many cases, as with presynaptic modulation, this is caused by changes in calcium and/or potassium channel function. We give only a few examples here.

- The slow excitatory effect produced by various mediators, including acetylcholine and peptides such

Neuromodulation and presynaptic interactions

- As well as functioning directly as neurotransmitters, chemical mediators may regulate:
  - presynaptic transmitter release
  - neuronal excitability.
- Both are examples of *neuromodulation* and generally involve second messenger regulation of membrane ion channels.
- Presynaptic receptors may inhibit or increase transmitter release, the former being more important.
- Inhibitory *presynaptic autoreceptors* occur on noradrenergic and cholinergic neurons, causing each transmitter to inhibit its own release (*autoinhibitory feedback*).
- Many endogenous mediators (e.g. GABA, prostaglandins, opioid and other peptides), as well as the transmitters themselves, exert presynaptic control (mainly inhibitory) over autonomic transmitter release.

as **substance P** (see Ch. 19), results mainly from a decrease in K^+ permeability. Conversely, the inhibitory effect of various opioid peptides in the gut is mainly due to increased K^+ permeability.

- **Neuropeptide Y** (**NPY**), which is released as a co-transmitter with noradrenaline at many sympathetic nerve endings and acts on smooth muscle cells to enhance the vasoconstrictor effect of noradrenaline, thus greatly facilitating transmission.

The pre- and postsynaptic effects described above are often described as *neuromodulation*, because the mediator acts to increase or decrease the efficacy of synaptic transmission without participating directly as a transmitter. Many neuropeptides, for example, affect membrane ion channels in such a way as to increase or decrease excitability and thus control the firing pattern of the cell. Neuromodulation is loosely defined but, in general, involves slower processes (taking seconds to days) than neurotransmission (which occurs in milliseconds), and operates through cascades of intracellular messengers (see Ch. 3) rather than directly on ligand-gated ion channels.

TRANSMITTERS OTHER THAN ACETYLCHOLINE AND NORADRENALINE

As mentioned above, acetylcholine or noradrenaline are not the only autonomic transmitters. The rather grudging realisation that this was so dawned many years ago when it was noticed that autonomic transmission in many organs could not be completely blocked by drugs that abolish responses to these transmitters. The dismal but tenacious term *non-adrenergic non-cholinergic* (NANC) transmission was coined. Later, fluorescence and immunocytochemical methods showed that neurons, including autonomic neurons, contain many potential transmitters, often several in the same cell. Compounds now known to function as NANC transmitters include ATP, vasoactive intestinal peptide (VIP), NPY and nitric oxide (Fig. 13.5 and Table 13.2), which function at postganglionic nerve terminals, as

well as substance P, 5-hydroxytryptamine, GABA and dopamine, which play a role in ganglionic transmission (see Lundberg, 1996, for a comprehensive review).

CO-TRANSMISSION

It is the rule rather than the exception that neurons release more than one transmitter or modulator (see Lundberg, 1996), each of which interacts with specific receptors and produces effects, often both pre- and postsynaptically. The example of noradrenaline/ATP co-transmission at sympathetic nerve endings is shown in Fig. 13.5, and the best-studied examples and mechanisms are summarised in Table 13.2 and Figs 13.6 and 13.7.

What, one might well ask, could be the functional advantage of co-transmission, compared with a single transmitter acting on various different receptors? The possible advantages include the following:

- One constituent of the cocktail (e.g. a peptide) may be removed or inactivated more slowly than the other (e.g. a monoamine), and therefore reach targets further from the site of release and produce longer-lasting effects. This appears to be the case, for example, with acetylcholine and gonadotrophin-releasing hormone in sympathetic ganglia.
- The balance of the transmitters released may vary under different conditions. At sympathetic nerve terminals, for example, where noradrenaline and NPY are stored in separate vesicles, NPY is preferentially released at high stimulation frequencies, so that differential release of one or other mediator may result from varying impulse patterns. Differential effects of presynaptic modulators are also possible; for example, activation of β adrenoceptors inhibits ATP release while enhancing noradrenaline release from sympathetic nerve terminals.

TERMINATION OF TRANSMITTER ACTION

Chemically transmitting synapses other than the peptidergic variety (Ch. 19) invariably incorporate a mechanism for disposing rapidly of the released transmitter, so that its action remains brief and localised. At cholinergic synapses (Ch. 14), the released acetylcholine is inactivated very rapidly in the synaptic cleft by *acetylcholinesterase*. In most other cases (see Fig. 13.8), transmitter action is terminated by active reuptake into the presynaptic nerve, or into supporting cells such as glia. Such reuptake depends on transporter proteins (see Ch. 4), each being specific for a particular transmitter. The major class (Na^+/Cl^- co-transporters) whose molecular structure and function are well understood (see Torres et al., 2003; Gether et al., 2006), consists of a family of membrane proteins, each possessing 12 transmembrane helices. Different members of the family show selectivity for each of the main monoamine transmitters (e.g. the noradrenaline [norepinephrine] transporter; NET, the serotonin transporter; SERT, which transports 5-hydroxytryptamine; and the dopamine transporter, DAT) (see Manepalli et al., 2012). These transporters are important targets for psychoactive drugs, particularly antidepressants (Ch. 48), anxiolytic drugs (Ch. 45) and stimulants (Ch. 49). Transporters for glycine and GABA belong to the same family.

Vesicular transporters (Ch. 4), which load synaptic vesicles with transmitter molecules, are closely related to plasma membrane transporters. Membrane transporters

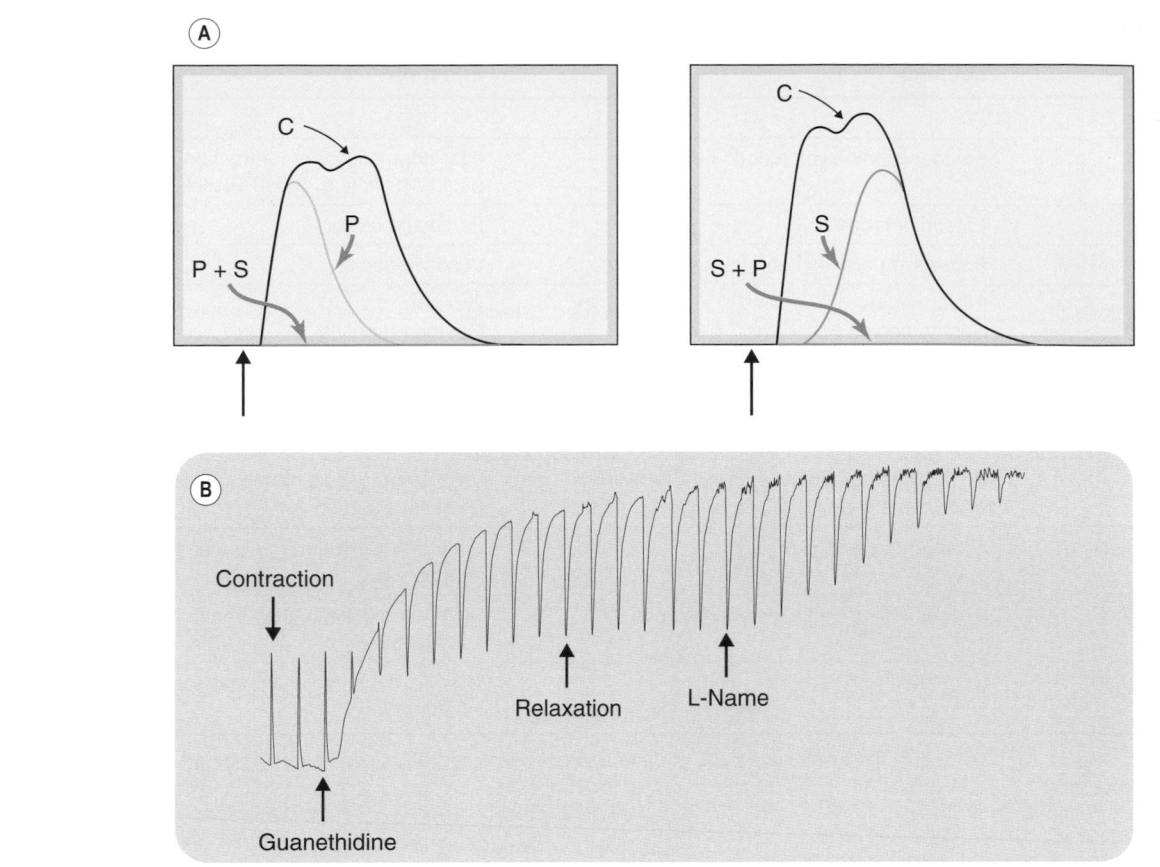

Fig. 13.5 **ATP and nitric oxide as neurotransmitters.** (A) Noradrenaline and ATP are co-transmitters released from the same nerves in the guinea pig vas deferens. Contractions of the tissue are shown in response to a single electrical stimulus causing excitation of sympathetic nerve endings. With no blocking drugs present, a twin-peaked response is produced *(C)*. The early peak is selectively abolished by the ATP antagonist suramin *(S)*, while the late peak is blocked by the α_1-adrenoceptor antagonist prazosin *(P)*. The response is completely eliminated when both drugs are present. (B) Noradrenaline and nitric oxide are neurotransmitters in the rat anococcygeus muscle but are probably released from different nerves. The nerves innervating the muscle were stimulated with brief trains of pulses. Initially, nerve stimulation evoked rapid contractions by releasing noradrenaline. Application of guanethidine blocked stimulus-evoked noradrenaline release and raised the tone of the preparation revealing nerve-evoked relaxations that were blocked by L-NAME, an inhibitor of nitric oxide synthesis. (Panel [A] reproduced with permission from von Kugelglen, I., Starke, K., 1991. Trends Pharmacol. Sci. 12, 319–324; data in panel [B] are from a student practical class at Glasgow Caledonian University, courtesy A. Corbett.)

usually act as co-transporters of Na^+, Cl^- and transmitter molecules, and it is the inwardly directed 'downhill' gradient for Na^+ that provides the energy for the inward 'uphill' movement of the transmitter. The simultaneous transport of ions along with the transmitter means that the process generates a net current across the membrane, which can be measured directly and used to monitor the transport process. Very similar mechanisms are responsible for other physiological transport processes, such as glucose uptake (Ch. 32) and renal tubular transport of amino acids. Because it is the electrochemical gradient for sodium that drives the inward transport of transmitter molecules, a reduction of this gradient can reduce or even reverse the flow of transmitter. This is probably not important under physiological conditions, but when the nerve terminals are depolarised or abnormally loaded with sodium (e.g. in ischaemic conditions), the resulting non-vesicular release of transmitter (and inhibition of the normal synaptic reuptake mechanism) may play a significant role in the effects of ischaemia on tissues such as heart and brain (see Chs 22

and 41). Studies with transgenic 'knockout' mice (see Torres et al., 2003) show that the store of releasable transmitter is substantially depleted in animals lacking the membrane transporter, showing that synthesis is unable to maintain the store if the recapture mechanism is disabled. As with receptors (see Ch. 3), many genetic polymorphisms of transporter genes occur in humans, finding associations with various neurological, cardiovascular and psychiatric disorders has provided insight into their aetiology and may explain altered responsiveness to drugs (see Reynolds et al., 2014).

As we shall see in subsequent chapters, both plasma membrane and vesicular transporters are targets for various drugs, and defining the physiological role and pharmacological properties of these molecules has been the focus of much research.

DENERVATION SUPERSENSITIVITY

It is known, mainly from the work of Cannon on the sympathetic system, that if a nerve is cut and its terminals

Table 13.2 **Examples of non-adrenergic non-cholinergic transmitters and co-transmitters in the peripheral nervous system**

Transmitter	Location	Function
Non-peptides		
ATP	Postganglionic sympathetic neurons	Fast depolarisation/contraction of smooth muscle cells (e.g. blood vessels, vas deferens)
GABA, 5-HT	Enteric neurons	Peristaltic reflex
Dopamine	Some sympathetic neurons (e.g. kidney)	Vasodilatation
Nitric oxide	Pelvic nerves Gastric nerves	Erection Gastric emptying
Peptides		
Neuropeptide Y	Postganglionic sympathetic neurons	Facilitates constrictor action of noradrenaline; inhibits noradrenaline release (e.g. blood vessels)
VIP	Parasympathetic nerves to salivary glands NANC innervation of airways smooth muscle	Vasodilatation; co-transmitter with acetylcholine Bronchodilatation
Gonadotrophin-releasing hormone	Sympathetic ganglia	Slow depolarisation; co-transmitter with acetylcholine
Substance P	Sympathetic ganglia, enteric neurons	Slow depolarisation; co-transmitter with acetylcholine
Calcitonin gene-related peptide	Non-myelinated sensory neurons	Vasodilatation; vascular leakage; neurogenic inflammation

5-HT, 5-hydroxytryptamine; *ATP*, adenosine triphosphate; *GABA*, gamma-aminobutyric acid; *NANC*, non-adrenergic non-cholinergic; *VIP*, vasoactive intestinal peptide.

Fig. 13.6 **The main co-transmitters at postganglionic parasympathetic and sympathetic neurons.** The different mediators generally give rise to fast, intermediate and slow responses of the target organ. *ACh*, acetylcholine; *ATP*, adenosine triphosphate; *NA*, noradrenaline; *NO*, nitric oxide; *NPY*, neuropeptide Y; *VIP*, vasoactive intestinal peptide.

is evidence that pathways in the CNS show the same phenomenon.

▼ Several mechanisms contribute to denervation supersensitivity, and the extent and mechanism of the phenomenon varies from organ to organ. Reported mechanisms include the following (see Luis & Noel, 2009).

- *Proliferation of receptors.* This is particularly marked in skeletal muscle, in which the number of acetylcholine receptors increases 20-fold or more after denervation; the receptors, normally localised to the endplate region of the fibres (Ch. 14), spread over the whole surface. Elsewhere, increases in receptor number are much smaller, or absent altogether.
- *Loss of mechanisms for transmitter removal.* At noradrenergic synapses, the loss of neuronal uptake of noradrenaline (see Ch. 15) contributes substantially to denervation supersensitivity. At cholinergic synapses, a partial loss of cholinesterase occurs (see Ch. 14).
- *Increased postjunctional responsiveness.* Smooth muscle cells become partly depolarised and hyperexcitable after denervation (due in part to reduced Na^+-K^+-ATPase activity; see Ch. 4) and this phenomenon contributes appreciably to their supersensitivity. Increased Ca^{2+} signalling, resulting in enhanced excitation–contraction coupling, may also occur.

allowed to degenerate, the structure supplied by it becomes supersensitive to the transmitter substance released by the terminals. Thus skeletal muscle, which normally responds to injected acetylcholine only if a large dose is given directly into the arterial blood supply, will, after denervation, respond by contracture to much smaller amounts. Other organs, such as salivary glands and blood vessels, show similar supersensitivity to acetylcholine and noradrenaline when the postganglionic nerves degenerate, and there

Supersensitivity can occur, but is less marked, when transmission is interrupted by processes other than nerve section. Pharmacological block of ganglionic transmission, for example, if sustained for a few days, causes some degree of supersensitivity of the target organs, and long-term blockade of postsynaptic receptors also causes receptors to proliferate, leaving the cell supersensitive when the blocking agent is removed. Phenomena such as this

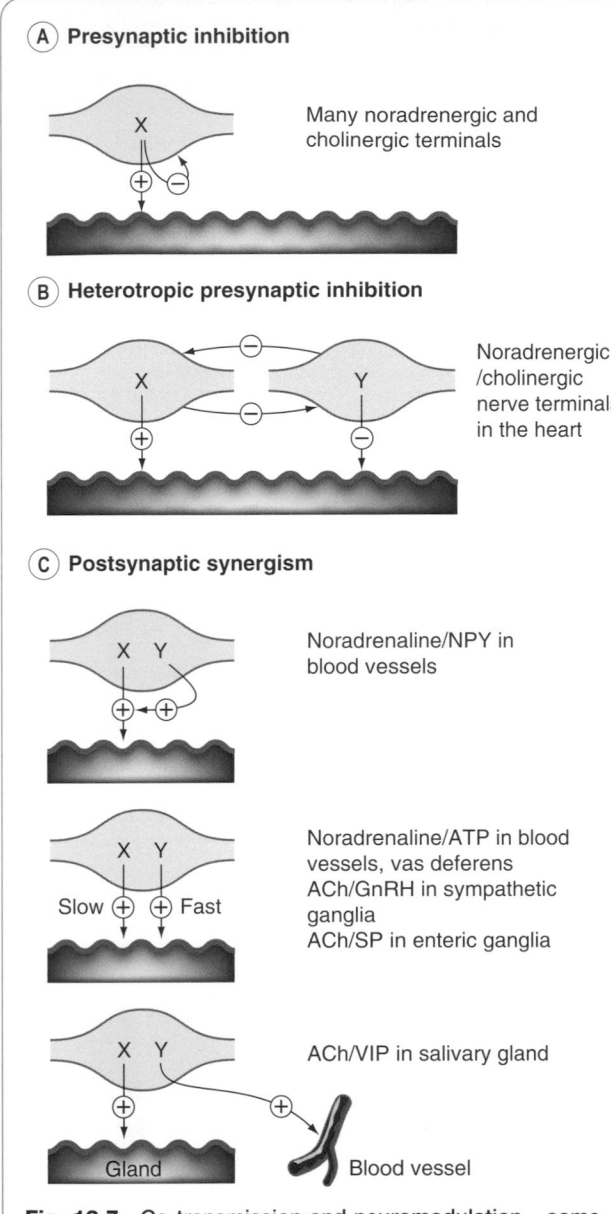

Fig. 13.7 Co-transmission and neuromodulation – some examples. (A) Presynaptic inhibition. (B) Heterotropic presynaptic inhibition. (C) Postsynaptic synergism. *ACh*, acetylcholine; *ATP*, adenosine triphosphate; *GnRH*, gonadotrophin-releasing hormone (luteinising hormone-releasing hormone); *NPY*, neuropeptide Y; *SP*, substance P; *VIP*, vasoactive intestinal peptide.

Fig. 13.8 The main processes involved in synthesis, storage and release of amine and amino acid transmitters. *1*, Uptake of precursors; *2*, synthesis of transmitter; *3*, uptake/transport of transmitter into vesicles; *4*, degradation of surplus transmitter; *5*, depolarisation by propagated action potential; *6*, influx of Ca^{2+} in response to depolarisation; *7*, release of transmitter by exocytosis; *8*, diffusion to postsynaptic membrane; *9*, interaction with postsynaptic receptors; *10*, inactivation of transmitter; *11*, reuptake of transmitter or degradation products by nerve terminals; *12*, uptake and release of transmitter by non-neuronal cells; and *13*, interaction with presynaptic receptors. The transporters *(11 and 12)* can release transmitter under certain conditions by working in reverse. These processes are well characterised for many transmitters (e.g. acetylcholine, monoamines, amino acids, ATP). Peptide mediators (see Ch. 18) differ in that they may be synthesised and packaged in the cell body rather than the terminals.

are of importance in the CNS, where such supersensitivity can cause 'rebound' effects when drugs that impair synaptic transmission are given for some time and then discontinued.

BASIC STEPS IN NEUROCHEMICAL TRANSMISSION: SITES OF DRUG ACTION

Fig. 13.8 summarises the main processes that occur in a classical chemically transmitting synapse, and provides a useful basis for understanding the actions of the many different classes of drug, discussed in later chapters, that act by facilitating or blocking neurochemical transmission.

All the steps shown in Fig. 13.8 (except for transmitter diffusion, step 8) can be influenced by drugs. For example, the enzymes involved in synthesis or inactivation of the transmitter can be inhibited, as can the transport systems responsible for the neuronal and vesicular uptake of the transmitter or its precursor. The actions of the great majority of drugs that act on the peripheral nervous system (Chs 14 and 15) and the CNS fit into this general scheme.

REFERENCES AND FURTHER READING

General references

Bacq, Z.M., 1975. Chemical Transmission of Nerve Impulses: A Historical Sketch. Pergamon Press, Oxford. (*Lively account of the history of the discovery of chemical transmission*)

Burnstock, G., 2009. Autonomic neurotransmission: 60 years since Sir Henry Dale. Ann. Rev. Pharmacol. 49, 1–30. (*Elegant and well-illustrated account of many of the topics discussed in this chapter. Recommended*)

Furness, J.B., Callaghan, B.P., Rivera, L.R., Cho, H.J., 2014. The enteric nervous system and gastrointestinal innervation: integrated local and central control. Adv. Exp. Med. Biol. 817, 39–71. (*Excellent review of the anatomy and physiology of the enteric nervous system*)

Iversen, L.L., Iversen, S.D., Bloom, F.E., Roth, R.H., 2009. Introduction to Neuropsychopharmacology. Oxford University Press, New York. (*Excellent general account covering many aspects of neuropharmacology*)

Luis, E.M.Q., Noel, F., 2009. Mechanisms of adaptive supersensitivity in vas deferens. Auton. Neurosci. 146, 38–46. (*Summarises mechanisms contributing to denervation supersensitivity in a typical organ supplied by the sympathetic nervous system*)

Robertson, D.W., Biaggioni, I., Burnstock, G., Low, P.A., Paton, J.F.R. (Eds.), 2012. Primer on the Autonomic Nervous System, third ed. Academic Press, London. (*An excellent comprehensive textbook on all aspects, including pharmacology, of the autonomic nervous system. By no means elementary despite its title*)

Valenstein, E.S., 2005. The War of the Soups and the Sparks. Columbia University Press, New York. (*Readable and informative account of origins of the theory of chemical transmission*)

Presynaptic modulation

Boehm, S., Kubista, H., 2002. Fine tuning of sympathetic transmitter release via ionotropic and metabotropic receptors. Pharm. Rev. 54, 43–99. (*Comprehensive review of presynaptic modulation, focusing on sympathetic neurons though mechanisms are widespread*)

Dorostkar, M.M., Boehm, S., 2008. Presynaptic ionotropic receptors. Handb. Exp. Pharmacol. 184, 479–527. (*Review of how presynaptic ionotropic receptors modify transmitter release*)

Kubista, H., Boehm, S., 2006. Molecular mechanisms underlying the modulation of exocytotic noradrenaline release via presynaptic receptors. Pharm. Ther. 112, 213–242. (*Describes the wide variety of mechanisms by which presynaptic receptors affect transmitter release*)

Starke, K., Gothert, M., Kilbinger, H., 1989. Modulation of neurotransmitter release by presynaptic autoreceptors. Physiol. Rev. 69, 864–989. (*Comprehensive review article*)

Co-transmission

Lundberg, J.M., 1996. Pharmacology of co-transmission in the autonomic nervous system: integrative aspects on amines, neuropeptides, adenosine triphosphate, amino acids and nitric oxide. Pharmacol. Rev. 48, 114–192. (*Detailed and informative review article*)

Transporters

Gether, U., Andersen, P.H., Larsson, O.M., et al., 2006. Neurotransmitter transporters: molecular function of important drug targets. Trends Pharmacol. Sci. 27, 375–383. (*Useful short review article*)

Manepalli, S., Surratt, C.K., Madura, J.D., Nolan, T.L., 2012. Monoamine transporter structure, function, dynamics, and drug discovery: a computational perspective. AAPS J. 14, 820–831. (*Complex review concentrating on molecular modelling of substrate and drug interactions with monoamine transporters*)

Reynolds, G.P., McGowan, O.O., Dalton, C.F., 2014. Pharmacogenomics in psychiatry: the relevance of receptor and transporter polymorphisms. Br. J. Clin. Pharmacol. 77, 654–672. (*Reviews the role of polymorphisms in membrane transporters in altered responses to drugs*)

Torres, G.E., Gainetdinov, R.R., Caron, M.G., 2003. Plasma membrane monoamine transporters: structure, regulation and function. Nat. Rev. Neurosci. 4, 13–25. (*Describes molecular, physiological and pharmacological aspects of transporters*)

Cholinergic transmission

OVERVIEW

This chapter is concerned mainly with cholinergic transmission in the periphery, and the ways in which drugs affect it. Here we describe the different types of acetylcholine (ACh) receptors and their functions, as well as the synthesis and release of ACh. Drugs that act on ACh receptors, many of which have clinical uses, are described in this chapter. Cholinergic mechanisms in the central nervous system (CNS) and their relevance to dementia are discussed in Chapters 40 and 41.

MUSCARINIC AND NICOTINIC ACTIONS OF ACETYLCHOLINE

▼ The discovery of the pharmacological action of ACh came, paradoxically, from work on adrenal glands, extracts of which were known to produce a rise in blood pressure owing to their content of adrenaline (epinephrine). In 1900, Reid Hunt found that after adrenaline had been removed from such extracts, they produced a fall in blood pressure instead of a rise. He attributed the fall to the presence of choline, but later concluded that a more potent derivative of choline must be responsible. With Taveau, he tested a number of choline derivatives and discovered that ACh was some 100,000 times more active than choline in lowering the rabbit's blood pressure. The physiological role of ACh was not apparent at that time, and it remained a pharmacological curiosity until Loewi, Dale and their colleagues discovered its transmitter role in the 1930s.

Analysing the pharmacological actions of ACh in 1914, Dale distinguished two types of activity, which he designated as *muscarinic* and *nicotinic* because they mimicked, respectively, the effects of **muscarine**, the active principle of the poisonous mushroom *Amanita muscaria*, and of **nicotine**. Muscarinic actions closely resemble the effects of parasympathetic stimulation (Table 13.1). After the muscarinic effects have been blocked by **atropine**, larger doses of ACh produce nicotine-like effects, which include:

* stimulation of all autonomic ganglia
* stimulation of voluntary muscle
* secretion of adrenaline from the adrenal medulla

The muscarinic and nicotinic actions of ACh are demonstrated in Fig. 14.1. Small and medium doses of ACh produce a transient fall in blood pressure due to arteriolar vasodilatation and slowing of the heart – muscarinic effects that are abolished by atropine. A large dose of ACh given after atropine produces nicotinic effects: an initial rise in blood pressure due to a stimulation of sympathetic ganglia and consequent vasoconstriction, and a secondary rise resulting from secretion of adrenaline.

Dale's pharmacological classification corresponds closely to the main physiological functions of ACh in the body. The muscarinic actions correspond to those of ACh released at

postganglionic parasympathetic nerve endings, with two significant exceptions:

1. ACh causes generalised vasodilatation, even though most blood vessels have no parasympathetic innervation. This is an indirect effect: ACh (like many other mediators) acts on vascular endothelial cells to release **nitric oxide** (see Ch. 21), which relaxes smooth muscle. The physiological function of this is uncertain, because ACh is not normally present in circulating blood.
2. ACh evokes secretion from sweat glands, which are innervated by cholinergic fibres of the sympathetic nervous system (see Table 13.1).

The nicotinic actions correspond to those of ACh acting on autonomic ganglia of the sympathetic and parasympathetic systems, the motor endplate of voluntary muscle and the secretory cells of the adrenal medulla.

ACETYLCHOLINE RECEPTORS

Although Dale himself dismissed the concept of receptors as sophistry rather than science, his functional classification provided the basis for distinguishing muscarinic and nicotinic receptors, the two major classes of ACh receptor (see Ch. 3 and Southan et al., 2016). Many important therapeutic drugs target these receptors, and despite their long and distinguished history, recent advances continue to open new opportunities for drug development in both muscarinic (Kruse et al., 2014; Carruthers et al., 2015) and nicotinic (Dinely et al., 2015) fields.

NICOTINIC RECEPTORS

Nicotinic ACh receptors (nAChRs) fall into three main classes – the muscle, ganglionic and CNS types – whose subunit compositions are summarised in Table 14.1. Muscle receptors are confined to the skeletal neuromuscular junction; ganglionic receptors are responsible for fast transmission at sympathetic and parasympathetic ganglia; and CNS-type receptors are widespread in the brain, and are heterogeneous with respect to their molecular composition and location (see Ch. 40). Most of the CNS-type nAChRs are located presynaptically and serve to facilitate or inhibit the release of other mediators, such as glutamate and dopamine.

▼ All nAChRs are pentameric structures that function as ligand-gated ion channels (see Fig. 3.4). The five subunits that form the receptor–channel complex are similar in structure, and so far 17 different members of the family have been identified and cloned, designated α (ten types), β (four types), γ, δ and ε (one of each). The five subunits each possess four membrane-spanning helical domains, and one of these helices (M_2) from each subunit defines the central pore

175

Fig. 14.1 Dale's experiment showing that acetylcholine (ACh) produces two kinds of effect on the cat's blood pressure. Arterial pressure was recorded with a mercury manometer from a spinal cat. (A) ACh causes a fall in blood pressure due to vasodilatation. (B) A larger dose also produces bradycardia. Both (A) and (B) are muscarinic effects. (C) After atropine (muscarinic antagonist), the same dose of ACh has no effect. (D) Still under the influence of atropine, a much larger dose of ACh causes a rise in blood pressure due to stimulation of sympathetic ganglia, accompanied by tachycardia, followed by a secondary rise (due to release of adrenaline from the adrenal gland). These effects result from its action on nicotinic receptors. (From Burn, J.H., 1963. Autonomic Pharmacology. Blackwell, Oxford.)

Table 14.1 Nicotinic receptor subtypes[a]

	Muscle type	Ganglion type	CNS type		Notes
Main molecular form	$(\alpha1)_2\beta1\delta\epsilon$ (adult form)	$(\alpha3)_2(\beta2)_3$	$(\alpha4)_2(\beta2)_3$	$(\alpha7)_5$	—
Main synaptic location	Skeletal neuromuscular junction: mainly postsynaptic	Autonomic ganglia: mainly postsynaptic	Many brain regions: pre- and postsynaptic	Many brain regions: pre- and postsynaptic	—
Membrane response	Excitatory Increased cation permeability (mainly Na^+, K^+)	Excitatory Increased cation permeability (mainly Na^+, K^+)	Pre- and postsynaptic excitation Increased cation permeability (mainly Na^+, K^+)	Pre- and postsynaptic excitation Increased cation permeability	$(\alpha7)_5$ receptor produces large Ca^{2+} entry, evoking transmitter release
Agonists	Acetylcholine Carbachol Succinylcholine	Acetylcholine Carbachol Nicotine Epibatidine Dimethylphenyl-piperazinium	Nicotine Epibatidine Acetylcholine Cytosine Varenicline[b]	Epibatidine Dimethylphenyl-piperazinium Varenicline[b]	—
Antagonists	Tubocurarine Pancuronium Atracurium Vecuronium α-Bungarotoxin α-Conotoxin	Mecamylamine Trimetaphan Hexamethonium α-Conotoxin	Mecamylamine Methylaconitine	α-Bungarotoxin α-Conotoxin Methylaconitine	—

[a]This table shows only the main subtypes expressed in mammalian tissues. Several other subtypes are expressed in selected brain regions, and also in the peripheral nervous system and in non-neuronal tissues. For further details, see Ch. 40 and review by Kalamida et al. (2007).
[b]Varenicline is used as an aid to smoking cessation. It acts as a partial agonist on $(\alpha4)_2(\beta2)_3$ receptors and a full agonist on $(\alpha7)_5$ receptors (see Ch. 50).

(see Ch. 3). nAChR subtypes generally contain both α and β subunits, the exception being the homomeric $(\alpha 7)_5$ subtype found mainly in the brain (Ch. 40). The adult muscle receptor has the composition $\alpha 2\beta 1\epsilon 1\delta 1$, while the main ganglionic subtype is $\alpha 2\beta 3$ (for more detail on which subunits are present in the different subtypes see Southan et al., 2016). The two binding sites for ACh (both of which need to be occupied to cause the channel to open) reside at the interface between the extracellular domain of each of the α subunits and its neighbour. The diversity of the nAChR family (for details see Kalamida et al., 2007), which emerged from cloning studies in the 1980s, took pharmacologists somewhat by surprise. Although they knew that the neuromuscular and ganglionic synapses differed pharmacologically, and suspected that cholinergic synapses in the CNS might be different again, the molecular diversity goes far beyond this, and its functional significance is only slowly emerging.

The different action of agonists and antagonists on neuromuscular, ganglionic and brain synapses is of practical importance and mainly reflects the differences between the muscle and neuronal nAChRs (Table 14.1).

MUSCARINIC RECEPTORS

Muscarinic receptors (mAChRs) are typical G protein–coupled receptors (see Ch. 3), and five molecular subtypes $(M_1–M_5)$ are known. The odd-numbered members of the group (M_1, M_3, M_5) couple with G_q to activate the inositol phosphate pathway (Ch. 3), while the even-numbered receptors (M_2, M_4) act through G_i to open potassium (K_{ir}) channels causing membrane hyperpolarisation; they also inhibit adenylyl cyclase but intracellular cAMP is usually low. Muscarinic agonists with either transduction mechanism also activate the mitogen-activated protein kinase pathway. The location and pharmacology of the various receptor subtypes are summarised in Table 14.2.

M_1 *receptors* ('*neural*') are found mainly on CNS and peripheral neurons and on gastric parietal cells. They mediate excitatory effects, for example, the slow muscarinic excitation mediated by ACh in sympathetic ganglia (Ch. 13) and central neurons. This excitation is produced by a decrease in K^+ conductance, which causes membrane depolarisation. Deficiency of this kind of ACh-mediated effect in the brain is possibly associated with dementia (see Ch. 41), although transgenic M_1-receptor knockout mice show only slight cognitive impairment. M_1 receptors are also involved in the increase of gastric acid secretion following vagal stimulation (see Ch. 31).

Table 14.2 Muscarinic receptor subtypes[a]

	M₁ ('neural')	M₂ ('cardiac')	M₃ ('glandular/smooth muscle')	M₄	M₅
Main locations	Autonomic ganglia (including intramural ganglia in stomach) gastric oxyntic glands (acid secretion) Glands: salivary, lacrimal, etc. Cerebral cortex	Heart: atria CNS: widely distributed	Exocrine glands: salivary, etc. Smooth muscle: gastrointestinal tract, eye, airways, bladder Blood vessels: endothelium	CNS	CNS: very localised expression in substantia nigra Salivary glands Iris/ciliary muscle
Cellular response	↑ IP₃, DAG Depolarisation Excitation (slow epsp) ↓ K⁺ conductance	↓ cAMP Inhibition ↓ Ca²⁺ conductance ↑ K⁺ conductance	↑ IP₃ Stimulation ↑ [Ca²⁺]ᵢ	↓ cAMP Inhibition	↑ IP₃ Excitation
Functional response	CNS excitation (? improved cognition) Gastric secretion	Cardiac inhibition Neural inhibition Central muscarinic effects (e.g. tremor, hypothermia)	Gastric, salivary secretion Gastrointestinal smooth muscle contraction Ocular accommodation Vasodilatation	Enhanced locomotion	Not known
Non-selective agonists (see also Table 14.3)	Acetylcholine Carbachol Oxotremorine Pilocarpine **Bethanechol**				
Selective agonists	McNA343		**Cevimeline**		
Non-selective antagonists (see also Table 14.5)	**Atropine** **Dicycloverine** **Tolterodine** **Oxybutynin** **Ipratropium**				
Selective antagonists	**Pirenzepine** Mamba toxin MT7	Gallamine (see p. 178)	**Darifenacin**		Mamba toxin MT3

[a]This table shows only the predominant subtypes expressed in mammalian tissues. For further details, see Ch. 40 and review by Kalamida et al. (2007).
Drugs in clinical use are shown in **bold**.
DAG, diacylglycerol; *epsp*, excitatory postsynaptic potential; *IP₃*, inositol trisphosphate.

M_2 receptors ('cardiac') occur in the heart, and also on the presynaptic terminals of peripheral and central neurons. They exert inhibitory effects, mainly by increasing K^+ conductance and by inhibiting calcium channels (see Ch. 4). M_2-receptor activation is responsible for cholinergic inhibition of the heart, as well as presynaptic inhibition in the CNS and periphery (Ch. 13). They are also co-expressed with M_3 receptors in visceral smooth muscle, and contribute to the smooth-muscle-stimulating effect of muscarinic agonists in several organs.

M_3 receptors (*glandular/smooth muscle*) produce mainly excitatory effects, i.e. stimulation of glandular secretions (salivary, bronchial, sweat, etc.) and contraction of visceral smooth muscle. M_3 receptor activation also causes relaxation of some smooth muscles (mainly vascular) via the release of nitric oxide from neighbouring endothelial cells (Ch. 21). M_3 receptors occur also in specific locations in the CNS (see Ch. 40).

M_4 and M_5 receptors are largely confined to the CNS, and their functional role is not well understood, although mice lacking these receptors do show behavioural changes.

Cytokine secretion from lymphocytes and other cells is regulated by M_1 and M_3 receptors, while M_2 and M_4 receptors affect cell proliferation in various situations, opening up the possibility of new therapeutic roles for mAChR ligands (see Wessler & Kirkpatrick, 2008).

The agonist binding region is highly conserved between the different subtypes, so attempts to develop selective agonists and antagonists have had limited success. Most known agonists are non-selective, though an experimental compound, **McNA343**, is selective for M_1 receptors. **Cevimeline**, a relatively selective M_3-receptor agonist, is used to improve salivary and lacrimal secretion in Sjögren's syndrome, an autoimmune disorder characterised by dryness of mouth and eyes. It is possible that new allosteric mAChR ligands, such as positive allosteric modulators (PAMs, see Ch. 3, Fig. 3.7), which are the focus of much current interest (see Nickols & Conn, 2014), will allow better subtype selectivity for drugs acting on this important class of receptors, for example, by targeting CNS muscarinic receptors without producing unwanted cardiovascular effects (see Ch. 41).

There is more subtype selectivity among antagonists. Although most of the classic muscarinic antagonists (e.g. **atropine**, **hyoscine**) are non-selective, **pirenzepine** (previously used for peptic ulcer disease) is selective for M_1 receptors, and **darifenacin** (used for urinary incontinence in adults with detrusor muscle instability, known as 'overactive bladder') is selective for M_3 receptors. **Gallamine**, once used as a neuromuscular-blocking drug, is also a selective, although weak, allosteric M_2 receptor antagonist.[1] Toxins from the venom of the green mamba have been discovered to be highly selective mAChR antagonists (see Table 14.2).

PHYSIOLOGY OF CHOLINERGIC TRANSMISSION

The physiology of cholinergic neurotransmission is described in detail by Nicholls et al. (2012). The main ways in which drugs can affect cholinergic transmission are shown in Fig. 14.2.

[1]Unlike most other antagonists, gallamine acts *allosterically* (i.e. at a site distinct from the ACh binding site).

Acetylcholine receptors

- Main subdivision is into nicotinic (nAChR) and muscarinic (mAChR) subtypes.
- nAChRs are directly coupled to cation channels, and mediate fast excitatory synaptic transmission at the neuromuscular junction, autonomic ganglia and various sites in the CNS. Muscle and neuronal nAChRs differ in their molecular structure and pharmacology.
- mAChRs and nAChRs occur presynaptically as well as postsynaptically, and function to regulate transmitter release.
- mAChRs are G protein–coupled receptors causing:
  - activation of phospholipase C (hence formation of inositol trisphosphate and diacylglycerol as second messengers)
  - inhibition of adenylyl cyclase
  - activation of potassium channels and/or inhibition of calcium channels.
- mAChRs mediate acetylcholine effects at postganglionic parasympathetic synapses (mainly heart, smooth muscle and glands), and contribute to ganglionic excitation. They occur in many parts of the CNS.
- Three main types of mAChR occur:
  - M_1 receptors ('neural') producing slow excitation of ganglia. They are selectively blocked by **pirenzepine**.
  - M_2 receptors ('cardiac') causing decrease in cardiac rate and force of contraction (mainly of atria). They are selectively blocked by **gallamine**. M_2 receptors also mediate presynaptic inhibition.
  - M_3 receptors ('glandular') causing secretion, contraction of visceral smooth muscle, vascular relaxation. **Cevimeline** is a selective M_3 agonist.
- Two further molecular mAChR subtypes, M_4 and M_5, occur mainly in the CNS.
- All mAChRs are activated by acetylcholine and blocked by **atropine**. There are also subtype-selective agonists and antagonists.

ACETYLCHOLINE SYNTHESIS AND RELEASE

ACh is synthesised within the nerve terminal from choline, which is taken up into the nerve terminal by a specific transporter (Ch. 13), similar to those that operate for many transmitters but which transports the precursor, choline, not ACh, so it is not important in terminating the action of the transmitter. The concentration of choline in the blood and body fluids is normally about 10 µmol/L, but in the immediate vicinity of cholinergic nerve terminals it increases, probably to about 1 mmol/L, when the released ACh is hydrolysed, and more than 50% of this choline is normally recaptured by the nerve terminals. Free choline within the nerve terminal is acetylated by a cytosolic enzyme, *choline acetyltransferase* (CAT), which transfers the acetyl group from acetyl coenzyme A. The rate-limiting process in ACh synthesis appears to be choline transport, which is determined by the extracellular choline concentration and hence is linked to the rate at which ACh is being released (see Fig. 14.2). *Cholinesterase* is present in the presynaptic nerve

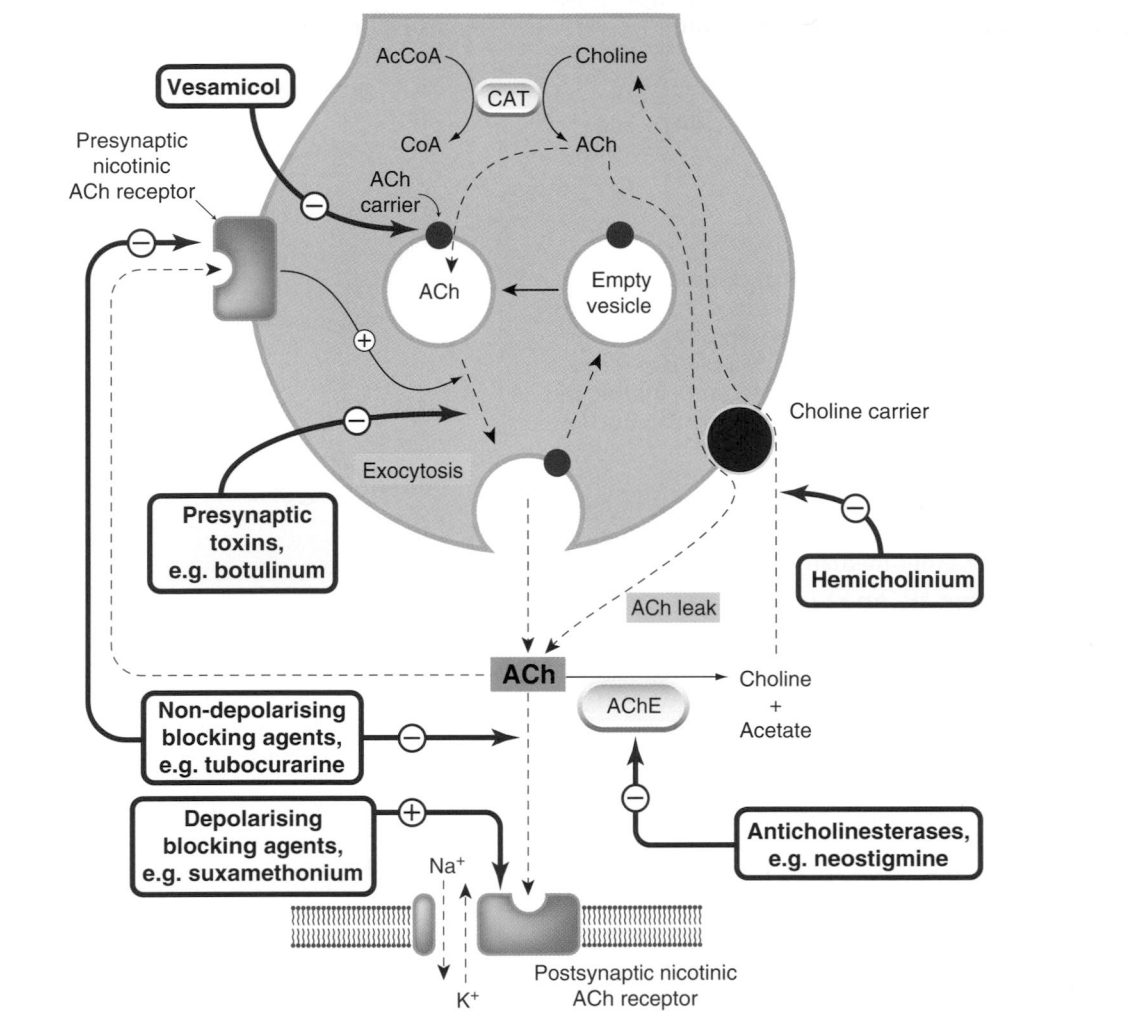

Fig. 14.2 **Events and sites of drug action at a nicotinic cholinergic synapse.** Acetylcholine (ACh) is shown acting postsynaptically on a nicotinic receptor controlling a cation channel (e.g. at the neuromuscular or ganglionic synapse), and also on a presynaptic nicotinic receptor that acts to facilitate ACh release during sustained synaptic activity. The nerve terminal also contains acetylcholinesterase (not shown); when this is inhibited, the amount of free ACh, and the rate of leakage of ACh via the choline carrier, is increased. Under normal conditions, this leakage of ACh is insignificant. At muscarinic cholinergic junctions (e.g. heart, smooth muscle and exocrine glands), both postsynaptic and presynaptic (inhibitory) receptors are of the muscarinic type. *AcCoA*, acetyl coenzyme A; *AChE*, acetylcholinesterase; *CAT*, choline acetyltransferase; *CoA*, coenzyme A.

terminals, and ACh is continually being hydrolysed and resynthesised. Inhibition of the nerve terminal cholinesterase causes the accumulation of surplus ACh in the cytosol, which is not available for release by nerve impulses (although it is able to leak out via the choline carrier). Most of the ACh synthesised, however, is packaged into synaptic vesicles, in which its concentration is extraordinarily high (about 100 mmol/L), and from which release occurs by exocytosis triggered by Ca^{2+} entry into the nerve terminal (see Ch. 4).

Cholinergic vesicles accumulate ACh actively, by means of a specific transporter belonging to the family of amine transporters described in Chapter 13. Accumulation of ACh is coupled to the large electrochemical gradient for protons that exists between acidic intracellular organelles and the cytosol; it is blocked selectively by the experimental drug **vesamicol**. Following its release, ACh diffuses across the synaptic cleft to combine with receptors on the postsynaptic cell. Some of it succumbs on the way to hydrolysis by *acetylcholinesterase* (AChE), an enzyme that is bound to

the basement membrane that lies between the pre- and postsynaptic membranes. At fast cholinergic synapses (e.g. the neuromuscular and ganglionic synapses), but not at slow ones (smooth muscle, gland cells, heart, etc.), the released ACh is hydrolysed very rapidly (within 1 ms), so that it acts only very briefly.

▼ At the neuromuscular junction, which is a highly specialised synapse, a single nerve impulse releases about 300 synaptic vesicles (altogether about 3 million ACh molecules) from the nerve terminals supplying a single muscle fibre, which contain altogether about 3 million synaptic vesicles. The synaptic vesicles are the structural basis for the release of ACh from the nerve terminal in packets ('quanta'). Approximately 2 million ACh molecules combine with receptors, of which there are about 30 million on each muscle fibre, the rest being hydrolysed without reaching a receptor. The ACh molecules remain bound to receptors for, on average, about 2 ms, and are quickly hydrolysed after dissociating. The result is that transmitter action is very rapid and very brief, which is important for a synapse that initiates speedy muscular responses and transmits signals faithfully at high frequency. Muscle cells are much larger than neurons and require much more synaptic current to generate an action potential. Thus all the chemical events happen on a larger scale than at a neuronal synapse; the number of transmitter molecules in a quantum, the number of quanta released, and the number of receptors activated by each quantum are all 10–100 times greater. Our brains would be huge, but not very clever, if their synapses were built on the industrial scale of the neuromuscular junction.

PRESYNAPTIC MODULATION

ACh release is regulated by mediators, including ACh itself, acting on presynaptic receptors, as discussed in Chapter 13. At postganglionic parasympathetic nerve endings, inhibitory M_2 receptors participate in autoinhibition of ACh release; other mediators, such as noradrenaline, also inhibit the release of ACh (see Ch. 13). At the neuromuscular junction, however, presynaptic nAChRs facilitate ACh release, a mechanism that may allow the synapse to function reliably during prolonged high-frequency activity. In the brain, as mentioned above, presynaptic nAChRs either facilitate or inhibit the release of other mediators.

ELECTRICAL EVENTS IN TRANSMISSION AT FAST CHOLINERGIC SYNAPSES

ACh, acting on the postsynaptic membrane of a nicotinic (neuromuscular or ganglionic) synapse, causes a large increase in its permeability to cations, particularly to Na^+ and K^+, and to a lesser extent Ca^{2+}. The resulting inflow of Na^+ depolarises the postsynaptic membrane. This transmitter-mediated depolarisation is called an *endplate potential* (*epp*) in a skeletal muscle fibre, or a *fast excitatory postsynaptic potential* (*fast epsp*) at the ganglionic synapse. In a muscle fibre, the localised epp spreads to adjacent, electrically excitable parts of the muscle fibre; if its amplitude reaches the threshold for excitation, an action potential is initiated, which propagates to the rest of the fibre and evokes a contraction (Ch. 4).

In a nerve cell, depolarisation of the soma or a dendrite by the fast epsp causes a local current to flow. This depolarises the axon hillock region of the cell, where, if the epsp is large enough, an action potential is initiated. Fig. 14.3 shows that **tubocurarine**, a drug that blocks postsynaptic nACh receptors, reduces the amplitude of the fast epsp until it no longer initiates an action potential, although the cell is still capable of responding when it is stimulated electrically. Most ganglion cells are supplied by several presynaptic axons, and it requires simultaneous activity in more than one to make the postganglionic cell fire (integrative action). At the neuromuscular junction, only one nerve fibre supplies each muscle fibre – like a relay station in a telegraph line the synapse ensures faithful 1:1 transmission despite the impedance mismatch between the fine nerve fibre and the much larger muscle fibre. The amplitude of the epp is normally more than enough to initiate an action potential – indeed, transmission still occurs when the epp is reduced by 70%–80%, showing a large margin of safety so that fluctuations in transmitter release (e.g. during repetitive stimulation) do not affect transmission.

▼ Transmission at the ganglionic synapse is more complex than at the neuromuscular junction. Although the primary event at both is the depolarisation (fast epsp or epp, respectively) produced by ACh acting on nAChRs, this is followed in the ganglion by a succession of much slower postsynaptic responses:

- A *slow inhibitory (hyperpolarising) postsynaptic potential* (*slow ipsp*), lasting 2–5 s. This mainly reflects a muscarinic

Fig. 14.3 **Cholinergic transmission in an autonomic ganglion cell.** Records were obtained with an intracellular microelectrode from a guinea pig parasympathetic ganglion cell. The artefact at the beginning of each trace shows the moment of stimulation of the preganglionic nerve. Tubocurarine (TC), an acetylcholine antagonist, causes the excitatory postsynaptic potential (epsp) to become smaller. In record (C), it only just succeeds in triggering the action potential, and in (D) it has fallen below the threshold. Following complete block, antidromic stimulation (not shown) will still produce an action potential (cf. depolarisation block, Fig. 14.4). (From Blackman, J.G. et al., 1969. J Physiol 201, 723.)

(M_2)-receptor-mediated increase in K^+ conductance, but other transmitters, such as dopamine and adenosine, also contribute.
- A *slow epsp*, which lasts for about 10 s. This is produced by ACh acting on M_1 receptors, which close K^+ channels.
- A *late slow epsp*, lasting for 1–2 min. This is thought to be mediated by a peptide co-transmitter, substance P in some ganglia, and a gonadotrophin-releasing hormone-like peptide in others (see Ch. 13). Like the slow epsp, it is produced by a decrease in K^+ conductance.

DEPOLARISATION BLOCK

▼ Depolarisation block occurs at cholinergic synapses when the excitatory nAChRs are persistently activated, and it results from a decrease in the electrical excitability of the postsynaptic cell. This is shown in Fig. 14.4. Application of nicotine to a sympathetic ganglion activates nAChRs, causing a depolarisation of the cell, which at first initiates action potential discharge. After a few seconds, this discharge ceases and transmission is blocked. The loss of electrical excitability is shown by the fact that electrical stimuli also fail to produce an action potential. The main reason for the loss of electrical excitability during a period of maintained depolarisation is that the voltage-sensitive sodium channels (see Ch. 4) become inactivated (i.e. refractory) and no longer able to open in response to a brief depolarising stimulus.

A second type of effect is also seen in the experiment shown in Fig. 14.4. After nicotine has acted for several minutes, the cell partially repolarises and its electrical excitability returns but, despite this,

Cholinergic transmission

- Acetylcholine (ACh) synthesis:
  - requires choline, which enters the neuron via carrier-mediated transport
  - choline is acetylated to form ACh by choline acetyl transferase, a cytosolic enzyme found only in cholinergic neurons. Acetyl coenzyme A is the source of acetyl groups.
- ACh is packaged into synaptic vesicles at high concentration by carrier-mediated transport.
- ACh release occurs by Ca^{2+}-mediated exocytosis. At the neuromuscular junction, one presynaptic nerve impulse releases 100–500 vesicles.
- At the neuromuscular junction, ACh acts on nicotinic receptors to open cation channels, producing a rapid depolarisation (endplate potential), which normally initiates an action potential in the muscle fibre. Transmission at other 'fast' cholinergic synapses (e.g. ganglionic) is similar.
- At 'fast' cholinergic synapses, ACh is hydrolysed within about 1 ms by acetylcholinesterase, so a presynaptic action potential produces only one postsynaptic action potential.
- Transmission mediated by muscarinic receptors is much slower in its time course, and synaptic structures are less clearly defined. In many such situations, ACh functions as a *modulator* (i.e. where the mediator acts indirectly to alter the efficiency of transmission rather than as a direct transmitter – see Ch. 13).
- Main mechanisms of pharmacological block: inhibition of choline uptake, inhibition of ACh release, block of postsynaptic receptors or ion channels, persistent postsynaptic depolarisation.

transmission remains blocked. This type of secondary, *non-depolarising block* occurs also at the neuromuscular junction if repeated doses of the depolarising drug **suxamethonium**[2] (see below) are used. The main factor responsible for the secondary block (known clinically as *phase II block*) appears to be receptor desensitisation (see Ch. 2). This causes the depolarising action of the blocking drug to subside, but transmission remains blocked because the receptors are desensitised to ACh.

EFFECTS OF DRUGS ON CHOLINERGIC TRANSMISSION

As shown in Fig. 14.2, drugs can influence cholinergic transmission either by acting on postsynaptic ACh receptors as agonists or antagonists (see Tables 14.1 and 14.2), or by affecting the release or destruction of endogenous ACh.

In the rest of this chapter, we describe the following groups of drugs, subdivided according to their site of action:

- muscarinic agonists
- muscarinic antagonists
- ganglion-stimulating drugs
- ganglion-blocking drugs

[2]Also known as **succinylcholine**.

- neuromuscular-blocking drugs
- anticholinesterases and other drugs that enhance cholinergic transmission

DRUGS AFFECTING MUSCARINIC RECEPTORS
MUSCARINIC AGONISTS

Structure–activity relationships
Muscarinic agonists, as a group, are often referred to as *parasympathomimetic*, because the main effects that they produce in the whole animal resemble those of parasympathetic stimulation. The structures of ACh and related choline esters are given in Table 14.3. They are agonists at

Fig. 14.4 Depolarisation block of ganglionic transmission by nicotine. (A) System used for intracellular recording from sympathetic ganglion cells of the frog, showing the location of orthodromic *(O)* and antidromic *(A)* stimulating *(stim)* electrodes. Stimulation at *O* excites the cell via the cholinergic synapse, whereas stimulation at *A* excites it by electrical propagation of the action potential. (B) The effect of nicotine. *(a)* Control records. The membrane potential is −55 mV (dotted line = 0 mV), and the cell responds to both *O* and *A*. *(b)* Shortly after adding nicotine, the cell is slightly depolarised and spontaneously active, but still responsive to *O* and *A*. *(c and d)* The cell is further depolarised, to −25 mV, and produces only a vestigial action potential. The fact that it does not respond to A shows that it is electrically inexcitable. *(e and f)* In the continued presence of nicotine, the cell repolarises and regains its responsiveness to *A*, but it is still unresponsive to *O* because the ACh receptors are desensitised by nicotine. (From Ginsborg, B.L., Guerrero, S., 1964. J. Physiol. 172, 189.)

Table 14.3 Muscarinic agonists

Compound	Structure	Receptor specificity		Hydrolysis by cholinesterase	Clinical uses
		Muscarinic	Nicotinic		
Acetylcholine		+++	+++	+++	None
Carbachol		++	+++	—	None
Methacholine		+++	+	++	None
Bethanechol		+++	—	—	Treatment of bladder and gastrointestinal hypotonia[a]
Muscarine		+++	—	—	None[b]
Pilocarpine		++	—	—	Glaucoma
Oxotremorine		++	—	—	None
Cevimeline		++[c]	—	—	Sjögren's syndrome (to increase salivary and lacrimal secretion)

[a]Essential to check that bladder neck is not obstructed.
[b]Cause of one type of mushroom poisoning.
[c]Selective for M_3 receptors.

both mAChRs and nAChRs, but act more potently on mAChRs (see Fig. 14.1). **Bethanechol, pilocarpine** and **cevimeline** are the main ones used clinically.

The key features of the ACh molecule that are important for its activity are the quaternary ammonium group, which bears a positive charge, and the ester group, which bears a partial negative charge and is susceptible to rapid hydrolysis by cholinesterase. Variants of the choline ester structure (see Table 14.3) have the effect of reducing the susceptibility of the compound to hydrolysis by cholinesterase, and altering the relative activity on mAChRs and nAChRs.

Carbachol and **methacholine** are less rapidly hydrolysed by cholinesterase enzymes than is ACh. They are used as experimental tools. Bethanechol, which is a hybrid of these two molecules, is stable to hydrolysis and selective for mAChRs, and is occasionally used clinically (see clinical box, p. 184). Pilocarpine is a partial agonist and shows some selectivity in stimulating secretion from sweat, salivary, lacrimal and bronchial glands, and contracting iris smooth muscle (see later), with weak effects on gastrointestinal smooth muscle and the heart.

Effects of muscarinic agonists

The main actions of muscarinic agonists are readily understood in terms of the parasympathetic nervous system.

Cardiovascular effects. These include cardiac slowing and a decrease in cardiac output due both to the reduced heart rate and to a decreased force of contraction of the atria (the ventricles have only a sparse parasympathetic innervation and a low sensitivity to muscarinic agonists). Generalised vasodilatation also occurs (mediated by nitric oxide, NO; see Ch. 21) and, combined with the reduced cardiac output, produces a sharp fall in arterial pressure (see Fig. 14.1). Parasympathetic regulation of the heart is discussed in Chapter 22 (see Fig. 22.7).

Smooth muscle. Smooth muscle generally *contracts* in direct response to muscarinic agonists, in contrast to their indirect effect via NO on vascular smooth muscle. Peristaltic activity of the gastrointestinal tract is increased, which can cause colicky pain, and the bladder and bronchial smooth muscle also contract.

Sweating, lacrimation, salivation and bronchial secretion. Muscarinic agonists stimulate exocrine glands. The combined effect of bronchial secretion and constriction can interfere with breathing. **Methacholine** is used as an inhaled challenge agent in the investigation of airways responsiveness.

Effects on the eye. Ocular effects of muscarinic agents are clinically important. The parasympathetic nerves to the eye supply the constrictor pupillae muscle, which runs circumferentially in the iris, and the ciliary muscle, which adjusts the curvature of the lens (Fig. 14.5). Contraction of the ciliary muscle in response to activation of mAChRs pulls the ciliary body forward and inward, thus relaxing the tension on the suspensory ligament of the lens, allowing the lens to bulge more and reducing its focal length. This parasympathetic reflex is thus necessary to accommodate the eye for near vision. The constrictor pupillae is important not only for adjusting the pupil in response to changes in light intensity, but also in regulating the intraocular pressure. Aqueous humour is secreted slowly and continuously by the cells of the epithelium covering the ciliary body, and drains into the *canal of Schlemm* (see Fig. 14.5), which

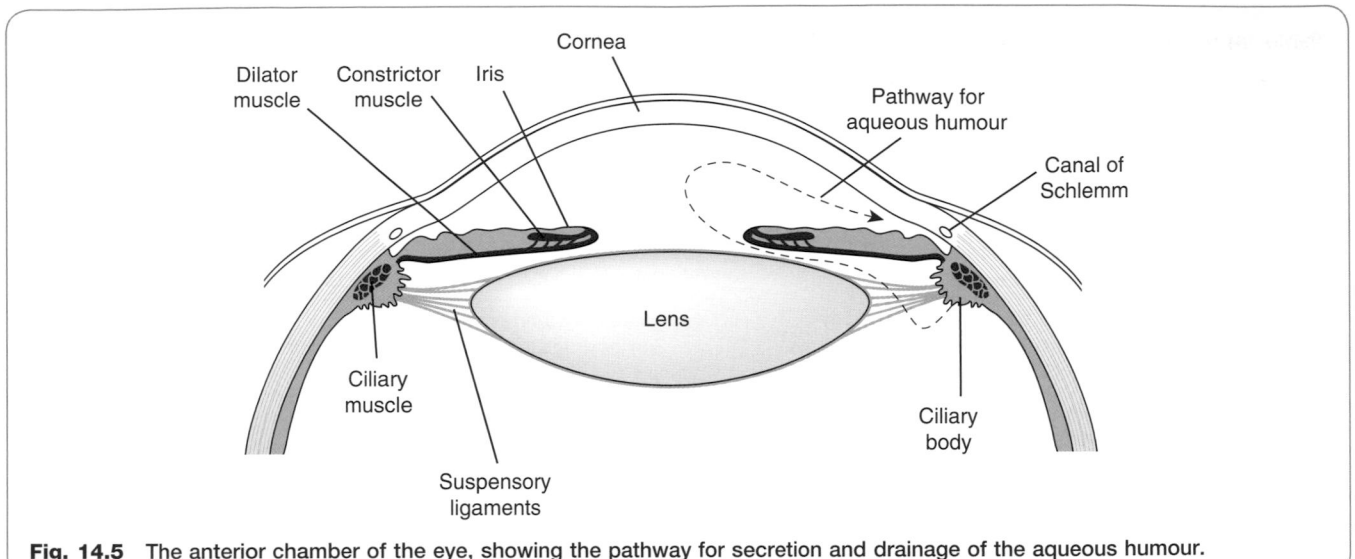

Fig. 14.5 The anterior chamber of the eye, showing the pathway for secretion and drainage of the aqueous humour.

Table 14.4 Drugs that lower intraocular pressure

Drug[a]	Mechanism	Notes	See Chapter
Timolol, carteolol	β-adrenoceptor antagonist	Given as eye drops but may still cause systemic side effects: bradycardia, bronchoconstriction	15
Acetazolamide, dorzolamide	Carbonic anhydrase inhibitor	Acetazolamide is given systemically Side effects include diuresis, loss of appetite, tingling, neutropenia Dorzolamide is used as eye drops Side effects include bitter taste and burning sensation	30
Clonidine, apraclonidine	α_2-adrenoceptor agonist	Used as eye drops	15
Latanoprost	Prostaglandin analogue	Can alter iris pigmentation	18
Pilocarpine	Muscarinic agonist	Used as eye drops	This chapter
Ecothiophate	Anticholinesterase	Used as eye drops Can cause muscle spasm and systemic effects	This chapter

[a]The most important drugs are shown in **bold**.

runs around the eye close to the outer margin of the iris. The intraocular pressure is normally 10–15 mmHg above atmospheric, which keeps the eye slightly distended. Abnormally raised intraocular pressure (which leads to the pathological condition of *glaucoma*) damages the eye and is one of the commonest preventable causes of blindness. In acute glaucoma, drainage of aqueous humour becomes impeded when the pupil is dilated, because folding of the iris tissue occludes the drainage angle, causing the intraocular pressure to rise. Activation of the constrictor pupillae muscle by muscarinic agonists in these circumstances lowers the intraocular pressure, whereas in a healthy individual it has little effect on intraocular pressure. Drugs used in the treatment of glaucoma are summarised in Table 14.4.

In addition to these peripheral effects, muscarinic agonists that penetrate the blood–brain barrier produce marked central effects due to activation of muscarinic (mainly M_1)

receptors in the brain. These include tremor, hypothermia and increased locomotor activity (see also Ch. 41 for effects of cholinesterase inhibitors in improving cognition in Alzheimer's disease).

Clinical use

Currently there are few important uses for muscarinic agonists (though there are still hopes that new, more selective agents may prove useful in various CNS disorders). Current clinical uses are summarised in the clinical box (p. 184).

MUSCARINIC ANTAGONISTS

mAChR antagonists (*parasympatholytic drugs*; Table 14.5) are competitive antagonists whose chemical structures usually contain ester and basic groups in the same relationship as ACh, but they have a bulky aromatic group in place of the acetyl group. The two naturally occurring compounds, **atropine** and **hyoscine** (also known as **scopolamine**),

Table 14.5   Muscarinic antagonists[a]

Compound	Pharmacological properties	Notes
Atropine	Non-selective antagonist Well absorbed orally CNS stimulant	Belladonna alkaloid Main side effects: urinary retention, dry mouth, blurred vision Dicycloverine (dicyclomine) is similar and used mainly as an antispasmodic agent
Hyoscine	Similar to atropine CNS depressant	Belladonna alkaloid (also known as scopolamine) Causes sedation; other side effects as atropine
Hyoscine butylbromide	Similar to atropine but poorly absorbed and lacks CNS effects Significant ganglion-blocking activity	Quaternary ammonium derivative Similar drugs include atropine methonitrate, propantheline
Tiotropium	Similar to atropine methonitrate Does not inhibit mucociliary clearance from bronchi	Quaternary ammonium compound Ipratropium similar
Tropicamide	Similar to atropine May raise intraocular pressure	—
Cyclopentolate	Similar to tropicamide	—
Darifenacin	Selective for M_3 receptors	Used to treat unstable bladder and associated urge incontinence. Causes fewer adverse effects than unselective muscarinic antagonists

Other non-selective muscarinic antagonists in clinical use, with very similar actions and side effects, include oxybutynin, tolterodine, fesoterodine, solifenacin and trospium – an example of me-too development by pharmaceutical companies.
[a]For chemical structures, see Southan et al. (2016).
CNS, central nervous system.

Clinical uses of muscarinic agonists and related drugs

- **Pilocarpine** eye drops cause constriction of the pupils (miosis) and have been used to treat glaucoma (raised pressure within the eye).
- **Pilocarpine** or **cevimeline**, a selective M_3 agonist, can be used to increase salivation and lacrimal secretion in patients with dry mouth or dry eyes (e.g. following irradiation, or in patients with autoimmune damage to the salivary or lacrimal glands as in Sjögren's syndrome).
- **Bethanechol** or **distigmine** (a cholinesterase inhibitor) are now seldom used as stimulant laxatives or to stimulate bladder emptying.

are alkaloids found in solanaceous plants. The deadly nightshade (*Atropa belladonna*) contains mainly atropine, whereas the thorn apple (*Datura stramonium*) contains mainly hyoscine. These are tertiary ammonium compounds that are sufficiently lipid-soluble to be readily absorbed from the gut or conjunctival sac and, importantly, to penetrate the blood–brain barrier. Analogues containing quaternary rather than tertiary ammonium groups have peripheral actions very similar to those of atropine but, because of their exclusion from the brain, lack central actions. Clinically important examples include **hyoscine butylbromide** and **propantheline**. Other muscarinic antagonists in clinical use are described below.

Effects of muscarinic antagonists

All the muscarinic antagonists produce similar peripheral effects, although some show a degree of selectivity, for example, for the heart or bladder, reflecting heterogeneity among mAChRs.

The main effects of atropine are:

Inhibition of secretions. Salivary, lacrimal, bronchial and sweat glands are inhibited by very low doses of atropine, producing uncomfortably dry eyes, mouth and skin. Gastric secretion is only slightly reduced. Mucociliary clearance in the bronchi is inhibited, so that residual secretions tend to accumulate in the lungs. **Ipratropium** lacks this effect.

Effects on heart rate. Atropine causes tachycardia through block of cardiac mAChRs. The tachycardia is modest, up to 80–90 beats/min in humans, since it has no effect on the sympathetic system, but only inhibition of tonic parasympathetic tone. Tachycardia is most pronounced in young people, in whom vagal tone at rest is highest; it is often absent in the elderly. At very low doses, atropine causes a paradoxical bradycardia, possibly due to a central action. Arterial blood pressure and the response of the heart to exercise are unaffected.

Effects on the eye. The pupil is dilated (*mydriasis*) by atropine administration, and becomes unresponsive to light. Relaxation of the ciliary muscle causes paralysis of accommodation (*cycloplegia*), so that near vision is impaired. Intraocular pressure may rise; although this is unimportant in normal individuals, it is dangerous in patients suffering from narrow-angle glaucoma due to impaired drainage of aqueous humour into the canal of Schlemm (see earlier). **Cyclopentolate** and **tropicamide** are tertiary amine muscarinic antagonists developed for ophthalmic use and administered as eye drops to facilitate fundoscopy (looking at the back of the eye with an ophthalmoscope, a key part of the examination of the eye).

Effects on the gastrointestinal tract. Gastrointestinal motility is inhibited by atropine, although this requires larger doses than the other effects listed, and is not complete since excitatory transmitters other than ACh are important in normal function of the myenteric plexus (see Ch. 13). Atropine-like drugs such as **hyoscine butylbromide** (a quaternary ammonium antimuscarinic agent) relax intestinal spasm and are used for symptomatic relief in pathological conditions in which there is gastrointestinal spasm, as well as in gastrointestinal imaging to improve resolution. **Pirenzepine**, owing to its selectivity for M_1 receptors, inhibits gastric acid secretion in doses that do not affect other systems.

Effects on other smooth muscle. Bronchial, biliary and urinary tract smooth muscle are all relaxed by atropine. Reflex bronchoconstriction (e.g. during anaesthesia) is prevented by atropine, whereas bronchoconstriction caused by local mediators, such as histamine and leukotrienes (e.g. in asthma; Ch. 29) is unaffected. **Ipratropium** and **tiotropium**, quaternary ammonium antimuscarinic drugs, are administered by inhalation as bronchodilators (Ch. 29). Biliary and urinary tract smooth muscle are only slightly affected in normal individuals, probably because transmitters other than ACh (see Ch. 13) are important in these organs; nevertheless, atropine and similar drugs commonly precipitate urinary retention in elderly men with prostatic enlargement. **Oxybutynin**, **tolterodine** and **darifenacin** (M_3-selective) act on the bladder to inhibit micturition, and are used for treating overactive bladder. They produce unwanted effects typical of muscarinic antagonists, such as dry mouth, constipation and blurred vision, but these are less severe than with less selective drugs.

Effects on the CNS. Atropine produces mainly excitatory effects on the CNS. At low doses, this causes mild restlessness; higher doses cause agitation and disorientation. In atropine poisoning, which occurs in young children who eat deadly nightshade berries, marked excitement and irritability result in hyperactivity and a considerable rise in body temperature, which is accentuated by the loss of sweating. These central effects are the result of blocking mAChRs in the brain, and are less marked or absent with quaternary ammonium drugs such as hyoscine butylbromide, propantheline, ipratropium and tiotropium that have limited access beyond the blood–brain barrier. The central effects of muscarinic antagonists are opposed by anticholinesterase drugs such as **physostigmine**, which have been used to treat atropine poisoning. Hyoscine in low doses causes marked sedation, but has similar effects to atropine in high dosage. Hyoscine additionally has a central anti-emetic effect and is used to prevent motion sickness. Muscarinic antagonists also affect the extrapyramidal system, reducing the involuntary movement and rigidity of patients with Parkinson's disease (Ch. 41) and counteracting the extrapyramidal side effects of many antipsychotic drugs (Ch. 47).

Clinical use

The main uses of muscarinic antagonists are summarised in the clinical box (p. 186).

DRUGS AFFECTING AUTONOMIC GANGLIA
GANGLION STIMULANTS

Most nAChR agonists act on either neuronal (ganglionic and CNS) nAChRs or on striated muscle (motor endplate)

receptors but not, apart from nicotine and ACh, on both (Table 14.6).

Nicotine and **lobeline** are tertiary amines found in the leaves of tobacco and lobelia plants, respectively. Nicotine belongs in pharmacological folklore, as it was the substance on the tip of Langley's paintbrush causing stimulation of muscle fibres when applied to the endplate region, leading him to postulate in 1905 the existence of a 'receptive substance' on the surface of the fibres (Ch. 13). **Epibatidine**, found in the skin of poisonous frogs, is a highly potent nicotinic agonist selective for ganglionic and CNS receptors. It was found, unexpectedly, to be a powerful analgesic (see Ch. 43), though its autonomic side effects ruled out its clinical use. **Varenicline**, a synthetic agonist relatively selective for CNS receptors, is used (as is nicotine itself) to treat nicotine addiction (Ch. 50). Otherwise these drugs are used only as experimental tools.

They cause complex peripheral responses associated with generalised stimulation of autonomic ganglia. The effects of nicotine on the gastrointestinal tract and sweat glands are familiar to neophyte smokers (see Ch. 50), although usually insufficient to act as an effective deterrent.

Clinical uses of muscarinic antagonists

Cardiovascular

- Treatment of sinus bradycardia (e.g. after myocardial infarction; see Ch. 22): for example, **atropine**.

Ophthalmic

- To dilate the pupil: for example **tropicamide** or **cyclopentolate** eye drops.

Neurological

- Prevention of motion sickness: for example, **hyoscine**.
- Parkinsonism (see Ch. 41), especially to counteract movement disorders caused by antipsychotic drugs (see Ch. 47): for example, **benzhexol, benztropine**.

Respiratory

- Asthma and chronic obstructive pulmonary disease (see Ch. 29): **ipratropium** or **tiotropium** by inhalation.

Palliative care

- Bowel colic and excessive salivation/respiratory secretion: hyoscine or glycopyrronium.

Anaesthetic premedication

- To dry secretions: for example, **atropine**, **hyoscine**. (Current anaesthetics are relatively non-irritant, see Ch. 42, so this is less important than in the past.)

Gastrointestinal

- To facilitate endoscopy and gastrointestinal radiology by relaxing gastrointestinal smooth muscle (antispasmodic action; see Ch. 31): for example, **hyoscine butylbromide**.
- As an antispasmodic in irritable bowel syndrome or colonic diverticular disease: for example, **dicycloverine** (**dicyclomine**).

Urinary tract

- To relieve symptoms of overactive bladder: for example, **oxybutynin, tolterodine, darifenacin.**

GANGLION-BLOCKING DRUGS

Ganglion-blocking drugs are used experimentally to study autonomic function, but their clinical use is obsolete. Ganglion block can occur by several mechanisms:

- By interference with ACh release, as at the neuromuscular junction (Ch. 13).
- By prolonged depolarisation. Nicotine (see Fig. 14.4) can block ganglia, after initial stimulation, in this way, as can ACh itself if cholinesterase is inhibited, thereby prolonging its action on the postsynaptic membrane.
- Interfering with the postsynaptic action of ACh, by blocking neuronal nAChRs or the associated ion channels.

▼ In the middle of the last century, Paton and Zaimis investigated a series of linear bisquaternary compounds. Compounds with five or six carbon atoms (**hexamethonium** is obsolete clinically but famous as the first effective antihypertensive agent) in the methylene chain linking the two quaternary groups produced ganglionic block.[3]

[3]Based on their structural similarity to ACh, these compounds were originally assumed to compete with ACh for its binding site. However, they are now known to act mainly by blocking the ion channel rather than the receptor itself.

Effects of ganglion-blocking drugs

The effects of ganglion-blocking drugs are diverse, because both divisions of the autonomic nervous system are blocked indiscriminately. The description by Paton of 'hexamethonium man' cannot be bettered:

▼ He is a pink-complexioned person, except when he has stood in a queue for a long time, when he may get pale and faint. His handshake is warm and dry. He is a placid and relaxed companion; for instance he may laugh but he can't cry because the tears cannot come. Your rudest story will not make him blush, and the most unpleasant circumstances will fail to make him turn pale. His collars and socks stay very clean and sweet. He wears corsets and may, if you meet him out, be rather fidgety (corsets to compress his splanchnic vascular pool, fidgety to keep the venous return going from his legs). He dislikes speaking much unless helped with something to moisten his dry mouth and throat. He is long-sighted and easily blinded by bright light. The redness of his eyeballs may suggest irregular habits and in fact his head is rather weak. But he always behaves like a gentleman and never belches or hiccups. He tends to get cold and keeps well wrapped up. But his health is good; he does not have chilblains and those diseases of modern civilisation, hypertension and peptic ulcer, pass him by. He gets thin because his appetite is modest; he never feels hunger pains and his stomach never rumbles. He gets rather constipated so that his intake of liquid paraffin is high. As old age comes on, he will suffer from retention of urine and impotence, but frequency, precipitancy and strangury (i.e. an intensely painful sensation of needing to pass urine coupled with an inability to do so) will not worry him. One is uncertain how he will end, but perhaps if he is not careful, by eating less and less and getting colder and colder, he will sink into a symptomless, hypoglycaemic coma and die, as was proposed for the universe, a sort of entropy death.
(From Paton, W.D.M., 1954. The principles of ganglion block. Lectures on the Scientific Basis of Medicine, Vol. 2.)

In practice, the main effect is a marked fall in arterial blood pressure resulting mainly from block of sympathetic ganglia, which causes arteriolar vasodilatation, and the block of cardiovascular reflexes. Venoconstriction, which occurs normally when a subject stands up and prevents a fall in central venous pressure and cardiac output, is reduced. Standing thus causes a sudden fall in arterial pressure (*postural hypotension*) that can cause fainting. The vasodilatation of skeletal muscle that occurs during exercise is normally accompanied by vasoconstriction elsewhere (e.g. splanchnic area) produced by sympathetic activity. Ganglion blockers prevent this adjustment, so the overall peripheral resistance falls leading to *postexercise hypotension*.

NEUROMUSCULAR-BLOCKING DRUGS

Drugs can block neuromuscular transmission either by acting presynaptically to inhibit ACh synthesis or release, or by acting postsynaptically.

Neuromuscular block is an important adjunct to general anaesthesia (Ch. 42). The drugs used for this purpose all work postsynaptically, either (a) by blocking ACh receptors (or in some cases the ion channel) or (b) by activating ACh receptors and thus causing persistent depolarisation of the motor endplate. **Suxamethonium** (see pp. 189–190) is the only depolarising blocker in clinical use, while all of the other drugs used clinically are *non-depolarising agents*.

NON-DEPOLARISING BLOCKING AGENTS

In 1856, Claude Bernard, in a famous experiment, showed that 'curare' causes paralysis by blocking neuromuscular transmission, rather than by abolishing nerve conduction or muscle contractility. Curare is a mixture of naturally

Table 14.6 Nicotinic receptor agonists and antagonists

Drug	Main site	Type of action	Notes
Agonists			
Nicotine	Autonomic ganglia CNS	Stimulation then block Stimulation	See Ch. 50
Lobeline	Autonomic ganglia Sensory nerve terminals	Stimulation Stimulation	—
Epibatidine	Autonomic ganglia CNS	Stimulation	Isolated from frog skin Highly potent No clinical use
Varenicline	CNS Autonomic ganglia	Stimulation	Used for nicotine addiction (see Ch. 50)
Suxamethonium	Neuromuscular junction	Depolarisation block	Used clinically as muscle relaxant
Decamethonium	Neuromuscular junction	Depolarisation block	No clinical use
Antagonists			
Hexamethonium	Autonomic ganglia	Transmission block	No clinical use
Trimetaphan	Autonomic ganglia	Transmission block	Blood pressure-lowering in surgery (rarely used)
Tubocurarine	Neuromuscular junction	Transmission block	Now rarely used
Pancuronium Atracurium Vecuronium	Neuromuscular junction	Transmission block	Widely used as muscle relaxants in anaesthesia

CNS, central nervous system.

Drugs acting on autonomic ganglia

Ganglion-stimulating drugs

- Compounds include **nicotine**, **dimethylphenyl-piperazinium** (**DMPP**).
- Both sympathetic and parasympathetic ganglia are stimulated, so effects are complex, including tachycardia and increase of blood pressure; variable effects on gastrointestinal motility and secretions; increased bronchial, salivary and sweat secretions. Additional effects result from stimulation of other neuronal structures, including sensory and noradrenergic nerve terminals.
- Ganglion stimulation may be followed by depolarisation block.
- **Nicotine** also has important central nervous system effects.
- Therapeutic uses are limited to assisting smoking cessation (**nicotine**, **varenicline**).

Ganglion-blocking drugs

- Compounds include **hexamethonium**, **tubocurarine** (also **nicotine**; see p. 185).
- Block all autonomic ganglia and enteric ganglia. Main effects: hypotension and loss of cardiovascular reflexes, inhibition of secretions, gastrointestinal paralysis, impaired micturition.
- Clinically obsolete (historically: the first therapeutic drugs for treating hypertension).

occurring alkaloids found in various South American plants and used as arrow poisons by South American Indians. The most important component is **tubocurarine**, itself now rarely used in clinical medicine, being superseded by synthetic drugs with improved properties. The most important are **pancuronium**, **vecuronium**, **cisatracurium** and **mivacurium** (Table 14.7), which differ mainly in their duration of action. These substances are all quaternary ammonium compounds, so are poorly absorbed[4] (they are administered intravenously) and generally are efficiently excreted by the kidneys. They do not cross the placenta, which is important in relation to their use in obstetric anaesthesia.

Mechanism of action

Non-depolarising blocking agents act as competitive antagonists (see Ch. 2) at the ACh receptors of the endplate.

▼ The amount of ACh released by a nerve impulse normally exceeds by several-fold what is needed to elicit an action potential in the muscle fibre. It is therefore necessary to block 70%–80% of the receptor sites before transmission actually fails. In any individual muscle fibre, transmission is all-or-nothing, so graded degrees of block represent a varying proportion of muscle fibres failing to respond. In this situation, where the amplitude of the epp in all the fibres is close to threshold (just above in some, just below in others), small variations in the amount of transmitter released, or in the rate at which it is destroyed, will have a large effect on the proportion of fibres contracting, so the degree of block is liable to vary according to various physiological circumstances (e.g. stimulation frequency, temperature and cholinesterase activity), which otherwise have little effect on the efficiency of transmission.

[4]Animals killed by curare-tipped arrows are safe to eat because of this.

Table 14.7 Characteristics of neuromuscular-blocking drugs[a]

Drug	Speed of onset	Duration of action	Main side effects	Notes
Tubocurarine	Slow (>5 min)	Long (1–2 h)	Hypotension (ganglion block plus histamine release) Bronchoconstriction (histamine release)	Plant alkaloid, now rarely used Alcuronium is a semisynthetic derivative with similar properties but fewer side effects
Pancuronium	Intermediate (2–3 min)	Long (1–2 h)	Slight tachycardia Hypertension	The first steroid-based compound Better side effect profile than tubocurarine Widely used Pipecuronium is similar
Vecuronium	Intermediate	Intermediate (30–40 min)	Few side effects	Widely used Occasionally causes prolonged paralysis, probably owing to active metabolite Rocuronium is similar, with faster onset
Atracurium	Intermediate	Intermediate (<30 min)	Transient hypotension (histamine release)	Unusual mechanism of elimination (spontaneous non-enzymic chemical degradation in plasma); degradation slowed by acidosis Widely used Doxacurium is chemically similar but stable in plasma, giving it long duration of action Cisatracurium is the pure active isomeric constituent of atracurium, more potent but with less histamine release
Mivacurium	Fast (~2 min)	Short (~15 min)	Transient hypotension (histamine release)	Chemically similar to atracurium but rapidly inactivated by plasma cholinesterase (therefore longer acting in patients with liver disease or with genetic cholinesterase deficiency [see p. 189 and Ch. 12])
Suxamethonium	Fast	Short (~10 min)	Bradycardia (muscarinic agonist effect) Cardiac dysrhythmias (increased plasma K^+ concentration – avoid in patients with burns or severe trauma) Raised intraocular pressure (nicotinic agonist effect on extraocular muscles) Postoperative muscle pain	Acts by depolarisation of endplate (nicotinic agonist effect) – the only drug of this type still in use Paralysis is preceded by transient muscle fasciculations Short duration of action owing to hydrolysis by plasma cholinesterase (prolonged action in patients with liver disease or genetic deficiency of plasma cholinesterase) Used for brief procedures (e.g. tracheal intubation, electroconvulsive shock therapy) Rocuronium has similar speed of onset and recovery, with fewer unwanted effects

[a]For chemical structures, see Hardman, J.G., Limbird, L.E., Gilman, A.G., Goodman-Gilman A. et al., 2001. Goodman and Gilman's Pharmacological Basis of Therapeutics, 10th ed. McGraw–Hill, New York.

Non-depolarising blocking agents also block facilitatory presynaptic autoreceptors, and thus inhibit the release of ACh during repetitive stimulation of the motor nerve, resulting in the phenomenon of 'tetanic fade', used by anaesthetists to monitor postoperative recovery of neuromuscular transmission.

Effects of non-depolarising blocking drugs
The effects of non-depolarising neuromuscular-blocking agents are mainly due to motor paralysis, although some of the drugs also produce clinically significant autonomic effects.

▼ The first muscles to be affected are the extrinsic eye muscles (causing double vision), reminiscent of the disease myasthenia gravis, which is caused by autoantibodies directed against nAChR (see pp. 195–196), and the small muscles of the face, limbs and pharynx (causing difficulty in swallowing). Respiratory muscles are the last to be affected and the first to recover. An experiment in 1947 in which a heroic volunteer was fully curarised while conscious under artificial ventilation established this orderly paralytic march, and showed that consciousness and awareness of pain were quite normal even when paralysis was complete.[5]

Unwanted effects

An important unwanted effect of tubocurarine is a fall in arterial pressure, due to (a) sympathetic ganglion block and (b) histamine release from mast cells (see Ch. 18), which can also give rise to bronchospasm in sensitive individuals. This is unrelated to nAChRs but also occurs with **atracurium** and **mivacurium** (as well as with some pharmacologically unrelated drugs such as morphine; see Ch. 43). Other non-depolarising blocking drugs lack these adverse effects.

[5]The risk of patients waking up paralysed during surgery, and subsequently recalling this (awareness during anaesthesia) is a serious concern.

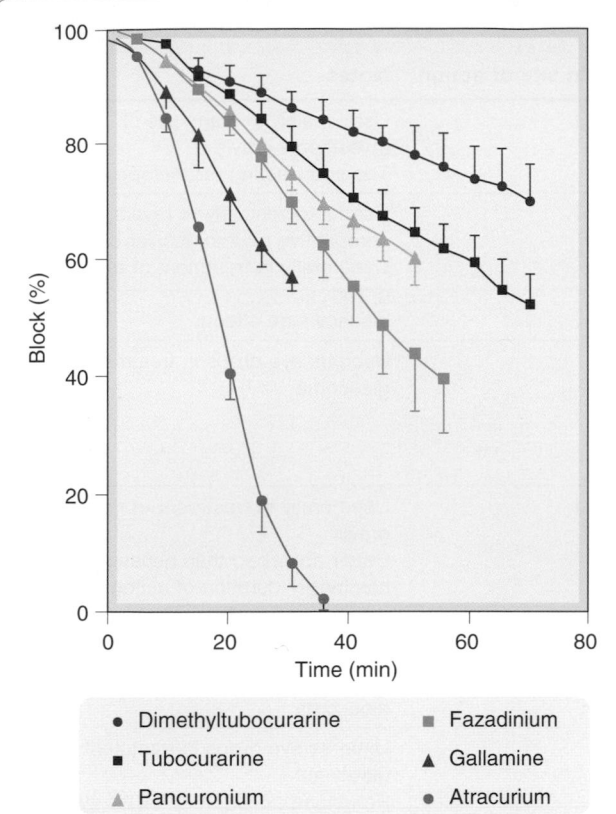

Fig. 14.6 Rate of recovery from various non-depolarising neuromuscular-blocking drugs in humans. Drugs were given intravenously to patients undergoing surgery, in doses just sufficient to cause 100% block of the tetanic tension of the indirectly stimulated adductor pollicis muscle. Recovery of tension was then followed as a function of time. (From Payne, J.P., Hughes, R., 1981. Br. J. Anaesth. 53, 45.)

Legend: Dimethyltubocurarine, Tubocurarine, Pancuronium, Fazadinium, Gallamine, Atracurium

Pancuronium also blocks mAChRs, particularly in the heart, causing tachycardia.

Pharmacokinetic aspects
Neuromuscular-blocking drugs are given intravenously. They differ in their rates of onset and recovery (Fig. 14.6 and Table 14.7).

Most non-depolarising blocking agents are metabolised by the liver or excreted unchanged in the urine, exceptions being **atracurium**, which hydrolyses spontaneously in plasma, and **mivacurium**, which, like **suxamethonium** (see later), is hydrolysed by plasma cholinesterase. Their duration of action varies between about 15 min and 1–2 h (see Table 14.7), by which time the patient regains enough strength to cough and breathe properly. The route of elimination is important, because many patients undergoing anaesthesia have impaired renal or hepatic function, which can enhance or prolong paralysis to an important degree.

Atracurium was designed to be chemically unstable at physiological pH (splitting into two inactive fragments by cleavage at one of the quaternary nitrogen atoms), although stable when stored at an acid pH. It has a short duration of action, which is unaffected by renal or hepatic function. Because of the marked pH dependence of its degradation, however, its action becomes considerably briefer during respiratory alkalosis caused by hyperventilation.

Rapid postoperative recovery of muscle strength after surgery is important to minimise respiratory complications. The cholinesterase inhibitor, **neostigmine** (Table 14.8) is often used to reverse the action of non-depolarising drugs postoperatively. Co-administration of atropine is necessary to prevent unwanted parasympathomimetic effects.

▼ Anticholinesterase drugs *overcome* the blocking action of non-depolarising agents because released ACh, protected from hydrolysis, can diffuse further within the synaptic cleft and so access a wider area of postsynaptic membrane. The chances of an ACh molecule finding an unoccupied receptor before being hydrolysed are thus increased. This diffusional effect seems to be more important than a truly competitive interaction, for it is unlikely that appreciable dissociation of the antagonist can occur in the short time for which the ACh is present. In contrast, depolarisation block is unaffected by anticholinesterase drugs, or even increased via potentiation of the depolarising action of endogenous ACh.

An alternative approach for reversal of neuromuscular blockade induced by **rocuronium** or **vecuronium** is the use of a synthetic cyclodextrin, **sugammadex**, a macromolecule that selectively binds steroidal neuromuscular-blocking drugs as an inactive complex in the plasma (Nicholson et al., 2007). The complex is excreted unchanged in the urine. Sugammadex rapidly reverses block with few unwanted effects.

DEPOLARISING BLOCKING AGENTS

Suxamethonium is the only depolarising agent used clinically. There are several differences in the pattern of neuromuscular block produced by depolarising and non-depolarising mechanisms:

- Fasciculation, seen with suxamethonium (see Table 14.7) as a prelude to paralysis, does not occur with non-depolarising drugs. Its severity is linked to postoperative muscle pain experienced after suxamethonium.
- *Tetanic fade* (see earlier) occurs with non-depolarising blocking drugs, but not with suxamethonium, which does not block presynaptic nAChRs.

Unwanted effects and dangers of suxamethonium
Suxamethonium has several adverse effects (see Table 14.7), but remains in use for short-lasting procedures because of the rapid recovery that follows its intravenous administration.

Bradycardia. This is preventable by atropine and is due to a direct muscarinic action.

Potassium release. The increase in cation permeability of the motor endplates causes a net loss of K^+ from muscle, and thus a small rise in plasma K^+ concentration. This is not usually important, but may be an issue following trauma, burns or injuries causing muscle denervation (Fig. 14.7). Denervation increases the rise in plasma K^+ caused by suxamethonium because it causes ACh receptors to spread to regions of the muscle fibre away from the endplates (see Ch. 13), so that a much larger area of membrane is sensitive to suxamethonium. The resulting hyperkalaemia can be enough to cause ventricular dysrhythmia or cardiac arrest.

Increased intraocular pressure. Extraocular muscles are unusual in containing a population of fibres with nAChRs distributed along their length, rather than localised at motor endplates; these respond to suxamethonium with a sustained contracture, applying pressure to the eyeball. It is particularly important to avoid this if the eyeball has been injured.

Table 14.8 Anticholinesterase drugs

Drug	Structure	Duration of action	Main site of action	Notes
Edrophonium		Short	NMJ	Used mainly in diagnosis of myasthenia gravis Too short-acting for therapeutic use
Neostigmine		Medium	NMJ	Used intravenously to reverse competitive neuromuscular block Used orally in treatment of myasthenia gravis Visceral side effects
Physostigmine		Medium	P	Used as eye drops in treatment of glaucoma
Pyridostigmine		Medium	NMJ	Used orally in treatment of myasthenia gravis Better absorbed than neostigmine and has longer duration of action
Dyflos		Long	P	Highly toxic organophosphate, with very prolonged action Has been used as eye drops for glaucoma
Ecothiophate		Long	P	Used as eye drops in treatment of glaucoma Prolonged action; may cause systemic effects
Parathion		Long	–	Converted to active metabolite by replacement of sulfur by oxygen Used as insecticide but also causes poisoning in humans

Other anticholinesterase drugs developed for the treatment of dementia are described in Chapter 41.
NMJ, neuromuscular junction; *P*, postganglionic parasympathetic junction.

Prolonged paralysis. The action of suxamethonium, given as an intravenous bolus to achieve relaxation during tracheal intubation, normally lasts for only 2–6 min, because the drug is hydrolysed by plasma cholinesterase. Its action is prolonged by various factors that reduce the activity of this enzyme:

- Genetic variants of plasma cholinesterase with reduced activity (see Ch. 12). Severe deficiency, enough to increase the duration of action to 2 h or more, occurs in approximately 1 in 3500 individuals. Rarely, the enzyme is completely absent and paralysis lasts for many hours. Biochemical testing of enzyme activity in the plasma and its sensitivity to inhibitors is used clinically to diagnose this problem; genotyping is possible but as yet not practicable for routine screening to prevent the problem.
- Anticholinesterase drugs. The use of organophosphates to treat glaucoma (see Table 14.4) can inhibit plasma cholinesterase and prolong the action of suxamethonium. Competing substrates for plasma cholinesterase (e.g. **procaine**, **propanidid**) can also have this effect.

- Neonates may have low plasma cholinesterase activity and experience prolonged paralysis if treated with suxamethonium.

Malignant hyperpyrexia. This is a rare inherited condition, due to a mutation of the Ca^{2+} release channel of the sarcoplasmic reticulum (the ryanodine receptor, see Ch. 4), which results in intense muscle spasm and a dramatic rise in body temperature when certain drugs are given (see Ch. 12). Suxamethonium is now the commonest culprit, although an episode of malignant hyperpyrexia can also be precipitated by a variety of other drugs. The condition carries a high mortality (about 65%) and is treated by administration of **dantrolene**, a drug that inhibits muscle contraction by preventing Ca^{2+} release from the sarcoplasmic reticulum.

DRUGS THAT ACT PRESYNAPTICALLY
DRUGS THAT INHIBIT ACETYLCHOLINE SYNTHESIS

The steps in the synthesis of ACh in the presynaptic nerve terminals are shown in Fig. 14.2. The rate-limiting process appears to be the transport of choline into the nerve terminal. **Hemicholinium** blocks this transport and thereby inhibits ACh synthesis. It is useful as an experimental tool but has

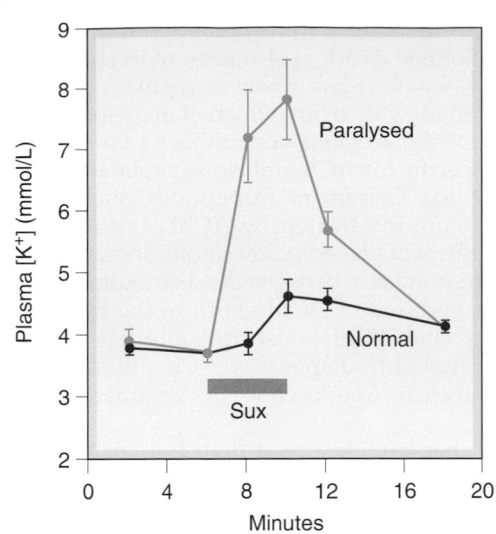

Fig. 14.7 **Effect of suxamethonium (Sux) on plasma potassium concentration in humans.** Blood was collected from veins draining paralysed and non-paralysed limbs of seven injured patients undergoing surgery. The injuries had resulted in motor nerve degeneration, and hence denervation supersensitivity of the affected muscles. (From Tobey, R.E. et al., 1972. Anaesthesiology 37, 322.)

Neuromuscular-blocking drugs

- Substances that block choline uptake: for example, **hemicholinium** (not used clinically).
- Substances that block acetylcholine release: **aminoglycoside antibiotics**, **botulinum toxin**.
- Drugs used to cause paralysis during anaesthesia comprise:
  - Depolarising neuromuscular-blocking agents: **suxamethonium**, short-acting and used during induction of anaesthesia and intubation of the airway.
  - Non-depolarising neuromuscular-blocking agents: **tubocurarine**, **pancuronium**, **atracurium**, **vecuronium**, **mivacuronium**. These block nicotinic acetylcholine receptors and differ mainly in duration of action; they are used to maintain neuromuscular relaxation throughout a surgical operation, or in patients in an intensive care unit who may otherwise experience muscular spasm or involuntary movement.
- Important characteristics of non-depolarising and depolarising blocking drugs:
  - Non-depolarising block is reversible by anticholinesterase drugs, depolarising block is not.
  - Steroidal ('curonium') drugs (**rocuronium**, **vecuronium**) are reversed by **sugammadex**.
  - Depolarising block produces initial fasciculations and often postoperative muscle pain.
  - **Suxamethonium** is hydrolysed by plasma cholinesterase and is normally very short-acting, but may cause long-lasting paralysis in congenitally cholinesterase-deficient individuals.
- Main side effects: early curare derivatives caused ganglion block, histamine release and hence hypotension and bronchoconstriction; newer non-depolarising blocking drugs have fewer side effects; **suxamethonium** may cause bradycardia, cardiac dysrhythmias due to K^+ release (especially in burned or injured patients), increased intraocular pressure, or (in rare genetically susceptible individuals) malignant hyperthermia.

no clinical applications. Its blocking effect on transmission develops slowly, as the existing stores of ACh become depleted. **Vesamicol**, which acts by blocking ACh transport into synaptic vesicles, has a similar effect.

DRUGS THAT INHIBIT ACETYLCHOLINE RELEASE

ACh release by a nerve impulse involves the entry of Ca^{2+} into the nerve terminal; the increase in $[Ca^{2+}]_i$ stimulates exocytosis and increases the rate of quantal release (see Fig. 14.2). Agents that inhibit Ca^{2+} entry include Mg^{2+} and various aminoglycoside antibiotics (e.g. **streptomycin** and **neomycin**; see Ch. 52), which can unpredictably prolong muscle paralysis when used clinically in patients treated with neuromuscular-blocking agents as an adjunct to general anaesthesia.

Two potent neurotoxins, namely **botulinum toxin** and **β-bungarotoxin**, act specifically to inhibit ACh release. Botulinum toxin is a protein produced by the anaerobic bacillus *Clostridium botulinum*, an organism that can multiply in preserved food and can cause botulism, an extremely serious type of food poisoning.[6]

▼ The potency of botulinum toxin is extraordinary, the minimum lethal dose in a mouse being less than 10^{-12} g – only a few million molecules. It belongs to the group of potent bacterial exotoxins that includes tetanus and diphtheria toxins. They possess two subunits, one of which binds to a membrane receptor and is responsible for cellular specificity. By this means, the toxin enters the cell, where the other subunit produces the toxic effect. Botulinum toxin contains several components (A–G, see Zhongxing Peng Chen et al., 2012). They are peptidases that cleave specific proteins involved in exocytosis (*synaptobrevins*, *syntaxins*, etc.; see Ch. 4), thereby producing a long-lasting block of synaptic function. Each toxin component inactivates a different functional protein – a remarkably coordinated attack by a humble bacterium on a vital component of mammalian physiology.

Botulinum poisoning causes progressive parasympathetic and motor paralysis, with dry mouth, blurred vision and difficulty in swallowing, followed by progressive respiratory paralysis. Treatment with antitoxin is effective only if given before symptoms appear, for once the toxin is bound its action cannot be reversed. Mortality is high, and recovery takes several weeks. Anticholinesterases and drugs that increase transmitter release are ineffective in restoring transmission. **Botulinum toxin**, given by local injection, has a number of clinical and cosmetic uses (a testament to

---

[6]Among the more spectacular outbreaks of botulinum poisoning was an incident on Loch Maree in Scotland in 1922, when all eight members of a fishing party died after eating duck pâté for their lunch. Their ghillies, consuming humbler fare no doubt, survived. The innkeeper committed suicide.

Paracelsus' dictum that all drugs are poisons, the distinction lying in the dose), including:

- *blepharospasm* (persistent and disabling eyelid spasm) and other forms of unwanted movement disorder including *torsion dystonia* and *spasmodic torticollis* (twisting movements of, respectively, limbs or neck);
- *spasticity* (excessive extensor muscle tone, associated with developmental brain abnormalities or birth injury);
- *urinary incontinence* associated with bladder overactivity (given by intravesical injection);
- *squint* (given by injection into extraocular muscles);
- *hyperhidrosis* (injected intradermally into axillary skin), for excessive sweating resistant to other treatment;
- *sialorrhoea* (excessive salivary secretion);
- *headache prophylaxis* (in adults with chronic migraine and frequent headaches);
- *forehead wrinkles* (injected intradermally it removes frown lines by paralysing the superficial muscles that pucker the skin).

Injections need to be repeated every few months. Botulinum toxin is antigenic, and may lose its effectiveness due to its immunogenicity. There is a risk of more general muscle paralysis if the toxin spreads beyond the injected region.

▼ β-Bungarotoxin is a protein contained in the venom of various snakes of the cobra family, and has a similar action to botulinum toxin, although its active component is a phospholipase rather than a peptidase. The same venoms also contain α-bungarotoxin (Ch. 3), which blocks postsynaptic ACh receptors. These snakes evidently cover all eventualities as far as causing paralysis of their victims is concerned.

DRUGS THAT ENHANCE CHOLINERGIC TRANSMISSION

Drugs that enhance cholinergic transmission act either by inhibiting cholinesterase (the main group) or by increasing ACh release. In this chapter, we focus on the peripheral actions of such drugs; drugs affecting cholinergic transmission in the CNS, used to treat senile dementia, are discussed in Chapter 41, which also mentions *spinal muscular atrophy* – a rare disorder characterised by degeneration of the anterior horn cells in the spinal cord and motor nuclei in the lower brainstem resulting in clinical features reminiscent of infant botulism and caused by loss of a survival protein in the motoneurones. Such patients may be treated with **nusinersen**, an antisense oligonucleotide designed to increase expression of the survival protein and administered intrathecally (see Chs 9, 40, 41).

DISTRIBUTION AND FUNCTION OF CHOLINESTERASE

There are two distinct types of cholinesterase, namely *acetylcholinesterase* (*AChE*) and *butyrylcholinesterase* (BuChE, sometimes called pseudocholinesterase), closely related in molecular structure but differing in their distribution, substrate specificity and functions. Both consist of globular catalytic subunits, which constitute the soluble forms found in plasma (BuChE) and cerebrospinal fluid (AChE). Elsewhere, the catalytic units are linked to accessory proteins, which tether them like a bunch of balloons to the basement membrane (at the neuromuscular junction) or to the neuronal membrane at neuronal synapses (and also, oddly, the erythrocyte membrane, where the function of the enzyme is unknown).

The bound AChE at cholinergic synapses serves to hydrolyse the released transmitter and terminate its action rapidly. Soluble AChE is also present in cholinergic nerve terminals, where it has a role in regulating the free ACh concentration, and from which it may be secreted; the function of the secreted enzyme is so far unclear. AChE is quite specific for ACh and closely related esters such as methacholine. Certain neuropeptides, such as substance P (Ch. 19) are inactivated by AChE, but it is not known whether this is of physiological significance. Overall, there is poor correspondence between the distribution of cholinergic synapses and that of AChE, both in the brain and in the periphery, and AChE most probably has synaptic functions additional to disposal of ACh, although the details remain unclear (see review by Zimmerman & Soreq, 2006).

BuChE has a widespread distribution, being found in tissues such as liver, skin, brain and gastrointestinal smooth muscle, as well as in soluble form in the plasma. It is not particularly associated with cholinergic synapses, and its physiological function is unclear. It has a broader substrate specificity than AChE. It hydrolyses the synthetic substrate butyrylcholine more rapidly than ACh, as well as other esters, such as **procaine**, **suxamethonium** and **propanidid** (a short-acting anaesthetic agent; see Ch. 42). The plasma enzyme is important in relation to the inactivation of the drugs listed previously. Genetic variants of BuChE causing significantly reduced enzymic activity occur rarely (see Ch. 12), and these partly account for the variability in the duration of action of these drugs. The short duration of action of ACh given intravenously (see Fig. 14.1) results from its rapid hydrolysis in the plasma. Normally, AChE and BuChE between them keep the plasma ACh at an undetectably low level, so ACh is strictly a neurotransmitter and not a hormone.

▼ Both AChE and BuChE belong to the class of serine hydrolases, which includes many proteases such as trypsin. The active site of AChE comprises two distinct regions (Fig. 14.8): an *anionic site* (glutamate residue), which binds the basic (choline) moiety of ACh; and an *esteratic (catalytic) site* (histidine + serine). As with other serine hydrolases, the acidic (acetyl) group of the substrate is transferred to the serine hydroxyl group, leaving (transiently) an acetylated enzyme molecule and a molecule of free choline. Spontaneous hydrolysis of the serine acetyl group occurs rapidly, and the overall turnover number of AChE is extremely high (over 10,000 molecules of ACh hydrolysed per second by a single active site).

DRUGS THAT INHIBIT CHOLINESTERASE

Peripherally acting anticholinesterase drugs, summarised in Table 14.8, fall into three main groups according to the nature of their interaction with the active site, which determines their duration of action. Most of them inhibit AChE and BuChE about equally. Centrally acting anticholinesterases, developed for the treatment of dementia, are discussed in Chapter 41.

Short-acting anticholinesterases

The only important drug of this type is **edrophonium**, a quaternary ammonium compound that binds to the anionic site of the enzyme only. The ionic bond formed is readily reversible, and the action of the drug is very brief. It is used mainly for diagnostic purposes, because improvement of muscle strength by an anticholinesterase is characteristic of myasthenia gravis (see pp. 195–196) but does not occur when muscle weakness is due to other causes.

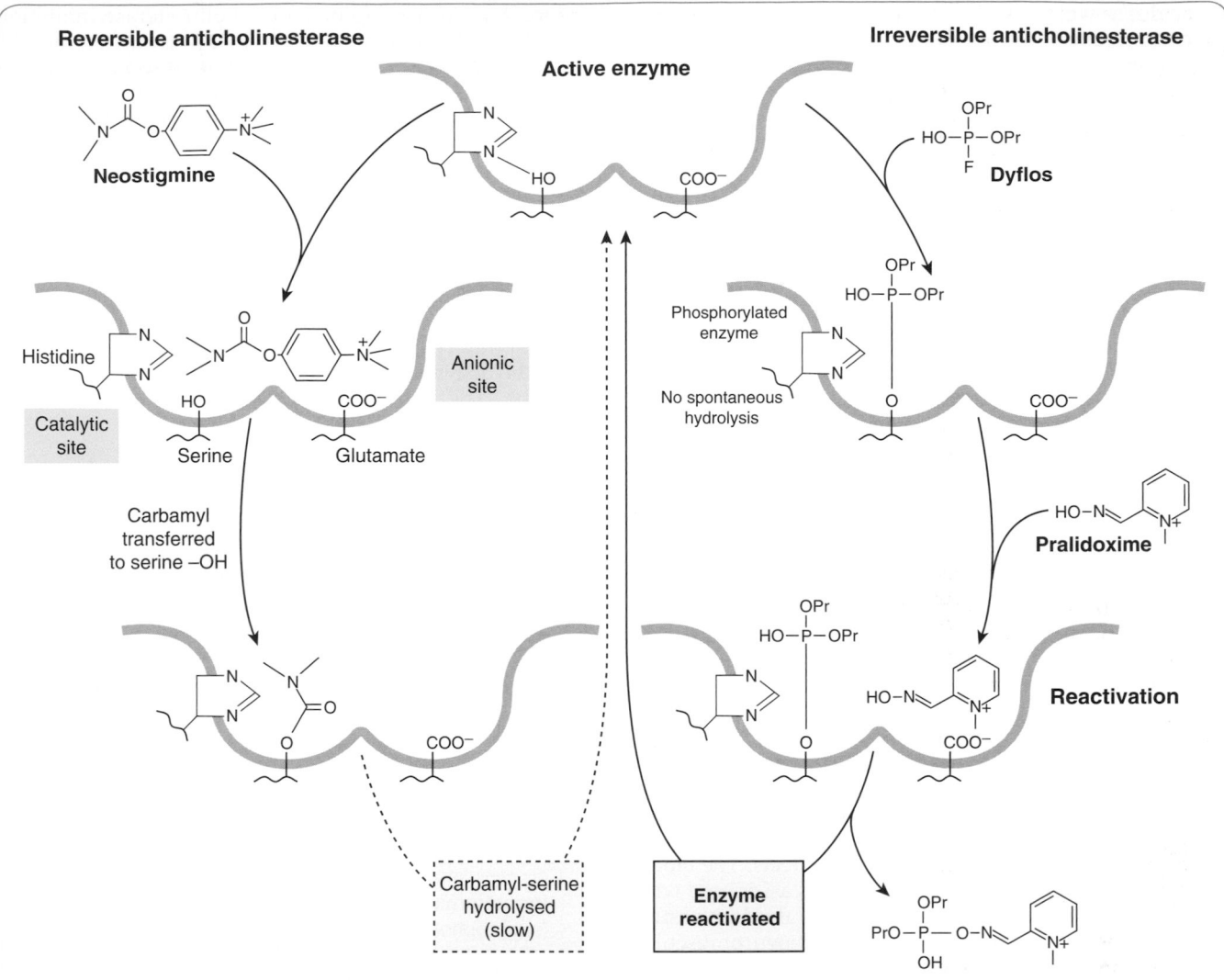

Fig. 14.8 Action of anticholinesterase drugs. Reversible anticholinesterase (neostigmine): recovery of activity by hydrolysis of the carbamylated enzyme takes many minutes. Irreversible anticholinesterase (dyflos): reactivation of phosphorylated enzyme by pralidoxime. The representation of the active site is purely diagrammatic and by no means representative of the actual molecular structure.

Medium-duration anticholinesterases

These include **neostigmine** and **pyridostigmine**, which are quaternary ammonium compounds of clinical importance, and **physostigmine** (eserine), a tertiary amine, which occurs naturally in the Calabar bean.[7]

These drugs are all carbamyl, as opposed to acetyl, esters and all possess basic groups that bind to the anionic site. Transfer of the carbamyl group to the serine hydroxyl group of the esteratic site occurs as with ACh, but the carbamylated enzyme is very much slower to hydrolyse (see Fig. 14.8), taking minutes rather than microseconds. The anticholinesterase drug is therefore hydrolysed, but at a negligible rate compared with ACh, and the slow recovery of the carbamylated enzyme means that the action of these drugs is quite long-lasting.

Donepezil is a CNS-active drug developed for the treatment of Alzheimer's disease (Ch. 41).

Irreversible anticholinesterases

Irreversible anticholinesterases (see Table 14.8) are pentavalent phosphorus compounds containing a labile group such as fluoride (in **dyflos**) or an organic group (in **parathion** and **ecothiophate**). This group is released, leaving the serine hydroxyl group of the enzyme phosphorylated (see Fig. 14.8). Most of these organophosphate compounds, of which there are many, were developed as weapons, such as **sarin,** and the more potent **VX** (10 mg of which through skin contact is said to be fatal) which acquired notoriety as an agent of state-sponsored assassination.[8] Some are used as

[7]Otherwise known as the ordeal bean. In the Middle Ages, extracts of these beans were used to determine the guilt or innocence of those accused of crime or heresy. Death implied guilt.

[8]On February 13, 2017, Kin Jong-nam, half-brother of North Korean leader Kim Jong-un, died after an assault in Kuala Lumpur International Airport. According to the authorities he was murdered by poisoning with VX, which was found on his face. The authorities further reported that one of the women suspected of applying the nerve agent experienced some physical symptoms of VX poisoning. The director of a research program of the Middlebury Institute of International Studies at Monterey stated that VX fumes would have killed the suspected attackers even if they had been wearing gloves, suggesting that the VX was applied as two non-lethal components that would mix to form VX only on the victim's face. (Wikipedia, accessed July 30, 2017).

pesticides as well as for clinical use; they interact only with the esteratic site of the enzyme and have no cationic group. **Ecothiophate** is an exception in having a quaternary nitrogen group designed to bind also to the anionic site.

The inactive phosphorylated enzyme is usually very stable. With drugs such as dyflos, no appreciable hydrolysis occurs, and recovery of enzymic activity depends on the synthesis of new enzyme molecules, a process that may take weeks. With other drugs, such as ecothiophate, hydrolysis occurs over the course of a few days, so that their action is not strictly irreversible. Dyflos and parathion are volatile non-polar substances of very high lipid solubility, and are rapidly absorbed through mucous membranes and even through unbroken skin and insect cuticles; the use of these agents as war gases or insecticides relies on this property. The lack of a specificity-conferring quaternary group means that most of these drugs block other serine hydrolases (e.g. trypsin, thrombin), although their pharmacological effects result mainly from cholinesterase inhibition.

Effects of anticholinesterase drugs
Cholinesterase inhibitors affect peripheral as well as central cholinergic synapses.

Some organophosphate compounds can produce, in addition, a severe form of neurotoxicity.

Effects on autonomic cholinergic synapses. These mainly reflect enhancement of ACh activity at parasympathetic postganglionic synapses (i.e. increased secretions from salivary, lacrimal, bronchial and gastrointestinal glands; increased peristaltic activity; bronchoconstriction; bradycardia and hypotension; pupillary constriction; fixation of accommodation for near vision; fall in intraocular pressure). Large doses can stimulate, and later block, autonomic ganglia, producing complex autonomic effects. The block, if it occurs, is a depolarisation block and is associated with a build-up of ACh in the plasma and body fluids. Neostigmine and pyridostigmine tend to affect neuromuscular transmission more than the autonomic system, whereas physostigmine and organophosphates show the reverse pattern. The reason is not clear, but therapeutic usage takes advantage of this partial selectivity.

Acute anticholinesterase poisoning (e.g. from contact with insecticides or war gases) causes severe bradycardia, hypotension and difficulty in breathing. Combined with a depolarising neuromuscular block and central effects (see below), the result may be fatal.

Effects on the neuromuscular junction. The twitch tension of a muscle stimulated via its motor nerve is increased by anticholinesterases, owing to repetitive firing in the muscle fibre associated with prolongation of the epp. Normally, the ACh is hydrolysed so quickly that each stimulus initiates only one action potential in the muscle fibre, but when AChE is inhibited this is converted to a short train of action potentials in the muscle fibre, and hence greater tension. Much more important is the effect produced when transmission has been blocked by a non-depolarising blocking agent such as pancuronium. In this case, addition of an anticholinesterase can dramatically restore transmission. If a large proportion of the receptors is blocked, the majority of ACh molecules will normally encounter, and be destroyed by, an AChE molecule before reaching a vacant receptor; inhibiting AChE gives the ACh molecules a greater chance of finding a vacant receptor before being destroyed, and thus increase the epp so that it reaches threshold. In myasthenia gravis (see pp. 195–196), transmission fails because there

are too few ACh receptors, and cholinesterase inhibition improves transmission just as it does in curarised muscle.

In large doses, such as can occur in poisoning, anticholinesterases initially cause twitching of muscles. This is because spontaneous ACh release can give rise to endplate potentials that reach the firing threshold. Later, paralysis may occur due to depolarisation block, which is associated with the build-up of ACh.

Effects on the CNS. Tertiary compounds, such as physostigmine, and the non-polar organophosphates penetrate the blood–brain barrier freely and affect the brain. The result is an initial excitation, which can result in convulsions, followed by depression, which can cause unconsciousness and respiratory failure. These central effects result mainly from the activation of mAChRs, and are antagonised by atropine. The use of anticholinesterases to treat senile dementia is discussed in Chapter 41.

Cholinesterase and anticholinesterase drugs

- There are two main forms of cholinesterase: *acetylcholinesterase* (AChE), which is mainly membrane-bound, relatively specific for acetylcholine, and responsible for rapid acetylcholine hydrolysis at cholinergic synapses; and *butyrylcholinesterase* (BuChE) or pseudocholinesterase, which is relatively non-selective and occurs in plasma and many tissues. Both enzymes belong to the family of serine hydrolases.
- Anticholinesterase drugs are of three main types: short-acting (**edrophonium**); medium-acting (**neostigmine**, **physostigmine**); irreversible (organophosphates, **dyflos**, **ecothiophate**). They differ in the nature of their chemical interaction with the active site of cholinesterase.
- Effects of anticholinesterase drugs are due mainly to enhancement of cholinergic transmission at cholinergic autonomic synapses and at the neuromuscular junction. Anticholinesterases that cross the blood–brain barrier (e.g. **physostigmine**, organophosphates) also have marked central nervous system effects. Autonomic effects include bradycardia, hypotension, excessive secretions, bronchoconstriction, gastrointestinal hypermotility and decrease of intraocular pressure. Neuromuscular action causes muscle fasciculation and increased twitch tension, and can produce depolarisation block.
- Anticholinesterase poisoning may occur from exposure to insecticides or nerve gases.

Toxicity of organophosphates. Many organophosphates can cause a severe type of delayed peripheral nerve degeneration, leading to progressive weakness and sensory loss. This is not a problem with clinically used anticholinesterases but occasionally results from poisoning with insecticides or nerve gases. In 1931, an estimated 20,000 Americans were affected, some fatally, by contamination of fruit juice with an organophosphate insecticide, and other similar outbreaks have been recorded. The mechanism of this reaction is only partly understood, but it seems to result from inhibition of a *neuropathy target esterase* distinct from cholinesterase. Chronic low-level exposure of agricultural and other workers to organophosphorous pesticides has been associated with neurobehavioural disorders (Blanc-Lapierre et al., 2013). Other serine hydrolases apart from acetylcholinesterase can be secondary organophosphate targets including neuropathy target esterase, lipases, and endocannabinoid hydrolases (Casida, 2017).

The main uses of anticholinesterases are summarised in the clinical box (see below).

Clinical uses of anticholinesterase drugs

- To reverse the action of non-depolarising neuromuscular-blocking drugs after surgery (**neostigmine**). **Atropine** must be given to limit parasympathomimetic effects.
- To treat myasthenia gravis (**neostigmine** or **pyridostigmine**).
- As a test for myasthenia gravis and to distinguish weakness caused by anticholinesterase overdosage ('cholinergic crisis') from the weakness of myasthenia itself ('myasthenic crisis'): **edrophonium**, a short-acting drug given intravenously.
- Alzheimer's disease (e.g. **donepezil**; see Ch. 41).
- Glaucoma (**ecothiophate** eye drops).

CHOLINESTERASE REACTIVATION

Spontaneous hydrolysis of phosphorylated cholinesterase is extremely slow, so poisoning with organophosphates necessitates prolonged supportive care. **Pralidoxime** (see Fig. 14.8) reactivates the enzyme by bringing an oxime group into close proximity with the phosphorylated esteratic site. This group is a strong nucleophile and lures the phosphate group away from the serine hydroxyl group of the enzyme. The effectiveness of pralidoxime in reactivating plasma cholinesterase activity in a poisoned subject is shown in Fig. 14.9. The main limitation to its use as an antidote

Fig. 14.9 Reactivation of plasma cholinesterase (ChE) in a volunteer subject by intravenous injection of pralidoxime.

to organophosphate poisoning is that, within a few hours, the phosphorylated enzyme undergoes a chemical change ('ageing') that renders it no longer susceptible to reactivation, so that pralidoxime must be given early in order to work. Pralidoxime does not enter the brain, but related compounds have been developed to treat the central effects of organophosphate poisoning.

Myasthenia gravis

▼ The neuromuscular junction is a robust structure that very rarely fails, myasthenia gravis and the Lambert–Eaton myasthenic syndrome (see p. 196) being two of the few disorders that specifically affect it. Myasthenia gravis affects about 1 in 2000 individuals, often, but by no means always, young women who are particularly susceptible to autoimmune disorders. It is characterised by weakness and increased fatigability of skeletal muscles resulting from impaired neuromuscular transmission. The tendency for transmission to fail during repetitive activity can be seen in Fig. 14.10. Muscles cannot produce prolonged contractions, resulting in the characteristic drooping eyelids and double vision on attempting to sustain lateral gaze. The effectiveness of anticholinesterase drugs in improving muscle strength in myasthenia was discovered in 1931, long before the pathophysiology of the disease was understood.

The cause of the transmission failure is an autoimmune response to nAChRs of the neuromuscular junction, first revealed in studies showing that the number of bungarotoxin-binding sites at the endplates of myasthenic patients was reduced by about 70% compared with normal. It had been suspected that myasthenia had an immunological basis, because the disease is sometimes accompanied by a tumour of the thymus gland and removal of the thymus improves the motor symptoms. Immunisation of rabbits with purified ACh receptor causes, after a delay, a disorder very similar to human myasthenia gravis. The presence of antibody directed against the ACh receptor protein can be detected in the serum of myasthenic patients, but the reason

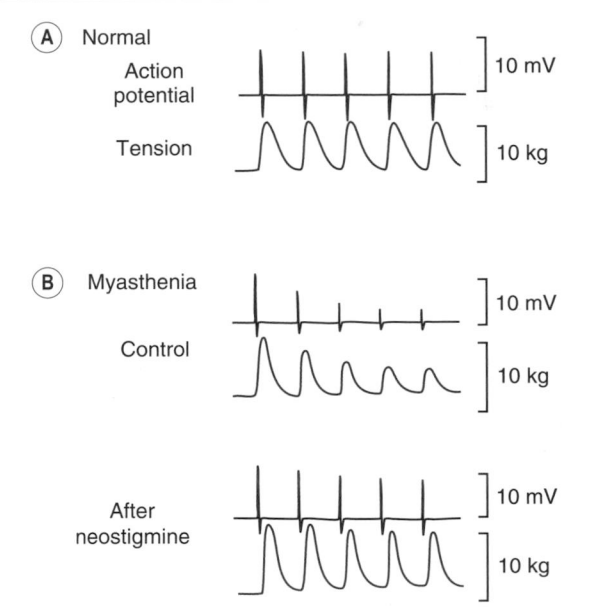

Fig. 14.10 Neuromuscular transmission in a normal and a myasthenic human subject. Electrical activity was recorded with a needle electrode in the adductor pollicis muscle, in response to ulnar nerve stimulation (3 Hz) at the wrist. In a normal subject, electrical and mechanical response is well sustained. In a myasthenic patient, transmission fails rapidly when the nerve is stimulated. Treatment with neostigmine improves transmission. (From Desmedt, J.E., 1962. Bull. Acad. R. Med. Belg. VII 2, 213.)

for the development of the autoimmune response in humans is unknown (Gilhus, 2016).

The improvement of neuromuscular function by anticholinesterase treatment (shown in Fig. 14.10) can be dramatic, but if the disease progresses too far, the number of receptors remaining may be insufficient to produce an adequate epp, and anticholinesterase drugs will then cease to be effective.

Alternative approaches to the treatment of myasthenia are to remove circulating antibody by plasma exchange, which is transiently effective, or, for a more prolonged effect, to inhibit antibody production with immunosuppressant drugs (e.g. **prednisolone, azathioprine, mycophenolate, cyclosporine** and **tacrolimus**; see Ch. 27) or thymectomy.

OTHER DRUGS THAT ENHANCE CHOLINERGIC TRANSMISSION

It was observed many years ago that **tetraethylammonium**, a potassium-channel blocker and ganglion-blocking drug, could reverse the neuromuscular-blocking action of tubocurarine by prolonging the action potential in the nerve terminal and hence increasing the release of transmitter evoked by nerve stimulation. Subsequently, more potent and selective potassium-channel blocking drugs, such as **amifampridine**, were developed. These drugs are not selective for cholinergic nerves but increase the evoked release of many different transmitters. Amifampridine is used to treat the muscle weakness associated with Lambert–Eaton myasthenic syndrome, a complication of certain neoplastic diseases in which ACh release is inhibited because antitumour antibodies cross react with Ca^{2+} channels on the prejunctional membrane.

REFERENCES AND FURTHER READING

Further reading

Changeux, J.P., 2012. The nicotinic acetylcholine receptor: the founding father of the pentameric ligand-gated ion channel superfamily. J. Biol. Chem. 287, 40207–40215. (*Min-review describing how electrophysiology, pharmacology, and biochemistry joined forces to identify the mechanisms that transduce a chemical signal into an electrical one. The nicotinic receptor is the founding father of the family of pentameric membrane receptors – see Fig. 3.4*)

Fagerlund, M.J., Eriksson, L.I., 2009. Current concepts in neuromuscular transmission. Br. J. Anaesth. 103, 108–114. (*Concentrates on findings of potential clinical importance*)

Nicholls, J.G., Martin, A.R., Fuchs, P.A., Brown, D.A., Diamond, M.E., Weisblat, D., 2012. From neuron to brain, fifth ed. Sinauer, Sunderland. (*Excellent general textbook*)

Acetylcholine receptors

Carruthers, S.P., Gurrich, C.T., Rossell, S.L., 2015. The muscarinic system, cognition and schizophrenia. Neurosci. Biobehav. Rev. 55, 393–402. (*M1 and M4 receptor manipulation has promise in treatment of cognitive impairment in schizophrenia*)

Dinely, K.T., Pandya, A.A., Yakel, J.L., 2015. Nicotinic ACh receptors as therapeutic targets in CNS disorders. Trends Pharmacol. Sci. 36, 96–108. (*nACh receptors are widely distributed in CNS neurons and non-neuronal cells, and participate in anxiety, the central processing of pain, food intake, nicotine-seeking behavior, and cognitive function. Nine different subunits occur in mammalian brain, assembled into diverse pentameric complexes*)

Kalamida, D., Poulas, K., Avramopoulou, V., et al., 2007. Muscle and neuronal nicotinic acetylcholine receptors: structure, function and pathogenicity. FEBS J. 274, 3799–3845. (*Excellent comprehensive review*)

Kruse, A.C., Kobilka, B.K., Gautam, D., et al., 2014. Muscarinic acetylcholine receptors: novel opportunities for drug development. Nat. Rev. Drug Discov. 13, 549–560. (*Solution of resting and active receptor structures and insight into allosteric control should lead to new muscarinic receptor subtype-selective drugs*)

Nickols, H.H., Conn, P.J., 2014. Development of allosteric modulators of GPCRs for the treatment of CNS disorders. Neurobiol. Dis. 61 (Special Issue), SI 55–SI 71. (*Describes development of novel allosteric modulators [including modulators of muscarinic receptors] as potential therapeutic agents*)

Southan, C., Sharman, J.L., Benson, H.E., et al., 2016. The IUPHAR/BPS Guide to Pharmacology in 2016: towards curated quantitative interactions between 1300 protein targets and 6000 ligands. Nucl. Acids Res. 44 (Database Issue), D1054–D1068. (*See Acetylcholine receptors (muscarinic), Nicotinic acetylcholine receptors*)

Wessler, I., Kirkpatrick, C.J., 2008. Acetylcholine beyond neurons: the non-neuronal cholinergic system in humans. Br. J. Pharmacol. 154, 1558–1571. (*Summarises findings that reveal surprisingly diverse roles for acetylcholine*)

Cholinergic transmission

Gilhus, N.E., 2016. Myasthenia gravis. N. Engl. Med. 375, 2570–2581. (*Recent review*)

Drugs affecting the neuromuscular junction

Peng Chen, Z., Morris, J.G., Rodriguez, R.L., Shukla, A.W., Tapia-Nunez, J., Okun, M.S., 2012. Emerging opportunities for serotypes of botulinum neurotoxins. Toxins (Basel) 4, 1196–1222. (*Reviews current research on botulinum serotypes A-G*)

Nicholson, W.T., Sprung, J., Jankowski, C.J., 2007. Sugammadex: a novel agent for the reversal of neuromuscular blockade. Pharmacotherapy 27, 1181–1188. (*An alternative to neostigmine*)

Cholinesterase

Blanc-Lapierre, A., Bouvier, G., Gruber, A., 2013. Cognitive disorders and occupational exposure to organophosphates: results from the PHYTONER Study. Am. J. Epidemiol. 177, 1086–1096. (*Cognitive disorders in vine workers may be associated with specific organophosphate exposure over long periods.*)

Casida, J., 2017. Organophosphate xenobiotic toxicology. Ann. Rev. Pharmacol. Toxicol. 57, 309–327. (*Topical review: other serine hydrolases than acetylcholinesterase can be secondary targets. "The organophosphate herbicides glyphosate and glufosinate act in plants but not animals to block aromatic amino acid and glutamine biosynthesis, respectively, with safety for crops conferred by their expression of herbicide-tolerant targets and detoxifying enzymes from bacteria."*)

Zimmerman, G., Soreq, H., 2006. Termination and beyond: acetylcholinesterase as a modulator of synaptic transmission. Cell Tissue Res. 326, 655–669. (*Review of evidence suggesting functions for AChE other than ACh hydrolysis*)

Noradrenergic transmission

OVERVIEW

Peripheral noradrenergic neurons and the structures that they innervate are fundamental components of autonomic function, and are the targets of many therapeutic drugs. In this chapter we describe the physiology of noradrenergic neurons and the properties of adrenoceptors (the receptors on which noradrenaline and adrenaline act), and discuss the various classes of drugs that affect them. For convenience, much of the pharmacological information is summarised in tables later in the chapter.

CATECHOLAMINES

Catecholamines contain a catechol moiety (a benzene ring with two adjacent hydroxyl groups) and an amine side chain (Fig. 15.1). The most important are:

- *noradrenaline (norepinephrine),* a transmitter released by sympathetic nerve terminals;
- *adrenaline (epinephrine),* a hormone secreted by chromaffin cells in the adrenal medulla;
- *dopamine,* the metabolic precursor of noradrenaline and adrenaline, also a transmitter/neuromodulator in the central nervous system (CNS);
- *isoprenaline (isoproterenol),* a synthetic derivative of noradrenaline and pharmacological tool.

CLASSIFICATION OF ADRENOCEPTORS

In 1896, Oliver and Schafer discovered that intravenous injection of extracts of adrenal gland in anaesthetised cats caused a rise in arterial pressure. Adrenaline was identified as the active principle, and was shown by Dale in 1913 to cause two distinct kinds of vascular effect, namely vasoconstriction in certain vascular beds and vasodilatation in others. Dale showed that the vasoconstrictor component disappeared if the animal was first injected with an ergot derivative[1] (see Ch. 16), and noticed that adrenaline then caused a fall, instead of a rise, in arterial pressure, reminiscent of his demonstration of the separate muscarinic and

nicotinic components of the action of acetylcholine (see Ch. 14). He avoided interpreting it in terms of different types of receptor, but later pharmacological work, beginning with that of Ahlquist, showed clearly the existence of several subclasses of adrenoceptor with distinct tissue distributions and actions (Table 15.1).

In 1948 Ahlquist found that the rank order of the potencies of various catecholamines, including adrenaline, noradrenaline and isoprenaline, fell into two distinct patterns, depending on what response was being measured. He postulated the existence of two kinds of receptor, α and β, defined in terms of agonist potencies as follows:

α: noradrenaline > adrenaline > isoprenaline
β: isoprenaline > adrenaline > noradrenaline

It was then recognised that certain ergot alkaloids, which Dale had studied, act as selective α-receptor antagonists and that Dale's adrenaline reversal experiment reflected the unmasking of the β effects of adrenaline by α-receptor blockade. Selective β-receptor antagonists were not developed until 1955, when their effects fully confirmed Ahlquist's original classification and also suggested the existence of further subdivisions of both α and β receptors. Subsequently it has emerged that there are two α-receptor subtypes (α_1 and α_2), each comprising three further subclasses (α_{1A}, α_{1B}, α_{1D} and α_{2A}, α_{2B}, α_{2C}) and three β-receptor subtypes (β_1, β_2 and β_3) – altogether nine distinct subtypes – all of which are typical G protein–coupled receptors (Table 15.2). Genetic variants of both β_1 and β_2 receptors occur in humans, and influence the effects of agonists and antagonists (see Ahles & Engelhardt, 2014). Evidence from specific agonists and antagonists, as well as studies on receptor knockout mice (Philipp & Hein, 2004), has shown that α_1 receptors are particularly important in the cardiovascular system and lower urinary tract, while α_2 receptors are predominantly neuronal, acting to inhibit transmitter release both in the brain and at autonomic nerve terminals in the periphery. The α_{2B} subtype appears to be involved in neurotransmission in the spinal cord and α_{2C} in regulating catecholamine release from adrenal medulla (Alexander et al., 2015), but the distinct functions of the different subclasses of α_1 and α_2 adrenoceptors remain for the most part unclear; they are frequently co-expressed in the same tissues, and may form heterodimers, making pharmacological analysis difficult.

Each of the three main receptor subtypes is associated with a specific second messenger system (see Table 15.2). Thus α_1 receptors are coupled through Gq to phospholipase C and produce their effects mainly by the release of intracellular Ca^{2+}; α_2 receptors couple through Gi/Go to inhibit adenylyl cyclase, and thus reduce cAMP formation as well as inhibiting Ca^{2+} channels and activating K^+ channels; and all three types of β receptor couple through Gs to stimulate adenylyl cyclase. β-Adrenoceptor agonists may act not only through cAMP formation, but also through other signal transduction pathways (e.g. the mitogen-activated protein [MAP] kinase

---

[1]Dale was a new recruit in the laboratories of the Wellcome pharmaceutical company, given the job of checking the potency of batches of adrenaline coming from the factory. He tested one batch at the end of a day's experimentation on a cat that he had earlier injected with an ergot preparation. Because it produced a fall in blood pressure rather than the expected rise, he advised that the whole expensive consignment should be rejected. Unknown to him, he was given the same sample to test a few days later, and reported it to be normal. How he explained this to Wellcome's management is not recorded.

197

Fig. 15.1 Structures of the major catecholamines.

Classification of adrenoceptors

- Main pharmacological classification into α and β subtypes, based originally on order of potency among agonists, later on selective antagonists.
- Adrenoceptor subtypes:
  - two main α-adrenoceptor subtypes, α_1 and α_2, each divided into three further subtypes (α_{1A}, α_{1B}, α_{1D} and α_{2A}, α_{2B}, α_{2C})
  - three β-adrenoceptor subtypes (β_1, β_2, β_3)
  - all belong to the superfamily of G protein–coupled receptors (see Ch. 3).
- Second messengers:
  - α_1 receptors activate phospholipase C, producing inositol trisphosphate and diacylglycerol as second messengers
  - α_2 receptors inhibit adenylyl cyclase (but cAMP is usually low), and also modulate Ca^{2+} and K^+ channels.
  - all types of β receptor stimulate adenylyl cyclase.
- The main effects of receptor activation are as follows:
  - α_1 receptors: vasoconstriction, relaxation of gastrointestinal smooth muscle, salivary secretion and hepatic glycogenolysis
  - α_2 receptors: inhibition of: transmitter release (including noradrenaline and acetylcholine release from autonomic nerves) caused by opening of K^+ channels and inhibition of Ca^{2+} channels; platelet aggregation; vascular smooth muscle contraction; inhibition of insulin release
  - β_1 receptors: increased cardiac rate and force
  - β_2 receptors: bronchodilatation; vasodilatation; relaxation of visceral smooth muscle; hepatic glycogenolysis; muscle tremor
  - $\beta3$ receptors: lipolysis and thermogenesis; bladder detrusor muscle relaxation.

pathway which may be important in trophic actions; see Ch. 3 and p. 212, later). The major effects that are produced by adrenoceptors, and the main drugs that act on them, are shown in Tables 15.1 and 15.2.

The distinction between β_1 and β_2 receptors is an important one, because β_1 receptors are found mainly in the heart, where they are responsible for the positive inotropic and chronotropic effects of catecholamines (see Ch. 22), whereas β_2 receptors are responsible for causing smooth muscle relaxation in many organs, most importantly in the lungs, where they relax the bronchioles and relieve bronchoconstriction in asthmatics, a useful therapeutic effect (see Ch. 29). The cardiac effects can be harmful, predisposing to cardiac dysrhythmia and increasing myocardial oxygen demand (see Ch. 22); consequently, considerable efforts have been made to discover selective β_2 agonists to relax smooth muscle without affecting the heart, and selective β_1 antagonists to exert a useful blocking effect on the heart without blocking β_2 receptors at the same time (see Table 15.1). The available drugs are not completely specific, and marketed selective β_1 antagonists have some action on β_2 receptors as well, which can cause unwanted effects such as bronchoconstriction.

In relation to vascular control, it is important to note that both α- and β-receptor subtypes are expressed in smooth muscle cells, nerve terminals and endothelial cells, and

their role in physiological regulation and pharmacological responses of the cardiovascular system is only partly understood (see Guimaraes & Moura, 2001).

PHYSIOLOGY OF NORADRENERGIC TRANSMISSION

THE NORADRENERGIC NEURON

Noradrenergic neurons in the periphery are postganglionic sympathetic neurons whose cell bodies are situated in sympathetic ganglia (see Ch. 13). They generally have long[2] axons that end in a series of varicosities strung along the branching terminal network. These varicosities contain numerous synaptic vesicles, which are the sites of synthesis and release of noradrenaline and of co-released mediators such as ATP and neuropeptide Y (see Ch. 13), which are

---

[2]Just how long may be appreciated by scaling up the 20 μm diameter of a neuronal cell body to that of a golf ball (~40,000 μm diameter, a scaling factor of about 2000); proportionately the axon (length from sympathetic chain ganglion to, say, a blood vessel in the calf, (approximately 1 metre in humans, never mind giraffes) will now reach about 2 km – some challenge in terms of command and control!

Table 15.1 Distribution and actions of adrenoceptors

Tissues and effects	α_1	α_2	β_1	β_2	β_3
Smooth muscle					
Blood vessels	Constrict	Constrict/dilate	—	Dilate	—
Bronchi	Constrict	—	—	Dilate	—
Gastrointestinal tract	Relax	Relax (presynaptic effect)	—	Relax	—
Gastrointestinal sphincters	Contract	—	—	—	—
Uterus	Contract	—	—	Relax	—
Bladder detrusor	—	—	—	Relax	Relax
Bladder sphincter	Contract	—	—	—	—
Seminal tract	Contract	—	—	Relax	—
Iris (radial muscle)	Contract	—	—	—	—
Ciliary muscle	—	—	—	Relax	—
Heart					
Rate	—	—	Increase	Increase[a]	—
Force of contraction	—	—	Increase	Increase[a]	—
Other tissues/cells					
Skeletal muscle	—	—	—	Tremor Increased muscle mass and speed of contraction Glycogenolysis	Thermogenesis
Liver (hepatocytes)	Glycogenolysis	—	—	Glycogenolysis	—
Fat (adipocytes)	—	—	—	—	Lipolysis Thermogenesis
Pancreatic islets (B cells)	—	Decrease insulin secretion	—	—	—
Salivary gland	K^+ release	—	Amylase secretion	—	—
Platelets	—	Aggregation	—	—	—
Mast cells	—	—	—	Inhibition of histamine release	—
Brain stem	—	Inhibits sympathetic outflow	—	—	—
Nerve terminals					
Adrenergic	—	Decrease release	—	Increase release	—
Cholinergic	—	Decrease release	—	—	—

[a]Minor component normally but may become significant in heart failure.

Table 15.2 Characteristics of adrenoceptors

	$\alpha_{1(A,B,D)}$	$\alpha_{2(A,B,C)}$	β_1	β_2	β_3
G protein coupling	Gq	Gi/Go	GS	GS	GS
Second messengers and effectors	Phospholipase C activation ↑ Inositol trisphosphate ↑ Diacylglycerol ↑ Ca^{2+}	↓ cAMP ↓ Calcium channels ↑ Potassium channels	↑ cAMP	↑ cAMP	↑ cAMP
Agonist potency order	NA > A ≫ ISO	A > NA ≫ ISO	ISO > NA > A	ISO > A > NA	ISO > NA = A
Selective agonists	Phenylephrine Methoxamine	Clonidine	Dobutamine Xamoterol	Salbutamol Terbutaline Salmeterol Formoterol Clenbuterol	Mirabegron
Selective antagonists	Prazosin Doxazocin	Yohimbine Idazoxan	Atenolol Metoprolol	Butoxamine	—

A, adrenaline; *ISO*, isoprenaline; *NA*, noradrenaline.

stored in vesicles and released by exocytosis (Ch. 4). In most peripheral tissues, the tissue content of noradrenaline closely parallels the density of the sympathetic innervation. With the exception of the adrenal medulla, sympathetic nerve terminals account for all the noradrenaline content of peripheral tissues. Organs such as the heart, spleen, vas deferens and some blood vessels are particularly rich in noradrenaline (5–50 nmol/g of tissue) and have been widely used for studies of noradrenergic transmission. For detailed information on noradrenergic neurons, see Robertson (2004) and Cooper et al. (2002).

NORADRENALINE SYNTHESIS

The biosynthetic pathway for noradrenaline synthesis is shown in Fig. 15.1 and drugs that affect noradrenaline synthesis are summarised in Table 15.6 (p. 206). The metabolic precursor for noradrenaline is *L-tyrosine*, an aromatic amino acid that is present in body fluids and is taken up by adrenergic neurons. *Tyrosine hydroxylase*, a cytosolic enzyme that catalyses the conversion of tyrosine to *dihydroxyphenylalanine* (dopa), is found only in catecholamine-containing cells. It is a rather selective enzyme; unlike other enzymes involved in catecholamine metabolism, it does not accept indole derivatives as substrates, and is not involved in 5-hydroxytryptamine (5-HT) synthesis This first hydroxylation step is the main control point for noradrenaline synthesis. Tyrosine hydroxylase is inhibited by the end product of the biosynthetic pathway, noradrenaline, and this provides the mechanism for the moment-to-moment regulation of the rate of synthesis; much slower regulation, taking hours or days, occurs by changes in the rate of production of the enzyme.

The tyrosine analogue **α-methyltyrosine** strongly inhibits tyrosine hydroxylase and has been used experimentally to block noradrenaline synthesis.

The next step, conversion of dopa to dopamine, is catalysed by *dopa decarboxylase*, a cytosolic enzyme that is not confined to catecholamine-synthesising cells. It is relatively non-specific, and catalyses the decarboxylation of various other L-aromatic amino acids, such as *L-histidine* and *L-tryptophan*, which are precursors in the synthesis of histamine (Ch. 18) and 5-HT (Ch. 16), respectively. Dopa decarboxylase activity is not rate-limiting for noradrenaline synthesis and its activity does not regulate noradrenaline synthesis.

Dopamine-β-hydroxylase (DBH) is also a relatively non-specific enzyme, but is restricted to catecholamine-synthesising cells. It is located in synaptic vesicles, mainly in membrane-bound form. A small amount of the enzyme is released from adrenergic nerve terminals in company with noradrenaline, representing the small proportion in a soluble form within the vesicle. Unlike noradrenaline, the released DBH is not subject to rapid degradation or uptake, so its concentration in plasma and body fluids can be used as an index of overall sympathetic nerve activity.

Many drugs inhibit DBH, including copper-chelating agents and **disulfiram** (a drug used mainly for its effect on ethanol metabolism; see Ch. 49). Such drugs can cause a partial depletion of noradrenaline stores and interference with sympathetic transmission. A rare genetic disorder, DBH deficiency, causes failure of noradrenaline synthesis resulting in severe orthostatic hypotension (see Ch. 23).

Phenylethanolamine N-*methyl transferase* (PNMT) catalyses the *N*-methylation of noradrenaline to form adrenaline. The main location of this enzyme is in the adrenal medulla,

which contains a population of adrenaline-releasing (A) cells separate from the smaller proportion of noradrenaline-releasing (N) cells. The A cells, which appear only after birth, lie adjacent to the adrenal cortex, and the production of PNMT is induced by an action of the steroid hormones secreted by the adrenal cortex (see Ch. 34). PNMT is also found in certain parts of the brain, where adrenaline may function as a transmitter, but little is known about its role in the CNS.

In peripheral tissues, the turnover time of noradrenaline is generally about 5–15 h, but it becomes much shorter if sympathetic nerve activity is increased. Under normal circumstances, the rate of synthesis closely matches the rate of release, so that the noradrenaline content of tissues is constant regardless of how fast it is being released.

NORADRENALINE STORAGE

Most of the noradrenaline in nerve terminals and adrenal medulla is contained in vesicles; only a little is free in the cytoplasm under normal circumstances. The concentration in the vesicles is very high (0.3–1.0 mol/L) and is maintained by the *vesicular monoamine transporter* (VMAT), which shares some features of the amine transporter responsible for noradrenaline uptake into the nerve terminal (see Ch. 13), but uses the transvesicular proton gradient as its driving force. Certain drugs, such as **reserpine** (see p. 213; Table 15.3) block this transport and cause nerve terminals to become depleted of their vesicular noradrenaline stores. The vesicles contain two major constituents besides noradrenaline, namely ATP (about four molecules per molecule of noradrenaline) and a protein called *chromogranin A*. These substances are released along with noradrenaline, and it is generally assumed that a reversible complex, depending partly on the opposite charges on the molecules of noradrenaline and ATP, is formed within the vesicle. This would serve both to reduce the osmolarity of the vesicle contents and to reduce the tendency of noradrenaline to leak out of the vesicles within the nerve terminal.

ATP itself has a transmitter function at sympathetic nerve synapses (see Fig. 13.5; Ch. 17), being responsible for the fast-excitatory synaptic potential and the rapid phase of contraction produced by sympathetic nerve activity in many smooth muscle tissues.

NORADRENALINE RELEASE

The processes linking the arrival of a nerve impulse at a nerve terminal, Ca^{2+} entry, and the release of transmitter are described in Chapter 4. Drugs that affect noradrenaline release are summarised in Table 15.6 (p. 206).

An unusual feature of the release mechanism at the varicosities of noradrenergic nerves is that the probability of release, even of a single vesicle, when a nerve impulse arrives at a varicosity is very low (less than 1 in 50). A single neuron possesses many thousand varicosities, so one impulse leads to the discharge of a few hundred vesicles, scattered over a wide area. This contrasts sharply with the neuromuscular junction (Ch. 14), where the release probability at a single terminal is high, and release of acetylcholine is sharply localised.

Regulation of noradrenaline release

Noradrenaline release is affected by a variety of substances that act on presynaptic receptors (see Ch. 13). Many different types of nerve terminal (cholinergic, noradrenergic, dopaminergic, 5-HT-ergic, etc.) are subject to this type of control,

Table 15.3 Characteristics of noradrenaline (norepinephrine) transport systems

	Neuronal (NET)	Extraneuronal (EMT)	Vesicular (VMAT)
Transport of NA (rat heart) V_{max} (nmol g^{-1} min^{-1})	1.2	100	—
K_m (µmol/L)	0.3	250	~0.2
Specificity	NA > A > ISO	A > NA > ISO	NA = A = ISO
Location	Neuronal membrane	Non-neuronal cell membrane (smooth muscle, cardiac muscle, endothelium)	Synaptic vesicle membrane
Other substrates	Tyramine Methylnoradrenaline Adrenergic neuron-blocking drugs (e.g. guanethidine) Amphetamine[a]	(+)-Noradrenaline Dopamine 5-Hydroxytryptamine Histamine	Dopamine 5-Hydroxytryptamine Guanethidine MPP$^+$ (see Ch. 41)
Inhibitors	Cocaine Tricyclic antidepressants (e.g. desipramine) Phenoxybenzamine Amphetamine[a]	Normetanephrine Steroid hormones (e.g. corticosterone) Phenoxybenzamine	Reserpine Tetrabenazine

[a]Amphetamine is transported slowly, so acts both as a substrate and as an inhibitor of noradrenaline uptake. For details, see Gainetdinov & Caron, 2003.
A, adrenaline; *EMT*, extraneuronal monoamine transporter; *ISO*, isoprenaline; *MPP$^+$*, toxic metabolite of MPTP (see p. 213 and Ch 41); *NA*, noradrenaline; *NET*, norepinephrine transporter; *VMAT*, vesicular monoamine transporter.

and many different mediators (acetylcholine acting through muscarinic receptors, catecholamines acting through α and β receptors, angiotensin II, prostaglandins, purine nucleotides, neuropeptides, etc.) can act on presynaptic terminals. Presynaptic modulation represents an important physiological control mechanism throughout the nervous system.

▼ Noradrenaline, by acting on presynaptic α$_2$ receptors, can regulate its own release, and also that of co-released ATP (see Ch. 13). This is believed to occur physiologically, so that released noradrenaline exerts a local inhibitory effect on the terminals from which it came – the so-called *autoinhibitory feedback* mechanism (Fig. 15.2; see Gilsbach & Hein, 2012). Agonists or antagonists affecting presynaptic receptors can have large effects on sympathetic transmission. However, the physiological significance of presynaptic autoinhibition in the sympathetic nervous system is still somewhat contentious, and there is evidence that, in most tissues, it is less influential than biochemical measurements of transmitter overflow would seem to imply. Thus, although blocking autoreceptors causes large changes in noradrenaline *overflow* – the amount of noradrenaline released into the bathing solution or the bloodstream when sympathetic nerves are stimulated – the associated changes in the tissue response are often rather small. This suggests that what is measured in overflow experiments may not be the physiologically important component of transmitter release.

The inhibitory feedback mechanism operates through α$_2$ receptors, which inhibit adenylyl cyclase and prevent the opening of calcium channels (see Fig. 15.2). Sympathetic nerve terminals also possess β$_2$ receptors, coupled to activation of adenylyl cyclase, which *increase* noradrenaline release. Whether they have any physiological function is not clear.

UPTAKE AND DEGRADATION OF CATECHOLAMINES

The action of released noradrenaline is terminated mainly by reuptake of the transmitter into noradrenergic nerve terminals. Some is also sequestered by other cells in the vicinity. Circulating adrenaline and noradrenaline are degraded

Fig. 15.2 Feedback control of noradrenaline (NA) release. The presynaptic α$_2$ receptor inhibits Ca^{2+} influx in response to membrane depolarisation via an action of the βγ subunits of the associated G protein on the voltage-dependent Ca^{2+} channels (Ch. 3).

enzymically, but much more slowly than acetylcholine (see Ch. 14), where synaptically located acetylcholinesterase inactivates the transmitter in milliseconds. The two main catecholamine-metabolising enzymes are located intracellularly, so uptake into cells necessarily precedes metabolic degradation.

UPTAKE OF CATECHOLAMINES

About 75% of the noradrenaline released by sympathetic neurons is recaptured and repackaged into vesicles. This serves to cut short the action of the released noradrenaline, as well as recycling it. The remaining 25% is captured by non-neuronal cells in the vicinity, limiting its local spread. These two uptake mechanisms depend on distinct transporter molecules. Neuronal uptake is performed by the plasma membrane noradrenaline transporter (generally known as NET, the *norepinephrine transporter*), which belongs to the family of neurotransmitter transporter proteins (NET, DAT, SERT, etc.) specific for different amine transmitters, described in Chapter 13; these act as co-transporters of Na^+, Cl^- and the amine in question, using the electrochemical gradient for Na^+ as a driving force. Packaging into vesicles occurs through the VMAT, driven by the proton gradient between the cytosol and the vesicle contents. Extraneuronal uptake is performed by the *extraneuronal monoamine transporter* (EMT), which belongs to a large and widely distributed family of organic cation transporters (OCTs, see Ch. 9). NET is relatively selective for noradrenaline, with high affinity and a low maximum rate of uptake, and it is important in maintaining releasable stores of noradrenaline. NET is blocked by tricyclic antidepressant drugs and **cocaine**. EMT has lower affinity and higher transport capacity than NET, and transports adrenaline and isoprenaline as well as noradrenaline. The effects of several important drugs that act on noradrenergic neurons depend on their ability either to inhibit NET or to enter the nerve terminal with its help. Table 15.3 summarises the properties of neuronal and extraneuronal uptake.

METABOLIC DEGRADATION OF CATECHOLAMINES

Endogenous and exogenous catecholamines are metabolised mainly by two intracellular enzymes: *monoamine oxidase* (MAO) and *catechol-O-methyl transferase* (COMT). MAO (of which there are two distinct isoforms, MAO-A and MAO-B; see Chs 40 and 48) is bound to the surface membrane of mitochondria. It is abundant in noradrenergic nerve terminals but is also present in liver, intestinal epithelium and other tissues. MAO converts catecholamines to their corresponding aldehydes,[3] which, in the periphery, are rapidly metabolised by *aldehyde dehydrogenase* to the corresponding carboxylic acid (3,4-dihydroxyphenylglycol being formed from noradrenaline; Fig. 15.3). MAO can also oxidise other monoamines, including dopamine and 5-HT. It is inhibited by various drugs which are used mainly for their antidepressant effects in the CNS (see Ch. 48), where these three amines all have transmitter functions (see Ch. 40). These drugs have important harmful effects that are related to disturbances of peripheral noradrenergic transmission. Within sympathetic neurons, MAO controls the content of dopamine and noradrenaline, and the releasable store of

noradrenaline increases if the enzyme is inhibited. MAO and its inhibitors are discussed in more detail in Chapter 48.

The second major pathway for catecholamine metabolism involves methylation of one of the catechol hydroxyl groups by COMT to give a methoxy derivative. COMT is absent from noradrenergic neurons but present in the adrenal medulla and many other tissues. The final product formed by the sequential action of MAO and COMT is *3-methoxy-4-hydroxyphenylglycol* (MHPG; see Fig. 15.3). This is partly conjugated to sulfate- or glucuronide- derivatives, which are excreted in the urine and reflect noradrenaline release in brain, but most of it is converted to *vanillylmandelic acid* (VMA; see Fig. 15.3) and excreted in the urine in this form. In patients with tumours of chromaffin tissue that secrete these amines (a rare cause of high blood pressure), the urinary excretion of VMA is markedly increased, this being used as a diagnostic test for such tumours.

In the periphery, neither MAO nor COMT is primarily responsible for the termination of transmitter action, most of the released noradrenaline being quickly recaptured by NET. Circulating catecholamines are sequestered and inactivated by a combination of NET, EMT and COMT, the relative importance of these processes varying according to the agent concerned. Thus circulating noradrenaline is removed mainly by NET, whereas adrenaline is more dependent on EMT. Isoprenaline, however, is not a substrate for NET, and is removed by a combination of EMT and COMT.

In the CNS (see Ch. 40), MAO is more important as a means of terminating transmitter action than it is in the periphery, and MAO knockout mice show a greater enhancement of noradrenergic transmission in the brain than do NET knockouts, in which neuronal stores of noradrenaline are much depleted (see Gainetdinov & Caron, 2003). The main excretory product of noradrenaline released in the brain is MHPG.

DRUGS ACTING ON NORADRENERGIC TRANSMISSION

Many clinically important drugs, particularly those used to treat cardiovascular, respiratory and psychiatric disorders (see Chs 22, 23, 29, 48 and 49), act by affecting noradrenergic neuron function, acting on adrenoceptors, transporters or catecholamine-metabolising enzymes. The properties of the most important drugs in this category are summarised in Tables 15.4–15.6.

DRUGS ACTING ON ADRENOCEPTORS

The overall activity of these drugs is governed by their affinity, efficacy and selectivity with respect to different types of adrenoceptor, and intensive research has been devoted to developing drugs with the right properties for specific clinical indications. As a result, the pharmacopoeia is awash with adrenoceptor ligands. Many clinical needs are met, it turns out, by drugs that relax smooth muscle in different organs of the body[4] and those that block the cardiac

---

[3]Aldehyde metabolites are potentially neurotoxic, and are thought to play a role in certain degenerative CNS disorders (see Ch. 41).

[4]And conversely, contracting smooth muscle is often bad news. This bald statement must not be pressed too far, but the exceptions (such as nasal decongestants and drugs acting on the eye) are surprisingly few. Even adrenaline (potentially life-saving in cardiac arrest) dilates some vessels while constricting others to less immediately essential tissues such as skin).

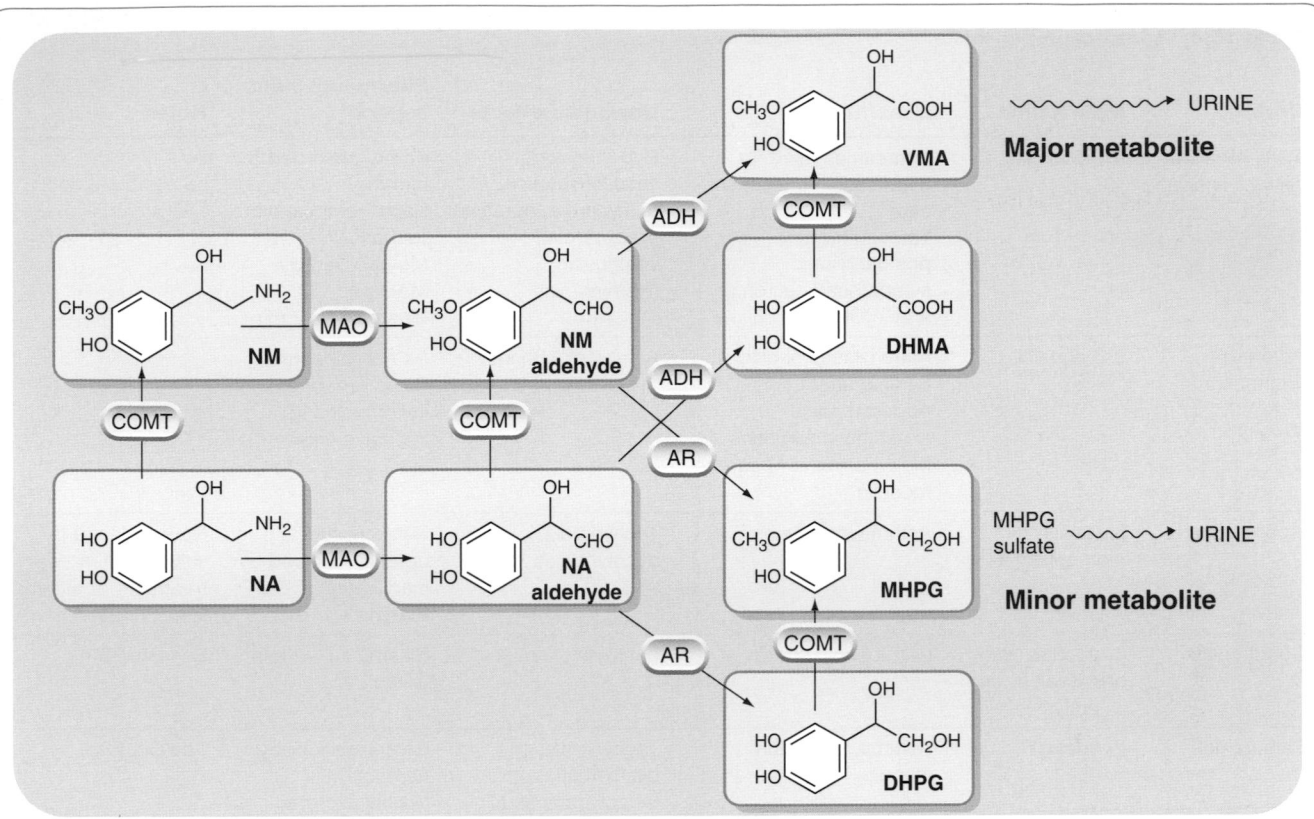

Fig. 15.3 **The main pathways of noradrenaline metabolism.** The oxidative branch (catalysed by aldehyde dehydrogenase [ADH]) predominates, giving vanillylmandelic acid (VMA) as the main urinary metabolite. The reductive branch (catalysed by aldehyde reductase [AR]) produces the less abundant metabolite, 3-methoxy-4-hydroxyphenylglycol (MHPG), which is conjugated to MHPG sulfate before being excreted; MHPG sulfate excretion reflects noradrenaline (NA) release in brain. *COMT,* catechol-*O*-methyl transferase; *DHMA,* 3,4-dihydroxymandelic acid; *DHPG,* 3,4-dihydroxyphenylglycol; *MAO,* monoamine oxidase; *NM,* normetanephrine.

Noradrenergic transmission

- Transmitter synthesis involves the following:
  - L-tyrosine is converted to dihydroxyphenylalanine (dopa) by tyrosine hydroxylase (rate-limiting step). Tyrosine hydroxylase occurs only in catecholaminergic neurons.
  - Dopa is converted to dopamine by dopa decarboxylase.
  - Dopamine is converted to noradrenaline by dopamine-β-hydroxylase (DBH), located in synaptic vesicles.
  - In the adrenal medulla, noradrenaline is converted to adrenaline by phenylethanolamine N-methyltransferase.
- Transmitter storage: noradrenaline is stored at high concentration in synaptic vesicles, together with ATP, chromogranin and DBH, which are co-released by exocytosis. Transport of noradrenaline into vesicles occurs by a reserpine-sensitive transporter, vesicular monoamine transporter (VMAT). Noradrenaline content of cytosol is normally low due to monoamine oxidase in nerve terminals.

- Transmitter release occurs normally by Ca^{2+}-mediated exocytosis from varicosities on the terminal network. Non-exocytotic release occurs in response to indirectly acting sympathomimetic drugs (e.g. **tyramine** and **amphetamine**), which displace noradrenaline from vesicles. Noradrenaline escapes via the norepinephrine transporter (NET; reverse transport).
- Transmitter action is terminated mainly by reuptake of noradrenaline into nerve terminals via the NET transporter. NET is blocked by tricyclic antidepressant drugs and **cocaine**.
- Noradrenaline release is controlled by autoinhibitory feedback mediated by α_2 receptors.
- Co-transmission occurs at many noradrenergic nerve terminals, ATP and neuropeptide Y being frequently co-released with NA. ATP mediates the early phase of smooth muscle contraction in response to sympathetic nerve activity.

stimulant effects of the sympathetic nervous system; on the other hand, cardiac stimulation is generally undesirable in chronic disease.

Broadly speaking, β_2-adrenoceptor agonists are useful as smooth muscle relaxants (especially in the airways), while β_1-adrenoceptor antagonists (often called β blockers) are used mainly for their cardiodepressant effects. α_1-Adrenoceptor antagonists are used mainly for their vasodilator effects in cardiovascular indications and also for the treatment of prostatic hyperplasia. Adrenaline, with its mixture of cardiac

Table 15.4 Adrenoceptor agonists

Drug	Main action	Uses/function	Unwanted effects	Pharmacokinetic aspects	Notes
Noradrenaline (Norepinephrine)	α/β agonist	Sometimes used for hypotension in intensive care Transmitter at postganglionic sympathetic neurons, and in CNS	Hypertension, vasoconstriction, tachycardia (or reflex bradycardia), ventricular dysrhythmias	Poorly absorbed by mouth Rapid removal by tissues Metabolised by MAO and COMT Plasma $t_{1/2}$ ~2 min	—
Adrenaline (Epinephrine)	α/β agonist	Anaphylactic shock, cardiac arrest Added to local anaesthetic solutions Main hormone of adrenal medulla	As norepinephrine	As norepinephrine Given i.m. or s.c. (i.v. infusion in intensive care settings)	
Isoprenaline	β agonist (non-selective)	Asthma (obsolete)	Tachycardia, dysrhythmias	Some tissue uptake, followed by inactivation (COMT) Plasma $t_{1/2}$ ~2 h	Now replaced by salbutamol in treatment of asthma (see Ch. 29)
Dobutamine	β_1 agonist (also has weak β_2 and α_1 activity)	Cardiogenic shock	Dysrhythmias	Plasma $t_{1/2}$ ~2 min Given i.v.	See Ch. 22
Salbutamol	β_2 agonist	Asthma, premature labour	Tachycardia, dysrhythmias, tremor, peripheral vasodilatation	Given orally or by aerosol Mainly excreted unchanged Plasma $t_{1/2}$ ~4 h	See Ch. 29
Salmeterol	β_2 agonist	Asthma	As salbutamol	Given by aerosol Long acting	Formoterol is similar
Terbutaline	β_2 agonist	Asthma Delay of parturition	As salbutamol	Poorly absorbed orally Given by aerosol Mainly excreted unchanged Plasma $t_{1/2}$ ~4 h	See Ch. 29
Clenbuterol	β_2 agonist	'Anabolic' action to increase muscle strength	As salbutamol	Active orally Long acting	Illicit use in sport, see Ch. 59
Mirabegron	β_3 agonist	Symptoms of overactive bladder	Tachycardia	Active orally, given once daily	See Ch. 30
Phenylephrine	α_1 agonist	Nasal decongestion	Hypertension, reflex bradycardia	Given intranasally Metabolised by MAO Short plasma $t_{1/2}$	—
Methoxamine	α agonist (non-selective)	Nasal decongestion	As phenylephrine	Given intranasally Plasma $t_{1/2}$ ~1 h	—
Clonidine, lofexidine	α_2 partial agonist	Hypertension, migraine prophylaxis, vasomotor instability ('hot flushes'); lofexidine is used to reduce symptoms during opioid withdrawal	Drowsiness, hypotension, oedema and weight gain, rebound hypertension	Well absorbed orally Excreted unchanged and as conjugate Plasma $t_{1/2}$ ~12 h	—

CNS, central nervous system; *COMT*, catechol-O-methyl transferase; *MAO*, monoamine oxidase.

Table 15.5 Adrenoceptor antagonists

Drug	Main action	Uses/function	Unwanted effects	Pharmacokinetic aspects	Notes
α-Adrenoceptor antagonists					
Phenoxybenzamine	α antagonist (non-selective, irreversible) Uptake 1 inhibitor	Phaeochromocytoma	Postural hypotension, tachycardia, nasal congestion, impotence	Absorbed orally Plasma $t_{1/2}$ ~12 h	Action outlasts presence of drug in plasma, because of covalent binding to receptor
Phentolamine	α antagonist (non-selective), vasodilator	Rarely used	As phenoxybenzamine	Usually given i.v. Metabolised by liver Plasma $t_{1/2}$ ~2 h	
Prazosin	α_1 antagonist	Hypertension	As phenoxybenzamine	Absorbed orally Metabolised by liver Plasma $t_{1/2}$ ~4 h	Doxazosin, terazosin are similar but longer acting See Ch. 23
Tamsulosin	α_{1A} antagonist ('uroselective')	Prostatic hyperplasia	Failure of ejaculation	Absorbed orally Plasma $t_{1/2}$ ~5 h	Selective for α_{1A}-adrenoceptor
Yohimbine	α_2 antagonist	Not used clinically Claimed to be aphrodisiac	Excitement, hypertension	Absorbed orally Metabolised by liver Plasma $t_{1/2}$ ~4 h	
β-Adrenoceptor antagonists					
Propranolol	β antagonist (non-selective)	Angina, hypertension, cardiac dysrhythmias, anxiety, tremor, glaucoma	Bronchoconstriction, cardiac failure, cold extremities, fatigue and depression, hypoglycaemia	Absorbed orally Extensive first-pass metabolism About 90% bound to plasma protein Plasma $t_{1/2}$ ~4 h	Timolol is similar and used mainly to treat glaucoma See Ch. 22
Alprenolol	β antagonist (non-selective) (partial agonist)	As propranolol	As propranolol	Absorbed orally Metabolised by liver Plasma $t_{1/2}$ ~4 h	Oxprenolol and pindolol are similar See Ch. 22
Metoprolol	β_1 antagonist	Angina, hypertension, dysrhythmias	As propranolol, less risk of bronchoconstriction	Absorbed orally Mainly metabolised in liver Plasma $t_{1/2}$ ~3 h	Atenolol is similar, with a longer half-life See Ch. 22
Nebivolol	β_1 antagonist Enhances nitric oxide synthesis	Hypertension	Fatigue, headache	Absorbed orally $t_{1/2}$ ~10 h	—
Butoxamine	β_2-selective antagonist Weak α agonist	No clinical uses	—	—	—
Mixed (α-/β-) antagonists					
Labetalol	α/β antagonist	Hypertension in pregnancy	Postural hypotension, bronchoconstriction	Absorbed orally Conjugated in liver Plasma $t_{1/2}$ ~4 h	See Chs 22 and 23
Carvedilol	β/α_1 antagonist	Heart failure	As for other β blockers Initial exacerbation of heart failure Renal failure	Absorbed orally $t_{1/2}$ ~10 h	Additional actions may contribute to clinical benefit. See Ch. 22

Table 15.6 Drugs that affect noradrenaline synthesis, release or uptake

Drug	Main action	Uses/function	Unwanted effects	Pharmacokinetic aspects	Notes
Drugs affecting NA synthesis					
α-Methyl-p-tyrosine	Inhibits tyrosine hydroxylase	Occasionally used in phaeochromocytoma	Hypotension, sedation	—	—
Carbidopa	Inhibits dopa decarboxylase	Used as adjunct to levodopa to prevent peripheral effects	—	Absorbed orally Does not enter brain	See Ch. 41
Methyldopa	False transmitter precursor	Hypertension in pregnancy	Hypotension, drowsiness, diarrhoea, impotence, hypersensitivity reactions	Absorbed slowly by mouth Excreted unchanged or as conjugate Plasma $t_{1/2}$ ~6 h	See Ch. 23
Droxidopa (L-dihydroxyphenylserine, L-DOPS)	Converted to NA by dopa decarboxylase, thus increasing NA synthesis and release	Neurogenic orthostatic hypotension	Not known	Absorbed orally Duration of action ~6 h	FDA approved
Drugs that release NA (indirectly acting sympathomimetic amines)					
Tyramine	NA release	No clinical uses Present in various foods	As norepinephrine	Normally destroyed by MAO in gut Does not enter brain	See Ch. 48 for interaction with MAO inhibitors
Amphetamine	NA release, MAO inhibitor, NET inhibitor, CNS stimulant	Used as CNS stimulant in narcolepsy, also (paradoxically) in hyperactive children Appetite suppressant Drug of abuse	Hypertension, tachycardia, insomnia Acute psychosis with overdose Dependence	Well absorbed orally Penetrates freely into brain Excreted unchanged in urine Plasma $t_{1/2}$ ~12 h, depending on urine flow and pH	See Ch. 49 Methylphenidate and atomoxetine are similar (used for CNS effects; see Ch. 49)
Ephedrine	NA release, β agonist, weak CNS stimulant action	Nasal decongestion	As amphetamine but less pronounced	Similar to amphetamine aspects	Interacts with MAO inhibitors, Ch. 48
Drugs that inhibit NA release					
Reserpine	Depletes NA stores by inhibiting VMAT	Hypertension (obsolete)	As methyldopa Also depression, parkinsonism, gynaecomastia	Poorly absorbed orally Slowly metabolised Plasma $t_{1/2}$ ~100 h Excreted in milk	Antihypertensive effect develops slowly and persists when drug is stopped
Guanethidine	Inhibits NA release Also causes NA depletion and can damage NA neurons irreversibly	Hypertension (obsolete)	As methyldopa Hypertension on first administration	Poorly absorbed orally Mainly excreted unchanged in urine Plasma $t_{1/2}$ ~100 h	Action prevented by NET inhibitors
Drugs affecting NA uptake					
Imipramine	Blocks neuronal transporter (NET) Also has atropine-like action	Depression	Atropine-like side effects Cardiac dysrhythmias in overdose	Well absorbed orally 95% bound to plasma protein Converted to active metabolite (desmethylimipramine) Plasma $t_{1/2}$ ~4 h	Desipramine and amitriptyline are similar See Ch. 48
Cocaine	Local anaesthetic; blocks NET CNS stimulant	Rarely used local anaesthetic Major drug of abuse	Hypertension, excitement, convulsions, dependence	Well absorbed orally or intranasally	See Chs 44 and 50

CNS, central nervous system; MAO, monoamine oxidase; NA, noradrenaline; NET, norepinephrine transporter; VMAT, vesicular monoamine transporter.

stimulant, vasodilator and vasoconstrictor actions is uniquely important in cardiac arrest (Ch. 22). α_1-adrenoceptor agonists are widely used intranasally as decongestants.

ADRENOCEPTOR AGONISTS

Examples of adrenoceptor agonists (also known as *directly-acting sympathomimetic* drugs) are given in Table 15.2, and the characteristics of individual drugs are summarised in Table 15.4.

Actions

The major physiological effects mediated by different types of adrenoceptor are summarised in Table 15.1.

Smooth muscle

All types of smooth muscle, except that of the gastrointestinal tract, contract in response to stimulation of α_1 adrenoceptors, through activation of the signal transduction mechanism, leading to intracellular Ca^{2+} release described in Chapter 4. Although vascular smooth muscle possesses both α_1 and α_2 receptors, it appears that α_1 receptors lie close to the sites of noradrenaline release (and are mainly responsible for neurally mediated vasoconstriction), while α_2 receptors lie elsewhere on the muscle fibre surface.

When α_1 agonists are given systemically to experimental animals or humans, the most important action is on vascular smooth muscle, particularly in the small arteries and arterioles in skin and splanchnic vascular beds, which are strongly constricted increasing total peripheral vascular resistance. Smooth muscle cells in the walls of large arteries and veins, also contract, resulting in decreased arterial compliance and increased central venous pressure, which contribute to an increase in arterial and venous pressure and increased cardiac work. Some vascular beds (e.g. cerebral, coronary and pulmonary) are relatively little affected.

In the whole animal, baroreceptor reflexes are activated by the rise in arterial pressure produced by α_1 agonists, causing reflex bradycardia and inhibition of respiration.

Smooth muscle in the vas deferens, spleen capsule and eyelid retractor muscles (or nictitating membrane, in some species) is also stimulated by α_1 agonists, and these organs were once widely used for pharmacological studies.

Stimulation of β receptors causes relaxation of most kinds of smooth muscle by increasing cAMP formation (see Ch. 4). Additionally, β-receptor activation enhances Ca^{2+} extrusion and intracellular Ca^{2+} binding, both effects acting to reduce intracellular Ca^{2+} concentration. In the vascular system, β_2-mediated vasodilatation is (particularly in humans) mainly endothelium dependent and mediated by nitric oxide release (see Ch. 21). It occurs in many vascular beds and is especially marked in skeletal muscle.

The powerful inhibitory effect of the sympathetic system on gastrointestinal smooth muscle is produced by both α and β receptors, this tissue being unusual in that α receptors cause relaxation in most regions. Part of the effect is due to stimulation of presynaptic α_2 receptors (see later), which inhibit the release of excitatory transmitters (e.g. acetylcholine) from intramural nerves, but there are also α_1 and α_2 receptors on the muscle cells, stimulation of which hyperpolarises the cell (by increasing the membrane permeability to K^+) and inhibits action potential discharge. The sphincters of the gastrointestinal tract are contracted by α-receptor activation.

Bronchial smooth muscle is relaxed by activation of β_2 adrenoceptors, and selective β_2 agonists are important in the treatment of asthma (see Ch. 29). Uterine smooth muscle responds similarly, and these drugs are also used to delay premature labour (Ch. 36). Bladder detrusor muscle is relaxed by activation of β_3 adrenoceptors, and selective β_3 agonists are used to treat symptoms of overactive bladder (see Sacco & Bientinesi, 2012).

α_1 adrenoceptors have long-lasting trophic effects stimulating smooth muscle proliferation in various tissues, for example, in blood vessels and in the prostate gland, which is of pathological importance. *Benign prostatic hyperplasia* (see Ch. 36) is commonly treated with α_1-adrenoceptor antagonists. 'Cross-talk' between the α_1 adrenoceptor and the growth factor signalling pathways (see Ch. 3) probably contributes to the clinical effect, in addition to immediate symptomatic improvement which is probably mediated by smooth muscle relaxation.

Nerve terminals

Presynaptic adrenoceptors are present on both cholinergic and noradrenergic nerve terminals (see Chs 4 and 13). As mentioned previously, the main effect (α_2-mediated) is inhibitory, but a weaker facilitatory action of β receptors on noradrenergic nerve terminals has also been described.

Heart

Catecholamines, acting on β_1 receptors, exert a powerful stimulant effect on the heart (see Ch. 22). Both the heart rate (*chronotropic effect*) and the force of contraction (*inotropic effect*) are increased, resulting in a markedly increased cardiac output and cardiac oxygen consumption. Cardiac efficiency (see Ch. 22) is reduced. Catecholamines can also disturb cardiac rhythm, culminating in ventricular fibrillation. (Paradoxically, but importantly, adrenaline is also used to treat ventricular fibrillation arrest as well as other forms of cardiac arrest; Ch. 22). Fig. 15.4 shows the overall pattern of cardiovascular responses to catecholamine infusions in humans, reflecting their actions on both the heart and vascular system.

Cardiac hypertrophy occurs in response to activation of both β_1 and α_1 receptors, probably by a mechanism similar to the hypertrophy of vascular and prostatic smooth muscle. This may be important in the pathophysiology of hypertension and of cardiac failure (which is associated with sympathetic overactivity); see Chapters 22 and 23.

Metabolism

Catecholamines encourage the conversion of energy stores (glycogen and fat) to freely available fuels (glucose and free fatty acids), and cause an increase in the plasma concentration of the latter substances. The detailed biochemical mechanisms (see review by Nonogaki, 2000) vary from species to species, but in most cases the effects on carbohydrate metabolism of liver and muscle (Fig. 15.5) are mediated through β_1 receptors and the stimulation of lipolysis and thermogenesis is produced by β_3 receptors (see Table 15.1). Activation of α_2 receptors inhibits insulin secretion, an effect that further contributes to the hyperglycaemia. The production of *leptin* by adipose tissue (see Ch. 33) is also inhibited. Adrenaline-induced hyperglycaemia in humans is blocked completely by a combination of α and β antagonists but not by either on its own.

Other effects

Skeletal muscle is affected by adrenaline, acting on β_2 receptors, although the effect is far less dramatic than that

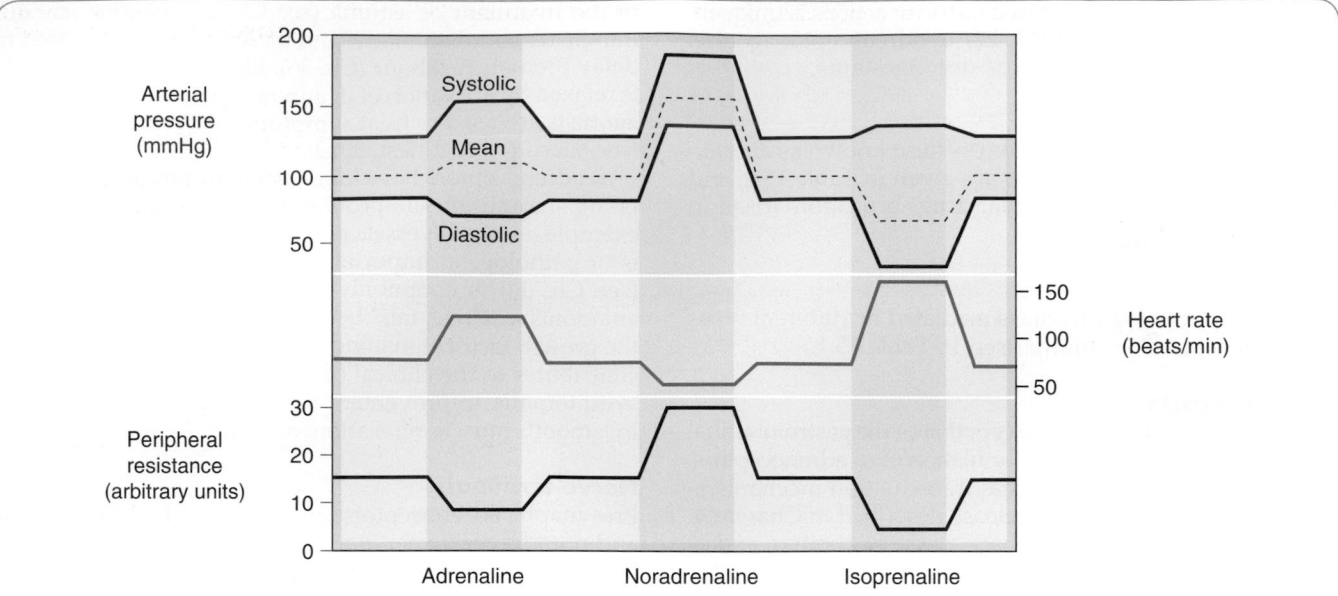

Fig. 15.4 **Schematic representation of the cardiovascular effects of intravenous infusions of adrenaline, noradrenaline and isoprenaline in humans.** Noradrenaline (predominantly α agonist) causes vasoconstriction and increased systolic and diastolic pressure, with a reflex bradycardia. Isoprenaline (β agonist) is a vasodilator, but strongly increases cardiac force and rate. Mean arterial pressure falls. Adrenaline combines both actions.

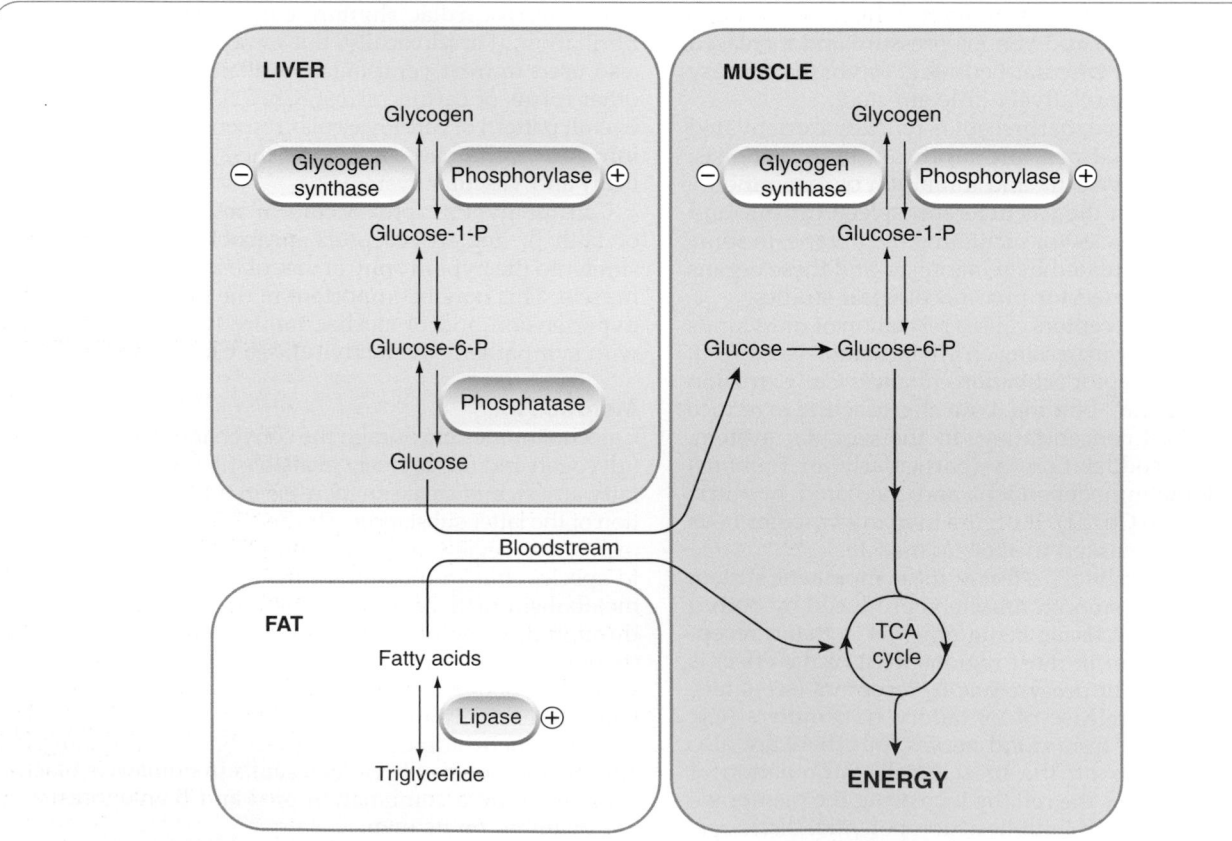

Fig. 15.5 **Regulation of energy metabolism by catecholamines.** The main enzymic steps that are affected by β-adrenoceptor activation are indicated by + and – signs, denoting stimulation and inhibition, respectively. The overall effect is to mobilise glycogen and fat stores to meet energy demands. *TCA*, tricarboxylic acid.

on the heart. The twitch tension of fast-contracting fibres (white muscle) is increased by adrenaline, particularly if the muscle is fatigued, whereas the twitch of slow (red) muscle is reduced. These effects depend on an action on the contractile proteins, rather than on the membrane, and the mechanism is poorly understood. In humans, adrenaline and other β_2 agonists cause a marked tremor, the shakiness that accompanies fear, excitement, withdrawal from alcohol (Ch. 49) or the excessive use of β_2 agonists (e.g. **salbutamol**) in the treatment of asthma being examples of this. It probably results from an increase in muscle spindle discharge, coupled with an effect on the contraction kinetics of the fibres, these effects combining to produce an instability in the reflex control of muscle length. β-receptor antagonists are sometimes used to control pathological tremor. Increased susceptibility to cardiac dysrhythmias associated with β_2 agonists is thought to be partly due to hypokalaemia, caused by an increase in K^+ uptake by skeletal muscle. β_2 agonists also cause long-term changes in the expression of sarcoplasmic reticulum proteins that control contraction kinetics, and thereby increase the rate and force of contraction of skeletal muscle. **Clenbuterol**, an 'anabolic' drug used illicitly by athletes to improve performance (see Ch. 59), is a β_2 agonist that acts in this way.

Histamine release by human and guinea pig lung tissue in response to anaphylactic challenge (see Ch. 18) is inhibited by catecholamines, acting on β_2 receptors.

Lymphocytes and other cells of the immune system also express adrenoceptors (mainly β adrenoceptors). Lymphocyte proliferation, lymphocyte-mediated cell killing, and production of many cytokines are inhibited by β-adrenoceptor agonists. The physiological and clinical importance of these effects has not yet been established. For a review of the effects of the sympathetic nervous system on immune function, see Elenkov et al., 2000.

Adrenoceptor agonists

- **Noradrenaline** and **adrenaline** show relatively little receptor selectivity.
- Selective α_1 agonists include **phenylephrine** and **oxymetazoline**.
- Selective α_2 agonists include clonidine and **α-methylnoradrenaline**. They cause a fall in blood pressure, partly by inhibition of noradrenaline release and partly by a central action. Methylnoradrenaline is formed as a false transmitter from **methyldopa**, developed as a hypotensive drug (now largely obsolete, except during pregnancy).
- Selective β_1 agonists include **dobutamine**. Increased cardiac contractility may be useful clinically, but all β_1 agonists can cause cardiac dysrhythmias.
- Selective β_2 agonists include **salbutamol**, **terbutaline** and **salmeterol**; used mainly for their bronchodilator action in asthma.
- A selective β_3 agonist, **mirabegron**, is used to treat overactive bladder; β_3 agonists promote lipolysis and have potential in the treatment of obesity.

Clinical use

The main clinical uses of adrenoceptor agonists are summarised in the clinical box (below) and Table 15.4, the most

important being the use of β-adrenoceptor agonists for the treatment of asthma (Ch. 29).

Clinical uses of adrenoceptor agonists

- Cardiovascular system:
  - cardiac arrest: adrenaline
  - cardiogenic shock (see Chs 22 and 23): **dobutamine** (β_1 agonist).
- Anaphylaxis (acute hypersensitivity, see Chs 18 and 29): **adrenaline**.
- Respiratory system:
  - asthma (Ch. 29): selective β_2-receptor agonists (**salbutamol**, **terbutaline**, **salmeterol**, **formoterol**)
  - nasal decongestion: drops containing **xylometazoline** or **ephedrine** for short-term use.
- Miscellaneous indications:
  - **adrenaline**: with local anaesthetics to prolong their action (see Ch. 44).
  - premature labour (salbutamol; see Ch. 36).
  - α_2 agonists (e.g. **clonidine**, **lofexidine**): to lower blood pressure, but are now seldom prescribed for this other than in specialist situations (Ch. 23) and intraocular pressure; lofexidine is used as an adjunct during opioid withdrawal, to reduce menopausal flushing, especially when **oestrogen** is contraindicated as in patients with breast cancer; and to reduce frequency of migraine attacks (Ch. 16). Tourette syndrome, characterised by multiple tics and outbursts of foul language, is an unlicensed indication.
  - A β_3 agonist, **mirabegron**: to treat urgency, increased micturition frequency and incontinence (overactive bladder symptoms).

ADRENOCEPTOR ANTAGONISTS

The main drugs are listed in Table 15.2, and further information is given in Table 15.5. Most are selective for α or β receptors, and many are also subtype-selective.

α-Adrenoceptor antagonists

The main groups of α-adrenoceptor antagonists are:

- non-selective between subtypes (e.g. **phenoxybenzamine**, **phentolamine**)
- α_1-selective (e.g. **prazosin**, **doxazosin**, **terazosin**)
- α_2-selective (e.g. **yohimbine**, **idazoxan**)

In addition, *ergot derivatives* (e.g. **ergotamine**, **dihydroergotamine**) block α receptors as well as having many other actions, notably on 5-HT receptors. They are described in Chapter 16. Their action on α adrenoceptors is of pharmacological interest but not used therapeutically.

Non-selective α-adrenoceptor antagonists

Phenoxybenzamine is not specific for α receptors, and also antagonises the actions of acetylcholine, histamine and 5-HT. It is long lasting because it binds covalently to the receptor. **Phentolamine** is more selective, but it binds reversibly and its action is short lasting. In humans, these drugs cause a fall in arterial pressure (because of block of α-receptor-mediated vasoconstriction) and postural hypotension. The cardiac output and heart rate are increased. This is a reflex response to the fall in arterial pressure, mediated through β receptors. The concomitant block of α_2 receptors tends to increase noradrenaline release, which has the effect of enhancing the reflex tachycardia that occurs with any blood pressure-lowering agent. Phenoxybenzamine retains a niche use in preparing patients with *phaeochromocytoma* (Ch. 23, and below) for surgery.

Labetalol and **carvedilol**[5] are mixed α_1- and β-receptor-blocking drugs, although at doses used clinically they act predominantly on β receptors. Carvedilol is used mainly to treat hypertension and heart failure (see Chs 21 and 22); labetalol is used to treat hypertension in pregnancy.

Selective α_1 antagonists

Prazosin was the first selective α_1 antagonist/inverse agonist; it acts on all three subtypes of α_1 receptor (Alexander et al., 2016). Similar drugs with longer half-lives (e.g. **doxazosin**, **terazosin**), which have the advantage of allowing once-daily dosing, are now preferred. They are highly selective for α_1 adrenoceptors and cause vasodilatation and fall in arterial pressure, but less tachycardia than occurs with non-selective α-receptor antagonists, presumably because they do not increase noradrenaline release from sympathetic nerve terminals. Mild postural hypotension is common, but is less problematic than with shorter-acting prazosin.

The α_1-receptor antagonists cause relaxation of the smooth muscle of the bladder neck and prostate capsule, and inhibit hypertrophy of these tissues, and are therefore useful in treating urinary retention associated with *benign prostatic hypertrophy*. **Tamsulosin**, an α_{1A}-receptor antagonist, shows some selectivity for the bladder, and causes less hypotension than the less selective α_1-receptor antagonists.

It is believed that α_{1A} receptors play a part in the pathological hypertrophy not only of prostatic and vascular smooth muscle, but also in the cardiac hypertrophy that occurs in hypertension and heart failure (Papay et al., 2013), and the use of selective α_{1A}-receptor antagonists to treat these chronic conditions is under investigation.

Selective α_2 antagonists

Yohimbine is a naturally occurring alkaloid; various synthetic analogues have been made, such as **idazoxan**. These drugs are used experimentally to analyse α-receptor subtypes, and yohimbine, possibly by virtue of its vasodilator effect, historically enjoyed notoriety as an aphrodisiac, but they are not used therapeutically.

Clinical uses and unwanted effects of α-adrenoceptor antagonists

The main uses of α-adrenoceptor antagonists are related to their cardiovascular actions, and are summarised in the clinical box (below) These drugs have only limited therapeutic applications. Non-selective α-blocking drugs are unsatisfactory in treating hypertension, because of their tendency to produce tachycardia, postural hypotension and gastrointestinal symptoms. Selective α_1-receptor antagonists (especially the longer-acting compounds **doxazosin** and

[5]Carvedilol is also a biased agonist, acting through the arrestin pathway (Ch. 3).

α-Adrenoceptor antagonists

- Selective α_1 antagonists (e.g. **prazosin**, **doxazosin**, **terazosin**) are used in treating hypertension and for benign prostatic hypertrophy. Postural hypotension, stress incontinence and impotence are unwanted effects.
- **Tamsulosin** is α_{1A} selective and acts mainly on the urogenital tract. It is used to treat benign prostatic hypertrophy and may cause less postural hypotension than other α_1 agonists.
- **Yohimbine** is a selective α_2 antagonist. It is not used clinically.

terazosin) are, however, useful. They do not directly affect cardiac function appreciably, and postural hypotension is less troublesome than with prazosin or non-selective α-receptor antagonists. They have a place in treating severe hypertension, where they are added to treatment with first- and second-line drugs, but are not used as first-line agents (see Ch. 23). Unlike other antihypertensive drugs, they cause a modest decrease in low-density lipoprotein, and an increase in high-density lipoprotein cholesterol (see Ch. 24), although the clinical importance of these potentially beneficial effects is uncertain. They are also used to control obstructive symptoms in patients with benign prostatic hypertrophy.

Phaeochromocytoma is a catecholamine-secreting tumour of chromaffin tissue, which causes severe and initially episodic hypertension. A combination of α- and β-receptor antagonists is the most effective way of controlling the blood pressure. The tumour may be surgically removable, and it is essential to block α and β receptors before surgery is begun, to avoid the effects of a sudden release of catecholamines when the tumour is disturbed. Phenoxybenzamine, an irreversible α antagonist which reduces the maximum of the agonist dose–response curve (see Ch. 2, Fig. 2.4B) is combined with a β-adrenoceptor antagonist for this purpose.

Clinical uses of α-adrenoceptor antagonists

- Severe hypertension (see Ch. 23): α_1-selective antagonists (e.g. **doxazosin**) in combination with other drugs.
- Benign prostatic hypertrophy (e.g. **tamsulosin**, a selective α_{1A}-receptor antagonist).
- Phaeochromocytoma: **phenoxybenzamine** (irreversible antagonist) in preparation for surgery.

β-Adrenoceptor antagonists

β-Adrenoceptor antagonists are therapeutically important. They were first discovered in 1958, 10 years after Ahlquist had postulated the existence of β adrenoceptors. The first compound, **dichloroisoprenaline**, was a partial agonist. Further development led to **propranolol**, which is much more potent and a pure antagonist that blocks β_1 and β_2

receptors equally. The potential clinical advantages of drugs with some partial agonist activity, and/or with selectivity for β₁ receptors, led to the development of **practolol** (selective for β₁ receptors but withdrawn because of its off-target toxicity), **oxprenolol** and **alprenolol** (non-selective with considerable partial agonist activity), and **atenolol** (β₁-selective with no agonist activity). Two newer drugs are **carvedilol** (a non-selective β-adrenoceptor antagonist with additional α₁-blocking activity) and **nebivolol** (a β₁-selective antagonist with vasodilator nitric oxide-mediated activity; see Ch. 21). Both these drugs have proven more effective than conventional β-adrenoceptor antagonists in treating heart failure (see Chs 22 and 23). The characteristics of the most important compounds are set out in Table 15.5. Most clinically available β-receptor antagonists are inactive on β₃ receptors so do not affect lipolysis.

Actions
The main pharmacological actions of β-receptor antagonists can be deduced from Table 15.1. The acute effects produced in humans depend on the degree of sympathetic activity and are modest in subjects at rest. The most important effects are on the cardiovascular system and on bronchial smooth muscle (see Chs 22, 23 and 29).

In a healthy subject at rest, propranolol causes modest changes in heart rate, cardiac output or arterial pressure, but β-blockade markedly reduces the effect of exercise or excitement on these variables (Fig. 15.6). Drugs with partial agonist activity, such as oxprenolol, increase the heart rate at rest but reduce it during exercise. Maximum exercise tolerance is considerably reduced in normal subjects, partly because of the limitation of the cardiac response, and partly because the β-mediated vasodilatation in skeletal muscle is reduced. Coronary flow is reduced, but relatively less

than the myocardial oxygen consumption, so oxygenation of the myocardium is improved, an effect of importance in the treatment of angina pectoris (see Ch. 22). In healthy subjects, the reduction of the force of contraction of the heart is not important, in contrast to patients with heart disease (see further in chapter).

An important, and somewhat unexpected, effect of β-receptor antagonists is their antihypertensive action (see Ch. 23). Patients with hypertension show a gradual fall in arterial pressure that takes several days to develop fully. The mechanism is complex and involves the following:

- reduction in cardiac output;
- reduction of renin release from the juxtaglomerular cells of the kidney;
- a central action, reducing sympathetic activity.

Vasodilatation may contribute to the antihypertensive action of drugs (e.g. carvedilol and nebivolol, see earlier) with such properties.

Blockade of the facilitatory effect of presynaptic β receptors on noradrenaline release (see Table 15.1) may also contribute to the antihypertensive effect. The antihypertensive effect of β-receptor antagonists is clinically useful. Because reflex vasoconstriction is preserved, postural and exercise-induced hypotension are less troublesome than with many other antihypertensive drugs.

Many β-receptor antagonists have an important antidysrhythmic effect on the heart (see Ch. 22).

Airways resistance in normal subjects is only slightly increased by β-receptor antagonists, and this is of no consequence. In asthmatic subjects, however, non-selective β-receptor antagonists (such as propranolol) can cause severe bronchoconstriction, which does not, of course, respond to the usual doses of drugs such as salbutamol or adrenaline.

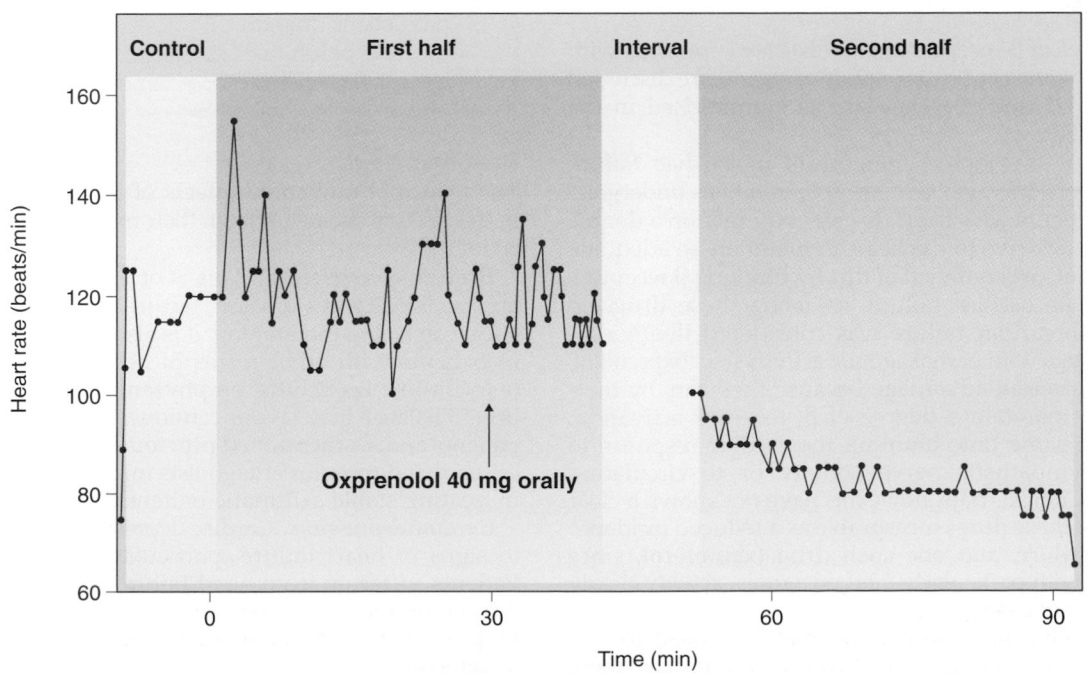

Fig. 15.6 Heart rate recorded continuously in a spectator watching a live football match, showing the effect of the β-adrenoceptor antagonist oxprenolol. (From Taylor, S.H., Meeran, M.K., 1973. In: Burley et al. (Eds) New Perspectives in Beta-Blockade. CIBA Laboratories, Horsham.)

This danger is less with β_1-selective antagonists, but none is so selective that this danger can be ignored.

Despite the involvement of β receptors in the hyperglycaemic actions of adrenaline, β-receptor antagonists cause only minor metabolic changes in normal subjects. They do not affect the onset of hypoglycaemia following an injection of insulin, but somewhat delay the recovery of blood glucose concentration. In diabetic patients, the use of β-receptor antagonists increases the likelihood of exercise-induced hypoglycaemia, because the normal adrenaline-induced release of glucose from the liver is diminished. Furthermore, β-receptor antagonists may alter the awareness of hypoglycaemia by blunting its symptoms (see Ch. 32 and later, p. 213).

β-Adrenoceptor antagonists

- Non-selective between β_1 and β_2 adrenoceptors: **propranolol**, **alprenolol**, **oxprenolol**.
- β_1-selective: **atenolol**, **nebivolol**.
- **Alprenolol** and **oxprenolol** have partial agonist activity.
- Many clinical uses (see clinical box, see later).
- Important hazards are bronchoconstriction, and bradycardia and cardiac failure (when administered to unstable patients with deteriorating cardiac function).
- Adverse effects include cold extremities, insomnia, depression, fatigue.
- Some (e.g. propranolol) show rapid first-pass metabolism, hence poor bioavailability.
- Some drugs (e.g. **labetalol**, **carvedilol**) block both α and β adrenoceptors.

Clinical use

The main uses of β-receptor antagonists are connected with their effects on the cardiovascular system, and are discussed in Chapters 22 and 23. They are as summarised in the clinical box below.

The use of β-receptor antagonists in cardiac failure deserves special mention, as clinical opinion has undergone a U-turn. Patients with heart disease may rely on a degree of sympathetic drive to the heart to maintain an adequate cardiac output, and removal of this by blocking β receptors can exacerbate cardiac failure, so using these drugs in patients with cardiac failure was considered ill-advised. In theory, drugs with partial agonist activity (e.g. oxprenolol, alprenolol) offer an advantage because they can, by their own action, maintain a degree of β_1-receptor activation, while at the same time blunting the cardiac response to increased sympathetic nerve activity or to circulating adrenaline. Clinical trials, however, have not shown a clear advantage of these drugs measurable as a reduced incidence of cardiac failure, and one such drug (**xamoterol**, since withdrawn) with particularly marked agonist activity clearly made matters worse.

Paradoxically, β-receptor antagonists are used in low doses to treat well-compensated cardiac failure and there is strong evidence that this improves survival in carefully selected patients (Ch. 23), although at the outset there is a danger of exacerbating the problem (Bristow, 2011). **Carvedilol** is often used for this purpose.

Infantile haemangioma is the commonest soft-tissue tumour in children, occurring in 3%–10% of infants and usually regressing without treatment. Approximately 12% are complicated by, for example, impingement on vital organs such as the eye, and require intervention. In 2008 a chance observation that treatment of heart failure with propranolol in two young children with severe haemangiomas was associated with their regression led to clinical trials that confirmed the effectiveness of propranolol for this indication. Such use has been approved by the FDA as well as in Europe, and propranolol is now standard therapy for severe infantile haemangioma. The evidence of such marked efficacy (Léauté-Labrèze et al., 2015) highlights the probable importance of β-adrenoceptor-mediated trophic actions, at the least in this paediatric endothelial tumour. Milder uncomplicated forms of infantile haemangioma are sometimes treated with topical timolol or propranolol.

Clinical uses of β-adrenoceptor antagonists

- Cardiovascular (see Chs 22 and 23):
  - angina pectoris
  - myocardial infarction, and following infarction
  - prevention of recurrent dysrhythmias (especially if triggered by sympathetic activation)
  - heart failure (in well-compensated patients)
  - hypertension (no longer first choice; Ch. 23).
- Other uses:
  - severe/complicated infantile haemangioma
  - glaucoma (e.g. **timolol** eye drops)
  - thyrotoxicosis (Ch. 35), as adjunct to definitive treatment (e.g. preoperatively and during initiation of carbimazole treatment)
  - anxiety (Ch. 45), to control somatic symptoms (e.g. palpitations, tremor)
  - migraine prophylaxis (Ch. 16)
  - benign essential tremor (a familial disorder).

Unwanted effects

The principal unwanted effects of β-receptor antagonists in therapeutic use result from their main (receptor-blocking) action.

Bronchoconstriction. This is of little importance in the absence of airways disease, but in asthmatic patients the effect can be life-threatening. It is also of clinical importance in patients with other forms of obstructive lung disease (e.g. chronic bronchitis, emphysema), although the risk–benefit balance may favour cautious treatment in individual patients and, as mentioned previously, it has been hypothesised that β-receptor antagonists might actually be of value in treating stable asthmatic patients.

Cardiac depression. Cardiac depression can occur, leading to signs of heart failure, particularly in elderly people. Patients suffering from heart failure who are treated with β-receptor antagonists (see earlier) often deteriorate symptomatically in the first few weeks before the beneficial effect develops.

Bradycardia. Sinus bradycardia can progress to life-threatening heart block, particularly if β-adrenoceptor antagonists are co-administered with other antidysrhythmic drugs that impair cardiac conduction (see Ch. 22).

Hypoglycaemia. Glucose release in response to adrenaline is a safety device that may be important to diabetic patients and to other individuals prone to hypoglycaemic attacks. The sympathetic response to hypoglycaemia produces symptoms (especially tachycardia) that warn patients of the urgent need for carbohydrate (usually in the form of a sugary drink). β-Receptor antagonists reduce these symptoms, so incipient hypoglycaemia is more likely to go unnoticed by the patient. There is a theoretical advantage in using β₁-selective agents, because glucose release from the liver is controlled by β₂ receptors.

Fatigue. This is probably due to reduced cardiac output and reduced muscle perfusion in exercise. It is a frequent complaint of patients taking β-receptor-blocking drugs.

Cold extremities. This is common, due to a loss of β-receptor-mediated vasodilatation in cutaneous vessels. Theoretically, β₁-selective drugs are less likely to produce this effect, which may also be less marked in patients treated with β-adrenoceptor antagonists with additional vasodilating properties, but it is not clear that this is so in practice.

Other adverse effects associated with β-receptor antagonists are not obviously the result of β-receptor blockade. One is the occurrence of bad dreams, which occur mainly with highly lipid-soluble drugs such as propranolol, which enter the brain easily.

DRUGS THAT AFFECT NORADRENERGIC NEURONS

Emphasis in this chapter is placed on peripheral sympathetic transmission. The same principles, however, are applicable to the CNS (see Ch. 40, where many of the drugs mentioned here also act). The major drugs and mechanisms are summarised in Table 15.6.

DRUGS THAT AFFECT NORADRENALINE SYNTHESIS

α-Methyltyrosine, which inhibits tyrosine hydroxylase, has been used experimentally but is no longer used clinically. Indeed, very few clinically important drugs affect noradrenaline synthesis directly. **Carbidopa**, a hydrazine derivative of dopa, which inhibits dopa decarboxylase is one example and is used in the treatment of parkinsonism (see Ch. 41).

Methyldopa, still used in the treatment of hypertension during pregnancy (see Ch. 23), is taken up by noradrenergic neurons, where it is converted to the false transmitter α-methylnoradrenaline. This substance is not deaminated within the neuron by MAO, so it accumulates and displaces noradrenaline from the synaptic vesicles. α-Methylnoradrenaline is released in the same way as noradrenaline, but is less active than noradrenaline on α₁ receptors and thus is less effective in causing vasoconstriction. However, it is more active on presynaptic (α₂) receptors, so the autoinhibitory feedback mechanism operates more strongly than normal, thus reducing transmitter release. Both of these effects (as well as a central effect, probably caused by the same cellular mechanism) contribute to the hypotensive action. It produces side effects typical of centrally acting antiadrenergic drugs (e.g. sedation), as well as carrying 'off-target' risks of immune haemolytic reactions and liver toxicity, so it is now little used, except for hypertension in the second half of pregnancy where there is considerable experience of its use and no suggestion of harm to the unborn baby.

6-Hydroxydopamine (identical with dopamine except for an extra hydroxyl group) is a neurotoxin of the Trojan horse kind. It is taken up selectively by noradrenergic nerve terminals, where it is converted to a reactive quinone, which destroys the nerve terminal, producing a 'chemical sympathectomy'. The cell bodies survive, and eventually the sympathetic innervation recovers. The drug is useful for experimental purposes but has no clinical uses. If injected directly into the brain, it selectively destroys those nerve terminals (i.e. dopaminergic, noradrenergic and adrenergic) that take it up, but it does not reach the brain if given systemically.

MPTP (1-methyl-4-phenyl-1,2,3,5-tetrahydropyridine; see Ch. 41) is a similar selective neurotoxin acting on dopaminergic neurons.

Droxidopa (dihydroxyphenylserine, L-DOPS) is under investigation for treating hypotension. It penetrates the blood–brain barrier and is a prodrug being converted to noradrenaline by dopa decarboxylase, bypassing the DBH-catalysed hydroxylation step. It raises blood pressure by increasing noradrenaline release.

DRUGS THAT AFFECT NORADRENALINE STORAGE

Reserpine is an alkaloid from the shrub *Rauwolfia*, which has been used in India for centuries for the treatment of mental disorders. Reserpine potently blocks the transport of noradrenaline and other amines into storage vesicles, by blocking the VMAT. Noradrenaline accumulates instead in the cytoplasm, where it is degraded by MAO. The noradrenaline content of tissues drops, and sympathetic transmission is blocked. Reserpine also depletes 5-HT and dopamine from neurons in the brain, where these amines are transmitters (see Ch. 40). Reserpine is now used only experimentally, but was at one time used as an antihypertensive drug. Its central effects, especially depression, which probably result from impairment of noradrenergic and 5-HT-mediated transmission in the brain (see Ch. 48), were a serious problem when its dose was increased.

DRUGS THAT AFFECT NORADRENALINE RELEASE

Drugs can affect noradrenaline release in four main ways:

- by directly blocking release (noradrenergic neuron-blocking drugs)
- by evoking noradrenaline release in the absence of nerve terminal depolarisation (indirectly acting sympathomimetic drugs)
- by acting on presynaptic receptors that indirectly inhibit or enhance depolarisation-evoked release; examples include α₂ agonists (see pp. 200–201), angiotensin II, dopamine and prostaglandins
- by increasing or decreasing available stores of noradrenaline (e.g. reserpine, see p. 213; MAO inhibitors, see Ch. 48).

NORADRENERGIC NEURON-BLOCKING DRUGS

Noradrenergic neuron-blocking drugs (e.g. **guanethidine**) were discovered in the mid-1950s when alternatives to ganglion-blocking drugs were being sought for use in the treatment of hypertension. The main effect of guanethidine is to inhibit the release of noradrenaline from sympathetic nerve terminals. It has little effect on the adrenal medulla, and none on nerve terminals that release transmitters other than noradrenaline. Related drugs include **bretylium**, **bethanidine** and **debrisoquin** (now of interest mainly as a tool for studying drug metabolism; see Ch. 12).

Actions

Drugs of this class reduce or abolish the response of tissues to sympathetic nerve stimulation.

▼ The action of guanethidine on noradrenergic transmission is complex. It is selectively accumulated by noradrenergic nerve terminals, being a substrate for NET (see Table 15.6). Its initial activity is due to block of impulse conduction in the nerve terminals that selectively accumulate the drug – acting as a local anaesthetic selective for noradrenergic nerves, the selectivity being down to its uptake by NET in the terminals of these axons. Consequently, its action is prevented by drugs such as *tricyclic antidepressants* (see Ch. 48) that block NET.

Guanethidine is also concentrated in synaptic vesicles by means of the vesicular transporter VMAT, possibly interfering with their ability to undergo exocytosis, and displacing noradrenaline. In this way, it causes a gradual and long-lasting depletion of noradrenaline in sympathetic nerve endings, similar to the effect of reserpine.

Large doses of guanethidine cause structural damage to noradrenergic neurons, probably due to its accumulation in high concentration in the nerve terminals. It can therefore be used experimentally as a neurotoxin selective for sympathetic neurons.

Guanethidine, bethanidine and debrisoquin are no longer used clinically, now that better antihypertensive drugs are available. Although extremely effective in lowering standing blood pressure, they produce severe side effects associated with the loss of sympathetic reflexes. The most troublesome include postural hypotension, diarrhoea, nasal congestion and failure of ejaculation. They also fail to lower blood pressure effectively at night, when patients are lying flat.

INDIRECTLY ACTING SYMPATHOMIMETIC AMINES

Mechanism of action and structure–activity relationships

Tyramine, **amphetamine** and **ephedrine** are structurally related to noradrenaline and, although much less potent, have qualitatively similar effects. However, rather than acting directly on adrenoceptors they mainly act indirectly by releasing endogenous noradrenaline from the sympathetic nerve endings. Drugs that act similarly and are used for their central effects (see Ch. 49) include **methylphenidate** and **atomoxetine**.

These drugs have only weak actions on adrenoceptors, but sufficiently resemble noradrenaline to be transported into nerve terminals by NET. Once inside the nerve terminals, they are taken up into the vesicles by VMAT, in exchange for noradrenaline, which escapes into the cytosol. Cytosolic noradrenaline escapes via NET, in exchange for the foreign monoamine, to act on postsynaptic receptors (Fig. 15.7). Exocytosis is not involved in the release process, so their actions do not require the presence of Ca^{2+}. They are not completely specific in their actions, and act partly by a direct effect on adrenoceptors, partly by inhibiting NET (thereby enhancing the effect of the released noradrenaline) and partly by inhibiting MAO.

As would be expected, the effects of these drugs are strongly influenced by other drugs that modify noradrenergic transmission. Thus reserpine and 6-hydroxydopamine abolish their effects by depleting the terminals of noradrenaline. MAO inhibitors, on the other hand, strongly potentiate their effects by preventing inactivation, within the terminals, of the transmitter displaced from the vesicles. MAO inhibition particularly enhances the action of tyramine, because this substance is itself a substrate for MAO. Normally, dietary tyramine is destroyed by MAO in the gut wall and liver before reaching the systemic circulation. When MAO is inhibited this is prevented, and ingestion of tyramine-rich foods such as fermented cheese (e.g. ripe

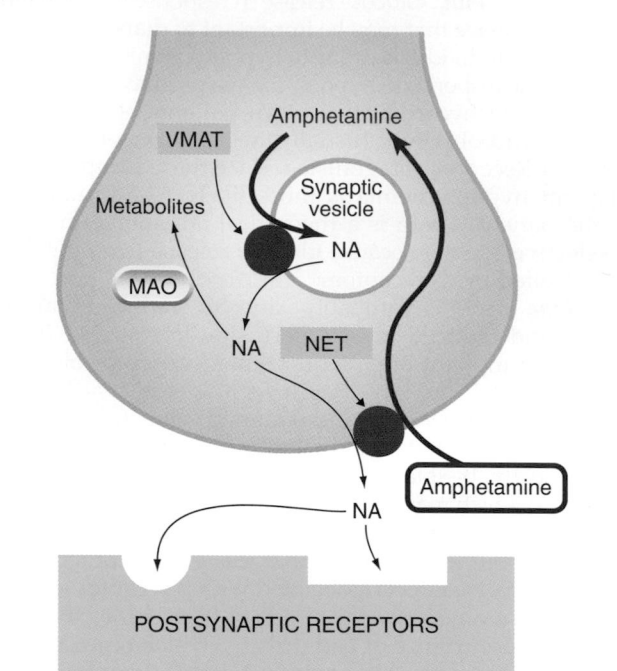

Fig. 15.7 **The mode of action of amphetamine, an indirectly acting sympathomimetic amine.** Amphetamine enters the nerve terminal via the noradrenaline transporter (NET) and enters synaptic vesicles via the vesicular monoamine transporter (VMAT), in exchange for noradrenaline (NA), which accumulates in the cytosol. Some of the NA is degraded by monoamine oxidase (MAO) within the nerve terminal and some escapes, in exchange for amphetamine via the noradrenaline transporter, to act on postsynaptic receptors. Amphetamine also reduces NA reuptake via the transporter, so enhancing the action of the released NA.

Brie) can then provoke a sudden and dangerous rise in blood pressure. Inhibitors of NET, such as **imipramine** (see Table 15.6), interfere with the effects of indirectly acting sympathomimetic amines by preventing their uptake into the nerve terminals.

These drugs, especially amphetamine, have important effects on the CNS (see Chs 49 and 50) that depend on their ability to release not only noradrenaline, but also 5-HT and dopamine from nerve terminals in the brain. An important characteristic of the effects of indirectly acting sympathomimetic amines is that marked tolerance develops. Repeated doses of amphetamine or tyramine, for example, produce progressively smaller pressor responses. This is probably caused by depletion of the releasable store of noradrenaline. Tolerance to the central effects also develops with repeated administration.

Actions

The peripheral actions of the indirectly acting sympathomimetic amines include bronchodilatation, raised arterial pressure, peripheral vasoconstriction, increased heart rate and force of myocardial contraction, and inhibition of gut motility. Their central actions account for their significant abuse potential and for limited therapeutic applications (see Chs 49, 50 and 59). Apart from ephedrine, which is still used as a nasal decongestant because its central action is minor, these drugs are no longer used for their peripheral sympathomimetic effects.

INHIBITORS OF NORADRENALINE UPTAKE

Reuptake of released noradrenaline by NET is the most important mechanism by which its action is terminated. Many drugs inhibit NET, and thereby enhance the effects of both sympathetic nerve activity and circulating noradrenaline. NET is not responsible for clearing circulating adrenaline, so these drugs do not affect responses to this amine.

The main class of drugs whose primary action is inhibition of NET are the *tricyclic antidepressants* (see Ch. 48), for example **imipramine**. These drugs have their major effect on the CNS but also cause tachycardia and cardiac dysrhythmias, reflecting their peripheral effect on sympathetic transmission. **Cocaine**, known mainly for its abuse liability (Chs 49 and 50) and local anaesthetic activity (Ch. 44), enhances sympathetic transmission, causing tachycardia and increased arterial pressure (and, with chronic use, cardiomyopathy and cardiac hypertrophy).

Its central effects of euphoria and excitement (Ch. 49) are probably a manifestation of the same mechanism acting via dopamine and 5-HT in the brain. It strongly potentiates the actions of noradrenaline in experimental animals or in isolated tissues provided the sympathetic nerve terminals are intact.

Many drugs that act mainly on other steps in sympathetic transmission also inhibit NET to some extent, presumably because the carrier molecule has structural features in common with other noradrenaline recognition sites, such as receptors and degradative enzymes.

The extraneuronal monoamine transporter EMT, which is important in clearing circulating adrenaline from the bloodstream, is not affected by most of the drugs that block NET. It is inhibited by **phenoxybenzamine**, however, and by various *corticosteroids* (see Ch. 27). This action of corticosteroids may have some relevance to their therapeutic effect in conditions such as asthma, but is probably of minor importance.

The main sites of action of drugs that affect adrenergic transmission are summarised in Fig. 15.8.

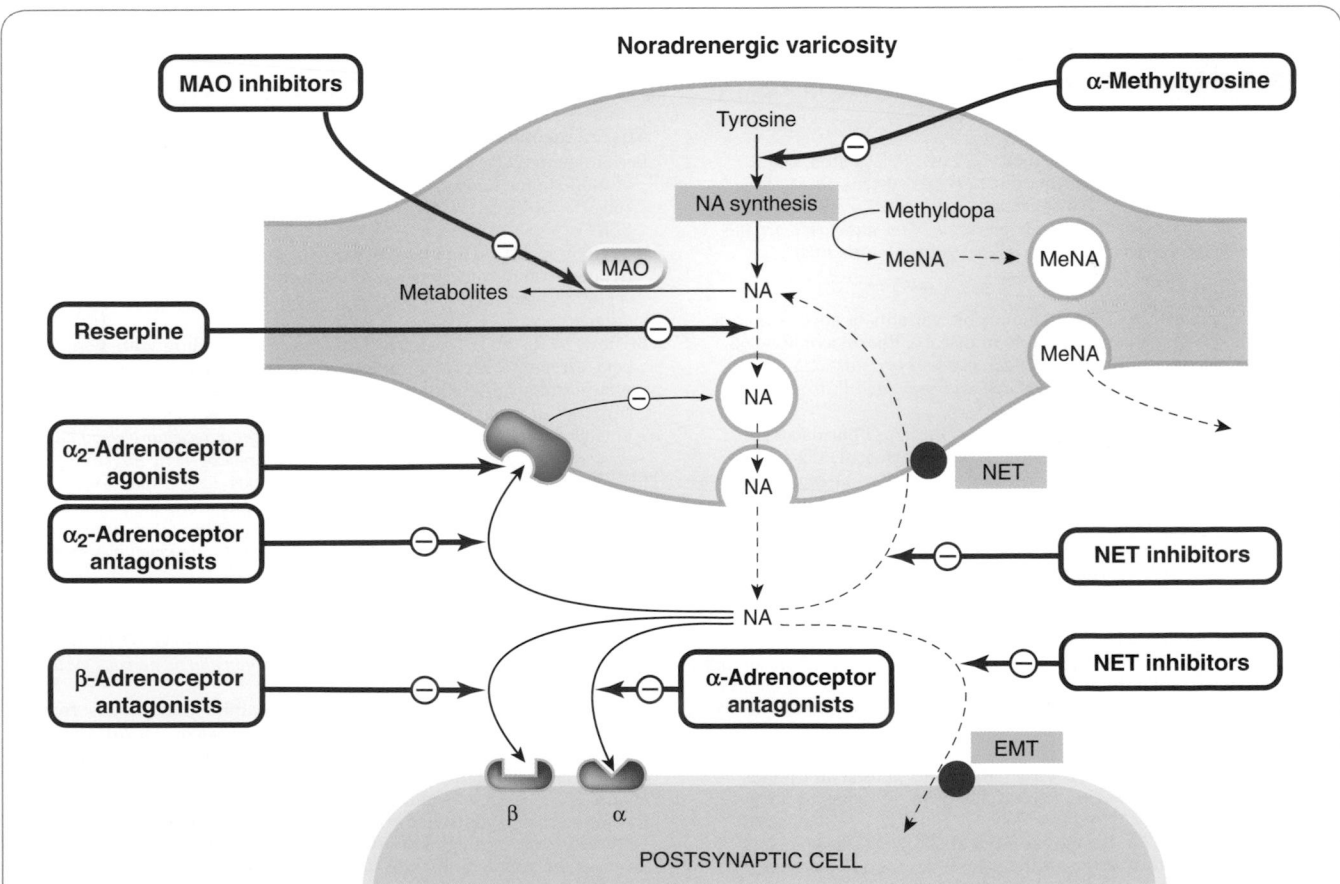

Fig. 15.8 Generalised diagram of a noradrenergic nerve terminal, showing sites of drug action. *EMT*, extraneuronal monoamine transporter; *MAO*, monoamine oxidase; *MeNA*, methylnoradrenaline; *NA*, noradrenaline; *NET*, neuronal noradrenaline transporter.

Drugs acting on noradrenergic nerve terminals

- Drugs that inhibit noradrenaline synthesis include:
  - **α-methyltyrosine**: blocks tyrosine hydroxylase; not used clinically
  - **carbidopa**: blocks dopa decarboxylase and is used in treatment of parkinsonism (see Ch. 41); little effect on noradrenaline synthesis.
- **α-Methyldopa** gives rise to false transmitter (α-methylnoradrenaline), which is a potent α_2 agonist, thus causing powerful presynaptic inhibitory feedback (also central actions). Its use as an antihypertensive agent is now limited mainly to during pregnancy.
- **Reserpine** blocks noradrenaline accumulation in vesicles by vesicular monoamine transporter (VMAT), thus depleting noradrenaline stores and blocking transmission. Effective in hypertension but may cause severe depression. Clinically obsolete.
- Noradrenergic neuron-blocking drugs (e.g. **guanethidine**, **bethanidine**) are selectively concentrated in terminals and in vesicles (by norepinephrine transporter [NET] and VMAT respectively), and block transmitter release, partly by local anaesthetic action. Effective in

hypertension but cause severe side effects (postural hypotension, diarrhoea, nasal congestion, etc.), so now little used.
- **6-Hydroxydopamine** is selectively neurotoxic for noradrenergic neurons, because it is taken up and converted to a toxic metabolite. Used experimentally to eliminate noradrenergic neurons, not used clinically.
- Indirectly acting sympathomimetic amines (e.g. **amphetamine**, **ephedrine**, **tyramine**) are accumulated by NET and displace noradrenaline from vesicles, allowing it to escape. Effect is much enhanced by monoamine oxidase (MAO) inhibition, which can lead to severe hypertension following ingestion of tyramine-rich foods by patients treated with MAO inhibitors.
- Indirectly acting sympathomimetic agents are central nervous system stimulants. **Methylphenidate** and **atomoxetine** are used to treat attention deficit–hyperactivity disorder.
- Drugs that inhibit NET include cocaine and **tricyclic antidepressant** drugs. Sympathetic effects are enhanced by such drugs.

REFERENCES AND FURTHER READING

General

Robertson, D., Biaggioni, I., Burnstock, G., Low, P.A., Paton, G.F.R. (Eds.), 2012. Primer on the autonomic nervous system, third ed. Academic Press, Elsevier, Amsterdam. (*An excellent comprehensive textbook on all aspects, including pharmacology, of the autonomic nervous system. By no means elementary despite the "primer" in its title*)

Adrenoceptors

Ahles, A., Engelhardt, S., 2014. Polymorphic variants of adrenoceptors: pharmacology, physiology, and role in disease. Pharmacol. Rev. 66, 598–637. (*Comprehensive overview of adrenoceptor variants with respect to the modulation of receptor function and expression and their role in physiology and disease*)

Alexander, S.P.H., et al., 2015. The Concise Guide to Pharmacology 2015/16: G protein-coupled receptors. Br. J. Pharmacol. 172, 5744–5869. (*Summary articles on drug targets including adrenoceptors*)

Baker, J.G., Hall, I.P., Hill, S.J., 2003. Agonist and inverse agonist actions of β-blockers at the human β_2-adrenoceptor provide evidence for agonist-directed signalling. Mol. Pharmacol. 64, 1357–1369. (*β-blockers differ in their ability to activate and block cAMP and mitogen-activated protein kinase pathways, pointing to possible differences in clinical efficacy between different members of the class*)

Gilsbach, R., Hein, L., 2012. Are the pharmacology and physiology of α_2 adrenoceptors determined by α_2-heteroreceptors and autoreceptors respectively? Br. J. Pharmacol. 165, 90–102. (*Argues for the significance of auto- versus heteroreceptors in mediating the physiological functions of α_2-adrenoceptors and the pharmacological functions of α_2-adrenoceptor agonist drugs respectively*)

Guimaraes, S., Moura, D., 2001. Vascular adrenoceptors: an update. Pharmacol. Rev. 53, 319–356. (*Review describing the complex roles of different adrenoceptors in blood vessels*)

Kahsai, A.W., Xiao, K.H., Rajagopal, S., et al., 2011. Multiple ligand-specific conformations of the beta(2)-adrenergic receptor. Nature Chem. Biol. 7, 692–700. (*Contrary to two-state models for receptor activity, there is significant variability in receptor conformations induced by different ligands, with implications for the design of new therapeutic agents*)

Papay, R.S., Ting, S., Piascik, M.T., Prasad, S.V.N., Perez, D.M., 2013. α_{1A}-Adrenergic receptors regulate cardiac hypertrophy in vivo through interleukin-6 secretion. Mol. Pharmacol. 83, 939–948. (*Evidence that, in the mouse, IL-6 is a major mediator of α_{1A}-AR cardiac hypertrophy*)

Philipp, M., Hein, L., 2004. Adrenergic receptor knockout mice: distinct functions of 9 receptor subtypes. Pharm. Ther. 101, 65–74.

Miscellaneous topics

Bermingham, D.P., Blakely, R.D., 2016. Kinase-dependent regulation of monoamine neurotransmitter transporters. Pharmacol. Rev. 68, 888–953. (*Reviews evidence for kinase-dependent control of DAT, NET and SERT*)

Biaggioni, I., 2017. The pharmacology of autonomic failure: from hypotension to hypertension. Pharmacol. Rev. 69, 53–62. (*Fascinating applied pharmacology of a relatively uncommon but highly informative disorder*)

Bristow, M.R., 2011. Treatment of chronic heart failure with beta-adrenergic receptor antagonists: a convergence of receptor pharmacology and clinical cardiology. Circ. Res. 109, 1176–1194. (*Argues that there is: 'ample room to improve antiadrenergic therapy, through novel approaches exploiting the nuances of receptor biology and/or intracellular signaling, as well as through pharmacogenetic targeting'*)

Eisenhofer, G., Kopin, I.J., Goldstein, D.S., 2004. Catecholamine metabolism: a contemporary view with implications for physiology and medicine. Pharmacol. Rev. 56, 331–349. (*Review that dismisses a number of fallacies concerning the routes by which catecholamines from different sources are metabolised and excreted*)

Elenkov, I.J., Wilder, R.L., Chrousos, G.P., et al., 2000. The sympathetic nerve – an integrative interface between two supersystems: the brain and the immune system. Pharmacol. Rev. 52, 595–638. (*Detailed catalogue of effects of catecholamines and the sympathetic nervous system on the immune system*)

Gainetdinov, R.R., Caron, M.G., 2003. Monoamine transporters: from genes to behaviour. Annu. Rev. Pharmacol. Toxicol. 43, 261–284. (*Review article focusing on the characteristics of transgenic mice lacking specific monoamine transporters*)

Léauté-Labrèze, C., Hoeger, P., Mazereeuw-Hautier, J., et al., 2015. A randomized, controlled trial of oral propranolol in infantile hemangioma. N. Engl. J. Med. 372, 735–746. (*Randomised controlled trial with adaptive design elegantly identifying a highly effective dose regimen. Will this stimulate more "basic" research on b-adrenoceptor mechanisms in endothelial cell growth and development?*)

Nonogaki, K., 2000. New insights into sympathetic regulation of glucose and fat metabolism. Diabetologia 43, 533–549. (*Review of the complex adrenoceptor-mediated effects on the metabolism of liver, muscle and adipose tissue*)

Sacco, E., Bientinesi, R., 2012. Mirabegron: a review of recent data and its prospects in the management of overactive bladder. Ther. Adv. Urol. 4, 315–324. (*Pharmacology of a selective β_3-adrenoceptor agonist, licensed to treat symptoms of overactive bladder*)

5-Hydroxytryptamine and the pharmacology of migraine

16

OVERVIEW

5-Hydroxytryptamine (5-HT) is an important neuro-transmitter in the brain and periphery. It is also a local hormone and is important in platelet function. We describe its synthesis, storage and release as well as its role in the pathophysiology of three disorders (migraine, carcinoid syndrome and pulmonary hypertension). We also review the pharmacology of the numerous drugs that act at 5-HT receptors.

5-HYDROXYTRYPTAMINE

A biologically active, low molecular-weight factor originally detected in extracts of gut ('enteramine') and in blood serum ('serotonin') was eventually identified chemically as *5-hydroxytryptamine* (Fig. 16.1). Today, the terms '5-HT' and 'serotonin' are used interchangeably. 5-HT was subsequently found in the central nervous system (CNS) and shown to function both as a neurotransmitter and as a local hormone in the peripheral vascular system. This chapter deals with the metabolism, distribution and physiological roles of 5-HT in the periphery, and with the different types of 5-HT receptor and the drugs that act on them. Further information on the role of 5-HT in the brain, its relationship to psychiatric disorders and the actions of psychotropic drugs, is presented in Chapters 40, 47 and 48. The use of drugs that modulate 5-HT in the gut is dealt with in Chapter 31.

DISTRIBUTION, BIOSYNTHESIS AND DEGRADATION

The highest concentrations of 5-HT are found in three organs:

- *In the wall of the intestine.* Over 90% of the total amount in the body is present in the *enterochromaffin* cells (endocrine cells with distinctive staining properties) in the gut. These cells are derived from the neural crest and resemble those of the adrenal medulla. They are found mainly in the stomach and small intestine interspersed with mucosal cells. Some 5-HT also occurs in nerve cells of the myenteric plexus, where it functions as an excitatory neurotransmitter (see Chs 13 and 31).
- *In blood.* Platelets contain high concentrations of 5-HT. They accumulate it from the plasma by an active transport system and release it from cytoplasmic granules when they aggregate (hence the high concentration of 5-HT in serum from clotted blood, see Ch. 25).
- *In the CNS.* 5-HT is a transmitter in the CNS and is present in high concentrations in localised regions

of the midbrain. Its functional role is discussed in Chapter 40.

Although 5-HT is present in the diet, most of this is metabolised before entering the bloodstream. Endogenous 5-HT arises from a biosynthetic pathway similar to that of noradrenaline (see Ch. 15), except that the precursor amino acid is *tryptophan* instead of tyrosine (see Fig. 16.1). Tryptophan is converted to 5-hydroxytryptophan in chromaffin cells and neurons by the action of *tryptophan hydroxylase*, an enzyme confined to 5-HT-producing cells (but not present in platelets). The 5-hydroxytryptophan is then decarboxylated to 5-HT by the ubiquitous *L-aromatic acid decarboxylase,* which also participates in the synthesis of catecholamines (Ch. 15) and histamine (Ch. 18). Platelets (and neurons) possess a high-affinity 5-HT uptake mechanism. They become loaded with 5-HT as they pass through the intestinal circulation, where the local concentration is relatively high. Because the mechanisms of synthesis, storage, release and reuptake of 5-HT are very similar to those of noradrenaline, many drugs affect both processes indiscriminately (see Ch. 15). However, *selective serotonin reuptake inhibitors* (SSRIs) have been developed and are important therapeutically as anxiolytics and antidepressants (Chs 45 and 48). 5-HT is often stored in neurons and chromaffin cells as a co-transmitter, together with various peptide hormones, such as *somatostatin, substance P* or *vasoactive intestinal polypeptide* (Ch. 19).

Degradation of 5-HT (see Fig. 16.1) occurs mainly through oxidative deamination, catalysed by *monoamine oxidase A,* followed by oxidation to *5-hydroxyindoleacetic acid* (5-HIAA), the pathway again being the same as that of noradrenaline catabolism. 5-HIAA is excreted in the urine and serves as an indicator of 5-HT production in the body. This is used, for example, in the diagnosis of carcinoid syndrome.

CLASSIFICATION OF 5-HT RECEPTORS

▼ It was realised long ago that the actions of 5-HT are not all mediated by receptors of the same type, and various pharmacological classifications have come and gone. The current system is summarised in Table 16.1 and full details are available at <www.guidetopharmacology.org>. This classification takes into account sequence data derived from cloning, signal transduction mechanisms and pharmacological specificity as well as the phenotypes of 5-HT receptor 'knock-out' mice.

Their diversity is astonishing. Currently, there are some 14 known receptor subtypes (together with an extra gene in mouse). These are divided into seven classes (5-HT$_{1-7}$), one of which (5-HT$_3$) is a ligand-gated cation channel while the remainder are G protein–coupled receptors (GPCRs; see Ch. 3). The six GPCR families are further subdivided into some 13 receptor subtypes based on their sequence and pharmacology. Most subtypes are found in all species so far examined, but there are some exceptions (the 5-HT$_{5B}$ gene is found in mouse but has not been found in humans). The sequences of 5-HT$_1$ and 5-HT$_2$ receptors are highly conserved among species, but the 5-HT$_{4-7}$ receptors are more diverse and are grouped together largely

217

Tryptophan

Tryptophan hydroxylase

5-Hydroxytryptophan

L-Aromatic acid decarboxylase (= dopa decarboxylase)

5-Hydroxytryptamine (serotonin)

Monoamine oxidase

Aldehyde dehydrogenase

5-Hydroxyindoleacetic acid (5-HIAA)

Fig. 16.1 Biosynthesis and metabolism of 5-hydroxytryptamine.

Actions and functions of 5-hydroxytryptamine (5-HT)

- Important actions are:
  - increased gastrointestinal motility (direct excitation of smooth muscle and indirect action via enteric neurons)
  - contraction of other smooth muscle (bronchi, uterus)
  - mixture of vascular constriction (direct and via sympathetic innervation) and dilatation (endothelium dependent)
  - platelet aggregation
  - stimulation of peripheral nociceptive nerve endings
  - excitation/inhibition of central nervous system neurons.
- Postulated physiological and pathophysiological roles include:
  - in periphery: peristalsis, vomiting, platelet aggregation and haemostasis, inflammation, sensitisation of nociceptors and microvascular control
  - in central nervous system: many postulated functions, including control of appetite, sleep, mood, hallucinations, stereotyped behaviour, pain perception and vomiting.
- Clinical conditions associated with disturbed 5-hydroxytryptamine (5-HT) include:
  - migraine, carcinoid syndrome, pulmonary hypertension, mood disorders and anxiety.

Distribution, biosynthesis and degradation of 5-hydroxytryptamine (5-HT)

- Tissues rich in 5-HT are:
  - gastrointestinal tract (chromaffin cells and enteric neurons)
  - platelets
  - central nervous system.
- Metabolism closely parallels that of noradrenaline.
  - 5-HT is formed from dietary tryptophan, which is converted to 5-hydroxytryptophan by tryptophan hydroxylase, then to 5-HT by a non-specific decarboxylase.
- 5-HT is transported into cells by a specific serotonin uptake transporter (SERT).
  - Degradation occurs mainly by monoamine oxidase, forming 5-hydroxyindoleacetic acid (5-HIAA), which is excreted in urine.

on pharmacological grounds. Most 5-HT GPCRs signal through adenylyl cyclase/cAMP, but some (the 5-HT$_2$ subtype) activate phospholipase C to generate phospholipid-derived second messengers (see Ch. 3).

In addition to these main subtypes, many genetic isoforms have been found, giving rise to four or more variants of some of these receptors. The pharmacological and pathophysiological relevance of these genetic isoforms is unclear.

With the exception of 5-HT$_3$-selective agents, 5-HT receptor agonists and antagonists are relatively non-selective with respect to different receptor subtypes. This makes their pharmacology difficult to interpret and summarise.

Many transgenic mice lacking functional members of this receptor family have been produced (see for example Bonasera & Tecott, 2000). The functional deficits in such animals are generally quite subtle, suggesting that these receptors may serve to modulate, rather than to enable, physiological responses. Table 16.1 gives an overview of the most important receptors. Some of the more significant drug targets include the following:

5-HT$_1$ receptors. Those of pharmacological significance occur mainly in the brain, the subtypes being distinguished on the basis of their regional distribution and their pharmacological specificity. Their function is mainly inhibitory. The 5-HT$_{1A}$ subtype is particularly important in relation to mood and behaviour (see Chs 45, 47) and 5-HT$_1$ 'knock-out' mice exhibit defects in sleep regulation, learning ability and other CNS functions. Receptor polymorphisms may be associated with increased susceptibility to substance abuse. The 5-HT$_{1B}$ and 5-HT$_{1D}$ subtypes, which are expressed in neurones innervating cerebral blood vessels, are believed to be important in migraine and are the target for *triptans* (e.g. **sumatriptan**), an important group of drugs used to treat acute attacks (Fig. 16.2). Unfortunately, the 5-HT$_{1B}$ receptor is also present in the vasculature of the heart and elsewhere, explaining some of the unwanted effects associated with triptan

Table 16.1   Some significant drugs acting at the main 5-HT receptor subtypes

Receptor	Location	Main function	Primary signalling system	Significant drugs	
				Agonists	Antagonists
5-HT$_{1A}$	Chiefly CNS	Neuronal inhibition. Behavioural effects: sleep, feeding, thermoregulation, anxiety	G protein (G$_i$/G$_o$) ↓ cAMP (may also modulate Ca^{2+} channels)	8-OH-DPAT, triptans, clozapine, buspirone (PA), cabergoline	Methiothepin, yohimbine, ketanserin, pizotifen, spiperone
5-HT$_{1B}$	CNS, vascular smooth muscle, many other sites	Presynaptic inhibition. Behavioural effects. Pulmonary vasoconstriction	G protein (G$_i$/G$_o$) ↓ cAMP (may also modulate Ca^{2+} channels)	8-OH-DPAT, triptans (PA), clozapine, cabergoline, dihydroergotamine	Methiothepin (IA), yohimbine, ketanserin, spiperone
5-HT$_{1D}$	CNS, blood vessels	Cerebral vasoconstriction. Behavioural effects: locomotion	G protein (G$_i$/G$_o$) ↓ cAMP (may also modulate Ca^{2+} channels)	8-OH-DPAT, triptans, clozapine, cabergoline (PA), dihydroergotamine/ ergotamine	Methiothepin (IA), yohimbine, ketanserin, methysergide, spiperone
5-HT$_{1E}$	CNS	—	G protein (G$_i$/G$_o$) ↓ cAMP (may also modulate Ca^{2+} channels)	8-OH-DPAT, triptans; clozapine, dihydroergotamine	Methiothepin, yohimbine, methysergide
5-HT$_{1F}$	CNS, uterus, heart, GI tract	—	G protein (G$_i$/G$_o$) ↓ cAMP (may also modulate Ca^{2+} channels)	8-OH-DPAT, triptans; clozapine dihydroergotamine/ ergotamine, lamistidan	Yohimbine, methysergide
5-HT$_{2A}$	CNS, PNS, smooth muscle, platelets	Neuronal excitation. Behavioural effects. Smooth muscle contraction (gut, bronchi, etc.). Platelet aggregation. Vasoconstriction/vasodilatation	G protein (G$_q$/G$_{11}$) ↑ IP$_3$, Ca^{2+}	LSD, cabergoline, methysergide (PA), 8-OH-DPAT, ergotamine (PA)	Ketanserin, clozapine, methysergide
5-HT$_{2B}$	Gastric fundus	Contraction	G protein (G$_q$/G$_{11}$) ↑ IP$_3$, Ca^{2+}	LSD, cabergoline, methysergide (PA), 8-OH-DPAT, ergotamine (PA)	Ketanserin, clozapine, yohimbine
5-HT$_{2C}$	CNS, lymphocytes	—	G protein (G$_q$/G$_{11}$) ↑ IP$_3$, Ca^{2+}	LSD, cabergoline, methysergide (PA), 8-OH-DPAT, ergotamine (PA)	Ketanserin, clozapine (IA), methysergide
5-HT$_3$ (recently renamed 5-HT$_{3A}$)	PNS, CNS	Neuronal excitation (autonomic, nociceptive neurons). Emesis. Behavioural effects: anxiety	Ligand-gated cation channel	2-Me-5-HT, chloromethyl biguanide	Granisetron, ondansetron, palonosetron.
5-HT$_4$	PNS (GI tract), CNS	Neuronal excitation. GI motility	G protein (G$_s$) ↑ cAMP	Metoclopramide, tegaserod (PA), cisapride	Tropisetron
5-HT$_{5A}$	CNS	Modulation of exploratory behaviour (rodents)?	G protein (G$_s$) ↑ cAMP	Triptans, 8-OH-DPAT	Clozapine, methysergide, yohimbine, ketanserin
5-HT$_6$	CNS, leukocytes	Learning and memory, modulation of neurotransmission.	G protein (G$_s$) ↑ cAMP	LSD, ergotamine	Clozapine (IA), spiperone, methysergide, dihydroergotamine
5-HT$_7$	CNS, GI tract, blood vessels	Thermoregulation? Circadian rhythm?	G protein (G$_s$) ↑ cAMP	Buspirone (PA), bromocriptine, cisapride, 8-OH-DPAT, LSD,	Clozapine (IA), methysergide, buspirone, dihydroergotamine, ketanserin, yohimbine

The receptor classification system is based upon the IUPHAR database at <www.guidetopharmacology.org>
Many drugs here are not used clinically or are not currently available in the United Kingdom (e.g. tropisetron), but are included as they are often used experimentally or referred to in the literature.
The list of agonists and antagonists is not exhaustive.
2-Me-5-HT, 2-methyl-5-hydroxytryptamine; *8-OH-DPAT*, 8-hydroxy-2-(di-n-propylamino) tetraline; *CNS*, *central nervous system*; *GI*, gastrointestinal; *IA*, inverse agonist; *IP$_3$*, inositol trisphosphate; *LSD*, lysergic acid diethylamide; *PA*, partial agonist; *PNS*, peripheral nervous system.

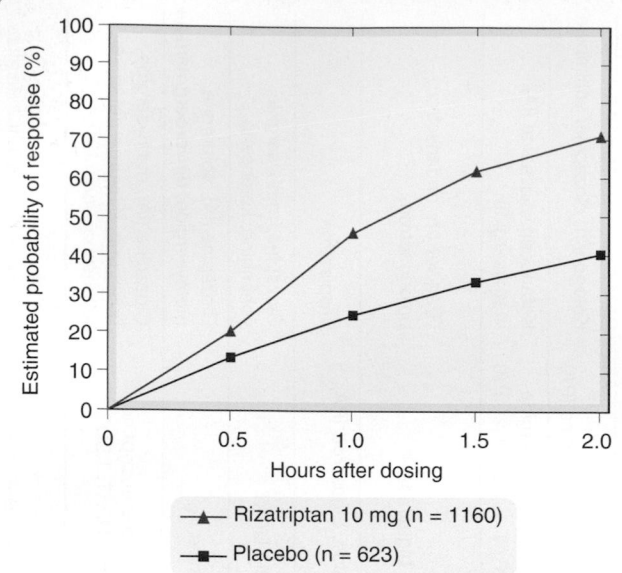

Fig. 16.2 The triptan, rizatriptan, relieves the pain associated with attacks of migraine. The graph is a Kaplan–Meir plot showing the probability of experiencing relief from the pain of the attack after treatment with placebo or with 10 mg rizatriptan. (Modified from Dahlof et al., 1999).

therapy. The hapless '$5\text{-}HT_{1C}$' receptor – actually the first to be cloned – has been officially declared non-existent, having been ignominiously reclassified as the $5\text{-}HT_{2C}$ receptor when it was found to be linked to inositol trisphosphate production rather than adenylyl cyclase.

$5\text{-}HT_2$ receptors. These are present in the CNS but are also particularly important in the periphery. The effects of 5-HT on smooth muscle and platelets, which have been known for many years, are mediated by the $5\text{-}HT_{2A}$ receptor, as are some of the behavioural effects of agents such as **lysergic acid diethylamide** (LSD; see Table 16.1 and Ch. 49). $5\text{-}HT_2$ receptors are linked to phospholipase C and thus stimulate inositol trisphosphate formation. The $5\text{-}HT_{2A}$ subtype is functionally the most important, the others having a much more limited distribution and functional role. The role of $5\text{-}HT_2$ receptors in normal physiology is probably a minor one, but it becomes more prominent in pathological conditions such as asthma and vascular thrombosis (see Chs 25 and 29). Mice lacking $5\text{-}HT_2$ receptors exhibit defects in colonic motility ($5\text{-}HT_{2A}$), heart defects ($5\text{-}HT_{2B}$) and CNS disorders ($5\text{-}HT_{2C}$).

$5\text{-}HT_3$ receptors. $5\text{-}HT_3$ receptors are exceptional in being membrane ion channels (Ch. 3) and cause excitation directly, without involvement of any second messenger. The receptor itself consists of a homo- or hetero-pentameric assembly of distinct subunits which are designated by further subscript letters (e.g. $5\text{-}HT_{3A\text{-}E}$ in humans). $5\text{-}HT_3$ receptors occur mainly in the peripheral nervous system, particularly on nociceptive sensory neurons (see Ch. 43) and on autonomic and enteric neurons, where 5-HT exerts a strong excitatory effect. 5-HT evokes pain when injected locally; when given intravenously, it elicits a fine display of autonomic reflexes, which result from excitation of many types of vascular, pulmonary and cardiac sensory nerve fibres. $5\text{-}HT_3$ receptors also occur in the brain, particularly in the *area postrema*, a region of the medulla involved in the vomiting reflex, and selective $5\text{-}HT_3$ antagonists are used as antiemetic drugs (see Ch. 31). Polymorphisms in the subunits are associated with increased susceptibility to nausea and vomiting.

$5\text{-}HT_4$ receptors. These occur in the brain, as well as in peripheral organs such as the gastrointestinal tract, bladder and heart. Their main physiological role appears to be in the gastrointestinal tract, where they produce neuronal excitation and mediate the effect of 5-HT in stimulating peristalsis. Mice deficient in the $5\text{-}HT_4$ receptor

exhibit a complex phenotype including abnormal feeding behaviour in response to stress.

$5\text{-}HT_5$, $5\text{-}HT_6$ and $5\text{-}HT_7$ receptors. Little is known about these receptors. All are present in the CNS as well as other tissues. There are two genes for $5\text{-}HT_5$ isoforms but only one codes for a functional receptor in humans although both may be functional in rodents. In addition to its action on $5\text{-}HT_{1B/D}$ receptors, sumatriptan is also an antagonist at the $5\text{-}HT_7$ receptor suggesting this receptor may also be a significant target for migraine treatment (Agosti, 2007).

5-Hydroxytryptamine (5-HT) receptors

- There are seven families ($5\text{-}HT_{1\text{-}7}$), with further subtypes of $5\text{-}HT_1$ (A–F) and $5\text{-}HT_2$ (A–C). Many polymorphisms and splice variants have also been observed.
- All are G protein–coupled receptors, except $5\text{-}HT_3$, which are ligand-gated cation channels.
  - $5\text{-}HT_1$ receptors occur mainly in the central nervous system (CNS) (all subtypes) and some blood vessels ($5\text{-}HT_{1B/D}$ subtypes). Some effects are mediated through inhibition of adenylyl cyclase, include neural inhibition and vasoconstriction. Specific agonists include triptans (used in migraine therapy) and **buspirone** (used in anxiety). Specific antagonists include **spiperone** and **methiothepin**.
  - $5\text{-}HT_2$ receptors occur in the CNS and many peripheral sites (especially blood vessels, platelets, autonomic neurons). Neuronal and smooth muscle effects are excitatory and some blood vessels are dilated as a result of nitric oxide release from endothelial cells. $5\text{-}HT_2$ receptors act through the phospholipase C/inositol trisphosphate pathway. Ligands include lysergic acid diethylamide (**LSD**; agonist in CNS, antagonist in periphery). Specific antagonists include **ketanserin**.
  - $5\text{-}HT_3$ receptors occur in the peripheral nervous system, especially nociceptive afferent neurons and enteric neurons, and in the CNS. Effects are excitatory, mediated through direct receptor-coupled ion channels. **2-Methyl-5-HT** is a specific agonist. Specific antagonists include **ondansetron** and **palonosetron**. Antagonists are used mainly as antiemetic drugs but may also be anxiolytic.
  - $5\text{-}HT_4$ receptors occur mainly in the enteric nervous system (also in the CNS). Effects are excitatory, through stimulation of adenylyl cyclase, causing increased gastrointestinal motility. Specific agonists include **metoclopramide** (used to stimulate gastric emptying).
  - $5\text{-}HT_5$ receptors (one subtype in humans) are located in the CNS. Little is known about their role in humans.
  - $5\text{-}HT_6$ receptors are located in the CNS and on leukocytes. Little is known about their role in humans.
  - $5\text{-}HT_7$ receptors are located in the CNS and the gastrointestinal tract. Little is known about their role in humans but emerging data shows they may also be important in migraine.

PHARMACOLOGICAL EFFECTS

The actions of 5-HT are numerous and complex and there is considerable species variation. This complexity reflects the profusion of 5-HT receptor subtypes. The main sites of action are as follows.

Gastrointestinal tract. Most 5-HT receptor subtypes are present in the gut with the exception of those of the $5\text{-HT}_{5/6}$ family. Only about 10% of 5-HT in the intestine is located in neurons, where it acts as a neurotransmitter, while the remainder is located in the enterochromaffin cells, which act as sensors to transduce information about the state of the gut, and release 5-HT into the *lamina propria*. Broadly speaking, 5-HT receptors are present on most neuronal components of the enteric nervous system as well as smooth muscle, secretory and other cells. Their main function is to regulate peristalsis, intestinal motility, secretion and visceral sensitivity; the responses observed are complex and the reader is referred to Beattie and Smith (2008) for a more comprehensive account.

The importance of 5-HT in the gut is underlined by the widespread distribution in the enteric nervous system and the intestinal mucosa, of the *serotonin uptake transporter* (SERT) which rapidly and efficiently removes extracellular 5-HT, thus limiting its action. Inhibitors of this transporter such as the SSRIs (Ch. 48) exaggerate the action of 5-HT in the gut, explaining some of the common side effects of these drugs, which include diarrhoea. Interestingly, there is evidence for genetic defects in this reuptake system in irritable bowel syndrome, which might explain the rather bewildering symptoms of the disease (Ch. 31).

Smooth muscle. In many species (although only to a minor extent in humans), smooth muscle outside of the gastrointestinal tract (e.g. uterus and bronchial tree) is also contracted by 5-HT.

Blood vessels. The effect of 5-HT on blood vessels depends on various factors, including the size of the vessel, the species and the prevailing sympathetic activity. Large vessels, both arteries and veins, are usually constricted by 5-HT, although the sensitivity varies greatly. This is the result of a direct action on vascular smooth muscle cells, mediated through 5-HT_{2A} receptors. Dilatation of large intracranial vessels contributes to headache whereas activation of 5-HT_1 receptors causes constriction, perhaps contributing to the antimigraine action of these drugs. 5-HT can also cause vasodilatation indirectly by releasing nitric oxide from vascular endothelial cells (see Ch. 21) and inhibiting noradrenaline release from sympathetic nerve terminals. If 5-HT is injected intravenously, the blood pressure initially rises, owing to the constriction of large vessels, and then falls, owing to arteriolar dilatation. 5-HT may play a role in the pathology of *pulmonary hypertension* (see later in this chapter and Ch. 23).

Platelets. 5-HT causes platelet aggregation (see Ch. 25) by acting on 5-HT_{2A} receptors, and the platelets that collect in the vessel release further 5-HT. If the endothelium is intact, 5-HT release from adherent platelets causes vasodilatation, which helps to sustain blood flow; if it is damaged (e.g. by atherosclerosis), 5-HT causes constriction and impairs blood flow further. These effects of platelet-derived 5-HT are thought to be important in vascular disease.

Nerve endings. 5-HT stimulates nociceptive (pain-mediating) sensory nerve endings, an effect mediated mainly by 5-HT_3 receptors. If injected into the skin, 5-HT causes pain; when given systemically, it elicits a variety of autonomic reflexes through stimulation of afferent fibres in the heart and lungs, which further complicate the cardiovascular response. In some species, mast cells release 5-HT when stimulated and nettle stings contain 5-HT among other mediators. 5-HT also inhibits transmitter release from adrenergic neurons in the periphery.

Central nervous system. 5-HT is an important neurotransmitter in the CNS and several important antipsychotic and antidepressant drugs act on these pathways (Chs 47 and 48). LSD is a relatively non-selective 5-HT receptor agonist/partial agonist, which acts centrally as a potent hallucinogen. However, its actions are complex: 5-HT excites some neurons and inhibits others; it also acts presynaptically to inhibit transmitter release from nerve terminals and this might underlie some of the actions of serotonergic drugs in migraine. Different receptor subtypes mediate these effects. The role of 5-HT in the CNS is discussed in Chapter 40.

Ergot alkaloids

- These active substances are produced by a fungus that infects cereal crops and are responsible for occasional poisoning incidents. The most important compounds are:
  - **ergotamine** used in migraine prophylaxis, and **dihydroergotamine**
  - **ergometrine**, used in obstetrics to prevent postpartum haemorrhage
  - **methysergide**, formerly used to treat carcinoid syndrome, and migraine prophylaxis
  - **bromocriptine**, used in parkinsonism and endocrine disorders.
- Main sites of action are 5-hydroxytryptamine (5-HT) receptors, dopamine receptors and adrenoceptors (mixed agonist, antagonist and partial agonist effects).
- Unwanted effects include nausea and vomiting, vasoconstriction (ergot alkaloids are contraindicated in patients with peripheral vascular disease).

DRUGS ACTING AT 5-HT RECEPTORS

Table 16.1 lists some significant agonists and antagonists at the different receptor types. Many are only partly selective. Our increasing understanding of the location and function of the different receptor subtypes has raised the possibility of developing compounds with improved receptor selectivity.

Important drugs that act on 5-HT receptors in the periphery include the following:

- Although not clinically useful, selective 5-HT_{1A} agonists, such as 8-hydroxy-2-(di-*n*-propylamino) tetralin (8-OH-DPAT), are potent hypotensive agents, acting through a central mechanism. They are useful experimental drugs.
- $5\text{-HT1}_{B/D}$-receptor agonists (e.g. the triptans) are used for treating migraine.
- 5-HT_2-receptor antagonists (e.g. **methysergide, ketanserin**) act mainly on 5-HT_{2A} receptors but may also block other 5-HT receptors, as well as α adrenoceptors and histamine receptors (Ch. 27). **Ergotamine** and methysergide belong to the ergot family and have been used mainly for migraine prophylaxis (although methysergide is rarely used

Table 16.2 Properties of ergot alkaloids and related compounds

| Drug | Actions at receptors | | | Uterus | Main uses | Side effects, etc. |
	5-HT	α Adrenoceptor	Dopamine			
Ergotamine	Antagonist/partial agonist (5-HT$_1$) Antagonist (other sites)	Partial agonist (blood vessels)	Inactive	Contracts ++	Migraine (largely obsolete)	Emesis, vasospasm (avoid in peripheral vascular disease and pregnancy)
Dihydroergotamine	Antagonist/partial agonist (5-HT$_1$)	Antagonist	Inactive	Contracts +	Migraine (largely obsolete)	Less emesis than with ergotamine
Ergometrine	Weak antagonist/partial agonist (5-HT$_1$)	Weak antagonist/partial agonist	Weak	Contracts +++	Prevention of postpartum haemorrhage (Ch. 36)	Nausea, vomiting
Bromocriptine	Inactive	Weak antagonist	Agonist/partial agonist	—	Parkinson's disease (Ch. 41) Endocrine disorders (Ch. 32)	Drowsiness, emesis
Methysergide	Antagonist/partial agonist at several subtypes	—	—	—	Carcinoid syndrome Migraine prophylaxis (rarely used)	Retroperitoneal and mediastinal fibrosis Emesis

5-HT, 5-hydroxytryptamine.

these days). Other 5-HT$_2$ antagonists are used to control the symptoms of carcinoid tumours.

- 5-HT$_3$-receptor antagonists (e.g. **granisetron**, **ondansetron**, **palonosetron**) are used as antiemetic drugs (see Chs 31 and 57), particularly for controlling the severe nausea and vomiting that occurs with many forms of cancer chemotherapy.
- 5-HT$_4$-receptor agonists that stimulate coordinated peristaltic activity (known as a 'prokinetic action') could be used for treating gastrointestinal disorders (see Ch. 31). **Metoclopramide** acts in this way, as well as by blocking dopamine receptors. Similar but more selective drugs such as **cisapride** and **tegaserod** were introduced to treat irritable bowel syndrome, but were withdrawn on account of adverse cardiovascular side effects.

ERGOT ALKALOIDS

Ergot alkaloids have preoccupied pharmacologists for more than a century. As a group, they stubbornly resist classification. Many act on 5-HT receptors, but not selectively, so that their effects are complex and diverse.

▼ Ergot, an extract of the fungus *Claviceps purpurea* that infests cereal crops, contains many active substances, and it was the study of their pharmacological properties that led Dale to many important discoveries concerning acetylcholine, histamine and catecholamines. Epidemics of ergot poisoning have occurred, and still occur, when contaminated grain is used for food. The symptoms include mental disturbances and intensely painful peripheral vasoconstriction leading to gangrene[1].

Ergot alkaloids are complex molecules derived from lysergic acid. The

important members of the group (Table 16.2) include various naturally occurring and synthetic derivatives with different substituent groups arranged around a common nucleus. These compounds display diverse pharmacological actions and it is difficult to discern any clear relationship between chemical structure and pharmacological properties.

Actions

Most of the effects of ergot alkaloids appear to be mediated through adrenoceptors, 5-HT or dopamine receptors, although some may be produced through other mechanisms. All alkaloids stimulate smooth muscle, some being relatively selective for vascular smooth muscle while others act mainly on the uterus. Ergotamine and **dihydroergotamine** are, respectively, a partial agonist and an antagonist at α adrenoceptors. **Bromocriptine** is an agonist of dopamine receptors, particularly in the CNS (Ch. 40), and methysergide is an antagonist at 5-HT$_{2A}$ receptors.

The clinical use of ergot agents has diminished as more selective and safer drugs have been introduced but nevertheless, they remain important for pharmacologists. Their main actions and uses are summarised in Table 16.2. As one would expect of agents having so many actions, their physiological effects are complex and often rather poorly understood. Ergotamine, dihydroergotamine and methysergide are discussed here; further information on **ergometrine** and bromocriptine is given in Chapters 34, 36 and 41.

Vascular effects. When injected into an anaesthetised animal, ergotamine activates α adrenoceptors, causing vasoconstriction and a sustained rise in blood pressure. At the same time, ergotamine reverses the pressor effect of adrenaline (epinephrine; see Ch. 15). The vasoconstrictor effect of ergotamine is responsible for the peripheral gangrene of St Anthony's fire, and probably also for some of the effects of ergot on the CNS. Methysergide and dihydroergotamine have much less vasoconstrictor effect. Methysergide is a potent 5-HT$_{2A}$-receptor antagonist,

---

[1]This came to be known in the Middle Ages as *St Anthony's fire*, because it was believed that it could be cured by a visit to the Shrine of St Anthony (which conveniently happened to be in an ergot-free region of France).

whereas ergotamine and dihydroergotamine act on 5-HT$_1$ receptors, which may account for their antimigraine activity.

Clinical use. The only use of ergotamine is in the treatment of attacks of migraine unresponsive to simple analgesics (see Chs 27 and 43). Methysergide was formerly used for migraine prophylaxis, and for treating the symptoms of carcinoid tumours, but is seldom used today. All these drugs can be used orally or by injection.

Unwanted effects. Ergotamine often causes nausea and vomiting, and it must be avoided in patients with peripheral vascular disease because of its vasoconstrictor action. Methysergide also causes nausea and vomiting, but its most serious side effect, which considerably restricts its clinical usefulness, is *retroperitoneal* and *mediastinal fibrosis*, which impairs the functioning of the gastrointestinal tract, kidneys, heart and lungs. The mechanism of this is unknown, but it is noteworthy that similar fibrotic reactions also occur in carcinoid syndrome, in which there is a high circulating level of 5-HT.

MIGRAINE AND OTHER CLINICAL CONDITIONS IN WHICH 5-HT PLAYS A ROLE

In this section, we discuss three situations where the peripheral actions of 5-HT are believed to be important, namely *migraine, carcinoid syndrome* and *pulmonary hypertension*. The use of 5-HT$_3$ antagonists for treating drug-induced emesis is discussed in Chapter 31. Modulation of 5-HT-mediated transmission in the CNS is an important mechanism of action of antidepressant and antipsychotic drugs (see Chs 40, 45 and 48).

MIGRAINE AND ANTIMIGRAINE DRUGS

Migraine[2] is a common and debilitating condition affecting 10%–15% of people and is often stated to be the third most common disease in the world. Although the causes are not well understood, both genetic and environmental factors seem to be important. The frequency of attacks varies, with about three-quarters of *migraineurs* (as they are called) having more than one episode per month. Generally, the onset of attacks begins at puberty and wanes with increasing age. Women are twice as likely as men to suffer from the disorder and the attacks are often linked to the menstrual cycle or other reproductive events. It appears that rapidly falling oestrogen levels can precipitate bouts of migraine in susceptible subjects.

Migraine can be *episodic*, when the attacks are relatively infrequent, or *chronic*, when the frequency and severity become a major burden to the patient and is possibly accompanied by comorbidities such as gastrointestinal problems or mental health issues. The treatment of the two manifestations is a little different. It is likely that episodic attacks eventually transform into a more chronic illness unless treated.

In the United Kingdom, some 25 million work or school days are lost each year because of the incapacitating effects of the disease, with an economic cost of more than £3 billion. The WHO has classified migraine as amongst the 20 most disabling lifetime conditions.

Migraine can be differentiated from other types of headache (e.g. cluster headaches, tension headaches) based on strict diagnostic guidelines. The onset of an attack is heralded by a *premonitory phase*, with symptoms including nausea, mood changes and often sensitivity to light and sound (photophobia and phonophobia). These may occur hours before the onset, in some patients, of the *aura* phase during which phonophobia and photophobia are more common, and may be accompanied by more specific visual symptoms such as a slowly moving blind spot with associated flashing lights ('scintillating scotoma') or geometric patterns of coloured lights ('fortification spectra') or the illusion of looking through the wrong end of a telescope. The *headache* phase proper is characterised by a moderate or severe headache, starting unilaterally, but then usually spreading to both sides of the head. It may have a pulsating or throbbing quality accompanied by nausea, vomiting and prostration. This phase may persist for hours or even days. Following resolution of the headache, *postdromal* phase. may include feelings of fatigue, altered cognition or mood changes. Whilst these different phases probably represent discrete biological events, in practice they overlap and may run in parallel. A good account of these is given by Charles (2013).

PATHOPHYSIOLOGY

The causes of migraine are incompletely understood. Historically there have been three main hypotheses advanced to account for the symptoms (see Eadie, 2005).

The classic *'vascular' theory*, first proposed around 50 years ago by Wolff, implicated an initial humorally mediated intracerebral vasoconstriction as the cause of the aura, followed by an extracerebral vasodilatation causing the headache. This idea is not supported by the current evidence, although vascular events are certainly involved in the disease.

The *'brain' hypothesis* (see Lauritzen, 1987) linked the symptoms to the phenomenon of *cortical spreading depression*. This is a dramatic, although poorly understood, phenomenon, triggered in experimental animals by local application of K$^+$ to the cortex and also thought to occur in humans after (for example) concussion. An advancing wave of profound neural inhibition progresses slowly over the cortical surface at a rate of about 2 mm/min. In the affected area, the ionic balance is grossly disturbed, with an extremely high extracellular K$^+$ concentration, and the blood flow is reduced.

The *inflammation hypothesis* (see Waeber & Moskowitz, 2005) proposes that activation of trigeminal nerve terminals in the meninges and extracranial vessels is the primary event in a migraine attack. This would cause pain directly and also induce inflammatory changes through the release of neuropeptides and other inflammatory mediators from the sensory nerve terminals (neurogenic inflammation; see Chs 19 and 43). One such peptide (*calcitonin gene-related peptide* (CGRP); see Ch. 19) is indeed released into the meningeal circulation during a migraine attack and an antagonist of this peptide, **telcagepant** – an investigational drug (discontinued because of liver toxicity) – as well as a CGRP-neutralising monoclonal antibody were extremely effective in aborting attacks (Farinelli et al., 2008; Dodick et al., 2014; Pellesi et al., 2017; Hershey, 2017).

In practice, elements of all these phenomena seem to play a role in the pathogenesis of migraine but increasingly, attention is focusing on the *trigeminovascular system* – the sensory neurones that innervate the cerebral vessels (see

[2]The word is apparently of French origin and is probably a corruption of *hemicrania*, the Latin name for the disease.

Charles, 2013; Buture et al., 2016; Aurora & Brin, 2017) as the source of the pain. The symptoms associated with the premonitory phase are largely dopaminergic in origin. The onset of the aura phase coincides with the cortical spreading depression and imaging studies have indicated widespread changes in brain perfusion during this phase. There may be hypoperfusion of some brain areas as well as hyperperfusion in others, suggesting that the physiological mechanisms that normally regulate the relationship between brain activity and blood flow become disengaged. Such *neurovascular uncoupling* is a feature of cortical spreading depression.

During the headache phase, there are again vascular changes in (for example) the meningeal and middle cerebral arteries, but once again, these are not consistent and in any case not directly responsible for the pain and other symptoms. What does seem to be important is *central sensitisation*, which increases the migraineur's sensitivity to sound, light, cutaneous sensations and other normally non-painful stimuli. This is accompanied by a release of inflammatory or nociceptive mediators such as CGRP, nitric oxide (NO) and prostaglandins. Many of the observed vascular and other changes may persist into the postdromal phase, which may last for hours or days.

It is noteworthy that none of these mechanisms offer a totally conclusive explanation, at the biochemical level, for what initiates a migraine attack or define the underlying abnormality that predisposes particular individuals to suffer such attacks. In some rare types of familial migraine, inherited mutations affecting calcium channels and Na^+-K^+-ATPase have been found, suggesting that abnormal membrane function may be responsible, but in most forms of migraine there is no clear genetic cause.

Whether one inclines to the view that migraine is primarily a vascular disorder, a type of spontaneous concussion, an inflammatory disease or just a bad headache, there are two important factors that implicate 5-HT in its pathogenesis:

1. There is a sharp increase in the urinary excretion of the main 5-HT metabolite, 5-HIAA, during the attack. The blood concentration of 5-HT falls, probably because of depletion of platelet 5-HT.
2. Many of the drugs that are effective in treating migraine are 5-HT receptor agonists or antagonists. See Fig. 16.3 and the clinical box below for further information.

ANTIMIGRAINE DRUGS

The main drugs currently used to treat migraine are summarised in Table 16.3, and their postulated sites of action are shown in Fig. 16.3. It is important to distinguish between drugs used *therapeutically* to treat acute attacks of migraine (appropriate when the attacks are fairly infrequent) and drugs that are used *prophylactically*. Apart from 5-HT₂ receptor antagonists, the drugs used prophylactically are rather a mixed bag, and include the anticonvulsant agent **topimarate** (not UK), the potassium-sparing diuretic **amiloride** and **botulinum toxin**. Non-steroidal anti-inflammatory drugs (NSAIDs) (Ch. 27) seem to have a variable effect, being useful for some patients but not others.

The most important agents for the treatment of acute attacks are currently the triptans. These are 5-HT₁ agonists and are usually classified as 5-HT₁ᵦ/₁ᴅ agonists, largely because it is difficult to distinguish between actions at these two receptors. However, selective high-affinity 5-HT₁ᴅ subtype agonists have proved disappointing in the clinic.

Drugs used for migraine

Acute attack
- Simple analgesics (e.g. **aspirin**, **paracetamol**; see Ch. 27) with or without **metoclopramide** (see Ch. 31) to hasten absorption.
- **Ergotamine** (5-HT₁ᴅ receptor partial agonist).
- **Sumatriptan**, **zolmitriptan** (5-HT₁ᴅ agonists).

Prophylaxis
- β-Adrenoceptor antagonists (e.g. **propranolol**, **metoprolol**; see Ch. 15).
- **Pizotifen** (5-HT₂ receptor antagonist).
- Other 5-HT₂ receptor antagonists:
  - **cyproheptadine**: also has antihistamine actions
  - **methysergide**: rarely used because of risk of retroperitoneal fibrosis.
- Tricyclic antidepressants (e.g. **amitriptyline**; see Ch. 48).
- **Clonidine**, an α₂ adrenoceptor agonist (see Ch. 15).
- Calcium antagonists (e.g. dihydropyridines, **verapamil**; see Ch. 22): headache is a side effect of these drugs but, paradoxically, they may reduce frequency of migraine attacks.

Sumatriptan also has high affinity for the 5-HT₁ꜰ receptor (see Agosti, 2007) and **lasmiditan**, an investigational nontriptan drug that is a selective 5HT₁ꜰ-receptor agonist, is highly effective in aborting migraine attacks (Tfelt-Hansen, 2012). Interestingly, this receptor subtype is scarce in the vasculature, casting further doubt on the role of vascular changes *per se* in the pain experienced by patients. This is significant because a major drawback to triptan therapy is vasoconstriction in other peripheral vascular beds, including the heart. Lasmiditan would be expected to be free of such effects; however, it commonly causes other adverse effects (e.g. dizziness and nausea) that can be severe. It is postulated that the antimigraine action of the triptans is through activation of presynaptic 5-HT₁ receptors which inhibit the release of CGRP (and other neuropeptides) from neurones of the trigeminovascular system (Juhasz et al., 2015). This theory is consistent with the reported efficacy of telagepant and anti-CGRP antibodies mentioned above.

CARCINOID SYNDROME

Carcinoid syndrome (see Creutzfeld & Stockmann, 1987) is a rare disorder associated with malignant tumours of enterochromaffin cells, which usually arise in the small intestine and metastasise to the liver. These tumours secrete a variety of chemical mediators: 5-HT is the most important, but neuropeptides such as substance P (Ch. 19), and other agents such as prostaglandins and bradykinin (Ch. 18), are also produced. The sudden release of these substances (*carcinoid crisis*) into the bloodstream results in several unpleasant symptoms, including flushing, abdominal cramps, diarrhoea, bronchoconstriction and hypotension, which may cause dizziness or fainting. More insidiously, cognitive impairment may develop and sometimes fibrotic stenosis of heart valves, leading to cardiac failure. It is reminiscent of the retroperitoneal and mediastinal fibrosis seen with methysergide and some other serotonergic agents, and appears to be related to overproduction of 5-HT acting

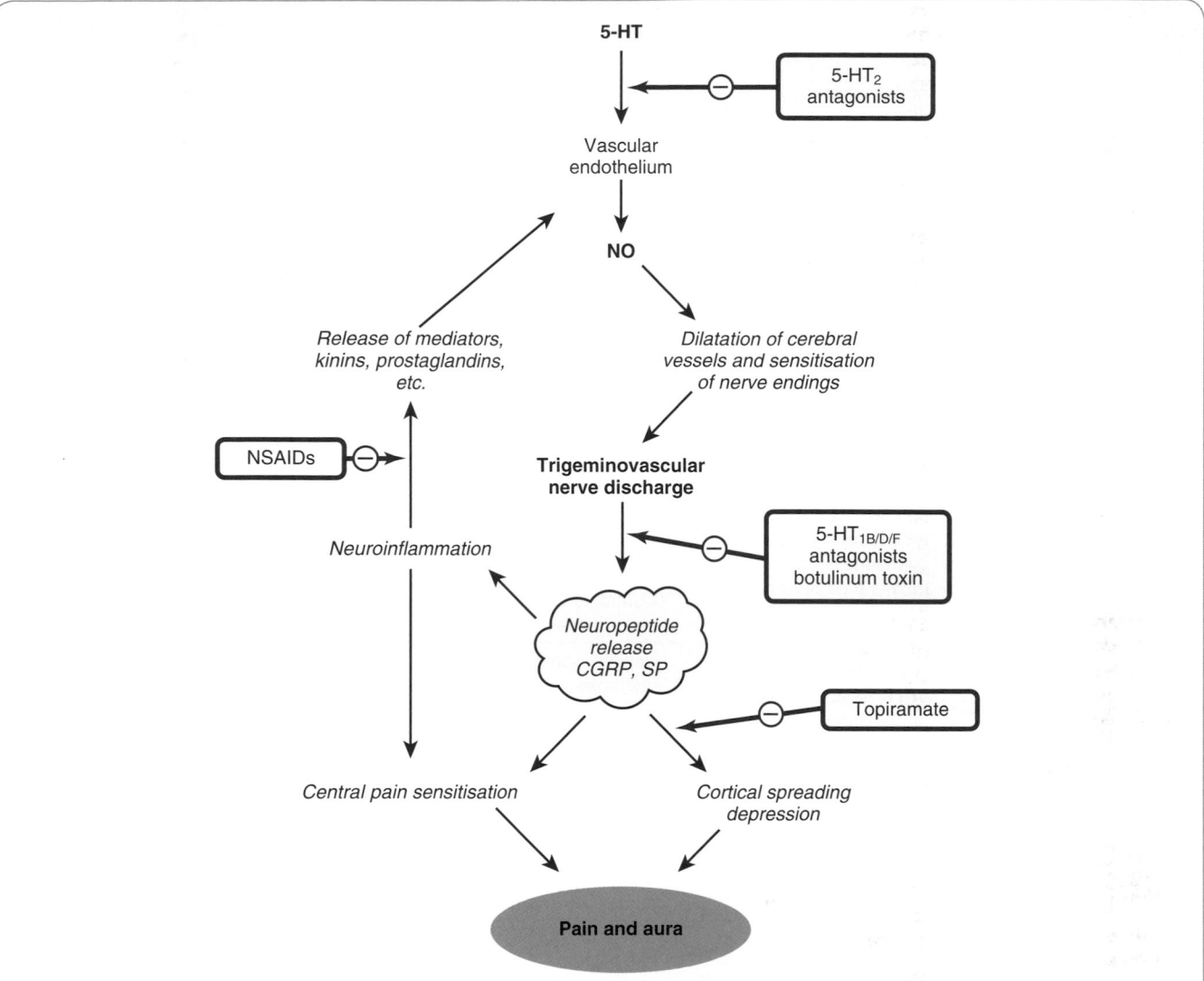

Fig. 16.3 **Postulated sites of drug action in migraine pain.** The initiating event is uncertain but may be an abnormal neuronal discharge set off by emotional or biochemical disturbances. The release of 5-HT, directly or indirectly, dilates cranial vessels and stimulates trigeminovascular nerve terminals in the meningeal vessels. This triggers a cycle of neurogenic inflammation, producing a cortical 'spreading depression', an uncoupling of neurovascular perfusion and sensitisation of central pain pathways. *5-HT*, 5-hydroxytryptamine; *CGRP*, calcitonin gene-related peptide; *NO*, nitric oxide; *NSAIDs*, non-steroidal anti-inflammatory drugs; *SP*, substance P.

through 5-HT$_{2B}$ receptors to drive the proliferation of connective tissue (Mota et al., 2016).

Clinical diagnosis can be confirmed by measuring the urinary excretion of the main metabolite of 5-HT, 5-HIAA. This may increase by as much as 20-fold when the disease is active and is raised even when the tumour is asymptomatic. 5-HT$_2$ antagonists, and the mixed 5-HT/histamine antagonist **cyproheptadine**, are effective in controlling some of the symptoms of carcinoid syndrome, but a more useful drug is **octreotide** (a long-acting agonist at somatostatin receptors), which suppresses hormone secretion from neuroendocrine, including carcinoid, cells (see Ch. 34).

PULMONARY HYPERTENSION

Pulmonary hypertension (see also Ch. 23) is an extremely serious disease characterised by the progressive remodelling of the pulmonary vascular tree leading to stiffening and narrowing of the vascular tree. This leads to an inexorable rise in pulmonary arterial pressure which, if untreated (and

treatment is difficult), inevitably leads to right heart failure and death. There are several types of pulmonary hypertension and the role of 5-HT was suggested by the fact that at least one form of the condition was precipitated by appetite suppressants (e.g. **dexfenfluramine** and **fenfluramine**) that were at one time widely prescribed as 'weight loss' or 'slimming' aids. These drugs apparently blocked SERT and since 5-HT promotes the growth and proliferation of pulmonary arterial smooth muscle cells and also produces a net vasoconstrictor effect in this vascular bed, the hypothesis seemed reasonable. The use of SSRI antidepressants (Ch. 48) in late pregnancy may lead to pulmonary hypertension in the newborn (Grigoriadis et al., 2014).

Some types of pulmonary hypertension (idiopathic and familial) are more prevalent in females and sex hormones may therefore be of relevance in the pathogenesis. The interested reader is referred to MacLean and Dempsie (2010) for an accessible account of the current thinking in this area, and to Chapter 23, where this topic is also discussed.

Table 16.3 Antimigraine drugs[a]

Use	Drug(s)	Mode of action	Side effects	Pharmacokinetic aspects	Notes
Acute	Sumatriptan	$5-HT_{1B/1D/1F}$ receptor agonist. Constricts large arteries, inhibits trigeminal nerve transmission.	Coronary vasoconstriction, dysrhythmias.	Poor oral absorption, hence delayed response. Can be given s.c. Does not cross blood–brain barrier. Plasma half-life 1.5 h.	Effective in ~70% of migraine attacks. Short duration of action is a drawback. Contraindicated in coronary disease.
Acute	Almotriptan Eletriptan Frovatriptan Naratriptan Rizatriptan Zolmitriptan	As above; additional actions on CNS.s	Side effects less than with sumatriptan.	Improved bioavailability and duration of action. Able to cross blood–brain barrier.	Similar to sumatriptan; but improved pharmacokinetics and reduced cardiac side effects.
Acute	Ergotamine	$5-HT_1$ receptor partial agonist; also affects α adrenoceptors. Vasoconstrictor. Blocks trigeminal nerve transmission.	Peripheral vasoconstriction, including coronary vessels. Nausea and vomiting. Contracts uterus and may damage fetus.	Poorly absorbed. Can be given by suppository, inhalation, etc. Duration of action 12–24 h.	Effective, but use limited by side effects.
Prophylaxis	Methysergide	$5-HT_2$ receptor antagonist/ partial agonist.	Nausea, vomiting, diarrhoea. Retroperitoneal or mediastinal fibrosis (rare but serious).	Used orally	Effective, but rarely used because of side effects and insidious toxicity.
Prophylaxis	Pizotifen	$5-HT_2$ and histamine receptor antagonist.	Weight gain, anti-muscarinic side effects.	Used orally	–
Prophylaxis	Topiramate	Acts on ion channels (e.g. Na^+) and possibly the $GABA_A$ receptor (see Ch. 46)	Sedation, dizziness, weight loss, nausea, paraesthesia, diarrhoea.	Used orally	Used for treating chronic migraine
Prophylaxis	Propranolol and similar drugs.	β-adrenoceptor antagonists. Mechanism of antimigraine effect not clear.	Fatigue, bronchoconstriction.	Used orally	Effective and widely used for migraine. Other anti-epileptics may also be of value.
Prophylaxis	Botulinum toxin A	Probably acts by preventing the neuronal release of CGRP and other neuropeptides.	Muscle paralysis and other neuromuscular disorders if used incorrectly.	Administered by s.c., i.m. or i.d. injection.	A single treatment can act for up to a year.

[a]Other drugs used for the *acute* treatment of migraine include non-steroidal anti-inflammatory drugs (NSAIDs) or opiate analgesic drugs (see Chs 27, 43 and 48). Other drugs used for migraine *prophylaxis* include calcium channel blockers (e.g. nifedipine, see Ch. 23), antidepressants (e.g. amitriptyline; see Ch. 48), and the antihypertensives, clonidine and amiloride (Ch. 15). Their efficacy is limited. *5-HT*, 5-hydroxytryptamine; *CNS*, central nervous system. *CGRP*, calcitonin gene-related peptide.

REFERENCES AND FURTHER READING

5-Hydroxytryptamine

Agosti, R.M., 2007. 5HT$_{1F}$- and 5HT$_7$-receptor agonists for the treatment of migraines. CNS Neurol. Disord. Drug Targets 6, 235–237. (*Describes research in the field of migraine treatment utilising agonists at cloned 5-HT receptors*)

Barnes, N.M., Sharp, T., 1999. A review of central 5-HT receptors and their function. Neuropharmacology 38, 1083–1152. (*Useful general review focusing on CNS*)

Beattie, D.T., Smith, J.A., 2008. Serotonin pharmacology in the gastrointestinal tract: a review. Naunyn Schmiedebergs Arch. Pharmacol. 377, 181–203. (*Very comprehensive review dealing with a complex topic. Easy to read*)

Bonasera, S.J., Tecott, L.H., 2000. Mouse models of serotonin receptor function: towards a genetic dissection of serotonin systems.

Pharmacol. Ther. 88, 133–142. (*Review of studies on transgenic mice lacking 5-HT$_1$ or 5-HT$_2$ receptors; shows how difficult it can be to interpret such experiments*)

Branchek, T.A., Blackburn, T.P., 2000. 5-HT$_6$ receptors as emerging targets for drug discovery. Annu. Rev. Pharmacol. Toxicol. 40, 319–334. (*Emphasises potential therapeutic opportunities in this area*)

Gershon, M.D., 2004. Review article: serotonin receptors and transporters – roles in normal and abnormal gastrointestinal motility. Aliment. Pharmacol. Ther. 20 (Suppl. 7), 3–14.

Spiller, R., 2008. Serotonergic agents and the irritable bowel syndrome: what goes wrong? Curr. Opin. Pharmacol. 8, 709–714. (*A very interesting account of the development – and withdrawal – of 5-HT$_{3/4}$ antagonists in irritable bowel syndrome and a discussion of the role of SERT* *polymorphisms in the disease. Illustrates the type of problems encountered when trying to develop useful drugs that act at 5-HT receptors)*

Migraine and other pathologies

Aurora, S.K., Brin, M.F., 2017. Chronic migraine: an update on physiology, imaging, and the mechanism of action of two available pharmacologic therapies. Headache 57, 109–125. (*This paper, together with the one below, summarise recent views on the causes of migraine and discuss the mechanism of action of some drugs. Both are quite clinical in outlook but easy to read*)

Buture, A., Gooriah, R., Nimeri, R., Ahmed, F., 2016. Current understanding on pain mechanism in migraine and cluster headache. Anesth. Pain. Med. 6, e35190. (*Excellent concise review of these two pathologies focusing on the latest ideas about pain mechanisms*)

Charles, A., 2013. The evolution of a migraine attack – a review of recent evidence. Headache 53, 413–419. (*An excellent and easily readable account of modern thinking about the causes of migraine*)

Creutzfeld, W., Stockmann, F., 1987. Carcinoids and carcinoid syndrome. Am. J. Med. 82 (Suppl. 58), 4–16.

Dahlof, C.G., Rapoport, A.M., Sheftell, F.D., Lines, C.R., 1999. Rizatriptan in the treatment of migraine. Clin. Ther. 21, 1823–1836.

Dodick, D.W., Goadsby, P.J., Spierings, E.L., Scherer, J.C., Sweeney, S.P., Grayzel, D.S., 2014. Safety and efficacy of LY2951742, a monoclonal antibody to calcitonin gene-related peptide, for the prevention of migraine: a phase 2, randomised, double-blind, placebo-controlled study. Lancet Neurol. 13, 885–892.

Eadie, M.J., 2005. The pathogenesis of migraine – 17th to early 20th century understandings. J. Clin. Neurosci. 12, 383–388. (*Fascinating account of the historical development of theories of causes of migraine. Good if you are interested in the history of medicine!*)

Farinelli, I., Missori, S., Martelletti, P., 2008. Proinflammatory mediators and migraine pathogenesis: moving towards CGRP as a target for a novel therapeutic class. Expert Rev. Neurother. 8, 1347–1354.

Grigoriadis, S., Vonderporten, E.H., Mamisashvili, L., et al., 2014. Prenatal exposure to antidepressants and persistent pulmonary hypertension of the newborn: systematic review and meta-analysis. BMJ 348, f6932.

Goadsby, P.J., 2005. Can we develop neurally acting drugs for the treatment of migraine? Nat. Rev. Drug Discov. 4, 741–750. (*Useful review of the causes and treatments of migraine*)

Hershey, A.D., 2017. CGRP - the next frontier for migraine. N. Engl. J. Med. 377, 2190–2191.

Juhasz, G., Zsombok, T., Jakab, B., Nemeth, J., Szolcsanyi, J., Bagdy, G., 2005. Sumatriptan causes parallel decrease in plasma calcitonin gene-related peptide (CGRP) concentration and migraine headache during nitroglycerin induced migraine attack. Cephalalgia 25, 179–183.

Lauritzen, M., 1987. Cerebral blood flow in migraine and cortical spreading depression. Acta Neurol. Scand. Suppl. 113, 1–40. (*Review of clinical measurements of cerebral blood flow in migraine, which overturned earlier hypotheses*)

Maclean, M.R., Dempsie, Y., 2010. The serotonin hypothesis of pulmonary hypertension revisited. Adv. Exp. Med. Biol. 661, 309–322. (*An account of the evidence supporting a role for 5-HT in pulmonary hypertension by one of the leaders in this field*)

Mota, J.M., Sousa, L.G., Riechelmann, R.P., 2016. Complications from carcinoid syndrome: review of the current evidence. Ecancermedicalscience 10, 662. (*Good account of carcinoid syndrome written from a clinical viewpoint. Easy to read*)

Pellesi, L., Guerzoni, S., Pini, L.A., 2017. Spotlight on anti-CGRP monoclonal antibodies in migraine: the clinical evidence to date. Clin. Pharmacol. Drug Dev. 6, 534–547. (*Lists a number of anti-CGRP monoclonals undergoing clinical trials for migraine treatment*)

Tfelt-Hansen, P., 2012. Clinical pharmacology of current and future drugs for the acute treatment of migraine: a review and an update. Curr. Clin. Pharmacol. 7, 66–72. (*A good account of anti-migraine drugs. Recommended*)

Waeber, C., Moskowitz, M.A., 2005. Migraine as an inflammatory disorder. Neurology 64, S9–S15. (*Useful review of the 'inflammation' hypothesis of migraine*)

Books

Sjoerdsma, A.G., 2008. Starting With Serotonin: How a High-Rolling Father of Drug Discovery Repeatedly Beat the Odds. Improbable Books, Silver Spring, MD. (*Biography of an astonishing pharmacologist, by his daughter. Very well reviewed*)

17 Purines

OVERVIEW

In addition to their role in the energy economy of the cell, purine nucleosides and nucleotides function as extracellular chemical mediators subserving a wide range of functions. In this chapter we describe the mechanisms responsible for their synthesis and release, the drugs that act through purinergic signalling pathways and the receptors that transduce these effects.

INTRODUCTION

Nucleosides (especially adenosine) and nucleotides (especially ADP and ATP) will already be familiar to you because of their crucial role in DNA/RNA synthesis and energy metabolism, but it may come as a surprise to learn that they also function extracellularly as signalling molecules that produce a wide range of unrelated pharmacological effects.

The finding, in 1929, that adenosine injected into anaesthetised animals caused bradycardia, hypotension, vasodilatation and inhibition of intestinal movements, foreshadowed the current interest in purines. But the true origins of the field can really be traced to the crucial observations in 1970 by Burnstock and his colleagues, who provided strong evidence that ATP is a neurotransmitter (see Ch. 2). After a period during which this radical idea was treated with scepticism, it has become clear that the 'purinergic' signalling system is not only of ancient evolutionary origin but participates in many physiological control mechanisms, including the regulation of coronary blood flow and myocardial function (Chs 22 and 23), platelet aggregation and immune responses (Chs 18 and 25), as well as neurotransmission in both the central and peripheral nervous system (Chs 13 and 40).

The full complexity of purinergic control systems, their importance in many pathophysiological mechanisms and the therapeutic relevance of the various receptor subtypes is now emerging. As a result, there is an increasing interest in purine pharmacology and the prospect of developing 'purinergic' drugs for the treatment of pain and a variety of other disorders, particularly of thrombotic and inflammatory origin. There is no doubt that such drugs will assume growing significance but, recognising that the overall picture is still developing, we will focus our discussion in this chapter on a few prominent areas.

Fig. 17.1 summarises the mechanisms by which purines are stored, released and interconverted, and the main receptor types on which they act.

PURINERGIC RECEPTORS

Purines exert their biological actions through three families of receptors. Table 17.1 (and the Box on p. 229) list these and summarises what is currently known about their signalling systems, their endogenous ligands and antagonists of pharmacological interest. It should be noted, however, that the action of drugs and ligands at purinergic receptors can be confusing. In part, this is because nucleotides are rapidly degraded by ecto-enzymes and there is also evidence of interconversion by phosphate exchange. Thus ATP may produce effects at all three receptor subclasses depending upon the extent of its enzymatic conversion to ADP, AMP and adenosine.

The three main families of purine receptor are:

- Adenosine receptors (A_1, A_{2A}, A_{2B} and A_3), formerly known as *P1* receptors before the agonist was discovered to be adenosine. These are G protein–coupled receptors that act through adenylyl cyclase/cAMP, or by direct effects on Ca^{2+} and K^+ channels, as described in Ch 3.
- P2Y metabotropic receptors ($P2Y_{1-14}$), which are G protein–coupled receptors that utilise either phospholipase C activation or cAMP as their signalling system (see Ch. 3); they respond to various adenine nucleotides, generally preferring ATP over ADP or AMP. Some also recognise pyrimidines such as UTP.
- P2X ionotropic receptors ($P2X_{1-7}$) which are trimeric (in many cases heterotrimeric) ATP-gated cation channels. In the presence of ATP, the channels become permeable to Ca^{2+} and Na^+ ions, activating Ca^{2+}-sensitive pathways and causing membrane depolarisation.

The subtypes in each family are distinguished on the basis of their molecular structure as well as their agonist and antagonist selectivity. The P2Y group is particularly problematic: several receptors have been cloned on the basis of homology with other family members, but their ligands have yet to be identified (in other words they are 'orphan receptors'). In addition, since some members of this group also recognise pyrimidines such as UTP and UDP as well as purines, they are sometimes classed as pyrimidinoceptors. However, little is currently known about the role of pyrimidines in cell signalling.

We will now discuss some prominent and interesting aspects of purinergic pharmacology; the reading list provides further information.

ADENOSINE AS A MEDIATOR

The simplest of the purines, adenosine, is found in biological fluids throughout the body. It exists free in the cytosol

Fig. 17.1 Purines as mediators. ATP (and, in platelets, ADP) is present in the cytosol of cells (and released following cellular damage) or concentrated into vesicles by the vesicular nucleotide transporter (VNUT). Nucleotides may be released by exocytosis or through membrane channels such an pannexins (Pnx) or transporters (NtT). Once released, ATP can be converted to ADP and to adenosine by the action of ectonucleotidases. Adenosine is present in the cytosol of all cells and is released and taken up via a specific membrane transporter(s) (NsT), which is blocked by dipyramidole. Adenosine itself can be hydrolysed to inosine by the enzyme adenosine deaminase. ATP acts directly upon the P2X receptors (ligand-gated ion channels) but also upon P2Y receptors (GPCRs; G protein coupled receptors), the principal target for ADP. Adenosine itself acts on A receptors (also called P1 receptors), which are also GPCRs. Ch. 4 contains more details of exocytotic and other secretory mechanisms.

Purines as mediators

- *Adenosine* acts through A_1, A_{2A}, A_{2B} and A_3 G protein receptors, coupled to inhibition or stimulation of adenylyl cyclase. Adenosine receptors are blocked by methylxanthines such as **caffeine** and **theophylline**. **Dipyramidole** blocks adenosine uptake.
  - *Adenosine* affects many cells and tissues, including smooth muscle and nerve cells. It is not a conventional transmitter but may be important as a local hormone and 'homeostatic modulator'.
  - Important sites of action include the heart and the lung. Adenosine is very short-acting and is sometimes used for its antidysrhythmic effect.
- *ADP* acts through the $P2Y_{1-14}$ 'metabotropic' G protein–receptor family. These are coupled to cAMP or PLCβ.
  - Important sites of action include platelets where ADP released from granules promotes aggregation by

acting on the PY_{12} receptor. This is antagonised by the drugs **clopidogrel**, **prasugrel**, **ticagrelor** and **cangrelor**.
- *ATP* is stored in vesicles and released by exocytosis or through membrane channels when cells are damaged. It also functions as an intracellular mediator, inhibiting the opening of membrane potassium channels.
  - ATP acts on P2X receptors: these are ligand-gated ion channels. It can also act on P2Y receptors.
  - **Suramin** blocks the ATP actions at most receptors.
  - Important sites of ATP action include the central nervous system (CNS), peripheral and central pathways and inflammatory cells.
  - When released, ATP is rapidly converted to ADP and adenosine yielding products that may act on other purinergic receptors.

Table 17.1 Purinergic receptors

Receptor subtype	Mechanism	Principal endogenous ligands	Notes
Adenosine (also called P1)			
A_1	G protein coupled ($G_{i/o}$) Lowers cAMP	Adenosine (high affinity)	Caffeine, theophylline (antagonists)
A_{2A}	G protein coupled (G_s) Raises cAMP		
A_{2B}	G protein coupled (G_s) Raises cAMP	Adenosine (low affinity)	
A_3	G protein coupled ($G_{i/o}$) Lowers cAMP		
P2Y 'metabotropic'[a]			
$P2Y_1$	G protein coupled (mainly $G_{q/11}$). Activates PLCβ mobilises Ca^{2+} Sometimes alters cAMP	ATP (antagonist or partial agonist) ADP (agonist)	Suramin (antagonist)
$P2Y_2$		UTP and ATP	Suramin (antagonist)
$P2Y_4$		ATP, GTP, UTP (partial agonists)	Pyrimidinoceptor
$P2Y_6$		UDP	Pyrimidinoceptor
$P2Y_{11}$		ATP > ADP	Suramin (antagonist)
$P2Y_{12}$	G protein coupled (mainly $G_{i/o}$) Reduces cAMP	ADP>ATP	Platelet ADP receptor. Clopidigrel, prasugrel, cangrelor and ticagrelor (antagonists)
$P2Y_{13}$		ADP	Suramin
$P2Y_{14}$		UDP-glucose	UDP
P2X 'ionotropic'			
$P2X_1$ $P2X_2$ $P2X_3$ $P2X_4$ $P2X_5$ $P2X_6$ $P2X_7$	Receptor-gated cation-selective ion channels	ATP	Suramin (antagonist; rather non-selective)

[a]Only functional human receptors are listed. The missing numbers in the sequence indicate that these receptors have been cloned, but their ligands have not yet been identified. A further family of related receptors that binds extracellular cAMP (CAR_{1-4}) is omitted as little is known about their biology.

of all cells and is transported in (by active transport against a concentration gradient) and out mainly by a membrane transporter (of which there are several types). Little is known about the way in which this is controlled, but the extracellular concentrations are usually quite low compared with intracellular levels. Extracellular adenosine in tissues comes partly from this intracellular source and partly from hydrolysis of released ATP or ADP by nucleotidases such as CD39 and CD73 (see Fig. 17.1). Adenosine can be inactivated by *adenosine deaminase*, yielding *inosine*, providing yet another level of control of this biologically active molecule, and another potential drug target.

Virtually all cells express one or more adenosine receptors and so adenosine produces many pharmacological effects, both in the periphery and in the central nervous system (CNS). Based on its ability to minimise the metabolic requirements of cells, one of its functions may be as an 'acute' defensive agent that is released immediately when tissue integrity is threatened (e.g. by coronary or cerebral

ischaemia; see Chs 22 and 41). Under less extreme conditions, variations in adenosine release play a role in controlling blood flow and (through effects on the carotid bodies) respiration, matching them to the metabolic needs of the tissues.

ADENOSINE AND THE CARDIOVASCULAR SYSTEM

Adenosine inhibits cardiac pacemaker activity and atrioventricular node conduction and it is likely that all four of the adenosine receptors are involved in these effects. Because of this, adenosine is used therapeutically, being given as an intravenous bolus injection to terminate supraventricular tachycardia (Ch. 22). Because of its short duration of action (it is destroyed or taken up within a few seconds of intravenous administration) it is considered safer than alternatives such as β-adrenoceptor antagonists or **verapamil**. **Regadenoson**, a powerful vasodilator used for diagnostic tests of cardiac function, is a selective A_{2A} agonist. **Dipyramidole** (a vasodilator and antiplatelet drug: Ch. 25) blocks adenosine uptake by cells, thus effectively increasing its extracellular concentration.

ADENOSINE IN ASTHMA

Adenosine receptors are found on all the cell types involved in asthma (Ch. 29) and the overall pharmacology is complex. For example, activation of the A_{2A} subtype exerts a largely protective and anti-inflammatory effect, but acting through its A_1 receptor, adenosine promotes mediator release from mast cells, and causes enhanced mucus secretion, bronchoconstriction and leukocyte activation. Methylxanthines, especially analogues of **theophylline** (Ch. 29), are adenosine receptor antagonists. Theophylline has been used for the treatment of asthma and part of its beneficial activity may be ascribed to its antagonism of the A_1 receptor; however, methylxanthines also increase cAMP by inhibiting phosphodiesterase, which underwrites some of their pharmacological actions independently of adenosine receptor antagonism. Certain derivatives of theophylline are claimed to show greater selectivity for adenosine receptors over phosphodiesterase.

Activation of the A_{2B} receptor also promotes mast cell mediator release, while the role of the A_3 receptor has yet to be fully elucidated. An antagonist of the A_1 and A_{2B} receptor or an agonist of the A_{2A} receptor could therefore represent a significant advance in this therapeutic area (see Brown et al., 2008; Burnstock et al., 2012).

ADENOSINE IN INFLAMMATION

Adenosine also regulates the inflammatory response elsewhere and A receptors at various locations in the eye (particularly A_{2A} receptors) have been identified as potential targets in ocular diseases (Guzman-Aranguez et al., 2014). Experimental A_3 antagonists have been observed to produce a beneficial effect in experimental models of colitis and may be useful in other inflammatory disorders, including rheumatoid arthritis, psoriasis and dry eye syndrome (Ochoa-Cortes et al., 2014). Interestingly, **sulfasalazine** and **methotrexate**, which are used to treat inflammatory bowel disease (Ch. 31) and have other anti-inflammatory properties, stimulate the hydrolysis of ATP and AMP by ectonucleotidases to produce adenosine thereby increasing its effective local concentration.

ADENOSINE IN THE CNS

Acting through A_1 and A_{2A} receptors, adenosine has an inhibitory effect on many CNS neurons, and the stimulation experienced after consumption of methylxanthines such as **caffeine** and theophylline. Antagonism of adenosine receptors by the methylxanthines, (which share the purine structure), explains part of their stimulatory effects (see Ch. 49).

ADP AS A MEDIATOR

ADP is usually stored in vesicles in cells and released by exocytosis (see Ch. 4). It exerts its direct biological effects predominantly through the P2Y family of receptors but once released it can be converted to adenosine by ectonucleotidases.

ADP AND PLATELETS

The secretory vesicles of blood platelets store both ATP and ADP in high concentrations, and release them when the platelets are activated (see Ch 25). One of the many effects of ADP is to promote platelet aggregation, so this system provides positive feedback – an important mechanism for controlling this process. The receptor involved is $P2Y_{12}$. Exploitation of this finding has provided the best examples to date of the value of purinergic drugs. **Ticlopidine** (no longer used in UK), **clopidogrel** and **prasugrel** (prodrugs), **cangrelor** and **ticagrelor** (allosteric antagonist), all antagonise platelet $P2Y_{12}$ receptors inhibiting the aggregation response. They are used, often alongside aspirin, for preventing arterial thromboembolic disorders (Ch. 25). The $P2Y_1$ receptor may also play a part in the regulation of platelet reactivity (Hechler & Gachet, 2015).

ATP AS A MEDIATOR

ATP exerts its action primarily through the P2X receptors. The extracellular domain of these trimeric receptors can bind three molecules of ATP. When activated by binding of two or three ATP molecules, the receptor gates the cation-selective ion channels that trigger ongoing intracellular signalling. Some other actions of ATP in mammals are mediated through the P2Y receptors. **Suramin** (a drug originally developed to treat trypanosome infections) antagonises ATP and has broad-spectrum inhibitory activity at P2X and P2Y receptors. More selective ATP antagonists are in development.

ATP is present in all cells in millimolar concentrations and is released if the cells are damaged (e.g. by ischaemia). The mechanism of release can be through exocytosis of vesicles containing ATP, through ATP transporters or through *pannexin* or *connexin* channels in the cell membrane. Dying cells may release ATP, which may serve as a 'danger signal' alerting immune cells to potential local tissue damage (see Ch. 7).

ATP released from cells is rapidly dephosphorylated by tissue-specific nucleotidases, producing ADP and adenosine (see Fig. 17.1), both of which may produce further receptor-mediated effects. The role of intracellular ATP in regulating membrane potassium channels to control vascular smooth muscle (Ch. 23) and insulin secretion (Ch. 32), is quite distinct from this transmitter function.

ATP AS A NEUROTRANSMITTER

The idea that such a workaday metabolite as ATP might be a member of the neurotransmitter elite was resisted for a long time, but is now firmly established. ATP is a transmitter in the periphery, both as a primary mediator and as a co-transmitter in noradrenergic nerve terminals. $P2X_2$, $P2X_4$ and $P2X_6$ are the predominant receptor subtypes expressed in neurons. $P2X_1$ predominates in smooth muscle.

ATP is contained in synaptic vesicles of both adrenergic and cholinergic neurons, and it accounts for many of the actions produced by stimulation of autonomic nerves that are not caused by acetylcholine or noradrenaline (see Ch. 13). These effects include the relaxation of intestinal smooth muscle evoked by sympathetic stimulation, and contraction of the bladder produced by parasympathetic nerves. Burnstock and his colleagues have shown that ATP is released on nerve stimulation in a Ca^{2+}-dependent fashion, and that exogenous ATP, in general, mimics the effects of nerve stimulation in various preparations. ATP may function as a conventional 'fast' transmitter in autonomic ganglia and possibly the CNS, or as an inhibitory presynaptic transmitter.

Adenosine, produced following hydrolysis of ATP, exerts presynaptic inhibitory effects on the release of excitatory transmitters in the CNS and periphery.

ATP IN NOCICEPTION

ATP causes pain when injected (for example) subdermally, as a result of activation of $P2X_2$ and/or $P2X_3$ heteromeric receptors on afferent neurons involved in the transduction of nociception (see Ch. 43). The pain can be blocked by aspirin (see Ch. 27) suggesting the involvement of prostaglandins. There is considerable interest in the potential role of purinergic receptors (mainly P2Y and P2X receptors), in various aspects of nociceptive pain transmission and in particular the development of neuropathic pain, which is difficult to treat (see Ch. 43). Interestingly, purinergic receptors are found not just on neurons, but also on glial cells, suggesting a role for these 'support' cells in modulating the chain of nociceptive transmission. It has been suggested that both types of receptors could be useful targets for analgesic and anti-migraine drugs (Tsuda et al., 2012; Magni & Ceruti, 2013).

Oddly, perhaps, the same receptors seem to be involved in taste perception on the tongue.

ATP IN INFLAMMATION

ATP is released from stimulated, damaged or dying cells and P2X receptors are widely distributed on cells of the immune system; P2Y receptors less so. Acting through these receptors, ATP can regulate neutrophil and phagocyte chemotaxis and provoke the release from macrophages and mast cells of cytokines and other mediators of the inflammatory response (Hechler & Gachet, 2015). Mice in which the $P2X_7$ receptor is deleted show a reduced capacity to develop chronic inflammation. Purinergic signalling also plays an important role in T-cell signalling. A good account of the role of autocrine signalling in the immune system is given by Junger (2011).

FUTURE PROSPECTS

The area of purinergic pharmacology as a whole holds considerable promise for future therapeutic exploitation. Space does not permit a comprehensive listing but some of the papers cited below will enable the reader to follow up these.

REFERENCES AND FURTHER READING

(A note of caution: the nomenclature of these receptors has changed several times and this can make for difficulties when reading some older papers. For the latest version of the nomenclature, as well as information about ligands etc., always refer to www.guidetopharmacology.org/)

Antonioli, L., Colucci, R., Pellegrini, C., et al., 2013. The role of purinergic pathways in the pathophysiology of gut diseases: pharmacological modulation and potential therapeutic applications. Pharmacol. Ther. 139, 157–188. (*Very comprehensive survey of the distribution and function of purinergic receptors in the gut and their relevance to normal physiological function and disease*)

Brown, R.A., Spina, D., Page, C.P., 2008. Adenosine receptors and asthma. Br. J. Pharmacol. 153 (Suppl. 1), S446–S456. (*Excellent review of the pharmacology of adenosine in the lung. Very accessible*)

Burnstock, G., 2006. Purinergic P2 receptors as targets for novel analgesics. Pharmacol. Ther. 110, 433–454. (*This paper, and the reviews that follow by the same author, cover various aspects of purinergic signalling and its therapeutic application*)

Burnstock, G., 2008. Purinergic receptors as future targets for treatment of functional GI disorders. Gut 57, 1193–1194.

Burnstock, G., 2012. Purinergic signalling: Its unpopular beginning, its acceptance and its exciting future. Bioessays 34, 218–225. (*Interesting account of the entire field of purinergic signalling written by the scientist who really pioneered the field. Easy to read and informative*)

Burnstock, G., Brouns, I., Adriaensen, D., Timmermans, J.P., 2012. Purinergic signalling in the airways. Pharmacol. Rev. 64, 834–868. (*A substantial and authoritative review for those who want to delve into this area of purinergic pharmacology*)

Burnstock, G., 2017. Purinergic signalling: therapeutic developments. Front. Pharmacol. 8, 1–55. (*A very comprehensive review of this area highlighting the potential therapeutic opportunities for purinergic agents in many therapeutic areas*)

Chen, J.F., Eltzschig, H.K., Fredholm, B.B., 2013. Adenosine receptors as drug targets–what are the challenges? Nat. Rev. Drug Discov. 12, 265–286. (*Excellent and comprehensive coverage of adenosine receptors*)

Cunha, R.A., 2001. Adenosine as a neuromodulator and as a homeostatic regulator in the nervous system: different roles, different sources and different receptors. Neurochem. Int. 38, 107–125. (*Speculative review on the functions of adenosine in the nervous system*)

Guzman-Aranguez, A., Gasull, X., Diebold, Y., Pintor, J., 2014. Purinergic receptors in ocular inflammation. Mediators Inflamm. 2014, 320906. (*This is a relatively new area and this paper details receptor distribution in the eye and discusses the potential therapeutic uses of purinergic agents in ocular disorders. Some diagrams. A bit specialised, but interesting*)

Hechler, B., Gachet, C., 2015. Purinergic receptors in thrombosis and inflammation. Arterioscler. Thromb. Vasc. Biol. 35, 2307–2315. (*An excellent review of the role of purinergic receptors in these particular indications and prospects for future drug therapy. Focuses mainly on P2X receptors. Well written, useful diagrams. Recommended*)

Junger, W.G., 2011. Immune cell regulation by autocrine purinergic signalling. Nat. Rev. Immunol. 11, 201–212. (*An excellent, and well illustrated, overview of the role of the pruinergic system in immune cells. Focuses on T cells and neutrophil autocrine signalling. Recommended reading*)

Khakh, B.S., North, R.A., 2006. P2X receptors as cell-surface ATP sensors in health and disease. Nature 442, 527–532. (*Excellent and very readable review on P2X receptors. Recommended*)

Magni, G., Ceruti, S., 2013. P2Y purinergic receptors: new targets for analgesic and antimigraine drugs. Biochem. Pharmacol. 85, 466–477. (*Very thorough review of the potential for new analgesics that act at these receptors. Useful diagrams and structural information about P2Y receptor agonists*)

Ochoa-Cortes, F., Linan-Rico, A., Jacobson, K.A., Christofi, F.L., 2014. Potential for developing purinergic drugs for gastrointestinal diseases. Inflamm. Bowel Dis. 20, 1259–1287. (*Comprehensive and easy-to-read review of this topic. Includes data on herbal products containing purinergic drugs also. Recommended*)

Tsuda, M., Tozaki-Saitoh, H., Inoue, K., 2012. Purinergic system, microglia and neuropathic pain. Curr. Opin. Pharmacol. 12, 74–79. (*A short overview of the role of the purinergic system in microglia and the implications for the pathogenesis and treatment of neuropathic pain*)

Local hormones 1: histamine and the biologically active lipids

18

OVERVIEW

In Chapter 7 we discussed the function of cellular players in host defence and alluded to the crucial role of soluble chemical regulators of inflammation. In this chapter, and the next, we take a closer look at these substances. We begin with some small molecule mediators. While also having a physiological role, these are also pressed into service by host defence mechanisms when necessary, and are therefore important targets for anti-inflammatory drug action.

INTRODUCTION

The growth of pharmacology as a discipline was attended by the discovery of numerous biologically active substances. Many were initially described as uncharacterised smooth muscle contracting (or relaxing) 'factors', which appeared in blood or tissues during particular physiological or pathological events. Sometimes, these factors were identified comparatively quickly but others resisted analysis for many years and so the development of a particular pharmacological area was often tied to progress in analytical methodology. For example, 5-hydroxytryptamine (5-HT; Ch. 16) and histamine, which are quite simple compounds, were identified soon after their biological properties were described. However, the structural elucidation of the more complex prostaglandins, which were first discovered in the 1930s, had to await the development of the mass spectrometer some 30 years later before the field could really progress. Peptide and protein structures took even longer to solve. Substance P (11 amino acids) was also discovered in the 1930s, but was not characterised until 1970 when peptide sequencing techniques had been developed. By the 1980s however, molecular biology had greatly enhanced our analytical proficiency; for example, the 21 amino acid peptide, endothelin, was discovered and fully characterised, with the sequences of the gene and peptide published within about a year and the complete information published in a single paper (Yanagisawa et al., 1988).

WHAT IS A 'MEDIATOR'?

Like regular hormones, such as thyroxine (Ch. 35) or insulin (Ch. 32), a *local hormone* is simply a chemical messenger that conveys information from one cell to another.[1]

Hormones such as thyroxine and insulin are released from a single endocrine gland, circulate in the blood and produce their action on other 'target' tissues. In contrast, local hormones are usually produced by cells to operate within their immediate microenvironment. The distinction is not actually completely clear-cut however. For example, one of the 'classical' hormones, hydrocortisone, is normally released by the adrenal gland but, surprisingly, can also be produced by, and act locally upon, some other tissues such as the skin. Conversely, some cytokines (see Ch. 19), which are usually regarded as local hormones, can circulate in the blood and produce systemic actions as well.

When, in response to a stimulus of some kind, a local hormone is released and produces a particular biological effect (such as contraction of smooth muscle in response to allergen challenge), it is said to be a *mediator* of this response. Traditionally, a putative mediator[2] had to satisfy certain criteria before gaining official recognition. In the 1930s, Sir Henry Dale proposed a set of five rules to validate the credentials of mediators and these guidelines have been used as a point of reference ever since. Originally formulated as a test for putative neurotransmitters however, these criteria cannot easily be applied to mediators of other responses and have been modified on several occasions.

Currently, the experimental criteria that establish a substance as a mediator are:

- that it is released from local cells in sufficient amounts to produce a biological action on the target cells within an appropriate time frame;
- that application of an authentic sample of the mediator reproduces the original biological effect;
- that interference with the synthesis, release or action (e.g. using receptor antagonists, enzyme inhibitors, 'knock-down' or 'knock-out' techniques) ablates or modulates the original biological response.

HISTAMINE

In a classic study, Dale and his colleagues demonstrated that a local anaphylactic reaction (a type I or 'immediate hypersensitivity reaction' such as the response to egg albumin in a previously sensitised animal; see Ch. 7) was caused by antigen–antibody reactions in sensitised tissue, and found that histamine mimicked this effect both in vitro and in vivo. Later studies confirmed that histamine is present in tissues, and released (along with other mediators) during anaphylaxis.

---

[1]The term 'autocrine' is sometimes used to denote a local mediator that acts on the cell from which it is released, whereas a 'paracrine' mediator acts on other neighbouring cells.

[2]To add to the lexicographical confusion, the term 'bioregulator' has recently crept into use. As this portmanteau word could cover just about any biologically active substance, it is not much use for our purposes.

SYNTHESIS AND STORAGE OF HISTAMINE

Histamine is a basic amine formed from histidine by histidine decarboxylase (Fig. 18.1). It is found in most tissues but is present in high concentrations in tissues in contact with the outside world (lungs, skin and gastrointestinal tract). At the cellular level, it is found largely in mast cells (approximately 0.1–0.2 pmol/cell) and basophils (0.01 pmol/cell), but non-mast cell histamine also occurs in 'histaminocytes' in the stomach and in histaminergic neurons in the brain (see Ch. 40). In mast cells and basophils, histamine is complexed in intracellular granules with an acidic protein and a high molecular-weight heparin termed *macroheparin*.

HISTAMINE RELEASE

Histamine is released from mast cells by exocytosis during inflammatory or allergic reactions. Stimuli include complement components C3a and C5a (see Ch. 7), which interact with specific surface receptors, and the combination of antigen with cell-fixed immunoglobulin (Ig)E antibodies. In common with many secretory processes (Ch. 4), histamine release is initiated by a rise in cytosolic $[Ca^{2+}]$. Various basic drugs, such as **morphine** and **tubocurarine**, release histamine, as does **compound 48/80**, an experimental tool often used to investigate mast cell biology. Agents that increase cAMP formation (e.g. β-adrenoceptor agonists; see Ch. 15) inhibit histamine secretion. Replenishment of secreted histamine by mast cells or basophils is a slow process, which may take days or weeks, whereas turnover of histamine in the gastric histaminocyte is very rapid. Histamine is metabolised by histaminase and/or by the methylating enzyme imidazole *N*-methyltransferase.

HISTAMINE RECEPTORS

Four types of histamine receptor have been identified, H_{1-4}. All are G protein–coupled receptors but their downstream signalling systems differ. H_1 and H_3 receptors, for example, elevate cAMP, whereas H_2 and H_4 receptors stimulate PLC. Splice variants of H_3 and H_4 receptors have been reported. All four are implicated in the inflammatory response in some capacity. A good account of the role of histamine in inflammation has been given by Jutel et al. (2009).

Fig. 18.1 **The synthesis of histamine.** Histamine is synthesised by histidine decarboxylas, which removes the carboxyl group *(in shaded box)* from histidine. Histamine can be metabolised to inactive products by several enzymes, including histaminase (diamine oxidase), and/or by the methylating enzyme imidazole *N*-methyltransferase.

Selective antagonists at H_1, H_2 and H_3 receptors include mepyramine, cimetidine and thioperamide, respectively. Selective agonists for H_2 and H_3 receptors are, respectively, dimaprit and (R)-methylhistamine. Histamine H_1 antagonists are the principal antihistamines used in the treatment or prevention of inflammation (notably allergic inflammation such as hay fever). Other clinical uses of subtype antagonists may be found in Chapters 27, 28 and 40. The pharmacology of H_4 receptors is less well developed but strongly suggests that the receptor has a significant role in the inflammatory response. Eosinophils seem to be a prominent target. Panula et al. (2015) have compiled a comprehensive review of histamine receptors and their pharmacology.

ACTIONS

Smooth muscle effects. Histamine, acting on H_1 receptors, contracts the smooth muscle of the ileum, bronchi, bronchioles and uterus. The effect on the ileum is not as marked in humans as it is in the guinea pig (this tissue remains the *de facto* standard preparation for histamine bioassay). Histamine reduces air flow in the first phase of bronchial asthma (see Ch. 29) but H_1 antagonists are not of much benefit in the human disease. It is possible that H_4 receptors are more important (Thurmond, 2015) in mediating these resistant histamine effects.

Cardiovascular effects. Histamine dilates human blood vessels and increases permeability of postcapillary venules, by an action on H_1 receptors, the effect being partly endothelium-dependent in some vascular beds. It also increases the rate and the output of the heart mainly by an action on cardiac H_2 receptors. It seems that this mediator is involved mainly in regulation of cardiovascular system in pathological, rather than physiological, states. Hattori et al. (2017) have reviewed the area in detail.

Gastric secretion. Histamine stimulates the secretion of gastric acid by action on H_2 receptors. In clinical terms, this is the most important action of histamine, because it is implicated in the pathogenesis of peptic ulcer. It is considered in detail in Chapter 31.

Effects on skin. When injected intradermally, histamine causes a reddening of the skin, accompanied by a weal with a surrounding flare. This mimics the *triple response* to scratching of the skin, described by Sir Thomas Lewis over 80 years ago. The reddening reflects vasodilatation of the small arterioles and precapillary sphincters and the weal, the increased permeability of the postcapillary venules. These effects are mainly mediated through activation of H_1 receptors. The flare is an *axon reflex*: stimulation of sensory nerve fibres evokes antidromic impulses through neighbouring branches of the same nerve, releasing vasodilators such as calcitonin gene-related peptide (CGRP; see Chs 19 and 27). Histamine causes intense itch if injected into the skin or applied to a blister base, because it stimulates sensory nerve endings through an H_1-dependent mechanism. H_1 antagonists are used to control itch caused by allergic reactions, insect bites, etc.

Even though histamine release is manifestly capable of reproducing many of the inflammatory signs and symptoms, H_1 antagonists do not have much clinical utility in the acute inflammatory response per se, because other mediators are more important. Histamine is, however, important in type I hypersensitivity reactions such as allergic rhinitis and urticaria. Other significant actions of histamine in inflammation include effects on B and T cells, modulating the acquired immune response (Jutel et al., 2009). The use of

H_1 antagonists in these conditions is dealt with in Chapter 27. It is possible that the developing field of H_4 receptor pharmacology will fill in some significant gaps in our understanding of the role of histamine in inflammation in the near future (Thurmond, 2015).

Histamine

- Histamine is a basic amine, stored in mast cell and basophil granules, and secreted when C3a and C5a interact with specific membrane receptors or when antigen interacts with IgE fixed on cells triggering the high affinity IgE receptor.
- Histamine produces effects by acting on H_1, H_2, H_3 or H_4 receptors on target cells.
- The main actions in humans are:
  - stimulation of gastric secretion (H_2)
  - contraction of most smooth muscle, except blood vessels (H_1)
  - cardiac stimulation (H_2)
  - vasodilatation (H_1)
  - increased vascular permeability (H_1)
- Injected intradermally, histamine causes the 'triple response': *reddening* (local vasodilatation), *weal* (increased permeability of postcapillary venules) and *flare* (from an 'axon' reflex in sensory nerves releasing a peptide mediator).
- The main pathophysiological roles of histamine are:
  - as a stimulant of gastric acid secretion (treated with H_2-receptor antagonists)
  - as a mediator of type I hypersensitivity reactions such as urticaria and hay fever (treated with H_1-receptor antagonists)
  - CNS functions (see Ch. 40).

EICOSANOIDS

GENERAL REMARKS

The term *eicosanoid* refers to a group of mediators that are generated from specific fatty acid precursors. They are implicated in the control of many physiological processes, are among the most important mediators and modulators of the inflammatory reaction (Figs 18.2 and 18.3) and are a significant target for drug action.

Interest in eicosanoids first arose in the 1930s after reports that semen contained a lipid substance, apparently originating from the prostate gland, which contracted uterine smooth muscle. Later, it became clear that *prostaglandin* (as the factor was named[3]) was not a single substance but a whole family of compounds generated by virtually all cells from 20-carbon unsaturated fatty acid precursors.

---

[3]The name arose through an anatomical error. In some species it is difficult to differentiate the prostaglandin-rich seminal vesicles from the prostate gland which (ironically as we now know) contains relatively little. Nevertheless, the name stuck, outlasting the more appropriate term *vesiglandin*, which was suggested later.

STRUCTURE AND BIOSYNTHESIS

In land-dwelling mammals, the main eicosanoid precursor is arachidonic acid (5,8,11,14-eicosatetraenoic acid), a 20-carbon unsaturated fatty acid containing four unsaturated double bonds (hence the prefix *eicosa-*, referring to the 20 carbon atoms, and *tetra*-enoic, referring to the four double bonds; see Fig. 18.2). The principal groups of eicosanoids are prostaglandins, *thromboxanes*, *leukotrienes*, *lipoxins* and *resolvins*. The common term *prostanoids* refers to prostaglandins and thromboxanes only.

In most cell types, arachidonic acid is a component of phospholipids and the intracellular concentration of the free acid is low. Eicosanoids are not stored in cells (like histamine, for example) but are synthesised and released immediately. The initial and rate-limiting step in eicosanoid synthesis is therefore the liberation of arachidonate. Usually this is a one-step process catalysed by the enzyme *phospholipase A_2* (PLA_2; see Fig. 18.3) but an alternative multi-step process involving phospholipases C or D in conjunction with diacylglycerol lipase is sometimes utilised. Several types of PLA_2 exist, but the most important is probably the highly-regulated *cytosolic PLA_2* (cPLA_2). This enzyme not only generates arachidonic acid (and thus eicosanoids) but also lysoglyceryl-phosphorylcholine (lyso-PAF), the precursor of *platelet-activating factor* (PAF), another inflammatory mediator (see Figs 18.2 and 18.3).

Cytosolic PLA_2 is activated by phosphorylation and this may be triggered by signal transduction systems activated by many stimuli, such as thrombin action on platelets, C5a on neutrophils, bradykinin on fibroblasts and antigen–antibody reactions on mast cells. General cell damage also triggers cPLA_2 activation. The free arachidonic acid (which normally exists as *arachidonate* in solution) is metabolised separately (or sometimes jointly) by several pathways, including the following.

- *Fatty acid cyclo-oxygenase* (COX). Two main isoforms exist, COX-1 and COX-2. These are highly homologous enzymes but are regulated in different and tissue-specific ways. They enzymatically combine arachidonic (and some other unsaturated fatty acid) substrates with molecular oxygen to form unstable intermediates, *cyclic endoperoxides*, which can subsequently be transformed by other enzymes to different *prostanoids*.
- *Lipoxygenases*. There are several subtypes, which often work sequentially, to synthesise leukotrienes, lipoxins and other compounds (Figs 18.2–18.4).

Chapter 27 deals in detail with the way inhibitors of these pathways (including non-steroidal anti-inflammatory drugs [NSAIDs] and glucocorticoids) produce their anti-inflammatory effects.

PROSTANOIDS

COX-1 is present in most cells as a constitutive enzyme. It produces prostanoids that act mainly as homeostatic regulators (e.g. modulating vascular responses, regulating gastric acid secretion). COX-2 is not normally present (at least in most tissues – CNS and renal tissue are important exceptions) but it is strongly induced by inflammatory stimuli and therefore believed to be more relevant as a target for anti-inflammatory drugs (see Ch. 27). Both enzymes catalyse the incorporation of two molecules of oxygen into two of the unsaturated double bonds in each arachidonate molecule,

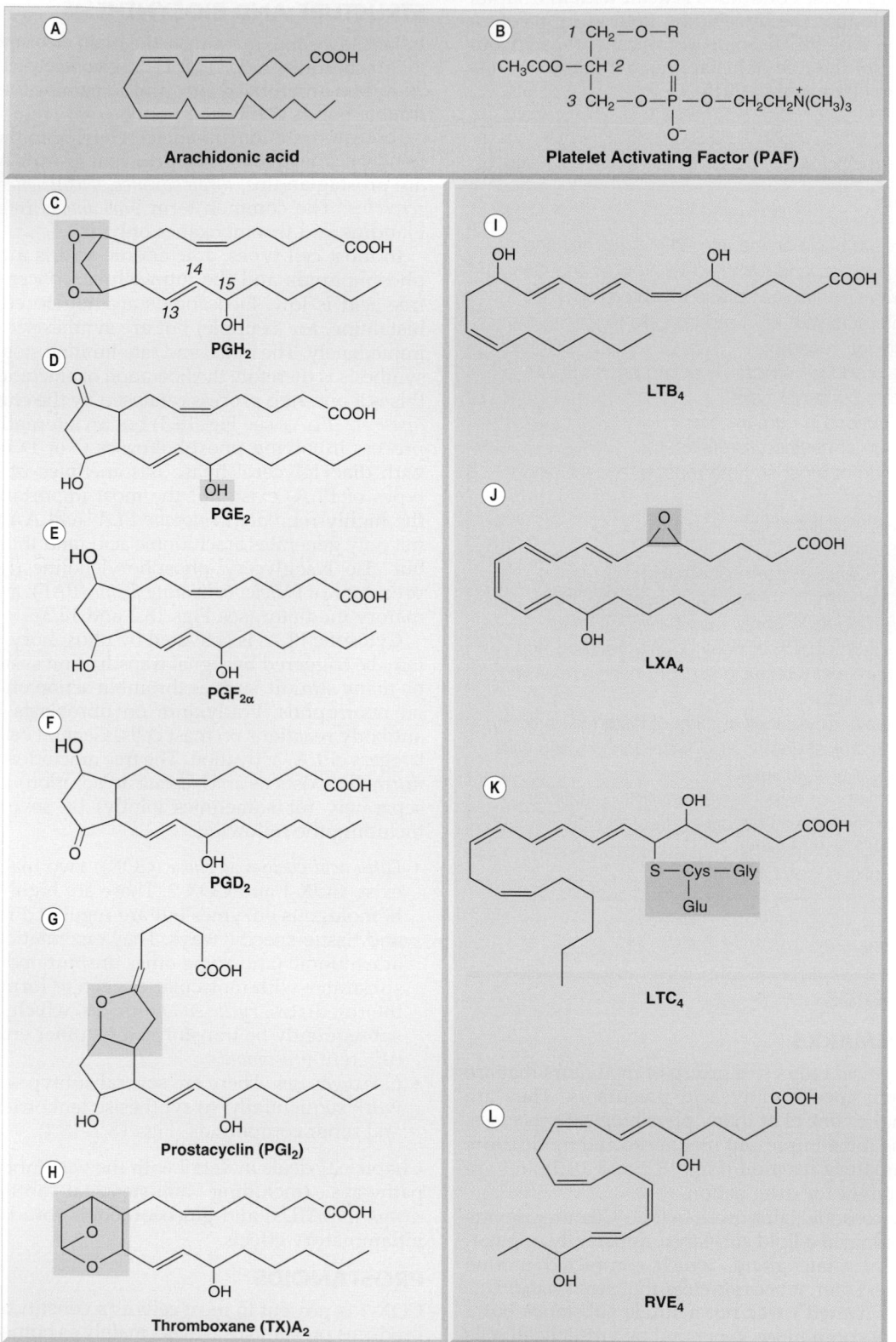

Fig. 18.2 Some key lipid mediators involved in the host defence response. (A) Arachidonic acid, an important precursor of prostanoids, leukotrienes and (some) lipoxins and resolvins. Note the conjugated double bonds *(in shaded box)*. (B) Platelet-activating factor (PAF): the location of the acetyl group at C2 is shown in the *shaded box*. R is a 6- or 8-carbon saturated fatty acid attached by an ether linkage to the carbon backbone. (C) Prostaglandin (PG)H$_2$, one of the labile intermediates in the synthesis of prostaglandins; note unstable ring structure *(in shaded box)* which can spontaneously hydrolyse in biological fluids if not enzymatically changed. (D) PGE$_2$, the 15-hydroxyl group *(in shaded box)* is crucial for the biological activity of prostaglandins and its removal is the first step in their inactivation. (E) and (F) PGF$_{2\alpha}$ and PGD$_2$. (G) Prostacyclin (PGI$_2$); note unstable ring structure *(in shaded box)*. (H) Thromboxane (TX)A$_2$; note unstable oxane structure *(in shaded box)*. (I) Leukotriene (LT)B$_4$. (J) Lipoxin (LX)A$_4$; note unstable and highly reactive oxygen bridge structure *(in shaded box)*. (K) Leukotriene (LT)C$_4$; note conjugated glutathione moiety *(in shaded box)*. (L) Resolvin (Rv)E$_4$.

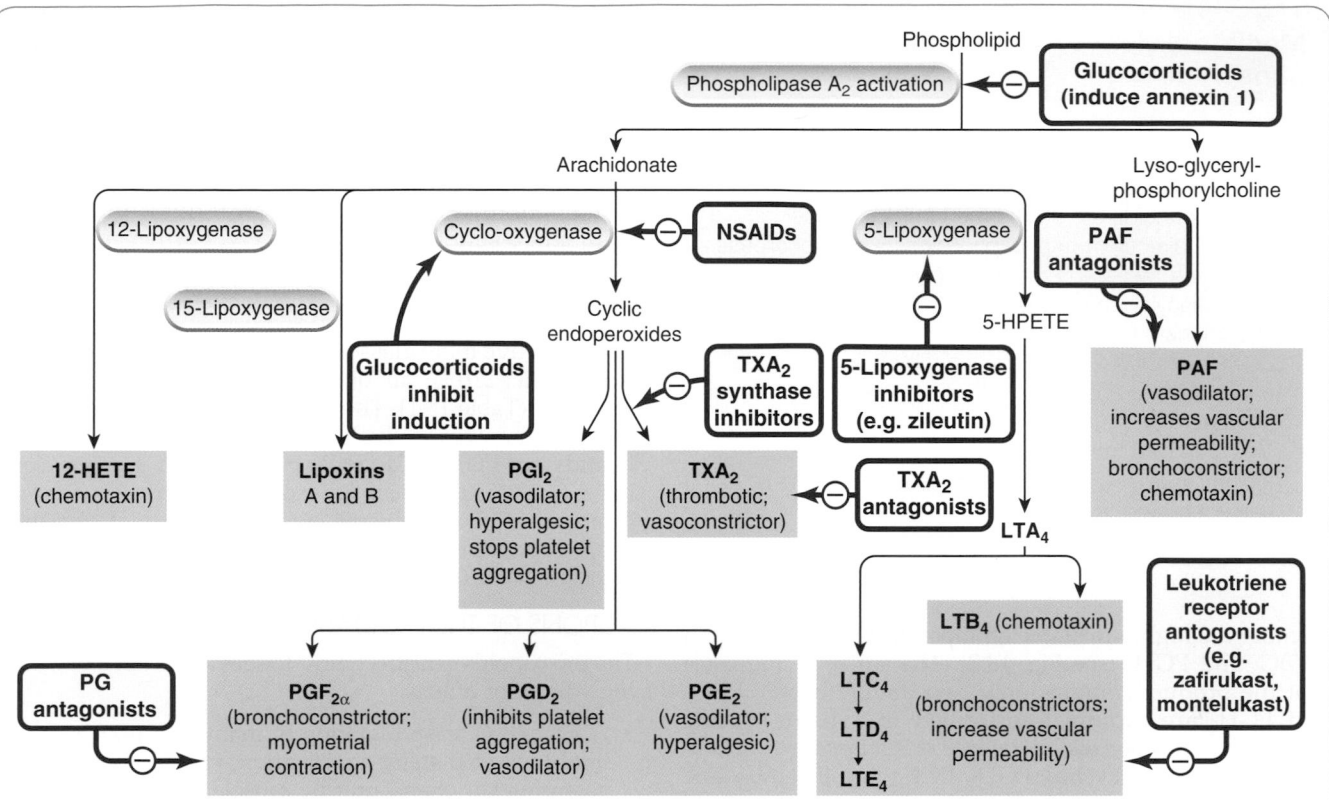

Fig. 18.3 **Summary diagram of the inflammatory mediators derived from phospholipids, with an outline of their actions and the sites of action of anti-inflammatory drugs.** Arachidonate metabolites are known as eicosanoids. The glucocorticoids inhibit transcription of the gene for cyclo-oxygenase (COX)-2, which is induced in cells by inflammatory mediators and induce and release Annexin A1 which down-regulates phospholipase A_2 activity thereby limiting arachidonate release. The effects of prostaglandin (PG)E_2 depend on which of the four receptors it activates. *HETE,* hydroxyeicosatetraenoic acid; *HPETE,* hydroperoxyeicosatetraenoic acid; *LT,* leukotriene; *NSAID,* non-steroidal anti-inflammatory drug; *PAF,* platelet-activating factor; *PGI₂,* prostacyclin; *TX,* thromboxane.

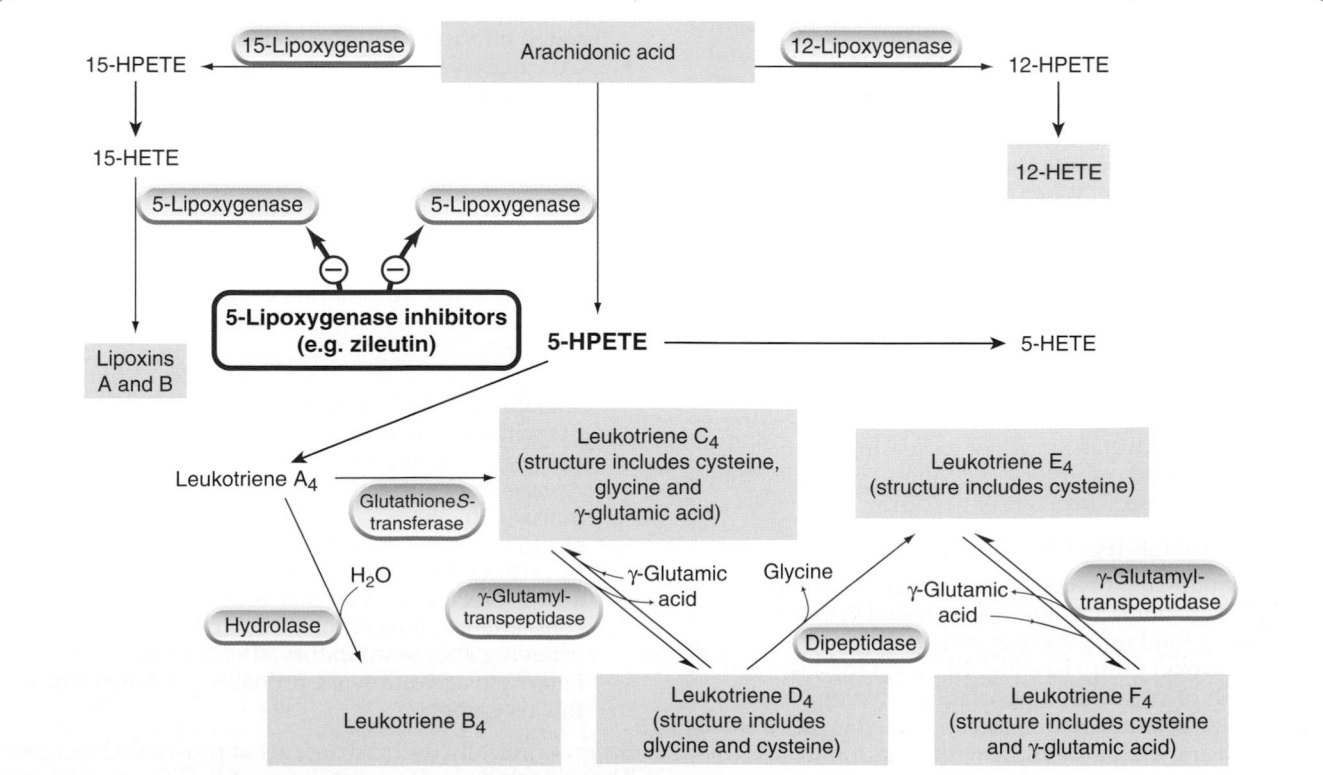

Fig. 18.4 **The biosynthesis of leukotrienes from arachidonic acid.** Compounds with biological action are shown in *grey boxes. HETE,* hydroxyeicosatetraenoic acid; *HPETE,* hydroperoxyeicosatetraenoic acid.

Mediators derived from phospholipids

- The principal phospholipid-derived mediators are the eicosanoids (prostanoids and leukotrienes) and platelet-activating factor (PAF).
- The eicosanoids are synthesised from arachidonic acid released directly from phospholipids by phospholipase A_2, or by a two-step process involving phospholipase C and diacylglycerol lipase.
- Arachidonate is metabolised by cyclo-oxygenases (COX)-1 or COX-2 to prostanoids, by 5-lipoxygenase to leukotrienes and, after further conversion, to lipoxins and other compounds.
- PAF is derived from phospholipid precursors by phospholipase A_2, giving rise to lyso-PAF, which is then acetylated to give PAF.

forming the highly unstable endoperoxides prostaglandin (PG)G_2 and PGH$_2$ (see Fig. 18.2). The suffix '2' indicates that the product contains only two double bonds. PGG$_2$ and PGH$_2$ are rapidly transformed in a tissue-specific manner by endoperoxide *isomerase* or *synthase* enzymes to PGE$_2$, PGI$_2$ (prostacyclin), PGD$_2$, PGF$_{2\alpha}$ and thromboxane (TX)A$_2$, which are the principal bioactive end products of this reaction. The mix of eicosanoids thus produced varies between cell types, depending on the particular endoperoxide isomerases or synthases present. In platelets, for example, TXA$_2$ predominates, whereas in vascular endothelium PGI$_2$ is the main product. Macrophages, neutrophils and mast cells synthesise a mixture of products. If *eicosatrienoic acid* (three double bonds) rather than arachidonic acid is the substrate for these enzymes, the resulting prostanoids have only a single double bond, for example PGE$_1$, while *eicosapentaenoic acid*, which contains five double bonds, yields PGE$_3$. Eicosapentaenoic acid is abundant in diets rich in oily fish and may, if present in sufficient amounts, represent a significant fraction of cellular fatty acids and thus constitute the major source of precursors for the COX enzyme. When this occurs, the production of the pro-inflammatory PGE$_2$ is diminished and, more significantly, the generation of TXA$_2$ as well. This may partly underlie the beneficial anti-inflammatory and cardiovascular actions that are ascribed to diets rich in this type of marine product (see also Resolvins, later).

The endocannabinoid *anandamide* (see Ch. 20) is an ethanolamine derivative of arachidonic acid and, surprisingly, it can also be oxidised by COX-2 to form a range of *prostamides*. These substances are of increasing interest. They act at prostanoid receptors but often exhibit a unique pharmacology (see Urquhart et al., 2015).

CATABOLISM OF THE PROSTANOIDS

This is a multi-step process. After carrier-mediated uptake, most prostaglandins are rapidly inactivated by prostaglandin *dehydrogenase* and *reductase* enzymes. These enzymes oxidise the 15-hydroxyl group (see Fig. 18.2) and the 13-14 double bond, both of which are important for biological activity. The inactive products are further degraded by general fatty acid-oxidising enzymes and excreted in the urine. These dehydrogenase enzymes are present in high concentration

in the lung, and 95% of infused PGE$_2$, PGE$_1$ or PGF$_{2\alpha}$ is inactivated after a single passage through the lungs, meaning that little normally reaches the arterial circulation and for this reason the half-life of most prostaglandins in the circulation is less than 1 minute.

TXA$_2$ and PGI$_2$ are slightly different. Both are inherently unstable and decay rapidly and spontaneously (within 30 s and 5 min, respectively) in biological fluids into inactive TXB$_2$ and 6-keto-PGF$_{1\alpha}$, respectively. Further metabolism then occurs, but it is not really relevant to us here.

PROSTANOID RECEPTORS

There are five main classes of prostanoid receptor (Woodward et al., 2011), all of which are G protein–coupled receptors (Table 18.1). They are termed DP, FP, IP, EP and TP receptors, respectively, depending on whether their ligands are PGD, PGF, PGI, PGE or TXA species. Some have further subtypes; for example, there are four EP receptors. Polymorphisms and other variants of these enzymes have been implicated in the pathogenesis of various diseases (see Cornejo-Garcia et al., 2016).

ACTIONS OF THE PROSTANOIDS

The prostanoids can affect most tissues and exert a bewildering variety of effects.

- PGD$_2$ causes vasodilatation in many vascular beds, inhibition of platelet aggregation, relaxation of gastrointestinal and uterine muscle, and modification of release of hypothalamic/pituitary hormones. It has a bronchoconstrictor effect through a secondary action on TP receptors. It may also activate chemoattractant receptors on some leukocytes.
- PGF$_{2\alpha}$ causes uterine contraction in humans (see Ch. 36), luteolysis in some species (e.g. cattle) and bronchoconstriction in others (e.g. cats and dogs).
- PGI$_2$ causes vasodilatation, inhibition of platelet aggregation (see Ch. 25), renin release and natriuresis through effects on tubular reabsorption of Na$^+$.
- TXA$_2$ causes vasoconstriction, platelet aggregation (see Ch. 25) and bronchoconstriction (more marked in guinea pig than in humans).
- PGE$_2$, the predominant 'inflammatory' prostanoid has the following actions:
  - at EP$_1$ receptors, it causes contraction of bronchial and gastrointestinal smooth muscle;
  - at EP$_2$ receptors, it causes bronchodilatation, vasodilatation, stimulation of intestinal fluid secretion and relaxation of gastrointestinal smooth muscle;
  - at EP$_3$ receptors, it causes contraction of intestinal smooth muscle, inhibition of gastric acid (see Ch. 31) with increased mucus secretion, inhibition of lipolysis, inhibition of autonomic neurotransmitter release and contraction of the pregnant human uterus (Ch. 36);
  - at EP$_4$ receptors, it causes similar effects to those of EP$_2$ stimulation (these were originally thought to be a single receptor). Vascular relaxation is one consequence of receptor activation, as is cervical 'ripening'. Some inhibitory effects of PGE$_2$ on leukocyte activation are probably mediated through this receptor.

Several clinically useful drugs act at prostanoid receptors. These include **misoprostol,** an EP$_2$/EP$_3$ agonist that

Table 18.1 A simplified scheme of prostanoid and leukotriene receptor classification based upon their physiological effects

Receptor	Physiological ligands	Distribution	General physiological effects	Signalling system
IP	$PGI_2 \gg PGD_2$	Abundant in cardiovascular system, platelets, neurons and elsewhere	Generally inhibitory: e.g. smooth muscle relaxation, anti-inflammatory and anti-aggregatory effects	G_s ↑cAMP
DP_1	$PGD_2 \gg PGE_2$	Low abundance; vascular smooth muscle, platelets, CNS, airways, the eye		
EP_2	$PGE_2 > PG F_{2\alpha}$	Widespread distribution		
EP_4	$PGE_2 > PGF_{2\alpha}$	Widespread distribution		
TP	$TxA_2 = H_2 > D_2$	Abundant in cardiovascular system, platelets and immune cells. Two subtypes known with opposing actions	Generally excitatory: e.g. smooth muscle contraction, pro-inflammatory and platelet aggregatory actions	G_q/G_{11} $[PLC]^a$ ↑Ca^{2+}
FP	$PGF_{2\alpha} > PGD_2$	Very high expression in female reproductive organs		
EP_1	$PGE_2 > PGF_{2\alpha}$	Myometrium, intestine and lung		
EP_3	$PGE_2 > PGF_{2\alpha}$	Widespread distribution throughout body; many isoforms with different G protein coupling	Generally inhibitory: e.g. smooth muscle relaxation, anti-inflammatory and anti-aggregatory effects	G_i/G_o ↓cAMP
DP_2	$PGD_2 > PGF_{2\alpha}$	Different structure to other prostanoid receptors. Widely distributed especially in immune cells		
BLT_1	$LTB_4 > 20$ hydroxy LTB_4	Widely distributed in leukocytes and in some endothelial cells	'High-affinity' LTB_4 receptor. Activates leukocytes and stimulates chemotaxis	G_i/G_o↓ cAMP G_q/G_{11} ↑PLC
BLT_2	$LTB_4 > 20$ hydroxy LTB_4	Several tissues intestine, skin and some lesions	'Low-affinity' LTB_4 receptor. Maybe important in GI barrier formation and airway inflammation	G_i/Gq↓ cAMP
$CysLT_1$	$LTD_4 > LTC_4 > LTE_4$	Several tissues including leukocytes, mast cells, lung, intestinal and vascular tissue	Bronchoconstriction and leukocyte activation	G_q/G_{11} ↑PLC
$CysLT_2$	$LTC_4 > LTD_4 > LTE_4$	Several tissues including leukocytes, mast cells, nasal mucosa and vascular tissue	PMN activation, inflammation, contracts some vascular smooth muscle	G_q/G_{11} ↑PLC

^{a}PLC may not be involved in EP_1 signalling.
(Data derived from Woodward et al., 2011 and the IUPHAR/BPS Guide to Pharmacology.)

suppresses gastric acid secretion (see Ch. 31), the FP agonists **bimatoprost**,[4] **latanoprost, tafluprost** and **travoprost** which are used for the treatment of glaucoma (see Ch. 14) and **iloprost** and **epoprostanol** which are IP agonists used for the treatment of pulmonary hypertension (see Ch. 23).

THE ROLE OF PROSTANOIDS IN INFLAMMATION

The inflammatory response is inevitably accompanied by the release of prostanoids. PGE_2 predominates, although PGI_2 is also important. In areas of acute inflammation, PGE_2 and PGI_2 are generated by the local tissues and blood vessels, while mast cells release mainly PGD_2. In chronic inflammation, cells of the monocyte/macrophage series also release PGE_2 and TXA_2. Together, the prostanoids exert a sort of yin–yang effect in inflammation, stimulating some responses and decreasing others. The most striking effects are as follows.

- PGE_2, PGI_2 and PGD_2 are themselves powerful vasodilators but they also synergise with other inflammatory vasodilators, such as histamine and bradykinin. It is this combined dilator action on precapillary arterioles that contributes to the redness and increased blood flow in areas of acute inflammation. Prostanoids do not directly increase the permeability of the postcapillary venules, but potentiate the effects on vascular leakage caused by histamine and bradykinin. Similarly, they do not themselves produce pain, but sensitise afferent C fibres (see Ch. 43) to the effects of bradykinin and other noxious stimuli. The anti-inflammatory and analgesic effects of aspirin-like drugs (NSAIDs, see Ch. 27) stem largely from their ability to block these actions.

---

[4]Women being treated with bimatoprost eye drops for glaucoma were delighted with a side effect of this drug – stimulation of eyelash growth. It wasn't long before a thriving 'off-label' market had been established for its use in beauty spas. Eventually, the FDA licensed a preparation specifically for this cosmetic indication.

- Prostaglandins of the E series are also pyrogenic (i.e. they induce fever). High concentrations are found in cerebrospinal fluid during infection, and the increase in temperature (attributed to cytokines) is actually mediated by the release of PGE_2. NSAIDs exert antipyretic actions (Ch. 27) by inhibiting PGE_2 synthesis in the hypothalamus.
- Some prostaglandins have anti-inflammatory effects which are important during the resolution phase of inflammation. For example, PGE_2 decreases lysosomal enzyme release and the generation of toxic oxygen metabolites from neutrophils, as well as the release of histamine from mast cells.

Prostanoids

- The term *prostanoids* encompass prostaglandins and thromboxanes.
- Cyclo-oxygenases (COX) oxidise arachidonate, producing the unstable intermediates PGG_2 and PGH_2. These are enzymatically transformed to the different prostanoid species.
- There are two main COX isoforms: COX-1, a constitutive enzyme, and COX-2, which is often induced by inflammatory stimuli.
- The principal prostanoids are:
  - PGI_2 (prostacyclin), predominantly from vascular endothelium, acts on IP receptors, producing vasodilatation and inhibition of platelet aggregation.
  - Thromboxane (TX)A_2, predominantly from platelets, acts on TP receptors, causing platelet aggregation and vasoconstriction.
  - PGE_2 is an important mediator of the inflammatory responses and causes fever and pain.
- Other effects of PGE_2 include:
  - at EP_1 receptors: contraction of bronchial and gastrointestinal (GI) tract smooth muscle;
  - at EP_2 receptors: relaxation of bronchial, vascular and GI tract smooth muscle;
  - at EP_3 receptors: inhibition of gastric acid secretion, increased gastric mucus secretion, contraction of pregnant uterus and of gastrointestinal smooth muscle, inhibition of lipolysis and of autonomic neurotransmitter release.
- $PGF_{2\alpha}$ acts on FP receptors, found in uterine (and other) smooth muscle, and corpus luteum, producing contraction of the uterus and luteolysis (in some species).
- PGD_2 is abundant in activated mast cells. It acts on DP receptors, causing vasodilatation and inhibition of platelet aggregation.

LEUKOTRIENES

Leukotrienes (*leuko*- because they are made by white cells, and *-trienes* because they contain a conjugated triene system of double bonds; see Fig. 18.2) comprise two main categories, chemoattractant (LTB_4) and cysteinyl (or *sufidopeptide*) leukotrienes (LTC_4, D_4, E_4 and F_4). Both types

are synthesised from arachidonic acid by lipoxygenases. These soluble cytosolic enzymes are mainly found in lung, platelets, mast cells and white blood cells. The main enzyme in this group is *5-lipoxygenase*. On cell activation, this enzyme translocates to the nuclear membrane, where it associates with a crucial accessory protein, affectionately termed FLAP (**F**ive-**L**ipoxygenase **A**ctivating **P**rotein). The 5-lipoxygenase incorporates a hydroperoxy group at C5 in arachidonic acid to form *5-hydroperoxytetraenoic acid* (5-HPETE, see Fig. 18.4), which is further converted to the unstable leukotriene (LT)A_4. This may be converted enzymatically to LTB_4 or, utilising a separate pathway involving conjugation with glutathione, to the cysteinyl-containing leukotrienes LTC_4, LTD_4, LTE_4 and LTF_4. These cysteinyl leukotrienes are produced mainly by eosinophils, mast cells, basophils and macrophages. Mixtures of these substances constitute the biological activity historically ascribed to *slow-reacting substance of anaphylaxis* (SRS-A), an elusive bronchoconstrictor factor shown many years ago to be generated in guinea pig lung during anaphylaxis, and consequently predicted to be important in asthma.

Clinical uses of prostanoids

- Gynaecological and obstetric (see Ch. 36):
  - termination of pregnancy: **gemeprost** or **misoprostol** (a metabolically stable prostaglandin [PG]E analogue)
  - induction of labour: **dinoprostone** or **misoprostol**
  - postpartum haemorrhage: **carboprost**.
- Gastrointestinal:
  - to prevent ulcers associated with non-steroidal anti-inflammatory drug use: **misoprostol** (see Ch. 31).
- Cardiovascular:
  - to maintain the patency of the ductus arteriosus until surgical correction of the defect in babies with certain congenital heart malformations: **alprostadil** (PGE_1);
  - to inhibit platelet aggregation (e.g. during haemodialysis): **epoprostenol** (PGI_2), especially if **heparin** is contraindicated;
  - primary pulmonary hypertension: **epoprostenol** (see Ch. 23).
- Ophthalmic:
  - open-angle glaucoma: **latanoprost** eye drops.

LTB_4 is produced mainly by neutrophils. Lipoxins and other active products, some of which have anti-inflammatory properties, are also produced from arachidonate by this pathway (see Figs 18.2 and 18.4).

LTB_4 is metabolised by a unique membrane-bound cytochrome P450 enzyme in neutrophils, and then further oxidised to 20-carboxy-LTB_4. LTC_4 and LTD_4 are metabolised to LTE_4, which is excreted in the urine.

LEUKOTRIENE RECEPTORS

Leukotriene receptors are all GPCRs. They are termed BLT (two subtypes) if the ligand is LTB_4, and CysLT (two subtypes) for the cysteinyl leukotrienes (see Table 18.1). They are all of the G_q/G_{11} family that activates PLC signalling mechanisms, although there may be further receptors that respond to these potent mediators. Genetic variations in these receptors or the enzymes that synthesise leukotrienes may contribute to allergy and asthma, or to the failure of drug treatment in those disorders (Thompson et al., 2016).

LEUKOTRIENE ACTIONS

Cysteinyl leukotrienes have important actions on the respiratory and cardiovascular systems, and the CysLT-receptor antagonists **zafirlukast** and **montelukast** are now in use in the treatment of asthma (see Ch. 29), often in conjunction with a corticosteroid. Cysteinyl leukotrienes may mediate the cardiovascular changes of acute anaphylaxis. Agents that inhibit 5-lipoxygenase are therefore obvious candidates for anti-asthmatic (see Ch. 29) and anti-inflammatory agents. One such drug, **zileuton**, is available in some parts of the world for the treatment of asthma.

The respiratory system. Cysteinyl leukotrienes are potent spasmogens, causing dose-related contraction of human bronchiolar muscle in vitro. LTE_4 is less potent than LTC_4 and LTD_4, but its effect is much longer lasting. All cause an increase in mucus secretion. Given by aerosol to human volunteers, they reduce specific airway conductance and maximum expiratory flow rate, the effect being more protracted than that produced by histamine (Fig. 18.5).

The cardiovascular system. Small amounts of LTC_4 or LTD_4 given intravenously cause a rapid, short-lived fall in blood pressure, and significant constriction of small coronary resistance vessels. Given subcutaneously, they are equipotent with histamine in causing weal and flare. Given topically in the nose, LTD_4 increases nasal blood flow and local vascular permeability.

The role of leukotrienes in inflammation. LTB_4 is a potent chemotactic agent for neutrophils and macrophages (see Fig. 7.2). It upregulates membrane adhesion molecule expression on neutrophils, and increases the production of superoxide anions and the release of granule enzymes. On macrophages and lymphocytes, it stimulates proliferation and cytokine release. It is found in inflammatory exudates and tissues in many inflammatory conditions, including rheumatoid arthritis, psoriasis and ulcerative colitis.

The cysteinyl leukotrienes are present in the sputum of chronic bronchitis patients in amounts that are biologically active. On antigen challenge, they are released from samples of human asthmatic lung in vitro, and into nasal lavage fluid in subjects with allergic rhinitis. There is evidence that they contribute to the underlying bronchial hyper-reactivity in asthmatics, and it is thought that they are among the main mediators of both the early and late phases of asthma (see Fig. 29.2). Liu and Yokomizo (2015) have reviewed the role of these mediators in allergic diseases.

Leukotrienes

- 5-Lipoxygenase oxidises arachidonate to give 5-hydroperoxyeicosatetraenoic acid (5-HPETE), which is converted to leukotriene (LT)A_4. This, in turn, can be converted to either LTB_4 or to a series of glutathione adducts, the cysteinyl leukotrienes LTC_4, LTD_4 and LTE_4.
- LTB_4, acting on specific receptors, causes adherence, chemotaxis and activation of polymorphs and monocytes, and stimulates proliferation and cytokine production from macrophages and lymphocytes.
- The cysteinyl leukotrienes cause:
  - contraction of bronchial muscle
  - vasodilatation in most vessels, but coronary vasoconstriction
- LTB_4 is an important mediator in all types of inflammation; the cysteinyl leukotrienes are of importance in asthma.

OTHER IMPORTANT FATTY ACID DERIVATIVES

Unsaturated fatty acids such as arachidonic acid, eicosapentaenoic acid and *docosahexaenoic acid* can be enzymatically transformed into other important lipid mediators. Trihydroxy arachidonate metabolites termed *lipoxins* (see Figs 18.2 and 18.4) are formed by the concerted action of the 5- and the 12- or 15-lipoxygenase enzymes during inflammation. Lipoxins (abbreviation Lx) act on polymorphonuclear leukocytes, through G protein–coupled receptors such as ALX (also known as formyl peptide receptor 2 (FPR2) this receptor also recognises other anti-inflammatory factors such as annexin A1), to oppose the action of pro-inflammatory stimuli, providing what might be called 'stop signals' to halt inflammation (see Chandrasekharan & Sharma-Walia, 2015). Aspirin (a COX inhibitor, see Ch. 27) stimulates the synthesis of lipoxins because COX-2 can still produce hydroxy fatty acids even when inhibited by aspirin and unable to synthesise prostaglandins. The formation of lipoxins probably contributes to aspirin's anti-inflammatory effects, some of which are not completely explained through inhibition of prostaglandin generation (see Gilroy & Perretti, 2005; Serhan, 2005).

Resolvins (abbreviation Rv) are, as the name implies, a series of compounds that fulfil a similar function, but unlike

Fig. 18.5 The time course of action on specific airways conductance of the cysteinyl leukotrienes and histamine, in six normal subjects. Specific airways conductance was measured in a constant volume whole-body plethysmograph, and the drugs were given by inhalation. (From Barnes et al., 1984.)

lipoxins, their precursor fatty acid is eicosapentaenoic acid (RvE_{1-4}) or docosahexaenoic acid (RvD_{1-4}). Fish oils are rich in these fatty acids and it is likely that at least some of their claimed anti-inflammatory benefit is produced through conversion to these highly active species (see Zhang & Spite, 2012, for a review of this fascinating area). RvD_1 acts through the ALX/FPR2 receptor system whereas RvE_1 acts through a GPCR called the *chemerin receptor*. This signals through the G1/Gq system to lower cAMP and release intracellular calcium. Resolvins can counteract inflammatory pain (Xu et al., 2010) and analogues are undergoing trials for the treatment of a variety of inflammatory conditions (Lee & Surh, 2012). *Maresins* (abbreviation Ma) and *protectins* are dihydroxy acids generated from docosahexaenoic acid, also by the actions of lipoxygenases. Maresins are predominately synthesised by macrophages and have a role in inflammatory resolution. Protectins (abbreviation P) are produced by lymphocytes and probably act to modulate the operation of the immune system amongst other functions. The area, which can be confusing until you come to terms with lipid structures, has been well reviewed by Sansbury and Spite (2016), Duvall and Levy (2016) and Serhan et al. (2015).

PLATELET-ACTIVATING FACTOR

Platelet-activating factor, also variously termed PAF-acether and AGEPC (acetyl-glyceryl-ether-phosphorylcholine), is a biologically active lipid that can produce effects at exceedingly low concentrations (less than 10^{-10} mol/L) through its G protein–coupled PAF receptor (G_q/G_{11}; stimulates cAMP production). The name, PAF, is somewhat misleading because it acts on many different target cells and, in particular, is believed to be an important mediator in both acute and chronic allergic and inflammatory phenomena.

BIOSYNTHESIS

PAF (see Fig. 18.2) is produced by platelets in response to thrombin, and also by activated inflammatory cells. It is synthesised from phospholipids which have an ether-linked hexadecyl or octadecyl fatty acid at C1, an unsaturated fatty acid such as arachidonic acid ester-linked at C2 and a phosphoryl choline base at C3. The action of PLA_2 removes the arachidonic acid yielding *lyso-PAF*, which is then acetylated by an *acetyltransferase* to yield the biologically active PAF. The reaction is reversible and PAF, in turn, can be inactivated by an *acetylhydrolase* yielding lyso-PAF ready for recycling.

ACTIONS AND ROLE IN INFLAMMATION

PAF can reproduce many of the signs and symptoms of inflammation. Injected locally, it produces vasodilatation (and thus erythema), increased vascular permeability and weal formation. Higher doses produce hyperalgesia. It is a potent chemotaxin for neutrophils and monocytes, and recruits eosinophils into the bronchial mucosa in the late

phase of asthma (see Fig. 29.3). PAF contracts both bronchial and ileal smooth muscle.

Acting through its receptor, PAF activates $cPLA_2$ and stimulates arachidonate turnover in many cells. In platelets it increases TXA_2 generation, producing a shape change and the release of the granule contents. This is important in haemostasis and thrombosis (see Ch. 25).

The anti-inflammatory actions of the glucocorticoids may be caused, at least in part, by inhibition of PAF synthesis (see Fig. 18.2). Competitive antagonists of PAF and/or specific inhibitors of *lyso-PAF acetyltransferase* could well be useful anti-inflammatory drugs and/or anti-asthmatic agents. The PAF antagonist **lexipafant** is approved for the treatment of acute pancreatitis in some countries (see Leveau et al., 2005). Two other antagonists, **modipafant** and **apafant** are also undergoing trials. **Rupatadine** is a combined H_1 and PAF antagonist that is available in some parts of the world for treating allergic symptoms, but it is not clear what (if anything) its anti-PAF action adds clinically to its effect as an H_1 antagonist.

CONCLUDING REMARKS

In this chapter we have focused on histamine and lipid mediators, but in some species (i.e. rodents) 5-HT (Ch. 16) also has pro-inflammatory properties. Other low molecular-weight factors also have inflammogenic actions, including some purines (Ch. 17) and nitric oxide (Ch. 21).

Perhaps the most surprising development in this area is the extraordinary proliferation of lipid mediators. It is a feature that would have surprised Dale and his colleagues, as lipids were regarded for many years simply as inert building blocks for membranes or as a source of metabolic fuel. However, this has become one of the fastest growing and most exciting areas of small molecular-weight mediator research and has already yielded several novel therapeutic leads.

Platelet-activating factor (PAF)

- PAF precursors are released from activated inflammatory cells by phospholipase A_2. After acetylation, the resultant PAF is released and acts on specific receptors in target cells.
- Pharmacological actions include vasodilatation, increased vascular permeability, chemotaxis and activation of leukocytes (especially eosinophils), activation and aggregation of platelets, and smooth muscle contraction.
- PAF is implicated in bronchial hyper-responsiveness and in the delayed phase of asthma.
- A PAF antagonist, **lexipafant**, is used to treat pancreatitis.

REFERENCES AND FURTHER READING

Ariel, A., Serhan, C.N., 2007. Resolvins and protectins in the termination program of acute inflammation. Trends Immunol. 28, 176–183. (*Very accessible review on these unusual lipid mediators which promote inflammatory resolution and the link with fish oils*)

Barnes, N.C., Piper, P.J., Costello, J.F., 1984. Comparative effects of inhaled leukotriene C4, leukotriene D4, and histamine in normal human subjects. Thorax 39, 500–504.

Di Gennaro, A., Haeggstrom, J.Z., 2012. The leukotrienes: immune-modulating lipid mediators of disease. Adv. Immunol. 116,

51–92. (*Useful update on leukotriene actions in inflammation. Recommended*)

Chandrasekharan, J.A., Sharma-Walia, N., 2015. Lipoxins: nature's way to resolve inflammation. J Inflamm Res 8, 181–192. (*Recent review and update on the role of these lipids in inflammatory resolution. A good introduction and easy to read*)

Cornejo-Garcia, J.A., Perkins, J.R., Jurado-Escobar, R., et al., 2016. Pharmacogenomics of prostaglandin and leukotriene receptors. Front. Pharmacol. 7, 316. (*This paper details some of the genetic variants of eicosanoid receptors and reviews the evidence linking them to disease pathologies*)

Duvall, M.G., Levy, B.D., 2016. DHA- and EPA-derived resolvins, protectins, and maresins in airway inflammation. Eur. J. Pharmacol. 785, 144–155.

Gilroy, D.W., Perretti, M., 2005. Aspirin and steroids: new mechanistic findings and avenues for drug discovery. Curr. Opin. Pharmacol. 5, 405–411. (*A very interesting review of the anti-inflammatory substances that are released during the inflammatory response and that bring about resolution; it also deals with a rather odd effect of aspirin – its ability to boost the production of anti-inflammatory lipoxins. Easy to read and informative*)

Hattori, Y., Hattori, K., Matsuda, N., 2017. Regulation of the cardiovascular system by histamine. Handb. Exp. Pharmacol. 241, 239–258.

Jutel, M., Akdis, M., Akdis, C.A., 2009. Histamine, histamine receptors and their role in immune pathology. Clin. Exp. Allergy 39, 1786–1800. (*Excellent review. Easy to read*)

Kim, N., Luster, A.D., 2007. Regulation of immune cells by eicosanoid receptors. ScientificWorld J. 7, 1307–1328. (*Useful overview of eicosanoids, their biology and receptor family*)

Larsson, B.M., Kumlin, M., Sundblad, B.M., et al., 2006. Effects of 5-lipoxygenase inhibitor zileuton on airway responses to inhaled swine house dust in healthy subjects. Respir. Med. 100, 226–237. (*A paper describing the effects of zileuton, a 5-lipoxygenase inhibitor, on the allergic response in humans; the results are not unequivocally positive, but the study is an interesting one*)

Lee, H.N., Surh, Y.J., 2012. Therapeutic potential of resolvins in the prevention and treatment of inflammatory disorders. Biochem. Pharmacol. 84, 1340–1350. (*Good review and easy to read*)

Leveau, P., Wang, X., Sun, Z., et al., 2005. Severity of pancreatitis-associated gut barrier dysfunction is reduced following treatment with the PAF inhibitor lexipafant. Biochem. Pharmacol. 69, 1325–1331. (*An experimental study using a rat model but provides a useful insight into the potential clinical role of such an antagonist in pancreatitis*)

Liu, M., Yokomizo, T., 2015. The role of leukotrienes in allergic diseases. Allergol. Int. 64, 17–26. (*Comprehensive and very readable account of this area. Some useful diagrams and tables. Recommended*)

Panula, P., Chazot, P.L., Cowart, M., et al., 2015. International Union of Basic and Clinical Pharmacology. XCVIII. Histamine receptors.

Pharmacol. Rev. 67, 601–655. (*Very comprehensive review of histamine pharmacology for those who want to dig deep into this area*)

Sansbury, B.E., Spite, M., 2016. Resolution of acute inflammation and the role of resolvins in immunity, thrombosis, and vascular biology. Circ. Res. 119, 113–130.

Serhan, C.N., 2005. Lipoxins and aspirin-triggered 15-epi-lipoxins are the first lipid mediators of endogenous anti-inflammation and resolution. Prostaglandins Leukot. Essent. Fatty Acids 73, 141–162. (*A paper reviewing the lipoxins – anti-inflammatory substances formed by the 5-lipoxygenase enzyme; also discusses the action of aspirin in boosting the synthesis of these compounds and the receptors on which they act. A good review that summarises a lot of work*)

Serhan, C.N., Dalli, J., Colas, R.A., Winkler, J.W., Chiang, N., 2015. Protectins and maresins: New pro-resolving families of mediators in acute inflammation and resolution bioactive metabolome. Biochim. Biophys. Acta 1851, 397–413. (*Very good account of these new families of mediators detailing their discovery, biosynthesis and biology. Many useful tables summarising their main actions for those who are intimidated by the, often complex, biochemistry*)

Thompson, M.D., Capra, V., Clunes, M.T., et al., 2016. Cysteinyl leukotrienes pathway genes, atopic asthma and drug response: from population isolates to large genome-wide association studies. Front. Pharmacol. 7, 1–17. (*This is for you if you want to know the latest thinking on the genetic basis of atopic asthma and its relevance to leukotriene biology*)

Thurmond, R.L., 2015. The histamine H4 receptor: from orphan to the clinic. Front. Pharmacol. 6, 65.

Urquhart, P., Nicolaou, A., Woodward, D.F., 2015. Endocannabinoids and their oxygenation by cyclo-oxygenases, lipoxygenases and other oxygenases. Biochim. Biophys. Acta 1851, 366–376. (*The coming together of the cannabinoid and eicsanoid fields was unexpected and an exciting development. This is useful paper if you want to understand the biochemistry of these unusual compounds. Many pathway diagrams*)

Woodward, D.F., Jones, R.L., Narumiya, S., 2011. International Union of Basic and Clinical Pharmacology. LXXXIII: classification of prostanoid receptors, updating 15 years of progress. Pharmacol. Rev. 63, 471–538. (*Definitive and comprehensive review by the leaders in the field*)

Xu, Z.Z., Zhang, L., Liu, T., et al., 2010. Resolvins RvE$_1$ and RvD$_1$ attenuate inflammatory pain via central and peripheral actions. Nat. Med. 16, 592–597. (*Fascinating paper reporting the ability of these anti-inflammatory lipids to reduce pain*)

Yanagisawa, M., Kurihara, H., Kimura, S., et al., 1988. A novel potent vasoconstrictor peptide produced by vascular endothelial cells. Nature 332, 411–415. (*The discovery of endothelin – a remarkable tour de force*)

Zhang, M.J., Spite, M., 2012. Resolvins: anti-inflammatory and proresolving mediators derived from omega-3 polyunsaturated fatty acids. Annu. Rev. Nutr. 32, 203–227. (*Explores the link between 'fish oils' and anti-inflammatory resolving production*)

19 Local hormones 2: peptides and proteins

OVERVIEW

Having discussed small-molecule local hormones in the previous chapter, we now turn our attention to peptides and proteins, which are orders of magnitude larger in molecular terms. This constitutes a very diverse group and, unlike others described in Chapter 18, includes compounds (e.g. cytokines) that seem to be exclusively concerned with host defence. We begin with some general introductory observations on protein and peptide synthesis and secretion. We then discuss bradykinin, neuropeptides, cytokines (interleukins, chemokines and interferons) in more detail. Finally, we conclude with a few remarks on other proteins and peptides that down-regulate inflammation.

INTRODUCTION

Despite the fact that several mediators discovered early in the history of our discipline were recognised to be peptides, understanding of their pharmacology was limited until the 1970s, when the techniques for purifying, sequencing and synthesising peptides and proteins were first developed. The development of high-performance liquid chromatography and solid-phase peptide synthesis, for example, have greatly accelerated the development of the area, and while proteins containing 50 or more amino acids were (and are still) difficult to synthesise chemically, molecular biology techniques have provided a rapid alternative synthetic route. Indeed, the use of recombinant proteins as therapeutic agents – a development driven mainly by the emergent biotechnology industry – is rapidly gaining ground (see Ch. 5).

The use of molecular biology has helped understanding of peptide and protein pharmacology in many other ways as well. The availability of monoclonal antibodies for radioimmunoassay and immunocytochemistry has solved many quantitative problems. Transgenic animals with peptide or receptor genes deleted, overexpressed or mutated provide valuable clues about their functions, as has the use of antisense oligonucleotides, siRNA and gene editing (CRISPR-Cas9) technologies (see also Ch. 5) to silence these genes for experimental purposes. The control of precursor synthesis can be studied indirectly by measuring mRNA, for which highly sensitive and specific assays have been developed, which are even able to analyse mRNA in a single cell. The technique of in situ hybridisation enables the location and abundance of the mRNA to be mapped at microscopic resolution.

In summary, the molecular landscape has changed completely. Whereas the discovery of new 'small-molecule' mediators has slowed, the discovery of new protein and peptide mediators continues apace (Schulze et al., 2014).

More than 100 cytokines have been discovered since interleukin 2 (IL-2) was first characterised in 1982.

GENERAL PRINCIPLES OF PROTEIN AND PEPTIDE PHARMACOLOGY

STRUCTURE

Peptide and protein mediators generally vary from three to about 200 amino acid residues in length, the arbitrary dividing line between peptides and proteins being about 50 residues. An important difference is that proteins need to adopt a complex folded structure to exert their specific function, whereas short peptides are in most cases flexible. Specific residues in proteins and peptides often undergo post-translational modifications, such as *amidation, glycosylation, acetylation, carboxylation, sulfation* or *phosphorylation*.[1] They also may contain *intramolecular* disulfide bonds, such that the molecule adopts a partially cyclic conformation, or they may comprise two or more separate chains linked by *intermolecular* disulfide bonds.

Generally speaking, larger proteins adopt restricted conformations that expose functional groups in fixed locations on their surface, which interact with multiple sites on their receptors in 'lock-and-key' mode. To envisage flexible peptides fitting into a receptor site this way is to imagine that you can unlock your front door with a length of cooked spaghetti. These features have greatly impeded the rational design of non-peptide analogues that mimic the action of proteins and peptides at their receptors (peptidomimetics). The use of random screening methods has (somewhat to the chagrin of the rationalists) nevertheless led in recent years to the discovery of many non-peptide *antagonists* – although few *agonists* – for peptide receptors.

TYPES OF PROTEIN AND PEPTIDE MEDIATOR

Protein and peptide mediators that are secreted by cells and act on surface receptors of the same or other cells can be very broadly divided into four groups:

- neurotransmitters (e.g. endogenous opioid peptides, Ch. 43) and neuroendocrine mediators (e.g. vasopressin, somatostatin, hypothalamic releasing hormones, adrenocorticotrophic hormone [ACTH], luteinising hormone (LH), follicle-stimulating hormone (FSH) and thyroid-stimulating hormone (TSH), see Chs 34–36), not discussed further in this chapter);
- hormones from non-neural sources: these comprise plasma-derived peptides, notably angiotensin (Ch. 23) and bradykinin, as well as other hormones such as insulin (Ch. 32), endothelin (Ch. 23), atrial natriuretic peptide (Ch. 22) and leptin (Ch. 33);

---

[1]Bacteria are poor at post-translational modifications, hence over half of all protein drugs (biopharmaceuticals) are generated using mammalian cell cultures.

- growth factors: produced by many different cells and tissues that control cell growth and differentiation (especially, in adults, in the haemopoietic system; see Ch. 26);
- mediators of the immune system (cytokines, see later).

BIOSYNTHESIS AND REGULATION OF PEPTIDES

Peptide structure is, of course, directly coded in the genome, in a manner that the structure of (say) acetylcholine is not,

so intracellular manufacture is a matter of conventional protein synthesis. This often begins with the manufacture of a precursor protein in which the desired final peptide sequence is embedded. Specific proteolytic enzymes excise the mature active peptide from within this peptide sequence, a process of sculpture rather than synthesis. The precursor protein is packaged into vesicles at the point of synthesis, and the active peptide is formed *in situ* ready for release (Fig. 19.1). Thus there is no need for specialised biosynthetic pathways, or for the uptake or recapturing mechanisms, that are important for the synthesis and release of most non-peptide mediators (e.g. 5-hydroxytryptamine [5-HT]; Ch. 16).

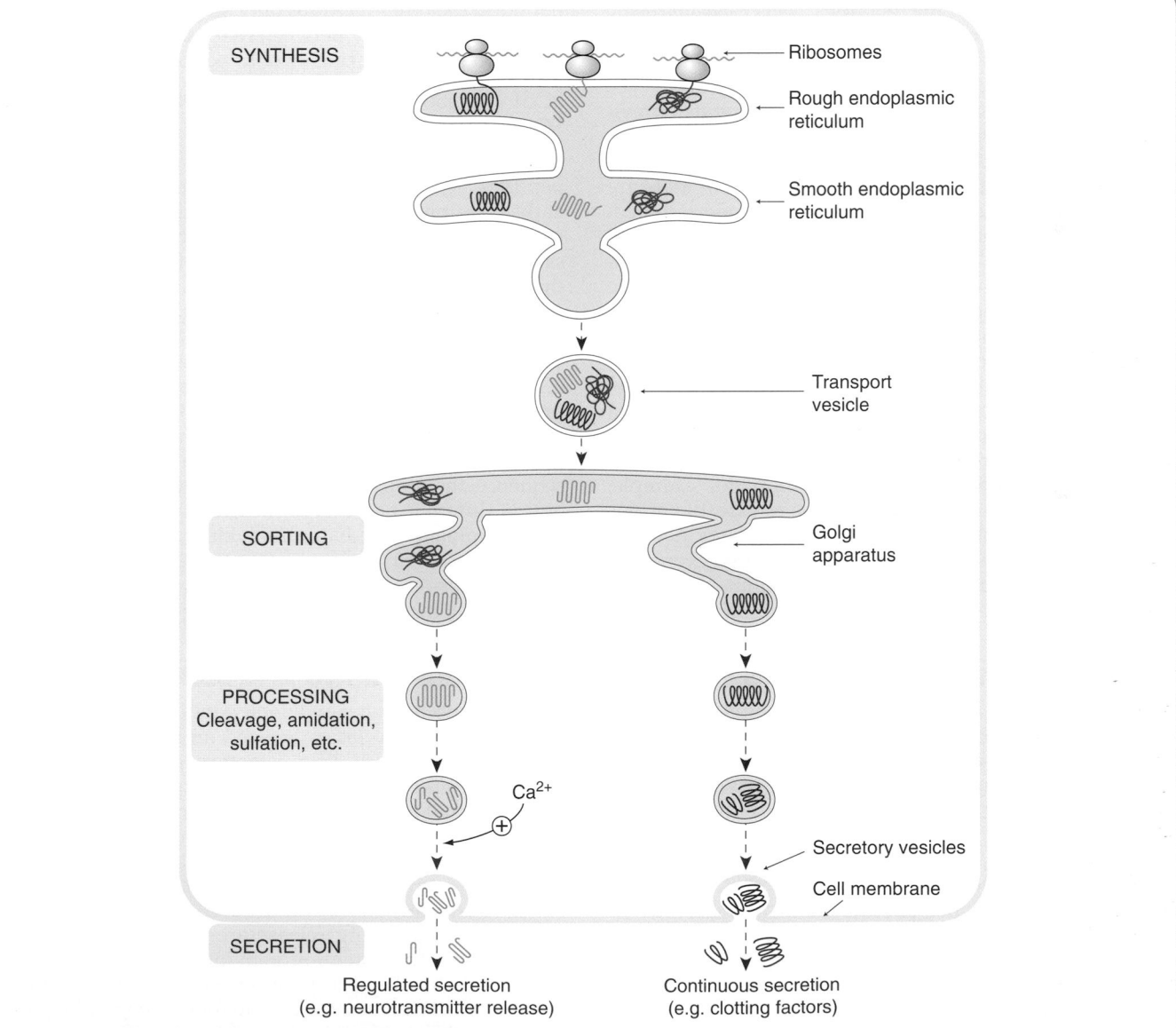

Fig. 19.1 Cellular mechanisms for peptide synthesis and release. Proteins synthesised by ribosomes are threaded through the membrane of the rough endoplasmic reticulum, from where they are conveyed in transport vesicles to the Golgi apparatus. Here, they are sorted and packaged into secretory vesicles. Processing (cleavage, glycosylation, amidation, sulfation, etc.) occurs within the transport and secretory vesicles, and the products are released from the cell by exocytosis. Constitutive secretion (e.g. of plasma proteins and clotting factors by liver cells) occurs continuously, and little material is stored in secretory vesicles. Regulated secretion (e.g. of neuropeptides or cytokines) occurs in response to increased intracellular Ca^{2+} or other intracellular signals, and material is typically stored in significant amounts in secretory vesicles awaiting release.

PEPTIDE PRECURSORS

The precursor protein, or *pre-prohormone*, usually 100–250 residues in length, consists of an N-terminal *signal sequence* (peptide), followed by a variable stretch of unknown function, and a peptide-containing region that may contain several copies of active peptide fragments. Often, several different peptides are found within one precursor, but sometimes there are multiple copies of a single peptide.[2] The *signal sequence*, which is strongly hydrophobic, facilitates insertion of the protein into the endoplasmic reticulum and is then cleaved off at an early stage, yielding the *prohormone*.

The active peptides are usually demarcated within the prohormone sequence by pairs of basic amino acids (Lys-Lys or Lys-Arg), which are cleavage points for the trypsin-like proteases that release the peptides. This *endoproteolytic cleavage* generally occurs in the Golgi apparatus or the secretory vesicles. The enzymes responsible are known as *prohormone convertases*. Scrutiny of the prohormone sequence often reveals likely cleavage points that distinguish previously unknown peptides. In some cases (e.g. calcitonin gene-related peptide [CGRP]; see later), new peptide mediators have been discovered in this way, but there are many examples where no function has yet been assigned. Whether these peptides are, like strangers at a funeral, waiting to declare their purpose or merely functionless mournful relics, remains a mystery. There are also large stretches of the prohormone sequence of unknown function lying between the active peptide fragments.[3]

The abundance of mRNA coding for particular pre-prohormones, which reflects the level of gene expression, is very sensitive to physiological conditions. This type of *transcriptional control* is one of the main mechanisms by which peptide expression and release are regulated over the medium to long term. Inflammation, for example, increases the expression, and hence the release, of various cytokines by immune cells (see Ch. 7). Sensory neurons respond to peripheral inflammation by increased expression of tachykinins (substance P and neurokinins A and B), which is important in the genesis of inflammatory pain (see Ch. 43).

DIVERSITY WITHIN PEPTIDE FAMILIES

Peptides commonly occur in families with similar or related sequences and actions. For example, the pro-opiomelanocortin (POMC) serves as a source of ACTH, melanocyte-stimulating hormones (MSH) and β-endorphin, all of which have a role in controlling the inflammatory response (as well as other processes).

GENE SPLICING AS A SOURCE OF DIVERSITY

Diversity of members of a peptide family can also arise by gene splicing or during post-translational processing of the prohormone. Genes contain coding regions (*exons*) interspersed with intervening non-coding regions (*introns*)

and when the gene is transcribed, the ensuing RNA (*heterologous nuclear RNA* [*hnRNA*]) is spliced to remove the introns and some of the exons, forming the final mature mRNA that is translated. Control of the splicing process allows a measure of cellular control over the peptides that are produced.

For example, the calcitonin gene codes for calcitonin itself, important in bone metabolism (Ch. 37), and also for a completely dissimilar peptide (CGRP, involved in migraine pathogenesis, Ch. 16). Alternative splicing allows cells to produce either pro-calcitonin (expressed in thyroid cells) or pro-CGRP (expressed in many neurons) from the same gene. Substance P and neurokinin A are two closely related tachykinins belonging to the same family, and are encoded on the same gene. Alternative splicing results in the production of two precursor proteins; one of these includes both peptides, the other includes only substance P. The ratio of the two varies widely between tissues, which correspondingly produce either one or both peptides.

POST-TRANSLATIONAL MODIFICATIONS AS A SOURCE OF PEPTIDE DIVERSITY

Many peptides, such as tachykinins and ACTH-related peptides (see Ch. 34), must undergo enzymatic amidation at the C-terminus to acquire full biological activity. Tissues may also generate peptides of varying length from the same primary sequence by the action of specific peptidases that cut the chain at different points. For example, pro-cholecystokinin (pro-CCK) contains the sequences of at least five CCK-like peptides ranging in length from 4 to 58 amino acid residues, all with the same C-terminal sequence. CCK itself (33 residues) is the main peptide produced by the intestine, whereas the brain produces mainly CCK-8. The opioid precursor *prodynorphin* similarly gives rise to several peptides with a common terminal sequence, the proportions of which vary in different tissues and in different neurons in the brain. In some cases (e.g. the inflammatory mediator bradykinin, see p. 247), peptide cleavage occurring after release generates a new active peptide (des-Arg^9-bradykinin), which acts on a different receptor, both peptides contributing differently to the combined inflammatory response.

PEPTIDE TRAFFICKING AND SECRETION

The basic mechanisms by which peptides are synthesised, packaged into vesicles, processed and secreted are summarised in Fig. 19.1. Two secretory pathways exist, for *constitutive* and *regulated* secretion, respectively. Constitutively secreted proteins (e.g. plasma proteins, some clotting factors) are not stored in appreciable amounts, and secretion is coupled to synthesis. Regulated secretion is, as with many hormones and transmitters, controlled by receptor-activated signals that lead to a rise in intracellular Ca^{2+} (see Ch. 4), and peptides awaiting release are stored in cytoplasmic vesicles. Specific protein–protein interactions appear to be responsible for the sorting of different proteins and their routing into different vesicles, and for choreographing their selective release. Identification of the specific 'trafficking' proteins involved in particular secretory pathways may eventually yield novel drug targets for the selective control of secretion.

Having described the general mechanisms by which peptides are synthesised, processed and released, we now describe some significant mediators that fall into this category.

---

[2] In the case of the invertebrate *Aplysia*, one protein precursor contains no fewer than 28 copies of the same short peptide.

[3] When these large sequences of unknown function were discovered in our DNA, they were termed 'junk DNA', not because they were rubbish, but arrogantly because we didn't understand it. It turns out 'junk DNA' is actually very important in controlling cell function and in diseases, etc. Likewise with unknown function 'junk peptide', watch this space for uncovering its true role.

BRADYKININ

Bradykinin and lysyl-bradykinin (*kallidin*) are active peptides formed by proteolytic cleavage of circulating proteins termed *kininogens* through a protease cascade pathway (see Fig. 7.1).

SOURCE AND FORMATION OF BRADYKININ

An outline of the formation of bradykinin from high molecular-weight *kininogen* in plasma by the serine protease *kallikrein* is given in Fig. 19.2. Kininogen is a plasma α-globulin that exists in both high (M_r 110,000) and low (M_r 70,000) molecular-weight forms. Kallikrein is derived from the inactive precursor *prekallikrein* by the action of *Hageman factor* (factor XII; see Fig. 7.1 and Ch. 25). Hageman factor is activated by contact with negatively charged surfaces such as collagen, basement membrane, bacterial lipopolysaccharides, urate crystals and so on. Hageman factor, prekallikrein and the kininogens leak out of the vessels during inflammation because of increased vascular permeability, and exposure to negatively charged surfaces promotes the interaction of Hageman factor with prekallikrein. The activated enzyme then 'clips' bradykinin from its kininogen precursor. Kallikrein can also activate the complement system and can convert plasminogen to plasmin (see Fig. 7.1 and Ch. 25).

In addition to plasma kallikrein, there are other kinin-generating isoenzymes found in pancreas, salivary glands, colon and skin. These *tissue kallikreins* act on both high and low molecular-weight kininogens and generate mainly kallidin, a peptide with actions similar to those of bradykinin.

METABOLISM AND INACTIVATION OF BRADYKININ

Specific enzymes that inactivate bradykinin and related kinins are called *kininases* (see Fig. 19.2). One of these, *kininase II*, is a peptidyl dipeptidase that inactivates kinins by removing the two C-terminal amino acids. This enzyme, which is bound to the luminal surface of endothelial cells, is identical to *angiotensin-converting enzyme* (ACE; see Ch. 23), which cleaves the two C-terminal residues from the inactive peptide angiotensin I, converting it to the active vasoconstrictor peptide angiotensin II. Thus kininase II inactivates a vasodilator and activates a vasoconstrictor. Potentiation of bradykinin actions by ACE inhibitors may contribute to some side effects of these drugs (e.g. cough). Kinins are also metabolised by various less specific peptidases, including a serum carboxypeptidase that removes the C-terminal arginine, generating des-Arg^9-bradykinin, a specific agonist at one of the two main classes of bradykinin receptor.

BRADYKININ RECEPTORS

There are two bradykinin receptors, designated B_1 and B_2. Both are G protein–coupled receptors and mediate very similar effects. B_1 receptors are normally expressed at very low levels but are strongly induced in inflamed or damaged tissues by cytokines such as IL-1. B_1 receptors respond to des-Arg^9-bradykinin but not to bradykinin itself. A number of selective peptide and non-peptide antagonists are known. It is likely that B_1 receptors play a significant role in inflammation and hyperalgesia (see Ch. 43), and antagonists could be used in cough and neurological disorders (Rodi et al., 2005).

B_2 receptors are constitutively present in many normal cells and are activated by bradykinin and kallidin, but not by des-Arg^9-bradykinin. Peptide and non-peptide antagonists have been developed, the best known being the bradykinin analogue **icatibant**, used to treat acute attacks in patients with *hereditary angio-oedema* (an uncommon disorder caused by deficiency of C1-esterase inhibitor that normally restrains complement activation).

ACTIONS AND ROLE IN INFLAMMATION

Bradykinin causes vasodilatation and increased vascular permeability. Its vasodilator action is partly a result of

Fig. 19.2 The structure of bradykinin and some bradykinin antagonists. The sites of proteolytic cleavage of high molecular-weight kininogen by kallikrein involved in the formation of bradykinin are shown in the upper half of the figure; the sites of cleavage associated with bradykinin and kallidin inactivation are shown in the lower half. The B_2-receptor antagonist icatibant (Hoe 140) has a pA_2 of 9, and the competitive B_1-receptor antagonist des-Arg Hoe 140 has a pA_2 of 8. The Hoe compounds contain unnatural amino acids: Thi, δ-Tic and Oic, which are analogues of phenylalanine and proline.

generation of prostaglandin-I_2 (PGI_2) and release of nitric oxide (NO). It causes pain by stimulating nociceptive nerve terminals, and its action here is potentiated by prostaglandins (Ch. 18), which are released by bradykinin. Bradykinin also contracts intestinal, uterine and bronchial smooth muscle in some species. The contraction is slow and sustained in comparison with that produced by tachykinins such as substance P (*brady-* means slow; *tachy-* means rapid).

Although bradykinin reproduces many inflammatory signs and symptoms, its role in inflammation and allergy is not clear, partly because its effects are often component parts of a complex cascade of events triggered by other mediators. However, excessive bradykinin production contributes to the diarrhoea of gastrointestinal disorders, and in allergic rhinitis it stimulates nasopharyngeal secretion. Bradykinin also contributes to the clinical picture in pancreatitis,[4] although, disappointingly, B_2 antagonists worsen rather than alleviate this disorder. Physiologically, the release of bradykinin by tissue kallikrein may regulate blood flow to certain exocrine glands, and influence secretions. Bradykinin also stimulates ion transport and fluid secretion by some epithelia, including intestine, airways and gall bladder.

Bradykinin

- Bradykinin (BK) is a nonapeptide 'clipped' from a plasma α-globulin, *kininogen*, by *kallikrein*.
- It is converted by *kininase I* to an active octapeptide, BK_{1-8} (des-Arg^9-BK), and inactivated by the removal of an additional amino acid by *kininase II* (angiotensin-converting enzyme) in the lung.
- Pharmacological actions:
  - vasodilatation (largely dependent on endothelial cell nitric oxide and PGI_2);
  - increased vascular permeability;
  - stimulation of pain nerve endings;
  - stimulation of epithelial ion transport and fluid secretion in airways and gastrointestinal tract;
  - contraction of intestinal and uterine smooth muscle.
- There are two main subtypes of BK receptors: B_2, which is constitutively present, and B_1, which is induced in inflammation.
- **Icatibant**, a peptide analogue of BK, is a selective competitive antagonist for B_2 receptors and is used to treat acute attacks of hereditary angioedema. Other, non-peptide antagonists for both B_1 and B_2 receptors are known, and may be developed for treating inflammatory disorders.

NEUROPEPTIDES

Neuropeptides constitute a large (>100) and diverse family of small to medium-sized peptides. Many are found in the central nervous system (CNS), the autonomic nervous system, and peripheral sensory neurons, as well as in many peripheral tissues. They are often released as co-transmitters (Chs 13, 40), along with non-peptide neurotransmitters.

When released from peripheral endings of nociceptive sensory neurons (see Ch. 43), neuropeptides in some species cause *neurogenic inflammation* (Maggi, 1996). The main peptides involved are *substance P, neurokinin A* and *CGRP*. Substance P and neurokinin A are small (about 1100 Da) members of the *tachykinin* family with partly homologous structures, which act on mast cells, releasing histamine and other mediators, and producing smooth muscle contraction, neural activation, mucus secretion and vasodilatation. CGRP is a member of the calcitonin family (37 amino acids in length) shares these properties and is a particularly potent vasodilator. Tachykinins released from the central endings of nociceptive neurons also modulate transmission in the dorsal horn of the spinal cord, affecting sensitivity to pain (see Ch. 43). All these neuropeptides act on specific G protein–coupled receptors to produce their effects.

Neurogenic inflammation is implicated in the pathogenesis of several inflammatory conditions, including the delayed phase of asthma, allergic rhinitis, inflammatory bowel disease and some types of arthritis as well as migraine (Ch. 16 and Pisi et al., 2009). Antagonists at the neurokinin NK_1 receptor, such as **aprepitant** and **fosaprepitant**, are used to treat emesis, particularly that associated with some forms of cancer chemotherapy (see Ch. 57). Other important members of the neuropeptide family include enkephalins/endorphins (Ch. 43) and orexins (Ch. 33).

CYTOKINES

'Cytokine' is an all-purpose functional term that is applied to protein or polypeptide mediators synthesised and released by cells of the immune system during inflammation. They are crucial for the overall coordination of the inflammatory response. Cytokines act locally by autocrine or paracrine mechanisms. Unlike conventional hormones such as insulin, concentrations in blood and tissues are almost undetectable under normal circumstances, but are massively up-regulated (100–1000-fold) during inflammatory episodes. All these mediators are usually active at very low (sub-nanomolar) concentrations.

On the target cell, cytokines bind to and activate specific, high-affinity receptors that, in most cases, are also up-regulated during inflammation. Except for *chemokines*, which act on G protein–coupled receptors, most cytokines act on kinase-linked receptors, regulating phosphorylation cascades that affect gene expression, such as the Jak/Stat pathway (Chs 3 and 7).

In addition to their own direct actions on cells, some cytokines amplify inflammation by inducing the formation of other inflammatory mediators. Others can induce receptors for other cytokines on their target cell, or engage in synergistic or antagonistic interactions with other cytokines. Cytokines constitute a complex chemical signalling language, with the final response of a particular cell involved being determined by the strength and number of different messages received concurrently at the cell surface.

Systems for classifying cytokines abound in the literature, as dodiagrams depicting complex networks of cytokines interacting with each other and with a range of target cells.

---

[4]A serious and painful condition in which proteolytic enzymes are released from damaged pancreatic cells, initiating cascades that release, among other things, bradykinin.

No one system of classification does justice to the complexity of cytokine biology. The terminology and nomenclature are horrendous, and a comprehensive coverage of this area is beyond the scope of this book. Table 19.1 lists some of the more significant cytokines and their biological actions. The would-be cytokine aficionado can find further classification tables in Murphy et al. (2011) and the IUPHAR/BPS Guide to Pharmacology.

More than 100 cytokines have been identified. These may be broadly categorised into four main functional groups, namely *interleukins, chemokines, interferons* and *colony-stimulating factors* (discussed separately in Ch. 26), but these demarcations are of limited use because many cytokines have multiple roles.

Using biopharmaceuticals (see Ch. 5) to interfere with cytokine action has proved to be a particularly fertile area of drug development: several successful strategies have been adopted, including direct antibody neutralisation of cytokines or the use of 'decoy' receptor proteins that remove the biologically active pool from the circulation (See Chs. 5 and 27).

INTERLEUKINS AND RELATED COMPOUNDS

The name was originally coined to describe mediators that signalled between leukocytes but, like so much else in the cytokine lexicography, it has become rather redundant, not to say misleading. The primary pro-inflammatory species are *tumour necrosis factor* (TNF)-α and *interleukin 1* (IL-1). The principal members of the latter cytokine group consist of two agonists, IL-1α, IL-1β and, surprisingly, an endogenous IL-1-receptor antagonist (IL-1ra).[5] Mixtures of these are released from macrophages and many other cells during inflammation and can initiate the synthesis and release of a cascade of secondary cytokines, among which are the chemokines. TNF and IL-1 are key regulators of almost all manifestations of the inflammatory response. A long-standing debate about which of the two is really the prime mover of inflammation ended when it was found that this varies according to the disease type. In auto-*immune* disease (e.g. rheumatoid arthritis, where the adaptive immune system is activated), TNF appears to be the predominant influence and blocking its action is therapeutically effective. In auto-*inflammatory* diseases (e.g. gout, where only the innate system is involved), IL-1 seems to be the key mediator (Dinarello et al., 2012). Both TNF-α and IL-1 are important targets for anti-inflammatory biopharmaceuticals (Chs 5 and 27).

Not all interleukins are pro-inflammatory: some, including *transforming growth factor (TGF)-β*, IL-4, IL-10 and IL-13 are potent anti-inflammatory substances. They inhibit chemokine production, and the responses driven by T-helper (Th) 1 cells, whose inappropriate activation is involved in the pathogenesis of several diseases.

CHEMOKINES

Chemokines are defined as *chemo*attractant cyto*kines* that control the migration of leukocytes, functioning as traffic coordinators during immune and inflammatory reactions. Again, the nomenclature (and the classification) is confusing, because some non-cytokine mediators also control leukocyte movement (C5a, LTB$_4$, fMet-Leu-Phe, etc; see Fig. 7.2) and many chemokines have more than one name. Furthermore, many chemokines have other actions, causing mast cell degranulation or promoting angiogenesis, for example.

More than 40 chemokines have been identified. They are all highly homologous peptides of 8–10 kDa, which are usually grouped according to the configuration of key cysteine residues in their polypeptide chain. Chemokines with one cysteine are known as *C chemokines*. If there are two adjacent residues they are called *C–C chemokines*. Other members have cysteines separated by one (*C–X–C chemokines*) or three other residues (*C–XXX–C chemokines*).

The C–X–C chemokines (main example IL-8; see Fig. 7.2) act on neutrophils and are predominantly involved in acute inflammatory responses. The C–C chemokines (main examples eotaxin, MCP-1 and RANTES)[6] act on monocytes, eosinophils and other cells, and are involved predominantly in chronic inflammatory responses.

▼ Chemokines generally act through G protein–coupled receptors, and alteration or inappropriate expression of these is implicated in multiple sclerosis, cancer, rheumatoid arthritis and some cardiovascular diseases (Gerard & Rollins, 2001). Some types of virus (herpes virus, cytomegalovirus, pox virus and members of the retrovirus family) can exploit the chemokine system and subvert the host's defences (Murphy, 2001). Some produce proteins that mimic host chemokines or chemokine receptors, some act as antagonists at chemokine receptors and some masquerade as growth or angiogenic factors. The AIDS-causing HIV virus is responsible for the most audacious exploitation of the host chemokine system. This virus has a protein (gp120) in its envelope that recognises and binds T-cell receptors for CD4 and a chemokine co-receptor that allows it to penetrate the T cell (see Ch. 53). These chemokine co-receptors, CCR5 (blocked by the HIV drug **maraviroc**) and CXCR4, are hijacked by HIV virus to enter a cell.

INTERFERONS

So called because they interfere with viral replication, there are three main types of interferon, termed IFN-α, IFN-β and IFN-γ. 'IFN-α' is not a single substance but a family of approximately 20 proteins with similar activities. IFN-α and IFN-β have antiviral activity whereas IFN-α also has some antitumour action. Both are released from virus-infected cells and activate antiviral mechanisms in neighbouring cells. IFN-γ has a role in induction of Th1 responses (Fig. 7.3).

CLINICAL USE OF INTERFERONS

IFN-α is used in the treatment of chronic hepatitis B and C, and has some action against herpes zoster and in the prevention of the common cold. Antitumour action against some lymphomas and solid tumours has been reported. Dose-related side effects, including influenza-like symptoms, may occur. IFN-β is used in patients with the relapsing–remitting form of multiple sclerosis, whereas IFN-γ is used in chronic granulomatous disease, an uncommon chronic disease of childhood in which neutrophil function is impaired, in conjunction with antibacterial drugs (see clinical box below for more details).

---

[5]One might have expected evolution to generate more examples of endogenous receptor antagonists as physiological regulators, but apart from IL-1ra, they are only exploited as toxins directed against other species.

---

[6]MCP, monocyte chemoattractant protein; RANTES, **R**egulated on **A**ctivation **N**ormal **T** cell **E**xpressed and **S**ecreted. (Don't blame us!)

Table 19.1 Some examples of significant cytokines and their actions

Cytokine	Main cell source	Main target cell or biological effect	Comments
IL-1	Monocyte/macrophages, dendritic and other cells	Regulates cell migration to sites of infection, produces inflammation, fever and pain	Two original subtypes IL-1α and IL-1β, and IL-1ra – a receptor antagonist. Target for anti-inflammatory therapy (Ch. 27)
IL-2	T cells	Stimulates proliferation, maturation and activation of T, B and NK cells	First interleukin to be discovered
IL-4	Th2 cells	Stimulates proliferation, maturation of T and B cells and promotes IgG and E synthesis. Promotes an anti-inflammatory phenotype	A key cytokine in the regulation of the Th2 response (Ch. 27)
IL-5	Th2 cells, mast cells	Important for eosinophil activation. Stimulates proliferation, maturation of B cells and IgA synthesis	Particularly important in allergic disease
IL-6	Monocyte/macrophages and T cells	Pro-inflammatory actions including fever. Stimulation of osteoclast activity	Target for anti-inflammatory drugs (Ch. 27)
IL-8	Macrophages, endothelial cells	Neutrophil chemotaxis, phagocytosis and angiogenesis	C–X–C chemokine (CXCL8)
IL-10	Monocytes and Th2 cells	Inhibits cytokine production and down-regulates inflammation	A predominately anti-inflammatory cytokine
IL-17	T cells and others	Stimulates Th17 cells, involved in allergic response and autoimmunity	Several subtypes. Target for anti-inflammatory drugs (Ch. 27)
GM–CSF	Macrophages, T cells, mast cells and others	Stimulates growth of leukocyte progenitor cells. Increases numbers of blood-borne leukocytes	Used therapeutically to stimulate myeloid cell growth (e.g. after bone marrow transplantation)
MIP-1	Macrophages/lymphocytes	Activation of neutrophils and other cells. Promotes cytokine release	C–C chemokine (CCL3). Two subtypes
TGF-β	T cells, monocytes	Induces apoptosis. Regulates cell growth	Three isoforms. Predominately anti-inflammatory action
TNF-α	Mainly macrophages but also many immune and other cells	Kills tumour cells. Stimulates macrophage cytokine expression and is a key regulator of many aspects of the immune response	A major target for anti-inflammatory drugs (Ch. 7)
TNF-β	Th1 cells	Initiates a variety of immune-stimulatory and pro-inflammatory actions in the host defence system	Now often called lymphotoxin α (LTA)
Eotaxin	Airway epithelial and other cells	Activation and chemotaxis of eosinophils. Allergic inflammation	C–C chemokine (CCL11). Three subtypes
MCP-1	Monocytes, osteoblasts/clasts, neurons and other cells	Promotes recruitment of monocytes and T cells to sites of inflammation	C–C chemokine (CC2)
RANTES	T cells	Chemotaxis of T cells. Chemotaxis and activation of other leukocytes	(CCL5)
IFN-α	Leukocytes	Activates NK cells and macrophages. Inhibits viral replication and has antitumour actions	Multiple molecular species
IFN-γ	Th1, NK cells	Stimulates Th1, and inhibits Th2, cell proliferation. Activates NK cells and macrophages	Crucial to the Th1 response (Ch. 7)

GM–CSF, granulocyte-macrophage colony-stimulating factor; *IFN,* interferon; *Ig,* immunoglobulin; *IL,* interleukin; *MCP,* monocyte chemoattractant protein; *MIP,* macrophage inflammatory protein; *NK,* natural killer (cell); *RANTES,* regulated on activation normal T cell expressed and secreted; *TGF,* transforming growth factor; *Th,* T-helper (cell); *TNF,* tumour necrosis factor.

Clinical uses of interferons

- α: chronic hepatitis B or C (ideally combined with **ribavirin**).
    - Malignant disease (alone or in combination with other drugs, e.g. **cytarabine**): chronic myelogenous leukaemia (CML), hairy cell leukaemia, follicular lymphoma, metastatic carcinoid, multiple myeloma, malignant melanoma (as an adjunct to surgery), myelodysplastic syndrome.
    - Conjugation with polyethylene glycol ('pegylation') results in preparations that are more slowly eliminated and are administered intermittently subcutaneously.
- β: multiple sclerosis (especially the relapsing–remitting form of this disease).
- γ: to reduce infection in children with chronic granulomatous disease.

Cytokines

- Cytokines are polypeptides that are rapidly induced and released during inflammation. They regulate the action of inflammatory and immune system cells.
- The cytokine superfamily includes the *interferons*, *interleukins*, *chemokines* and *colony-stimulating factors*.
- Utilising both autocrine or paracrine mechanisms, they exert complex effects on leukocytes, vascular endothelial cells, mast cells, fibroblasts, haemopoietic stem cells and osteoclasts, controlling proliferation, differentiation and/or activation.
- Interleukin 1 (IL-1) and tumour necrosis factor α (TNF-α) are important primary inflammatory cytokines, inducing the formation of other cytokines.
- Chemokines, such as IL-8, are mainly involved in the regulation of cell trafficking.
- Interferons IFN-α and IFN-β have antiviral activity, and IFN-α is used as an adjunct in the treatment of viral infections. IFN-γ has significant immunoregulatory function and is used in the treatment of multiple sclerosis.

THE 'CYTOKINE STORM'

Many cytokines release further cytokines in what is essentially a positive feedback loop. There are times when this feedback system becomes unstable, perhaps as a result of the absence of balancing anti-inflammatory factors. The result can be a massive overproduction of cytokines in response to infection or other injury. This is known as a *cytokine storm* (also called *hypercytokinemia*) and can lead to a particularly dangerous – potentially catastrophic – development called *systemic inflammatory response syndrome* (SIRS; Jaffer et al., 2010). Cytokine storms may be responsible for deaths in septic shock as well as in some pandemic diseases. A tragic case of volunteers suffering cytokine storms after receiving an experimental drug is related in Ch. 5.

PROTEINS AND PEPTIDES THAT DOWN-REGULATE INFLAMMATION

Inflammation is not regulated solely by factors that cause or enhance it: it has become increasingly evident that there is another panel of mediators that function at every step to down-regulate inflammation, to check its progress and limit its duration and scope. It is the dynamic balance between these two systems that regulates the onset and resolution of inflammatory episodes, and when this breaks down, may lead also to inflammatory disease or, in extreme cases, to the cytokine storm phenomenon. Some of these are peptidic in nature and we have already encountered IL-1ra, TGF-β and IL-10, which are important negative regulators of inflammation. There are two other systems that are significant here because common anti-inflammatory drugs exploit their action.

Annexin-A1 (Anx-A1) is a 37 kDa protein produced by many cells and especially abundant in cells of the myeloid lineage. When released, it exerts potent anti-inflammatory actions, down-regulating cell activation, cell transmigration and mediator release. It does this by acting through a G protein–coupled receptor called ALX/FPR2 a member of the formyl peptide receptor family: the same receptor that binds the anti-inflammatory lipoxins (see Ch. 18).

The significance of the Anx-A1 system is that it is activated by anti-inflammatory glucocorticoids (see Ch. 27), which increase Anx-A1 gene transcription and promote its release from cells. Interestingly, the anti-allergic *cromones* (cromoglicate, etc.; see Ch. 29) also promote the release of this protein from cells. Anx-A1 gene 'knock-out' studies have shown that this protein is important for restraining the inflammatory response and for its timely resolution. The anti-inflammatory glucocorticoids cannot develop their full inhibitory actions without it. An account of this field is given by Perretti and D'Acquisto (2009).

The *melanocortin* system also plays an important part in regulating inflammation. There are five G protein–coupled melanocortin receptors, MC_{1-5}. Endogenous ligands for these receptors, such as MSH (three types), are derived from the POMC gene, and serve a number of purposes, including regulating the development of a suntan, penile erection and the control of appetite through an action on various MC receptors.

From the point of view of host defence, the MC_3 receptor is the most important. Again, gene deletion studies have highlighted the importance of this receptor in a variety of inflammatory conditions. Interestingly, another product of the POMC gene, ACTH was formerly used as an anti-inflammatory agent, but it was thought that its action was secondary to its ability to release endogenous cortisol from the adrenals (an MC_2 action, see Ch. 34). It is now known that it is a ligand at the MC_3 receptor and it is likely that it owes some of its activity to this action.

An account of the importance of this field is given by Patel et al. (2011).

CONCLUDING REMARKS

Even from the superficial sketch presented here and in Chapter 7 it must be evident that the host defence response is among the most intricate of all physiological responses. Perhaps that is not surprising, given its central importance to survival. For the same reason, it is also understandable that so many different mediators orchestrate its operation. That the activity of many of these mediators can be blocked in experimental models with little or no obvious effect on the initiation and outcome of inflammation points to

redundancy amongst the many component systems and goes some way to explaining why, until the advent of highly specific antibody-based therapies for inflammatory conditions (see Ch. 27), our ability to curb the worst ravages of chronic inflammatory disease was so limited.

REFERENCES AND FURTHER READING

Chung, K.F., 2005. Drugs to suppress cough. Expert. Opin. Invest. Drugs 14, 19–27. (*Useful review of cough treatments, including a section on the role of neurokinin and bradykinin receptor antagonists*)

Dinarello, C.A., Simon, A., van der Meer, J.W., 2012. Treating inflammation by blocking interleukin-1 in a broad spectrum of diseases. Nat. Rev. Drug Discov. 11, 633–652. (*An extremely comprehensive survey of the role of IL1 in disease and the therapeutic benefits that can be gained by blocking its action. Written by pioneers of the field. Good diagrams*)

Gerard, C., Rollins, B., 2001. Chemokines and disease. Nat. Immunol. 2, 108–115. (*Discusses diseases associated with inappropriate activation of the chemokine network, and discusses some therapeutic implications; describes how viruses evade the immune responses by mimicry of the chemokines or their receptors*)

Horuk, R., 2001. Chemokine receptors. Cytokine Growth Factor Rev. 12, 313–335. (*Comprehensive review focusing on chemokine receptor research; describes the molecular, physiological and biochemical properties of each chemokine receptor*)

IUPHAR/BPS. Guide to Pharmacology. www.guidetopharmacology.org/. (*Comprehensive guide to pharmacological targets and the substances that act on them*)

Jaffer, U., Wade, R.G., Gourlay, T., 2010. Cytokines in the systemic inflammatory response syndrome: a review. HSR Proc. Intensive Care Cardiovasc. Anesth. 2, 161–175. (*An easy to read review dealing mainly with the role of cytokines in SIRS, but also has a good general review of cytokine biology. Some good diagrams*)

Luster, A.D., 1998. Mechanisms of disease: chemokines – chemotactic cytokines that mediate inflammation. N. Engl. J. Med. 338, 436–445. (*Excellent review; outstanding diagrams*)

Mackay, C.R., 2001. Chemokines: immunology's high impact factors. Nat. Immunol. 2, 95–101. (*Clear, elegant coverage of the role of chemokines in leukocyte–endothelial interaction, control of primary immune responses and T/B cell interaction, T cells in inflammatory diseases and viral subversion of immune responses*)

Maggi, C.A., 1996. Pharmacology of the efferent function of primary sensory neurones. In: Geppetti, P., Holzer, P. (Eds.), Neurogenic Inflammation. CRC Press, London. (*Worthwhile. Covers neurogenic inflammation, the release of neuropeptides from sensory nerves and inflammatory mediators. Discusses agents that inhibit release and the pharmacological modulation of receptor-mediated release*)

Murphy, P.M., 2001. Viral exploitation and subversion of the immune system through chemokine mimicry. Nat. Immunol. 2, 116–122. (*Excellent description of viral/immune system interaction*)

Patel, H.B., Montero-Melendez, T., Greco, K.V., Perretti, M., 2011. Melanocortin receptors as novel effectors of macrophage responses in inflammation. Front. Immunol. 2, 41–46. (*Succinct and easy-to-read review of the role of melanocortins in inflammatory resolution focusing on the role of the MC3 receptor. Useful diagrams*)

Pease, J.E., Williams, T.J., 2006. The attraction of chemokines as a target for specific anti-inflammatory therapy. Br. J. Pharmacol. 147 (Suppl. 1), S212–S221. (*Very good review of the history of chemokine research with particular emphasis on their potential role as drug targets*)

Perretti, M., D'Acquisto, F., 2009. Annexin A1 and glucocorticoids as effectors of the resolution of inflammation. Nat. Rev. Immunol. 9, 62–70. (*Explores the role of the glucocorticoid-regulated protein annexin 1 in the control of inflammatory resolution. Easy to read and good diagrams*)

Pisi, G., Olivieri, D., Chetta, A., 2009. The airway neurogenic inflammation: clinical and pharmacological implications. Inflamm. Allergy Drug Targets 8, 176–181.

Rodi, D., Couture, R., Ongali, B., et al., 2005. Targeting kinin receptors for the treatment of neurological diseases. Curr. Pharm. Des. 11, 1313–1326. (*An overview of the potential role of kinin receptor antagonists in neurological diseases, dealing particularly with those of immunological origin*)

Schulze, U., Baedeker, M., Chen, Y.T., Greber, D., 2014. R&D productivity: on the comeback trail. Nat. Rev. Drug Discov. 13, 331–332. (*Interesting overview of the decline of new small molecule drugs making it onto the market compared to biotherapeutics. Compares the historical cost effectiveness of the drug discovery process*)

Schulze-Topphoff, U., Prat, A., 2008. Roles of the kallikrein/kinin system in the adaptive immune system. Int. Immunopharmacol. 8, 155–160. (*Excellent overview of these mediators particularly with respect to their involvement in the adaptive response*)

Books

Murphy, K.M., Travers, P., Walport, M., 2011. Janeway's Immunobiology, eighth ed. Taylor & Francis, London. (*A classic textbook now completely updated and available as an e-book also. Excellent diagrams*)

Cannabinoids

OVERVIEW

Modern pharmacological interest in cannabinoids dates from the discovery that Δ^9-tetrahydrocannabinol (THC) is the main active principle of cannabis, and took off with the discovery of specific cannabinoid receptors – termed CB receptors – and endogenous ligands (endocannabinoids), together with mechanisms for their synthesis and elimination. Drugs that act on this endocannabinoid system have considerable therapeutic potential. Here we consider plant-derived cannabinoids, cannabinoid receptors, endocannabinoids, physiological functions, pathological mechanisms, synthetic ligands and potential clinical applications. More detailed information is given by Ligresti et al. (2016) and by Pertwee (2014; 2015). The pharmacology of cannabinoids in the central nervous system (CNS) is discussed in Chapters 40, 49 and 50.

PLANT-DERIVED CANNABINOIDS AND THEIR PHARMACOLOGICAL EFFECTS

Cannabis sativa, the hemp plant, has been used for its psychoactive properties for thousands of years (Ch. 49). Its medicinal use was advocated in antiquity, but serious interest resurfaced only in 1964 with the identification of Δ^9-*tetrahydrocannabinol* (THC, Fig. 20.1) as the main psychoactive component. Cannabis extracts contain numerous related compounds, called cannabinoids, most of which are insoluble in water. The most abundant cannabinoids are THC, its precursor *cannabidiol*, and *cannabinol*, a breakdown product formed spontaneously from THC. Cannabidiol and cannabinol lack the psychoactive properties of THC, but can exhibit anticonvulsant activity (Ch. 46) and induce hepatic drug metabolism (see Ch. 10).

PHARMACOLOGICAL EFFECTS

THC acts mainly on the CNS, producing a mixture of psychotomimetic and depressant effects, together with various centrally mediated autonomic effects. The main subjective effects in humans consist of:

- Sensations of relaxation and well-being, similar to the effect of ethanol but without the accompanying recklessness and aggression. (Insensitivity to risk is an important feature of alcohol intoxication and is often a factor in road accidents. Cannabis users are less accident prone in general – although cannabis does contribute to a significant number of road deaths each year – even though their motor performance is similarly impaired.)

- Feelings of sharpened sensory awareness, with sounds and sights seeming more intense and fantastic.
- These effects are similar to, but usually less pronounced than, those produced by psychotomimetic drugs such as lysergic acid diethylamide (LSD; see Ch. 49). Subjects report that time passes extremely slowly. The alarming sensations and serious paranoid delusions that often occur with LSD are seldom experienced after cannabis, except in high doses. However epidemiological studies support a connection between heavy cannabis use in adolescence and subsequent psychiatric disorder (Rubino et al., 2012).

Central effects that can be directly measured in human and animal studies include:

- impairment of short-term memory and simple learning tasks – subjective feelings of confidence and heightened creativity are not reflected in actual performance;
- impairment of motor coordination (e.g. driving performance);
- catalepsy – the adoption of fixed unnatural postures;
- hypothermia;
- analgesia;
- antiemetic action (see Ch. 31);
- increased appetite (see Ch. 33).

The main peripheral effects of cannabis are:

- tachycardia, which can be prevented by drugs that block sympathetic transmission;
- vasodilatation, which is particularly marked in superficial blood vessels of the eye (scleral and conjunctival vessels), producing a bloodshot appearance which is characteristic of cannabis smokers;
- reduction of intraocular pressure;
- bronchodilatation.

PHARMACOKINETIC ASPECTS

The effect of cannabis, taken by smoking, takes about 1 hour to develop fully and lasts for 2–3 hours. A small fraction of THC is converted to 11-hydroxy-THC, which is more active than THC itself and probably contributes to the pharmacological effect of smoking cannabis, but most is converted to inactive metabolites that are subject to conjugation and enterohepatic recirculation. Being highly lipophilic, THC and its metabolites are sequestered in body fat, and detectable urinary excretion continues for several weeks after a single dose.

ADVERSE EFFECTS

In overdose, THC is relatively safe, producing drowsiness and confusion but not life-threatening respiratory or

253

CH₃

OH

H₃C
CH₃   O   C₅H₁₁

Δ⁹-Tetrahydrocannabinol (THC)

O

N   OH

Anandamide

C—OH
O   C
O   C—OH

2-Arachidonoyl glycerol (2-AG)

Fig. 20.1 Structures of δ⁹-tetrahydrocannabinol and two endocannabinoids.

Cannabis

- Main active constituent is Δ⁹-tetrahydrocannabinol (THC) which generates a pharmacologically active 11-hydroxy metabolite.
- Actions on the central nervous system include both depressant and psychotomimetic effects.
- Subjective experiences include euphoria and a feeling of relaxation, with sharpened sensory awareness.
- Objective tests show impairment of learning, memory and motor performance, including impaired driving ability.
- THC also shows analgesic and antiemetic activity, as well as causing catalepsy and hypothermia in animal tests.
- Peripheral actions include vasodilatation, reduction of intraocular pressure and bronchodilatation.
- Cannabinoids are less liable than opiates, **nicotine** or **alcohol** to cause dependence but may have long-term psychological effects.

cardiovascular depression. In this respect, it is safer than most abused substances, particularly opiates and ethanol. Even in low doses, THC and synthetic derivatives such as **nabilone** (licensed for nausea and vomiting caused by cytotoxic chemotherapy) produce euphoria and drowsiness, sometimes accompanied by sensory distortion and

hallucinations. These effects, together with legal restrictions on the use of cannabis[1] have limited the widespread therapeutic use of cannabinoids, although recent regulatory approval in several countries for a cannabis extract administered by buccal spray as an adjunct in treating spasticity in multiple sclerosis may herald an expansion of potential clinical indications, several of which are being investigated.

In rodents, THC produces teratogenic and mutagenic effects, and an increased incidence of chromosome breaks in circulating white cells has been reported in humans. Such breaks are, however, by no means unique to cannabis, and epidemiological studies have not shown an increased risk of fetal malformation or cancer among cannabis users.

TOLERANCE AND DEPENDENCE

Tolerance to cannabis, and physical dependence, occur only to a minor degree and mainly in heavy users. Abstinence symptoms are similar to those of ethanol or opiate withdrawal, namely nausea, agitation, irritability, confusion, tachycardia and sweating, but are relatively mild and do not result in a compulsive urge to take the drug. Psychological dependence does occur with cannabis, but it is less compelling than with the major drugs of addiction (Ch. 50), although dependence is increasing in parallel with use of more potent material (Maldonado et al., 2011).

CANNABINOID RECEPTORS

Cannabinoids, being highly lipid-soluble, were originally thought to act in a similar way to general anaesthetics. However, in 1988, saturable high-affinity binding of a tritiated cannabinoid was demonstrated in membranes prepared from homogenised rat brain. This led to the identification of specific cannabinoid receptors in brain. These are now termed CB₁ receptors to distinguish them from the CB₂ receptors subsequently identified in peripheral tissues. Cannabinoid receptors are typical members of the family of G protein–coupled receptors (Ch. 3). CB₁ receptors are linked via $G_{i/o}$ to inhibition of adenylyl cyclase and of voltage-operated calcium channels, and to activation of G protein-sensitive inwardly rectifying potassium (GIRK) channels, causing membrane hyperpolarisation (Fig. 20.2). These effects are similar to those mediated by opioid receptors (Ch. 43). CB₁ receptors are located in the plasma membrane of nerve endings and inhibit transmitter release from presynaptic terminals, which is caused by depolarisation and Ca^{2+} entry (Ch. 4). CB receptors also influence gene expression, both directly by activating mitogen-activated protein kinase, and indirectly by reducing the activity of protein kinase A as a result of reduced adenylyl cyclase activity (see Ch. 3).

CB₁ receptors are abundant in the brain, with similar numbers to receptors for glutamate and GABA – the main central excitatory and inhibitory neurotransmitters (Ch. 39). They are not homogeneously distributed, being concentrated in the hippocampus (relevant to effects of cannabinoids on memory), cerebellum (relevant to loss of coordination), hypothalamus (important in control of appetite and body temperature; see Ch. 33 and further in this chapter), substantia nigra, mesolimbic dopamine pathways that have

---

[1]Past legal restrictions on the personal use of cannabis in the USA have been relaxed in some states, so this is an evolving scene.

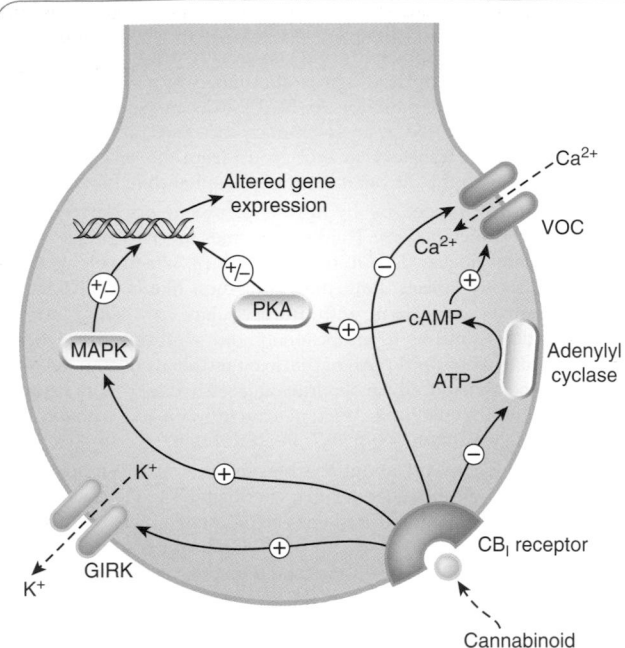

Fig. 20.2 Cellular actions of cannabinoids. CB$_1$ receptor activation inhibits neurotransmitter release via inhibition of Ca^{2+} entry and hyperpolarisation due to activation of potassium channels. It also alters gene expression. *GIRK*, G protein-sensitive inward-rectifying potassium channel; *MAPK*, mitogen-activated protein kinase; *PKA*, protein kinase A; *VOC*, voltage-operated calcium channel. (Redrawn from Devane et al., 1992.)

Table 20.1 Definite and possible endocannabinoids

Endocannabinoid	Selectivity
Definite endocannabinoids	
Anandamide	CB$_1$ > CB$_2$
2-Arachidonoyl glycerol	CB$_1$ = CB$_2$
Less well-established endocannabinoid candidates	
Virodhamine	CB$_2$ > CB$_1$
Noladin	CB$_1$ ≫ CB$_2$
N-Arachidonoyl dopamine	CB$_1$ ≫ CB$_2$

been implicated in psychological 'reward' (Ch.50), and in association areas of the cerebral cortex. There is a relative paucity of CB$_1$ receptors in the brain stem, consistent with the lack of serious depression of respiratory or cardiovascular function by cannabinoids. At a cellular level, CB$_1$ receptors are mainly localised presynaptically, and inhibit transmitter release as depicted in Fig. 20.2. Like opioids, they can, however, increase the activity of some neuronal pathways by inhibiting inhibitory connections, including GABA-ergic interneurons in the hippocampus and amygdala.

In addition to their well-recognised location in the CNS, CB$_1$ receptors are also expressed in peripheral tissues, for example on endothelial cells, adipocytes and peripheral nerves. Cannabinoids promote lipogenesis through activation of CB$_1$ receptors, an action that could contribute to their effect on body weight (see DiPatrizio & Piomele, 2012).

The CB$_2$ receptor has only approximately 45% amino acid homology with CB$_1$ and is located mainly in lymphoid tissue (spleen, tonsils and thymus as well as circulating lymphocytes, monocytes and tissue mast cells). CB$_2$ receptors are also present on microglia – immune cells in the CNS which, when activated, contribute to chronic pain (Ch. 38). The localisation of CB$_2$ receptors on cells of the immune system was unexpected, but may account for inhibitory effects of cannabis on immune function. CB$_2$ receptors differ from CB$_1$ receptors in their responsiveness to cannabinoid ligands (see Table 20.1). They are linked via G$_{i/o}$ to adenylyl cyclase, GIRK channels and mitogen-activated protein kinase similarly to CB$_1$, but not to voltage-operated calcium channels (which are not expressed in immune cells). So far,

rather little is known about their function. They are present in atherosclerotic lesions (see Ch. 24), and CB$_2$ agonists have potentially anti-atherosclerotic effects on macrophages and foam cells (Chiurchiu et al., 2014).

Some endocannabinoids turned out, surprisingly,[2] to bind to sites on the cytoplasmic side of transient receptor potential channels (TRP channels), activating these ionotropic receptors and thereby stimulating nociceptive nerve endings (see Ch. 43). Other as-yet-unidentified G protein–coupled receptors are also implicated, because cannabinoids exhibit analgesic actions and activate G proteins in the brain of CB$_1$ knock-out mice, despite the absence of CB$_1$ receptors.

ENDOCANNABINOIDS

The discovery of specific cannabinoid receptors led to a search for endogenous mediators. The first success was chalked up by a team that screened fractions of extracted pig brain for ability to compete with a radiolabelled cannabinoid receptor ligand (Devane et al., 1992). This led to the purification of N-*arachidonylethanolamide*, an eicosanoid mediator (see Ch. 19), the structure of which is shown in Fig. 20.1. This was christened *anandamide*.[3] Anandamide not only displaced labelled cannabinoid from synaptosomal membranes in the binding assay, but also inhibited electrically evoked twitches of mouse vas deferens, a bioassay for psychotropic cannabinoids (Fig. 20.3). A few years later, a second endocannabinoid, *2-arachidonoyl glycerol* (2-AG, see Fig. 20.1), was identified, and more recently at least three further endocannabinoid candidates – all arachidonic acid derivatives - with distinct CB$_1$/CB$_2$ receptor selectivities have been added to the list (see Table 20.1). Endocannabinoids are made 'on demand', like eicosanoids (see Ch. 19), rather than being presynthesised and stored for release when needed.

BIOSYNTHESIS OF ENDOCANNABINOIDS

Biosynthesis of anandamide and of 2-AG is summarised in Fig. 20.4. A fuller account of biosynthesis and degradation is given by Di Marzo (2008).

---

[2]Surprising, because capsaicin, the active principle of chili peppers, causes intense burning pain via activation of these receptors, whereas the endocannabinoid anandamide is associated with pleasure, or even bliss … so perhaps not so surprising after all!
[3]From a Sanskrit word meaning 'bliss' + amide.

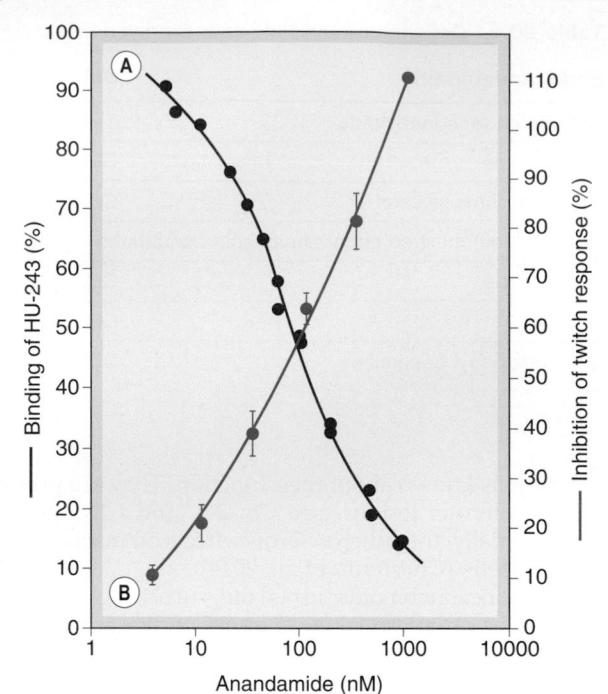

Fig. 20.3 Anandamide as an endocannabinoid. Anandamide is an endogenous cannabinoid. (A) Competitive inhibition of tritiated HU-243 (a cannabinoid receptor ligand) binding to synaptosomal membranes from rat brain by natural anandamide *(red circles, left-hand ordinate axis)*. (B) Inhibition of vas deferens twitch response (a bioassay for cannabinoids) by natural anandamide *(blue symbols, right-hand ordinate)*. Note the similarity between the binding and bioactivity. (Redrawn from Devane et al., 1992.)

▼ Anandamide is formed by a distinct phospholipase D (PLD) selective for N-acyl-phosphatidylethanolamine (NAPE) but with low affinity for other membrane phospholipids, and known as NAPE-PLD. NAPE-PLD is a zinc metallohydrolase that is stimulated by Ca^{2+} and also by polyamines. Selective inhibitors for NAPE-PLD are being sought. The precursors are produced by an as-yet-uncharacterised but Ca^{2+}-sensitive transacylase that transfers an acyl group from the *sn*-1 position of phospholipids to the nitrogen atom of phosphatidylethanolamine.

2-AG is also produced by hydrolysis of precursors derived from phospholipid metabolism. The key enzymes are two *sn*-1-selective diacylglycerol lipases (DAGL-α and DAGL-β), which belong to the family of serine lipases. Both these enzymes, like NAPE-PLD, are Ca^{2+} sensitive, consistent with intracellular Ca^{2+} acting as the physiological stimulus to endocannabinoid synthesis. The DAGLs are located in axons and presynaptic axon terminals during development, but postsynaptically in dendrites and cell bodies of adult neurons, consistent with a role for 2-AG in neurite growth, and with a role as a retrograde mediator (see p. 257) in adult brain.

Little is known as yet about the biosynthesis of the more recent endocannabinoid candidates noladin, virodhamine and N-arachidonoyl dopamine. pH-dependent non-enzymatic interconversion of virodhamine and anandamide is one possibility, and could result in a switch between CB_2- and CB_1-mediated responses (see Table 20.1).

TERMINATION OF THE ENDOCANNABINOID SIGNAL

Endocannabinoids are rapidly taken up from the extracellular space. Being lipid-soluble, they diffuse through plasma membranes down a concentration gradient. There is also evidence for a saturable, temperature-dependent, facilitated transport mechanism for anandamide and 2-AG, dubbed the 'endocannabinoid membrane transporter', for which selective uptake inhibitors (e.g. UCM-707) have been developed. Pathways of endocannabinoid metabolism are summarised in Fig. 20.4. The key enzyme for anandamide

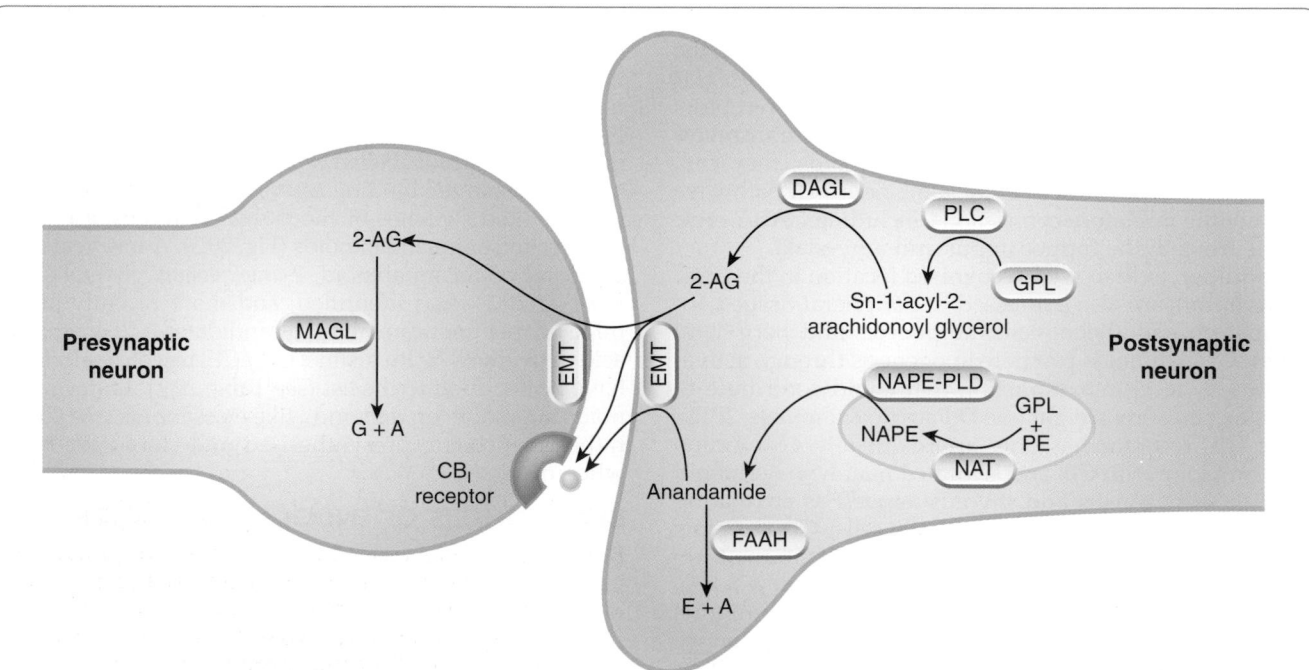

Fig. 20.4 Biosynthesis and inactivation of endocannabinoids. *2-AG*, 2-arachidonoyl glycerol; *A*, arachidonic acid; *DAGL*, diacylglycerol lipase; *E*, ethanolamine; *EMT*, endocannabinoid membrane transporter; *FAAH*, fatty acid amide hydrolase; *G*, glycerol; *GPL*, glycerophospholipid; *MAGL*, monoacyl glycerol lipase; *NAPE*, N-acyl-phosphatidylethanolamine; *NAPE-PLD*, N-acyl phosphatidylethanolamine-specific phospholipase D; *NAT*, N-acyl-transferase; *PE*, phosphatidylethanolamine; *PLC*, phospholipase C.

metabolism is a microsomal serine hydrolase known as fatty acid amide hydrolase (FAAH). FAAH converts anandamide to arachidonic acid plus ethanolamine and also hydrolyses 2-AG, yielding arachidonic acid and glycerol.

The phenotype of FAAH 'knock-out' mice gives some clues to endocannabinoid physiology; such mice have an increased brain content of anandamide and an increased pain threshold. Selective inhibitors of FAAH[4] have analgesic and anxiolytic properties in mice (see Ch. 45 for an explanation of how drugs are tested for anxiolytic properties in rodents). In contrast to anandamide, brain content of 2-AG is not increased in FAAH knock-out animals, indicating that another route of metabolism of 2-AG is likely to be important. Other possible routes of metabolism include esterification, acylation and oxidation by cyclo-oxygenase-2 to prostaglandin ethanolamides ('prostamides'), or by 12- or 15-lipoxygenase (see Ch. 18).

PHYSIOLOGICAL MECHANISMS

Stimuli that release endocannabinoids, leading to activation of CB_1 receptors and the linkage to downstream events including behavioural or psychological effects, are incompletely defined. Increased intracellular Ca^{2+} concentration is probably an important cellular trigger because, as mentioned on p. 256, Ca^{2+} activates NAPE-PLD and other enzymes involved in endocannabinoid biosynthesis.

Activation of CB receptors is implicated in a phenomenon known as *depolarisation-induced suppression of inhibition* (DSI). DSI occurs in hippocampal pyramidal cells; when these are depolarised by an excitatory input, this suppresses the GABA-mediated inhibitory input to the pyramidal cells, implying a retrograde flow of information from the depolarised pyramidal cell to inhibitory axons terminating on it. Such a reverse flow of information from post- to presynaptic cell is a feature of other instances of neuronal plasticity, such as 'wind-up' in nociceptive pathways (Fig. 43.2) and long-term potentiation in the hippocampus (Fig. 39.7). DSI is blocked by the CB_1 antagonist **rimonabant.** The presynaptic location of CB_1 receptors and cellular distributions of the DAGL and monoacyl glycerol lipase (MAGL) enzymes (see Fig. 20.4) fit nicely with the idea that the endocannabinoid 2-AG could be a 'retrograde' messenger in DSI (see Fig. 40.7).

Neuromodulatory actions of endocannabinoids could influence a wide range of physiological activities, including nociception, cardiovascular, respiratory and gastrointestinal function. Interactions of endocannabinoids with hypothalamic hormones are believed to influence food intake and reproductive function. Mouse models lacking CB receptors support important and balanced roles of endocannabinoid signalling in male and female fertility and such signalling is implicated in spermatogenesis, fertilisation, preimplantation development of the early embryo, implantation and postimplantation growth of the embryo (see Battista et al., 2012). Effects of endocannabinoids on food intake

are of particular interest, because of the importance of obesity (Ch. 33).

> **The endocannabinoid system**
>
> - Cannabinoid receptors (CB_1, CB_2) are G protein coupled ($G_{i/o}$).
> - Activation of CB_1 inhibits adenylyl cyclase and calcium channels, and activates potassium channels, inhibiting synaptic transmission.
> - The CB_2 receptor is expressed in cells of the immune system, and its expression is also upregulated in the central nervous system (CNS) in some pathological conditions.
> - Selective agonists and antagonists have been developed.
> - Endogenous ligands for CB receptors are known as endocannabinoids. They are eicosanoid mediators (see Ch. 18).
> - The best-established endocannabinoids are anandamide and 2-arachidonoyl glycerol (2-AG), which have many roles, including functioning as 'retrograde' mediators passing information from postsynaptic to presynaptic neurons.
> - The main enzyme that inactivates anandamide is fatty acid amide hydrolase (FAAH).
> - A putative 'endocannabinoid membrane transporter' may transport cannabinoids from postsynaptic neurons, where they are synthesised, to the synaptic cleft, where they access presynaptic CB_1 receptors, and into presynaptic terminals, where 2-AG is metabolised.
> - FAAH 'knock-out' mice have an increased brain content of anandamide and an increased pain threshold; selective inhibitors of FAAH have analgesic and anxiolytic properties, implicating endocannabinoids in nociception and anxiety. One such drug caused catastrophic CNS injury in healthy human volunteers for unknown reasons.

PATHOLOGICAL INVOLVEMENT

There is evidence, both from experimental animals and from human tissue, that endocannabinoid signalling is abnormal in various neurodegenerative diseases (see Ch. 41). Other diseases where abnormalities of cannabinoid signalling have been reported in human tissue as well as experimental models include hypotensive shock (both haemorrhagic and septic; see Ch. 23), advanced cirrhosis of the liver (where there is evidence that vasodilatation is mediated by endocannabinoids acting on vascular CB_1 receptors – see Bátkai et al., 2001), miscarriage (see Battista et al., 2012) and malignant disease. It seems likely that in some disorders endocannabinoid activity is a compensatory mechanism limiting the progression of disease or occurrence of symptoms, whereas in others it may be 'too much of a good thing' and actually contribute to disease progression. Consequently, there may be a place in therapeutics for drugs that potentiate or inhibit the cannabinoid system (see Pertwee, 2015, for a fuller discussion).

[4]Several such drugs have been administered to humans but none has progressed in development. One such drug, BIA 10-2474 caused sudden severe CNS damage during a trial involving repeated dosing of healthy volunteers in Rennes, France. BIA 10-2474 is less selective than another FAAH inhibitor which was innocuous in earlier trials, inhibiting several lipases that are not targeted by the more selective drug. This suggests that promiscuous lipase inhibitors can cause metabolic dysregulation in the nervous system due to off-target toxicity (see van Esbroeck et al., 2017).

SYNTHETIC CANNABINOIDS

Cannabinoid receptor agonists were developed in the 1970s in the hope that they would prove useful non-opioid/non-NSAID (non-steroidal anti-inflammatory) analgesics (cf. Chs 43 and 27, respectively, for limitations of opioids and NSAIDs), but adverse effects, particularly sedation and memory impairment, were problematic. Nevertheless, one such drug, **nabilone**, is sometimes used clinically for nausea and vomiting caused by cytotoxic chemotherapy if this is unresponsive to conventional antiemetics (Ch. 31). Furthermore, synthetic cannabinoid agonists (i.e. spice) have been used as legal 'highs'.[5] More than 20 of these were introduced in the United Kingdom in 2012–13 in attempts to circumvent the law on cannabis possession. The cloning of CB_2 receptors, and their absence from healthy neuronal brain cells, led to the synthesis of CB_2-selective agonists in the hope that these would lack the CNS-related adverse effects of plant cannabinoids. Several such drugs are being investigated for possible use in inflammatory and neuropathic pain.

The first selective CB_1 receptor antagonist, **rimonabant**, also has inverse agonist properties in some systems. It was licensed in Europe for treating obesity, and there were hopes that it would help promote abstinence from tobacco, but it was withdrawn because it caused psychiatric problems including depression. Synthetic inhibitors of endocannabinoid uptake and/or metabolism have shown potentially useful effects in animal models of pain, epilepsy, multiple sclerosis, Parkinson's disease, anxiety and diarrhoea.

In addition to central CB_1 receptors, hepatocyte CB_1 receptors are also implicated in obesity and in non-alcoholic fatty liver disease, and research on selective peripheral antagonists continues (Klumpers et al., 2013).

CLINICAL APPLICATIONS

Clinical uses of drugs that act on the cannabinoid system remain controversial, but in both the United Kingdom and

the United States, cannabinoids have been used as antiemetics and to encourage weight gain in patients with chronic disease such as HIV/AIDS and malignancy. Cannabis extract (**sativex**) is used to treat spasticity in patients with multiple sclerosis (see Borgelt et al., 2013). Adverse events were generally mild at the doses used – see UK MS Research Group (2003). Endocannabinoids have been implicated in shock and hypotension in liver disease (Malinowska et al., 2008), and modulation of this system is a potential therapeutic target. Other potential clinical uses are given in the clinical box below.

Potential and actual clinical uses of cannabinoid agonists and antagonists

Cannabis extract is licensed as an adjunct for experts treating spasticity in multiple sclerosis and cannabinoid agonists and antagonists are undergoing evaluation for a wide range of possible indications, including:

- Agonists:
  - nausea/vomiting associated with cancer chemotherapy
  - cancer and AIDS (to reduce weight loss)
  - neuropathic pain
  - head injury
  - glaucoma
  - Tourette syndrome (to reduce tics – rapid involuntary movements that are a feature of this disorder)
  - Parkinson's disease (to reduce involuntary movements caused as an adverse effect of **levodopa**; see Ch. 41)
  - seizures.
- Antagonists:
  - obesity
  - tobacco dependence
  - drug addiction
  - alcoholism.

---

[5]Note the past tense: 'legal' highs are all illegal now – at least in the United Kingdom.

REFERENCES AND FURTHER READING

General reading

Freund, T.F., Katona, I., Piomelli, D., 2003. Role of endogenous cannabinoids in synaptic signaling. Physiol. Rev. 83, 1017–1066. (*The fine-grain anatomical distribution of the neuronal cannabinoid receptor CB_1 is described, and possible functions of endocannabinoids as retrograde synaptic signal molecules discussed in relation to synaptic plasticity and network activity patterns*)

Ligresti, A., de Petrocellis, L., di Marzo, V., 2016. From phytocannabinoids to cannabinoid receptors and endocannabinoids: pleiotropic physiological and pathological roles through complex pharmacology. Physiol. Rev. 96, 1593–1659. (*Reviews the pharmacology of major phytocannabinoids, and physiological and pathological, roles of the endocannabinoid system in mammalian cells, tissues, and organs*)

Pertwee, R.G. (Ed.), 2014. Handbook of Cannabis (Handbooks of Psychopharmacology). Oxford University Press. (*Excellent textbook on cannabis*)

Pertwee, R.G. (Ed.), 2015. Endocannabinoids and Their Pharmacological Actions (Handbook of Experimental Pharmacology). Springer International Publications, Switzerland. (*Excellent textbook on endocannabinoid pharmacology*)

Specific aspects

Bátkai, S., Járai, Z., Wagner, J.A., et al., 2001. Endocannabinoids acting at vascular CB_1 receptors mediate the vasodilated state in advanced liver cirrhosis. Nat. Med. 7, 827–832. (*Rats with cirrhosis have low blood pressure, which is elevated by a CB_1 receptor antagonist. Compared with non-cirrhotic controls, in cirrhotic human livers there was a three-fold increase in CB_1 receptors on isolated vascular endothelial cells*)

Battista, N., Meccariello, R., Cobellis, G., 2012. The role of endocannabinoids in gonadal function and fertility along the evolutionary axis. Mol. Cell. Endocrinol. 355, 1–14. (*Reviews the actions of endocannabinoids on the main male and female reproductive events*)

Benyo, Z., Ruisanchez, E., Leszl-Ishiguro, M., 2016. Endocannabinoids in cerebrovascular regulation. Am. J. Physiol. Heart Circ. Physiol. 310, H785–H801. (*Reviews the complex ways in which the endocannabinoid system modulates regulation of cerebral circulation*)

Borgelt, L.M., Franson, K.L., Nussbaum, A.M., Wang, G.S., 2013. The pharmacologic and clinical effects of medical cannabis. Pharmacotherapy 33, 195–209.

Chiurchiu, V., Lanuti, M., Catanzaro, G., et al., 2014. Detailed characterization of the endocannabinoid system in human macrophages and foam cells, and anti-inflammatory role of type-2 cannabinoid receptor. Atherosclerosis 233, 55–63. (*A fully active endocannabinoid system is present in human macrophages and foam cells. Selective activation of CB2R reduces CD36-dependent oxLDL accumulation and modulates production of inflammatory cytokines*)

Devane, W.A., Hanu, L., Breurer, A., et al., 1992. Isolation and structure of a brain constituent that binds to the cannabinoid receptor. Science 258, 1946–1949. (*Identification of arachidonylethanolamide, extracted from pig brain, both chemically and via a bioassay, as a natural ligand for the cannabinoid receptor; the authors named it anandamide*)

Di Marzo, V., 2008. Endocannabinoids: synthesis and degradation. Rev. Physiol. Biochem. Pharmacol. 160, 1–24. (*Reviews current knowledge*)

Di Marzo, V., Petrosino, S., 2007. Endocannabinoids and the regulation of their levels in health and disease. Curr. Opin. Lipidol. 18, 129–140. (*Gastrointestinal disorders, inflammation, neurodegeneration*)

DiPatrizio, N.V., Piomele, D., 2012. The thrifty lipids: endocannabinoids and the neural control of energy conservation. Trends Neurosci. 35, 403–411. (*Endocannabinoids increase energy intake and decrease energy expenditure by controlling the activity of peripheral and central neural pathways involved in the sensing and hedonic processing of sweet and fatty foods, as well as in the storage of their energy content for future use*)

Karst, M., Salim, K., Burstein, S., et al., 2003. Analgesic effect of the synthetic cannabinoid CT-3 on chronic neuropathic pain. A randomized controlled trial. JAMA 290, 1757–1762. (*CT-3, a potent cannabinoid, produces marked antiallodynic and analgesic effects in animals. In a preliminary randomised cross-over study in 21 patients with chronic neuropathic pain, CT-3 was effective in reducing chronic neuropathic pain compared with placebo*)

Klumpers, L.E., Fridberg, M., de Kam, M.L., et al., 2013. Peripheral selectivity of the novel cannabinoid receptor antagonist TM38837 in healthy subjects. Br. J. Clin. Pharmacol. 76, 846–857.

Maldonado, R., Berrendero, F., Ozaita, A., et al., 2011. Neurochemical basis of cannabis addiction. Neuroscience 181, 1–17. (*Describes the experimental methods now available to study the pharmacological responses of cannabinoids related to their addictive effects and the specific contribution of different neurochemical systems in cannabis addiction*)

Malinowska, B., Lupinski, S., Godlewski, G., et al., 2008. Role of endocannabinoids in cardiovascular shock. J. Physiol. Pharmacol. 59, 91–107.

Rubino, T., Zamberletti, E., Parolaro, D., 2012. Adolescent exposure to cannabis as a risk factor for psychiatric disorders. J. Psychopharmacol. (Oxford) 26, SI177–SI188. (*Available data support the hypothesis that heavy cannabis use in adolescence increases the risk of developing psychiatric disorders*)

Steffens, S., 2005. Low dose oral cannabinoid therapy reduces progression of atherosclerosis in mice. Nature 434, 782–786. (*Oral administration of THC (1 mg/kg per day) inhibits atherosclerosis in a mouse model by an action on CB₂ receptors. See also News and Views, p. 708 of the same issue, for comment by Roth, M.D.*)

Taber, K.H., Hurley, R.A., 2009. Endocannabinoids: stress, anxiety and fear. J. Neuropsychiat. Clin. Neurosci. 21, 108–113. (*Succinctly reviews the involvement of the endocannabinoid system in brain function, and potential therapeutic applications in treating mood/anxiety, degenerative disease and brain injury*)

UK MS Research Group, 2003. Cannabinoids for treatment of spasticity and other symptoms related to multiple sclerosis (CAMS study): multicentre randomised placebo-controlled trial. Lancet 362, 1517–1526. (*Randomised, placebo-controlled trial in 667 patients with stable multiple sclerosis and muscle spasticity. Trial duration was 15 weeks. There was no treatment effect of THC or cannabis extract on the primary outcome of spasticity assessed with a standard rating scale, but there was an improvement in patient-reported spasticity and pain, which might be clinically useful*)

van Esbroeck, A.C.M., Janssen, A.P.A., Cognetta, A.B., III, et al., 2017. Activity-based protein profiling reveals off-target proteins of the FAAH inhibitor BIA 10-2474. Science 356, 1084–1087. (*BIA 10-2474 inhibits several lipases that are not targeted by a more selective FAAH inhibitor and alters lipid networks in human cortical neurons, suggesting that promiscuous lipase inhibitors have the potential to cause metabolic dysregulation in the nervous system, possibly accounting for the serious adverse effects caused by BIA 10-2474*)

Van Gaal, L.F., Rissanen, A.M., Scheen, A.J., et al. for the RIO-Europe Study Group, 2005. Effects of the cannabinoid-1 receptor blocker rimonabant on weight reduction and cardiovascular risk factors in overweight patients: 1-year experience from the RIO-Europe study. Lancet 365, 1389–1397. (*A total of 1507 overweight patients treated with rimonabant 5 or 20 mg or with placebo daily for 1 year in addition to dietary advice: significant dose-related decrease in weight and improvement in cardiovascular risk factors in actively treated patients; adverse effects were mild, but subsequent work demonstrated that depression is an important adverse effect and the drug was withdrawn*)

21 Nitric oxide and related mediators

OVERVIEW

Nitric oxide (NO) is a ubiquitous mediator with diverse functions. It is generated from L-arginine by nitric oxide synthase (NOS), an enzyme that occurs in endothelial, neuronal and inducible isoforms. In this chapter, we concentrate on general aspects of NO, especially its biosynthesis, degradation and effects. We touch on evidence that it can act as a circulating as well as local mediator, and conclude with a brief consideration of the therapeutic potential of drugs that act on the L-arginine/NO pathway. Other gaseous mediators (carbon monoxide, hydrogen sulfide)[1] are described briefly: while they have yet to yield therapeutic drugs, their pathways are tempting drug targets.

INTRODUCTION

NO, a free radical gas, is formed in the atmosphere during lightning storms. Less dramatically, but with far-reaching biological consequences, it is also formed in an enzyme-catalysed reaction between molecular oxygen and L-arginine. The convergence of several lines of research led to the realisation that NO is a key signalling molecule in the cardiovascular and nervous systems, and that it has a role in host defence.

A physiological function of NO emerged when biosynthesis of this gas was shown to account for the *endothelium-derived relaxing factor* described by Furchgott and Zawadzki (1980) (Figs 21.1 and 21.2). NO is the endogenous activator of soluble guanylyl cyclase, leading to the formation of cyclic guanosine monophosphate (cGMP), an important 'second messenger' (Ch. 3) in many cells, including neurons, smooth muscle, monocytes and platelets. Nitrogen and oxygen are neighbours in the periodic table, and NO shares several properties with O_2, in particular a high affinity for haem and other iron–sulfur groups. This is important for activation of guanylyl cyclase, which contains a haem group, for the inactivation of NO by haemoglobin and for the regulation of diffusion of NO from endothelial cells (which express the alpha chain of haemoglobin) to vascular smooth muscle.

The role of NO in specific settings is described in other chapters: the endothelium in Chapter 23, the autonomic nervous system (Ch. 13), and as a chemical transmitter and mediator of excitotoxicity in the central nervous system (CNS) in Chapters 38–40. Therapeutic uses of organic nitrates and of nitroprusside (NO donors) are described in Chapters 22 and 23.

BIOSYNTHESIS OF NITRIC OXIDE AND ITS CONTROL

NOS enzymes are central to the control of NO biosynthesis. There are three isoforms: an *inducible* form (iNOS or NOS2) which is expressed in macrophages and Kupffer cells, neutrophils, fibroblasts, vascular smooth muscle and endothelial cells in response to pathological stimuli such as invading microorganisms; and two *constitutive* forms, which are present under physiological conditions in endothelium (eNOS or NOS3)[2] and in neurons (nNOS or NOS1).[3] The constitutive enzymes generate small amounts of NO, whereas NOS2 produces much greater amounts, both because of its high activity and because of its abundance in pathological states associated with cytokine release.

▼ All three NOS isoenzymes are dimers. They are structurally and functionally complex, bearing similarities to the cytochrome P450 enzymes (described in Ch. 10) that are so important in drug metabolism. Each isoform contains iron protoporphyrin IX (haem), flavin adenine dinucleotide (FAD), flavin mononucleotide (FMN) and tetrahydro-biopterin (H_4B) as bound prosthetic groups. They also bind L-arginine, reduced nicotinamide adenine dinucleotide phosphate (NADPH) and calcium–calmodulin. These prosthetic groups and ligands control the assembly of the enzyme into the active dimer. NOS3 is doubly acylated by *N*-myristoylation and cysteine palmitoylation; these post-translational modifications lead to its association with membranes in the Golgi apparatus and in *caveolae*, specialised cholesterol-rich microdomains in the plasma membrane derived from the Golgi apparatus. In the caveolae, NOS3 is held as an inactive complex with *caveolin*, the main membrane protein of caveolae. Dissociation from caveolin activates the enzyme.

The nitrogen atom in NO is derived from the terminal guanidino group of L-arginine. NOS enzymes combine oxygenase and reductase activities. The oxygenase domain contains haem, while the reductase domain binds calcium–calmodulin. In pathological states, the enzyme can undergo structural change leading to electron transfer between substrates, enzyme co-factors and products becoming 'uncoupled', so that electrons are transferred to molecular oxygen, leading to the synthesis of superoxide anion (O_2^-) rather than NO. This is important, as superoxide anion reacts with NO to form a toxic product (peroxynitrite anion; see p. 263). Reactive nitrogen species such as peroxynitrite act together with reactive oxygen species (ROS) to damage cells, causing *nitrosative stress*.

---

[1]The pure substances (NO, CO and H_2S) are gases at room temperature and usual atmospheric pressure, and when pure NO is administered therapeutically (see p. 265 and clinical box, p. 267), it is in the form of a gas; when formed endogenously, the gases are, of course, dissolved in intra- and extracellular fluids.

[2]NOS3 is not restricted to endothelium. It is also present in cardiac myocytes, renal mesangial cells, osteoblasts and osteoclasts, airway epithelium and, in small amounts, platelets, so the term eNOS is somewhat misleading.
[3]It is possible that some of the NO made in healthy animals under basal conditions is derived from the action of NOS2, just as the inducible form of cyclo-oxygenase is active under basal conditions (Ch. 18) – whether this is because there is some NOS2 expressed even when there is no pathology, or because there is enough 'pathology' in healthy mammals, for example in relation to gut microflora, to induce it, is a moot point.

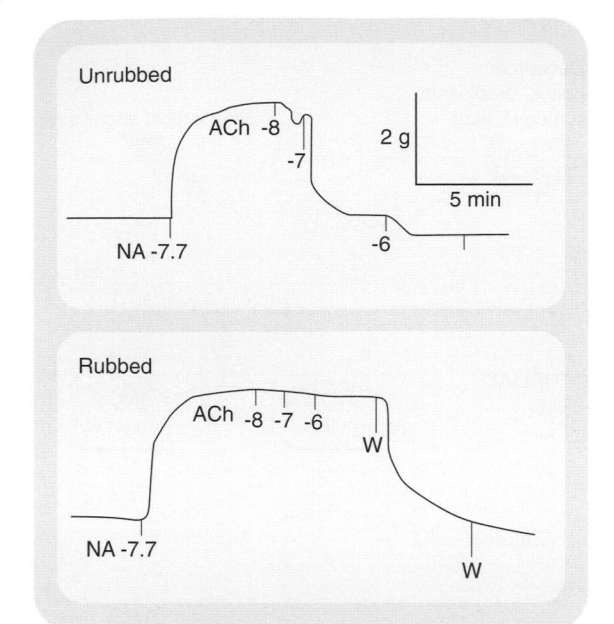

Fig. 21.1 Endothelium-derived relaxing factor.
Acetylcholine (ACh) relaxes a strip of rabbit aorta precontracted with noradrenaline (NA) if the endothelium is intact *('unrubbed': upper panel)*, but not if it has been removed by gentle rubbing *('rubbed': lower panel)*. The numbers are logarithms of molar concentrations of drugs. (From Furchgott & Zawadzki, 1980.)

The activity of constitutive isoforms of NOS is controlled by intracellular calcium–calmodulin (Fig. 21.3). L-Arginine, the substrate of NOS, is usually present in excess in endothelial cell cytoplasm, so the rate of production of NO is determined by the activity of the enzyme rather than by substrate availability. Nevertheless, very high doses of L-arginine can restore endothelial NO biosynthesis in some pathological states (e.g. hypercholesterolaemia) in which endothelial function is impaired. Possible explanations for this paradox include:

- compartmentation: i.e. existence of a distinct pool of substrate in a cell compartment with access to NOS, which can become depleted despite apparently plentiful total cytoplasmic arginine concentrations;
- competition by high concentrations of L-arginine with endogenous competitive inhibitors of NOS such as *asymmetric dimethylarginine* (ADMA; see p. 265 and Fig. 21.4), which is elevated in plasma from patients with hypercholesterolaemia;
- recoupling of electron transfer to L-arginine.

Control of constitutive NOS activity by calcium–calmodulin is exerted in two ways:

1. Many endothelium-dependent agonists (e.g. acetylcholine, bradykinin, substance P) increase the cytoplasmic concentration of calcium ions $[Ca^{2+}]_i$; the consequent increase in calcium–calmodulin activates NOS1 and NOS3.

Fig. 21.2 Endothelium-derived relaxing factor (EDRF) is closely related to nitric oxide (NO). (A) EDRF released from aortic endothelial cells (EC) by acetylcholine (ACh) *(right panel)* has the same effect on the absorption spectrum of deoxyhaemoglobin (Hb) as does authentic NO *(left panel)*. (B) EDRF is released from a column of cultured ECs by bradykinin (BK 3–100 nmol) applied through the column of cells (TC) and relaxes a de-endothelialised precontracted bioassay strip, as does authentic NO (upper trace). (C) A chemical assay of NO based on chemiluminescence shows that similar concentrations of NO are present in the EDRF released from the column of cells as in equiactive authentic NO solutions. (From Ignarro, L.J., Byrns,. RE., Buga, G.M. et al., 1987. Circ. Res. 61, 866–879; and Palmer, R.M.J., Ferrige, A.G., Moncada, S. et al., 1987. Nature 327, 524–526.)

Fig. 21.3 **Control of constitutive nitric oxide synthase (NOS) by calcium–calmodulin.** (A) Dependence on Ca^{2+} of nitric oxide (NO) and citrulline synthesis from L-arginine by rat brain synaptosomal cytosol. Rates of synthesis of NO from L-arginine were determined by stimulation of guanylyl cyclase (GC) *(upper panel)* or by synthesis of [^{3}H]-citrulline from L-[^{3}H]-arginine *(lower panel)*. (B) Regulation of GC in smooth muscle by NO formed in adjacent endothelium. Akt is a protein kinase that phosphorylates NOS, making it more sensitive to calcium–calmodulin. (Panel [A] from Knowles, R.G. et al., 1989. Proc. Natl. Acad. Sci. U. S. A. 86, 5159–5162.)

2. Phosphorylation of specific residues on NOS3 controls its sensitivity to calcium–calmodulin; this can alter NO synthesis in the absence of any change in $[Ca^{2+}]_i$.

Shear stress is an important physiological stimulus to endothelial NO synthesis in resistance vessels. This is sensed by endothelial mechanoreceptors and transduced via a serine–threonine protein kinase called Akt (see Ch. 3) which is also known as protein kinase B. Agonists that increase cAMP in endothelial cells (e.g. β_2-adrenoceptor agonists) increase NOS3 activity, via protein kinase A-mediated phosphorylation[4] whereas protein kinase C *reduces* NOS3 activity by phosphorylating residues in the calmodulin-binding domain, thereby reducing the binding of calmodulin. Insulin increases NOS3 activity via tyrosine kinase activation (and also increases the expression of NOS1 in diabetic mice).

In contrast to constitutive NOS isoforms, the activity of NOS2 is effectively independent of $[Ca^{2+}]_i$, being fully activated even at the low values of $[Ca^{2+}]_i$ present under resting conditions. The enzyme is induced by bacterial lipopolysaccharide and inflammatory cytokines, notably interferon-γ, the antiviral effect of which is due to this. Tumour necrosis factor-α and interleukin-1 do not alone induce NOS2, but they each synergise with interferon-γ in this regard (see Ch. 18). Induction of NOS2 is inhibited by glucocorticoids and by several cytokines, including transforming growth factor-β. There are important species differences in the inducibility of NOS2, which is less readily induced in human than in mouse cells.

DEGRADATION AND CARRIAGE OF NITRIC OXIDE

NO reacts with oxygen to form N_2O_4, which combines with water to produce a mixture of nitric and nitrous acids. Nitrite ions are oxidised to nitrate by oxyhaemoglobin. These reactions are summarised as follows:

$$2NO + O_2 \rightarrow N_2O_4 \tag{21.1}$$

$$N_2O_4 + H_2O \rightarrow NO_3^- + NO_2^- + 2H^+ \tag{21.2}$$

$$NO_2^- + HbO \rightarrow NO_3^- + Hb \tag{21.3}$$

---

[4]As explained in Chapter 4, β_2 agonists also act directly on smooth muscle cells, causing relaxation via cAMP.

Nitric oxide: synthesis, inactivation and carriage

- Nitric oxide (NO) is synthesised from L-arginine and molecular O_2 by NO synthase (NOS).
- NOS exists in three isoforms: inducible (NOS2), and constitutive 'endothelial' (NOS3, which is not restricted to endothelial cells) and neuronal (NOS1) forms. NOSs are dimeric flavoproteins, contain tetrahydrobiopterin and have homology with cytochrome P450. The constitutive enzymes are activated by calcium–calmodulin. Sensitivity to calcium–calmodulin is controlled by phosphorylation of specific residues on the enzymes.
- NOS2 is induced in macrophages and other cells by inflammatory cytokines, especially interferon-γ.
- NOS1 is present in the central nervous system (see Chs 38–41) and in some autonomic nerves.
- NOS3 is present in platelets and other cells in addition to endothelium.
- NO diffuses to sites of action in neighbouring cells. This is regulated by the redox state of haemoglobin alpha which is present in the myoendothelial junctions that act as diffusion corridors across the internal elastic lamina (and in other cells): signalling can occur when the haem is in the Fe^{3+} state, but is stopped – like at a red traffic light – when haem is in the Fe^{2+} state.
- NO is inactivated by combination with the haem of haemoglobin or by oxidation to nitrite and nitrate, which are excreted in urine; it is also present in exhaled air, especially in patients with inflammatory lung diseases such as bronchitis.
- NO can react reversibly with cysteine residues (e.g. in globin or albumin) to form stable nitrosothiols; as a result, red cells can act as an O_2-regulated source of NO. NO released in this way escapes inactivation by haem by being exported via cysteine residues in the anion exchange protein in red cell membranes.

Low concentrations of NO are relatively stable in air, because the rate of reaction shown in Eq. 21.1 depends on the square of the NO concentration, so small amounts of NO produced in the lung escape degradation and can be detected in exhaled air. Exhaled NO is increased in patients with lung diseases such as bronchitis, and is used as a biomarker of airway inflammation (Ch. 29). In contrast, NO reacts very rapidly with even low concentrations of superoxide anion (O_2^-) to produce peroxynitrite anion ($ONOO^-$), which is responsible for some of its toxic effects.

▼ Haem has an affinity for NO >10,000 times greater than for oxygen. In the absence of oxygen, NO bound to haem is relatively stable, but in the presence of oxygen NO is converted to nitrate and the haem iron (Fe^{2+}) oxidised to form methaemoglobin (Fe^{3+}).

Endothelium-derived NO acts locally on underlying vascular smooth muscle or on adherent monocytes or platelets. The internal elastic lamina of small arteries is a layer of elastic fibres between the endothelium and the smooth muscle, which represents a barrier to diffusion. It is penetrated by myoendothelial junctions where endothelial and smooth muscle cells kiss, forming a corridor along which NO can diffuse. Haemoglobin alpha is concentrated in these junctions and acts as a redox-sensitive stop/go signal. When the haem iron is in the oxidised Fe^{3+} state (methaemoglobin), NO can diffuse along the corridor and into the smooth muscle cell on which it acts; when the haem iron is in the Fe^{2+} state, however, NO is rapidly converted to nitrate and the diffusion pathway is effectively closed. Conversion of methaemoglobin to haemoglobin, preventing NO from crossing the barrier, is brought about by the enzyme cytochrome b5 reductase3 (also known as methaemoglobin reductase) and inhibition of this enzyme increases NO bioactivity in small arteries (Straub et al., 2012).

Distinct from the inactivation reaction between NO and haem, a specific cysteine residue (cys 93 of the β-chain) in globin combines reversibly with NO under physiological conditions. The resulting S-nitrosylated haemoglobin acts as a circulating oxygen-sensitive NO carrier that releases biologically active nitrosothiol (SNO) compounds such as cysteinyl-NO or glutathionyl-NO to mediate vasodilatation when haemoglobin transitions from the R (oxygenated) to the T (deoxygenated) state, thereby contributing to hypoxic vasodilatation. The biological importance of this mechanism is attested to by observations in mutant mice expressing humanised haemoglobin and lacking β-cys93 S-nitrosylation. Such mice are more susceptible to myocardial damage in experimental myocardial ischaemia and heart failure models than controls with humanised haemoglobin but intact β-cys93 S-nitrosylation (Zhang et al., 2015).

EFFECTS OF NITRIC OXIDE

NO reacts with various metals, thiols and oxygen species, thereby modifying proteins, DNA and lipids. One of its most important biochemical effects (see Ch. 3) is activation of soluble guanylyl cyclase, a heterodimer present in vascular and nervous tissue as two distinct isoenzymes. Guanylyl cyclase synthesises the second messenger cGMP. NO activates the enzyme by combining with its haem group, and many physiological effects of low concentrations of NO are mediated by cGMP. These effects are prevented by inhibitors of guanylyl cyclase (e.g. 1H-[1,2,4]-oxadiazole-[4,3-α]-quinoxalin-1-one, better known as 'ODQ'), which are useful investigational tools. NO activates soluble guanylyl cyclase in intact cells (neurons and platelets) extremely rapidly, and activation is followed by desensitisation to a steady-state level. This contrasts with its effect on the isolated enzyme, which is slower but more sustained. Guanylyl cyclase contains another regulatory site, which is NO independent. This is activated by **riociguat**, used to treat some forms of pulmonary hypertension (see Ch. 23).

Effects of cGMP are terminated by phosphodiesterase enzymes. **Sildenafil** and **tadalafil** are inhibitors of phosphodiesterase type V. They are used to treat erectile dysfunction and work by potentiating NO actions in the corpora cavernosa of the penis by this mechanism (see Ch. 36). NO also combines with haem groups in other biologically important proteins, notably cytochrome c oxidase, where it competes with oxygen, contributing to the control of cellular respiration (see Erusalimsky & Moncada, 2007). Cytotoxic and/or cytoprotective effects of higher concentrations of NO relate to its chemistry as a free radical (see Ch. 41). Some physiological and pathological effects of NO are shown in Table 21.1.

BIOCHEMICAL AND CELLULAR ASPECTS

Pharmacological effects of NO can be studied with NO gas dissolved in deoxygenated salt solution. More conveniently, but less directly, various donors of NO, such as **nitroprusside**, S-*nitrosoacetylpenicillamine* (SNAP) or S-*nitrosoglutathione*

Table 21.1 Postulated roles of endogenous nitric oxide

System	Physiological role	Pathological role	
		Excess production	Inadequate production or action
Cardiovascular			
Endothelium/vascular smooth muscle	Control of blood pressure and regional blood flow	Hypotension (septic shock)	Atherogenesis, thrombosis (e.g. in hypercholesterolaemia, diabetes mellitus)
Platelets	Limitation of adhesion/aggregation	—	—
Host defence			
Macrophages, neutrophils, leukocytes	Defence against viruses, bacteria, fungi, protozoa, parasites	—	—
Nervous system			
Central	Neurotransmission, long-term potentiation, plasticity (memory, appetite, nociception)	Excitotoxicity (Ch. 41) (e.g. ischaemic stroke, Huntington's disease, AIDS, dementia)	—
Peripheral	Neurotransmission (e.g. gastric emptying, penile erection)	—	Hypertrophic pyloric stenosis, erectile dysfunction

(SNOG), have been used as surrogates. This has pitfalls; for example, ascorbic acid potentiates SNAP but inhibits responses to authentic NO.[5]

NO can activate guanylyl cyclase in the same cells that produce it, giving rise to autocrine effects, for example on the barrier function of the endothelium. NO also diffuses from its site of synthesis and activates guanylyl cyclase in neighbouring cells. The resulting increase in cGMP affects protein kinase G, ion channels and possibly other proteins, inhibiting $[Ca^{2+}]_i$-induced smooth muscle contraction and platelet aggregation. NO hyperpolarises vascular smooth muscle as a consequence of potassium-channel activation, and inhibits monocyte adhesion and migration, adhesion and aggregation of platelets, and smooth muscle and fibroblast proliferation. These cellular effects probably underlie the anti-atherosclerotic action of NO (see Ch. 24).

Large amounts of NO (released following induction of NOS or excessive stimulation of NMDA receptors in the brain, see Chs 40 and 41) cause cytotoxic effects, either directly or via formation of peroxynitrite. Such cytotoxicity contributes to host defence, but also to the neuronal cell death that occurs when there is overstimulation of NMDA receptors by glutamate (see Chs 39 and 41). Paradoxically, NO is also cytoprotective under some circumstances (see Ch. 41).

VASCULAR EFFECTS (see also Ch. 23)

The L-arginine/NO pathway is tonically active in resistance vessels, reducing peripheral vascular resistance and hence systemic blood pressure. Mutant mice that lack the gene coding NOS3 are hypertensive, consistent with a role for NO biosynthesis in the physiological control of blood pressure. In addition, NO derived from NOS1 is implicated in the control of basal resistance vessel tone in human forearm and cardiac muscle vascular beds (Seddon et al., 2008, 2009). NO is believed to contribute to the generalised

vasodilatation that occurs during pregnancy. In addition to effects on basal resistance vessel tone and mediating the effects of endothelium-dependent vasodilator agonists such as acetylcholine and substance P, it has more recently been appreciated that NO promotes new vessel formation ('angiogenesis') and vascular remodelling (Kraehling & Sessa, 2017; Ghimire et al., 2017).

NEURONAL EFFECTS (see also Ch. 13)

NO is a non-noradrenergic non-cholinergic (NANC) neurotransmitter in many tissues (see Fig. 13.5), including the upper airways, gastrointestinal tract and corpora cavernosa of the penis (Chs 29, 31 and 36). It is implicated in the control of neuronal development and of synaptic plasticity in the CNS (Chs 38 and 41). Mice carrying a mutation that disrupts the gene coding NOS1 have grossly distended stomachs similar to those seen in human hypertrophic pyloric stenosis (a disorder in which deficient NO production has been implicated, characterised by pyloric hypertrophy causing gastric outflow obstruction, which occurs in approximately 1 in 150 male infants and is corrected surgically). NOS1 knock-out mice resist stroke damage caused by middle cerebral artery ligation but are aggressive and oversexed (characteristics that may not be unambiguously disadvantageous, at least in the context of natural selection!).

HOST DEFENCE (see Ch. 7)

Cytotoxic and/or cytostatic effects of NO are implicated in primitive non-specific host defence mechanisms against numerous pathogens, including viruses, bacteria, fungi, protozoa and parasites, and against tumour cells. The importance of this is evidenced by the susceptibility of mice lacking NOS2 to *Leishmania major* (to which wild-type mice are highly resistant). Mechanisms whereby NO damages invading pathogens include nitrosylation of nucleic acids and combination with haem-containing enzymes, including the mitochondrial enzymes involved in cell respiration.

[5]Ascorbic acid releases NO from SNAP but accelerates NO degradation in solution, which could explain this divergence.

Actions of nitric oxide

* Nitric oxide (NO) acts by:
  – combining with haem in guanylyl cyclase, activating the enzyme, increasing cGMP and thereby lowering $[Ca^{2+}]_i$;
  – combining with haem groups in other proteins (e.g. cytochrome C oxidase);
  – combining with superoxide anion to yield the cytotoxic peroxynitrite anion;
  – nitrosation of proteins, lipids and nucleic acids.
* Effects of NO include:
  – vasodilatation, inhibition of platelet and monocyte adhesion and aggregation, inhibition of smooth muscle proliferation, protection against atheroma, vascular remodelling and angiogenesis;
  – synaptic effects in the peripheral and central nervous system;
  – host defence and cytotoxic effects on pathogens;
  – cytoprotection.

THERAPEUTIC ASPECTS

Novel therapeutic approaches under investigation to increase bioavailability of NO include new ways to increase NO synthase activity, ways to amplify the nitrate-nitrite-NO pathway, novel classes of NO donors; drugs that limit NO inactivation by ROS; and ways to modulate phosphodiesterases and soluble guanylyl cyclases (reviewed by Lundberg et al. 2015).

NITRIC OXIDE

Inhaling high concentrations of NO (as occurred when cylinders of nitrous oxide, N_2O, for anaesthesia were accidentally contaminated) causes acute pulmonary oedema and methaemoglobinaemia, but concentrations below 50 ppm (parts per million) are not toxic. NO (5–300 ppm) inhibits bronchoconstriction (at least in guinea pigs), but the main action of low concentrations of inhaled NO in man is pulmonary vasodilatation. Inspired NO acts preferentially on ventilated alveoli, and is used therapeutically in respiratory distress syndrome, including acute hypoxic respiratory failure in newborn babies for which NO has been approved by the FDA. This is characterised by intrapulmonary 'shunting', that is, pulmonary arterial blood passing through non-ventilated alveoli and remaining deoxygenated. This causes arterial hypoxaemia, and, because hypoxaemia causes pulmonary arterial vasoconstriction, acute pulmonary arterial hypertension. Inhaled NO dilates blood vessels in ventilated alveoli (which are exposed to the inspired gas) and thus reduces shunting. NO is used in intensive care units to reduce pulmonary hypertension and to improve oxygen delivery in patients with respiratory distress syndrome, but it is not known whether this improves long-term survival in these severely ill patients.

NITRIC OXIDE DONORS/PRECURSORS

Nitrovasodilators have been used therapeutically for over a century. The common mode of action of these drugs is as a source of NO (Chs 22 and 23). There is interest in the potential for selectivity of nitrovasodilators; for instance, **glyceryl trinitrate** is more potent on vascular smooth muscle

than on platelets, whereas SNOG (see p. 264) selectively inhibits platelet aggregation. It was shown recently that dietary inorganic nitrate ions (contained in beetroot juice) acutely lower arterial blood pressure in parallel with a rise in plasma nitrite concentration and improved endothelial and platelet function. Interruption of the enterosalivary conversion of nitrate to nitrite prevents the rise in plasma nitrite, blocks the fall in blood pressure and abolishes the inhibitory effect on platelet aggregation (see review by Lidder & Webb, 2013).

INHIBITION OF NITRIC OXIDE SYNTHESIS

▼ Drugs can inhibit NO synthesis or action by several mechanisms. Certain arginine analogues compete with arginine for NOS. Several such compounds, for example, N^G-monomethyl-L-arginine (L-NMMA) and N^G-nitro-L-arginine methyl ester (L-NAME), have proved of great value as experimental tools. One such endogenous compound, ADMA (see earlier), is approximately equipotent with L-NMMA. It is present in human plasma and is excreted in urine. Its plasma concentration correlates with vascular mortality in patients receiving haemodialysis for chronic renal failure, and is increased in people with hypercholesterolaemia, possibly via changes in gene expression rather than direct inhibition (Caplin & Leiper, 2012). In addition to urinary excretion, ADMA is also eliminated by metabolism to a mixture of citrulline and methylamine by *dimethylarginine dimethylamino hydrolase* (DDAH), an enzyme that exists in two isoforms, each with a reactive cysteine residue in the active site that is subject to control by nitrosylation. Inhibition of DDAH by NO causes feedback inhibition of the L-arginine/NO pathway by allowing cytoplasmic accumulation of ADMA. Conversely, activation of DDAH could potentiate the L-arginine/NO pathway; see Fig. 21.4.

Infusion of the non-selective NOS inhibitor L-NMMA into the brachial artery causes local vasoconstriction (Fig. 21.5), owing to inhibition of the basal production of NO in the infused arm, probably partly by inhibiting NOS1 in autonomic nerve fibres (Seddon et al., 2008). A contribution of NOS3-derived NO to basal vasodilator tone is also possible, since NOS3 knock-out mice are hypertensive, as mentioned previously (p. 264). Intravenous L-NMMA causes vasoconstriction

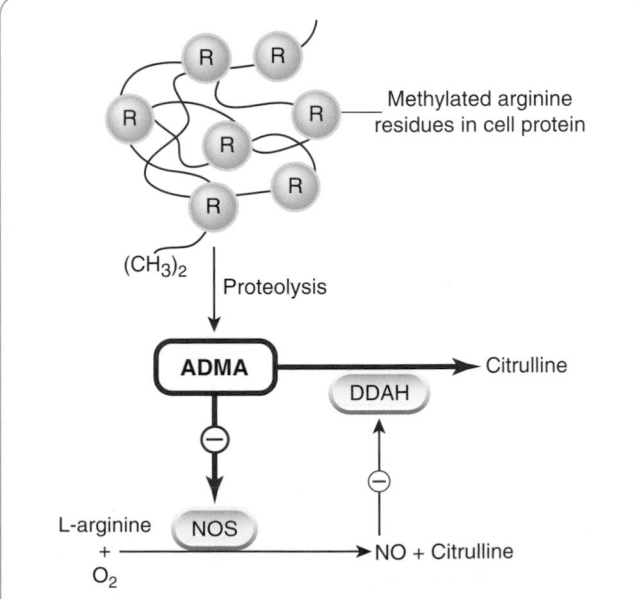

Fig. 21.4 **Control of NO synthesis by asymmetric dimethylarginine (ADMA).** *DDAH*, dimethylarginine dimethylamino hydrolase; *NO*, nitric oxide; *NOS*, nitric oxide synthase.

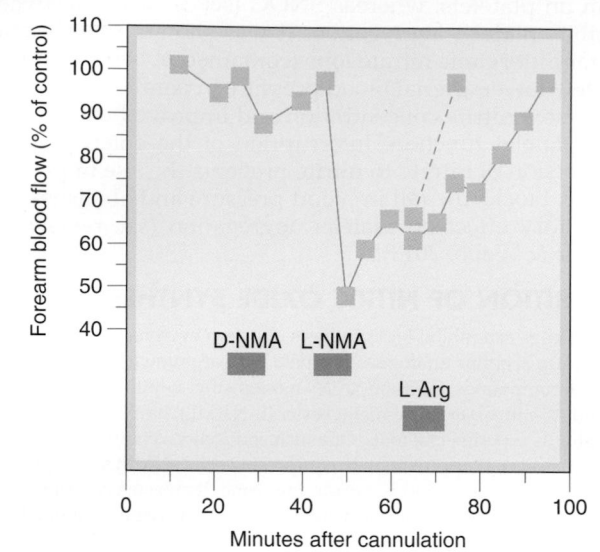

Fig. 21.5 Basal blood flow in the human forearm is influenced by nitric oxide (NO) biosynthesis. Forearm blood flow is expressed as a percentage of the flow in the non-cannulated control arm (which does not change). Brachial artery infusion of the D-isomer of the arginine analogue N^G-monomethyl-L-arginine (D-NMA) has no effect, while the L-isomer (L-NMA) causes vasoconstriction. L-Arginine (L-Arg) accelerates recovery from such vasoconstriction (dashed line). (From Vallance, P., Bhagat, K., MacAllister, R. et al., 1989. Lancet ii, 997–1000.)

in renal, mesenteric, cerebral and striated muscle resistance vessels, increases blood pressure and causes reflex bradycardia.

There is therapeutic interest in selective inhibitors of different isoforms of NOS. Selective inhibitors of NOS2 versus the constitutive enzymes have been described (e.g. N-iminoethyl-l-lysine), and have potential for the treatment of inflammatory and other conditions in which NOS2 has been implicated (e.g. asthma). 7-Nitroindazole selectively inhibits NOS1, the mechanism of selectivity being uncertain. S-methyl-L-thiocitrulline is a potent and selective inhibitor of human NOS1 (Furfine et al., 1994), and has recently provided new understanding of the importance of NOS1 in control of human resistance vessel tone in vivo as mentioned earlier.

Inhibition of the L-arginine/nitric oxide pathway

- Glucocorticoids inhibit biosynthesis of nitric oxide synthase 2 (NOS2).
- Synthetic arginine and citrulline analogues (e.g. L-NMMA, L-NAME; see text) compete with arginine and are useful experimental tools. Isoform-selective inhibitors include S-methyl-L-thiocitrulline (selective for NOS1).
- ADMA (asymmetric dimethylarginine) is an endogenous inhibitor of NOS.

NITRIC OXIDE REPLACEMENT OR POTENTIATION

Several means whereby the L-arginine/NO pathway could be enhanced are under investigation. Some of these rely on existing drugs of proven value in other contexts. The hope (as yet unproven) is that, by potentiating NO, they will prevent atherosclerosis or its thrombotic complications or have other beneficial effects attributed to NO. Possibilities include:

- selective NO donors as 'replacement' therapy (see clinical box, p. 267) or to protect against unwanted aspects of the action of another drug (e.g. **naproxinod**, Ch. 27);
- dietary supplementation with L-arginine or inorganic nitrate (see clinical box, p. 267);
- antioxidants (to reduce concentrations of ROS and hence stabilise NO and reduce toxic reaction products; Ch. 23);
- drugs that restore endothelial function in patients with metabolic risk factors for vascular disease (e.g. angiotensin-converting enzyme inhibitors, statins, insulin, oestrogens; Chs 23, 24, 32 and 36);
- β_2-adrenoceptor agonists and related drugs (e.g. **nebivolol**, a β_1-adrenoceptor antagonist that is metabolised to an active metabolite that potentiates the L-arginine/NO pathway);
- phosphodiesterase type V inhibitors (e.g. **sildenafil**; see clinical box, p. 267 and Ch. 36).

CLINICAL CONDITIONS IN WHICH NITRIC OXIDE MAY PLAY A PART

The wide distribution of NOS enzymes and diverse actions of NO suggest that abnormalities in the L-arginine/NO pathway could be important in disease. Either increased or reduced production could play a part, and hypotheses abound. Evidence is harder to come by but has been sought using various indirect approaches, including:

- Analysing nitrate and/or cGMP in urine: these studies are bedevilled, respectively, by dietary nitrate and by cGMP produced by membrane-bound guanylyl cyclase (which is stimulated by endogenous natriuretic peptides independently of NO; see Ch. 22).
- A refinement is to administer [^{15}N]-arginine and use mass spectrometry to measure the enrichment of ^{15}N over naturally abundant [^{14}N]-nitrate in urine.
- Measuring NO in exhaled air.
- Measuring effects of NOS inhibitors (e.g. L-NMMA),
- Comparing responses to endothelium-dependent agonists (e.g. **acetylcholine**) and endothelium-independent agonists that act by providing NO (e.g. **nitroprusside**).
- Measuring responses to increased blood flow ('flow-mediated dilatation'), which are largely mediated by NO.
- Comparing in vitro responses to pharmacological probes of tissue obtained at operation (e.g. coronary artery surgery) with histochemical data from the tissue (e.g. anatomical distribution of NOS isoforms).

All these methods have limitations, and the dust is far from settled. Nevertheless, it seems clear that the L-arginine/NO pathway is indeed a player in the pathogenesis of several important diseases, opening the way to new therapeutic approaches. Some pathological roles of excessive or reduced NO production are summarised in Table 21.1. We touch only briefly on these clinical conditions, and would caution the reader that not all of these exciting possibilities are likely to withstand the test of time!

Nitric oxide in pathophysiology

- Nitric oxide (NO) is synthesised under physiological and pathological circumstances.
- Either reduced or increased NO production can contribute to disease.
- Underproduction of neuronal NO is reported in babies with hypertrophic pyloric stenosis. Endothelial NO production is reduced in patients with hypercholesterolaemia and some other risk factors for atherosclerosis, and this may contribute to atherogenesis.
- Overproduction of NO may be important in neurodegenerative diseases (see Ch. 41) and in septic shock (Ch. 23).

Sepsis can cause multiple organ failure. Whereas NO benefits host defence by killing invading organisms, excessive NO causes harmful hypotension. Disappointingly, however, L-NMMA worsens survival in sepsis.

Chronic low-grade endotoxaemia occurs in patients with *hepatic cirrhosis*. Systemic vasodilatation is typical in such patients. Urinary excretion of cGMP is increased, and it is plausible (but unproven) that vasodilatation is a consequence of induction of NOS leading to increased NO synthesis.

Nitrosative stress (see earlier, p. 260) and nitration of proteins in airway epithelium are believed to contribute to steroid resistance in *asthma*, and the ineffectiveness of glucocorticoids in *chronic obstructive pulmonary disease* (see Ch. 29).

NO biosynthesis is reduced in patients with *hypercholesterolaemia* and some other precursors of atheromatous disease, including cigarette smoking and diabetes mellitus. In hypercholesterolaemia, evidence of blunted NO release in forearm and coronary vascular beds is supported by evidence that this can be corrected by lowering plasma cholesterol with a statin (see Ch. 25).

Endothelial dysfunction in individuals (e.g. diabetic patients) with *erectile dysfunction* occurs in tissue from the corpora cavernosum of the penis, as evidenced by blunted relaxation to acetylcholine despite preserved responses to nitroprusside (Fig. 21.6). Vasoconstrictor responses to intra-arterial L-NMMA are reduced in forearm vasculature of insulin-dependent diabetics, especially in patients with traces of albumin in their urine ('microalbuminuria' – early evidence of glomerular endothelial dysfunction).

It is thought that failure to increase endogenous NO biosynthesis during pregnancy contributes to *eclampsia*. This is a hypertensive disorder that accounts for many maternal deaths and in which the normal vasodilatation seen in healthy pregnancy fails to manifest itself.

Excessive NMDA receptor activation increases NO synthesis, contributing to consequent neurological damage (see Ch. 41).

NOS1 is absent in pyloric tissue from babies with idiopathic hypertrophic pyloric stenosis.

Established clinical uses of drugs that influence the L-arginine/NO system are summarised in the clinical box.

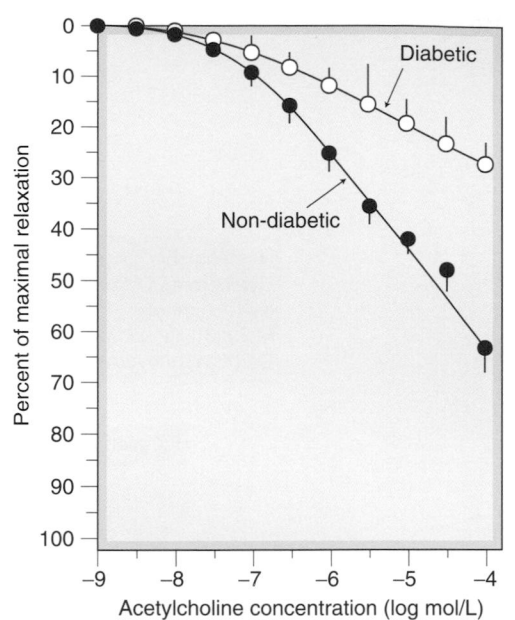

Fig. 21.6 Impaired endothelium-mediated relaxation of penile smooth muscle from diabetic men with erectile dysfunction. Mean (±SE) relaxation responses to acetylcholine in corpora cavernosa tissue (obtained at the time of performing surgical implants to treat impotence) from 16 diabetic men and 22 non-diabetic subjects. (Data from Saenz de Tejada, I., Carson, M.P., de las Morenas, A. et al., 1989. N. Engl. J. Med. 320, 1025–1030.)

Nitric oxide in therapeutics

- Nitric oxide (NO) donors (e.g. **nitroprusside** and organic nitrovasodilators) are well established (see Chs 22 and 23).
- Type V phosphodiesterase inhibitors (e.g. **sildenafil**, **tadalafil**) potentiate the action of NO. They are used to treat erectile dysfunction (Ch. 36).
- Other possible indications (e.g. pulmonary hypertension, gastric stasis) are being investigated.
- Inhaled NO is used in intensive care of adult and neonatal respiratory distress syndrome.
- Inhibition of NO biosynthesis is being investigated in disorders where there is overproduction of NO (e.g. inflammation and neurodegenerative disease). Disappointingly, *N*^{G}**-monomethyl-L-arginine (L-NMMA)** increases mortality in one such condition (sepsis).

RELATED MEDIATORS

NO, promoted from pollutant to 'molecule of the year',[6] was joined, similarly implausibly, by carbon monoxide (CO) – a potentially lethal exhaust gas – and by hydrogen sulfide

---

[6]By the American Association for the Advancement of Science in 1992.

Fig. 21.7 Synthesis, sites of action and disposition of H₂S. Endogenous biosynthesis from sulfur-containing amino acids (methionine, cycteine) via actions of the regulated enzymes methionine cystathionine γ-lyase (CSE) and cystathionine β-synthase (CBS) is shown; pharmacological H₂S donors *(red-rimmed box)* may be administered exogenously. Most H₂S is probably renally excreted as sulfate *(yellow box)*. Some is eliminated in exhaled air *(green box)*. Some molecular targets of H₂S are indicated in the *blue box*. (Adapted with permission from Ritter, J.M., 2010. Human pharmacology of hydrogen sulfide: putative gaseous mediator. Br. J. Clin. Pharmacol. 69, 573–575.)

(H₂S), which are also formed in mammalian tissues. There are striking similarities between these three gases, as well as some contrasts. All three are highly diffusible labile molecules that are rapidly eliminated from the body: NO as nitrite and nitrate in urine as well as NO in exhaled air (see pp. 262–263); CO in exhaled air; H₂S as thiosulfate, sulfite and sulfate in urine (Fig. 21.7) as well as in exhaled breath. All three react with haemoglobin, and all three affect cellular energetics via actions on cytochrome C oxidase. All have vasodilator effects (although chronic exposure to CO can cause vasoconstriction), and all have anti-inflammatory and cytoprotective effects at low concentrations but cause cellular injury at higher concentrations.

CARBON MONOXIDE (CO)

▼ CO is synthesised, together with biliverdin, by inducible and/or constitutive forms of haem oxygenase, and has been implicated as a signalling molecule in the cardiovascular and central nervous systems (especially olfactory pathways) and in controlling respiratory, gastrointestinal, endocrine and reproductive functions (see Wu & Wang, 2005). There is evidence that prostanoid-induced cerebral vasodilatation is mediated by CO, and that CO also interacts with NO in modulating cerebral vascular tone (Leffler et al., 2011). There are as yet no therapeutic drugs acting via this pathway, but CO (perhaps surprisingly for a gas associated with lethal effects in a domestic setting) has potentially beneficial effects on cell survival and CO-releasing molecules are under investigation (Motterlini & Foresti, 2017).

HYDROGEN SULFIDE (H₂S)

▼ H₂S has been known to generations of schoolboys as the source of the odour of rotten eggs and the proposal that it too is a gaseous

mediator was met with some scepticism. Its toxicology includes actions on enzymes including monoamine oxidase and carbonic anhydrase, but more recent work has demonstrated a diverse pharmacology consistent with functions as a signalling molecule under physiological conditions.

Endogenous H₂S is produced from l-cysteine by cystathionine γ-lyase (also known as cystathionase or CSE) and cystathionine β-synthase (CBS). Large amounts of CBS occur in mammalian brain (especially hippocampus and cerebellar Purkinje cells), whereas CSE activity is greatest in liver, kidney and media of blood vessels. These enzymes are regulated by lipopolysaccharide and by tumour necrosis factor α (TNF-α) and their expression is altered in pancreatitis and diabetes. Pharmacological inhibitors of H₂S synthesis are so far only of modest potency and specificity and have been of limited use in elucidating its physiological role. Several assays of H₂S in biological fluids grossly overestimate the true concentrations. Measuring thiosulfate excretion (see Fig. 21.7) may represent a better analytical approach than plasma sulfide to estimating overall turnover of H₂S; sulfite and sulfate (to which thiosulfate is converted) are not satisfactory, as their production from other sources of sulfur swamps the contribution of H₂S.

Pharmacological effects and therapeutic potential. H₂S has potent pharmacological effects in the cardiovascular system, including vasorelaxation secondary to activation of vascular smooth muscle K_{ATP} channels (see Ch. 4). It also acts on the nervous system and influences nociception, selectively modulating voltage dependent T-type Ca²⁺ channels (Elics et al., 2016). It also influences inflammatory processes. For a review of the effects of H₂S on ion channels and intracellular transduction systems see Li et al., 2011. Endocrine effects include inhibition of glucose-stimulated insulin secretion; actions on K_{ATP} channels may be important here also (see Ch. 32). One of the most striking effects of

H_2S is to induce a state of suspended animation and hypothermia, described first in nematode worms, but then also in rodents. Subsequently, a whole range of cytotoxic (high concentration) and cytoprotective (low concentration) effects of H_2S and H_2S donors have been described in a wide variety of cell types in many different tissues (reviewed by Szabo, 2007). These findings provided a rationale for studies of effects of H_2S donors in animal models of diseases as diverse as pulmonary vasoconstriction, ischaemic heart disease, pulmonary fibrosis and stroke. The results have been sufficiently encouraging to provide a rationale for studying H_2S donors in man. Several sulfide-releasing derivatives based on **naproxen**, **diclofenac** (Ch. 27) and on **mesalazine** (Ch. 31), as well as inorganic sodium sulfide, are under investigation as potential therapeutic agents. Again, a case of 'watch this space'.

REFERENCES AND FURTHER READING

Biochemical aspects

Derbyshire, E.R., Marletta, M.A., 2012. Structure and regulation of soluble guanylate cyclase. Annu. Rev. Biochem. 81, 533–559. (*Summarises sGC structure and regulation*)

Furfine, E.S., Harmon, M.F., Paith, J.E., et al., 1994. Potent and selective inhibition of human nitric oxide synthases: selective inhibition of neuronal nitric oxide synthase by S-methyl-L-thiocitrulline and S-ethyl-L-thiocitrulline. J. Biol. Chem. 269, 26677–26683.

Hill, B.G., Dranka, B.P., Shannon, M., et al., 2010. What part of NO don't you understand? Some answers to the cardinal questions in nitric oxide biology. J. Biol. Chem. 285, 19699–19704. (*Biochemistry of NO in a biological context*)

Kim-Shapiro, D.B., Schechter, A.N., Gladwin, M.T., 2006. Unraveling the reactions of nitric oxide, nitrite, and hemoglobin in physiology and therapeutics. Arterioscler. Thromb. Vasc. Biol. 26, 697–705. (*Reviews evidence that nitrite anion may be the main intravascular NO storage molecule; cf. Singel & Stamler, 2005*)

Matsubara, M., Hayashi, N., Jing, T., Titani, K., 2003. Regulation of endothelial nitric oxide synthase by protein kinase C. J. Biochem. 133, 773–781. (*Protein kinase C inhibits NOS3 activity by altering the affinity of calmodulin for the enzyme*)

Pawloski, J.R., Hess, D.T., Stamler, J.S., 2001. Export by red cells of nitric oxide bioactivity. Nature 409, 622–626. (*Movement of NO from red blood cells via anion exchange protein AE1; see also editorial by Gross, S.S., pp. 577–578*)

Ribiero, J.M.C., Hazzard, J.M.H., Nussenzveig, R.H., et al., 1993. Reversible binding of nitric oxide by a salivary haem protein from a blood sucking insect. Science 260, 539–541. (*Action at a distance*)

Shaul, P.W., 2002. Regulation of endothelial nitric oxide synthase: location, location, location. Annu. Rev. Physiol. 64, 749–774.

Zhang, R., Hess, D.T., Reynolds, J.D., Stamler, J.S., 2015. Hemoglobin S-nitrosylation plays and essential role in cardioprotection. J. Clin. Invest. 126, 4654–4658. (*Cardiac injury and mortality were substantially increased in models of myocardial infarction and heart failure in mice lacking β-cys93 S-nitrosylation. See also accompanying commentary on the cardioprotective role of S-nitrosylated haemoglobin from red blood cells aby Piantadosi C.A. pp. 4402–4403*)

Physiological aspects

Coggins, M.P., Bloch, K.D., 2007. Nitric oxide in the pulmonary vasculature. Arterioscler. Thromb. Vasc. Biol. 27, 1877–1885.

Diesen, D.L., Hess, D.T., Stamler, J.S., 2008. Hypoxic vasodilation by red blood cells evidence for an S-nitrosothiol-based signal. Circ. Res. 103, 545–553. (*An S-nitrosothiol originating from RBCs mediates hypoxic vasodilatation by RBCs*)

Erusalimsky, J.D., Moncada, S., 2007. Nitric oxide and mitochondrial signalling from physiology to pathophysiology. Arterioscler. Thromb. Vasc. Biol. 27, 2524–2531. (*Reviews the evidence that binding of NO to cytochrome c oxidase elicits intracellular signalling events*)

Furchgott, R.F., Zawadzki, J.V., 1980. The obligatory role of endothelial cells in the relaxation of arterial smooth muscle by acetylcholine. Nature 288, 3734ess reClassic.

Garthwaite, J., 2008. Concepts of neural nitric oxide-mediated transmission. Eur. J. Neurosci. 27, 2783–2802. (*Diverse ways in which NO receptor activation initiates changes in neuronal excitability and synaptic strength by acting at pre- and/or postsynaptic locations*)

Ghimire, K., et al., 2017. Nitric oxide: what's new to NO? Am. J. Physiol. Cell Physiol. 312, C254–C262. (*Wide-ranging discussion including vessel wall remodeling. "In microvessels and particularly capillaries, NO, along with growth factors, is important in promoting new vessel formation, a process termed angiogenesis."*)

Kraehling, J.R., Sessa, W.C., 2017. Contemporary approaches to modulating the nitric oxide-cGMP pathway in cardiovascular disease. Circ. Res. 120, 1174–1182. (*Discusses remodeling of blood vessels and approaches to improve endothelial NO generation and bioavailability. Also discusses therapeutic opportunities aimed at activation of soluble guanylate cyclase*)

Nelson, R.J., Demas, G.E., Huang, P.L., et al., 1995. Behavioural abnormalities in male mice lacking neuronal nitric oxide synthase. Nature 378, 383–386. ('*A large increase in aggressive behaviour and excess, inappropriate sexual behaviour in nNOS knock-out mice*')

Seddon, M.D., Chowienczyk, P.J., Brett, S.E., et al., 2008. Neuronal nitric oxide synthase regulates basal microvascular tone in humans in vivo. Circulation 117, 1991–1996. (*Paradigm shift? – very possibly; see next reference*)

Seddon, M., Melikian, N., Dworakowski, R., et al., 2009. Effects of neuronal nitric oxide synthase on human coronary artery diameter and blood flow in vivo. Circulation 119, 2656–2662. (*Local nNOS-derived NO regulates basal blood flow in the human coronary vascular bed, whereas substance P-stimulated vasodilatation is NOS3 mediated*)

Straub, A.C., Lohman, A.W., Billaud, M., et al., 2012. Endothelial cell expression of haemoglobin α regulates nitric oxide signalling. Nature 491, 473–477. (*See also accompanying editorial Gladwyn, M.T., Kim-Shapiro, D.B., 2012. Nitric oxide caught in traffic. Nature 491, 344–345*)

Toda, N., Okamura, T., 2003. The pharmacology of nitric oxide in the peripheral nervous system of blood vessels. Pharmacol. Rev. 55, 271–324.

Vallance, P., Leiper, J., 2004. Cardiovascular biology of the asymmetric dimethylarginine:dimethylaminohydrolase pathway. Arterioscler. Thromb. Vasc. Biol. 24, 1023–1030.

Victor, V.M., Núñez, C., D'Ocón, P., et al., 2009. Regulation of oxygen distribution in tissues by endothelial nitric oxide. Circ. Res. 104, 1178–1183. (*Endogenously released endothelial NO inhibits cytochrome c oxidase and can modulate tissue O_2 consumption and regulates O_2 distribution to the surrounding tissues*)

Pathological aspects

Caplin, B., Leiper, J., 2012. Endogenous nitric oxide synthase inhibitors in the biology of disease: markers, mediators, and regulators? Arterioscler. Thromb. Vasc. Biol. 32, 1343–1353. (*Review outlining the basic biochemistry and physiology of endogenous methylarginines, examining their role in disease pathogenesis, and the potential for therapeutic regulation of these molecules*)

Ricciardolo, F.L.M., Sterk, P.J., Gaston, B., et al., 2004. Nitric oxide in health and disease of the respiratory system. Physiol. Rev. 84, 731–765.

Clinical and therapeutic aspects

Griffiths, M.J.D., Evans, T.W., 2005. Drug therapy: inhaled nitric oxide therapy in adults. N. Engl. J. Med. 353, 2683–2695. (*Concludes that, on the available evidence, inhaled NO is not effective in patients with acute lung injury, but that it may be useful as a short-term measure in acute hypoxia ± pulmonary hypertension*)

Lidder, S., Webb, A.J., 2013. Vascular effects of dietary nitrate (as found in green leafy vegetables and beetroot) via the nitrate–nitrite–nitric oxide pathway. Br. J. Clin. Pharmacol. 75, 677–696.

Lundberg, J.O., Gladwin, M.T., Weitzberg, E., 2015. Strategies to increase nitric oxide signalling in cardiovascular disease. Nat. Rev. Drug Discov. 14, 623–641. (*Discusses new pathways for enhancing NO synthase activity; ways to amplify the nitrate-nitrite-NO pathway; novel classes of NO-donating drugs; drugs that limit NO metabolism through effects on reactive oxygen species; and ways to modulate downstream phosphodiesterases and soluble guanylyl cyclises, focusing on cardiovascular disease*)

Malmström, R.E., Törnberg, D.C., Settergren, G., et al., 2003. Endogenous nitric oxide release by vasoactive drugs monitored in exhaled air. Am. J. Respir. Crit. Care Med. 168, 114–120. (*In humans, acetylcholine evokes a dose-dependent increase of NO in exhaled air; NO release by vasoactive agonists can be measured online in the exhaled air of pigs and humans*)

Miller, M.R., Megson, I.L., 2007. Review – Recent developments in nitric oxide donor drugs. Br. J. Pharmacol. 151, 305–321. (*Explores some of the more promising recent advances in NO donor drug development and challenges associated with NO as a therapeutic agent*)

Pawloski, J.R., Hess, D.T., Stamler, J.S., 2005. Impaired vasodilation by red blood cells in sickle cell disease. Proc. Natl. Acad. Sci. U.S.A. 102, 2531–2536. (*Sickle red cells are deficient in membrane S-nitrosothiol and impaired in their ability to mediate hypoxic vasodilation; the magnitudes of these impairments correlate with the clinical severity of disease*)

Carbon monoxide as possible mediator

Leffler, C.W., Parfenova, H., Jaggar, J.H., 2011. Carbon monoxide as an endogenous vascular modulator. Am. J. Physiol. 301, H1–H11.

Motterlini, R., Foresti, R., 2017. Biological signaling by carbon monoxide and carbon monoxide-releasing molecules. Am. J. Physiol. Cell Physiol. 312, C302–C313.

Wu, L., Wang, R., 2005. Carbon monoxide: endogenous production, physiological functions and pharmacological applications. Pharmacol. Rev. 57, 585–630.

Hydrogen sulfide as possible mediator

Elies, J., Scragg, J.L., Boyle, J.P., 2016. Regulation of the T-type Ca^{2+} channel Cav3.2 by hydrogen sulfide: emerging controversies concerning the role of H_2S in nociception. J. Physiol. (Lond.) 594, 4119–4129. (*Evidence that H_2S modulates low voltage-activated T-type Ca^{2+} channels, and discriminates between the different subtypes of T-type Ca^{2+} channel, selectively modulating Cav3.2, whilst Cav3.1 and Cav3.3 are unaffected*)

Li, L., Rose, P., Moore, P.K., 2011. Hydrogen sulfide and cell signaling. Annu. Rev. Pharmacol. Toxicol. 51, 169–187. (*H2S inhibits cytochrome c oxidase and reduces cell energy production; it also activates K-ATP, and transient receptor potential (TRP) channels but usually inhibits big conductance Ca^{2+}-sensitive K^+ (BKCa) channels, T- and M-type calcium channels. H_2S may inhibit or activate NF-kappa B nuclear translocation while affecting the activity of numerous kinases including p38 mitogen-activated protein kinase (p38 MAPK), extracellular signal-regulated kinase (ERK), and Akt*)

Reiffenstein, R.J., Hulbert, W.C., Roth, S.H., 1992. Toxicology of hydrogen sulfide. Annu. Rev. Pharmacol. Toxicol. 32, 109–134.

Szabo, C., 2007. Hydrogen sulphide and its therapeutic potential. Nat. Rev. Drug Discov. 6, 917–935.

The heart 22

OVERVIEW

This chapter presents an overview of cardiac function in terms of electrophysiology, contraction, oxygen consumption and coronary blood flow, autonomic control and natriuretic peptides as a basis for understanding effects of drugs on the heart and their place in treating cardiac disease. We concentrate on drugs that act directly on the heart, namely antidysrhythmic drugs and drugs that increase the force of contraction (especially digoxin), as well as anti-anginal drugs that act indirectly by reducing cardiac work. The commonest form of heart disease is caused by atheroma in the coronary arteries, complicated by thrombosis on ruptured atheromatous plaques; drugs to treat and prevent these are considered in Chapters 24 and 25. Heart failure is mainly treated by drugs that work indirectly on the heart via actions on vascular smooth muscle, discussed in Chapter 23, by diuretics (Ch. 30) and β-adrenoceptor antagonists (Ch. 15).

INTRODUCTION

In this chapter we consider effects of drugs on the heart under three main headings:

1. Rate and rhythm.
2. Myocardial contraction.
3. Metabolism and blood flow.

The effects of drugs on these aspects of cardiac function are not, of course, independent of each other. For example, if a drug affects the electrical properties of the myocardial cell membrane, it is likely to influence both cardiac rhythm and myocardial contraction. Similarly, a drug that affects contraction will inevitably alter metabolism and blood flow as well. Nevertheless, from a therapeutic point of view, these three classes of effect represent distinct clinical objectives in relation to the treatment, respectively, of cardiac dysrhythmias, cardiac failure and coronary insufficiency (as occurs during angina pectoris or myocardial infarction).

PHYSIOLOGY OF CARDIAC FUNCTION

CARDIAC RATE AND RHYTHM

The chambers of the heart normally contract in a coordinated manner, pumping blood efficiently by a route determined by the valves. Coordination of contraction is achieved by a specialised conducting system. Normal *sinus rhythm* is generated by pacemaker impulses that arise in the sinoatrial (SA) node and are conducted in sequence through the atria, the atrioventricular (AV) node, bundle of His, Purkinje

fibres and ventricles. Cardiac cells owe their electrical excitability to voltage-sensitive plasma membrane channels selective for various ions, including Na^+, K^+ and Ca^{2+}, the structure and function of which are described in Chapter 4. Electrophysiological features of cardiac muscle that distinguish it from other excitable tissues include:

- pacemaker activity
- absence of fast Na^+ current in SA and AV nodes, where slow inward Ca^{2+} current initiates action potentials
- long action potential ('plateau') and refractory period
- influx of Ca^{2+} during the plateau

Several of these special features of cardiac rhythm relate to Ca^{2+} currents. The heart contains *intracellular* calcium channels (i.e. ryanodine receptors and inositol trisphosphate-activated calcium channels described in Chapter 4, which are important in myocardial contraction) and voltage-dependent calcium channels in the plasma membrane, which are important in controlling cardiac rate and rhythm. The main type of voltage-dependent calcium channel in adult working myocardium is the L-type channel, which is also important in vascular smooth muscle; L-type channels are important in specialised conducting regions as well as in working myocardium.

The action potential of an idealised cardiac muscle cell is shown in Fig. 22.1A and is divided into five phases: 0 (fast depolarisation), 1 (partial repolarisation), 2 (plateau), 3 (repolarisation) and 4 (pacemaker).

▼ Ionic mechanisms underlying these phases can be summarised as follows.

Phase 0, rapid depolarisation, occurs when the membrane potential reaches a critical firing threshold (about –60 mV), at which the inward current of Na^+ flowing through the voltage-dependent sodium channels becomes large enough to produce a regenerative ('all-or-nothing') depolarisation. This mechanism is the same as that responsible for action potential generation in neurons (see Ch. 4). Activation of sodium channels by membrane depolarisation is transient, and if the membrane remains depolarised for more than a few milliseconds, they close again (inactivation). They are therefore closed during the plateau of the action potential and remain unavailable for the initiation of another action potential until the membrane repolarises.

Phase 1, partial repolarisation, occurs as the Na^+ current is inactivated. There may also be a transient voltage-sensitive outward current.

Phase 2, the plateau, results from an inward Ca^{2+} current. Calcium channels show a pattern of voltage-sensitive activation and inactivation qualitatively similar to sodium channels, but with a much slower time course. The plateau is assisted by a special property of the cardiac muscle membrane known as *inward-going rectification*, which means that the K^+ conductance falls to a low level when the membrane is depolarised. Because of this, there is little tendency for outward K^+ current to restore the resting membrane potential during the plateau, so a relatively small inward Ca^{2+} current suffices to maintain the plateau. A persistent sodium current (I_{Nap}) also contributes to the plateau; it is very small compared with the fast component of sodium current, but as it flows throughout the action potential it makes a substantial contribution to sodium loading during each cardiac cycle, and is a major contributor to ischaemic arrhythmias and a drug target (see p. 284).

Fig. 22.1 **The cardiac action potential.** (A) Phases of the action potential: *(0)* rapid depolarisation; *(1)* partial repolarisation; *(2)* plateau; *(3)* repolarisation; *(4)* pacemaker depolarisation. The lower panel shows the accompanying changes in membrane conductance for Na^+, K^+ and Ca^{2+}. (B) Conduction of the impulse through the heart, with the corresponding electrocardiogram (ECG) trace. Note that the longest delay occurs at the atrioventricular (AV) node, where the action potential has a characteristically slow waveform. *SA*, sinoatrial.

Phase 3, repolarisation, occurs as the Ca^{2+} current inactivates and a delayed outwardly rectifying K^+ current (analogous to, but much slower than, the K^+ current that causes repolarisation in nerve fibres; Ch. 4) activates, causing outward K^+ current. This is augmented by another K^+ current, which is activated by high intracellular Ca^{2+} concentrations, $[Ca^{2+}]_i$ during the plateau, and sometimes also by other K^+ currents, including one through channels activated by acetylcholine (see p. 277) and another that is activated by arachidonic acid, which is liberated under pathological conditions such as myocardial infarction.

Phase 4, the *pacemaker potential*, is a gradual depolarisation during diastole. Pacemaker activity is normally found only in nodal and conducting tissue. The pacemaker potential is caused by a combination of increasing inward currents and declining outward currents during diastole. It is usually most rapid in cells of the SA node, which therefore acts as pacemaker for the whole heart. Cells in the SA node have a greater background Na^+-conductance than do atrial or ventricular myocytes, leading to a greater background inward current. In addition, inactivation of voltage-dependent calcium channels wears off during diastole, resulting in increasing inward Ca^{2+} current during late diastole. Activation of T-type calcium channels during late diastole contributes to pacemaker activity in the SA node. The negative membrane potential early in diastole activates a cation channel that is permeable to Na^+ and K^+, giving rise to another inward current, called I_f.[1] An inhibitor of this current, **ivabradine**, slows the heart and is used therapeutically (see later). Several voltage- and time-dependent outward currents play a part as well: delayed rectifier K^+ current (I_K), which is activated during the action potential, is turned off by the negative membrane potential early in diastole. Current from the electrogenic Na^+/K^+ pump also contributes to the outward current during the pacemaker potential.

Fig. 22.1B shows the action potential configuration in different parts of the heart. Phase 0 is absent in the nodal regions, where the conduction velocity is correspondingly slow

(~5 cm/s) compared with other regions such as the Purkinje fibres (conduction velocity ~200 cm/s), which propagate the action potential rapidly to the ventricles. Regions that lack a fast inward current have a much longer refractory period than fast-conducting regions. This is because recovery of the slow inward current following its inactivation during the action potential takes a considerable time (a few hundred milliseconds), and the refractory period outlasts the action potential. With fast-conducting fibres, inactivation of the Na^+ current recovers rapidly, and the cell becomes excitable again almost as soon as it is repolarised.

The orderly pattern of sinus rhythm can be disrupted either by heart disease or by the action of drugs or circulating hormones, and an important therapeutic use of drugs is to restore a normal cardiac rhythm where it has become disturbed. The commonest cause of cardiac dysrhythmia is ischaemic heart disease, and many deaths following myocardial infarction result from *ventricular fibrillation* rather than directly from failure of the contractile machinery due to death of cardiac myocytes. Fibrillation is a state where heart chambers stop contracting in a coordinated way because the rhythm is replaced by chaotic electrical activity, causing rapid uncoordinated contractions within ventricles or atria that do not support cardiac output from the affected chambers.

DISTURBANCES OF CARDIAC RHYTHM

Clinically, dysrhythmias are classified according to:

- the site of origin of the abnormality – atrial, junctional or ventricular;
- whether the rate is increased (*tachycardia*) or decreased (*bradycardia*).

They may cause palpitations (awareness of the heartbeat) or symptoms from cerebral hypoperfusion (faintness or

---

[1] 'f' for 'funny', because it is unusual for cation channels to be activated by hyperpolarisation; cardiac electrophysiologists have a peculiar sense of humour!

loss of consciousness). Their diagnosis depends on the surface electrocardiogram (ECG), and details are beyond the scope of this book – see Opie and Gersh (2013). The commonest types of tachyarrhythmia are *atrial fibrillation*, where the heartbeat is completely irregular, and *supraventricular tachycardia* (SVT), where the heartbeat is rapid but regular. Occasional ectopic beats (ventricular as well as supraventricular) are common. Sustained ventricular tachyarrhythmias are much less common but more serious; they include *ventricular tachycardia*, and *ventricular fibrillation* where the electrical activity in the ventricles is completely chaotic and cardiac output ceases. Bradyarrhythmias include various kinds of *heart block* (e.g. at the AV or SA node) and complete cessation of electrical activity ('*asystolic arrest*'). It is often unclear which of the various mechanisms discussed below are responsible. These cellular mechanisms nevertheless provide a useful starting point for understanding how antidysrhythmic drugs work. Four basic phenomena underlie disturbances of cardiac rhythm:

1. Delayed after-depolarisation.
2. Re-entry.
3. Ectopic pacemaker activity.
4. Heart block.

The main cause of delayed after-depolarisation is abnormally raised $[Ca^{2+}]_i$, which triggers inward current and hence a train of abnormal action potentials (Fig. 22.2). After-depolarisation is the result of a net inward current, known as the transient inward current. A rise in $[Ca^{2+}]_i$ activates Na^+/Ca^{2+} exchange. This transfers one Ca^{2+} ion out of the cell in exchange for entry of three Na^+ ions, resulting in a net influx of one positive charge and hence membrane depolarisation. Raised $[Ca^{2+}]_i$ also contributes to the depolarisation by opening non-selective cation channels in the plasma membrane. Consequently, hypercalcaemia (which increases the entry of Ca^{2+}) promotes after-depolarisation. Hypokalaemia also influences repolarisation, via an effect on the gating of cardiac delayed rectifier potassium channels. Many drugs, including ones whose principal effects are on

other organs, delay cardiac repolarisation by binding to potassium or other cardiac channels or by influencing electrolyte concentrations (see Roden, 2008). Delayed repolarisation, evidenced by prolongation of the QT interval on the ECG, increases Ca^{2+} entry during the prolonged action potential, leading to after-depolarisation, which carries a risk of causing dangerous ventricular dysrhythmias. QT prolongation is a concern in drug development (see section on antidysrhythmic drugs, pp. 279–283, and see Ch. 60).

Normally, a cardiac action potential dies out after it has activated the ventricles because it is surrounded by refractory tissue, which it has just traversed. *Re-entry* (Fig. 22.3) describes a situation in which the impulse re-excites regions of the myocardium after the refractory period has subsided, causing continuous circulation of action potentials. It can result from anatomical anomalies or, more commonly, from myocardial damage. Re-entry underlies many types of dysrhythmia, the pattern depending on the site of the re-entrant circuit, which may be in the atria, ventricles or nodal tissue. A simple ring of tissue can give rise to a re-entrant rhythm if a transient or unidirectional conduction block is present. Normally, an impulse originating at any point in the ring will propagate in both directions and die out when the two impulses meet, but if a damaged area causes either a transient block (so that one impulse is blocked but the second can get through; see Fig. 22.3) or a unidirectional block, continuous circulation of the impulse can occur. This is known as *circus movement* and was demonstrated experimentally on rings of jellyfish tissue many years ago.

Although the physiological pacemaker resides in the SA node, other cardiac tissues can take on pacemaker activity. This provides a safety mechanism in the event of failure of the SA node but can also trigger tachyarrhythmias. Ectopic pacemaker activity is encouraged by sympathetic activity and by partial depolarisation, which may occur during ischaemia. Catecholamines, acting on β_1 adrenoceptors (see p. 276), increase the rate of depolarisation during phase 4 and can cause normally quiescent parts of the heart to take

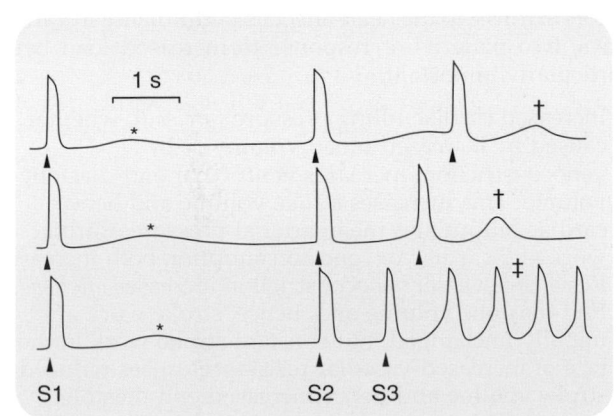

Fig. 22.2 **After-depolarisation in cardiac muscle recorded from a dog coronary sinus in the presence of noradrenaline (norepinephrine).** The first stimulus *(S1)* causes an action potential followed by a small after-depolarisation. As the interval *S2–S3* is decreased, the after-depolarisation gets larger *(†)* until it triggers an indefinite train of action potentials *(‡).* (Adapted from Wit, A.L., Cranefield, P.F., 1977. Circ. Res. 41, 435.)

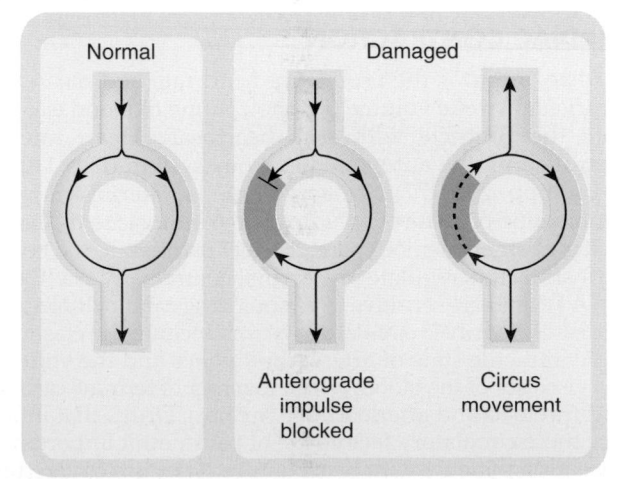

Fig. 22.3 **Generation of a re-entrant rhythm by a damaged area of myocardium.** The damaged area *(brown)* conducts in one direction only. This disturbs the normal pattern of conduction and permits continuous circulation of the impulse to occur.

on a spontaneous rhythm. Several tachyarrhythmias (e.g. paroxysmal atrial fibrillation) can be triggered by circumstances associated with increased sympathetic activity. Pain (e.g. during myocardial infarction) triggers sympathetic discharge and release of adrenaline (epinephrine) from the adrenal gland increasing myocardial excitability. Partial depolarisation resulting from ischaemic damage can also cause abnormal pacemaker activity.

Heart block results from fibrosis of, or ischaemic damage to, the conducting system (often in the AV node). In complete heart block, the atria and ventricles beat independently of one another, the ventricles beating at a slow rate determined by whatever pacemaker picks up distal to the block. Sporadic complete failure of AV conduction causes sudden periods of unconsciousness (Stokes–Adams attacks) and is treated by implanting an artificial pacemaker.

Cardiac dysrhythmias

- Dysrhythmias arise because of:
  - delayed after-depolarisation, which triggers ectopic beats
  - re-entry, resulting from partial conduction block
  - ectopic pacemaker activity
  - heart block.
- Delayed after-depolarisation is caused by an inward current associated with abnormally raised intracellular Ca^{2+}.
- Re-entry is facilitated when parts of the myocardium are depolarised as a result of disease.
- Ectopic pacemaker activity is encouraged by sympathetic activity.
- Heart block results from disease in the conducting system, especially the atrioventricular node.
- Clinically, dysrhythmias are divided:
  - according to their site of origin (supraventricular and ventricular)
  - according to whether the heart rate is increased or decreased (tachycardia or bradycardia).

CARDIAC CONTRACTION

Cardiac output is the product of heart rate and mean left ventricular stroke volume (i.e. the volume of blood ejected from the ventricle with each heartbeat). Heart rate is controlled by the autonomic nervous system (Chs 13–15, and see pp. 276–277). Stroke volume is determined by a combination of factors, including some intrinsic to the heart itself and other haemodynamic factors extrinsic to the heart. Intrinsic factors regulate myocardial contractility via $[Ca^{2+}]_i$ and ATP, and are sensitive to various drugs and pathological processes. Extrinsic circulatory factors include the elasticity and contractile state of arteries and veins, and the volume and viscosity of the blood, which together determine cardiac load (preload and afterload, see further). Drugs that influence these circulatory factors are of paramount importance in treating patients with heart failure. They are covered in Chapter 23.

MYOCARDIAL CONTRACTILITY AND VIABILITY

The contractile machinery of myocardial striated muscle is basically the same as that of voluntary striated muscle (Ch. 4). It involves binding of Ca^{2+} to troponin C; this changes the conformation of the troponin complex, permitting cross-bridging of myosin to actin and initiating contraction. **Levosimendan** (a drug used in some countries to treat acute decompensated heart failure; Ch. 23), increases the force of contraction of the heart by binding troponin C and sensitising it to the action of Ca^{2+}.

▼ Many effects of drugs on cardiac contractility can be explained in terms of actions on $[Ca^{2+}]_i$, via effects on calcium channels in plasma membrane or sarcoplasmic reticulum, or on the Na^+/K^+ pump, which indirectly influences the Na^+/Ca^{2+} pump (see p. 283). Other factors that affect the force of contraction are the availability of oxygen and a source of metabolic energy such as free fatty acids. Myocardial *stunning* – contractile dysfunction that persists after ischaemia and reperfusion despite restoration of blood flow and absence of cardiac necrosis – is incompletely understood but can be clinically important. Its converse is known as *ischaemic preconditioning*; this refers to an improved ability to withstand ischaemia following previous ischaemic episodes. This potentially beneficial state could be clinically important. There is some evidence that it is mediated by *adenosine* (see Ch. 17), which accumulates as ATP is depleted. Exogenous adenosine affords protection similar to that caused by ischaemic preconditioning, and blockade of adenosine receptors prevents the protective effect of preconditioning (see Eltzschig et al., 2012). There is considerable interest in developing strategies to minimise harmful effects of ischaemia while maximising preconditioning, but clinical trials have so far been negative and translation into therapeutics is fraught with difficulty (Heusch, 2017).

VENTRICULAR FUNCTION CURVES AND HEART FAILURE

The force of contraction of the heart is determined partly by its intrinsic contractility (which, as described above, depends on $[Ca^{2+}]_i$ and availability of ATP), and partly by extrinsic haemodynamic factors that affect end-diastolic volume and hence the resting length of the muscle fibres. The end-diastolic volume is determined by the end-diastolic pressure, and its effect on stroke work is expressed in the Frank–Starling law of the heart, which reflects an inherent property of the contractile system. The Frank–Starling law can be represented as a ventricular function curve (Fig. 22.4). The area enclosed by the pressure–volume curve during the cardiac cycle provides a measure of ventricular stroke work. It is approximated by the product of stroke volume and mean arterial pressure. As Starling showed, factors extrinsic to the heart affect its performance in various ways, two patterns of response to increased load being particularly important:

1. Increased cardiac filling pressure (*preload*), whether caused by increased blood volume or by venoconstriction, increases ventricular end-diastolic volume. This increases stroke volume and hence cardiac output and mean arterial pressure. Cardiac work and cardiac oxygen consumption both increase.
2. Resistance vessel vasoconstriction increases *afterload*. End-diastolic volume and, hence, stroke work are initially unchanged, but constant stroke work in the face of increased vascular resistance causes reduced stroke volume and hence increased end-diastolic volume. This in turn increases stroke work, until a steady state is re-established with increased end-diastolic volume and the same cardiac output as before. As with increased preload, cardiac work and cardiac oxygen consumption both increase.

Normal ventricular filling pressure is only a few centimetres of water, on the steep part of the ventricular function curve, so a large increase in stroke work can be achieved with

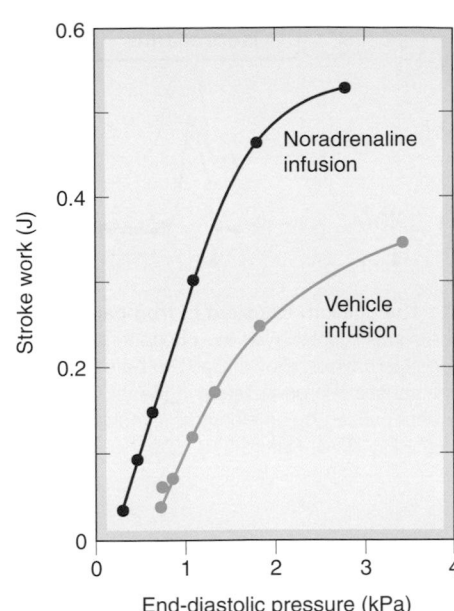

Fig. 22.4 Ventricular function curves in the dog. Infusion of physiological saline increases blood volume and hence end-diastolic pressure. This increases stroke work ('extrinsic' control) by increasing the force of contraction of the heart. This relationship is called the Starling curve. Noradrenaline has a direct action on the heart ('intrinsic' control), increasing the slope of the Starling curve. (Redrawn from Sarnoff, S.J. et al., 1960. Circ. Res. 8, 1108.)

Myocardial contraction

- Controlling factors are:
  - intrinsic myocardial contractility
  - extrinsic circulatory factors.
- Myocardial contractility depends critically on intracellular Ca^{2+}, and hence on:
  - Ca^{2+} entry across the cell membrane
  - Ca^{2+} storage in the sarcoplasmic reticulum.
- The main factors controlling Ca^{2+} entry are:
  - activity of voltage-gated calcium channels
  - intracellular Na^+, which affects Ca^{2+}/Na^+ exchange.
- Catecholamines, cardiac glycosides and other mediators and drugs influence these factors.
- Extrinsic control of cardiac contraction is through the dependence of stroke work on the end-diastolic volume, expressed in the Frank–Starling law.
- Cardiac work is affected independently by afterload (i.e. peripheral resistance and arterial compliance) and preload (i.e. central venous pressure).

only a small increase in filling pressure. The Starling mechanism plays little part in controlling cardiac output in healthy subjects (e.g. during exercise), because changes in contractility, mainly as a result of changes in sympathetic nervous activity, achieve the necessary regulation without any increase in ventricular filling pressure (see Fig. 22.4). In contrast, the denervated heart in patients who have received a heart transplant relies on the Starling mechanism to increase cardiac output during exercise.

In heart failure, the cardiac output is insufficient to meet the needs of the body, initially only when these are increased during exercise but ultimately, as disease progresses, also at rest. It has many causes, most commonly ischaemic heart disease. In patients with heart failure (see Ch. 23), the heart may be unable to deliver as much blood as the tissues require, even when its contractility is increased by sympathetic activity. Under these conditions, the basal (i.e. at rest) ventricular function curve is greatly depressed, and there is insufficient reserve, in the sense of extra contractility that can be achieved by sympathetic activity, to enable cardiac output to be maintained during exercise without a large increase in central venous pressure (see Fig. 22.4). Oedema of peripheral tissues (causing swelling of the legs) and the lungs (causing breathlessness) is an important consequence of cardiac failure. It is caused by the increased venous pressure, and retention of Na^+ (see Ch. 23).

MYOCARDIAL OXYGEN CONSUMPTION AND CORONARY BLOOD FLOW

Relative to its large metabolic needs, the heart is one of the most poorly perfused tissues in the body, and is therefore at greater risk of ischaemic damage. Coronary flow is, under normal circumstances, closely related to myocardial oxygen consumption, and both change over a nearly 10-fold range between conditions of rest and maximal exercise. Most drugs that influence cardiac metabolism do so indirectly by influencing coronary blood flow.[2]

PHYSIOLOGICAL FACTORS

The main physiological factors that regulate coronary flow are:

- physical factors
- vascular control by metabolites
- neural and humoral control

Physical factors

During systole, the pressure exerted by the myocardium on vessels that pass through it equals or exceeds the perfusion pressure, so coronary flow occurs only during diastole. Diastole is shortened more than systole during tachycardia, reducing the period available for myocardial perfusion. During diastole, the effective perfusion pressure is equal to the difference between the aortic and ventricular pressures (Fig. 22.5). If diastolic aortic pressure falls or diastolic ventricular pressure increases, perfusion pressure falls and so (unless other control mechanisms can compensate) does coronary blood flow. Stenosis of the aortic valve reduces aortic pressure but increases left ventricular pressure upstream of the narrowed valve and hence reducing coronary perfusion pressure and often causes ischaemic chest pain (angina), even in the absence of coronary artery disease, by this mechanism.

Vascular control by metabolites/mediators

Vascular control by metabolites is the most important mechanism by which coronary flow is regulated. A reduction

---

[2]**Trimetazidine,** used to treat angina in some European countries, is claimed to improve cardiac metabolism by blocking fatty acid oxidation, thereby increasing the use of glucose as an energy source, which requires less oxygen per unit of energy generated.

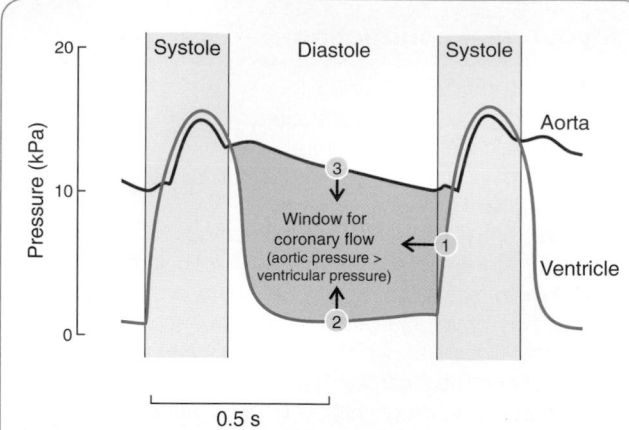

Fig. 22.5 Mechanical factors affecting coronary blood flow. The 'window' for coronary flow may be encroached on by: *(1)* shortening diastole, when heart rate increases; *(2)* increased ventricular end-diastolic pressure and *(3)* reduced diastolic arterial pressure.

Fig. 22.6 The calcium transient in frog cardiac muscle. A group of cells was injected with the phosphorescent Ca^{2+} indicator aequorin, which allows $[Ca^{2+}]_i$ to be monitored optically. Isoprenaline causes a large increase in the tension and in the $[Ca^{2+}]_i$ transient caused by an electrical stimulus (▲). (From Allen, D.G., Blinks, J.R., 1978. Nature 273, 509.)

in arterial partial pressure of oxygen (PO_2) causes marked vasodilatation of coronary vessels in situ but has little effect on isolated strips of coronary artery, suggesting that it is a change in the metabolites produced by the myocardial cells, rather than the change in PO_2 per se, that controls the state of the coronary vessels. *Adenosine* is a popular candidate for the dilator metabolite (see Ch. 17).

Neural and humoral control

Coronary vessels have a dense sympathetic innervation, but sympathetic nerves (like circulating catecholamines) exert only a small direct effect on the coronary circulation. Large coronary vessels possess α adrenoceptors that mediate vasoconstriction, whereas smaller vessels have $β_2$ adrenoceptors that have a dilator effect. Coronary vessels are also innervated by purinergic, peptidergic and nitrergic nerves, and basal coronary blood flow in patients with angiographically normal coronary arteries is reduced by about one-third by selective inhibition of NOS1 (Seddon et al., 2009). Coronary vascular responses to altered mechanical and metabolic activity during exercise or pathological events overshadow neural and endocrine effects.

AUTONOMIC CONTROL OF THE HEART

The sympathetic and parasympathetic systems (see Chs 13–15) each exert a tonic effect on the heart at rest and influence each of the aspects of cardiac function discussed above, namely rate and rhythm, myocardial contraction, and myocardial metabolism and blood flow.

SYMPATHETIC SYSTEM

The main effects of sympathetic activity on the heart are:

- increased force of contraction (positive *inotropic* effect; Fig. 22.6);
- increased heart rate (positive *chronotropic* effect; Fig. 22.7);
- increased *automaticity* (i.e. tendency to generate ectopic beats);

Coronary flow, ischaemia and infarction

- The heart has a smaller blood supply in relation to its oxygen consumption than most organs.
- Coronary flow is controlled mainly by:
  - physical factors, including transmural pressure during systole
  - vasodilator metabolites.
- Autonomic innervation is less important.
- Coronary ischaemia is usually the result of atherosclerosis and causes angina. Sudden ischaemia is usually caused by thrombosis and may result in cardiac infarction (death of a region of the myocardium).
- Coronary spasm sometimes causes angina (variant angina).
- Cellular Ca^{2+} overload results from ischaemia and may be responsible for:
  - cell death
  - dysrhythmias.

- repolarisation and *restoration of function* following generalised cardiac depolarisation
- reduced cardiac *efficiency* (i.e. oxygen consumption is increased more than cardiac work);
- cardiac hypertrophy (which seems to be directly mediated by stimulation of myocardial α and β adrenoceptors rather than by haemodynamic changes).

▼ These effects mainly result from activation of $β_1$ adrenoceptors. The $β_1$ effects of catecholamines on the heart, although complex, probably all occur through activation of adenylyl cyclase resulting in increased intracellular cAMP (see Ch. 3). cAMP activates protein kinase A, which phosphorylates sites on the $α_1$ subunits of calcium channels. This increases the probability that the channels will open, increasing inward Ca^{2+} current and hence force of cardiac contraction (see Fig. 22.6). Activation of $β_1$ adrenoceptors also increases the Ca^{2+} sensitivity of the contractile machinery, possibly by phosphorylating troponin C; furthermore, it facilitates Ca^{2+} capture by the sarcoplasmic reticulum, thereby increasing the amount of Ca^{2+} available for release

Fig. 22.7 Autonomic regulation of the heartbeat. (A) and (B) Effects of sympathetic stimulation and noradrenaline (NA). (C and D) Effects of parasympathetic stimulation and acetylcholine (ACh). Sympathetic stimulation (A) increases the slope of the pacemaker potential and increases heart rate, whereas parasympathetic stimulation (C) abolishes the pacemaker potential, hyperpolarises the membrane and temporarily stops the heart (frog sinus venosus). NA (B) prolongs the action potential, while ACh (D) shortens it (frog atrium). ([A] and [C] from Hutter, O.F., Trautwein, W., 1956. J. Gen. Physiol. 39, 715; [B] from Reuter, H., 1974. J. Physiol. 242, 429; [D] from Giles, W.R., Noble, S.J., 1976. J. Physiol. 261, 103.)

by the action potential. The net result of catecholamine action is to elevate and steepen the ventricular function curve (see Fig. 22.4). The increase in heart rate results from an increased slope of the pacemaker potential (see Figs 22.1 and 22.7A). Increased Ca^{2+} entry also increases automaticity because of the effect of $[Ca^{2+}]_i$ on the transient inward current, which can result in a train of action potentials following a single stimulus (see Fig. 22.2).

Activation of β_1 adrenoceptors repolarises damaged or hypoxic myocardium by stimulating the Na^+/K^+ pump. This can restore function if asystole has occurred following myocardial infarction, and **adrenaline** is one of the most important drugs used during cardiac arrest.

The reduction of cardiac efficiency by catecholamines is important because it means that the oxygen requirement of the myocardium increases. This limits the use of β agonists such as adrenaline and **dobutamine** for circulatory shock (Ch. 23). Myocardial infarction activates the sympathetic nervous system (see Fig. 22.8), which has the undesirable effect of increasing the oxygen needs of the damaged myocardium.

PARASYMPATHETIC SYSTEM

Parasympathetic activity produces effects that are, in general, opposite to those of sympathetic activation. However, in contrast to sympathetic activity, the parasympathetic nervous system has little effect on contractility, its main effects being on rate and rhythm, namely:

- cardiac slowing and reduced automaticity
- inhibition of AV conduction

▼ These effects result from activation of muscarinic (M_2) acetylcholine receptors, which are abundant in nodal and atrial tissue but spares in the ventricles. These receptors are negatively coupled to adenylyl

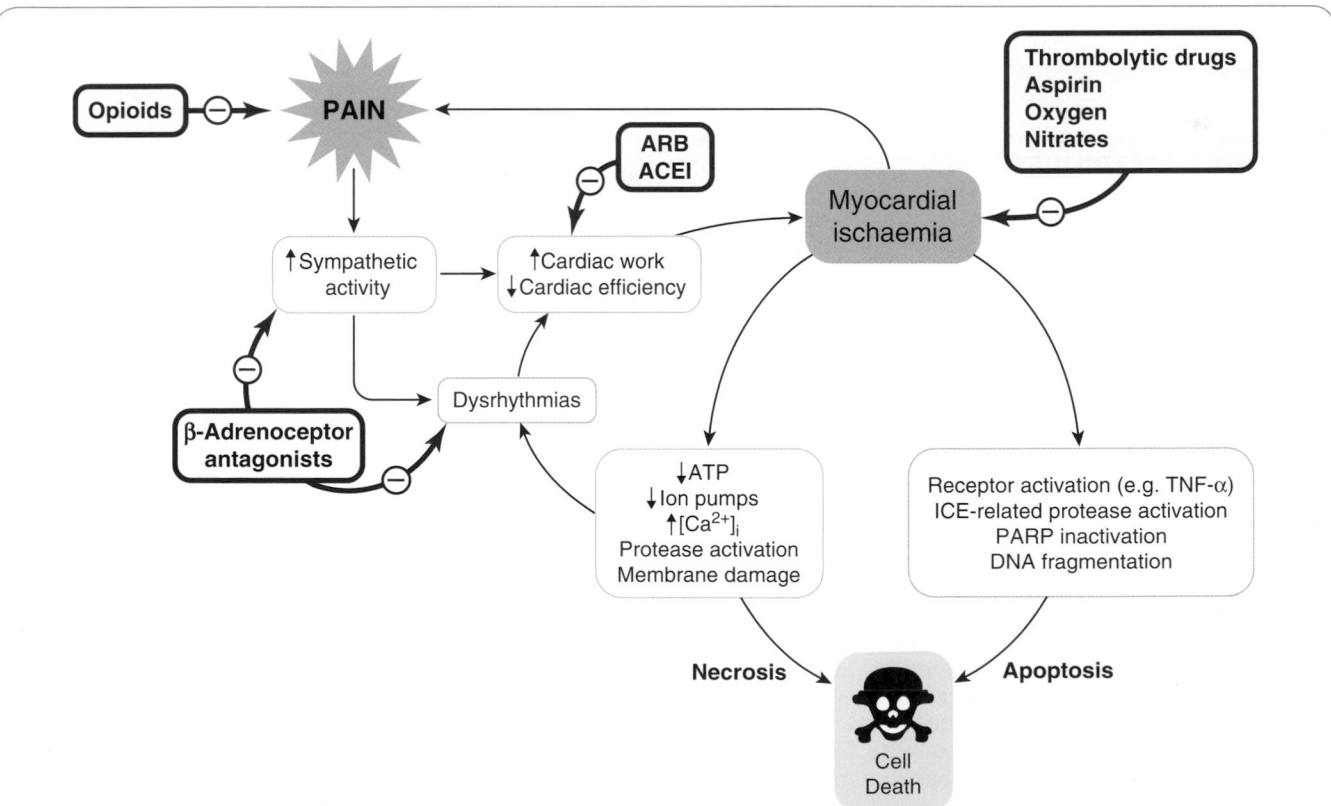

Fig. 22.8 Effects of myocardial ischaemia. This leads to cell death by one of two pathways: necrosis or apoptosis. *ACEI*, angiotensin-converting enzyme inhibitor; *ARB*, angiotensin AT₁ receptor antagonist; *ICE*, interleukin-1-converting enzyme; *PARP*, poly-[ADP-ribose]-polymerase; *TNF-α*, tumour necrosis factor-α.

cyclase and thus reduce cAMP formation, acting to inhibit the opening of L-type Ca^{2+} channels and reduce the slow Ca^{2+} current, in opposition to β_1 adrenoceptors. M_2 receptors also open a type of K^+ channel known as GIRK (G protein–activated inward rectifying K^+ channel) via production of G β/γ subunits (see Ch. 3). The resulting increase in K^+ permeability produces a hyperpolarising current that opposes the inward pacemaker current, slowing the heart and reducing automaticity (see Fig. 22.7C). Vagal activity is often increased during myocardial infarction, both in association with vagal afferent stimulation and as a side effect of opioids used to control the pain, and parasympathetic effects are important in predisposing to acute dysrhythmias.

Vagal stimulation decreases the force of contraction of the atria associated with marked shortening of the action potential (see Fig. 22.7D). Increased K^+ permeability and reduced Ca^{2+} current both contribute to conduction block at the AV node, where propagation depends on the Ca^{2+} current. Shortening the atrial action potential reduces the refractory period, which can lead to re-entrant arrhythmias. Coronary vessels lack cholinergic innervation; consequently, the parasympathetic nervous system has little effect on coronary artery tone (see Ch. 14).

Autonomic control of the heart

- Sympathetic activity, acting through β_1 adrenoceptors, increases heart rate, contractility and automaticity, but reduces cardiac efficiency (in relation to oxygen consumption).
- The β_1 adrenoceptors act by increasing cAMP formation, which increases Ca^{2+} currents.
- Parasympathetic activity, acting through muscarinic M_2 receptors, causes cardiac slowing, decreased force of contraction (atria only) and inhibition of atrioventricular conduction.
- M_2 receptors inhibit cAMP formation and also open potassium channels, causing hyperpolarisation.

CARDIAC NATRIURETIC PEPTIDES

Cardiac natriuretic peptides are an important family of mediators (see Potter et al., 2009, for a review). Atrial cells contain secretory granules, and store and release *atrial natriuretic peptide* (ANP). This has powerful effects on the kidney and vascular system. Release of ANP occurs during volume overload in response to stretching of the atria, and intravenous saline infusion is sufficient to stimulate its release. B-natriuretic peptide (BNP) is released from ventricular muscle and opposes ventricular fibrosis; its plasma concentration is increased in patients with heart failure and this (or the concentration of its precursor, N-terminal pro-BNP) is used as an aid to diagnosis. C-natriuretic peptide (CNP) is stored in endothelium and, in addition to vascular actions, influences the development of long bones. Both ANP and BNP are inactivated by neprilysin, also known as neutral endopeptidase (NEP) (see Ch. 23).

The main effects of natriuretic peptides are to increase Na^+ and water excretion by the kidney; relax vascular smooth muscle (except efferent arterioles of renal glomeruli; see below); increase vascular permeability; and inhibit the release and/or actions of several vasoconstrictor or salt-retaining hormones and mediators, including aldosterone, angiotensin II, endothelin and antidiuretic hormone. They exert their effects by combining with membrane receptors (natriuretic peptide receptors, NPRs, which exist in at least two subtypes, designated A and B).[3]

▼ Both NPR-A and NPR-B incorporate a catalytic guanylyl cyclase moiety (see Ch. 3), and, when activated, increase intracellular cGMP. Organic nitrates (discussed later) and endogenous nitric oxide (Ch. 21) also increase cGMP, though they interact with soluble rather than membrane-bound guanylyl cyclase. Renal glomerular afferent arterioles are dilated by ANP but efferent arterioles are constricted, so filtration pressure is increased, leading to increased glomerular filtration and enhanced Na^+ excretion. Elsewhere in the vasculature, natriuretic peptides cause vasorelaxation and reduce blood pressure. Recombinant BNP (**nesiritide**) had a yo-yo ride as a potential therapy for acute heart failure. After initial regulatory rejection, it was approved in 2001 by the US FDA. However, in 2011 a large study showed that it did not increase life expectancy or improve symptoms requiring re-hospitalisation in such acutely ill patients (O'Connor et al., 2011). This line of investigation took a happier turn when it was found that **sacubitril**, an inhibitor of neprilysin (see earlier), increases circulating BNP and ANP and, in fixed combination with **valsartan**, is effective in treating *chronic* heart failure (see Ch.23).

ISCHAEMIC HEART DISEASE

Atheromatous deposits are ubiquitous in the coronary arteries of adults living in developed countries. They are asymptomatic for most of the natural history of the disease (see Ch. 24), but can progress insidiously, culminating in acute myocardial infarction and its complications, including dysrhythmia and heart failure. Details of ischaemic heart disease are beyond the scope of this book, and excellent accounts (e.g. Mann et al., 2014) are available for those seeking pathological and clinical information. Here, we merely set the scene for understanding the place of drugs that affect cardiac function in treating this most common form of heart disease.

Important consequences of coronary atherosclerosis include:

- angina (chest pain caused by cardiac ischaemia)
- myocardial infarction

ANGINA

Angina occurs when the oxygen supply to the myocardium is insufficient for its needs. The pain has a characteristic distribution in the chest, arm and neck, and is brought on by exertion, cold or excitement. A similar type of pain occurs in skeletal muscle when it is made to contract while its blood supply is interrupted, and Lewis showed many years ago that chemical factors released by ischaemic muscle are responsible. Possible candidates include K^+, H^+ and adenosine (Ch. 17), all of which sensitise or stimulate nociceptors (see Ch. 43). It is possible that the same mediator that causes coronary vasodilatation is responsible, at higher concentration, for initiating pain.

Three kinds of angina are recognised clinically: stable, unstable and variant.

Stable angina. This is predictable chest pain on exertion. It is produced by an increased demand on the heart and is usually caused by fixed narrowing(s) of the coronary vessels

---

[3]The nomenclature of natriuretic peptides and their receptors is peculiarly obtuse. The peptides are named 'A' for atrial, 'B' for brain – despite being present mainly in cardiac ventricle – and 'C' for A, B, C …; NPRs are named NPR-A, which preferentially binds ANP; NPR-B, which binds CNP preferentially; and NPR-C for 'clearance' receptor, because until recently clearance via cellular uptake and degradation by lysosomal enzymes was the only definite known function of this binding site.

by atheroma, although, as explained above, narrowing of the aortic valve ('aortic stenosis') can cause angina by reducing coronary blood flow even in the absence of coronary artery narrowing. Symptomatic therapy is directed at reducing cardiac work with organic nitrates, β-adrenoceptor antagonists and/or calcium antagonists, together with treatment of the underlying atheromatous disease, usually including a statin (Ch. 24), and prophylaxis against thrombosis with an antiplatelet drug, such as **aspirin** (Ch. 25).

Unstable angina. This is characterised by pain that occurs with less and less exertion, culminating in pain at rest. The pathology is similar to that involved in myocardial infarction, namely platelet–fibrin thrombus associated with a ruptured atheromatous plaque, but without complete occlusion of the vessel. Treatment is similar to that for myocardial infarction and includes imaging and consideration of revascularisation procedures. Antiplatelet drugs (aspirin and/or an ADP antagonist such as **clopidogrel** or **prasugrel**, see Ch. 17) reduce the risk of myocardial infarction in this setting, and antithrombotic drugs add to this benefit (Ch. 25) at the cost of increased risk of haemorrhage. Organic nitrates (see later) are used to relieve ischaemic pain.

Variant angina. This is relatively uncommon. It can occur at rest and is caused by coronary artery spasm, often in association with atheromatous disease. Therapy is with coronary artery vasodilators (e.g. organic nitrates, calcium antagonists).

MYOCARDIAL INFARCTION

Myocardial infarction occurs when a coronary artery has been blocked by thrombus. This may be fatal and is a common cause of death, usually as a result of mechanical failure of the ventricle or from dysrhythmia. Cardiac myocytes rely on aerobic metabolism. If the supply of oxygen remains below a critical value, a sequence of events leading to cell death ensues, detected clinically by an elevation of circulating *troponin* (a biochemical marker of myocardial injury) as well as of cardiac enzymes (e.g. the cardiac isoform of creatinine kinase) and changes in the surface ECG. The sequences leading from vascular occlusion to cell death via necrosis or apoptosis (see Ch. 6) are illustrated in Fig. 22.8. The relative importance of these two pathways in causing myocardial cell death is unknown, but apoptosis may be an adaptive process in hypoperfused regions, sacrificing some jeopardised myocytes and thereby avoiding the disturbance of membrane function and risk of dysrhythmia inherent in necrosis. Consequently, it is currently unknown if pharmacological approaches to promote or inhibit this pathway could be clinically beneficial.

Prevention of irreversible ischaemic damage[4] following an episode of coronary thrombosis is crucial. Opening the occluded artery must be achieved as fast as possible. If logistically possible, *angioplasty* (performed using a catheter with an inflatable balloon near its tip, with administration of a glycoprotein IIb/IIIa antagonist – see Chapter 25 – to prevent reocclusion) is somewhat more effective than thrombolytic drugs, which are an effective alternative if angioplasty is unavailable. The main therapeutic drugs for myocardial infarction (see Fig. 22.8) include drugs to improve

cardiac function by maintaining oxygenation and reducing cardiac work, as well as treating pain and preventing further thrombosis. They are used in combination, and include:

- combinations of thrombolytic, antiplatelet (aspirin and clopidogrel) and antithrombotic (a heparin preparation) drugs to open the blocked artery and prevent reocclusion (see Ch. 25)
- oxygen if there is arterial hypoxia;
- opioids (given with an antiemetic) to prevent pain and reduce excessive sympathetic activity;
- organic nitrate;
- β-adrenoceptor antagonists;
- angiotensin-converting enzyme inhibitors (ACEIs) or angiotensin AT$_1$ receptor antagonists (ARBs; see Ch. 23).

β-Adrenoceptor antagonists reduce cardiac work and thereby the metabolic needs of the heart, and are used as soon as the patient is stable. ACEIs and ARBs also reduce cardiac work and improve survival, as does opening the coronary artery (with angioplasty or thrombolytic drug) and antiplatelet treatment.

DRUGS THAT AFFECT CARDIAC FUNCTION

Drugs that have a major action on the heart can be divided into three groups.

1. *Drugs that affect myocardial cells directly.* These include:
   a. autonomic neurotransmitters and related drugs
   b. antidysrhythmic drugs
   c. cardiac glycosides and other inotropic drugs
   d. miscellaneous drugs and hormones; these are dealt with elsewhere (e.g. **doxorubicin**, Ch. 57; thyroxine, Ch. 35; glucagon, Ch. 32)
2. *Drugs that affect cardiac function indirectly.* These have actions elsewhere in the vascular system. Some anti-anginal drugs (e.g. nitrates) fall into this category, as do many drugs that are used to treat heart failure (e.g. diuretics and ACEIs).
3. *Calcium antagonists.* These affect cardiac function by a direct action on myocardial cells and also indirectly by relaxing vascular smooth muscle.

ANTIDYSRHYTHMIC DRUGS

A classification of antidysrhythmic drugs based on their electrophysiological effects was proposed by Vaughan Williams in 1970 (Table 22.1). It provides a good starting point for discussing mechanisms, although many useful drugs do not fit neatly into this classification (Table 22.2). Furthermore, emergency treatment of serious dysrhythmias is usually by physical means (e.g. pacing or electrical cardioversion by applying a direct current shock to the chest or via an implanted device) rather than drugs.

There are four classes (see Table 22.1).

- Class I: drugs that block voltage-sensitive sodium channels. They are subdivided: Ia, Ib and Ic.
- Class II: β-adrenoceptor antagonists.
- Class III: drugs that substantially prolong the cardiac action potential.
- Class IV: calcium antagonists.

The phase of the action potential on which each of these classes of drug have their main effect is shown in Fig. 22.9.

---

[4]'Irreversible' by present technologies; cell therapies based on cardiac stem cells have been attempted therapeutically, and are a beacon of hope for the future.

Table 22.1   Summary of antidysrhythmic drugs (Vaughan Williams classification)

Class	Example(s)	Mechanism
Ia	Disopyramide	Sodium-channel block (intermediate dissociation)
Ib	Lidocaine	Sodium-channel block (fast dissociation)
Ic	Flecainide	Sodium-channel block (slow dissociation)
II	Propranolol	β-Adrenoceptor antagonism
III	Amiodarone, sotalol	Potassium-channel block
IV	Verapamil	Calcium-channel block

Table 22.2   Antidysrhythmic drugs unclassified in the Vaughan Williams system

Drug	Use
Atropine	Sinus bradycardia
Adrenaline (epinephrine)	Cardiac arrest
Isoprenaline	Heart block
Digoxin	Rapid atrial fibrillation
Adenosine	Supraventricular tachycardia
Calcium chloride	Ventricular tachycardia due to hyperkalaemia
Magnesium chloride	Ventricular fibrillation, digoxin toxicity

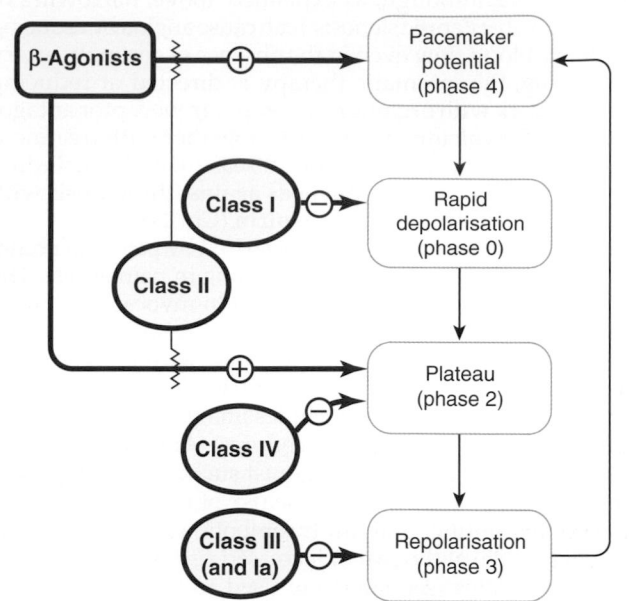

Fig. 22.9   Effects of antidysrhythmic drugs on the different phases (as defined in Fig. 22.1) of the cardiac action potential.

MECHANISMS OF ACTION

Class I drugs

Class I drugs block sodium channels, just as local anaesthetics do, by binding to sites on the α subunit (see Chs 4 and 44). Because this inhibits action potential propagation in many excitable cells, it has been referred to as a 'membrane-stabilising' activity, a phrase best avoided now that the ionic mechanism is understood. The characteristic effect on the action potential is to reduce the maximum rate of depolarisation during phase 0.

▼ The reason for further subdivision of these drugs into classes Ia, Ib and Ic is that the earliest examples, **quinidine** and **procainamide** (class Ia), have different effects from many of the more recently developed drugs, even though all share the same basic mechanism of action. A partial explanation for these functional differences comes from electrophysiological studies of the characteristics of the sodium-channel block produced by different class I drugs.

The central concept is of *use-dependent channel block*. It is this characteristic that enables all class I drugs to block the high-frequency excitation of the myocardium that occurs in tachyarrhythmias, without preventing the heart from beating at normal frequencies. Sodium channels exist in three distinct functional states: resting, open and inactivated (see Ch. 4). Channels switch rapidly from resting to open in response to depolarisation; this is known as *activation*. Maintained

depolarisation, as in ischaemic muscle, causes channels to change more slowly from open to inactivated, and the membrane, which is then refractory, must then be repolarised for a time to restore the channel to the resting state before it can be activated again. Class I drugs bind to channels most strongly when they are in either the open or the inactivated state, less strongly to channels in the resting state. Their action therefore shows the property of 'use dependence' (i.e. the more frequently the channels are activated, the greater the degree of block produced).

Class Ib drugs, for example, **lidocaine**, associate and dissociate rapidly within the timeframe of the normal heartbeat. The drug binds to open channels during phase 0 of the action potential (affecting the rate of rise very little, but leaving many of the channels blocked by the time the action potential reaches its peak). Dissociation occurs in time for the next action potential, provided the cardiac rhythm is normal. A premature beat, however, will be aborted because the channels are still blocked. Furthermore, class Ib drugs bind selectively to inactivated channels and thus block preferentially when the cells are depolarised, for example, in ischaemia.

Class Ic drugs, such as **flecainide** and **encainide**, associate and dissociate much more slowly, thus reaching a steady-state level of block that does not vary appreciably during the cardiac cycle. They markedly inhibit conduction through the His–Purkinje system.

Class Ia, the oldest group (e.g. **quinidine**, **procainamide**, **disopyramide**), lies midway in its properties between Ib and Ic but, in addition, prolongs repolarisation, albeit less markedly than class III drugs (see later).

Class II drugs

Class II drugs comprise the β-adrenoceptor antagonists (e.g. **metoprolol**).

Adrenaline can cause dysrhythmias by its effects on the pacemaker potential and on the slow inward Ca^{2+} current (see pp. 276–277). Ventricular dysrhythmias following myocardial infarction are partly the result of increased sympathetic activity (see Fig. 22.8), providing a rationale for using β-adrenoceptor antagonists in this setting. AV conduction depends critically on sympathetic activity; β-adrenoceptor antagonists increase the refractory period of the AV node and can therefore prevent recurrent attacks of SVT. The β-adrenoceptor antagonists are also used to prevent paroxysmal attacks of atrial fibrillation when these occur in the setting of sympathetic activation.

Class III drugs

The class III category was originally based on the unusual behaviour of a single drug, **amiodarone** (see p. 282), although others with similar properties (e.g. **sotalol**) have since been described. Both amiodarone and sotalol have more than one mechanism of antidysrhythmic action. The special feature that defines them as class III drugs is that they substantially prolong the cardiac action potential. The mechanism of this effect is not fully understood, but it involves blocking some of the potassium channels involved in cardiac repolarisation, including the outward (delayed) rectifier. Action potential prolongation increases the refractory period, accounting for powerful and varied antidysrhythmic activity, for example, by interrupting re-entrant tachycardias and suppressing ectopic activity. However, drugs that prolong the cardiac action potential (detected clinically as prolonged QT interval on the ECG; see earlier) can paradoxically also have *proarrhythmic* effects, notably a polymorphic form of ventricular tachycardia called (somewhat whimsically) *torsade de pointes* (because the appearance of the ECG trace is said to be reminiscent of this ballet sequence). This occurs particularly in patients taking other drugs that can prolong QT, including several antipsychotic drugs; those with disturbances of electrolytes involved in repolarisation (e.g. hypokalaemia, hypercalcaemia); or individuals with hereditary prolonged QT (Ward–Romano syndrome).[5] The mechanism of the dysrhythmia is not fully understood; possibilities include increased dispersion of repolarisation (i.e. lack of spatial homogeneity) and increased Ca^{2+} entry during the prolonged action potential, leading to increased after-depolarisation.

Class IV drugs

Class IV agents act by blocking voltage-sensitive calcium channels. Class IV drugs in therapeutic use as antidysrhythmic drugs (e.g. **verapamil**) act on L-type channels. Class IV drugs slow conduction in the SA and AV nodes where action potential propagation depends on inward Ca^{2+} current, slowing the heart and terminating SVT by causing partial AV block. They shorten the plateau of the action potential and reduce the force of contraction. Decreased Ca^{2+} entry reduces after-depolarisation and thus suppresses premature ectopic beats. Functionally distinct classes of L-type voltage-gated calcium channels are expressed in heart and vascular smooth muscle, and L-type calcium-channel blockers that act mainly on vascular smooth muscle (e.g. **nifedipine**) indirectly increase sympathetic tone via their hypotensive effect, causing reflex tachycardia.

---

[5]A 3-year-old girl began to have blackouts, which decreased in frequency with age. Her ECG showed a prolonged QT interval. When 18 years of age, she lost consciousness running for a bus. When she was 19, she became quite emotional as a participant in a live television audience and died suddenly. The molecular basis of this rare inherited disorder is now known. It is caused by a mutation in either the gene coding for a particular potassium channel – called *HERG* – or another gene, *SCN5A*, which codes for the sodium channel and disruption of which results in a loss of inactivation of the Na⁺ current (see Welsh & Hoshi, 1995, for a commentary).

DETAILS OF INDIVIDUAL DRUGS

Quinidine, procainamide and disopyramide (class Ia)

Quinidine and **procainamide**, now mainly of historical interest, are pharmacologically similar. **Disopyramide** resembles quinidine, possessing an atropine-like effect, distinct from its class Ia action, which can cause blurred vision, dry mouth, constipation and urinary retention. It has more negative inotropic action than quinidine but is less likely to cause hypersensitivity reactions.

Lidocaine (class Ib)

Lidocaine, also well known as a local anaesthetic (see Ch. 43), has been given by intravenous infusion, to treat and prevent ventricular dysrhythmias in the immediate aftermath of myocardial infarction, but is now seldom used. It is almost completely extracted from the portal circulation by hepatic presystemic metabolism (Ch. 10), and so cannot usefully be swallowed (although if administered into the mouth to produce local anaesthesia it can be absorbed directly into the systemic circulation and cause systemic effects). Its plasma half-life is normally about 2 h, but its elimination is slowed if hepatic blood flow is reduced, for example by reduced cardiac output following myocardial infarction or by drugs that reduce cardiac output (e.g. β-adrenoceptor antagonists). Dosage must be reduced accordingly to prevent accumulation and toxicity. Indeed, its clearance has been used to estimate hepatic blood flow, analogous to the use of *para*-aminohippurate (PAH) clearance to measure renal blood flow (Ch. 10).

The adverse effects of lidocaine are mainly due to its actions on the central nervous system and include drowsiness, disorientation and convulsions. Because of its relatively short half-life, the plasma concentration can be adjusted fairly rapidly by varying the infusion rate.

Flecainide and encainide (class Ic)

Flecainide and **encainide** suppress ventricular ectopic beats. They are long-acting and reduce the frequency of ventricular ectopic beats when administered orally. However, in clinical trials, they unexpectedly increased the incidence of sudden death associated with ventricular fibrillation after myocardial infarction, so they are no longer used in this setting. This counterintuitive result had a profound impact on the way clinicians and drug regulators view the use of seemingly reasonable intermediate end points (in this case, reduction of frequency of ventricular ectopic beats) as evidence of efficacy in clinical trials.

β-Adrenoceptor antagonists (class II)

β-Adrenoceptor antagonists are described in Chapter 15. Their clinical use for rhythm disorders is shown in the clinical box. **Propranolol**, like several other drugs of this type, has some class I action in addition to blocking β adrenoceptors. This may contribute to its antidysrhythmic effects, although probably not very much, because an isomer with little β-antagonist activity has little antidysrhythmic activity, despite similar activity as a class I agent.

Adverse effects include worsening bronchospasm in patients with asthma, a negative inotropic effect, bradycardia and fatigue. It was hoped that the use of β₁-selective drugs (e.g. **metoprolol, atenolol**) would remove the risk of bronchospasm, but their selectivity is insufficient to achieve this goal in clinical practice, although the once-a-day

Clinical uses of class I antidysrhythmic drugs

- Class Ia (e.g. disopyramide)
  - ventricular dysrhythmias
  - prevention of recurrent paroxysmal atrial fibrillation triggered by vagal overactivity.
- **Class Ib** (e.g. intravenous **lidocaine**)
  - now seldom used.
- **Class Ic**
  - to prevent paroxysmal atrial fibrillation (**flecainide**)
  - recurrent tachyarrhythmias associated with abnormal conducting pathways (e.g. Wolff–Parkinson–White syndrome).

convenience of several such drugs has led to their widespread use.

Clinical uses of class II antidysrhythmic drugs (e.g. propranolol, timolol)

- To reduce mortality following myocardial infarction.
- To prevent recurrence of tachyarrhythmias (e.g. paroxysmal atrial fibrillation) provoked by increased sympathetic activity.
- In managing hyperthyroidism while control with antithyroid drugs is being established (Ch. 35).

Class III

Amiodarone is highly effective at suppressing dysrhythmias (see the clinical box below). Like other drugs that interfere with cardiac repolarisation, it is important to monitor plasma electrolyte concentrations (especially of K^+). Unfortunately, several peculiarities complicate its use. It is extensively bound in tissues, has a long elimination half-life (10–100 days) and accumulates in the body during repeated dosing. For this reason, a loading dose is used, and for life-threatening dysrhythmias this is given intravenously via a central vein (it causes phlebitis if given into a peripheral vessel). Adverse effects are numerous and important; they include photosensitive rashes and a slate-grey/bluish discoloration of the skin; thyroid abnormalities (hypo- and hyper-, connected with its iodine content); pulmonary fibrosis, which is late in onset but may be irreversible; corneal deposits; and neurological and gastrointestinal disturbances, including hepatitis. Surprisingly (since it delays repolarisation and prolongs the QT interval) reports of *torsades de pointes* and ventricular tachycardia are very unusual. **Dronedarone** is a related benzofuran with somewhat different effects on individual ion channels. It does not incorporate iodine and was designed to be less lipophilic than amiodarone in hopes of reducing thyroid and pulmonary toxicities. Its elimination $t_{1/2}$ is shorter than that of amiodarone and it is indicated to maintain sinus rhythm after cardioversion of atrial fibrillation, but only as a last resort, due to safety concerns: it increased the rates of stroke, heart failure, and death from cardiovascular causes in patients with permanent atrial fibrillation and risk factors for vascular events and is hazardous in such patients (Connolly et al., 2011).

Sotalol is a non-selective β-adrenoceptor antagonist, this activity residing in the L isomer. Unlike other β antagonists, it prolongs the cardiac action potential and the QT interval by delaying the slow outward K^+ current. This class III activity is present in both L and D isomers. Racemic sotalol (the form prescribed) appears to be somewhat less effective than amiodarone in preventing chronic life-threatening ventricular tachyarrhythmias. It can cause torsades de pointes; it is valuable in patients in whom β-adrenoceptor antagonists are not contraindicated. Close monitoring of plasma K^+ is important.

Clinical uses of class III antidysrhythmic drugs

- **Amiodarone**: tachycardia associated with the Wolff–Parkinson–White syndrome. It is also effective in many other supraventricular and ventricular tachyarrhythmias but has serious adverse effects.
- (Racemic) **sotalol** combines class III with class II actions. It is used in paroxysmal supraventricular dysrhythmias and suppresses ventricular ectopic beats and short runs of ventricular tachycardia.

Verapamil and diltiazem (class IV)

Verapamil is given by mouth. (Intravenous preparations are available but are dangerous and almost never needed.) It has a plasma half-life of 6–8 h and is subject to quite extensive first-pass metabolism, which is more marked for the isomer that is responsible for its cardiac effects. A slow-release preparation is available for once-daily use, but it is less effective when used for prevention of dysrhythmia than the regular preparation because the bioavailability of the cardioactive isomer is reduced through the presentation of a steady low concentration to the drug-metabolising enzymes in the liver. If verapamil is added to **digoxin** in patients with poorly controlled atrial fibrillation, the dose of digoxin should be reduced and plasma digoxin concentration checked after a few days, because verapamil both displaces digoxin from tissue-binding sites and reduces its renal elimination, hence predisposing to digoxin accumulation and toxicity.

▼ Verapamil is contraindicated in patients with Wolff–Parkinson–White syndrome (a pre-excitation syndrome caused by a rapidly conducting pathway between atria and ventricles, anatomically distinct from the physiological conducting pathway, that predisposes to re-entrant tachycardia), and is ineffective and dangerous in ventricular dysrhythmias. Adverse effects of verapamil and diltiazem are described below in the section on calcium-channel antagonists.

Diltiazem is similar to verapamil but has relatively more effect on smooth muscle while producing less bradycardia (said to be 'rate neutral').

Adenosine (unclassified in the Vaughan Williams classification)

Adenosine is produced endogenously and is an important chemical mediator (Ch. 17) with effects on breathing, cardiac and smooth muscle, vagal afferent nerves and on platelets, in addition to the effects on cardiac conducting tissue that underlie its therapeutic use. The A_1 receptor is responsible for its effect on the AV node. These receptors are linked to the same cardiac potassium channel that is activated by acetylcholine, and adenosine hyperpolarises cardiac conducting tissue and slows the rate of rise of the pacemaker potential accordingly. It is administered intravenously to terminate SVT if this rhythm persists despite manoeuvres such as carotid artery massage to increase vagal tone. It has largely replaced verapamil for this purpose, because it is safer owing to its effect being short-lived. This is a consequence of its pharmacokinetics: it is taken up via a specific nucleoside transporter by red blood cells and is metabolised by enzymes on the lumenal surface of vascular endothelium. Consequently, the effects of an intravenous bolus dose of adenosine last only 20–30 s. Once SVT has terminated, the patient usually remains in sinus rhythm, even though adenosine is no longer present in plasma. Its short-lived unwanted effects include chest pain, shortness of breath, dizziness and nausea. **Regadenoson** is an A_{2A} adenosine receptor agonist that is used diagnostically in pharmacological cardiac stress testing (mentioned later, p. 285). It is claimed that its selectivity and short duration of action are advantages over adenosine for this indication. It has a 2- to 3-minute biological half-life and is administered as a bolus,

Theophylline and other xanthines (Chs 17 and 28) block adenosine receptors and inhibit the actions of intravenous adenosine, whereas **dipyridamole** (a vasodilator and antiplatelet drug; see p. 285 and Ch. 24) blocks the nucleoside uptake mechanism, potentiating adenosine and prolonging its adverse effects. Both these interactions are clinically important.

> ### Clinical uses of class IV antidysrhythmic drugs
>
> - **Verapamil** is the main drug. It is used:
>   - to prevent recurrence of paroxysmal supraventricular tachycardia (SVT)
>   - to reduce the ventricular rate in patients with atrial fibrillation, provided they do not have Wolff–Parkinson–White or a related disorder.
> - **Diltiazem** is similar
> - **Verapamil** was previously given intravenously to terminate SVT; it is now seldom used for this because **adenosine** is safer. (A slow-release preparation of verapamil is sometimes used to treat hypertension and/ or angina, especially where it is desired to slow the heart rate but a β-adrenoceptor antagonist is contraindicated.)

DRUGS THAT INCREASE MYOCARDIAL CONTRACTION

CARDIAC GLYCOSIDES

Cardiac glycosides come from foxgloves (*Digitalis* spp.) and related plants. Withering wrote on the use of the foxglove in 1775: 'it has a power over the motion of the heart to a degree yet unobserved in any other medicine …' Foxgloves contain several cardiac glycosides with similar actions. Their basic chemical structure consists of three components: a sugar moiety, a steroid and a lactone ring. The lactone is essential for activity, the other parts of the molecule mainly determining potency and pharmacokinetic properties. Therapeutically the most important cardiac glycoside is **digoxin**.

Endogenous digitalis-like factors, have been mooted for nearly half a century. There is evidence in mammals of an endogenous digitalis-like factor closely similar to **ouabain**, a short-acting cardiac glycoside implicated in cardiovascular function (see Schoner & Scheiner-Bobis, 2007; Blaustein et al., 2016). Endogenous cardiotonic steroids were first considered important in the regulation of renal sodium transport and arterial pressure, but have also been implicated in the regulation of cell growth, differentiation, apoptosis, fibrosis, the modulation of immunity and of carbohydrate metabolism, and the control of various central nervous functions (Bagrov et al., 2009).

Actions and adverse effects

The main actions of glycosides are on the heart, but some of their adverse effects are extracardiac, including nausea, vomiting, diarrhoea and confusion. The cardiac effects are:

- cardiac slowing and reduced rate of conduction through the AV node, due to increased vagal activity;
- increased force of contraction;
- disturbances of rhythm, especially:
  - block of AV conduction
  - increased ectopic pacemaker activity.

Adverse effects are common and can be severe. One of the main drawbacks of glycosides in clinical use is the narrow margin between effectiveness and toxicity.

Mechanism

The mechanism whereby cardiac glycosides increase the force of cardiac contraction (positive inotropic effect) is inhibition of the Na^+/K^+ pump in the cardiac myocytes. This causes increased $[Na^+]_i$, and a secondary rise in $[Ca^{2+}]_i$ (see later). Cardiac glycosides bind to a site on the extracellular aspect of the α subunit of the Na^+-K^+-ATPase, and are useful experimental tools for studying this important transporter. The molecular mechanism underlying increased vagal tone (negative chronotropic effect) is unknown, but could also be due to inhibition of the Na^+/K^+ pump.

Rate and rhythm

Cardiac glycosides slow, and in higher concentrations may block, AV conduction by increasing vagal outflow. Their beneficial effect in established rapid atrial fibrillation results partly from this. If ventricular rate is excessively rapid, the time available for diastolic filling is inadequate, so slowing heart rate by partly blocking AV conduction increases stroke volume and cardiac efficiency even if atrial fibrillation persists. Digoxin can terminate paroxysmal atrial tachycardia by its effect on AV conduction, although adenosine (see above) is usually preferred for this indication.

Toxic concentrations of glycosides disturb sinus rhythm. This can occur at plasma concentrations of digoxin within, or only slightly above, the therapeutic range. AV block can occur, and also ectopic beats. Because Na^+/K^+ exchange is electrogenic, inhibition of the pump by glycosides causes depolarisation, predisposing to disturbances of cardiac rhythm. Furthermore, the increased $[Ca^{2+}]_i$ causes increased after-depolarisation, leading first to coupled beats (bigeminy), in which a normal ventricular beat is followed by an ectopic beat; ventricular tachycardia and eventually ventricular fibrillation may ensue.

Force of contraction

Glycosides cause a large increase in twitch tension in isolated preparations of cardiac muscle. Unlike catecholamines, they do not accelerate relaxation (compare Fig. 22.6 with Fig. 22.10). Increased tension is caused by an increased $[Ca^{2+}]_i$ transient (see Fig. 22.10). The action potential is only slightly affected and the slow inward current little changed, so the increased $[Ca^{2+}]_i$ transient probably reflects a greater release of Ca^{2+} from intracellular stores. The most likely mechanism is as follows (see also Ch. 4):

1. Glycosides inhibit the Na^+/K^+ pump.
2. Increased $[Na^+]_i$ slows extrusion of Ca^{2+} via the Na^+/Ca^{2+} exchange transporter since increasing $[Na^+]_i$ reduces the inwardly directed gradient for Na^+ which drives extrusion of Ca^{2+} by Na^+/Ca^{2+} exchange.
3. Increased $[Ca^{2+}]_i$ is stored in the sarcoplasmic reticulum, and thus increases the amount of Ca^{2+} released by each action potential.

The effect of extracellular potassium

Effects of cardiac glycosides are increased if plasma $[K^+]$ decreases, because of reduced competition at the K^+-binding site on the Na^+-K^+-ATPase. This is clinically important, because many diuretics, which are often used to treat heart failure (Ch. 30), decrease plasma $[K^+]$ thereby increasing the risk of glycoside-induced dysrhythmia.

Pharmacokinetic aspects

Digoxin is administered by mouth or, in urgent situations, intravenously. It is a polar molecule; elimination is mainly by renal excretion and involves P-glycoprotein (Ch. 9), leading to clinically significant interactions with other drugs used to treat heart failure, such as **spironolactone**, and with antidysrhythmic drugs such as **verapamil** and **amiodarone**. Elimination half-time is approximately 36 h in patients with normal renal function, but considerably longer in elderly patients and those with overt renal failure, for whom the dose must be reduced. A loading dose is used in urgent situations. The therapeutic range of plasma concentrations, below which digoxin is unlikely to be effective and above which the risk of toxicity increases substantially, is rather narrow (1–2.6 nmol/L). Determination of plasma digoxin concentration is useful when lack of efficacy or toxicity is suspected.

> ### Clinical uses of cardiac glycosides (e.g. digoxin)
>
> - To slow ventricular rate in rapid persistent atrial fibrillation.
> - Treatment of heart failure in patients who remain symptomatic despite optimal use of diuretics and angiotensin-converting enzyme inhibitors (Ch. 23).

OTHER DRUGS THAT INCREASE MYOCARDIAL CONTRACTION

Certain β_1-adrenoceptor agonists, for example **dobutamine**, are used to treat acute but potentially reversible heart failure (e.g. following cardiac surgery or in some cases of cardiogenic or septic shock) because of their positive inotropic action. Dobutamine, for reasons that are not well understood, produces less tachycardia than other β_1 agonists. It is used intravenously for short-term treatment of acute heart failure, or for pharmacological cardiac stress testing and echocardiography. **Glucagon** also increases myocardial contractility by increasing synthesis of cAMP, and has been used in patients with acute cardiac dysfunction caused by overdosage of β-adrenoceptor antagonists.

Inhibitors of the heart-specific subtype (type III) of phosphodiesterase, the enzyme responsible for the intracellular degradation of cAMP, increase myocardial contractility. Consequently, like β-adrenoceptor agonists, they increase intracellular cAMP and can cause dysrhythmias for the same reason. Compounds in this group include **amrinone** and **milrinone**. They improve haemodynamic indices in patients with heart failure but paradoxically worsen survival, presumably because of dysrhythmias. As with the encainide/flecainide example (see p. 281) this disparity has had a sobering effect on clinicians and drug regulatory authorities.

ANTI-ANGINAL DRUGS

The mechanism of anginal pain is discussed previously. Angina is managed by using drugs that improve perfusion of the myocardium or reduce its metabolic demand, or both. Two of the main groups of drugs, organic nitrates and calcium antagonists, are vasodilators and produce both these effects. The third group, β-adrenoceptor antagonists, slow the heart and hence reduce metabolic demand. Organic nitrates and calcium antagonists are described below. The β-adrenoceptor antagonists are covered in Chapter 15, and their antidysrhythmic actions are described above. **Ivabradine** slows the heart by inhibiting the sinus node I_f current (see p. 272), and is an alternative to β-adrenoceptor antagonists in patients in whom these are not tolerated or are contraindicated. Combined use of ivabradine with a β-adrenoceptor antagonist is indicated in patients whose symptoms are not adequately controlled despite an optimal dose of the β-adrenoceptor antagonist. **Ranolazine** was introduced as an adjunct to other anti-anginal drugs: it inhibits late sodium current and hence indirectly reduces intracellular calcium and force of contraction (the opposite of the effects of cardiac glycosides), without affecting heart rate; more potent and selective inhibitors of the persistent sodium current are in development. Newer anti-anginal drugs are described by Jones et al. (2013).

Fig. 22.10 Effect of a cardiac glycoside (acetylstrophanthidin) on the Ca^{2+} transient and tension produced by frog cardiac muscle. The effect was recorded as in Fig. 22.6. (From Allen, D.G., Blinks, J.R., 1978. Nature 273, 509.)

Fig. 22.11 Comparison of the effects of organic nitrates and an arteriolar vasodilator (dipyridamole) on the coronary circulation. (A) Control. (B) Nitrates dilate the collateral vessel, thus allowing more blood through to the underperfused region (mostly by diversion from the adequately perfused area). (C) Dipyridamole dilates arterioles, increasing flow through the normal area at the expense of the ischaemic area (in which the arterioles are anyway fully dilated). *CAD*, coronary artery disease.

ORGANIC NITRATES

The ability of organic nitrates (see also Chs 21 and 24) to relieve angina was discovered by Lauder Brunton, a distinguished British physician, in 1867. He had found that angina could be partly relieved by bleeding, and knew that **amyl nitrite**, which had been synthesised 10 years earlier, caused flushing and tachycardia with a fall in blood pressure when its vapour was inhaled. He thought that the effect of bleeding resulted from hypotension, and found that amyl nitrite inhalation worked much better. Amyl nitrite has now been replaced by **glyceryl trinitrate** (GTN).[6] Several related organic nitrates, of which the most important is **isosorbide mononitrate**, have a prolonged action. **Nicorandil**, a potassium-channel activator with additional nitrovasodilator activity, is sometimes combined with other anti-anginal treatment in resistant cases.

Actions

Organic nitrates relax smooth muscle (especially vascular smooth muscle, but also oesophageal and biliary smooth muscle). They relax veins, with a consequent reduction in central venous pressure (reduced preload). In healthy subjects, this reduces stroke volume; venous pooling occurs on standing and can cause postural hypotension and dizziness. Therapeutic doses have less effect on small resistance arteries than on veins, but there is a marked effect on larger muscular arteries. This reduces pulse wave reflection from arterial branches (as appreciated in the 19th century by Murrell but neglected for many years thereafter), and

consequently reduces central (aortic) pressure and cardiac afterload (see Ch. 23 for the role of these factors in determining cardiac work). The direct dilator effect on coronary arteries opposes coronary artery spasm in variant angina. With larger doses, resistance arteries and arterioles dilate, and arterial pressure falls. Nevertheless, coronary flow increases because of coronary vasodilatation. Myocardial oxygen consumption is reduced because of the reductions in cardiac preload and afterload. This, together with the increased coronary blood flow, causes a large increase in the oxygen content of coronary sinus blood. Studies in experimental animals have shown that glyceryl trinitrate diverts blood from normal to ischaemic areas of myocardium. The mechanism involves dilatation of collateral vessels that bypass narrowed coronary artery segments (Fig. 22.11).

▼ It is interesting to compare this effect with that of other vasodilators, notably **dipyridamole**, which dilate arterioles but not collaterals. Dipyridamole is at least as effective as nitrates in increasing coronary flow in normal subjects but actually *worsens* angina. This is probably because arterioles in an ischaemic region are fully dilated by the ischaemia, and drug-induced dilatation of the arterioles in normal areas has the effect of diverting blood away from the ischaemic areas (see Fig. 22.11), producing what is termed a vascular steal. This effect is exploited in a pharmacological 'stress test' for coronary arterial disease, in which dipyridamole is administered intravenously to patients in whom this diagnosis is suspected but who cannot exercise, while monitoring myocardial perfusion and the ECG. **Regadenoson** is an A_{2A} adenosine receptor agonist that is used similarly in pharmacological cardiac stress testing (see earlier, p. 283).

In summary, the anti-anginal action of nitrates involves:

- reduced cardiac work, because of reduced cardiac preload (venodilatation) and afterload (reduced arterial wave reflection), leading to reduced myocardial oxygen requirement;

---

[6]Nobel discovered how to stabilise GTN with kieselguhr, enabling him to exploit its explosive properties in dynamite, the manufacture of which earned him the fortune with which he endowed the eponymous prizes.

- redistribution of coronary flow towards ischaemic areas via collaterals;
- relief of coronary spasm.

▼ In addition to its effects on smooth muscle, nitric oxide (NO) increases the rate of relaxation of cardiac muscle (dubbed a '*lusiotropic*' action). It is probable that organic nitrates mimic this action, which could be important in patients with impaired diastolic function, a common accompaniment of hypertension and of heart failure.

Mechanism of action

Organic nitrates are metabolised with release of NO. At concentrations achieved during therapeutic use, this involves an enzymic step and possibly a reaction with tissue sulf-hydryl (–SH) groups. NO activates soluble guanylyl cyclase (see Ch. 21), increasing formation of cGMP, which activates protein kinase G (Ch. 4) and leads to a cascade of effects in smooth muscle culminating in dephosphorylation of myosin light chains, sequestration of intracellular Ca^{2+} and consequent relaxation.

Tolerance and unwanted effects

Repeated administration of nitrates to smooth muscle preparations in vitro results in diminished relaxation, possibly partly because of depletion of free –SH groups, although attempts to prevent tolerance by agents that restore tissue –SH groups have not been clinically useful. Tolerance to the anti-anginal effect of nitrates does not occur to a clinically important extent with ordinary formulations of short-acting drugs (e.g. glyceryl trinitrate), but does occur with longer-acting drugs (e.g. isosorbide mononitrate) or when glyceryl trinitrate is administered by prolonged intravenous infusion or by frequent application of slow-release transdermal patches (see later).

The main adverse effects of nitrates are a direct consequence of their main pharmacological actions, and include postural hypotension and headache. This was the cause of 'Monday morning sickness' among workers in explosives factories. Tolerance to these effects develops quite quickly but wears off after a brief nitrate-free interval (which is why the symptoms appeared on Mondays and not later in the week). Formation of *methaemoglobin*, an oxidation product of haemoglobin that is ineffective as an oxygen carrier, seldom occurs when nitrates are used clinically but is induced deliberately with **amyl nitrite** in the treatment of *cyanide poisoning*, because methaemoglobin binds and inactivates cyanide ions.

Pharmacokinetic and pharmaceutical aspects

Glyceryl trinitrate is rapidly inactivated by hepatic metabolism. It is well absorbed from the mouth and is taken as a tablet under the tongue or as a sublingual spray, producing its effects within a few minutes. If swallowed, it is ineffective because of presystemic metabolism in the liver. Given sublingually, the trinitrate is converted to di- and mononitrates. Its effective duration of action is approximately 30 min. It is appreciably absorbed through the skin, and a more sustained effect can be achieved by applying it as a transdermal patch. Once a bottle of the tablets has been opened, its shelf-life is quite short because the volatile active substance evaporates; spray preparations avoid this problem.

Isosorbide mononitrate is longer acting than glyceryl trinitrate because it is absorbed and metabolised more slowly, but has similar pharmacological actions. It is swallowed rather than taken sublingually, and is taken twice a day for prophylaxis (usually in the morning and at lunch,

to allow a nitrate-free period during the night, when patients are not exerting themselves, to avoid tolerance). It is also available in slow-release form for once-daily use in the morning.

Organic nitrates

- Important compounds include **glyceryl trinitrate** and longer-acting **isosorbide mononitrate**.
- These drugs are powerful vasodilators, acting on veins to reduce cardiac preload and on arteries to reduce arterial wave reflection and hence afterload.
- Act via nitric oxide, to which they are metabolised. Nitric oxide stimulates formation of cGMP and hence activates protein kinase G, affecting contractile proteins (myosin light chains) and Ca^{2+} regulation.
- Tolerance occurs experimentally and is important clinically with frequent use of long-acting drugs or sustained-release preparations.
- Effectiveness in angina results partly from reduced cardiac load and partly from dilatation of collateral coronary vessels, causing more effective distribution of coronary flow. Dilatation of constricted coronary vessels is particularly beneficial in variant angina.
- Serious unwanted effects are uncommon; headache and postural hypotension may occur initially. Overdose can, rarely, cause methaemoglobinaemia.

Clinical uses of organic nitrates

- Stable angina:
  - prevention (e.g. daily **isosorbide mononitrate**, or **glyceryl trinitrate** sublingually immediately before exertion);
  - treatment (sublingual **glyceryl trinitrate**).
- Unstable angina: intravenous **glyceryl trinitrate**.
- Acute heart failure: intravenous **glyceryl trinitrate**.
- Chronic heart failure: **isosorbide mononitrate**, with **hydralazine** in patients of African origin (Ch. 23).

POTASSIUM-CHANNEL ACTIVATORS

Nicorandil combines activation of the potassium K_{ATP} channel (see Ch. 4) with nitrovasodilator (NO donor) actions. It is both an arterial and a venous dilator, and causes the expected unwanted effects of headache, flushing and dizziness. It is used for patients who remain symptomatic despite optimal management with other drugs, often while they await surgery or angioplasty.

β-ADRENOCEPTOR ANTAGONISTS

β-Adrenoceptor antagonists (see Ch. 15) are important in prophylaxis of stable angina, and in treating patients with unstable angina, acting by reducing cardiac oxygen consumption. They reduce the risk of death following myocardial infarction, possibly via their antidysrhythmic action. Any effects on coronary vessel diameter are of minor importance, although these drugs are avoided in variant angina because of the theoretical risk that they will increase coronary spasm. Their astonishingly diverse clinical uses are summarised in the clinical boxes earlier (p. 282) and in Chapter 15.

CALCIUM ANTAGONISTS

The term 'calcium antagonist' is used for drugs that block cellular entry of Ca^{2+} through calcium channels rather than preventing its intracellular actions (Ch. 4). Some authors use the term 'Ca^{2+} entry blockers' to make this distinction clearer. Therapeutically important calcium antagonists act on L-type channels. L-type calcium antagonists comprise three chemically distinct classes: *phenylalkylamines* (e.g. **verapamil**), *dihydropyridines* (e.g. **nifedipine, amlodipine**) and *benzothiazepines* (e.g. **diltiazem**).

Mechanism of action: types of calcium channel

The properties of voltage-gated calcium channels have been studied by voltage clamp and patch clamp techniques (see Ch. 3). Drugs of each of the three chemical classes mentioned above all bind the α_1 subunit of the L-type calcium channel but at distinct sites. These interact allosterically with each other and with the gating machinery of the channel to prevent its opening (see later and Fig. 22.12), thus reducing Ca^{2+} entry. Many calcium antagonists show properties of use dependence (i.e. they block more effectively in cells in which the calcium channels are most active; see the discussion of class I antidysrhythmic drugs earlier). For the same reason, they also show voltage-dependent blocking actions, blocking more strongly when the membrane is depolarised, causing calcium-channel opening and inactivation.

▼ Dihydropyridines affect calcium-channel function in a complex way, not simply by physical plugging of the pore. This became clear when some dihydropyridines, exemplified by BAY K 8644, were found to bind to the same site but to do the opposite; that is, to promote the opening of voltage-gated calcium channels. Thus BAY K 8644 *increases* the force of cardiac contraction, and *constricts* blood vessels; it is competitively antagonised by nifedipine. Calcium channels can exist in one of three distinct states, termed 'modes' (see Fig. 22.12). When a channel is in mode 0, it does not open in response to depolarisation; in mode 1, depolarisation produces a low opening probability, and each opening is brief. In mode 2, depolarisation produces a very high opening probability, and single openings are prolonged. Under normal conditions, about 70% of the channels at any one moment exist in mode 1, with only 1% or less in mode 0; each channel switches randomly and quite slowly between the three modes. Dihydropyridine antagonists bind selectively to channels in mode 0, thus favouring

this non-opening state, whereas agonists bind selectively to channels in mode 2 (see Fig. 22.12). This type of two-directional modulation resembles the phenomenon seen with the GABA/benzodiazepine interaction (Ch. 45), and invites speculation about possible endogenous dihydropyridine-like mediator(s) with a regulatory effect on Ca^{2+} entry.

Mibefradil blocks T- as well as L-type channels at therapeutic concentrations, but was withdrawn from therapeutic use because it caused adverse drug interactions by interfering with drug metabolism. **Ethosuximide** (a carbonic anhydrase inhibitor used to treat absence seizures, Ch. 46) also blocks T channels in thalamic and reticular neurones.

Pharmacological effects

The main effects of calcium antagonists, as used therapeutically, are on cardiac and smooth muscle. Verapamil preferentially affects the heart, whereas most of the dihydropyridines (e.g. nifedipine) exert a greater effect on smooth muscle than on the heart. Diltiazem is intermediate in its actions.

Cardiac actions

The antidysrhythmic effects of verapamil and diltiazem have been discussed earlier. Calcium antagonists can cause AV block and cardiac slowing by their actions on conducting tissues, but this is offset by a reflex increase in sympathetic activity secondary to their vasodilator action. For example, nifedipine typically causes reflex tachycardia; diltiazem causes little or no change in heart rate and verapamil slows the heart rate. Calcium antagonists also have a negative inotropic effect, from their inhibition of Ca^{2+} entry during the action potential plateau. Verapamil has the most marked negative inotropic action, and is contraindicated in heart failure, whereas amlodipine does not worsen cardiovascular mortality in patients with severe but stable chronic heart failure.

Vascular smooth muscle

Calcium antagonists cause generalised arterial/arteriolar dilatation, thereby reducing blood pressure, but do not much affect the veins. They affect all vascular beds, although regional effects vary considerably between different drugs. They cause coronary vasodilatation and are used in patients with coronary artery spasm (variant angina). Other types

Fig. 22.12 **Mode behaviour of calcium channels.** The traces are patch clamp recordings (see Ch. 3) of the opening of single calcium channels *(downward deflections)* in a patch of membrane from a cardiac muscle cell. A depolarising step is imposed close to the start of each trace, causing an increase in the opening probability of the channel. When the channel is in mode 1 *(centre)*, this causes a few brief openings to occur; in mode 2 *(right)*, the channel stays open for most of the time during the depolarising step; in mode 0 *(left)*, it fails to open at all. Under normal conditions, in the absence of drug, the channel spends most of its time in modes 1 and 2, and only rarely enters mode 0. *DHP*, dihydropyridine. (Redrawn from Hess, et al., 1984. Nature 311, 538–544.)

287

of smooth muscle (e.g. biliary tract, urinary tract and uterus) are also relaxed by calcium antagonists, but these effects are less important therapeutically than their actions on vascular smooth muscle.

Protection of ischaemic tissues

There are theoretical reasons (see Fig. 22.8) why calcium antagonists might exert a cytoprotective effect in ischaemic tissues (see Ch. 41) and thus be of use in treating heart attack and stroke. However, randomised clinical trials have been disappointing, with little or no evidence of beneficial (or harmful) effects of calcium antagonists on cardiovascular morbidity or mortality in patient groups other than patients with hypertension, in whom calcium antagonists have beneficial effects comparable with those of other drugs that lower blood pressure to similar extents (see Ch. 23). **Nimodipine** is partly selective for cerebral vasculature and there is some evidence that it reduces cerebral vasospasm following subarachnoid haemorrhage.

Pharmacokinetics

Calcium antagonists in clinical use are well absorbed from the gastrointestinal tract, and are given by mouth except for some special indications, such as following subarachnoid haemorrhage, for which intravenous preparations are available. They are extensively metabolised. Pharmacokinetic differences between different drugs and different pharmaceutical preparations are clinically important, because they determine the dose interval and the intensity of some of the unwanted effects, such as headache and flushing. Amlodipine has a long elimination half-life and is given once daily, whereas nifedipine, diltiazem and verapamil have shorter elimination half-lives and are either given more frequently or are formulated in various slow-release preparations to permit once-daily dosing.

Unwanted effects

Most of the unwanted effects of calcium antagonists are extensions of their main pharmacological actions. Short-acting dihydropyridines cause flushing and headache because of their vasodilator action, and in chronic use dihydropyridines often cause ankle swelling (oedema) related to arteriolar dilatation and increased permeability of postcapillary venules. Verapamil can cause constipation, probably because of effects on calcium channels in gastrointestinal nerves or smooth muscle. Effects on cardiac rhythm (e.g. heart block) and force of contraction (e.g. worsening heart failure) are discussed earlier.

Apart from these predictable effects, calcium-channel antagonists, as a class, have few idiosyncratic adverse effects.

Calcium antagonists

- Block Ca^{2+} entry by preventing opening of voltage-gated L-type calcium channels.
- There are three main L-type antagonists, typified by **verapamil**, **diltiazem** and dihydropyridines (e.g. **nifedipine**).
- Mainly affect heart and smooth muscle, inhibiting the Ca^{2+} entry caused by depolarisation in these tissues.
- Selectivity between heart and smooth muscle varies: **verapamil** is relatively cardioselective, **nifedipine** is relatively smooth muscle selective, and diltiazem is intermediate.
- Vasodilator effect (mainly dihydropyridines) is mainly on resistance vessels, reducing afterload. Calcium antagonists dilate coronary vessels, which is important in variant angina.
- Effects on heart (**verapamil**, **diltiazem**): antidysrhythmic action (mainly atrial tachycardias), because of impaired atrioventricular conduction; reduced contractility.
- Clinical uses:
  - antidysrhythmic (mainly **verapamil**)
  - angina (e.g. **diltiazem**)
  - hypertension (mainly dihydropyridines).
- Unwanted effects include headache, constipation (**verapamil**) and ankle oedema (dihydropyridines). There is a risk of causing cardiac failure or heart block, especially with **verapamil**.

Clinical uses of calcium antagonists

- Dysrhythmias (**verapamil**):
  - to slow ventricular rate in rapid atrial fibrillation
  - to prevent recurrence of supraventricular tachycardia (SVT) (intravenous administration of **verapamil** to terminate SVT attacks has been replaced by use of **adenosine**).
- Hypertension: usually a dihydropyridine drug (e.g. **amlodipine** or slow-release **nifedipine**; Ch. 23).
- To prevent angina (e.g. a dihydropyridine or **diltiazem**).

REFERENCES AND FURTHER READING

Further reading

Fink, M., Noble, D., 2010. Pharmacodynamic effects in the cardiovascular system: the modeller's view. Basic Clin. Pharmacol. Toxicol. 106, 243–249.

Jones, D.A., Timmis, A., Wragg, A., 2013. Novel drugs for treating angina. BMJ 347, 34–37. (*Useful summary*)

Mann, D.L., Zipes, D.P., Libby, P., Bonow, R.O., 2014. Braunwald's Heart Disease: A Textbook of Cardiovascular Medicine, tenth ed. Saunders/Elsevier, Philadelphia.

Opie, L.H., Gersh, B.J., 2013. Drugs for the Heart, eighth ed. Saunders/Elsevier, Philadelphia.

Specific aspects

Physiological and pathophysiological aspects

Bagrov, A.Y., Shapiro, J.I., Fedorova, O.V., 2009. Endogenous cardiotonic steroids: physiology, pharmacology, and novel therapeutic targets. Pharmacol. Rev. 61, 9–38. (*Reviews physiological interactions between CTS and other regulatory systems that may be important in the pathophysiology of essential hypertension, pre-eclampsia, end-stage renal disease, congestive heart failure and diabetes*)

Blaustein, M.P., Chen, L., Hamlyn, J.M., 2016. Pivotal role of alpha 2 Na^+ pumps and their high affinity ouabain binding site in cardiovascular health and disease. J. Physiol. 594, 6079–6103.

("Circulating endogenous ouabain modulates ouabain-sensitive 2 Na$^+$ pump activity and Ca^{2+} transporter expression and, via Na$^+$/Ca^{2+} exchange, Ca^{2+} homeostasis. This regulates sensitivity to sympathetic activity, Ca^{2+} signalling and arterial and cardiac contraction.")

Eltzschig, H.K., Sitkovsky, M.V., Robson, S.C., 2012. Purinergic signaling during inflammation. N. Engl. J. Med. 367, 2322–2333.

Noble, D., 2008. Computational models of the heart and their use in assessing the actions of drugs. J. Pharmacol. Sci. 107, 107–117. (*Models of cardiac cells are sufficiently well developed to answer questions concerning the actions of drugs such as ranolazine, a recently introduced blocker of persistent sodium current, on repolarisation and the initiation of arrhythmias*)

Potter, L.R., Yoder, A.R., Flora, D.R., et al., 2009. Natriuretic peptides: their structures, receptors, physiologic functions and therapeutic applications. Handb. Exp. Pharmacol. 191, 341–366. (*Reviews the history, structure, function and clinical applications of natriuretic peptides and their receptors*)

Rockman, H.A., Koch, W.J., Lefkowitz, R.J., 2002. Seven-transmembrane-spanning receptors and heart function. Nature 415, 206–212.

Schoner, W., Scheiner-Bobis, G., 2007. Endogenous and exogenous cardiac glycosides: their roles in hypertension, salt metabolism, and cell growth. Am. J. Physiol. Cell Physiol. 293, C509–C536. (*Review: touches on anticancer potential also*)

Seddon, M., Melikian, N., Dworakowski, R., et al., 2009. Effects of neuronal nitric oxide synthase on human coronary artery diameter and blood flow in vivo. Circulation 119, 2656–2662. (*Local nNOS-derived NO regulates basal blood flow in the human coronary vascular bed, whereas substance P-stimulated vasodilatation is eNOS mediated*)

Welsh, M.J., Hoshi, T., 1995. Molecular cardiology — ion channels lose the rhythm. Nature 376, 640–641. (*Commentary on Ward–Romano syndrome*)

Therapeutic aspects

COMMIT Collaborative Group, 2005. Early intravenous then oral metoprolol in 45 852 patients with acute myocardial infarction: randomised placebo-controlled trial. Lancet 366, 1622–1632. (*Early β blockade reduced ventricular fibrillation and reinfarction, benefits that were offset by increased cardiogenic shock in patients with signs of heart failure; see accompanying comment by Sabatine, M.S., pp. 1587–1589 in the same issue*)

Connolly, S.J., Camm, J., Halperin, J.L., et al., 2011. Dronedarone in high-risk permanent atrial fibrillation. N. Engl. J. Med. 365, 2268–2276. (*Dronedarone increased the rates of stroke, heart failure, and death from cardiovascular causes in patients with permanent atrial fibrillation and risk factors for vascular events and is hazardous in such patients*)

Fox, K., Ford, I., Steg, P.G., et al., 2008. Ivabradine for patients with stable coronary artery disease and left-ventricular systolic dysfunction (BEAUTIFUL): a randomised, double-blind, placebo-controlled trial. Lancet 372, 807–816. (*Ivabradine does not improve cardiac outcomes in all patients with stable coronary artery disease and left-ventricular systolic dysfunction, but improved outcome in patients with heart rates >70 bpm. See also adjacent paper: Fox, K., et al., 2008. Heart rate as a prognostic risk factor in patients with coronary artery disease and left-ventricular systolic dysfunction (BEAUTIFUL): a subgroup analysis of a randomised controlled trial. Lancet 372, 817–821*)

Heusch, G., 2017. Critical issues for the translation of cardioprotection. Circ. Res. 120, 1477–1486. (*"Future trials must focus on interventions/agents with robust preclinical evidence, have solid phase II dosing and timing data, and recruit patients who have truly a chance to benefit from adjunct cardioprotection"*)

ISIS-4 Collaborative Group, 1995. ISIS-4: a randomised factorial trial assessing early oral captopril, oral mononitrate, and intravenous magnesium sulphate in 58 050 patients with suspected acute myocardial infarction. Lancet 345, 669–685. (*Impressive trial: disappointing results! Magnesium was ineffective; oral nitrate did not reduce 1-month mortality*)

O'Connor, C.M., Starling, R.C., Hernandez, A.F., et al., 2011. Effect of nesiritide in patients with acute decompensated heart failure. N. Engl. J. Med. 365, 32–43. (*see also Topol, E.T., 2011. The lost decade of nesiritide. N. Engl. J. Med. 365, 81–82*)

Rahimtoola, S.H., 2004. Digitalis therapy for patients in clinical heart failure. Circulation 109, 2942–2946. (*Review*)

Roden, D.M., 2008. Cellular basis of drug-induced torsades de pointes. Br. J. Pharmacol. 154, 1502–1507. (*This adverse drug reaction occurs during therapy with some antidysrhythmic drugs and also several drugs not used for cardiovascular indications, including certain antibiotics, antipsychotics and antihistamines. The common mechanism is inhibition of a specific repolarizing potassium current, I-Kr*)

Ruskin, J.N., 1989. The cardiac arrhythmia suppression trial (CAST). N. Engl. J. Med. 321, 386–388. (*Enormously influential trial showing increased mortality with active treatment despite suppression of dysrhythmia*)

23 The vascular system

OVERVIEW

This chapter is concerned with the pharmacology of blood vessels. The walls of arteries, arterioles, venules and veins contain smooth muscle, the contractile state of which is controlled by circulating hormones and by mediators released locally from sympathetic nerve terminals (Ch. 15), endothelial cells and other cells resident in the vessel wall or visiting it from the circulating blood. These work mainly by regulating Ca²⁺ in vascular smooth muscle cells, as described in Chapter 4. In the present chapter, we first consider the control of vascular smooth muscle by the endothelium and by the renin–angiotensin system, followed by the actions of vasoconstrictor and vasodilator drugs. Finally, we consider briefly some of the clinical uses of vasoactive drugs in selected important diseases, namely hypertension (pulmonary as well as systemic), heart failure, shock, peripheral vascular disease and Raynaud's disease. The use of vasoactive drugs to treat angina is covered in Chapter 22.

INTRODUCTION

Actions of drugs on the vascular system can be broken down into effects on:

- total systemic ('peripheral') vascular resistance, one of the main determinants of arterial blood pressure;
- the resistance of individual vascular beds, which determines the local distribution of blood flow to and within different organs; such effects are relevant to the drug treatment of angina (Ch. 22), Raynaud's phenomenon, pulmonary hypertension and circulatory shock
- aortic compliance and pulse wave reflection, which are relevant to the treatment of hypertension, cardiac failure and angina;
- venous tone and blood volume (the 'fullness' of the circulation), which together determine the central venous pressure and are relevant to the treatment of cardiac failure and angina; diuretics (which reduce blood volume) are discussed in Chapter 30;
- atheroma (Ch. 24) and thrombosis (Ch. 25);
- new vessel formation (angiogenesis) – important, for example, in diabetic retinopathy (Ch. 32) and in treating malignant disease (Ch. 57).

Drug effects considered in this chapter are caused by actions on vascular smooth muscle cells. Like other muscles, vascular smooth muscle contracts when cytoplasmic Ca²⁺ ($[Ca^{2+}]_i$) rises, but the coupling between $[Ca^{2+}]_i$ and contraction is less tight than in striated voluntary or cardiac muscle (Ch. 4). Vasoconstrictors and vasodilators act by increasing

or reducing $[Ca^{2+}]_i$, and/or by altering the sensitivity of the contractile machinery to $[Ca^{2+}]_i$. Fig. 4.10 (see Ch. 4) summarises cellular mechanisms that are involved in the control of smooth muscle contraction and relaxation. The control of vascular smooth muscle tone by various mediators is described in other chapters (noradrenaline in Ch. 15, 5-HT in Ch. 16, prostanoids in Ch. 18, nitric oxide [NO] in Ch. 21, cardiac natriuretic peptides in Ch. 22, antidiuretic hormone in Ch. 34). Here we focus on endothelium-derived mediators and on the renin–angiotensin–aldosterone system, before describing the actions of vasoactive drugs and their uses in some important clinical disorders (hypertension, heart failure, shock, peripheral vascular disease and Raynaud's disease).

VASCULAR STRUCTURE AND FUNCTION

Blood is ejected with each heartbeat from the left ventricle into the aorta, whence it flows rapidly to the organs via large conduit arteries. Successive branching leads via muscular arteries to arterioles (endothelium surrounded by a layer of smooth muscle only one cell thick) and capillaries (naked tubes of endothelium), where gas and nutrient exchanges occur. Capillaries coalesce to form postcapillary venules, venules and progressively larger veins leading, via the vena cava, to the right heart. Deoxygenated blood ejected from the right ventricle travels through the pulmonary artery, pulmonary capillaries and pulmonary veins back to the left atrium.[1] Small muscular arteries and arterioles are the main resistance vessels, while veins are capacity vessels that contain a large fraction of the total blood volume. In terms of cardiac function, therefore, arteries and arterioles regulate the *afterload*, while veins and pulmonary vessels regulate the *preload* of the ventricles (see Ch. 22).

Viscoelastic properties of large arteries determine arterial compliance (i.e. the degree to which the volume of the arterial system increases as the pressure increases). This is an important factor in a circulatory system that is driven by an intermittent pump such as the heart. Blood ejected from the left ventricle is accommodated by distension of the aorta, which absorbs the pulsations and delivers a relatively steady flow to the tissues. The greater the compliance of the aorta, the more effectively are fluctuations damped out,[2] and the smaller the oscillations of arterial

---

[1]William Harvey (physician to King Charles I) inferred the circulation of the blood on the basis of superbly elegant quantitative experiments long before the invention of the microscope enabled visual confirmation of the tiny vessels he had predicted. This intellectual triumph did his medical standing no good at all, and Aubrey wrote that 'he fell mightily in his practice, and was regarded by the vulgar as 'crack-brained'. *Plus ça change …*
[2]This cushioning action is called the 'windkessel' effect. The same principle was used to deliver a steady rather than intermittent flow from old-fashioned fire pumps.

Fig. 23.1 Endothelium-derived mediators. The schematic shows some of the more important endothelium-derived contracting and relaxing mediators; many (if not all) of the vasoconstrictors also cause smooth muscle mitogenesis, while vasodilators commonly inhibit mitogenesis. *5-HT*, 5-hydroxytryptamine; *A*, angiotensin; *ACE*, angiotensin-converting enzyme; *ACh*, acetylcholine; *AT$_1$*, angiotensin AT$_1$ receptor; *BK*, bradykinin; *CNP*, C-natriuretic peptide; *DAG*, diacylglycerol; *EDHF*, endothelium-derived hyperpolarising factor; *EET*, epoxyeicosatetraenoic acid; *ET-1*, endothelin-1; *ET$_{A/B)}$*, endothelin A (and B) receptors; *G$_q$*, G protein; *IL-1*, interleukin-1; *IP*, I prostanoid receptor; *IP$_3$*, inosinol 1,4,5-trisphosphate; *K$_{IR}$*, inward rectifying potassium channel; *Na$^+$/K$^+$ ATPase*, electrogenic pump; *NO*, nitric oxide; *NPR*, natriuretic peptide receptor; *PG*, prostaglandin; *TP*, T prostanoid receptor.

pressure with each heartbeat (i.e. the difference between the systolic and diastolic pressure, known as the 'pulse pressure'). Reflection[3] of the pressure wave from branch points in the vascular tree also sustains arterial pressure during diastole. In young people, this helps to preserve a steady perfusion of vital organs, such as the kidneys, during diastole.

However, excessive reflection can pathologically augment aortic systolic pressure, because the less compliant the aorta, the greater the pulse wave velocity. Consequently, returning (reflected) pressure waves collide with the forward-going pulse wave from the next heartbeat earlier in the cardiac cycle. This results from stiffening of the aorta due to loss of elastin during ageing, especially in people with hypertension. Elastin is replaced by inelastic collagen. Cardiac work (see Ch. 22) can be reduced by increasing arterial compliance or by reducing arterial wave reflection (both of which decrease the pulse pressure), even if the cardiac output and mean arterial pressure are unchanged. Over the age of around 55 years, pulse pressure and aortic stiffness are important risk factors for cardiac disease.

---

[3]Think of the waves in your bath as you sit up: down the tub, a splash down the overflow but most comes back as reflections from the foot end under the taps and interferes with the forward waves.

CONTROL OF VASCULAR SMOOTH MUSCLE TONE

In addition to the sympathetic nervous system (Ch. 15), two important physiological systems that regulate vascular tone, namely the vascular endothelium and the renin–angiotensin system, deserve special attention.

THE VASCULAR ENDOTHELIUM

A new chapter in our understanding of vascular control opened with the discovery that vascular endothelium acts not only as a passive barrier between plasma and extracellular fluid, but also as a source of numerous potent mediators. These actively control the underlying smooth muscle as well as influencing platelet and mononuclear cell function: the roles of the endothelium in haemostasis and thrombosis are discussed in Chapter 25. Several distinct classes of mediator are involved (Fig. 23.1).

- *Prostanoids* (see Ch. 18). The discovery by Bunting, Gryglewski, Moncada and Vane (1976) of prostaglandin PGI$_2$ (prostacyclin) ushered in this era. This mediator, acting on IP receptors (Ch. 18), relaxes smooth muscle and inhibits platelet aggregation by activating adenylyl cyclase. Endothelial cells from

Vascular smooth muscle

- Vascular smooth muscle is controlled by mediators secreted by sympathetic nerves (Ch. 15) and vascular endothelium, and by circulating hormones.
- Smooth muscle cell contraction is initiated by a rise in $[Ca^{2+}]_i$, which activates myosin light-chain kinase, causing phosphorylation of myosin, or by sensitisation of the myofilaments to Ca^{2+} by inhibition of myosin phosphatase (see Ch. 4).
- Agents cause contraction via one or more mechanism:
  - release of intracellular Ca^{2+} via inositol trisphosphate
  - depolarising the membrane, opening voltage-gated calcium channels and causing Ca^{2+} entry
  - increasing sensitivity to Ca^{2+} via actions on myosin light-chain kinase and/or myosin phosphatase (Ch. 4, Fig. 4.9)
- Agents cause relaxation by:
  - inhibiting Ca^{2+} entry through voltage-gated calcium channels either directly (e.g. **nifedipine**) or indirectly by hyperpolarising the membrane (e.g. potassium-channel activators such as the active metabolite of **minoxidil**)
  - increasing intracellular cAMP or cGMP; cAMP inactivates myosin light-chain kinase and facilitates Ca^{2+} efflux, cGMP opposes agonist-induced increases in $[Ca^{2+}]_i$.

microvessels also synthesise PGE_2, which is a direct vasodilator and additionally inhibits noradrenaline release from sympathetic nerve terminals, while lacking the effect of PGI_2 on platelets. Prostaglandin endoperoxide intermediates (PGG_2, PGH_2) are endothelium-derived contracting factors acting via thromboxane (TX) T prostanoid (TP) receptors.

- *NO (see Ch. 21). Endothelium-derived relaxing factor (EDRF)* was described by Furchgott and Zawadzki in 1980, and identified as NO by the groups of Moncada and of Ignarro (see Fig. 21.2). These discoveries enormously expanded our understanding of the role of the endothelium. NO activates guanylyl cyclase. It is released continuously in resistance vessels, giving rise to vasodilator tone and contributing to the physiological control of blood pressure. As well as causing vascular relaxation, it inhibits vascular smooth muscle cell proliferation, inhibits platelet adhesion and aggregation, and inhibits monocyte adhesion and migration; consequently, it may protect blood vessels from atherosclerosis and thrombosis (see Chs 24 and 25).
- *Peptides.* The endothelium secretes several vasoactive peptides (see Ch. 19 for general mechanisms of peptide secretion). *C-natriuretic peptide* (CNP) (Ch. 22) and *adrenomedullin* (a vasodilator peptide originally discovered in an adrenal tumour – phaeochromocytoma – but expressed in many tissues, including vascular endothelium) are vasodilators working, respectively, through cGMP and cAMP. *Angiotensin II*, formed by angiotensin-converting enzyme (ACE) on the surface of endothelial cells (see p. 295), and *endothelin* are potent endothelium-derived vasoconstrictor peptides.

- *Endothelium-derived hyperpolarisation factors (EDHFs).* PGI_2 and NO each hyperpolarise vascular smooth muscle cells, which contributes to their relaxant effects. Endothelium-dependent dilatation and hyperpolarisation in response to several mediators (including acetylcholine and bradykinin) persists in some vessels in the absence of prostaglandin and NO synthesis. Several endothelium-derived mediators have been implicated, including *epoxyeicosatrienoic acids* (EETs – derived from endothelial cytochrome P450 enzymes), various lipoxygenase (LOX) products, *hydrogen peroxide* (H_2O_2), *carbon monoxide* (CO), *hydrogen sulfide* (H_2S), and CNP – see Félétou and Vanhoutte (2009). These authors define an additional EDHF distinct from these mediators, and dependent on calcium-activated potassium (K_{Ca}) channels in endothelial cells. As the name implies, these channels are activated by an increase in endothelial cell $[Ca^{2+}]_i$.

In addition to secreting vasoactive mediators, endothelial cells express several enzymes and transport mechanisms that act on circulating hormones and are important targets of drug action. ACE is a particularly important example (see pp. 295–296, including Figs 23.4 and 23.5).

Many endothelium-derived mediators are mutually antagonistic, conjuring an image of opposing rugby football players swaying back and forth in a scrum; in moments of exasperation, one sometimes wonders whether all this makes sense or whether the designer simply could not make up their mind! An important distinction is made between mechanisms that are tonically active in resistance vessels under basal conditions, as is the case with the noradrenergic nervous system (Ch. 15), NO (Ch. 21) and endothelin (see pp. 292–294), and those that operate mainly in response to injury, inflammation, etc., as with PGI_2. Some of the latter group may be functionally redundant, perhaps representing vestiges of mechanisms that were important to our evolutionary forebears, or they may simply be taking a breather on the touchline and are ready to rejoin the fray if called on by the occurrence of some vascular insult. Evidence for such a 'back-up' role comes, for example, from mice that lack the IP receptor for PGI_2; they have a normal blood pressure and do not develop spontaneous thrombosis, but are more susceptible to vasoconstrictor and thrombotic stimuli than their wild-type litter mates (Murata et al., 1997).

THE ENDOTHELIUM IN ANGIOGENESIS

As touched on in Chapter 9, the barrier function of vascular endothelium differs markedly in different organs, and its development during angiogenesis is controlled by several growth factors, including *vascular endothelial growth factor* (VEGF) and various tissue-specific factors such as endocrine gland VEGF. These are involved in repair processes and in pathogenesis (e.g. tumour growth and in neovascularisation in the eye – an important cause of blindness in patients with diabetes mellitus). These factors and their receptors are potentially fruitful targets for drug development and new therapies (including gene therapies; Ch. 5).

ENDOTHELIN

Discovery, biosynthesis and secretion

Hickey et al. described a vasoconstrictor factor produced by cultured endothelial cells in 1985. This was identified as *endothelin (ET)*, a 21-residue peptide, by Yanagisawa

Table 23.1 Distribution of endothelins and endothelin receptors in various tissues[a]

Tissues	Endothelin 1	Endothelin 2	Endothelin 3	Endothelin receptor ET$_A$	Endothelin receptor ET$_B$
Vascular tissue Endothelium	++++	—	—		+
Smooth muscle	+	—	—	++	—
Brain	+++		+	+	+++
Kidney	++	++	+	+	++
Intestines	+	+	+++	+	+++
Adrenal gland	+	—	+++	+	++

[a]Levels of expression of endothelins or the receptor mRNA and/or immunoreactive endothelins: ++++, highest; +++, high; ++, moderate; +, low.

(Adapted from Masaki, T., 1993. Endocr. Rev. 14, 256–268.)

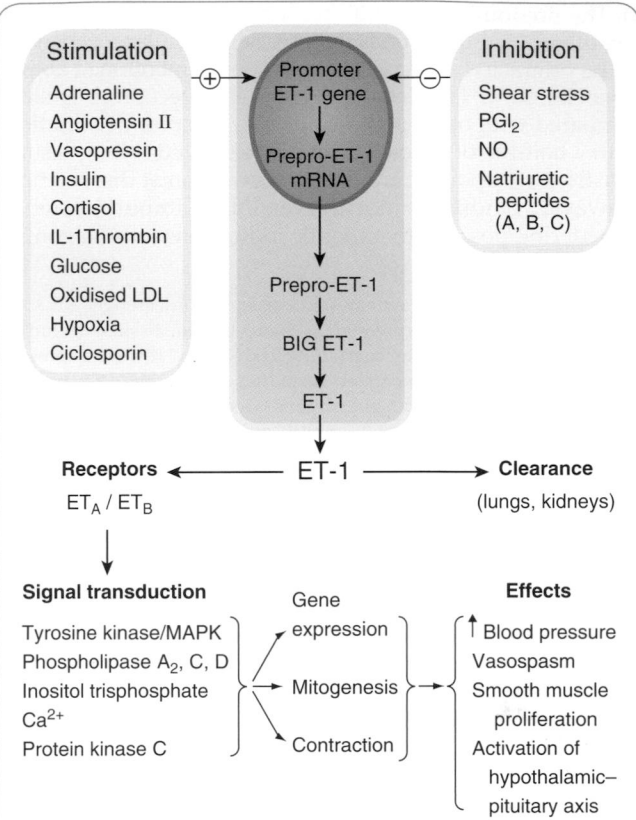

Fig. 23.2 Endothelin-1 (ET-1) synthesis and actions. The schematic shows some of the more important actions only. *IL-1*, interleukin-1; *LDL*, low-density lipoprotein; *MAPK*, mitogen-activated protein kinase; *NO*, nitric oxide; *PGI$_2$*, prostaglandin I$_2$.

et al. (1988), who achieved the isolation, analysis and cloning of the gene for this peptide, which at that time was the most potent vasoconstrictor known,[4] in an impressively short space of time.

▼ Three genes encode different sequences (ET-1, ET-2 and ET-3), each with a distinctive 'shepherd's crook' structure produced by two internal disulfide bonds. These isoforms are differently expressed in organs such as brain and adrenal glands (Table 23.1), suggesting that endothelins have functions beyond the cardiovascular system and this is supported by observations of mice in which the gene coding for ET-1 is disrupted (see later). ET-1 is the only endothelin present in endothelial cells, and is also expressed in many other tissues. Its synthesis and actions are summarised schematically in Fig. 23.2. ET-2 is much less widely distributed: it is present in kidney and intestine. ET-3 is present in brain, lung, intestine and adrenal gland. ET-1 is synthesised from a 212-residue precursor molecule (prepro-ET), which is processed to 'big ET-1' and finally cleaved by an endothelin-converting enzyme to yield ET-1. Cleavage occurs not at the usual Lys–Arg or Arg–Arg position (see Ch. 19), but at a Trp–Val pair, implying a very atypical endopeptidase. The converting enzyme is a metalloprotease and is inhibited by **phosphoramidon** (a pharmacological tool but not used therapeutically). Big ET-1 is converted to ET-1 intracellularly and also on the surface of endothelial and smooth muscle cells.

Stimuli of endothelin synthesis include many vasoactive mediators released by trauma or inflammation, including activated platelets, endotoxin, thrombin, various cytokines and growth factors, angiotensin II, antidiuretic hormone (ADH), adrenaline, insulin, hypoxia and low shear stress. Inhibitors of endothelin synthesis include NO, natriuretic peptides, PGE$_2$, PGI$_2$, heparin and high shear stress.

Release of ET-1 is poorly understood. Preformed ET-1 can be stored in endothelial cells, although probably not in granules. ET-1 concentration in plasma is too low (<5 pmol/L) to activate endothelin receptors, but concentrations in the extracellular space between endothelium and

Table 23.2 Endothelin receptors

Receptor	Affinity	Pharmacological response
ET$_A$	ET-1 = ET-2 > ET-3	Vasoconstriction, bronchoconstriction, stimulation of aldosterone secretion
ET$_B$	ET-1 = ET-2 = ET-3	Vasodilatation, inhibition of ex vivo platelet aggregation

(From Masaki, T., 1993. Endocr. Rev. 14, 256–268.)

vascular smooth muscle are presumably much higher, since endothelin receptor antagonists (see later) cause vasodilatation when infused directly into the brachial artery, implying tonic ET-1-mediated vasoconstrictor activity in resistance vasculature. ET-1 has a plasma elimination half-life of less than 5 min, despite a much longer duration of action following intravenous administration, and clearance occurs mainly in the lung and kidneys.

Endothelin receptors and responses

There are two types of endothelin receptor, designated ET$_A$ and ET$_B$ (Table 23.2), both of which are G protein–coupled (Ch.

---

[4]Subsequently, an 11-amino acid peptide (*urotensin*) was isolated from the brains of bony fish and found to be 50–100 times more potent than endothelin in some blood vessels. It and its receptor are expressed in human tissue but its function, if any, in man remains enigmatic.

3). The predominant overall response is vasoconstriction. A key unresolved question is the precise molecular mechanism of the protracted vasoconstrictor response mentioned above; dissociation of labelled ET-1 from ET_A receptors is slow compared with other peptide agonist/receptor dissociation, with a half-life of about 6 hours, as expected if long-lasting constrictor responses are due to slow agonist dissociation. However, binding is not irreversible – important when considering possible therapeutic indications for antagonists (Davenport et al., 2016).

▼ ET-1 preferentially activates ET_A receptors. Messenger RNA for the ET_A receptor is expressed in many human tissues, including vascular smooth muscle, heart, lung and kidney. It is not expressed in endothelium. ET_A-mediated responses include vasoconstriction, bronchoconstriction and aldosterone secretion. ET_A receptors are coupled to phospholipase C, which stimulates Na^+/H^+ exchange, protein kinase C and mitogenesis, as well as causing vasoconstriction through inositol trisphosphate-mediated Ca^{2+} release (Ch. 3). There are several partially selective ET_A-receptor antagonists, including BQ-123 (a cyclic pentapeptide) and several orally active non-peptide drugs (e.g. **bosentan**, a mixed ET_A/ET_B antagonist, and **ambrasentan**, ET_A-selective, both of which are used in treating pulmonary arterial hypertension – see pp. 307–308). ET_B receptors are activated to a similar extent by each of the three endothelin isoforms, but *sarafotoxin S6c* (a 21-residue peptide that shares the shepherd's crook structure of the endothelins and was isolated from the venom of the burrowing asp) is a selective agonist and has proved useful as a pharmacological tool for studying the ET_B receptor. Messenger RNA for the ET_B receptor is mainly expressed in brain (especially cerebral cortex and cerebellum), with moderate expression in aorta, heart, lung, kidney and adrenals. In contrast to the ET_A receptor, it is highly expressed in endothelium, where it causes *vasodilatation* by stimulating NO and PGI_2 production, but it is also present in vascular smooth muscle, where it initiates vasoconstriction like the ET_A receptor. ET_B receptors play a part in clearing ET-1 from the circulation, and ET antagonists with appreciable affinity for ET_B receptors consequently increase plasma concentrations of ET-1, complicating interpretation of such concentrations during experiments with these drugs.

Functions of endothelin

ET-1 is a local mediator rather than a circulating hormone, although it stimulates secretion of several hormones (see Table 23.1). Administration of an ET_A-receptor antagonist or of phosphoramidon into the brachial artery increases forearm blood flow, and ET_A-receptor antagonists lower arterial blood pressure, suggesting that ET-1 contributes to vasoconstrictor tone and the control of peripheral vascular resistance in man. Endothelins have several other possible functions, including roles in:

- release of various hormones, including atrial natriuretic peptide, aldosterone, adrenaline, and hypothalamic and pituitary hormones;
- natriuresis and diuresis via actions of collecting duct-derived ET-1 on ET_B receptors on tubular epithelial cells;
- thyroglobulin synthesis (the concentration of ET-1 in thyroid follicles is extremely high)
- control of uteroplacental blood flow (ET-1 is abundant in amniotic fluid)
- renal and cerebral vasospasm (Fig. 23.3);
- development of the cardiorespiratory systems (if the ET-1 gene is disrupted in mice, pharyngeal arch tissues develop abnormally and homozygotes die of respiratory failure at birth, and ET receptor antagonists are teratogenic, causing cardiorespiratory developmental disorders).

Fig. 23.3 In vivo effects of a potent non-peptide endothelin-1 ET_A- and ET_B-receptor antagonist, Ro 46-2005, in three animal models. (A) Prevention by Ro 46-2005 of post-ischaemic renal vasoconstriction in rats. (B) Prevention by Ro 46-2005 of the decrease in cerebral blood flow after subarachnoid haemorrhage (SAH) in rats treated with placebo *(blue)* or with Ro 46-2005 *(red)*. (C) Effect of orally administered Ro 46-2005 on mean arterial pressure in sodium-depleted squirrel monkeys treated with placebo *(blue)* or increasing doses of antagonist *(red: ● < ▲ < ◆)*. (From Clozel, M., et al., 1993. Nature 365, 759–761.)

The role of the endothelium in controlling vascular smooth muscle

- Endothelial cells release vasoactive mediators including prostacyclin (PGI₂), nitric oxide (NO) and distinct but incompletely characterised hyperpolarising factor(s) 'EDHF' (vasodilators), and endothelin and endoperoxide thromboxane receptor agonists (vasoconstrictors).
- Many vasodilators (e.g. acetylcholine and bradykinin) act via endothelial NO production. The NO derives from arginine and is produced when $[Ca^{2+}]_i$ increases in the endothelial cell, or the sensitivity of endothelial NO synthase to Ca^{2+} is increased (see Fig. 21.3).
- NO relaxes smooth muscle by increasing cGMP formation.
- Endothelin is a potent and long-acting vasoconstrictor peptide released from endothelial cells by many chemical and physical factors. It is not confined to blood vessels, and it has several functional roles.

THE RENIN–ANGIOTENSIN SYSTEM

The renin–angiotensin system synergises with the sympathetic nervous system, for example, by increasing the release of noradrenaline from sympathetic nerve terminals. It stimulates aldosterone secretion and plays a central role in the control of Na⁺ excretion and fluid volume, as well as of vascular tone.

The control of renin secretion (Fig. 23.4) is only partly understood. It is a proteolytic enzyme that is secreted by the *juxtaglomerular apparatus* (see Ch. 30, Fig. 30.2) in response to various physiological stimuli including reduced renal perfusion pressure, or reduced Na⁺ concentration in distal tubular fluid, which is sensed by the *macula densa* (a specialised part of the distal tubule apposed to the juxtaglomerular apparatus). Renal sympathetic nerve activity, β-adrenoceptor agonists and PGI₂ all stimulate renin secretion directly, whereas angiotensin II causes feedback inhibition. Atrial natriuretic peptide (Ch. 22) also inhibits renin secretion. Renin is cleared rapidly from plasma. It acts on *angiotensinogen* (a plasma globulin made in the liver), splitting off a decapeptide, *angiotensin I*.

Angiotensin I is inactive, but is converted by *ACE* to an octapeptide, *angiotensin II*, which is a potent vasoconstrictor. Angiotensin II is a substrate for enzymes (aminopeptidase A and N) that remove single amino acid residues, giving rise, respectively, to angiotensin III and angiotensin IV (Fig. 23.5). Angiotensin III stimulates aldosterone secretion and is involved in thirst. Angiotensin IV also has distinct actions, probably via its own receptor, including release of *plasminogen activator inhibitor-1* from the endothelium (Ch. 25). Receptors for angiotensin IV have a distinctive distribution, including the hypothalamus.

ACE is a membrane-bound enzyme on the surface of endothelial cells, and is particularly abundant in the lung, which has a vast surface area of vascular endothelium.[5]

[5]Approximately that of a football field.

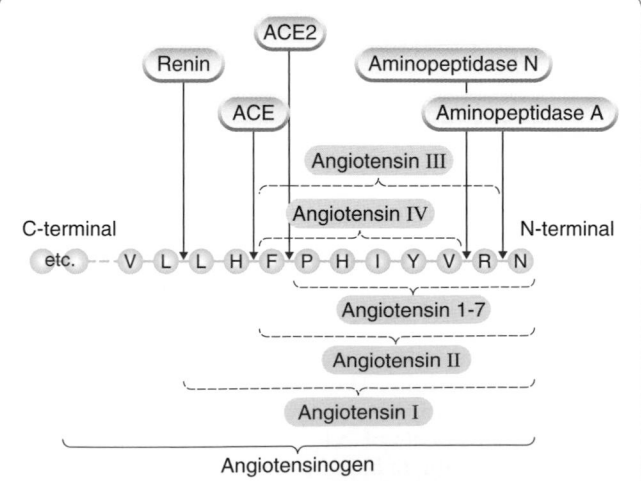

Fig. 23.4 Control of renin release and formation, and action of angiotensin II. Sites of action of drugs that inhibit the cascade are shown. *ACE*, angiotensin-converting enzyme; *AT₁*, angiotensin II receptor subtype 1; *PGI₂*, prostaglandin I₂.

Fig. 23.5 Formation of angiotensins I–IV from the N-terminal of the precursor protein angiotensinogen. Also shown is angiotensin 17 which is a product of the action of angiotensin-converting enzyme 2 (ACE2) and opposing actins to angiotensin II.

Table 23.3 Classification of vasoactive drugs that act indirectly

Site	Mechanism	Examples	See chapter
Vasoconstrictors			
Sympathetic nerves	Noradrenaline (norepinephrine) release	Tyramine	15
	Blocks noradrenaline reuptake	Cocaine	15
Endothelium	Endothelin release	Angiotensin II (in part)	This chapter
Vasodilators			
Sympathetic nerves	Inhibits noradrenaline release	Prostaglandin E_2, guanethidine	18 15
Endothelium	Nitric oxide release	Acetylcholine, substance P	21
Central nervous system	Vasomotor inhibition	Anaesthetics	42
Enzymes	ACE inhibition	Captopril	This chapter

The common isoform of ACE is also present in other vascularised tissues, including heart, brain, striated muscle and kidney, and is not restricted to endothelial cells. Consequently, local formation of angiotensin II can occur in different vascular beds, and it provides local control independent of blood-borne angiotensin II. ACE inactivates bradykinin (see Ch. 19) and several other peptides. This may contribute to the pharmacological actions of ACE inhibitors (ACEIs), as discussed below.

▼ ACE2, a homologue of ACE, converts angiotensin II to angiotensin 1-7 (Ang 1-7) as shown in Fig. 23.5. Ang 1-7 acts on the Mas receptor (a G-protein–coupled receptor coded by the *MAS1*oncogene) opposing the effects of angiotensin II. ACE2 is widely expressed, including in cardiomyocytes and endothelial cells, and potentially protects against heart failure. Recombinant human ACE2 has been tested in humans without adverse effects while lowering plasma angiotensin II and increasing Ang 1-7 concentration. For a recent review of the therapeutic potential of enhancing ACE2/Ang 1-7 action for heart failure see Patel et al. (2016). ACE2 is expressed in Leydig cells of the testis and male mice lacking this ACE isoform have markedly reduced fertility. ACE2 is insensitive to conventional ACE inhibitors.

The main actions of angiotensin II are mediated via AT_1 and/or AT_2 receptors, which belong to the family of G protein–coupled receptors. Effects mediated by AT_1 receptors include:

- generalised vasoconstriction, especially marked in efferent arterioles of the renal glomeruli;
- increased noradrenaline release, reinforcing sympathetic effects;
- proximal tubular reabsorption of Na^+;
- secretion of aldosterone from the adrenal cortex (see Ch. 34);
- growth of cardiac and vascular cells.[6]

AT_2 receptors are expressed during fetal life and in distinct brain regions in adults. They are believed to be involved in growth, development and exploratory behaviour. Cardiovascular effects of AT_2 receptors (inhibition of cell growth and lowering of blood pressure) are relatively subtle and oppose those of AT_1 receptors.

The renin–angiotensin–aldosterone pathway contributes to the pathogenesis of heart failure, and several leading classes of therapeutic drug act on it at different points (see Fig. 23.4).

VASOACTIVE DRUGS

Drugs can affect vascular smooth muscle by acting either directly on smooth muscle cells, or indirectly, for example, on endothelial cells, on sympathetic nerve terminals or on the central nervous system (CNS) (Table 23.3). Mechanisms of directly acting vasoconstrictors and vasodilators are summarised in Fig. 4.10 (Ch. 4). Many indirectly acting drugs are discussed in other chapters (see Table 23.3). We concentrate here on agents that are not covered elsewhere.

VASOCONSTRICTOR DRUGS

The α_1-adrenoceptor agonists and drugs that release noradrenaline from sympathetic nerve terminals or inhibit its reuptake (sympathomimetic amines) are discussed in Chapter 15. Some eicosanoids (e.g. *thromboxane A_2*; see Chs 18 and 25) and several peptides, notably *endothelin, angiotensin* and *ADH*, are also predominantly vasoconstrictor. **Sumatriptan** and ergot alkaloids acting on certain 5-hydroxytryptamine receptors ($5\text{-}HT_2$ and $5\text{-}HT_{1D}$) also cause vasoconstriction (Ch. 16).

ANGIOTENSIN II

The physiological role of the renin–angiotensin system is described previously. Angiotensin II is roughly 40 times as potent as noradrenaline in raising blood pressure. Like α_1-adrenoceptor agonists, it constricts mainly cutaneous, splanchnic and renal vasculature, with less effect on blood flow to brain and skeletal muscle. It has no routine clinical uses, although it has promise in the treatment of vasodilatory shock (Khanna et al., 2017), its main therapeutic importance lying in the fact that other drugs (e.g. **captopril** and **losartan**, see pp. 300–301) affect the cardiovascular system by reducing its production or action.

ANTIDIURETIC HORMONE

ADH (also known as vasopressin) is a posterior pituitary peptide hormone (Ch. 34). It is physiologically important

---

[6]These effects are initiated by the G protein–coupled AT_1 receptor acting via the same intracellular tyrosine phosphorylation pathways as are used by cytokines, for example, the Jak/Stat pathway (Ch. 3).

for its antidiuretic action on the kidney (Ch. 30) but is also a powerful vasoconstrictor. Its effects are initiated by two distinct receptors (V_1 and V_2). Water retention is mediated through V_2 receptors, occurs at low plasma concentrations of ADH and involves activation of adenylyl cyclase in renal collecting ducts. Vasoconstriction is mediated through V_1 receptors (two subtypes, see Ch. 34), requires higher concentrations of ADH and involves activation of phospholipase C (see Ch. 3). ADH causes generalised vasoconstriction, including the skin, coeliac, mesenteric and coronary vessels. It also affects other (e.g. gastrointestinal and uterine) smooth muscle and causes abdominal cramps for this reason. Vasopressin or its analogue, **terlipressin**, is commonly used to treat patients with bleeding oesophageal varices and portal hypertension before more definitive endoscopic treatment; although gastroenterologists also have the option of using **octreotide** (unlicensed indication; see Ch. 34) for this. It may also have a place in treating vasodilatory shock (see p. 307).

ENDOTHELIN

Endothelins are discussed earlier in the context of their physiological roles; as explained above, they have vasodilator and vasoconstrictor actions, but vasoconstriction predominates. Intravenous administration causes transient vasodilatation followed by profound and long-lived vasoconstriction. The endothelins are even more potent vasoconstrictors than angiotensin II. As yet, they have no clinical uses, and endothelin antagonists are licensed only for primary pulmonary hypertension (see p. 308).

VASODILATOR DRUGS

Vasodilator drugs play a major role in the treatment of common conditions, including hypertension, cardiac failure and angina pectoris, as well as several less common but serious diseases, including pulmonary hypertension and Raynaud's disease.

DIRECT ACTING VASODILATORS

Targets on which drugs act to relax vascular smooth muscle include plasma membrane voltage-dependent calcium channels, sarcoplasmic reticulum channels (Ca^{2+} release or

> ### Vasoconstrictor substances
>
> - The main groups are sympathomimetic amines (direct and indirect; Ch. 15), certain eicosanoids (especially thromboxane A_2; Ch. 18), peptides (angiotensin II, antidiuretic hormone [ADH] and endothelin; Ch. 19) and a group of miscellaneous drugs (e.g. ergot alkaloids; Ch. 16).
> - Clinical uses include local applications (e.g. nasal decongestion, co-administration with local anaesthetics). Sympathomimetic amines and **ADH** are used in circulatory shock. **Adrenaline** is life-saving in anaphylactic shock and in cardiac arrest. **ADH** or **terlipressin** (an analogue) has been infused intravenously to stop bleeding from oesophageal varices before surgery in patients with portal hypertension caused by liver disease.

reuptake) and enzymes that determine Ca^{2+} sensitivity of the contractile proteins (see Fig. 4.10).

Calcium antagonists

L-type calcium antagonists are discussed in Chapter 22.

Drugs that activate potassium channels

Some drugs (e.g. **minoxidil**, **diazoxide**) relax smooth muscle by opening K_{ATP} channels (Fig. 23.6). This hyperpolarises the cells and switches off voltage-dependent calcium channels. Potassium-channel activators work by antagonising the action of intracellular ATP on these channels.

Minoxidil (acting through an active sulfate metabolite) is an especially potent and long-acting vasodilator, used as a drug of last resort in treating severe hypertension unresponsive to other drugs. It causes hirsutism (the active metabolite is actually used as a rub-on cream to treat baldness, see Ch. 28). It causes marked salt and water retention,

Fig. 23.6 **ATP-sensitive potassium channels.** Patch clamp (see Ch. 3) record from insulin-secreting pancreatic B cell: saponin permeabilised the cell, with loss of intracellular ATP, causing the channels to open (upward deflection) until they were inhibited by ATP. Addition of diazoxide, a vasodilator drug (which also inhibits insulin secretion; see text) reopens the channels. In smooth muscle, this causes hyperpolarisation and relaxation. (Redrawn from Dunne, et al., 1990. Br. J. Pharmacol. 99, 169.)

so is usually prescribed with a loop diuretic. It causes reflex tachycardia, and a β-adrenoceptor antagonist is used to prevent this. **Nicorandil** (Ch. 22) combines K_{ATP} channel activation with NO donor activity, and is used in refractory angina.

Drugs that act via cyclic nucleotides
Cyclase activation
Many drugs relax vascular smooth muscle by increasing the cellular concentration of either cGMP or cAMP. For example, NO, nitrates and the natriuretic peptides act through cGMP (see Chs 21 and 22); BAY41-2272, a pyrazolopyridine, activates soluble guanylyl cyclase via an NO-independent site (see Ch. 21). The *$β_2$ agonists, adenosine* and *PGI_2* increase cytoplasmic cAMP (see Chs 15, 17, 18). *Dopamine* has mixed vasodilator and vasoconstrictor actions. It selectively dilates renal vessels, where it increases cAMP by activating adenylyl cyclase. Dopamine, when administered as an intravenous infusion, produces a mixture of cardiovascular effects resulting from agonist actions on α and β adrenoceptors, as well as on dopamine receptors. Blood pressure increases slightly, but the main effects are vasodilatation in the renal circulation and increased cardiac output. Dopamine was widely used in intensive care units in patients in whom renal failure associated with decreased renal perfusion appeared imminent; despite its beneficial effect on renal haemodynamics, clinical trials have shown that it does not improve survival in these circumstances and this use is obsolete. **Nesiritide**, a recombinant form of human B-type natriuretic peptide (BNP) (see Ch. 22), was widely used in the United States for the treatment of acutely decompensated heart failure, but efficacy data have not been impressive (O'Connor et al., 2011). However, **sacubitril**, prodrug of an active metabolite sacubitilat, an inhibitor of neprilysin (which is also known as neutral endopeptidase, NEP), increases circulating natriuretic peptides (BNP and ANP) and, in fixed combination with **valsartan**, is effective in treating chronic heart failure (see later, p. 305).

Nitroprusside (nitroferricyanide) is a powerful vasodilator which acts by releasing NO (Ch. 21). Unlike the organic nitrates, it acts equally on arterial and venous smooth muscle. Its clinical usefulness is limited because it must be given intravenously. In solution, particularly when exposed to light, nitroprusside hydrolyses with formation of cyanide. The intravenous solution must therefore be made up freshly from dry powder and protected from light. Nitroprusside is rapidly converted to thiocyanate in the body, its plasma half-life being only a few minutes, so it must be given as a continuous infusion with careful monitoring to avoid hypotension. Prolonged use causes thiocyanate accumulation and toxicity (weakness, nausea and inhibition of thyroid function); consequently, nitroprusside is useful only for short-term treatment (usually up to 72 h maximum). It is used in intensive care units for hypertensive emergencies, to produce controlled hypotension during surgery, and to reduce cardiac work during the reversible cardiac dysfunction that occurs after cardiopulmonary bypass surgery.

Phosphodiesterase inhibition
Phosphodiesterases (PDEs; see Ch. 3) include at least 14 distinct isoenzymes. Methylxanthines (e.g. **theophylline**) and **papaverine** are non-selective PDE inhibitors (and have additional actions). Methylxanthines exert their main effects on bronchial smooth muscle and on the CNS, and are

discussed in Chapters 29 and 49. In addition to inhibiting PDE, some methylxanthines are also purine receptor antagonists (Ch. 17). Papaverine is produced by opium poppies (see Ch. 43) and relaxes vascular smooth muscle. Its mechanism is poorly understood but seems to involve a combination of PDE inhibition and block of calcium channels. Selective PDE type III inhibitors (e.g. **milrinone**) increase cAMP in cardiac muscle. They have a positive inotropic effect but, despite short-term haemodynamic improvement, increase mortality in patients with heart failure, possibly by causing dysrhythmias. **Dipyridamole**, as well as enhancing the actions of adenosine (see Ch. 17), also causes vasodilatation by inhibiting PDE. Selective *PDE type V* inhibitors (e.g. **sildenafil**) inhibit the breakdown of cGMP, thereby potentiating NO signalling. It revolutionised treatment of erectile dysfunction (see Ch. 36) and has therapeutic potential in other situations, including pulmonary hypertension (see clinical box, p. 308).

> ## Vasodilator drugs
>
> - Vasodilators act:
>   - to increase local tissue blood flow
>   - to reduce arterial pressure
>   - to reduce central venous pressure
> - Reduce cardiac work by reducing cardiac preload (reduced filling pressure) and afterload (reduced vascular resistance).
> - Main uses are:
>   - antihypertensive therapy (e.g. angiotensin II type 1 [AT_1] antagonists, calcium antagonists and $α_1$-adrenoceptor antagonists)
>   - treatment/prophylaxis of angina (e.g. calcium antagonists, nitrates)
>   - treatment of cardiac failure (e.g. angiotensin-converting enzyme inhibitors, AT_1 antagonists)
>   - treatment of erectile dysfunction.

VASODILATORS WITH UNCERTAIN MECHANISM OF ACTION

Hydralazine
Hydralazine acts mainly by relaxing arteries and arterioles, causing a fall in blood pressure accompanied by reflex tachycardia and increased cardiac output. It interferes with the action of inositol trisphosphate on Ca^{2+} release from the sarcoplasmic reticulum. Its original clinical use was in hypertension, and is still used for short-term treatment of severe hypertension in pregnancy but it can cause an immune disorder resembling systemic lupus erythematosus (SLE),[7] so alternative agents are now preferred for long-term treatment of hypertension. It has a place in treating heart failure in patients of African origin in combination with a long-acting organic nitrate (see clinical box, p. 306).

---

[7]An autoimmune disease affecting one or more tissues, including joints, kidneys, brain, blood platelets, skin and pleural membranes (Chs 27 and 58). The autoantibodies are directed against antigens that are intracellular in healthy cells but which become clustered in blebs at the surface of apoptotic cells. In SLE apoptotic waste may present these multiple antigens to cells of the immune system; hydralazine is one of several drugs that can mimic SLE but the mechanism is incompletely understood.

Ethanol

Ethanol (see Ch. 50) dilates cutaneous vessels, causing the familiar drunkard's flush. Several general anaesthetics (e.g. **propofol**) cause vasodilatation as an unwanted effect (Ch. 42).

INDIRECTLY ACTING VASODILATOR DRUGS

Indirectly acting vasodilator drugs work by inhibiting vasoconstrictor systems, namely the sympathetic nervous system (see Ch. 15) and the renin–angiotensin–aldosterone and endothelin systems or by potentiating endogenous vasodilators such as the natriuretic peptides (see Ch.22 and further in this chapter, p. 305).

The central control of sympathetically mediated vasoconstriction involves α_2 adrenoceptors and another class of receptor, termed the *imidazoline I_1 receptor*, present in the brain stem in the rostral ventrolateral medulla. **Clonidine** (an α_2-adrenoceptor agonist, now largely obsolete as an antihypertensive drug) and **moxonodine**, an I_1-receptor agonist, lower blood pressure by reducing sympathetic activity centrally. In addition, many vasodilators (e.g.

acetylcholine, bradykinin, substance P) exert some or all of their effects by stimulating biosynthesis of vasodilator prostaglandins or of NO (or of both) by vascular endothelium (see previously and Ch. 21), thereby causing functional antagonism of the constrictor tone caused by sympathetic nerves and angiotensin II.

Many useful drugs block the renin–angiotensin–aldosterone system (RAAS; see Table 23.4 for a summary of selective antagonists) at one of several points:

- renin release: β-adrenoceptor antagonists inhibit renin release (Ch. 15)
- renin activity: renin inhibitors inhibit conversion of angiotensinogen to angiotensin I
- ACE: ACEIs (see later) block conversion of angiotensin I to angiotensin II
- angiotensin II receptors: AT_1-receptor antagonists (ARBs, see later)
- aldosterone receptors: aldosterone-receptor antagonists (see later)

Table 23.4 Summary of drugs that inhibit the renin–angiotensin–aldosterone system

Class	Drug[a]	Pharmacokinetics	Adverse effects[b]	Uses	Notes
ACE inhibitors	Captopril	Short acting $t_{1/2}$ ~2 h Dose 2–3 times daily	Cough Hypotension Proteinuria Taste disturbance	Hypertension Heart failure After MI	ACEIs are cleared mainly by renal excretion
	Enalapril	Prodrug – active metabolite enalaprilat $t_{1/2}$ ~11 h Dose 1–2 times daily	Cough Hypotension Reversible renal impairment (in patients with renal artery stenosis)	As captopril	Lisinopril, perindopril, ramipril, trandolapril are similar Some are licensed for distinct uses (e.g. stroke, left ventricular hypertrophy)
ARBs	Valsartan	$t_{1/2}$ ~6 h	Hypotension Reversible renal impairment (in patients with renal artery stenosis)	Hypertension Heart failure	ARBs are cleared by hepatic metabolism
	Losartan	Long-acting metabolite $t_{1/2}$ ~8 h	As valsartan	As valsartan Diabetic nephropathy	Irbesartan is similar, with $t_{1/2}$ ~10–15 h
	Candesartan	$t_{1/2}$ 5–10 h Long-acting because receptor complex is stable	As valsartan	As valsartan	Given as prodrug ester (candesartan cilexetil)
Renin inhibitor	Aliskiren	Low oral bioavailability $t_{1/2}$ 24 h	As valsartan, also diarrhoea	Essential hypertension	The FDA has warned against combining with ACEI or ARB in patients with renal impairment + diabetes mellitus
Aldosterone antagonists	Eplerenone	$t_{1/2}$ 3–5 h	As valsartan, especially hyperkalaemia Nausea, diarrhoea	Heart failure after MI	Caution in renal impairment; monitor plasma potassium
	Spironolactone	Prodrug converted to canrenone, which has $t_{1/2}$ ~24 h	As eplerenone Also oestrogenic effects (gynaecomastia, menstrual irregularity, erectile dysfunction)	Primary hyperaldosteronism Heart failure Oedema and ascites (e.g. in hepatic cirrhosis)	

[a]All drugs listed are orally active.
[b]Adverse effects common to all drugs listed include hyperkalaemia (especially in patients with impaired renal function) and teratogenesis.
ACE, angiotensin-converting enzyme; *ACEI*, angiotensin-converting enzyme inhibitor; *ARB*, angiotensin receptor blocker; *MI*, myocardial infarction.

Fig. 23.7 **The active site of angiotensin-converting enzyme.** (A) Binding of angiotensin I. (B) Binding of the inhibitor captopril, which is an analogue of the terminal dipeptide of angiotensin I.

Renin inhibitors

Aliskiren, an orally active non-peptide renin inhibitor, was developed and registered as an antihypertensive drug. It is a triumph of drug design and lowers blood pressure, but has adverse effects that include diarrhoea (common), acute renal failure, cardiovascular events in patients with diabetes mellitus, and, rarely, angioedema and severe allergic reactions.

Angiotensin-converting enzyme inhibitors

The first ACEI to be marketed was **captopril** (Fig. 23.7), an early example of successful drug design based on a chemical knowledge of the target molecule. Various small peptides had been found to be weak inhibitors of the enzyme.[8] Captopril was designed to combine the steric properties of such peptide antagonists in a non-peptide molecule that was active when given by mouth. Captopril has a short plasma half-life (about 2 h) and must be given 2 or 3 times daily. Many of the ACEIs developed subsequently (see Table 23.4), which are widely used in the clinic, have a longer duration of action and are administered once daily.

Pharmacological effects

ACEIs cause only a small fall in arterial pressure in healthy human subjects who are consuming the amount of salt contained in a usual Western diet, but a much larger fall in hypertensive patients, particularly those in whom renin secretion is enhanced (e.g. in patients receiving diuretics).

ACEIs affect capacitance and resistance vessels, and reduce cardiac load as well as arterial pressure. They act preferentially on angiotensin-sensitive vascular beds, which include those of the kidney, heart and brain. This selectivity may be important in sustaining adequate perfusion of these vital organs in the face of reduced perfusion pressure. Critical renal artery stenosis[9] represents an exception to this, where ACE inhibition results in a fall in glomerular filtration rate (see later).

Clinical uses of ACEIs are summarised in the clinical box.

Clinical uses of angiotensin-converting enzyme inhibitors

- Hypertension
- Cardiac failure
- Following myocardial infarction (especially when there is ventricular dysfunction)
- In people at high risk of ischaemic heart disease
- Diabetic nephropathy
- Chronic renal insufficiency to prevent progression

Unwanted effects

Adverse effects (see Table 23.4) directly related to ACE inhibition are common to all drugs of this class. These include hypotension, especially after the first dose and especially in patients with heart failure who have been

---

[8]The lead compound was a nonapeptide derived from the venom of *Bothrops jacaraca* – a South American snake. It was originally characterised as a bradykinin-potentiating peptide (ACE inactivates bradykinin, Ch. 19).

[9]Severe narrowing of the renal artery caused, for example, by atheroma (Ch. 24).

treated with loop diuretics, in whom the renin–angiotensin system is activated. A dry cough, possibly the result of accumulation of bradykinin (Ch. 19), is the commonest persistent adverse effect. Kinin accumulation may also underlie *angioedema* (painful swelling in tissues which can be life-threatening if it involves the airway); this adverse effect aborted the introduction of **omapatrilat**, a combined ACEI/ NEP inhibitor, and can also occur, albeit less frequently, during treatment with **sacubitril**, a selective NEP inhibitor used for chronic heart failure (see later). Patients with severe bilateral renal artery stenosis predictably develop renal failure if treated with ACEIs, because glomerular filtration is normally maintained, in the face of low afferent arteriolar pressure, by angiotensin II, which selectively constricts *efferent* arterioles; hyperkalaemia may be severe owing to reduced aldosterone secretion. Such renal failure is reversible provided that it is recognised promptly and ACEI treatment discontinued.

Angiotensin II receptor antagonists

Losartan, **candesartan**, **valsartan** and **irbesartan** (sartans) are non-peptide, orally active AT_1 receptor antagonists (ARBs). ARBs differ pharmacologically from ACEIs (Fig. 23.8) but behave similarly to ACEIs apart from not causing cough – consistent with the 'bradykinin accumulation' explanation of this side effect, mentioned above; however, ACEIs have a more robust evidence base than ARBs, reducing cardiovascular morbidity and mortality (including stroke) compared with placebo in hypertension. For ethical reasons placebo-controlled outcome data are not available for ARBs used as single agents, since these were introduced after incontrovertible evidence was available for the efficacy of other drug classes. The situation has been clouded by evidence of fabricated clinical trial data in several studies of valsartan.

ACE is not the only enzyme capable of forming angiotensin II, *chymase* (which is not inhibited by ACEIs) providing one alternative route. It is not known if alternative pathways of angiotensin II formation are important in vivo, but if so, then ARBs could be more effective than ACEIs when such alternative pathways are active. Again, it is not known whether any of the beneficial effects of ACEIs are bradykinin/NO mediated. It is therefore unwise to assume that ARBs will necessarily share all the therapeutic properties of ACEIs, although there is considerable overlap in the clinical indications for these drugs (see Table 23.4).

Neutral endopeptidase (NEP, neprilysin) inhibition

▼ NEP (see also Ch. 22) is a zinc-dependent metalloprotease that inactivates several peptide mediators including not only natriuretic peptides (ANP and BNP) but also glucagon, enkephalins, substance P, neurotensin, oxytocin and bradykinin. It also degrades amyloid beta peptide (a suspect in the pathogenesis of Alzheimer's disease, see Ch 41). In health it is expressed in many tissues including kidney and lung. Several NEP inhibitors have been developed for possible indications including analgesia and hypertension; as mentioned above one such drug, **omapatrilat**, is a combined ACEI/ NEP inhibitor which was not introduced because it caused angioedema.

CLINICAL USES OF VASOACTIVE DRUGS

It is beyond the scope of this book to provide a detailed account of the clinical uses of vasoactive drugs, but it is

Fig. 23.8 Comparison of effects of angiotensin-converting enzyme inhibition and angiotensin receptor blockade in the human forearm vasculature. (A) Effect of brachial artery infusion of angiotensin II on forearm blood flow after oral administration of placebo, enalapril (10 mg) or losartan (100 mg). (B) Effect of brachial artery infusion of bradykinin, as in (A). (From Cockcroft, J.R. et al., 1993. J. Cardiovasc. Pharmacol. 22, 579–584.)

nonetheless useful to consider briefly the treatment of certain important disorders, namely:

* systemic hypertension
* heart failure
* vasodilatory shock
* peripheral vascular disease
* Raynaud's disease
* pulmonary hypertension

SYSTEMIC HYPERTENSION

Systemic hypertension is a common disorder that, if not effectively treated, increases the risk of coronary thrombosis, strokes and renal failure. Until about 1950, there was no effective treatment, and the development of antihypertensive

Types of vasodilator drug

Directly acting vasodilators

- Calcium antagonists (e.g. **nifedipine**, **diltiazem**, **verapamil**): block Ca^{2+} entry in response to depolarisation. Common adverse effects include ankle swelling and (especially with verapamil) constipation.
- K_{ATP} channel activators (e.g. **minoxidil**): open potassium channels, hyperpolarising vascular smooth muscle cells. Ankle swelling and increased hair growth are common.
- Drugs that increase cytoplasmic cyclic nucleotide concentrations by:
  – increasing adenylyl cyclase activity, for example prostacyclin (**epoprostenol**), $β_2$-adrenoceptor agonists, **adenosine**
  – increasing guanylyl cyclase activity: nitrates (e.g. **glyceryl trinitrate**, **nitroprusside**)
  – inhibiting phosphodiesterase activity (e.g. **sildenafil**)

Indirectly acting vasodilators

- Drugs that interfere with the sympathetic nervous system (e.g. $α_1$-adrenoceptor antagonists). Postural hypotension is a common adverse effect.
- Drugs that block the renin–angiotensin system:
  – renin inhibitors (e.g. **aliskiren**)
  – angiotensin-converting enzyme inhibitors (e.g. **ramipril**); dry cough may be troublesome
  – AT_1 receptor antagonists (e.g. **losartan**).
- Drugs or mediators that stimulate endothelial nitric oxide release (e.g. acetylcholine, bradykinin).
- Drugs that block the endothelin system:
  – endothelin synthesis (e.g. **phosphoramidon**)
  – endothelin receptor antagonists (e.g. **bosentan**)
- Drugs that potentiate vasodilator peptides by blocking their breakdown (e.g. **sacubitril**).

Vasodilators whose mechanism is uncertain

- Miscellaneous drugs including alcohol, **propofol** (Ch. 42) and **hydralazine**.

Clinical uses of angiotensin II subtype 1 receptor antagonists (sartans)

The AT_1 antagonists are extremely well tolerated but are teratogenic. Their uses include the following:
- Hypertension, especially in:
  – young men (circulating renin decreases with increasing age, and sartans are avoided during pregnancy)
  – diabetic patients
  – hypertension complicated by left ventricular hypertrophy
  – as an additional agent in hypertensive patients insufficiently responsive to a thiazide diuretic.
- Heart failure; especially the combination of valsartan with sacubitril (NEP inhibitor).
- Diabetic nephropathy.

drugs has been a major success story. Systemic blood pressure is an excellent 'surrogate marker' for increased cardiovascular risk in that there is good evidence from randomised controlled trials that common antihypertensive drugs (diuretics, ACEIs, calcium antagonists) combined with lifestyle changes not only lower blood pressure but also prolong life and reduce the extra risks of heart attacks and, especially, strokes associated with high blood pressure.

Correctable causes of hypertension include phaeochromocytoma,[10] steroid-secreting tumours of the adrenal cortex and narrowing (coarctation) of the aorta, but most cases involve no obvious cause and are grouped as *essential hypertension* (so-called because it was originally, albeit incorrectly, thought that the raised blood pressure was 'essential' to maintain adequate tissue perfusion). Increased cardiac output may be an early feature, but by the time essential hypertension is established (commonly in middle life) there is usually increased peripheral resistance and the cardiac output is normal. Blood pressure control is intimately related to the kidneys, as demonstrated in humans requiring renal transplantation: hypertension 'goes with' the kidney from a hypertensive donor, and donating a kidney from a normotensive to a hypertensive corrects hypertension in the recipient (see also Ch. 30). It seems likely that the cause of most cases of essential hypertension is a combination of inherited variations in renal tubular sodium ion handling and of dietary salt consumption (Meneton et al., 2005). Persistently raised arterial pressure leads to hypertrophy of the left ventricle and remodelling of resistance arteries, with narrowing of the lumen, and predisposes to atherosclerosis in larger conduit arteries.

Fig. 23.9 summarises physiological mechanisms that control arterial blood pressure and shows sites at which antihypertensive drugs act, notably the sympathetic nervous system, the renin–angiotensin–aldosterone system and endothelium-derived mediators. Remodelling of resistance arteries in response to raised pressure reduces the ratio of lumen diameter to wall thickness and increases the peripheral vascular resistance. The role of cellular growth factors (including angiotensin II) and inhibitors of growth (e.g. NO) in the evolution of these structural changes is of great interest to vascular biologists, and is potentially important for ACEIs and ARBs.

Reducing arterial blood pressure greatly improves the prognosis of patients with hypertension. Controlling hypertension (which is asymptomatic) without producing unacceptable side effects is therefore an important clinical need, which is, in general, well catered for by modern drugs. Treatment involves non-pharmacological measures (e.g. increased exercise, reduced dietary salt and saturated fat with increased fruit and fibre, and weight and alcohol reduction) followed by the staged introduction of drugs, starting with those of proven benefit and least likely to produce side effects. Some of the drugs that were used to lower blood pressure in the early days of antihypertensive therapy, including *ganglion blockers*, *adrenergic neuron blockers* and **reserpine** (see Ch. 15), produced a fearsome array of adverse effects and are now obsolete. The preferred regimens have changed progressively as better-tolerated drugs have become available. A rational strategy is to start treatment

---

[10]Catecholamine-secreting tumours of chromaffin tissue, usually the adrenal medulla (Ch. 13).

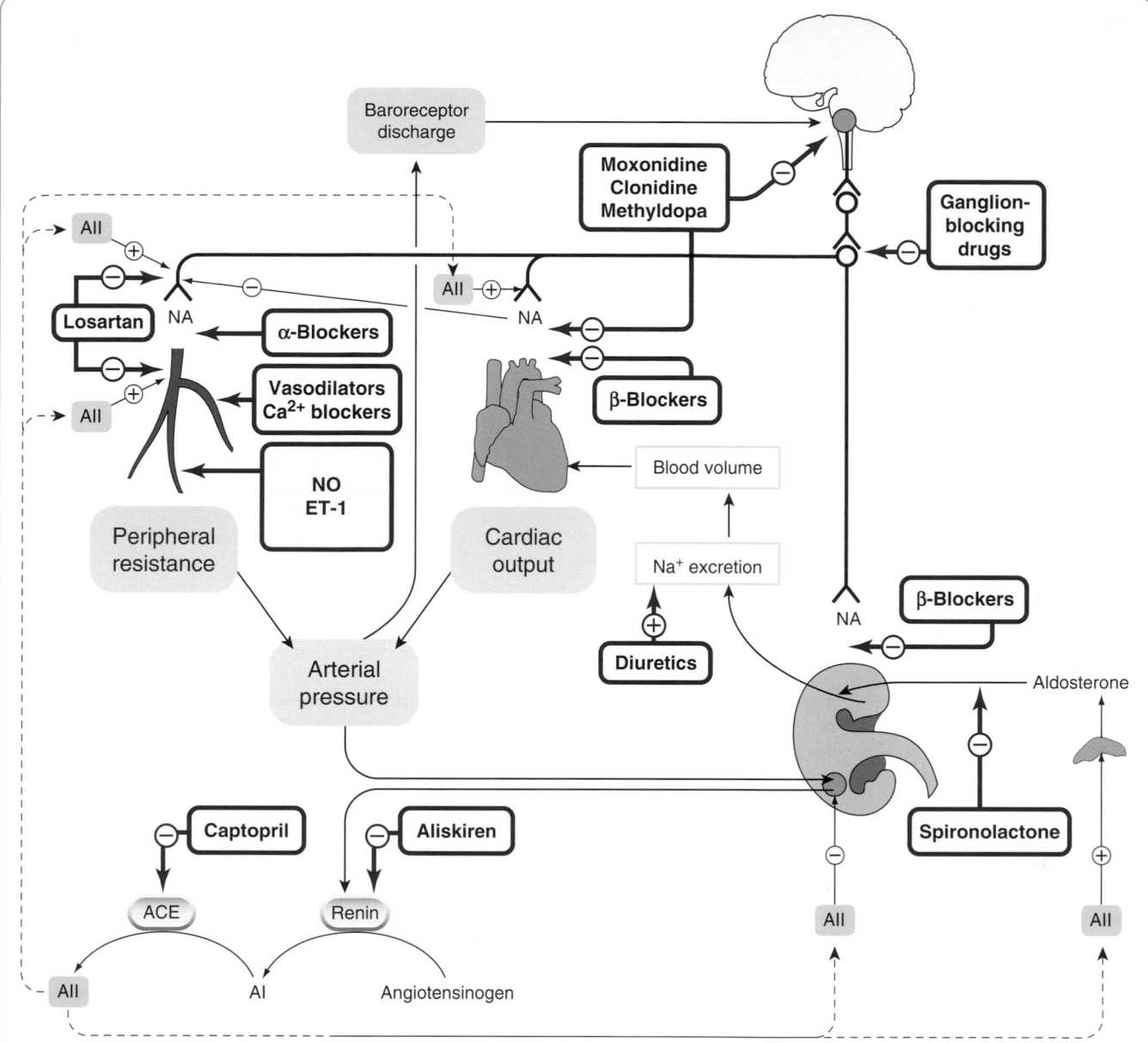

Fig. 23.9 Main mechanisms involved in arterial blood pressure regulation *(black lines)*, and the sites of action of antihypertensive drugs *(hatched boxes + orange lines)*. *ACE*, angiotensin-converting enzyme; *AI*, angiotensin I; *AII*, angiotensin II; *ET-1*, endothelin-1; *NA*, noradrenaline; *NO*, nitric oxide.

with either an ACEI or an ARB in patients who are likely to have normal or raised plasma renin (i.e. younger white people), and with either a thiazide diuretic or a calcium antagonist in older people and people of African origin (who are more likely to have low plasma renin). If the target blood pressure is not achieved but the drug is well tolerated, then a drug of the other group is added. It is best not to increase the dose of any one drug excessively, as this often causes adverse effects and engages homeostatic control mechanisms (e.g. renin release by a diuretic) that limit efficacy.

β-Adrenoceptor antagonists are less well tolerated than ACEIs or ARBs, and the evidence supporting their routine use is less strong than for other classes of antihypertensive drugs. They are useful for hypertensive patients with some additional indication for β blockade, such as angina or heart failure.

Addition of a third or fourth drug (e.g. to ARB/diuretic or ARB/calcium antagonist combination) is often needed, and a long-acting α_1-adrenoceptor antagonist (Ch. 15) such as once daily **doxazosin** is one option in this setting. The α_1 antagonists additionally improve symptoms of prostatic hyperplasia (also known as benign prostatic hypertrophy) (Chs 15, 30 and 36), which is common in older men, albeit at the risk of postural hypotension, which is the main unwanted effect of these agents. **Spironolactone**, whose active metabolite canrenone is a competitive antagonist of aldosterone (Ch. 30), has staged something of a comeback

Table 23.5 Common antihypertensive drugs and their adverse effects

Drug	Adverse effects[a]		
	Postural hypotension	Impotence	Other
Thiazide (e.g. bendroflumethiazide) and related (e.g. chlortalidone) diuretics	±	++	Urinary frequency, gout, glucose intolerance, hypokalaemia, hyponatraemia
ACE inhibitors (e.g. enalapril)	±	—	Cough, first-dose hypotension, teratogenicity, reversible renal dysfunction (in presence of renal artery stenosis)
AT$_1$ antagonists (e.g. losartan)	—	—	Teratogenicity, reversible renal dysfunction (in presence of renal artery stenosis)
Ca^{2+} antagonists (e.g. nifedipine)	—	±	Ankle oedema
β-Adrenoceptor antagonists (e.g. metoprolol)	—	+	Bronchospasm, fatigue, cold hands and feet, bradycardia
α$_1$-Adrenoceptor antagonists (e.g. doxazosin)	++	—	First-dose hypotension

[a]± indicates that the adverse effect occurs in special circumstances only (e.g. postural hypotension occurs with a thiazide diuretic only if the patient is dehydrated for some other reason, is taking some additional drug or suffers from some additional disorder).
ACE, angiotensin-converting enzyme; *AT$_1$*, angiotensin II type 1 receptor.

as an additional agent in treating severe hypertension. Careful monitoring of plasma K$^+$ concentration is required, because spironolactone inhibits urinary K$^+$ excretion as well as causing oestrogen-related adverse effects, but it is usually well tolerated in low doses. **Methyldopa** is now used mainly for hypertension during pregnancy because of the lack of documented adverse effects on the baby (in contrast to ACEIs, ARBs and standard β-adrenoceptor antagonists, which are contraindicated during pregnancy and therefore often avoided in women of child-bearing potential). **Clonidine** (a centrally acting α$_2$ agonist) is now seldom used. **Moxonidine**, a centrally acting agonist at imidazoline I$_1$ receptors that causes less drowsiness than α$_2$ agonists, is licensed for mild or moderate hypertension, but there is little evidence from clinical end-point trials to support its use. **Minoxidil**, combined with a diuretic and β-adrenoceptor antagonist, is sometimes effective where other drugs have failed in severe hypertension resistant to other drugs. **Fenoldopam**, a selective dopamine D$_1$ receptor agonist, is approved in the United States for the short-term management in hospital of severe hypertension. Its effect is similar in magnitude to that of intravenous nitroprusside, but it lacks thiocyanate-associated toxicity and is slower in onset and offset.

Commonly used antihypertensive drugs and their main adverse effects are summarised in Table 23.5.

HEART FAILURE

Heart failure is a clinical syndrome characterised by symptoms of breathlessness and/or fatigue, usually with signs of fluid overload (oedema, raised venous pressure and crackles heard when listening to the chest). The underlying physiological abnormality (see also Ch. 22) is a cardiac output that is inadequate to meet the metabolic demands of the body, initially during exercise but, as the syndrome progresses, also at rest. It may be caused by disease of the myocardium itself (most commonly secondary to coronary artery disease but also other pathologies

including cardiotoxic drugs such as **doxorubicin** and **trastuzumab** – Ch. 57), or by circulatory factors such as volume overload (e.g. leaky valves, or arteriovenous shunts caused by congenital defects) or pressure overload (e.g. stenosed – i.e. narrowed – valves, systemic or pulmonary hypertension). Some of these underlying causes are surgically correctable, and in some either the underlying disease (e.g. hyperthyroidism; Ch. 35), or an aggravating factor such as anaemia (Ch. 26) or atrial fibrillation (Ch. 22), is treatable with drugs. Here, we focus on drugs used to treat heart failure per se, irrespective of the underlying cause.

When cardiac output is insufficient to meet metabolic demand, an increase in fluid volume occurs, partly because increased venous pressure increases capillary pressure and hence formation of tissue fluid, and partly because reduced renal blood flow activates the renin–angiotensin–aldosterone system, causing Na$^+$ and water retention. Irrespective of the cause, the outlook for adults with cardiac failure is grim: 50% of those with the most severe grade are dead in 6 months, and of those with 'mild/moderate' disease, 50% are dead in 5 years. Non-drug measures, including dietary salt restriction and exercise training in mildly affected patients,[11] are important, but drugs are needed to improve symptoms of oedema, fatigue and breathlessness, and to improve prognosis.

A simplified diagram of the sequence of events is shown in Fig. 23.10. A common theme is that several of the feedbacks that are activated are 'counter-regulatory' – that is, they make the situation worse not better. This occurs because the body fails to distinguish the haemodynamic state of heart failure from haemorrhage, in which release of vasoconstrictors such as angiotensin II and ADH would

---

[11]Bed rest used to be recommended but results in deconditioning, and regular exercise has been shown to be beneficial in patients who can tolerate it.

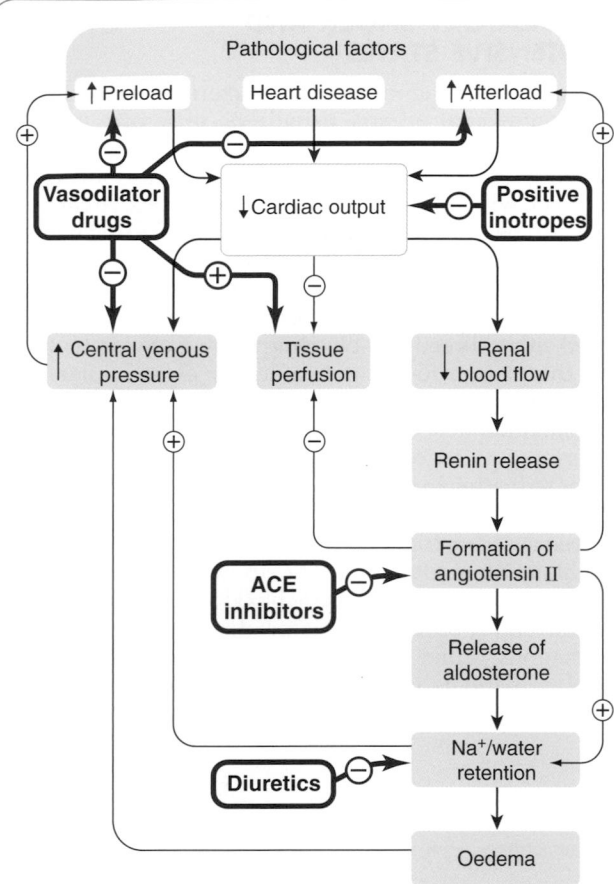

Fig. 23.10 Simplified scheme showing the pathogenesis of heart failure, and the sites of action of some of the drugs used to treat it. The symptoms of heart failure are produced by reduced tissue perfusion, oedema and increased central venous pressure. *ACE*, angiotensin-converting enzyme.

be appropriate.[12] ACEIs and ARBs, β-adrenoceptor and aldosterone antagonists interrupt these counter-regulatory neurohormonal mechanisms and have each been shown to prolong life in heart failure, although prognosis remains poor despite optimal management.

Drugs used to treat heart failure act in various complementary ways to do the following.

Increase natriuresis. Diuretics, especially loop diuretics (Ch. 30), are important in increasing salt and water excretion, especially if there is pulmonary oedema. In chronic heart failure, drugs that have been shown to improve survival were studied mainly in patients treated with diuretics.

Inhibit the renin–angiotensin–aldosterone system/ potentiate NEP. The renin–angiotensin–aldosterone system is inappropriately activated in patients with cardiac failure, especially when they are treated with diuretics. The β-adrenoceptor antagonists inhibit renin secretion and are used in clinically stable patients with chronic heart failure (see clinical box, p. 306). ACEIs and ARBs block the formation of angiotensin II and inhibit its action, respectively,

thereby reducing vascular resistance, improving tissue perfusion and reducing cardiac afterload. They also cause natriuresis by inhibiting secretion of aldosterone and by reducing the direct stimulatory effect of angiotensin II on reabsorption of Na^+ and HCO_3^- in the early part of the proximal convoluted tubule. Most important of all, they prolong life.

▼ Differences in the pharmacology of ACEIs and ARBs led to the hypothesis that co-administration of these drugs ('dual blockade') could confer additional benefit over increasing the dose of either given as a single agent. However, two large randomised controlled trials comparing monotherapy with ACEI or ARB with combined therapy both showed that the combined treatment produced more symptoms attributable to hypotension, and no survival benefit compared with monotherapy in patients with acute myocardial infarction (Pfeffer et al., 2003).

In contrast to the disappointing experience of combining ARBs with ACEI, a fixed combination of sacubitril with valsartan is used in patients symptomatic with chronic heart failure and reduced cardiac ejection. In comparison to an ACEI (enalapril), sacubitril/valsartan usefully reduced cardiac and all-cause mortality in such patients and Jhund and McMurray (2016) argue that this combination should therefore replace an ACEI as the foundation of treatment of symptomatic heart failure.

▼ The choice of valsartan as ARB in this combination is supported by its pharmacokinetic similarity to sacubitril. Sacubitril, sacubitrilat and valsartan are highly bound to plasma proteins (94%–97%) but sacubitril does cross the blood–brain barrier to a limited extent (0.28%). Cerebrospinal fluid (CSF) Aβ clearance in young cynomolgus monkeys is reduced by sacubitril/ valsartan. Administration of the combination for two weeks to healthy subjects increased CSF Aβ1-38 without change in Aβ1-40 and 1-42. The clinical relevance of this is not known, and the product is subject to ongoing safety monitoring.

Adverse effects and drug interactions observed during treatment with valsartan/sacubitril are in line with those of its two components. Hypotension, hyperkalaemia and renal impairment are the commonest observed adverse effects. Angioedema occurred during the pivotal controlled trial in 0.5% of patients treated with the combination, compared with 0.2% of patients treated with enalapril. Concomitant use of sacubitril with ACEIs is contraindicated since, consistent with the experience with omapatrilat mentioned above, the concomitant inhibition of NEP and ACE increases the risk of angioedema. PDE5 inhibitors (Ch. 22) including sildenafil that work through cGMP signalling are potentiated by sacubitril.

Angiotensin II is not the only stimulus to aldosterone secretion, and during chronic treatment with ACEIs, circulating aldosterone concentrations return towards pretreatment values (a phenomenon known as 'aldosterone escape'). This provides a rationale for combining **spironolactone** (an aldosterone antagonist; see Ch. 34) with ACEI treatment, which further reduces mortality. **Eplerenone** is an aldosterone antagonist with less oestrogen-like adverse effects than spironolactone; it too has been shown to improve survival in patients with heart failure when added to conventional therapy. Patients with impaired renal function were excluded from these trials, and careful monitoring of plasma K^+ concentration is important when they are treated with an ACEI or an ARB in combination with an aldosterone antagonist.

---

[12]Natural selection presumably favoured mechanisms that would benefit young hunter–gatherers at risk of haemorrhage; middle-aged or elderly people at high risk of heart failure are past their reproductive prime.

Block β adrenoceptors. Heart failure is accompanied by potentially harmful activation of the sympathetic nervous system as well as of the renin–angiotensin system, providing a rationale for using β-adrenoceptor antagonists. Most clinicians were very wary of this approach because of the negative inotropic action of these drugs, but when started in low doses that are increased slowly, **metoprolol, carvedilol** and **bisoprolol** each improve survival when added to optimal treatment in clinically stable patients with chronic heart failure.

Glyceryl trinitrate (Ch. 22) is infused intravenously to treat acute cardiac failure. Its venodilator effect reduces venous pressure, and its effects on arterial compliance and wave reflection further reduce cardiac work. The combination of **hydralazine** (to reduce afterload) with a long-acting organic nitrate (to reduce preload) in patients with chronic heart failure improved survival in a North American randomised controlled trial, but the results suggested that the benefit was restricted to patients of African origin. This ethnic group is genetically very heterogeneous, and it is unknown what other groups will benefit from such treatment, which is underutilised in African-origin patients (Taylor et al., 2004; Cole et al., 2014).

Increase the force of cardiac contraction. Cardiac glycosides (Ch. 22) are used either in patients with heart failure who also have chronic rapid atrial fibrillation (in whom it improves cardiac function by slowing ventricular rate and hence ventricular filling in addition to any benefit from its positive inotropic action), or in patients who remain symptomatic despite treatment with a diuretic and ACEI. **Digoxin** does not reduce mortality in heart failure patients in sinus rhythm who are otherwise optimally treated, but does improve symptoms and reduce the need for hospital admission. In contrast, PDE inhibitors (see Ch. 22) increase cardiac output, but increase mortality in heart failure, probably through cardiac dysrhythmias. **Dobutamine** (a β$_1$-selective adrenoceptor agonist; see Ch. 22) is used intravenously when a rapid response is needed in the short term, for example following heart surgery.

Drugs used in chronic heart failure

- Loop diuretics, for example **furosemide** (Ch. 30).
- Angiotensin-converting enzyme inhibitors (e.g. **ramipril**).
- Angiotensin II subtype 1 receptor antagonists (e.g. **valsartan, candesartan**) alone or, increasingly, in combination with an neutral endopeptidase (NEP) inhibitor (**valsartan/sacubitril**).
- β-adrenoceptor antagonists (e.g. **metoprolol, bisoprolol, carvedilol**), introduced in low dose in stable patients.
- Aldosterone-receptor antagonists (e.g. **spironolactone**, Ch. 30; and **eplerenone**).
- **Digoxin** (see Ch. 22), especially for heart failure associated with established rapid atrial fibrillation. It is also indicated in patients who remain symptomatic despite optimal treatment.
- Organic nitrates (e.g. **isosorbide mononitrate**) reduce preload, and **hydralazine** reduces afterload. Used in combination, these prolong life in African-Americans with heart failure.

VASODILATORY SHOCK AND HYPOTENSIVE STATES

Shock is a medical emergency characterised by inadequate perfusion of vital organs, usually because of a very low arterial blood pressure. This leads to anaerobic metabolism and hence to increased lactate production. Mortality is very high, even with optimal treatment in an intensive care unit. Shock can be caused by various insults, including haemorrhage, burns, bacterial infections, anaphylaxis (Ch. 18) and myocardial infarction (Fig. 23.11). The common factor is reduced effective circulating blood volume (hypovolaemia) caused either directly by bleeding or by movement of fluid from the plasma to the gut lumen or extracellular fluid. The physiological (homeostatic) response to this is complex: vasodilatation in a vital organ (e.g. brain, heart or kidney) favours perfusion of that organ, but at the expense of a further reduction in blood pressure, which leads to reduced perfusion of other organs. Survival depends on a balance between vasoconstriction in non-essential vascular beds and vasodilatation in vital ones. The dividing line between the normal physiological response to blood loss and clinical shock is that in shock tissue hypoxia produces secondary effects that magnify rather than correct the primary disturbance. Therefore patients with established shock have profound and inappropriate vasodilatation in non-essential organs,

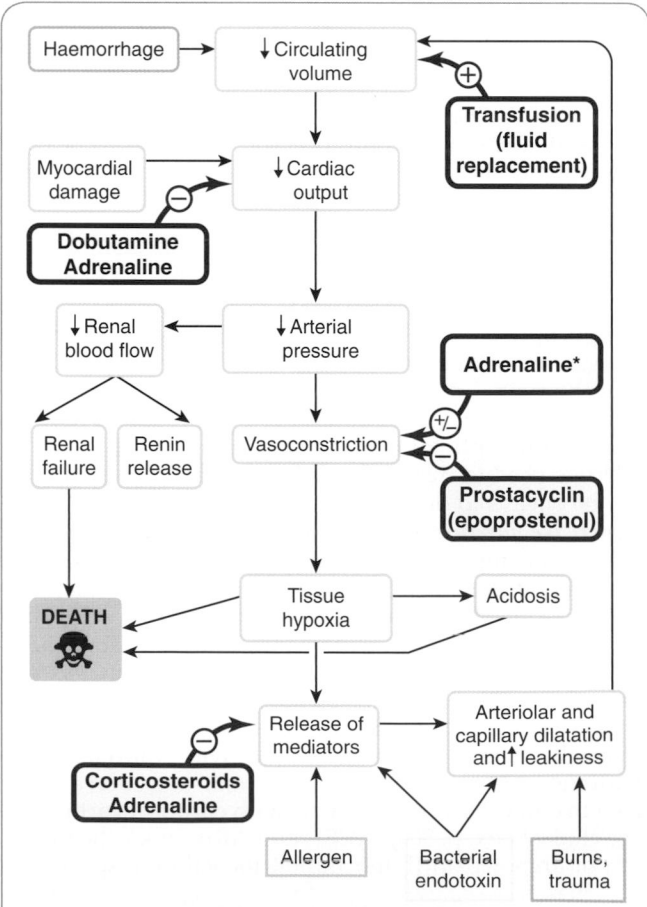

Fig. 23.11 Simplified scheme showing the pathogenesis of hypovolaemic shock. *Adrenaline causes vasodilatation in some vascular beds, vasoconstriction in others.

and this is difficult to correct with vasoconstrictor drugs. The release of mediators (e.g. histamine, 5-hydroxytryptamine, bradykinin, prostaglandins, cytokines including interleukins and tumour necrosis factor, NO and undoubtedly many more as-yet-unidentified substances) that cause capillary dilatation and leakiness is the opposite of what is required to improve function in this setting. Mediators promoting vasodilatation in shock converge on two main mechanisms:

1. Activation of ATP-sensitive potassium channels in vascular smooth muscle by reduced cytoplasmic ATP and increased lactate and protons.
2. Increased synthesis of NO, which activates myosin light-chain phosphatase and activates K_{Ca} channels.

A third important mechanism seems to be a relative *deficiency* of ADH, which is secreted acutely in response to haemorrhage but subsequently declines, probably because of depletion within the neurohypophysis (see Ch. 34).

Patients with shock are not a homogeneous population, making it hard to perform valid clinical trials, and in contrast to hypertension and heart failure there is very little evidence to support treatment strategies based on hard clinical end points (such as improved survival). *Volume replacement* is of benefit if there is hypovolaemia; *antibiotics* are essential if there is persistent bacterial infection; **adrenaline** can be life-saving in anaphylactic shock and is also used by intensivists in managing circulatory shock of other aetiologies. Hypoperfusion leads to multiple organ failure (including renal failure), and intensive therapy specialists spend much effort supporting the circulations of such patients with cocktails of vasoactive drugs in attempts to optimise flow to vital organs. Trials of antagonists designed to block or neutralise endotoxin, interleukins, tumour necrosis factor and the inducible form of NO synthase, and of recombinant human protein C have shown them to be ineffective or actually harmful. **Vasopressin** or angiotensin II may increase blood pressure even when there is resistance to adrenaline; *corticosteroids* suppress the formation of NO and of prostaglandins but are not of proven benefit once shock is established; **epoprostenol** (PGI₂) may be useful in patients with inappropriate platelet activation (e.g. *meningococcal sepsis*); positive inotropic agents, including adrenaline and **dobutamine**, may help in individual patients.

PERIPHERAL VASCULAR DISEASE

When atheroma involves peripheral arteries, the first symptom is usually pain in the calves on walking (claudication), followed by pain at rest, and in severe cases gangrene of the feet or legs. Other vascular beds (e.g. coronary, cerebral and renal) are often also affected by atheromatous disease in patients with peripheral vascular disease. Treatment is mainly mechanical (open surgery or endovascular procedures to open the stenosed artery), combined with drugs that reduce the risk of ischaemic heart disease and strokes. Drug treatment includes antiplatelet drugs (e.g. **aspirin**, **clopidogrel**; see Ch. 25), a statin (e.g. **simvastatin**; see Ch. 24) and an ACEI (e.g. **ramipril**; see p. 300).

RAYNAUD'S DISEASE

Inappropriate vasoconstriction of small arteries and arterioles gives rise to Raynaud's phenomenon (blanching of the fingers during vasoconstriction, followed by blueness owing to deoxygenation of the static blood and redness from reactive hyperaemia following return of blood flow).

This can be mild, but if severe causes ulceration and gangrene of the fingers. It can occur in isolation (Raynaud's disease) or in association with a number of other diseases, including several so-called connective tissue diseases (e.g. systemic sclerosis, systemic lupus erythematosus). Treatment of Raynaud's phenomenon hinges on stopping smoking (crucially) and on avoiding the cold; β-adrenoceptor antagonists are contraindicated. Vasodilators (e.g. **nifedipine**; see Ch. 22) are of some benefit in severe cases, and evidence from several small studies suggests sildenafil is helpful, as well as other vasodilators (e.g. PGI₂, calcitonin gene-related peptide (CGRP)) which can have surprisingly prolonged effects long outlasting their presence in the circulation, but are difficult to administer.

PULMONARY HYPERTENSION

After birth, pulmonary vascular resistance becomes much lower than systemic vascular resistance, and systolic pulmonary artery pressure in adults is normally approximately 20 mmHg.[13]

Pulmonary artery pressure is much less easy to measure than is systemic pressure, often requiring cardiac catheterisation, so only severe and symptomatic pulmonary hypertension tends to be diagnosed. Pulmonary hypertension usually causes some regurgitation of blood from the right ventricle to the right atrium. This tricuspid regurgitation can be used to estimate the pulmonary artery pressure indirectly by ultrasonography. Pulmonary hypertension may rarely be *idiopathic* (i.e. of unknown cause, a severe and progressive form), but is more commonly associated with some other disease. It can result from an increased cardiac output (such as occurs, for example, in patients with hepatic cirrhosis – where vasodilatation may accompany intermittent subclinical exposure to bacterial endotoxin – or in patients with congenital connections between the systemic and pulmonary circulations). Vasoconstriction and/or structural narrowing of the pulmonary resistance arteries increase pulmonary arterial pressure, even if cardiac output is normal. In some situations, both increased cardiac output and increased pulmonary vascular resistance are present.

Endothelial dysfunction (see pp. 291–295, and also Chs 24 and 25) is implicated in the aetiology of pulmonary hypertension. Drugs (e.g. anorexic drugs including **dexfenfluramine**, now withdrawn) and toxins (e.g. *monocrotaline*) can cause pulmonary hypertension. Occlusion of the pulmonary arteries, for example with *recurrent pulmonary emboli* (Ch. 25), is a further primary cause or exacerbating factor, and *anticoagulation* (see Ch. 25) is an important part of treatment. Aggregates of deformed red cells in patients with *sickle cell anaemia* (Ch. 26) can occlude small pulmonary arteries.

Increased pulmonary vascular resistance may, alternatively, result from vasoconstriction and/or structural changes in the walls of pulmonary resistance arteries. Many of the diseases (e.g. systemic sclerosis) associated with Raynaud's phenomenon mentioned in the section above

---

[13]In fetal life, pulmonary vascular resistance is high; failure to adapt appropriately at birth is associated with prematurity, lack of pulmonary surfactant and hypoxaemia. The resulting pulmonary hypertension is treated by paediatric intensive care specialists with measures including replacement of surfactant and ventilatory support, sometimes including inhaled NO – see Chapter 21.

are also associated with pulmonary hypertension. Vaso-constriction may precede cellular proliferation and medial hypertrophy which causes wall thickening in the pulmonary vasculature. Calcium antagonists (e.g. nifedipine) are used, but benefit is limited. Vasodilators with an antiproliferative action (e.g. epoprostenol, Fig. 23.12), drugs that potentiate NO such as **riociguat**, an allosteric activator of soluble guanylyl cyclase (see Ch. 21), approved for this indication in Europe and the United States, or antagonise endothelin – for example bosentan and **ambrisentan** – are considered to yield greater benefit.

Drugs used in treating pulmonary arterial hypertension and clinical disorders for which vasoactive drugs are important are shown in the clinical boxes.

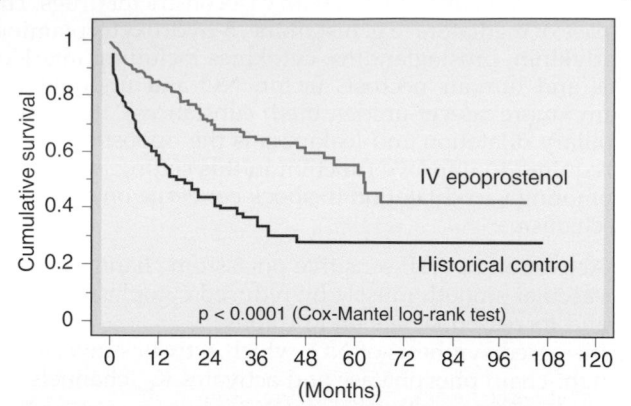

Fig. 23.12 Survival in primary pulmonary hypertension. Survival in 178 patients treated with intravenous epoprostenol versus a historical control group of 135 patients matched for disease severity. (Adapted from Sitbon, O. et al., 2002 Prog. Cardiovasc. Dis. 45, 115.)

Drugs used in pulmonary arterial hypertension

Drugs are used where indicated to treat any underlying cause; in addition, consider the following:
- Oral anticoagulants (Ch. 25).
- Diuretics (Ch. 30).
- **Oxygen**.
- **Digoxin** (Ch. 22).
- Calcium-channel blockers.
- Endothelin receptor antagonists (e.g. **bosentan**, **ambrisentan**, **sitaxentan**) by mouth for less severe stages of disease.
- Prostanoid analogues (**iloprost**, **treprostinil**, **beraprost**), subcutaneous or inhaled, are used for more severe stages of disease.

- **Epoprostenol** (Ch. 18) is given as a long-term intravenous infusion, and improves survival (see Fig. 23.12).
- Inhaled **NO** is administered in intensive care, for example for pulmonary hypertensive crises in newborn babies.
- Phosphodiesterase V inhibitor: **sildenafil** and **tadalafil** by mouth are licensed for pulmonary arterial hypertension (PAH)
- Riociguat (activator of guanylyl cyclase).

Clinical disorders for which vasoactive drugs are important

- Systemic hypertension:
  - secondary to underlying disease (e.g. renal or endocrine)
  - primary 'essential' hypertension, an important risk factor for atheromatous disease (Ch. 24). Treatment reduces the excess risk of stroke or myocardial infarction, the main classes of drugs being (a) angiotensin-converting enzyme inhibitor (ACEI) or AT_1 receptor antagonists; (b) β-adrenoceptor antagonists; (c) calcium antagonists; and (d) diuretics.
- Cardiac failure. Several diseases (most commonly ischaemic heart disease) impair the ability of the heart to deliver an output adequate to meet metabolic needs. Oedema can be improved with diuretics. Life expectancy is reduced but can be improved by treatment of haemodynamically stable patients with:
  - ACEIs and/or AT_1 receptor antagonists
  - β-adrenoceptor antagonists (e.g. **carvedilol**, **bisoprolol**)

  - aldosterone antagonists (e.g. **spironolactone**).
- Shock. Several diseases (e.g. overwhelming bacterial infections, Ch. 52; anaphylactic reactions, Ch. 28) lead to inappropriate vasodilatation, hypotension and reduced tissue perfusion with raised circulating concentrations of lactic acid. Pressors (e.g. **adrenaline**) are used.
- Peripheral vascular disease. Atheromatous plaques in the arteries of the legs are often associated with atheroma in other vascular territories. Statins (Ch. 23) and antiplatelet drugs (Ch. 24) are important.
- Raynaud's disease. Inappropriate vasoconstriction in small arteries in the hands causes blanching of the fingers followed by blueness and pain. **Nifedipine** or other vasodilators are used.
- Pulmonary hypertension, which can be:
  - idiopathic (a rare disorder): **epoprostenol**, **iloprost**, **bosentan** and **sildenafil** are of benefit in selected patients
  - associated with hypoxic lung disease.

REFERENCES AND FURTHER READING

Vascular endothelium (see Ch. 21 for further reading on nitric oxide)

Prostacyclin

Bunting, S., Gryglewski, R., Moncada, S., Vane, J.R., 1976. Arterial walls generate from prostaglandin endoperoxides a substance (*prostaglandin X*) which relaxes strips of mesenteric and celiac arteries and inhibits platelet aggregation. Prostaglandins 12, 897–913. (*Classic*)

Murata, T., Ushikubi, F., Matsuoka, T., et al., 1997. Altered pain perception and inflammatory response in mice lacking prostacyclin receptor. Nature 388, 678–682. (*I prostanoid receptor-deficient mice are viable, reproductive and normotensive; however, their susceptibility to thrombosis is increased … the results establish that prostacyclin is an endogenous antithrombotic agent*)

Endothelium-derived hyperpolarising factor

Ellinsworth, D.C., Sandow, S.L., Shukla, N., et al., 2016. Endothelium-derived hyperpolarization and coronary vasodilation: diverse and integrated roles of epoxyeicosatrienoic acids, hydrogen peroxide, and gap junctions. Micorocirculation 23, 15–32. (*Reviews the mechanisms by which EETs and H_2O_2 regulate vessel tone and examines the hypothesis that myoendothelial microdomain signaling facilitates EDH activity in the human heart*)

Endothelin

Hickey, K.A., Rubanyi, G., Paul, R.J., Highsmith, R.F., 1985. Characterization of a coronary vasoconstrictor produced by cultured endothelial cells. Am. J. Physiol. 248 (Pt 1), C550–C556. (*Key discovery*)

Yanagisawa, M., Kurihara, H., Kimura, S., et al., 1988. A novel potent vasoconstrictor peptide produced by vascular endothelial cells. Nature 332, 411–415. (*Tour de force*)

Davenport, A.P., Hyndman, K.A., Dhaun, N., et al., 2016. Endothelin. Pharmacol. Rev. 68, 357–418. (*Excellent review*)

Renin–angiotensin system

Lang, C.C., Struthers, A.D., 2013. Targeting the renin-angiotensin-aldosterone system in heart failure. Nat. Rev. Cardiol. 10, 125–134.

ONTARGET Investigators, 2008. Telmisartan, ramipril or both in patients at high risk for vascular events. N. Engl. J. Med. 358, 1547–1559.

Patel, V.B., Zhong, J.C., Grant, M.B., et al., 2016. Role of the ACE2/angiotensin 1-7 axis of the renin-angiotensin system in heart failure. Circ. Res. 118, 1313–1326. (*Reviews ACE2/Ang 1-7 limb of the renin-angiotensin axis and its therapeutic potential for heart failure*)

Circulation research

Pfeffer, M.A., McMurray, J.J.V., Velasquez, E.J., et al., 2003. The Valsartan in Acute Myocardial Infarction Trial I. Valsartan, captopril or both in myocardial infarction complicated by heart failure, left ventricular dysfunction, or both. N. Engl. J. Med. 349, 1839–1906.

Vasodilator drugs (see Ch. 22 for further reading on calcium antagonists)

Chan, C.K.S., Burke, S.L., Zhu, H., et al., 2005. Imidazoline receptors associated with noradrenergic terminals in the rostral ventrolateral medulla mediate the hypotensive responses of moxonidine but not clonidine. Neuroscience 132, 991–1007. (*The hypotensive and bradycardic actions of moxonidine but not clonidine are mediated through imidazoline receptors and depend on noradrenergic CNS pathways; noradrenergic innervation may be associated with imidazoline receptor protein*)

Hypertension

Meneton, P., Jeunemaitre, X., de Wardener, H.E., MacGregor, G.A., 2005. Links between dietary salt intake, renal salt handling, blood pressure, and cardiovascular diseases. Physiol. Rev. 85, 679–715. ("*The mechanisms by which dietary salt increases arterial pressure are not fully understood, but they seem related to the inability of the kidneys to excrete large amounts of salt. From an evolutionary viewpoint, the human species is adapted to ingest and excrete <1 g of salt per day, at least 10 times less than the average values currently observed in industrialized and urbanized countries.*")

Heart failure

Cole, R.T., Gupta, D., Butler, J., 2014. Current perspectives in hydralazine and nitrate therapies in heart failure. Heart Fail Clin 10, 565–575. (*Underutilised*)

Jhund, P.S., McMurray, J.J.V., 2016. The neprilysin pathway in heart failure: a review and guide on the use of sacubitril/valsartan. Heart 102, 1342–1347. (*Reviews the background to neprilysin inhibition in heart failure, the results of the PARADIGM-HF trial and describes the use of sacubitril/valsartan in clinical practice*)

O'Connor, C.M., Starling, R.C., Hernandez, A.F., et al., 2011. Effect of nesiritide in patients with acute decompensated heart failure. N. Engl. J. Med. 365, 32–43. (*see also Topol, E.T., 2011. The lost decade of nesiritide. N. Engl. J. Med. 365, 81–82*)

Task Force for the diagnosis and treatment of acute and chronic heart failure of the European Society of Cardiology (ESC), 2016. 2016 ESC Guidelines for the diagnosis and treatment of acute and chronic heart failure. Eur. Heart J. 37 (2016), 2129–2200.

Taylor, A.L., Ziesche, S., Yancy, C., et al., 2004. Combination of isosorbide dinitrate and hydralazine in blacks with heart failure. N. Engl. J. Med. 351, 2049–2057. (*Addition of a fixed dose of isosorbide dinitrate plus hydralazine to standard therapy for heart failure including neurohormonal blockers increased survival among black patients with advanced heart failure*)

Shock

Holmes, C.L., Russell, J.A., 2004. Vasopressin. Semin. Respir. Crit. Care Med. 25, 705–711. ('*A deficiency of vasopressin exists in some shock states and replacement of physiological levels of vasopressin can restore vascular tone. Vasopressin is therefore emerging as a rational therapy for vasodilatory shock.' Reviews rationale, evidence and uncertainties for using vasopressin in shock*)

Khanna, A., English, S.W., Wang, X.S., et al., for the ATHOS3 investigators, 2017. Angiotensin II for the treatment of vasodilatory shock. N. Engl. J. Med. 377, 419–430. ("*Angiotensin II effectively increased blood pressure in patients with vasodilatory shock that did not respond to high doses of conventional vasopressors*")

Landry, D.W., Oliver, J.A., 2001. Mechanisms of disease: the pathogenesis of vasodilatory shock. N. Engl. J. Med. 345, 588–595. (*Reviews mechanisms promoting inappropriate vasodilation in shock, including activation of ATP-sensitive potassium channels, increased synthesis of NO and depletion of ADH*)

Pulmonary arterial hypertension (PAH)

Higenbottam, T., Laude, L., Emery, C., Essener, M., 2004. Pulmonary hypertension as a result of drug therapy. Clin. Chest Med. 25, 123–131. (*Reviews anorectic drug-induced pulmonary arterial hypertension and considers mechanisms*)

Humbert, M., Ghofrani, H.A., 2016. The molecular targets of approved treatments for pulmonary arterial hypertension. Thorax 71, 73–83. (*This review describes how the four currently approved drug classes - prostanoids, endothelin receptor antagonists, phosphodiesterase type 5 inhibitors and the soluble guanylate cyclase stimulator riociguat - target the complex pathobiology of PAH*)

Mann, D.L., Zipes, D.P., Libby, P., Bonow, R.O. (Eds.), 2015. Braunwald's Heart Disease, tenth ed. Elsevier, Philadelphia. Ch. 74, Pulmonary hypertension.

Taichman, D.B., Ornelas, J., Chung, L., et al., 2014. Pharmacologic therapy for pulmonary arterial hypertension in adults: CHEST guideline and expert panel report. Chest 146, 449–475. (*Provides advice on drug therapy for adult patients with PAH based on available evidence*)

24 Atherosclerosis and lipoprotein metabolism

OVERVIEW

Atheromatous disease is ubiquitous and underlies the commonest causes of death (myocardial infarction caused by thrombosis – Ch. 25 – on ruptured atheromatous plaque in a coronary artery) and disability (stroke, heart failure) in industrial societies. Hypertension is one of the most important risk factors for atheroma, and is discussed in Chapter 23. Here, we consider other risk factors, especially dyslipidaemia,[1] which, like hypertension, is amenable to drug therapy. We describe briefly the processes of atherogenesis and of lipid transport as a basis for understanding the actions of lipid-lowering drugs. Agents employed therapeutically (statins, inhibitors of PCSK9,[2] fibrates, cholesterol absorption inhibitors, nicotinic acid derivatives) are described, with emphasis on the statins which, in selected patients, reduce the incidence of arterial disease and prolong life.

INTRODUCTION

In this chapter we summarise the pathological process of atherogenesis and approaches to the prevention of atherosclerotic disease. Lipoprotein transport forms the basis for understanding drugs used to treat dyslipidaemia. We emphasise the **statins**, which have been a major success story, not only lowering plasma cholesterol but also reducing cardiovascular events by approximately 25%–50% and prolonging life in people at increased risk of vascular disease. However, some patients do not tolerate them, and others fail to respond. Evidence that other drugs that influence dyslipidaemia improve clinical outcomes is less secure than for the statins, and there have been setbacks, described later, that call into question the universal reliability of changes in circulating lipid concentrations in response to drugs as surrogates predicting clinical improvement. In the absence of hard evidence of clinical improvement, other classes of lipid-lowering drugs remain second line to statins, so there is rather a lot of 'small print' in this section.

ATHEROGENESIS

Atheroma is a focal disease of the intima of large and medium-sized arteries. Lesions evolve over decades, during most of which time they are clinically silent, the occurrence of symptoms signalling advanced disease. Presymptomatic lesions are often difficult to detect non-invasively, although

ultrasound is useful in accessible arteries (e.g. the carotids), and associated changes such as reduced aortic compliance and arterial calcification can be detected by measuring, respectively, aortic pulse wave velocity and coronary artery calcification. There were no good animal models until transgenic mice (see Ch. 8) deficient in apolipoproteins or receptors that play key roles in lipoprotein metabolism transformed the scene. Nevertheless, most of our current understanding of atherogenesis comes from human epidemiology and pathology, and from clinical investigations.

Epidemiological studies have identified numerous risk factors for atheromatous disease. Some of these cannot be altered (e.g. a family history of ischaemic heart disease[3]), but others are modifiable (Table 24.1) and are potential targets for therapeutic drugs. Clinical trials have shown that improving risk factors can reduce the consequences of atheromatous disease. Many risk factors (e.g. type 2 diabetes, dyslipidaemia, cigarette smoking) cause endothelial dysfunction (see Ch. 23), evidenced by reduced vasodilator responses to acetylcholine or to increased blood flow (so-called flow-mediated dilatation), responses that are inhibited by drugs that block nitric oxide (NO) synthesis (Ch. 21). Healthy endothelium produces NO and other mediators that protect against atheroma, so it is likely that metabolic cardiovascular risk factors act by causing endothelial dysfunction.

Atherogenesis involves:

1. *Endothelial dysfunction*, with altered NO (Ch. 21) biosynthesis which predisposes to atherosclerosis.
2. *Injury* of dysfunctional endothelium, which leads to expression of adhesion molecules. This encourages monocyte attachment and migration of monocytes from the lumen into the intima. Lesions have a predilection for regions of disturbed flow such as the origins of aortic branches.
3. *Low-density lipoprotein (LDL) cholesterol* transport into the vessel wall. Endothelial cells and monocytes/macrophages generate free radicals that oxidise LDL (oxLDL), resulting in lipid peroxidation.
4. *oxLDL* uptake by macrophages via 'scavenger' receptors. Such macrophages are called *foam cells* because of their 'foamy' histological appearance, resulting from accumulation of cytoplasmic lipid, and are characteristic of atheroma. Uptake of oxLDL activates macrophages which release proinflammatory cytokines.
5. Subendothelial accumulation of foam cells and T lymphocytes to form *fatty streaks*.
6. Protective mechanisms, for example cholesterol *mobilisation from the artery wall* and transport in

---

[1]The term dyslipidaemia is preferred to hyperlipidaemia because a low plasma concentration of high-density lipoprotein cholesterol is believed to be harmful and is a potential therapeutic target.
[2]PCSK9 stands for proprotein convertase subtilisin/kexin type 9.

[3]As we learn how to tinker with the expression of genes even this seeming truism may turn out to be less immutable than it seemed (see Ch. 5 and later, p. 317.)

Table 24.1 Modifiable risk factors for atheromatous disease

Raised low-density lipoprotein cholesterol
Reduced high-density lipoprotein cholesterol
Hypertension (Ch. 23)
Diabetes mellitus (Ch. 32)
Cigarette smoking (Ch. 50)
Obesity (Ch. 33)
Physical inactivity
Raised C-reactive protein[a]
Raised coagulation factors (e.g. factor VII, fibrinogen)
Raised homocysteine
Raised lipoprotein(a)[b]

[a]Strongly associated with atheromatous disease but not causal of it.
[b]Potentially modifiable but strongly genetically determined: nicotinic acid does lower lipoprotein(a).

plasma as high-density lipoprotein (HDL) cholesterol, termed 'reverse cholesterol transport'.

7. Cytokine and growth factor release by activated platelets, macrophages and endothelial cells, causing proliferation of smooth muscle and deposition of connective tissue components. This *inflammatory fibroproliferative response* leads to a dense fibrous cap overlying a lipid-rich core, the whole structure comprising the atheromatous plaque.

8. Plaque *rupture*, which provides a substrate for *thrombosis* (see Ch. 25, Figs 25.1 and 25.10). The presence of large numbers of macrophages predisposes to plaque rupture, whereas vascular smooth muscle and matrix proteins stabilise the plaque.

To understand how drugs prevent atheromatous disease, it is necessary briefly to review lipoprotein transport.

LIPOPROTEIN TRANSPORT

Lipids and cholesterol are transported in the bloodstream as complexes of lipid and protein known as *lipoproteins*. These consist of a central core of hydrophobic lipid (including triglycerides and cholesteryl esters) encased in a hydrophilic coat of polar phospholipid, free cholesterol and *apoprotein*. There are four main classes of lipoprotein, differing in the relative proportion of the core lipids and in the type of apoprotein (various kinds of apoA and apoB). Apoproteins bind to specific receptors that mediate uptake of lipoprotein particles into liver, blood or other tissues. Lipoproteins differ in size and density, and this latter property, measured originally by ultracentrifugation but now commonly estimated by simpler methods, is the basis for their classification into:

- HDL particles (contain apoA1 and apoA2), diameter 7–20 nm
- LDL particles (contain apoB-100), diameter 20–30 nm

- very-low-density lipoprotein (VLDL) particles (contain apoB-100), diameter 30–80 nm
- chylomicrons (contain apoB-48), diameter 100–1000 nm

Each class of lipoprotein has a specific role in lipid transport, and there are different pathways for exogenous and endogenous lipids, as well as a pathway for reverse cholesterol transport (Fig. 24.1). In the *exogenous pathway*, cholesterol and triglycerides absorbed from the ileum are transported as chylomicrons in lymph and then blood, to capillaries in muscle and adipose tissue. Here, triglycerides are hydrolysed by lipoprotein lipase, and the tissues take up the resulting free fatty acids and glycerol. The chylomicron remnants, still containing their full complement of cholesteryl esters, pass to the liver, bind to receptors on hepatocytes and undergo endocytosis. Cholesterol liberated in hepatocytes is stored, oxidised to bile acids, secreted unaltered in bile, or can enter the endogenous pathway.

In the *endogenous pathway*, cholesterol and newly synthesised triglycerides are transported from the liver as VLDL to muscle and adipose tissue, where triglyceride is hydrolysed to fatty acids and glycerol; these enter the tissues as described above. During this process, the lipoprotein particles become smaller but retain a full complement of cholesteryl esters and become LDL particles. LDL provides the source of cholesterol for incorporation into cell membranes and for synthesis of steroids (see Chs 34 and 36) but is also key in atherogenesis. Cells take up LDL by endocytosis via *LDL receptors* that recognise apoB-100. LDL receptors are critically important in determining the concentration of circulating LDL, and hence the development and progression of atheromatous disease; the most widely used drugs for the prevention of such disease, the statins, act by blocking the synthesis of cholesterol within hepatocytes which respond by increasing LDL receptor expression on their surface membranes (see later, p. 312). A new class of drugs, the PCSK9 inhibitors, also influence LDL receptor density but by a different mechanism, namely reduced lysosomal degradation of internalised LDL receptors leading to increased recycling of functional LDL receptors to the surface membrane (see later, p. 315).

Cholesterol can return to plasma from the tissues in HDL particles (reverse cholesterol transport). Cholesterol is esterified with long-chain fatty acids in HDL particles, and the resulting cholesteryl esters are transferred to VLDL or LDL particles by a transfer protein present in the plasma and known as *cholesteryl ester transfer protein* (CETP). Lipoprotein(a), or Lp(a), is a species of LDL that is associated with atherosclerosis and is localised in atherosclerotic lesions. Lp(a) contains a unique apoprotein, apo(a), with structural similarities to plasminogen (Ch. 25). Lp(a) competes with plasminogen for its receptor on endothelial cells. Plasminogen is the substrate for plasminogen activator, which is secreted by, and bound to endothelial cells, generating the fibrinolytic enzyme *plasmin* (see Fig. 25.10). The effect of the binding of Lp(a) is that less plasmin is generated, fibrinolysis is inhibited and thrombosis promoted.

▼ Lipid transfer proteins have been implicated in atherogenesis (Stein & Stein, 2005). *ACAT* (acyl coenzyme A: cholesterol acyltransferase), which is expressed in two forms, catalyses the intracellular synthesis of cholesteryl ester in macrophages, adrenal cortex, gut and liver. **Tamoxifen**, used in the treatment and prevention of breast cancer (Chs 36 and 57), is a potent ACAT inhibitor (de Medina et al., 2004). *CETP* is involved in transfer of cholesterol between different classes of lipoprotein particle in plasma. Microsomal triglyceride transport

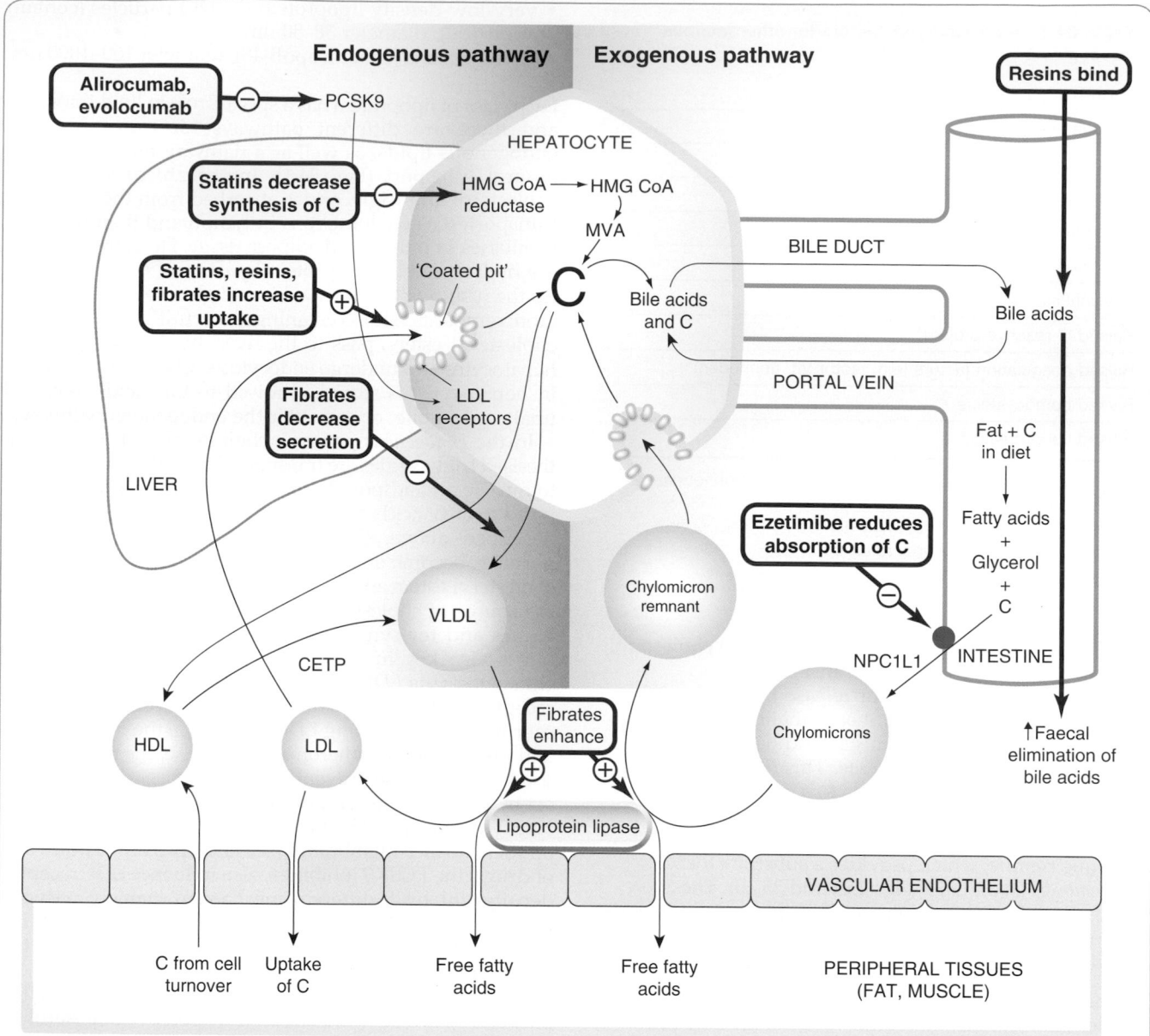

Fig. 24.1 Schematic diagram of cholesterol transport in the tissues, with sites of action of the main drugs affecting lipoprotein metabolism. *C*, cholesterol; *CETP*, cholesteryl ester transport protein; *HDL*, high-density lipoprotein; *HMG-CoA*, 3-hydroxy-3-methylglutaryl-coenzyme A; *LDL*, low-density lipoprotein; *MVA*, mevalonate; *NPC1L1*, a cholesterol transporter in the brush border of enterocytes; *PCSK9*, proprotein convertase subtilisin/kexin 9; *VLDL*, very-low-density lipoprotein.

protein (MTP) is a lipid-transfer protein present in the lumen of the endoplasmic reticulum responsible for binding and transfer of lipids between membranes. Inhibition of MTP interferes with apoB secretion and LDL assembly and **lomitapide,** one such inhibitor, is used in addition to diet and other measures in homozygous familial hypercholesterolaemia.

DYSLIPIDAEMIA

Dyslipidaemia may be primary or secondary. The *primary* forms are due to a combination of diet and genetics (often but not always polygenic). They are classified into six phenotypes (the Frederickson classification; Table 24.2). An especially great risk of ischaemic heart disease occurs in a subset of primary type IIa hyperlipoproteinaemia caused by single-gene defects of LDL receptors; this is known as

familial hypercholesterolaemia (FH), and the plasma total cholesterol concentration, normally <5 mmol/L, in affected adults is typically >8 mmol/L in heterozygotes and 12–25 mmol/L in homozygotes. Study of FH enabled Brown and Goldstein (1986) to define the LDL receptor pathway of cholesterol homeostasis (for which they shared a Nobel Prize). Further investigation of people with very low or very high circulating LDL cholesterol concentrations led to the discovery of inactivating and gain-of-function variants of the *PCSK9* gene (see Hall, 2013 for a popular account, and later, p. 315). Drugs used to treat primary dyslipidaemia are described below.

Secondary forms of dyslipidaemia are a consequence of other conditions, such as diabetes mellitus, alcoholism, nephrotic syndrome, chronic renal failure, hypothyroidism,

Table 24.2 Frederickson/World Health Organization classification of hyperlipoproteinaemia

Type	Lipoprotein elevated	Cholesterol	Triglycerides	Atherosclerosis risk	Drug treatment
I	Chylomicrons	+	+++	NE	None
IIa	LDL	++	NE	High	Statin ± ezetimibe
IIb	LDL + VLDL	++	++	High	Fibrates, statin, nicotinic acid
III	βVLDL	++	++	Moderate	Fibrates
IV	VLDL	+	++	Moderate	Fibrates
V	Chylomicrons + VLDL	+	++	NE	Fibrate, niacin, fish oil and statin combinations

+, increased concentration; *LDL*, low-density lipoprotein; *NE*, not elevated; *VLDL*, very-low-density lipoprotein; *βVLDL*, a qualitatively abnormal form of VLDL identified by its pattern on electrophoresis.

liver disease and administration of drugs, for example **isotretinoin** (an isomer of vitamin A given by mouth as well as topically in the treatment of severe acne, see Ch. 28), **tamoxifen**, **ciclosporine** (Ch. 27) and *protease inhibitors* used to treat infection with human immunodeficiency virus (Ch. 53). Secondary forms are treated where possible by correcting the underlying cause.

Lipoprotein metabolism and dyslipidaemia

Lipids, including cholesterol and triglycerides, are transported in the plasma as lipoproteins, of which there are four classes:

- Chylomicrons transport triglycerides and cholesterol from the gastrointestinal tract to the tissues, where triglyceride is split by lipoprotein lipase, releasing free fatty acids and glycerol which are taken up in muscle and adipose tissue. Chylomicron remnants are taken up in the liver, where cholesterol is stored, secreted in bile, oxidised to bile acids or converted into:
  - very-low-density lipoproteins (VLDLs), which transport cholesterol and newly synthesised triglycerides to the tissues, where triglycerides are removed as before, leaving:
  - intermediate-density and low-density lipoprotein (LDL) particles with a large component of cholesterol; some LDL cholesterol is taken up by the tissues and some by the liver, by endocytosis via specific LDL receptors.
- High-density lipoprotein (HDL) particles adsorb cholesterol derived from cell breakdown in tissues (including arteries) and transfer it to VLDL and LDL particles via cholesterol ester transport protein (CETP).
- Dyslipidaemias can be primary, or secondary to a disease (e.g. hypothyroidism). They are classified according to which lipoprotein particle is abnormal into six phenotypes (the Frederickson classification). The higher the LDL cholesterol and the lower the HDL cholesterol, the higher the risk of ischaemic heart disease.

PREVENTION OF ATHEROMATOUS DISEASE

Drug treatment is often justified, to supplement healthy habits. Treatment of hypertension (Ch. 23) and, to a lesser extent, diabetes mellitus (Ch. 32) reduces the incidence of symptomatic atheromatous disease, and antithrombotic drugs (Ch. 25) reduce arterial thrombosis. Reducing LDL is also effective and is the main subject of this present chapter, but several other steps in atherogenesis are also potential targets for pharmacological attack.

▼ *Angiotensin-converting enzyme inhibitors* (Ch. 23) improve endothelial function and prolong life in patients with atheromatous disease. Other drugs that also increase NO biosynthesis or availability are under investigation.

Measures to increase HDL: moderate alcohol consumption increases HDL, and epidemiological evidence favours moderate alcohol consumption in older people. Regular exercise also increases circulating HDL; drug treatment to increase HDL is of uncertain benefit. Fibrates and nicotinic acid derivatives – see below – modestly increase HDL, and reduce LDL and triglycerides. In subjects with low HDL, inhibition of CETP can markedly increase circulating HDL, but three such drugs have failed because of lack of clinical efficacy or adverse outcomes. Trials of a fourth, **anacetrapib,** showed that it increases HDL and lowers LDL, and is associated with a modest reduction in major coronary events, compared with placebo in patients at risk for cardiac events already receiving a statin, though no effect on overall mortality, and its development has been discontinued.

ApoA-I Milano is a variant of apolipoprotein A-I identified in individuals in rural Italy with very low levels of HDL but almost no cardiovascular disease. Infusion of recombinant ApoA-I Milano–phospholipid complexes causes rapid regression of atherosclerosis in animal models. It is expensive to produce and must be administered intravenously, but the strategy remains a possible future approach (see review by Ikenaga et al., 2016).

Antioxidants (e.g. vitamin C and vitamin E) are of interest, because of reports that they improve endothelial function in patients with increased oxidant stress, and because of epidemiological evidence that a diet rich in antioxidants is associated with reduced risk of coronary artery disease. Results from clinical trials have been negative, however, and several antioxidants reduce HDL. **Oestrogen**, used to prevent symptoms of the menopause (Ch. 36) and to prevent postmenopausal osteoporosis, has antioxidant properties and exerts other vascular effects that could be beneficial. Epidemiological evidence suggested that women who use such hormone replacement might be at reduced risk of atheromatous disease, but controlled trials showed significant *adverse* effects on cardiovascular mortality (Ch. 36).

Anti-inflammatory approaches: drug treatment to lower *C-reactive protein* (see Ch. 7) has been mooted, but it is likely that, while elevated C-reactive protein is a marker of vascular inflammation, it does not itself play a direct part in atherogenesis. Other anti-inflammatory measures are being investigated; for example, *ACAT inhibitors*.

Atheromatous disease

- Atheroma is a uniquely human focal disease of large and medium-sized arteries. Atheromatous plaques occur in most people, progress insidiously over many decades, and underlie the commonest causes of death (myocardial infarction) and disability (e.g. stroke) in industrialised countries.
- Fatty streaks are the earliest structurally apparent lesion and progress to fibrous and/or fatty plaques. Symptoms such as angina occur only when blood flow through the vessel is reduced below that needed to meet the metabolic demands of tissues downstream from the obstruction.
- Important modifiable risk factors include hypertension (Ch. 23), dyslipidaemia (this chapter) and smoking (Ch. 50).
- The pathophysiology is of chronic inflammation in response to injury. Endothelial dysfunction leads to loss of protective mechanisms, monocyte/macrophage and T-cell migration, uptake of low-density lipoprotein (LDL) cholesterol and its oxidation, uptake of oxidised LDL by macrophages, smooth muscle cell migration and proliferation, and deposition of collagen.
- Plaque rupture leads to platelet activation and thrombosis (Ch. 25) with the potential to cause downstream infarction of, for example, heart muscle or brain.

LIPID-LOWERING DRUGS

Several drugs decrease plasma lipoprotein concentrations. Drug therapy is used in addition to dietary measures and correction of other modifiable cardiovascular risk factors. The main agents used clinically are:

- statins: 3-hydroxy-3-methylglutaryl-coenzyme A (HMG CoA) reductase inhibitors
- PCSK9 inhibitors
- fibrates
- inhibitors of cholesterol absorption
- nicotinic acid or its derivatives

STATINS: HMG-COA REDUCTASE INHIBITORS

The rate-limiting enzyme in cholesterol synthesis is HMG-CoA reductase, which catalyses the conversion of HMG-CoA to mevalonic acid (see Fig. 24.1). **Simvastatin, lovastatin** and **pravastatin** are specific, reversible, competitive HMG-CoA reductase inhibitors with K_i values of approximately 1 nmol/L. **Atorvastatin** and **rosuvastatin** are long-lasting

inhibitors. Decreased hepatic cholesterol synthesis upregulates LDL receptor synthesis, increasing LDL clearance from plasma into liver cells. The main biochemical effect of statins is therefore to reduce plasma LDL. There is also some reduction in plasma triglyceride and increase in HDL. Several large randomised placebo-controlled trials of the effects of HMG-CoA reductase inhibitors on morbidity and mortality have been positive.

▼ The Scandinavian Simvastatin Survival Study (4S) recruited patients with ischaemic heart disease and plasma cholesterol of 5.5–8.0 mmol/L: simvastatin lowered serum LDL by 35% and death by 30% (Fig. 24.2). There was a 42% reduction in death from coronary disease. Other large trials have confirmed reduced mortality both in patients with established ischaemic heart disease and in apparently healthy people at high risk of coronary disease, with a wide range of plasma cholesterol values and other risk factors, and treated with different statins. Intensive lowering of LDL with atorvastatin 80 mg had a greater effect on event rate than did a 10-mg dose, but with a greater incidence of abnormally raised plasma transaminase activity (evidence of liver damage). In secondary prevention trials of statins, cardiovascular event rate has been approximately linearly related to the achieved plasma LDL over a concentration range from approximately 1.8–4.9 mmol/L, and the event rate falls on the same line in placebo- and statin-treated patients, suggesting that plasma LDL is a valid surrogate marker of cardiovascular risk in this context.

Other actions of statins

Products of the mevalonate pathway react with protein ('lipidation', which is the addition to a protein of hydrophobic groups such as prenyl or farnesyl moieties). Several important membrane-bound enzymes (e.g. endothelial NO synthase; see Ch. 21) are modified in this way. The fatty groups serve as anchors, localising the enzyme in organelles such as caveoli and Golgi apparatus. Consequently, there is interest in actions of statins that are unrelated, or indirectly related, to their effect on plasma LDL (sometimes referred to as *pleiotropic* effects). Some of these actions are undesirable (e.g. HMG-CoA reductase guides migrating primordial germ cells, and statin use is contraindicated during

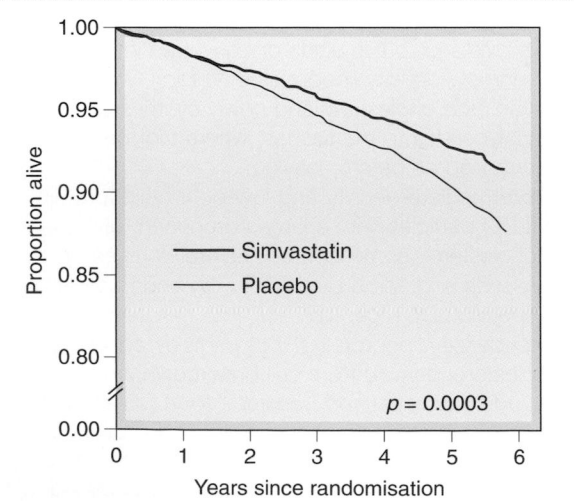

Fig. 24.2 Survival in patients with coronary heart disease and serum cholesterol 5.5–8.0 mmol/L treated either with placebo or with simvastatin. The relative risk of death in the simvastatin group was 0.70 (95% confidence intervals 0.58–0.85). (Based on 4S Study, 1994. Lancet 344, 1383–1389.)

pregnancy), but some offer therapeutic promise. Such potentially beneficial actions include:

- improved endothelial function
- reduced vascular inflammation
- reduced platelet aggregability
- increased neovascularisation of ischaemic tissue
- increased circulating endothelial progenitor cells
- stabilisation of atherosclerotic plaque
- antithrombotic actions
- enhanced fibrinolysis

The extent to which these effects contribute to the anti-atheromatous actions of statins is unknown.

Pharmacokinetics

Short-acting statins are given by mouth at night to reduce peak cholesterol synthesis in the early morning. They are well absorbed and extracted by the liver, their site of action, and are subject to extensive presystemic metabolism via cytochrome P450 and glucuronidation pathways. Simvastatin is an inactive lactone prodrug; it is metabolised in the liver to its active form, the corresponding β-hydroxy fatty acid.

Adverse effects

Statins are well tolerated; mild unwanted effects include muscle pain (myalgia), gastrointestinal disturbance, raised concentrations of liver enzymes in plasma, insomnia and rash. More serious adverse effects are rare but include skeletal muscle damage (myositis, which when severe is described as rhabdomyolysis) and angio-oedema. Myositis is a class effect of statins, occurring also with other lipid-lowering drugs (especially fibrates), and is dose-related.[4] It is more common in patients with low lean body mass or uncorrected hypothyroidism.

Clinical uses of HMG-CoA reductase inhibitors (statins, e.g. simvastatin, atorvastatin)

- Secondary prevention of myocardial infarction and stroke in patients who have symptomatic atherosclerotic disease (e.g. angina, transient ischaemic attacks, or following myocardial infarction or stroke).
- Primary prevention of arterial disease in patients who are at high risk because of elevated serum cholesterol concentration, especially if there are other risk factors for atherosclerosis such as diabetes (Ch. 32) or renal failure (Ch. 30). Tables (available, for example, in the British National Formulary) are used to target treatment to those at greatest risk.
- **Atorvastatin** lowers serum cholesterol in patients with homozygous familial hypercholesterolaemia.
- In severe drug-resistant dyslipidaemia (e.g. heterozygous familial hypercholesterolaemia), **ezetimibe,** which inhibits cholesterol absorption (see p. 316), is combined with statin treatment.
- Contraindicated in pregnancy.

PROPROTEIN CONVERTASE SUBTILISIN/KEXIN TYPE-9 (PCSK9) INHIBITORS

PCSK9 is synthesised in inactive form by many tissues, including brain and liver. It is activated autocatalytically by proteolytic cleavage, which removes a section of its peptide chain that blocks its activity. When activated, it binds to LDL receptors and promotes their lysosomal degradation following LDL uptake into hepatocyte cytoplasm (see Fig. 24.1), thereby preventing recycling of LDL receptors to the surface membrane and diminishing their ability to sequester LDL. Family members who inherit a hyperactive form of the *PCSK9* gene suffer from severe hypercholesterolaemia; conversely individuals with inactivating mutations in this gene have low circulating LDL and a low incidence of atheromatous disease. Individuals homozygous for inactivated PCSK9 have very low plasma concentrations of LDL and are healthy. This encouraged the development of monoclonal antibodies that block PCSK9, thereby preventing it from combining with LDL receptors and marking them down for lysosomal destruction. **Evolocumab** and **alirocumab** are now licensed in the United States and Europe for the treatment of primary hypercholesterolaemia in patients whose circulating LDL is not adequately controlled by a statin or statin/ezetimibe combination, as additional agents (or given alone to patients who do not tolerate treatment with a statin). Evolocumab is administered subcutaneously every 2–4 weeks, alirocumab every 2 weeks. Nasopharyngitis and influenza-like symptoms are common adverse effects of both agents. Other agents that work by inhibiting this pathway, for example, a small interfering RNA that causes long-lasting block of PCSK9 synthesis, are also being developed.

FIBRATES

Several fibric acid derivatives (fibrates) are available, including **bezafibrate**, **ciprofibrate**, **gemfibrozil**, **fenofibrate** and **clofibrate**. These markedly reduce circulating VLDL, and hence triglyceride, with a modest (approximately 10%) reduction in LDL and an approximately 10% increase in HDL. Their mechanism of action is complex (see Fig. 24.1). They are agonists at PPARα nuclear receptors[5] (Ch. 3); in humans, the main effects are to increase transcription of the genes for lipoprotein lipase, apoA1 and apoA5. They increase hepatic LDL uptake. In addition to effects on lipoproteins, fibrates reduce plasma C-reactive protein and fibrinogen, improve glucose tolerance and inhibit vascular smooth muscle inflammation by inhibiting the expression of the transcription factor nuclear factor κB (see Ch. 3). The relative importance of these effects is uncertain, and fibrates have not been demonstrated to improve survival.

Adverse effects

Rhabdomyolysis is unusual but severe, giving rise to acute renal failure associated with excretion of muscle proteins, especially myoglobin, by the kidney. It occurs particularly in patients with renal impairment, because of reduced protein binding and impaired drug elimination. Fibrates should be avoided in such patients and also in alcoholics,

---

[4]**Cerivastatin**, a potent statin introduced at relatively high dose, was withdrawn because of rhabdomyolysis occurring particularly in patients treated with gemfibrozil – discussed later in the chapter.

[5]Standing for peroxisome proliferator-activated receptors – don't ask! (Peroxisomes are organelles that are not present in human cells, so something of a misnomer!) Thiazolidinedione drugs used in treating diabetes act on related PPARγ receptors; see Ch. 31.

who are predisposed to hypertriglyceridaemia but are at risk of severe muscle inflammation and injury.[6] Rhabdomyolysis can also be caused (rarely) by statins (see p. 315), and the combined use of fibrates with this class of drugs is therefore generally inadvisable (although it is sometimes undertaken by specialists). Gastrointestinal symptoms, pruritus and rash are more common than with statins. Clofibrate predisposes to gallstones, and its use is therefore limited to patients who have had a cholecystectomy (i.e. removal of the gall bladder).

Clinical uses of fibrates (e.g. gemfibrozil, fenofibrate)

- Mixed dyslipidaemia (i.e. raised serum triglyceride as well as cholesterol), provided this is not caused by excessive alcohol consumption. **Fenofibrate** is uricosuric, which may be useful where hyperuricaemia coexists with mixed dyslipidaemia.
- In patients with low high-density lipoprotein and high risk of atheromatous disease (often type 2 diabetic patients; see Ch. 32).
- Combined with other lipid-lowering drugs in patients with severe treatment-resistant dyslipidaemia. This may, however, increase the risk of rhabdomyolysis.

DRUGS THAT INHIBIT CHOLESTEROL ABSORPTION

Historically, bile acid-binding resins (e.g. **colestyramine**, **colestipol**) were the only agents available to reduce cholesterol absorption and were among the few means to lower plasma cholesterol. Taken by mouth they sequester bile acids in the intestine and prevent their reabsorption and enterohepatic recirculation (see Fig. 24.1). The concentration of HDL is unchanged, and they cause an unwanted increase in triglycerides.

▼ The American Lipid Research Clinics' trial of middle-aged men with primary hypercholesterolaemia showed that addition of a resin to dietary treatment caused a fall in plasma cholesterol and a 20%–25% fall in coronary heart disease over 7 years, but no studies have shown improved survival.

Decreased absorption of exogenous cholesterol and increased metabolism of endogenous cholesterol into bile acids in the liver lead to increased expression of LDL receptors on hepatocytes, and hence to increased clearance of LDL from the blood and a reduced concentration of LDL in plasma. Resins are bulky, unpalatable and often cause diarrhoea. They interfere with the absorption of fat-soluble vitamins, and of thiazide diuretics (Ch 30), digoxin (Ch. 22) and warfarin (Ch. 25), which should therefore be taken at least 1 h before or 4–6 h after the resin. With the introduction of statins, their use in treating dyslipidaemia was relegated largely to additional treatment in patients with severe disease (e.g. FH) and (a separate use) treating bile salt-associated symptoms of pruritus (itch) and diarrhoea – see clinical box below. **Colesevelam** is available in tablet form and less bulky (daily dose up to 4 g compared with a dose up to 36 g for colestyramine) but more expensive. Subsequently, plant sterols and stanols

have been marketed; these are isolated from wood pulp and used to make margarines or yoghurts. They reduce plasma cholesterol to a small extent and are tastier than resins. Phytosterol and phytostanol esters interfere with the micellar presentation of sterols to the enterocyte surface, reducing cholesterol absorption and hence the exogenous pathway.

EZETIMIBE

Ezetimibe is one of a group of azetidinone cholesterol absorption inhibitors, and is used as an adjunct to diet and statins in hypercholesterolaemia. It inhibits absorption of cholesterol (and of plant stanols) from the duodenum by blocking a transport protein (NPC1L1) in the brush border of enterocytes, without affecting the absorption of fat-soluble vitamins, triglycerides or bile acids. Because of its high potency compared with resins (a daily dose of 10 mg), it represents a useful advance as a substitute for resins as supplementary treatment to statins in patients with severe dyslipidaemia.

Ezetimibe is administered by mouth and is absorbed into intestinal epithelial cells, where it localises to the brush border, which is its presumed site of action. It is also extensively (>80%) metabolised to an active metabolite. Enterohepatic recycling results in slow elimination. The terminal half-life is approximately 22 h. It enters milk (at least in animal studies) and is contraindicated for women who are breastfeeding. It is generally well tolerated but can cause diarrhoea, abdominal pain or headache; rash and angio-oedema have been reported.

Clinical use of drugs that reduce cholesterol absorption: ezetimibe or bile acid-binding resins (e.g. colestyramine, colesevelam)

- As an addition to a statin when response has been inadequate (**ezetimibe**).
- For hypercholesterolaemia when a statin is contraindicated.
- Uses unrelated to atherosclerosis, including:
  - pruritus in patients with partial biliary obstruction (bile acid-binding resin)
  - bile acid diarrhoea, for example, caused by diabetic neuropathy (bile acid-binding resin).

NICOTINIC ACID

▼ Nicotinic acid is a vitamin, and as such is essential for many important metabolic processes. Quite separately from this, it has been used in gram quantities as a lipid-lowering agent. It is converted to nicotinamide, which inhibits hepatic VLDL secretion (see Fig. 24.1), with consequent reductions in circulating triglyceride and LDL including Lp(a), and an increase in HDL. The mechanism is believed to be initiated by an effect on lipolysis via a G protein–coupled niacin receptor called HM74A and present in adipocyte membranes. Adverse effects include flushing, palpitations and gastrointestinal disturbance. Disappointingly, addition of nicotinic acid to a statin does not improve cardiovascular outcome, but does increase serious adverse effects (HSP2-THRIVE trial), and clinical use is dwindling.

FISH OIL DERIVATIVES

▼ Omega-3 marine triglycerides reduce plasma triglyceride concentrations but increase cholesterol. They are no longer generally recommended in clinical practice due to an absence of clinical benefit.

---

[6]For several reasons, including a tendency to lie immobile for prolonged periods followed by generalised convulsions – 'rum fits' – and delirium tremens.

MIPOMERSEN

Mipomersen is approved in the United States but not, at the time of writing, in Europe, for the 'orphan' indication of homozygous FH. It is an antisense oligonucleotide complementary to the coding region for apoB-100 of mRNA, which thereby inhibits synthesis of apoB-100 and LDL. Chemical modifications (see Ch. 5) make mipomersen resistant to degradation by nucleases, allowing it to be administered once weekly, as an adjunct to other treatment for homozygous FH. It accumulates in the liver, which is the site of its intended action but also of toxicity – hepatotoxicity being a serious problem that limits its use and necessitates careful monitoring. Other adverse effects include flu-like symptoms and oedema.

LOMITAPIDE

Lomitapide has also recently been approved as an adjunct to other treatment for homozygous FH. It is a small molecule inhibitor of MTP. MTP plays a key role in the assembly and release of apoB-containing lipoproteins into the circulation and inhibition of this protein significantly lowers plasma lipid levels. This action contrasts with other lipid-lowering drugs, which mainly work by increasing LDL uptake rather than by reducing hepatic lipoprotein secretion. Lomitapide is administered orally once a day and the dose individualised according to how it is tolerated. Gastrointestinal disturbances are common.

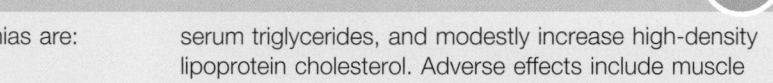

Drugs in dyslipidaemia

The main drugs used in patients with dyslipidaemias are:
- HMG-CoA reductase inhibitors (statins, e.g. **simvastatin**): inhibit synthesis of cholesterol, increasing expression of low-density lipoprotein (LDL) receptors on hepatocytes and hence increasing hepatic LDL cholesterol (LDL-C) uptake. They reduce cardiovascular events and prolong life in people at risk, and clinically are the most important class of drugs used in dyslipidaemias. Adverse effects include myalgias (rarely, severe muscle damage) and raised liver enzymes.
- Fibrates (e.g. **gemfibrozil**): activate PPARα receptors, increase activity of lipoprotein lipase, decrease hepatic very-low-density lipoprotein production and enhance clearance of LDL by the liver. They markedly lower serum triglycerides, and modestly increase high-density lipoprotein cholesterol. Adverse effects include muscle damage.
- Agents that interfere with cholesterol absorption, usually as an adjunct to diet plus statin:
  - **ezetimibe**
  - stanol-enriched foods
  - bile acid-binding resins (e.g. colestyramine, colesevelam).
- **Mipomersen**, **lomitapide**, **alirocumab** and **evolocumab** are used as adjuncts in treating patients with the rare homozygous form of familial hypercholesterolaemia.

REFERENCES AND FURTHER READING

Atherosclerosis and dyslipidaemia

Brown, M.S., Goldstein, J.L., 1986. A receptor-mediated pathway for cholesterol homeostasis. Science 232, 34–47. (*Classic from these Nobel Prize winners; see also Goldstein, J.L., Brown, M.S., 1990. Regulation of the mevalonate pathway. Nature 343, 425–430*)

Durrington, P.N., 2007. Hyperlipidaemia: Diagnosis and Management, third ed. Hodder Arnold, London. (*Extremely readable, authoritative book*)

Hall, S.H., 2013. Genetics: a gene of rare effect. Nature 496, 152–155. (*News feature describing the PCSK9 story as an example of a new paradigm for translational research*)

Ross, R., 1999. Atherosclerosis – an inflammatory disease. N. Engl. J. Med. 340, 115–126.

Stein, O., Stein, Y., 2005. Lipid transfer proteins (LTP) and atherosclerosis. Atherosclerosis 178, 217–230. (*Lipid transfer proteins – ACAT, CETP, LCAT and PLTP – and the therapeutic potential of modulating them*)

Statins

Hague, W., Emberson, J., Ridker, P.M., 2001. For the Air Force/Texas Coronary Atherosclerosis Prevention Study Investigators. Measurement of C-reactive protein for the targeting of statin therapy in the primary prevention of acute events. N. Engl. J. Med. 344, 1959–1965. (*Statins may be effective in preventing coronary events in people with unremarkable serum lipid concentrations but with elevated C-reactive protein, a marker of inflammation and risk factor for coronary disease*)

Liao, J.K., Laufs, U., 2005. Pleiotropic effects of statins. Annu. Rev. Pharmacol. Toxicol. 45, 89–118. ('*Many pleiotropic effects are mediated by inhibition of isoprenoids, which serve as lipid attachments for intracellular signalling molecules. In particular, inhibition of small GTP-binding proteins, Rho, Ras, and Rac, whose proper membrane localisation and function are dependent on isoprenylation, may play an important role in mediating the pleiotropic effects of statins*')

Merx, M.W., Liehn, E.A., Graf, J., et al., 2005. Statin treatment after onset of sepsis in a murine model improves survival. Circulation 112, 117–124. (*Statins offer the potential of effective sepsis treatment*)

Van Doren, M., Broihier, H.T., Moore, L.A., et al., 1998. HMG-CoA reductase guides migrating primordial germ cells. Nature 396, 466–469. (*Regulated expression of HMG-CoA reductase provides spatial guide to migrating primordial germ cells*)

Vasa, M., Fichtlscherer, S., Adler, K., et al., 2001. Increase in circulating endothelial progenitor cells by statin therapy in patients with stable coronary artery disease. Circulation 103, 2885–2890. (*May participate in repair after ischaemic injury*)

Other therapies
Nicotinic acid

Canner, P.L., Furberg, C.D., Terrin, M.L., et al., 2005. Benefits of niacin by glycemic status in patients with healed myocardial infarction (from the Coronary Drug Project). Am. J. Cardiol. 95, 254–257. (*The Coronary Drug Project, conducted during 1966 to 1974, was a randomised, double-blind, placebo-controlled trial in 8341 men with previous myocardial infarction; nicotinic acid significantly reduced total mortality during 6.2 years' treatment plus an additional 9 years of post-trial follow-up*)

HPS2-THRIVE Collaborative Group, 2013. HPS2-THRIVE randomized placebo-controlled trial in 25673 high-risk patients of ER niacin/laropiprant: trial design, pre-specified muscle and liver outcomes, and reasons for stopping study treatment. Eur. Heart J. 34, 1279–1291.

Fibrates
Bloomfield Rubins, H., Davenport, J., Babikian, V., et al., 2001. Reduction in stroke with gemfibrozil in men with coronary heart

disease and low HDL cholesterol. The Veterans Affairs HDL Intervention Trial (VA-HIT). Circulation 103, 2828–2833. (*Evidence that increasing HDL reduces stroke*)

Gervois, P., Torra, I.P., Fruchart, J.C., et al., 2000. Regulation of lipid and lipoprotein metabolism by PPAR activators. Clin. Chem. Lab. Med. 38, 3–11. (*Review*)

Fish oil

GISSI-Prevenzione Investigators (Gruppo Italiano per lo Studio della Sopravivenza nell'Infarto Miocardico), 1999. Dietary supplementation with n-3 polyunsaturated fatty acids and vitamin E after myocardial infarction: results of the GISSI-Prevenzione trial. Lancet 354, 447–455. (*11,324 patients surviving myocardial infarction were randomly assigned supplements of n-3 PUFA, 1 g daily, vitamin E, both or neither for 3.5 years. The primary end point was death, non-fatal myocardial infarction and stroke combined. Dietary supplementation with n-3 PUFA led to a clinically important and statistically significant benefit. Vitamin E had no benefit*)

Ezetimibe

Kosoglou, T., Statkevich, P., Johnson-Levonas, A.O., et al., 2005. Ezetimibe – a review of its metabolism, pharmacokinetics and drug interactions. Clin. Pharmacokinet. 44, 467–494.

Lomitapide

Cuchel, M., Meagher, E.A., du Toit Theron, H., et al., 2013. Efficacy and safety of a microsomal triglyceride transfer protein inhibitor in patients with homozygous familial hypercholesterolaemia: a single-arm, open-label, phase 3 study. Lancet 381, 40–46. (*See also accompanying editorial: Raal, F.J., pp. 7–8*)

Mipomersen

Merki, E., Graham, M.J., Mullick, A.E., 2008. Antisense oligonucleotide directed to human apolipoprotein B-100 reduces lipoprotein(a) levels and oxidized phospholipids on human apolipoprotein B-100 particles in lipoprotein(a) transgenic mice. Circulation 118, 743–753.

Potential therapies

de Medina, P., Payrá, B.L., Bernad, J., et al., 2004. Tamoxifen is a potent inhibitor of cholesterol esterification and prevents the formation of foam cells. J. Pharmacol. Exp. Ther. 308, 1542–1548. (*Molecular modelling revealed similarity between tamoxifen and ACAT inhibitor*)

Ikenaga, M., Higaki, Y., Saku, K., 2016. High-density lipoprotein mimetics: a therapeutic tool for atherosclerotic diseases. J. Atheroscler. Thromb. 23, 385–394. (*HDL therapies including reconstituted HDL, apolipoprotein (Apo) A-IMilano, ApoA-I mimetic peptides, or full-length ApoA-I, are highly effective in animal models. The ApoA-I-mimetic peptide FAMP enhances the function of HDL without elevating HDL cholesterol*)

25

Haemostasis and thrombosis

OVERVIEW

This chapter summarises the main features of blood coagulation, platelet function and fibrinolysis. These processes underlie haemostasis and thrombosis, and provide a basis for understanding haemorrhagic disorders (e.g. haemophilia) and thrombotic diseases both of arteries (e.g. thrombotic stroke, myocardial infarction) and of veins (e.g. deep vein thrombosis, pulmonary embolism). Anticoagulants, antiplatelet drugs and fibrinolytic drugs are especially important because of the prevalence of thrombotic disease.

INTRODUCTION

Haemostasis is the arrest of blood loss from damaged blood vessels and is essential to life. A wound causes vasoconstriction, accompanied by:

- adhesion and activation of platelets
- formation of fibrin

Platelet activation leads to the formation of a haemostatic plug, which stops the bleeding and is subsequently reinforced by fibrin. The relative importance of each process depends on the type of vessel (arterial, venous or capillary) that has been injured.

Thrombosis is the pathological formation of a 'haemostatic' plug within the vasculature in the absence of bleeding ('haemostasis in the wrong place'). Over a century ago, Rudolph Virchow defined three predisposing factors – 'Virchow triad': *injury to the vessel wall* – for example, when an atheromatous plaque ruptures or becomes eroded; *altered blood flow* – for example, in the left atrial appendage of the heart during atrial fibrillation, or in the veins of the legs while sitting awkwardly on a long journey; and *abnormal coagulability* of the blood – as occurs, for example, in the later stages of pregnancy or during treatment with certain oral contraceptives (see Ch. 36). Increased coagulability of the blood can be inherited and is referred to as *thrombophilia*. A *thrombus*, which forms in vivo, should be distinguished from a *clot*, which forms in blood in vitro (for example in a glass tube). Clots are amorphous, consisting of a diffuse fibrin meshwork in which red and white blood cells are trapped indiscriminately. By contrast, arterial and venous thrombi each have a distinct structure.

An *arterial thrombus* (Fig. 25.1) is composed of so-called white thrombus consisting mainly of platelets in a fibrin mesh. It is usually associated with atherosclerosis and can interrupt blood flow, causing ischaemia or death of tissue (infarction) downstream. Venous thrombus is composed of 'red thrombus' and consists of a small white head and a large jelly-like red tail, similar in composition to a blood

clot, which streams away in the flow. Thrombus can break away from its attachment and float through the circulation, forming an embolus; venous emboli usually lodge in a pulmonary artery ('pulmonary embolism'), while a thrombus that embolises from the left heart or a carotid artery usually lodges in an artery in the brain or other organs, causing death, stroke or other disaster.

Drug therapy to promote haemostasis (e.g. antifibrinolytic and haemostatic drugs; see p. 333) is indicated when this essential process is defective (e.g. defective or missing coagulation factors in haemophilia or following excessive anticoagulant therapy), or when it proves difficult to staunch haemorrhage following surgery or for menorrhagia (heavy menstrual periods). Drug therapy to treat or prevent thrombosis or thromboembolism is extensively used because such diseases are common as well as serious. Drugs affect haemostasis and thrombosis in three distinct ways, by influencing:

- blood coagulation (fibrin formation)
- platelet function
- fibrin removal (fibrinolysis)

BLOOD COAGULATION

COAGULATION CASCADE

Blood coagulation means the conversion of liquid blood to a clot. The main event is the conversion by thrombin of soluble *fibrinogen* to insoluble strands of *fibrin*, the last step in a complex enzyme cascade. The components (called factors) are present in blood as inactive precursors (zymogens) of proteolytic enzymes and co-factors. They are activated by proteolysis, the 'active' forms being designated by the suffix 'a'. Factors XIIa, XIa, Xa, IXa and thrombin (IIa) are all serine proteases. Activation of a small amount of one factor catalyses the formation of larger amounts of the next factor, which catalyses the formation of still larger amounts of the next, and so on; consequently, the cascade provides a mechanism of amplification.[1] As might be expected, this accelerating enzyme cascade has to be controlled by inhibitors, because otherwise all the blood in the body would solidify within minutes of the initiation of haemostasis. One of the most important inhibitors is *antithrombin III*, which neutralises all the serine proteases in the cascade. Vascular endothelium also actively limits thrombus extension (see pp. 321–322).

Two pathways of fibrin formation were described traditionally (termed 'intrinsic' – because all the components are present in the blood – and 'extrinsic' – because some

---

[1]Coagulation of 100 mL of blood requires 0.2 mg of factor VIII, 2 mg of factor X, 15 mg of prothrombin and 250 mg of fibrinogen.

319

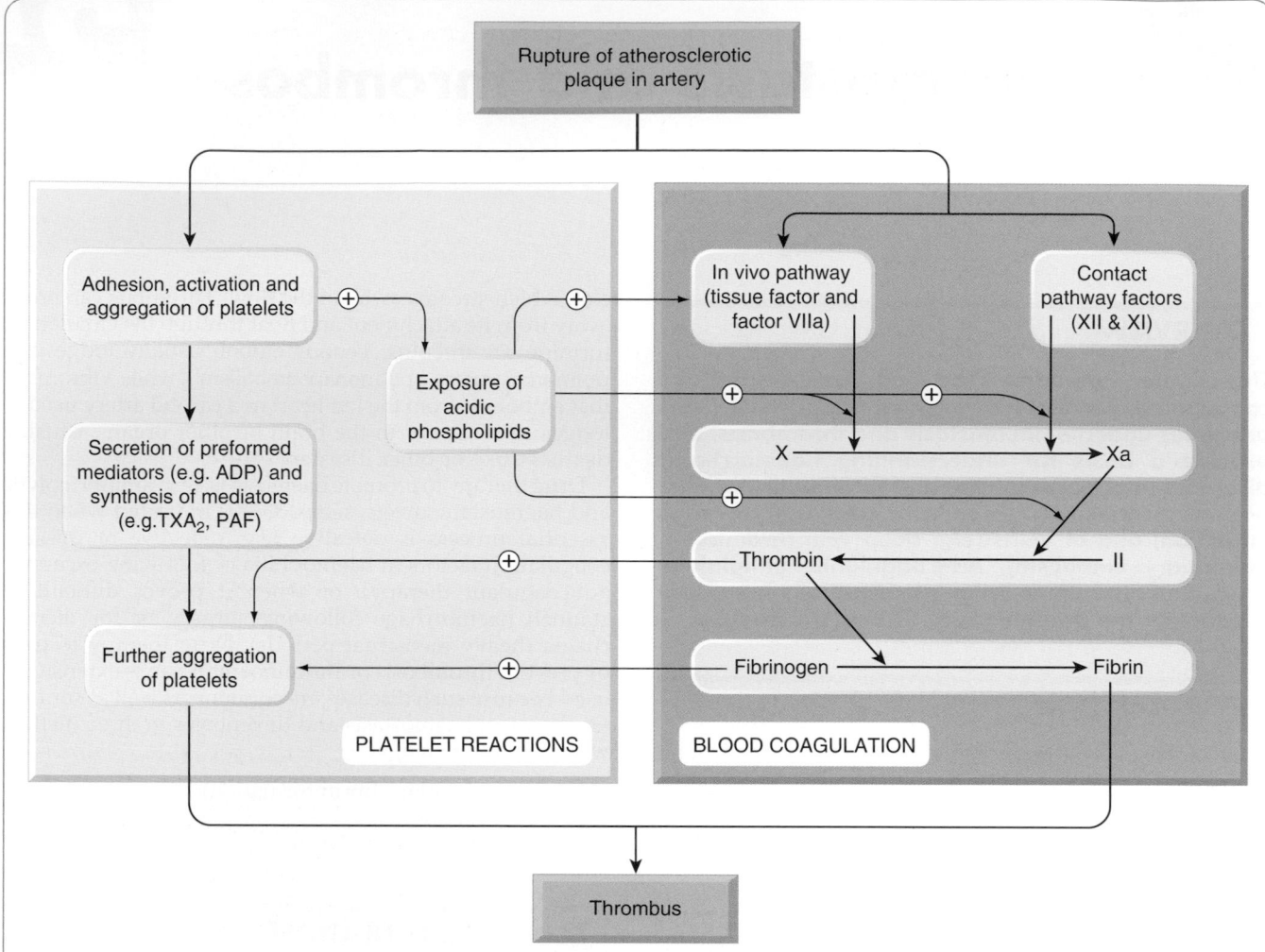

Fig. 25.1   The main events in the formation of an arterial thrombus. Exposure of acidic phospholipids during platelet activation provides a surface on which factors IXa and VIIa interact with factor X; factor Xa then interacts with factor II, as illustrated in more detail in Fig. 25.4. Activation of factor XII also initiates the fibrinolytic pathway, which is shown in Fig. 25.10. (A similar series of events occurs when there is vascular damage, leading to haemostasis.) *PAF*, platelet-activating factor; *TXA₂*, thromboxane A₂.

components come from outside the blood). The intrinsic or 'contact' pathway is activated when shed blood comes into contact with an artificial surface such as glass, but physiologically the system functions as a single in vivo *pathway* (Fig. 25.2). Tissue damage exposes blood to *tissue factor*, initiating the process and leading to production of a small amount of thrombin. This acts through several positive feedbacks (on Va, VIIIa and on platelets) that amplify and propagate the process with production of more thrombin.

▼ 'Tissue factor' is the cellular receptor for factor VII, which, in the presence of Ca^{2+}, undergoes an active site transition. This results in rapid autocatalytic activation of factor VII to VIIa. The tissue factor–VIIa complex activates factors IX and X. Acidic phospholipids function as *surface catalysts*. They are provided during platelet activation, which exposes acidic phospholipids (especially phosphatidylserine), on the platelets' outwardly facing membranes, and these activate various clotting factors, closely juxtaposing them in functional complexes. Platelets also contribute by secreting coagulation factors, including factor Va and fibrinogen. Coagulation is sustained by further generation of factor Xa by IXa–VIIIa–Ca^{2+}–phospholipid complex. This is needed because the tissue factor–VIIa complex is rapidly inactivated in plasma by tissue factor pathway inhibitor and by antithrombin III. Factor

Xa, in the presence of Ca^{2+}, phospholipid and factor Va, activates prothrombin to thrombin, the main enzyme of the cascade. The *contact* (intrinsic) pathway commences when factor XII (Hageman factor) adheres to a negatively charged surface and converges with the in vivo pathway at the stage of factor X activation (see Fig. 25.2). The proximal part of this pathway is not crucial for blood coagulation in vivo.[2] The two pathways are not entirely separate even before they converge, and various positive feedbacks promote coagulation.

THE ROLE OF THROMBIN

Thrombin (factor IIa) cleaves fibrinogen, producing fragments that polymerise to form fibrin. It also activates factor XIII, a *fibrinoligase*, which strengthens fibrin-to-fibrin links, thereby stabilising the coagulum. In addition to coagulation, thrombin also causes platelet aggregation, stimulates cell proliferation and modulates smooth muscle contraction. Paradoxically, it can inhibit as well as promote coagulation (see pp. 321–322). Effects of thrombin on platelets and

[2]Mr Hageman (the patient deficient in factor XII after whom it was named) died not from excessive bleeding but from a pulmonary embolism: factor XII deficiency does not give rise to a bleeding disorder.

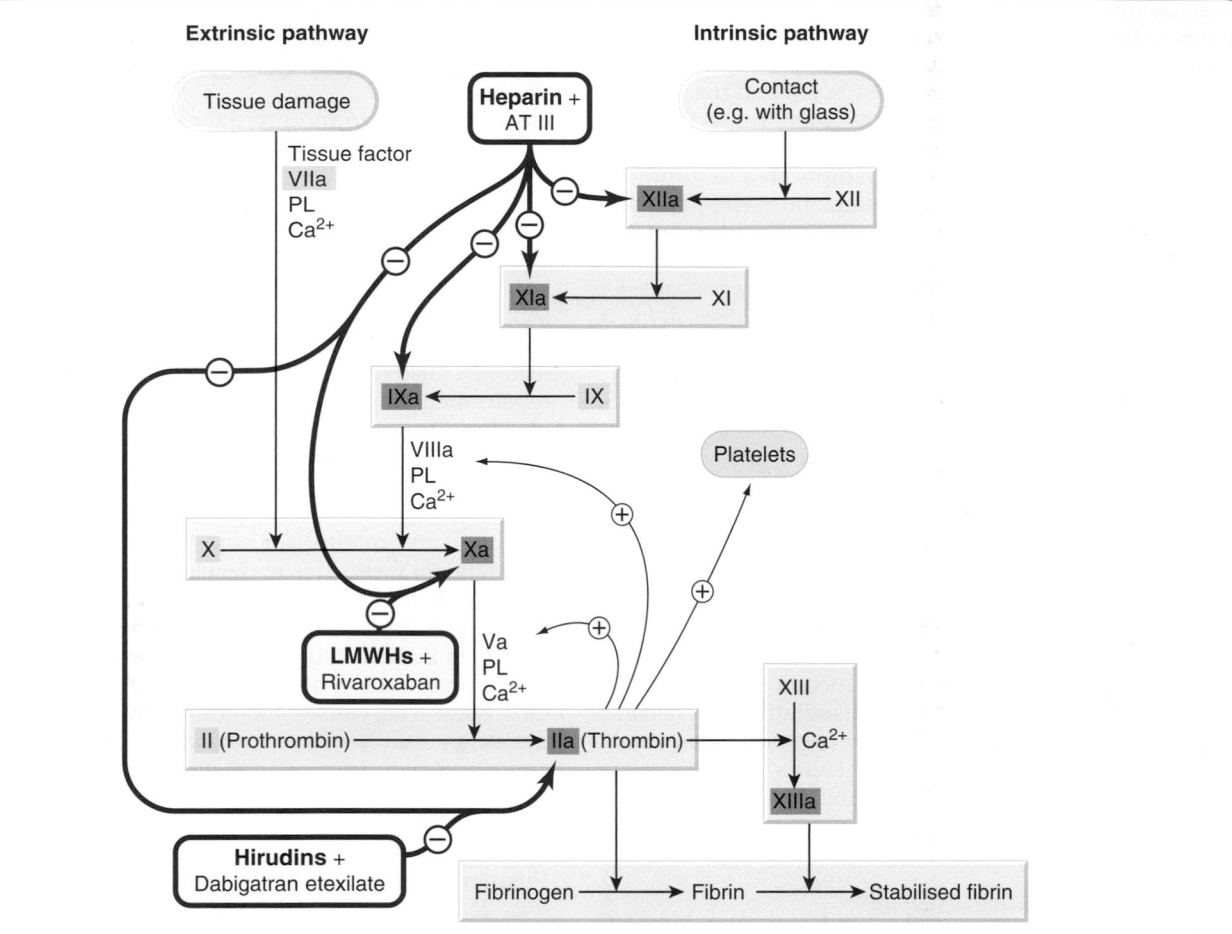

Fig. 25.2   The coagulation cascade: sites of action of anticoagulant drugs. Oral anticoagulants interfere with post-translational γ-carboxylation of factors II, VII, IX and X *(shown in blue boxes)*; see Fig. 25.4. Heparins activate antithrombin III. *AT III,* antithrombin III; *LMWHs,* low molecular-weight heparins; *PL,* negatively charged phospholipid supplied by activated platelets.

Haemostasis and thrombosis

- Haemostasis is the arrest of blood loss from damaged vessels and is essential to survival. The main phenomena are:
  - platelet adhesion and activation
  - blood coagulation (fibrin formation)
- Thrombosis is a pathological condition resulting from inappropriate activation of haemostatic mechanisms:
  - venous thrombosis is usually associated with stasis of blood; a venous thrombus has a small platelet component and a large component of fibrin.
  - arterial thrombosis is usually associated with atherosclerosis, and the thrombus has a large platelet component.
- A portion of a thrombus may break away, travel as an embolus and lodge downstream, causing ischaemia and/or infarction.

smooth muscle are initiated by interaction with specific protease-activated receptors (PARs; see Ch. 3), which belong to the superfamily of G protein–coupled receptors. PARs initiate cellular responses that contribute not only to haemostasis and thrombosis, but also to inflammation and

perhaps angiogenesis. The signal transduction mechanism is unusual: receptor activation requires cleavage by thrombin of the extracellular N-terminal domain of the receptor, revealing a new N-terminal sequence that acts as a 'tethered agonist' (see Fig. 3.7).

VASCULAR ENDOTHELIUM IN HAEMOSTASIS AND THROMBOSIS

Vascular endothelium, the container of the circulating blood, can change focally from a non-thrombogenic to a thrombogenic structure in response to different demands. Normally, it provides a non-thrombogenic surface by virtue of membrane *heparan sulfate,* a glycosaminoglycan related to heparin, which is, like heparin, a co-factor for antithrombin III. Endothelium thus plays an essential role in preventing intravascular platelet activation and coagulation. However, it also plays an active part in haemostasis, synthesising and storing several key haemostatic components; von Willebrand factor,[3] tissue factor and plasminogen

---

[3]von Willebrand factor is a glycoprotein that is missing in a hereditary haemorrhagic disorder called von Willebrand disease, which is the most common of the inherited bleeding disorders. It is synthesised by vascular endothelial cells (the presence of immunoreactive von Willebrand factor is an identifying feature of these cells in culture) and is also present in platelets.

activator inhibitor (PAI)-1 are particularly important. PAI-1 is secreted in response to *angiotensin IV*, receptors for which are present on endothelial cells, providing a link between the renin–angiotensin system (see Ch. 23) and thrombosis. These prothrombotic factors are involved, respectively, in platelet adhesion and in coagulation and clot stabilisation. However, the endothelium is also implicated in thrombus limitation. Thus it generates prostaglandin (PG) I_2 (prostacyclin; Ch. 18) and nitric oxide (NO; Ch. 21); converts ADP, which causes platelet aggregation, to adenosine, which inhibits it (Ch. 17); synthesises *tissue plasminogen activator* (tPA; see pp. 330–333); and expresses *thrombomodulin*, a receptor for thrombin. After combination with thrombomodulin, thrombin activates an anticoagulant, *protein C*. Activated protein C, helped by its co-factor protein S, inactivates factors Va and VIIa. This is known to be physiologically important, because a naturally occurring mutation of the gene coding for factor V (factor V Leiden), which confers resistance to activated protein C, results in the commonest recognised form of inherited thrombophilia.

Endotoxin and some cytokines, including tumour necrosis factor, tilt the balance of prothrombotic and antithrombotic endothelial functions towards thrombosis by causing loss of heparan (see earlier) and increased expression of tissue factor, and impair endothelial NO function. If other mechanisms limiting coagulation are also faulty or become exhausted, *disseminated intravascular coagulation* can result. This is a serious complication of sepsis and of certain malignancies, and the main treatment is to correct the underlying disease.

Blood coagulation (fibrin formation)

The clotting system consists of a cascade of proteolytic enzymes and co-factors.

- Inactive precursors are activated sequentially, each giving rise to more of the next.
- The last enzyme, thrombin, derived from prothrombin (II), converts soluble fibrinogen (I) to an insoluble meshwork of fibrin in which blood cells are trapped, forming the clot.
- There are two limbs in the cascade:
  – the in vivo (extrinsic) pathway
  – the contact (intrinsic) pathway
- Both pathways result in activation of factor X to Xa, which converts prothrombin to thrombin.
- Calcium ions and a negatively charged phospholipid (PL) are essential for three steps, namely the actions of:
  – factor IXa on X
  – factor VIIa on X
  – factor Xa on II
- PL is provided by activated platelets adhering to the damaged vessel.
- Some factors promote coagulation by binding to PL and a serine protease factor; for example, factor Va in the activation of II by Xa, or VIIIa in the activation of X by IXa.
- Blood coagulation is controlled by:
  – enzyme inhibitors (e.g. antithrombin III)
  – fibrinolysis

DRUGS THAT ACT ON THE COAGULATION CASCADE

Drugs are used to modify the cascade either when there is a defect in coagulation or when there is unwanted coagulation.

COAGULATION DEFECTS

Genetically determined deficiencies of clotting factors are not common. Examples are classic haemophilia, caused by lack of factor VIII, and an even rarer form of haemophilia (haemophilia B or Christmas disease) caused by lack of factor IX (also called Christmas factor). Intravenous factor replacement is given by specialists to prevent or to limit bleeding in such patients. Some patients develop factor inhibitors, and their management is particularly demanding (for example, by induction of immune tolerance, see Ch. 7). Plasma-derived concentrates are giving way to pure recombinant proteins (for example, of factors VIII and IX; recombinant factor II is in development) – this is a rapidly evolving field. A human recombinant form of factor VIIa is also available for bleeding in patients with severe bleeding disorders but can cause intravascular coagulation.

Acquired clotting defects are more common than hereditary ones. The causes include liver disease, vitamin K deficiency (universal in neonates) and excessive oral anticoagulant therapy, each of which may require treatment with vitamin K.

VITAMIN K

Vitamin K (for *Koagulation* in German) is a fat-soluble vitamin (Fig. 25.3) occurring naturally in plants (vitamin K_1) and as a series of bacterial menaquinones (vitamin K_2) formed in the gut (see Shearer & Newman, 2008, for a review). It is essential for the formation of clotting factors II, VII, IX and X, which are glycoproteins with γ-carboxyglutamic acid (Gla) residues. The interaction of factors Xa and prothrombin (factor II) with Ca^{2+} and phospholipid is shown in Fig. 25.4. γ-Carboxylation occurs after the synthesis of the amino acid chain, and the carboxylase enzyme requires reduced vitamin K as a co-factor (Fig. 25.5). Binding does not occur in the absence of γ-carboxylation. Similar considerations apply to the proteolytic activation of factor X by IXa and by VIIa (see Fig. 25.2).

Fig. 25.3 Vitamin K and warfarin. Warfarin, a vitamin K antagonist, is an oral anticoagulant. It competes with vitamin K (note the similarity in their structures) for the reductase enzyme (VKORC1) that activates vitamin K and is the site of its action (see Fig. 25.5).

Fig. 25.4 Activation of prothrombin (factor II) by factor Xa. The complex of factor Va with a negatively charged phospholipid surface (supplied by aggregating platelets) forms a binding site for factor Xa and prothrombin (II), which have peptide chains *(shown schematically)* that are similar to one another. Platelets thus serve as a localising focus. Calcium ions are essential for binding. Xa activates prothrombin, liberating thrombin *(shown in grey)*. (Modified from Jackson, C.M., 1978. Br. J. Haematol. 39, 1.)

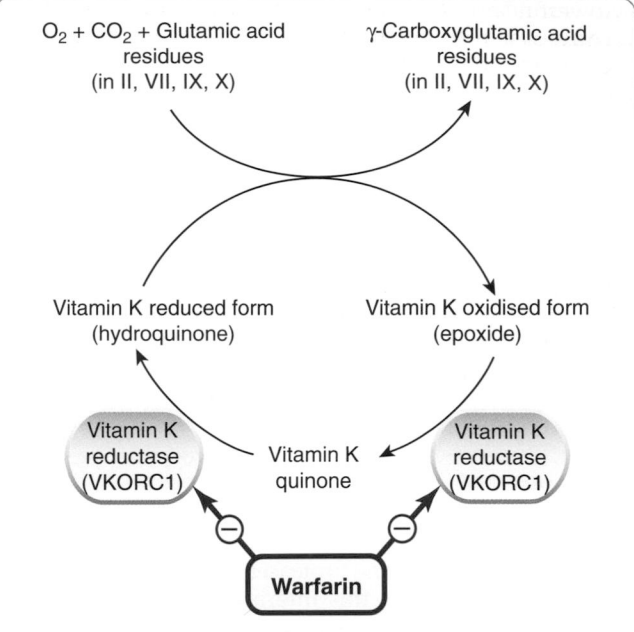

Fig. 25.5 Mechanism of vitamin K and of warfarin. After the peptide chains in clotting factors II, VII, IX and X have been synthesised, reduced vitamin K (the hydroquinone) acts as a co-factor in the conversion of glutamic acid to γ-carboxyglutamic acid. During this reaction, the reduced form of vitamin K is converted to the epoxide, which in turn is reduced to the quinone and then the hydroquinone by vitamin K epoxide reductase component 1 (VKORC1), the site of action of warfarin.

There are several other vitamin K-dependent Gla proteins, including proteins C and S and osteocalcin in bone.

Administration and pharmacokinetic aspects

Natural vitamin K_1 (**phytomenadione**) may be given orally or by injection. If given by mouth, it requires bile salts for absorption, and this occurs by a saturable energy-requiring process in the proximal small intestine. A synthetic preparation, **menadiol sodium phosphate**, is also available. It is water-soluble and does not require bile salts for its absorption. This synthetic compound takes longer to act than phytomenadione. There is very little storage of vitamin K in the body. It is metabolised to more polar substances that are excreted in the urine and the bile.

Clinical uses of vitamin K are summarised in the clinical box.

THROMBOSIS

Thrombotic and thromboembolic disease is common and has severe consequences, including myocardial infarction, stroke, deep vein thrombosis and pulmonary embolus. The main drugs used for platelet-rich 'white' arterial thrombi are the antiplatelet drugs and fibrinolytic drugs, which are considered below. The main drugs used to prevent or treat 'red' venous thrombi are:

Clinical uses of vitamin K

- Treatment and/or prevention of bleeding:
  - from excessive oral anticoagulation (e.g. by **warfarin**)
  - in babies: to prevent *haemorrhagic disease of the newborn*
- For vitamin K deficiencies in adults:
  - *sprue, coeliac disease, steatorrhoea*
  - lack of bile (e.g. with *obstructive jaundice*)

- injectable anticoagulants (**heparin** and newer thrombin inhibitors);
- oral anticoagulants (**warfarin** and related compounds; orally active thrombin inhibitors).

Heparins and thrombin inhibitors act immediately, whereas warfarin and other vitamin K antagonists take several days to exert their effect. Consequently, if warfarin is used to treat patients with venous thrombosis, an agent that acts immediately is also administered until the effect of warfarin has become established.

HEPARIN (INCLUDING LOW MOLECULAR-WEIGHT HEPARINS)

Heparin was discovered in 1916 by a second-year medical student at Johns Hopkins Hospital. He was attempting to extract thromboplastic (i.e. coagulant) substances from various tissues during a vacation project, but found instead a powerful anticoagulant activity.[4] This was named heparin, because it was first extracted from liver.

Heparin is not a single substance but a family of sulfated glycosaminoglycans (mucopolysaccharides). It is present together with histamine in the granules of mast cells. Commercial preparations are extracted from beef lung or hog intestine and, because preparations differ in potency, assayed biologically against an agreed international standard: doses are specified in units of activity rather than of mass.

Heparin fragments (e.g. **enoxaparin, dalteparin**) or a synthetic pentasaccharide (**fondaparinux**), referred to as low molecular-weight heparins (LMWHs), are longer acting than unfractionated heparin and are usually preferred, the unfractionated product being reserved for special situations such as patients with renal failure in whom LMWHs are contraindicated.

Mechanism of action

Heparin inhibits coagulation, both in vivo and in vitro, by activating antithrombin III. Antithrombin III inhibits thrombin and other serine proteases by binding to the active site. Heparin modifies this interaction by binding, via a unique pentasaccharide sequence, to antithrombin III, changing its conformation and increasing its affinity for serine proteases.

To inhibit thrombin, it is necessary for heparin to bind to the enzyme as well as to antithrombin III; to inhibit factor Xa, it is necessary only for heparin to bind to antithrombin III (Fig. 25.6). Antithrombin III deficiency is very rare but can cause thrombophilia and resistance to heparin therapy.

The LMWHs increase the action of antithrombin III on factor Xa but not its action on thrombin, because the molecules are too small to bind to both enzyme and inhibitor, essential for inhibition of thrombin but not for that of factor Xa (see Fig. 25.6).

Administration and pharmacokinetic aspects

Heparin is not absorbed from the gut because of its charge and high molecular-weight, and it is therefore given intravenously or subcutaneously (intramuscular injections would cause haematomas).

▼ After intravenous injection of a bolus dose, there is a phase of rapid elimination followed by a more gradual disappearance owing both to saturable processes (involving binding to sites on endothelial cells and macrophages) and to slower non-saturable processes including renal excretion. As a result, once the dose exceeds the saturating concentration, a greater proportion is dealt with by these slower processes, and the apparent half-life increases with increasing dose (saturation kinetics; see Ch. 11).

Heparin acts immediately following intravenous administration, but the onset is delayed by up to 60 min when it is given subcutaneously. The elimination half-life is approximately 40–90 min. In urgent situations, it is therefore usual to start treatment with a bolus intravenous dose, followed by a constant-rate infusion. The *activated partial thromboplastin time* (APTT), or some other in vitro clotting test, is measured and the dose of heparin adjusted to achieve a value within a target range (e.g. 1.5–2.5 times control).

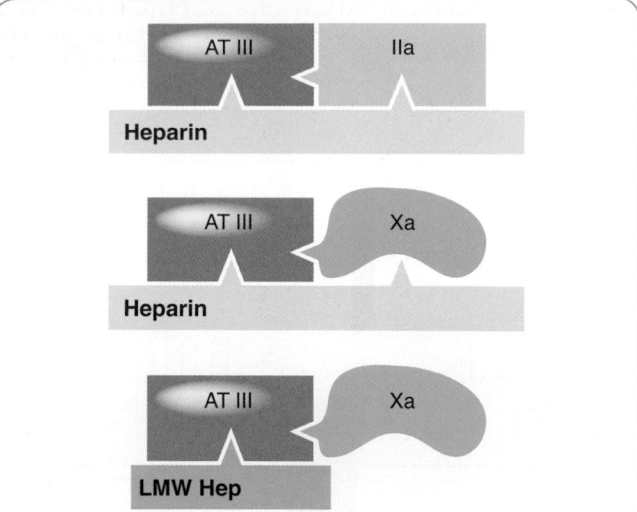

Fig. 25.6   Action of heparins. The schematic shows interactions of heparins, antithrombin III (AT III) and clotting factors. To increase the inactivation of thrombin (IIa) by AT III, heparin needs to interact with both substances *(top)*, but to speed up its effect on factor Xa it need only interact with AT III *(middle)*. Low molecular-weight heparins (LMW Hep) increase the action of AT III on factor Xa *(bottom)*, but cannot increase the action of AT III on thrombin because they cannot bind both simultaneously.

LMWHs are given subcutaneously. They have a longer elimination half-life than unfractionated heparin, and this is independent of dose (first-order kinetics), so the effects are more predictable and dosing less frequent (once or twice a day). LMWHs do not prolong the APTT. Unlike unfractionated heparin, the effect of a standard dose is sufficiently predictable that monitoring is not required routinely. LMWHs are eliminated mainly by renal excretion, and unfractionated heparin is preferred in renal failure, but with this exception LMWHs are at least as safe and effective as unfractionated heparin and are more convenient to use, because patients can be taught to inject themselves at home and there is generally no need for blood tests and dose adjustment.

Unwanted effects

Haemorrhage. The main hazard is haemorrhage, which is treated by stopping therapy and, if necessary, giving **protamine sulfate**. This heparin antagonist is a strongly basic protein that forms an inactive complex with heparin; it is given intravenously. The dose is estimated from the dose of heparin that has been administered recently, and it is important not to give too much, as this can itself cause bleeding. If necessary, an in vitro neutralisation test is performed first on a sample of blood from the patient to provide a more precise indication of the required dose.

Thrombosis. This is an uncommon but serious adverse effect of heparin and, as with warfarin necrosis, may be misattributed to the natural history of the disease for which heparin is being administered.

▼ Paradoxically, it is associated with *heparin-induced thrombocytopenia* (HIT). A transitory early decrease in platelet numbers is not uncommon after initiating heparin treatment, and is not clinically important. More serious thrombocytopenia occurring 2–14 days after the start

---

[4]This kind of good fortune also favoured Vane and his colleagues in their discovery of PGI$_2$ (Ch. 18), where they were looking for one kind of biological activity and found another. More specific chemical assays (Ch. 8), for all their strengths, cannot throw up this kind of unexpected discovery.

of therapy is uncommon and is referred to as type II HIT. This is caused by IgM or IgG antibodies against complexes of heparin and a platelet-derived chemokine, platelet factor 4. Circulating immune complexes bind to circulating platelets, and cause thrombocytopenia. Antibody also binds to platelet factor 4 attached to the surface of endothelial cells, leading to immune injury of the vessel wall, thrombosis and disseminated intravascular coagulation. LMWHs are less likely than unfractionated heparin to cause thrombocytopenia and thrombosis by this mechanism. HIT is usually treated by substituting **danaparoid** or a direct thrombin inhibitor such as **lepirudin** instead of the heparin preparation that caused the problem. Danaparoid is a low molecular-weight heparinoid consisting of a mixture of heparan, dermatan and chondroitin sulfates, with well-established antithrombotic activity.

Osteoporosis with spontaneous fractures has been reported with long-term (6 months or more) treatment with heparin (usually during pregnancy, when warfarin is contraindicated or problematic). Its explanation is unknown.

Hypoaldosteronism (with consequent hyperkalaemia) is uncommon, but increases with prolonged treatment. It is recommended to check plasma K^+ concentration if treatment is to be continued for >7 days.

Hypersensitivity reactions are rare with heparin but more common with protamine. (Protamine sensitivity also occurs in patients treated with protamine zinc insulin; Ch. 32. Protamine is extracted from fish roe, and sensitivity to protamine occurs in some people with fish allergy.)

DIRECT THROMBIN INHIBITORS AND RELATED DRUGS

Hirudins are polypeptides that act as direct thrombin inhibitors. They are derived from the anticoagulant present in saliva from the medicinal leech. Unlike the heparins, they do not depend on activation of antithrombin. **Lepirudin** is a recombinant hirudin that binds irreversibly to both the fibrin-binding and catalytic sites on thrombin and is used for thromboembolic disease in patients with type II HIT. It is administered intravenously, the dose being adjusted depending on the APTT, and can cause bleeding or hypersensitivity reactions (rash or fever). **Bivalirudin**, another hirudin analogue, is used in combination with **aspirin** and **clopidogrel** (see pp. 328–331) in patients undergoing percutaneous coronary artery surgery. Treatment is initiated with an intravenous bolus followed by an infusion during and up to 4 h after the procedure. It can cause bleeding and hypersensitivity reactions.

Orally active direct inhibitors. This field had more than one false dawn, but rapid progress has been made recently, and indications for such drugs have expanded considerably. In time, orally active direct inhibitors could come to replace warfarin, a venerable but troublesome drug that is a common cause of serious adverse effects. **Dabigatran** is a synthetic serine protease inhibitor; **dabigatran etexilate**, a prodrug with a hydrophobic tail, is orally active and is licensed for prevention of venous thromboembolism following hip or knee replacement and for the prevention of stroke and systemic embolism in atrial fibrillation (Ch. 21). It works rapidly and is administered 1–4 hours after surgery and then once daily for up to a month (depending on the type of surgery), or twice daily indefinitely for the prevention of stroke. The dose is reduced in patients aged over 75 or receiving concomitant verapamil or amiodarone. **Rivaroxaban**, an orally active direct inhibitor of factor Xa rather than of thrombin, but similar to dabigatran in other respects, is licensed for the same indications and in addition for the treatment (as well as prophylaxis) of deep vein thrombosis. **Apixiban** is similar. These drugs are administered in standard doses without laboratory monitoring of their anticoagulant effects. Their commonest adverse effects are predictable (bleeding, anaemia); rivaroxaban also commonly causes nausea. Other indications are being investigated, and if they prove safe and effective for a range of indications, this could transform the clinical management of the large group of patients currently maintained on warfarin (see the clinical box on the clinical use of anticoagulants, p. 327).

▼ Various other approaches are being explored. These include several naturally occurring anticoagulants (tissue factor pathway inhibitor, thrombomodulin and protein C) synthesised by recombinant technology. A particularly ingenious approach is the development of thrombin agonists that are selective for the anticoagulant properties of thrombin. One such modified thrombin, differing by a single amino acid substitution, has substrate specificity for protein C. It produces anticoagulation in monkeys without prolonging bleeding times, suggesting that it may be less likely than standard anticoagulants to cause bleeding (Bah et al., 2009).

WARFARIN

▼ Oral anticoagulants were discovered as an indirect result of a change in agricultural policy in North America in the 1920s. Sweet clover was substituted for corn in cattle feed, and an epidemic of deaths of cattle from haemorrhage ensued. This turned out to be caused by bishydroxycoumarin in spoiled sweet clover, and it led to the discovery of warfarin (named for the Wisconsin Alumni Research Foundation). One of the first uses to which this was put was as a rat poison, but for more than 50 years it was the standard anticoagulant for the treatment and prevention of thromboembolic disease.

Warfarin (see Fig. 25.3) is the most important oral anticoagulant; alternatives with a similar mechanism of action, for example **phenindione**, are now used only in rare patients who experience idiosyncratic adverse reactions to warfarin[5] (see Ch. 12). Warfarin and other vitamin K antagonists require frequent blood tests to individualise dose, and are consequently inconvenient as well as having a low margin of safety. Advances in the technology available for testing genomic DNA mutations in every patient (from less than £100 for each complete genome test), means that individualised pharmacology (so-called pharmacogenomics) may become more and more viable for even the cheapest drug. Tailoring drugs to a person's mutations to avoid such adverse reactions, is increasingly common.

Mechanism of action

Vitamin K antagonists act only in vivo and have no effect on clotting if added to blood in vitro. They interfere with the post-translational γ-carboxylation of glutamic acid residues in clotting factors II, VII, IX and X. They do this by inhibiting *vitamin K epoxide reductase component 1* (VKORC1), thus inhibiting the reduction of vitamin K epoxide to its active hydroquinone form (see Fig. 25.5). Inhibition is competitive (reflecting the structural similarity between warfarin and vitamin K; see Fig. 25.3). The *VKORC1* gene is polymorphic (see Ch. 12), and different haplotypes

---

[5]Warfarin is a good example for 'personalised medicine' or 'pharmacogenomics'. Prior to dosing with the anticoagulant, the patient can be checked by genotyping for mutations in their VKORC1 and CYP2C9 genes, which are involved in the coagulation cascade and metabolism of the drug. In patients possessing common mutations of these genes, standard doses of warfarin may cause potentially lethal bleeding or thromboembolism due to therapeutic failure.

have different affinities for warfarin. Genotyping to determine the haplotype, combined with genotyping *CYP2C9* (see later), while not yet routine, can be used to optimise the starting dose, reducing the variability in response to warfarin by around one-third. The effect of warfarin takes several days to develop because of the time taken for degradation of preformed carboxylated clotting factors. Onset of action thus depends on the elimination half-lives of the relevant factors. Factor VII, with a half-life of 6 h, is affected first, then IX, X and II, with half-lives of 24, 40 and 60 h, respectively.

Administration and pharmacokinetic aspects

Warfarin is absorbed rapidly and completely from the gut after oral administration. It has a small distribution volume, being strongly bound to plasma albumin (see Ch. 9). The peak concentration in the blood occurs within an hour of ingestion, but because of the mechanism of action this does not coincide with the peak pharmacological effect, which occurs about 48 h later. The effect on prothrombin time (PT, see later) of a single dose starts after approximately 12–16 h and lasts 4–5 days. Warfarin is metabolised by CYP2C9, which is polymorphic (see Ch. 12). Partly in consequence of this, its half-life is very variable, being of the order of 40 h in many individuals.

Warfarin crosses the placenta and is not given in the first months of pregnancy because it is teratogenic (see Table 58.2, Ch. 58), nor in the later stages because it can cause intracranial haemorrhage in the baby during delivery. It appears in milk during lactation. This could theoretically be important because newborn infants are naturally deficient in vitamin K. However, infants are routinely prescribed vitamin K to prevent haemorrhagic disease, so warfarin treatment of the mother does not generally pose a risk to the breastfed infant.

The therapeutic use of warfarin requires a careful balance between giving too little, leaving unwanted coagulation unchecked, and giving too much, thereby causing haemorrhage. Therapy is complicated not only because the effect of each dose is maximal some 2 days after its administration, but also because numerous medical and environmental conditions modify sensitivity to warfarin, including interactions with other drugs (see Chs 9 and 12). The effect of warfarin is monitored by measuring PT, which is expressed as an *international normalised ratio* (INR).

▼ The PT is the time taken for clotting of citrated plasma after the addition of Ca^{2+} and standardised reference thromboplastin; it is expressed as the ratio (PT ratio) of the PT of the patient to the PT of a pool of plasma from healthy subjects on no medication. Because of the variability of thromboplastins, different results are obtained in different laboratories. To standardise PT measurements internationally, each thromboplastin is assigned an international sensitivity index (ISI), and the patient's PT is expressed as an INR, where INR = (PT ratio)^{ISI}. This kind of inter-laboratory normalisation procedure shocks purists but provides similar results when a patient moves from, say, Birmingham to Baltimore. Pragmatic haematologists argue that the proof of the pudding is in the eating!

The dose of warfarin is usually adjusted to give an INR of 2–4, the precise target depending on the clinical situation. The duration of treatment also varies, but for several indications (e.g. to prevent thromboembolism in chronic atrial fibrillation), treatment is long term, with the logistical challenge of providing a worldwide network of anticoagulant clinics and demands on the patient in terms of repeat visits and blood tests.

FACTORS THAT POTENTIATE WARFARIN

Various diseases and drugs potentiate warfarin, increasing the risk of haemorrhage.

Disease

Liver disease interferes with the synthesis of clotting factors; conditions in which there is a high metabolic rate, such as fever and thyrotoxicosis, increase the effect of anticoagulants by increasing degradation of clotting factors.

Drugs (see also Ch. 10)

Many drugs potentiate warfarin.

Agents that inhibit hepatic drug metabolism. Examples include **co-trimoxazole, ciprofloxacin, metronidazole, amiodarone** and many antifungal azoles. Stereoselective effects (warfarin is a racemate, and its isomers are metabolised differently from one another) are described in Chapter 10.

Drugs that inhibit platelet function. Aspirin increases the risk of bleeding if given during warfarin therapy, although this combination can be used safely with careful monitoring. Other non-steroidal anti-inflammatory drugs (NSAIDs) also increase the risk of bleeding, partly by their effect on platelet thromboxane synthesis (Ch. 27) and, in the case of some NSAIDs, also by inhibiting warfarin metabolism as above. Some antibiotics, including **moxalactam** and **carbenicillin**, inhibit platelet function.

Drugs that displace warfarin from binding sites on plasma albumin. Some of the NSAIDs and **chloral hydrate** cause a transient increase in the concentration of free warfarin in plasma by competing with it for binding to plasma albumin. This mechanism seldom causes clinically important effects.

Drugs that inhibit reduction of vitamin K. Such drugs include the *cephalosporins*.

Drugs that decrease the availability of vitamin K. Broad-spectrum antibiotics and some *sulfonamides* (see Ch. 51) depress the intestinal flora that normally synthesise vitamin K_2; this has little effect unless there is concurrent dietary deficiency.

FACTORS THAT LESSEN THE EFFECT OF WARFARIN

Physiological state/disease

There is a decreased response to warfarin in conditions (e.g. pregnancy) where there is increased coagulation factor synthesis. Similarly, the effect of oral anticoagulants is lessened in hypothyroidism, which is associated with reduced degradation of coagulation factors.

Drugs (see also Ch. 10)

Several drugs reduce the effectiveness of warfarin; this leads to increased doses being used to achieve the target INR. Furthermore, the dose of warfarin must be reduced when the interacting drug is discontinued, to avoid haemorrhage.

Vitamin K. This vitamin is a component of some parenteral feeds and vitamin preparations.

Drugs that induce hepatic P450 enzymes. Enzyme induction (e.g. by **rifampicin, carbamazepine**) increases the rate of degradation of warfarin. Induction may wane only slowly after the inducing drug is discontinued, making it difficult to adjust the warfarin dose appropriately.

Drugs that reduce absorption. Drugs that bind warfarin in the gut, for example, **colestyramine**, reduce its absorption.

Drugs affecting blood coagulation

Procoagulant drugs: vitamin K
- Reduced vitamin K is a co-factor in the post-translational γ-carboxylation of glutamic acid (Glu) residues in factors II, VII, IX and X. The γ-carboxylated glutamic acid (Gla) residues are essential for the interaction of these factors with Ca^{2+} and negatively charged phospholipid.

Injectable anticoagulants (e.g. heparin, low molecular-weight heparins)
- Potentiate antithrombin III, a natural inhibitor that inactivates Xa and thrombin.
- Act both in vivo and in vitro.
- Anticoagulant activity results from a unique pentasaccharide sequence with high affinity for antithrombin III.
- **Heparin** therapy is monitored via activated partial thromboplastin time (APTT), and dose individualised. Unfractionated heparin (UFH) is used for patients with impaired renal function.
- **Low molecular-weight heparins** (LMWHs) have the same effect on factor X as heparin but less effect on thrombin; therapeutic efficacy is similar to **heparin** but monitoring and dose individualisation are not needed. Patients can administer them subcutaneously at home. They are preferred over UFH except for patients with impaired renal function.

Oral anticoagulants (e.g. warfarin, direct thrombin and Xa inhibitors)
- **Warfarin** is the main vitamin K antagonist.
- Vitamin K antagonists act on vitamin K epoxide reductase component 1 (VKORC1) to inhibit the reduction of vitamin K epoxide, thus inhibiting the γ-carboxylation of Glu in II, VII, IX and X.
- Vitamin K antagonists act only in vivo, and their effect is delayed until preformed clotting factors are depleted.
- Many factors modify the action of vitamin K antagonists; genetic factors (polymorphisms of CYP2C6 and VKORC1) and drug interactions are especially important.
- There is wide variation in response to vitamin K antagonists; their effect is monitored by measuring the international normalised ratio (INR) and the dose individualised accordingly.
- Orally active direct thrombin inhibitors (e.g. **dabigatran etexilate**) or factor Xa inhibitors (e.g. **rivaroxaban**, **apixaban**) are used increasingly and do not require laboratory monitoring/dose titration. They are licensed for preventing stroke in patients with atrial fibrillation and for preventing deep vein thrombosis after orthopaedic surgery.

or coagulation factor concentrates (for life-threatening bleeding).

Oral anticoagulants are *teratogenic*, causing disordered bone development which is believed to be related to binding to the vitamin K-dependent protein osteocalcin.

Hepatotoxicity occurs but is uncommon.

Necrosis of soft tissues (e.g. breast or buttock) owing to thrombosis in venules is a rare but serious effect that occurs shortly after starting treatment and is attributed to inhibition of biosynthesis of protein C, which has a shorter elimination half-life than do the vitamin K-dependent coagulation factors; this results in a procoagulant state soon after starting treatment. Treatment with a heparin is usually started at the same time as warfarin, avoiding this problem except in individuals experiencing HIT as an adverse effect of heparin (see p. 324).

The clinical use of anticoagulants is summarised in the box.

Clinical uses of anticoagulants

Heparin (often as **low molecular-weight heparin**) is used acutely. **Warfarin** or a direct thrombin or Xa inhibitor is used for more prolonged therapy. Anticoagulants are used to prevent:
- deep vein thrombosis (e.g. perioperatively)
- extension of established deep vein thrombosis
- pulmonary embolism
- thrombosis and embolisation in patients with atrial fibrillation (Ch. 22)
- thrombosis on prosthetic heart valves
- clotting in extracorporeal circulations (e.g. during haemodialysis)
- progression of myocardial damage in patients with unstable angina and during treatment of ST-elevation myocardial infarction

PLATELET ADHESION AND ACTIVATION

Platelets maintain the integrity of the circulation: a low platelet count results in *thrombocytopenic purpura*.[6] When platelets are activated, they undergo a sequence of reactions that are essential for haemostasis, important for the healing of damaged blood vessels, and play a part in inflammation (see Ch. 18). These reactions, several of which are redundant (in the sense that if one pathway of activation is blocked another is available) and several autocatalytic, include:

- *adhesion* following vascular damage (via von Willebrand factor bridging between subendothelial macromolecules and glycoprotein (GP) Ib receptors on the platelet surface)[7];
- *shape change* (from smooth discs to spiny spheres with protruding pseudopodia);

UNWANTED EFFECTS OF WARFARIN

Haemorrhage (especially into the bowel or the brain) is the main hazard. Depending on the urgency of the situation, treatment may consist of withholding warfarin (for minor problems), administration of vitamin K, or fresh plasma

---

[6]Purpura means a purple rash caused by multiple spontaneous bleeding points in the skin. When this is caused by reduced circulating platelets, bleeding can occur into other organs, including the gut and brain.
[7]Various platelet membrane glycoproteins act as receptors or binding sites for adhesive proteins such as von Willebrand factor or fibrinogen.

- *secretion* of the granule contents (including platelet agonists, such as ADP and 5-hydroxytryptamine, and coagulation factors and growth factors, such as platelet-derived growth factor);
- *biosynthesis of labile mediators* such as platelet-activating factor and thromboxane (TX)A$_2$ (see Ch. 18 and Fig. 25.7);
- *aggregation*, which is promoted by various agonists, including collagen, thrombin, ADP,

5-hydroxytryptamine and TXA$_2$, acting on specific receptors on the platelet surface; activation by agonists leads to expression of GPIIb/IIIa receptors that bind fibrinogen, which links adjacent platelets to form aggregates;

- *exposure of acidic phospholipid* on the platelet surface, promoting thrombin formation (and hence further platelet activation via thrombin receptors and fibrin formation via cleavage of fibrinogen; see earlier).

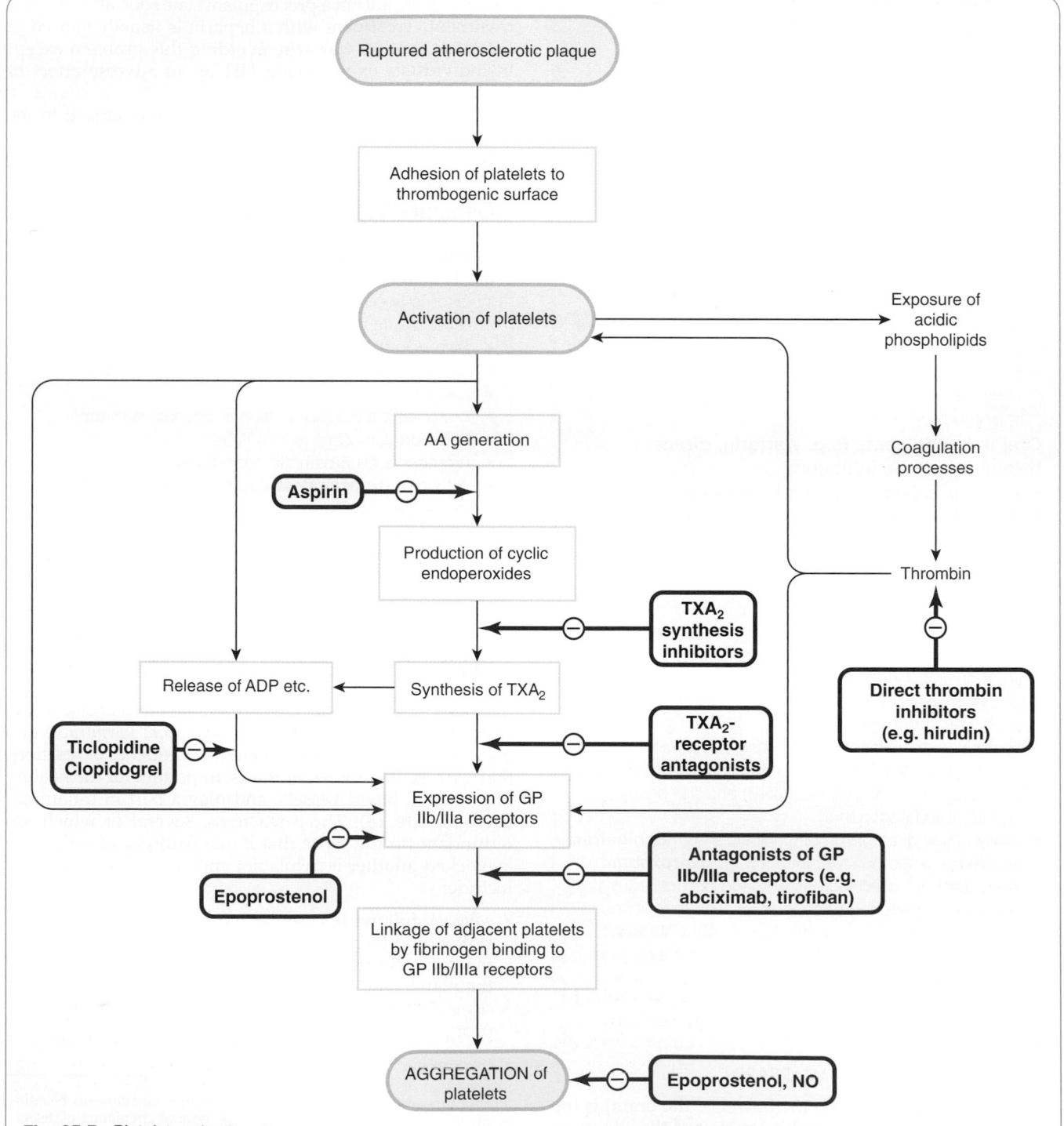

Fig. 25.7 **Platelet activation.** Events involved in platelet adhesion and aggregation are shown, with the sites of action of drugs and endogenous mediators. *AA*, arachidonic acid; *ADP*, adenosine bisphosphate; *GP*, glycoprotein; *NO*, nitric oxide; *TXA$_2$*, thromboxane A$_2$.

These processes are essential for haemostasis but may be inappropriately triggered if the artery wall is diseased, most commonly with atherosclerosis, resulting in thrombosis (see Fig. 25.7).

Platelet function

- Healthy vascular endothelium prevents platelet adhesion.
- Platelets adhere to diseased or damaged areas and become activated, changing shape and exposing negatively charged phospholipids and glycoprotein (GP) IIb/IIIa receptors, and synthesise and/or release various mediators, for example, thromboxane A_2 and ADP, which activate other platelets, causing aggregation.
- Aggregation entails fibrinogen binding to and bridging between GPIIb/IIIa receptors on adjacent platelets.
- Activated platelets constitute a focus for fibrin formation.
- Chemotactic factors and growth factors necessary for repair, but also implicated in atherogenesis, are released during platelet activation.

ANTIPLATELET DRUGS

Platelets play such a critical role in thromboembolic disease that it is no surprise that antiplatelet drugs are of great therapeutic value. Clinical trials of aspirin radically altered clinical practice, and more recently drugs that block ADP receptors and GPIIb/IIIa have also been found to be therapeutically useful. Sites of action of antiplatelet drugs are shown in Fig. 25.7.

ASPIRIN

Low-dose aspirin (see Ch. 27) in chronic use profoundly (>95%) inhibits platelet TXA_2 synthesis, by irreversible acetylation of a serine residue in the active site of cyclo-oxygenase I (COX-1). Oral administration is relatively selective for platelets partly because of presystemic drug elimination (Ch. 10). Unlike nucleated cells, platelets cannot synthesise proteins, so after administration of aspirin, TXA_2 synthesis does not recover fully until the affected cohort of platelets is replaced in 7–10 days. Clinical trials have demonstrated the efficacy of aspirin in several clinical settings (e.g. Fig. 25.8). For acute indications (progressing thrombotic stroke – so-called stroke-in-evolution – and acute myocardial infarction) treatment is started with a single dose of approximately 300 mg in order to achieve rapid substantial (>95%) inhibition of platelet thromboxane synthesis, followed by regular daily doses of 75 mg. For long-term thromboprophylaxis, a low dose (often 75 mg once daily) is used. At this dose, the risk of gastrointestinal bleeding is less than with the usual 300 mg dose given to control inflammation, but still significant, so thromboprophylaxis is reserved for people at high cardiovascular risk (e.g. survivors of myocardial infarction), in whom the benefit usually outweighs the risk of gastrointestinal bleeding.

▼ Treatment failure can occur despite taking aspirin, and there is current interest in the possibility that some patients exhibit a syndrome of 'aspirin resistance', although the mechanism and possible importance of this remains controversial (see Goodman et al., 2008). Other

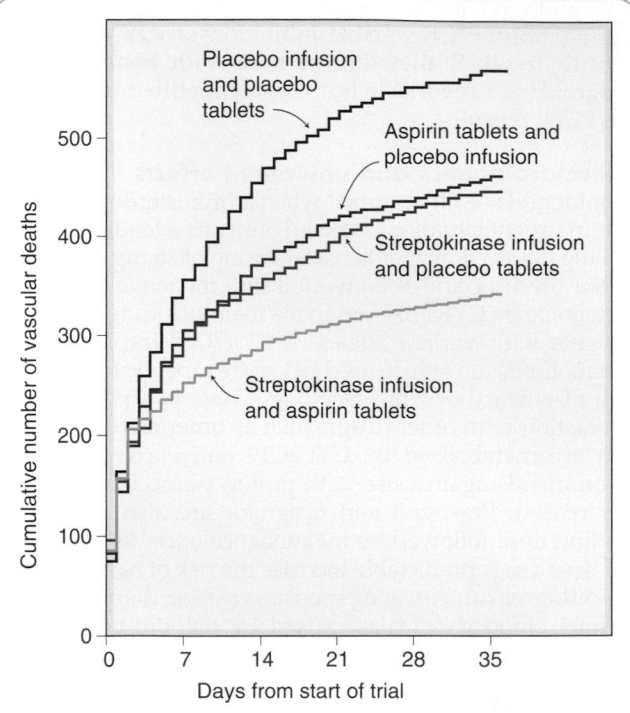

Fig. 25.8 **Efficacy of aspirin and streptokinase for myocardial infarction.** The curves show cumulative vascular mortality in patients treated with placebo, aspirin alone, streptokinase alone or a combined aspirin–streptokinase regimen. (ISIS-2 Trial, 1988. Lancet ii, 350–360.)

non-steroidal drugs that inhibit platelet TXA_2 synthesis >95% (e.g. **sulfinpyrazone**, for which there is also supportive clinical trial evidence, and **naproxen** – see Ch. 27) may have antithrombotic effects, but where inhibition of platelet TXA_2 synthesis does not reach this threshold there is evidence that such drugs are *proaggregatory*, related to inhibition of COX-2, possibly due to inhibition of antiaggregatory PGI_2 in blood vessels.

DIPYRIDAMOLE

Dipyridamole inhibits platelet aggregation by several mechanisms, including inhibition of phosphodiesterase, block of adenosine uptake into red cells (see Ch. 17) and inhibition of TXA_2 synthesis (see Ch. 27). Clinical effectiveness has been uncertain, but one study showed that a modified-release form of dipyridamole reduced the risk of stroke and death in patients with transient ischaemic attacks by around 15% – similar to aspirin (25 mg twice daily).[8] The beneficial effects of aspirin and dipyridamole were additive. The main side effects of dipyridamole are dizziness, headache and gastrointestinal disturbances; unlike aspirin, it does not increase the risk of bleeding.

ADENOSINE (P2Y$_{12}$) RECEPTOR ANTAGONISTS

Ticlopidine was the first to be introduced, but causes neutropenia and thrombocytopenia. The main agents are currently **clopidogrel**, **prasugrel** and **ticagrelor**, each of which is combined with low-dose aspirin in patients with unstable coronary artery disease, usually for up to 1 year.

---

[8]This dose regimen of aspirin is unconventional, being somewhat lower than the 75 mg once daily commonly used in thromboprophylaxis.

Clopidogrel and prasugrel inhibit ADP-induced platelet aggregation by irreversible inhibition of $P2Y_{12}$ receptors (Ch. 17) to which they link via a disulfide bond, whereas ticagrelor is a reversible but non-competitive inhibitor of the $P2Y_{12}$ receptor.

Pharmacokinetics and unwanted effects
Clopidogrel is well absorbed when administered by mouth, and in urgent situations is given orally as a loading dose of 300 mg followed by maintenance dosing of 75 mg once daily. It is a prodrug and is converted into its active sulfhydryl metabolite by CYP enzymes in the liver including CYP2C19. Patients with variant alleles of *CYP2C19* (rapid or poor metabolisers) are at increased risk of therapeutic failure from lack of efficacy or from bleeding. There is a potential for interaction with other drugs, such as **omeprazole** (Ch. 31), that are metabolised by CYP2C19 and current labelling recommends against use with proton pump inhibitors for this reason. Prasugrel and ticagrelor are also given as a loading dose followed by maintenance once daily dosing.

These drugs predictably increase the risk of haemorrhage. Clopidogrel can cause dyspepsia, rash or diarrhoea. The serious blood dyscrasias caused by ticlopidine are very rare with clopidogrel. Prasugrel can cause rash or, rarely hypersensitivity reactions and angioedema. Ticagrelor can cause dyspnoea (perhaps related to the role of adenosine signalling in the carotid bodies, Ch. 29) or, less commonly, gastrointestinal symptoms.

Clinical use
Clopidogrel was slightly more effective than aspirin as a single agent in reducing a composite outcome of ischaemic stroke, myocardial infarction or vascular death in one large trial; it can be used instead of aspirin in patients with symptomatic atheromatous disease, but is usually reserved for patients who are intolerant of aspirin. Clinical trials of adding clopidogrel to aspirin in patients with acute coronary syndromes (Fig. 25.9) and (in a megatrial of over 45,000 patients) in patients with acute myocardial infarction (COMMIT Collaborative Group, 2005) demonstrated that combined treatment reduces mortality. Treatment with clopidogrel for this indication is given for 4 weeks. Prasugrel

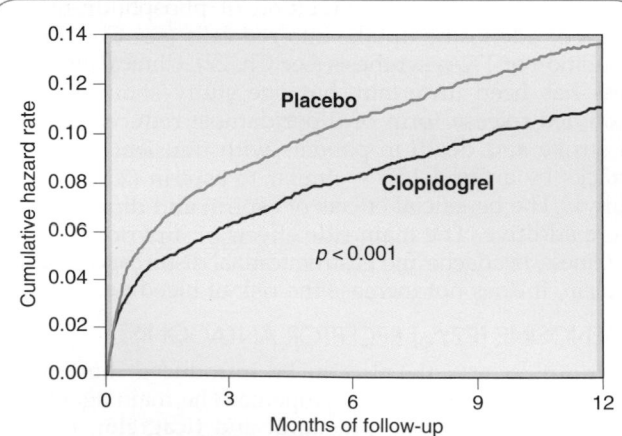

Fig. 25.9 Effect of adding clopidogrel to aspirin. The curves show cumulative hazard rates for major vascular events in patients with acute coronary syndromes treated either with placebo + aspirin or clopidogrel + aspirin. (Modified from CURE Investigators, 2001. N Engl J Med 345, 494–502.)

is more effective than clopidogrel in acute coronary syndromes, but more often causes serious bleeding. Pretreatment with clopidogrel and aspirin followed by longer-term therapy is also effective in patients with ischaemic heart disease undergoing percutaneous coronary interventions. Treatment of acute coronary syndrome with ticagrelor as compared with clopidogrel significantly reduces mortality for unknown reasons.

GLYCOPROTEIN IIB/IIIA RECEPTOR ANTAGONISTS
Antagonists of the GPIIb/IIIa receptor have the theoretical attraction that they inhibit all pathways of platelet activation (because these all converge on activation of GPIIb/IIIa receptors). A hybrid murine–human monoclonal antibody Fab fragment directed against the GPIIb/IIIa receptor, which rejoices in the catchy little name of **abciximab**,[9] is licensed for use in high-risk patients undergoing coronary angioplasty, as an adjunct to heparin and aspirin. It reduces the risk of restenosis at the expense of an increased risk of bleeding. Immunogenicity limits its use to a single administration.

Tirofiban is a synthetic non-peptide and **eptifibatide** is a cyclic peptide based on the Arg–Gly–Asp ('RGD') sequence that is common to ligands for GPIIb/IIIa receptors. Neither is absorbed if administered by mouth. Given intravenously as an adjunct to aspirin and a heparin preparation, they reduce early events in acute coronary syndrome, but long-term oral therapy with GPIIb/IIIa receptor antagonists is not effective and may be harmful. Unsurprisingly, they increase the risk of bleeding.

OTHER ANTIPLATELET DRUGS
Epoprostenol (PGI_2), an agonist at prostanoid IP receptors (see Ch. 18), causes vasodilatation as well as inhibiting platelet aggregation. It is added to blood entering the dialysis circuit in order to prevent thrombosis during haemodialysis, especially in patients in whom heparin is contraindicated. It is also used in severe pulmonary hypertension (Ch. 23) and circulatory shock associated with meningococcal septicaemia. It is unstable under physiological conditions and has a half-life of around 3 min, so it is administered as an intravenous infusion. Adverse effects related to its vasodilator action include flushing, headache and hypotension.

The clinical use of antiplatelet drugs is summarised in the clinical box (p. 331).

FIBRINOLYSIS (THROMBOLYSIS)
When the coagulation system is activated, the fibrinolytic system is also set in motion via several endogenous *plasminogen activators*, including tissue plasminogen activator (tPA), urokinase-type plasminogen activator, kallikrein and neutrophil elastase. tPA is inhibited by a structurally related lipoprotein, *lipoprotein(a)*, increased concentrations of which constitute an independent risk factor for myocardial infarction (Ch. 24). Plasminogen is deposited on the fibrin strands within a thrombus. Plasminogen activators are serine proteases and are unstable in circulating blood. They diffuse into thrombus and cleave plasminogen, a zymogen present

[9]The convention for naming monoclonals is: momab = **-mouse m**onoclonal **a**ntibody; -umab = human; -zumab = humanised; -ximab = chimeric – a kind of medieval mouse–man nightmare.

Antiplatelet drugs

- **Aspirin** inhibits cyclo-oxygenase irreversibly. In chronic use, low doses very effectively (>95%) inhibit platelet thromboxane (TX)A$_2$ synthesis and reduce the risk of thrombosis. Treatment is started with a larger dose (300 mg) in acute settings in order to achieve rapid inhibition of platelet thromboxane synthesis.[10]
- ADP antagonists are combined with low-dose aspirin in treating patients with unstable coronary artery disease. **Clopidogrel** is a prodrug. Given by mouth, it irreversibly inhibits P2Y$_{12}$ receptors and thereby inhibits platelet responses to ADP. Its clinical effect is additive with **aspirin**. **Prasugrel** has a similar mechanism. **Ticagrelor** is reversible but non-competitive. **Prasugrel** and **ticagrelor** are more effective than licensed doses of **clopidogrel**.
- Antagonists of GPIIb/IIIa receptors include a monoclonal antibody (**abciximab**) and several synthetic molecules (e.g. **tirofiban**). They inhibit diverse agonists, for example, ADP and TXA$_2$, because different pathways of activation converge on GPIIb/IIIa receptors. They are administered intravenously for short-term treatment.
- **Dipyridamole** inhibits phosphodiesterase and adenosine uptake. It is used in addition to aspirin in some patients with stroke or transient ischaemic attack.
- **Epoprostenol** (synthetic PGI$_2$) is chemically unstable. Given as an intravenous infusion, it acts on I prostanoid (IP) receptors on vascular smooth muscle and platelets (Ch. 18), stimulating adenylyl cyclase and thereby causing vasodilatation and inhibiting aggregation caused by any pathway (e.g. ADP or TXA$_2$).

Clinical uses of antiplatelet drugs

The main drug is **aspirin**. Other drugs with distinct actions (e.g. **dipyridamole**, **clopidogrel**, **ticagrelor**) can have additive effects, or be used in patients who are intolerant of **aspirin**. Uses of antiplatelet drugs relate mainly to arterial thrombosis and include:

- *acute myocardial infarction*
- prevention of myocardial infarction in patients at high risk, including a history of *myocardial infarction*, *angina* or *intermittent claudication* (see Ch. 23)
- following *coronary artery bypass grafting*
- *unstable coronary syndromes* (a P2Y12 antagonist such as **clopidogrel, prasugrel** or **ticagrelor** is added to **aspirin**)
- following coronary artery *angioplasty* and/or *stenting* (intravenous glycoprotein IIb/IIIa antagonists, e.g. **abciximab**, are used in some patients in addition to **aspirin**)
- *transient cerebral ischaemic attack* ('ministrokes') or *thrombotic stroke*, to prevent recurrence (**dipyridamole** can be added to **aspirin**)
- *atrial fibrillation*, if oral anticoagulation is contraindicated; or, by specialists, in high-risk situations in combination with anticoagulant Other antiplatelet drugs such as **epoprostenol** (PGI$_2$; see Ch. 18) have specialised clinical applications (e.g. in *haemodialysis* or *haemofiltration*, Ch. 29, or in *pulmonary hypertension*, Ch. 23).

in plasma, to release plasmin locally (Fig. 25.10). Plasmin is a trypsin-like protease that digests fibrin as well as fibrinogen, factors II, V and VIII, and many other proteins; any that escapes into the circulation is inactivated by plasmin inhibitors, including PAI-1 (see p. 321 and Ch. 23), which protect us from digesting ourselves from within.

Drugs affect this system by increasing or inhibiting fibrinolysis (*fibrinolytic* and *antifibrinolytic* drugs, respectively).

FIBRINOLYTIC DRUGS

Fig. 25.10 summarises the interaction of the fibrinolytic system with the coagulation cascade and platelet activation, and the action of drugs that modify this. Several fibrinolytic (thrombolytic) drugs are used clinically, principally to reopen the occluded arteries in patients with acute myocardial infarction[11] or stroke, less commonly in patients with life-threatening venous thrombosis or pulmonary embolism.

Streptokinase is a plasminogen activating protein extracted from cultures of streptococci. Infused intravenously, it reduces mortality in acute myocardial infarction, and this beneficial effect is additive with aspirin (see Fig. 25.8).

Its action is blocked by antibodies, which appear 4 days or more after the initial dose: its use should not be repeated after this time has elapsed.[12]

Alteplase and **duteplase** are, respectively, single- and double-chain recombinant tPA. They are more active on fibrin-bound plasminogen than on plasma plasminogen, and are therefore said to be 'clot selective'. Recombinant tPA is not antigenic, and can be used in patients likely to have antibodies to streptokinase. Because of their short half-lives, they must be given as intravenous infusions. **Reteplase** is similar but has a longer elimination half-life, allowing for bolus administration and making for simplicity of administration. It is available for clinical use in myocardial infarction.

UNWANTED EFFECTS AND CONTRAINDICATIONS

The main hazard of all fibrinolytic agents is bleeding, including gastrointestinal haemorrhage and haemorrhagic stroke. If serious, this can be treated with **tranexamic acid** (see p. 333), fresh plasma or coagulation factors. Streptokinase can cause allergic reactions and low-grade

[10]Its antithrombotic actions is the main reason for the saying 'An aspirin a day keeps the doctor away', although aspirin has also been found to have anti-cancer properties, particularly when it comes to colon cancer. If you're one of the unlucky individuals who is allergic to aspirin, please ignore the previous sentence.

[11]Fibrinolytic drugs are now less widely used in acute myocardial infarction since many units throughout the world provide an emergency angioplasty service (the blocked artery is identified angiographically, opened with a balloon catheter and, if necessary, kept open by means of a stent, Ch. 22). The important thing is to open up the thrombosed artery as swiftly as possible. If facilities are available to do this mechanically, this is at least as good as using a lytic drug. Surgical intra-arterial thrombectomy is also being introduced for acute stroke treatment.
[12]A once in a lifetime drug!

Fig. 25.10 **Fibrinolytic system.** The schematic shows interactions with coagulation and platelet pathways and sites of action of drugs that modify these systems. *LMWHs,* low molecular-weight heparins. For more details of platelet activation and the coagulation cascade, refer to Figs 25.1, 25.2 and 25.7.

fever. Streptokinase causes a burst of plasmin formation, generating kinins (see Ch. 18), and can cause hypotension by this mechanism.

Contraindications to the use of these agents are active internal bleeding, haemorrhagic cerebrovascular disease, bleeding diatheses, pregnancy, uncontrolled hypertension, invasive procedures in which haemostasis is important, and recent trauma – including vigorous cardiopulmonary resuscitation.

CLINICAL USE

Several large placebo-controlled studies in patients with myocardial infarction have shown convincingly that fibrinolytic drugs reduce mortality if given within 12 h of the onset of symptoms, and that the sooner they are administered the better is the result. Similar considerations apply to their use in thrombotic stroke. Scanning to exclude haemorrhagic stroke is advisable, though not always practicable in an emergency situation. Available fibrinolytic drugs, used in combination with aspirin, provide similar levels of benefit, generally less than that obtained by

mechanical (mainly angioplasty) unblocking procedures. Other uses of fibrinolytic agents are listed in the clinical box.

Fibrinolysis and drugs modifying fibrinolysis

- A fibrinolytic cascade is initiated concomitantly with the coagulation cascade, resulting in the formation within the coagulum of plasmin, which digests fibrin.
- Various agents promote the formation of plasmin from its precursor plasminogen, for example **streptokinase**, and tissue plasminogen activators (tPAs) such as **alteplase, duteplase** and **reteplase**. Most are infused; reteplase can be given as a bolus injection.
- Some drugs (e.g. **tranexamic acid**) inhibit fibrinolysis.

Clinical uses of fibrinolytic drugs

The main drugs are **streptokinase** and tissue plasminogen activators (tPAs), for example **alteplase**.

- The main use is in acute myocardial infarction, within 12 h of onset (the earlier the better!).
- Other uses include:
  - *acute thrombotic stroke* within 3 h of onset (tPA), in selected patients
  - clearing *thrombosed shunts* and *cannulae*
  - *acute arterial thromboembolism*
  - life-threatening *deep vein thrombosis* and *pulmonary embolism* (streptokinase, given promptly)

ANTIFIBRINOLYTIC AND HAEMOSTATIC DRUGS

Tranexamic acid inhibits plasminogen activation and thus prevents fibrinolysis. It can be given orally or by intravenous injection. It is used to treat various conditions in which there is bleeding or risk of bleeding, such as haemorrhage following prostatectomy or dental extraction, in menorrhagia (excessive menstrual blood loss) and for life-threatening bleeding following thrombolytic drug administration. It is also used in patients with the rare disorder of hereditary angio-oedema.

REFERENCES AND FURTHER READING

Blood coagulation and anticoagulants

Bah, A., Carrell, C.J., Chen, Z.W., et al., 2009. Stabilization of the E* form turns thrombin into an anticoagulant. J. Biol. Chem. 284, 20034–20040. (*The anticoagulant profile caused by a mutation of the thrombin gene is due to stabilisation of the inactive E* form of thrombin that is selectively shifted to the active E form upon thrombomodulin and protein C binding*)

Hirsh, J., O'Donnell, M., Weitz, J.I., 2005. New anticoagulants. Blood 105, 453–463. (*Review article on limitations of existing anticoagulants, vitamin K antagonist and heparins that have led to the development of newer anticoagulant therapies*)

Koenig-Oberhuber, M.F., 2016. New antiplatelet drugs and new oral anticoagulants V. Br. J. Anaesth. 117 (Suppl. 2), ii74–ii84.

Martin, F.A., Murphy, R.P., Cummins, P.M., 2013. Thrombomodulin and the vascular endothelium: insights into functional, regulatory, and therapeutic aspects. Am. J. Physiol. Heart Circ. Physiol. 304 (12), H1585–H1597.

Shearer, M.J., Newman, P., 2008. Metabolism and cell biology of vitamin K. Thromb. Haemost. 100, 530–547. (*Review*)

Endothelium, platelets and antiplatelet agents

Chew, D.P., Bhatt, D., Sapp, S., et al., 2001. Increased mortality with oral platelet glycoprotein IIb/IIIa antagonists: a meta-analysis of phase III multicenter trials. Circulation 103, 201–206.

COMMIT Collaborative Group, 2005. Addition of clopidogrel to aspirin in 45 852 patients with acute myocardial infarction: randomised placebo-controlled trial. Lancet 366, 1607–1621. (*Clopidogrel reduced the risk of death, myocardial infarction or stroke combined, and of mortality alone; see accompanying comment by Sabatine, M.S., pp. 1587–1589 in the same issue*)

Goodman, T., Ferro, A., Sharma, P., 2008. Pharmacogenetics of aspirin resistance: a comprehensive systematic review. Br. J. Clin. Pharmacol. 66, 222–232. (*Supports a genetic association between the PlA1/A2 molecular variant and aspirin resistance in healthy subjects, with the effect diminishing in the presence of cardiovascular disease*)

Patrono, C., Coller, B., FitzGerald, G.A., et al., 2004. Platelet-active drugs: the relationships among dose, effectiveness, and side effects. Chest 126, 234S–264S.

Wallentin, L., Becker, R.C., Budaj, A., et al., 2009. Ticagrelor versus clopidogrel in patients with acute coronary syndromes. N. Engl. J. Med. 361, 1045–1057.

Wiviott, S.D., Braunwald, E., McCabe, C.H., et al., 2007. For the TRITON-TIMI 38 Investigators. Prasugrel versus clopidogrel in patients with acute coronary syndromes. N. Engl. J. Med. 357, 2001–2015. (*Prasugrel reduced ischaemic events, including stent thrombosis, but with an increased risk of major bleeding, including fatal bleeding. Overall mortality did not differ significantly between treatment groups*)

Clinical and general aspects

Aster, R.H., 1995. Heparin-induced thrombocytopenia and thrombosis. N. Engl. J. Med. 332, 1374–1376. (*Succinct and lucid editorial; see also accompanying paper, pp. 1330–1335*)

Diener, H., Cunha, L., Forbes, C., et al., 1996. European Stroke Prevention Study 2. Dipyridamole and acetylsalicylic acid in the secondary prevention of stroke. J. Neurol. Sci. 143, 1–14. (*Slow-release dipyridamole 200 mg twice daily was as effective as aspirin 25 mg twice daily, and the effects of aspirin and dipyridamole were additive*)

Goldhaber, S.Z., 2004. Pulmonary embolism. Lancet 363, 1295–1305.

Kyrle, P.A., Eichinger, S., 2005. Deep vein thrombosis. Lancet 365, 1163–1174.

Levine, M., 1995. A comparison of low-molecular-weight heparin administered primarily at home with unfractionated heparin administered in the hospital for proximal deep vein thrombosis. N. Engl. J. Med. 334, 677–681. (*Concludes that LMWH can be used safely and effectively at home; this has potentially very important implications for patient care*)

Markus, H.S., 2005. Current treatments in neurology: stroke. J. Neurol. 252, 260–267.

26 Haematopoietic system and treatment of anaemia

OVERVIEW

This chapter summarises the different kinds of anaemia, caused by nutrient deficiencies, bone marrow depression or increased red cell destruction, and covers the main haematinic agents used to treat them. We describe haematopoietic growth factors for red and white blood cells, and conclude by mentioning two drugs (hydroxycarbamide and eculizumab) used in treating, respectively, sickle cell anaemia and paroxysmal nocturnal haemoglobinuria.

INTRODUCTION

In this chapter, we briefly review the haematopoietic system and different types of anaemia due to blood loss, deficiency of nutrients, depression of the bone marrow or increased destruction of red cells (haemolytic anaemias). Nutritional deficiencies of *iron*, *vitamin B$_{12}$* or *folic acid* are common and important, and most of the chapter is devoted to these haematinic agents (i.e. nutrients needed for healthy haematopoiesis, and related drugs). Treatment of many forms of bone marrow depression is mainly supportive, but *haematopoietic growth factors* (especially *epoietins* – preparations of the natural hormone erythropoietin) have a place, especially in patients with chronic renal failure, and are covered briefly, as are other haematopoietic factors, known as *colony-stimulating factors* (CSFs), which are used to increase numbers of circulating white blood cells. Treatment of haemolytic anaemias is again mainly supportive, but we mention two drugs (**hydroxycarbamide** and **eculizumab**) that provide mechanistic insights as well as clinical benefit in two specific haemolytic disorders.

THE HAEMATOPOIETIC SYSTEM

The main components of the haematopoietic system are the blood, bone marrow, lymph nodes and thymus, with the spleen, liver and kidneys as important accessory organs. Blood consists of formed elements (red and white blood cells and platelets) and plasma. This chapter deals mainly with red cells, which have the principal function of carrying oxygen. Their oxygen-carrying power depends on their haemoglobin content. The most important site of formation of red blood cells in adults is the bone marrow, whereas the spleen acts as their slaughterhouse. The lifetime of a red cell is normally about 120 days, and red cell loss in healthy adults – about 2×10^{10} cells per day – is precisely balanced by production of new cells. The liver stores vitamin B$_{12}$ and is involved in the process of breakdown of the haemoglobin liberated when red blood cells are destroyed. The kidney manufactures *erythropoietin*, a hormone that stimulates red cell production and is used in the anaemia of chronic kidney disease (Ch. 30) as well as (notoriously)

in competitive sport (Ch. 59). CSFs regulate the production of leukocytes and are also used therapeutically (e.g. in the supportive management of patients with haematological malignancies undergoing chemotherapy, Ch. 57). *Thrombopoietin*, produced by the liver and kidneys, stimulates platelet formation; attempts to develop it for therapeutic use are a cautionary tale, which is mentioned briefly later. Drugs used to treat leukaemias, malignant disorders of white blood cell precursors, are described in Chapter 57.

TYPES OF ANAEMIA

Anaemia is characterised by a reduced haemoglobin content in the blood. It may cause fatigue but, especially if it is chronic, is often surprisingly asymptomatic. The commonest cause is blood loss resulting from menstruation, drug treatment (e.g. with **aspirin** or other non-steroidal anti-inflammatory drugs; Ch. 27) or pathological processes such as colonic carcinoma or (especially in developing countries) parasitic infestation (Ch. 56). Pregnancy and child-bearing are important physiological drains on iron reserves. There are several different types of anaemia based on indices of red cell size and haemoglobin content and microscopical examination of a stained blood smear:

- *hypochromic, microcytic anaemia* (small red cells with low haemoglobin; caused by chronic blood loss giving rise to iron deficiency)
- *macrocytic anaemia* (large red cells, few in number)
- *normochromic normocytic anaemia* (fewer normal-sized red cells, each with a normal haemoglobin content)
- mixed pictures

Further evaluation may include determination of concentrations of ferritin, iron, vitamin B$_{12}$ and folic acid in serum, and microscopic examination of smears of bone marrow. This leads to more precise diagnostic groupings of anaemias into:

- Deficiency of nutrients necessary for haematopoiesis, most importantly:
  - iron
  - folic acid and vitamin B$_{12}$
  - pyridoxine and vitamin C
- Depression of the bone marrow, commonly caused by:
  - drug toxicity (e.g. anticancer drugs, **clozapine**)
  - exposure to radiation, including radiotherapy
  - diseases of the bone marrow (e.g. idiopathic aplastic anaemia, leukaemias)
  - reduced production of, or responsiveness to, erythropoietin (e.g. chronic renal failure, rheumatoid arthritis, AIDS)
- Excessive destruction of red blood cells (i.e. haemolytic anaemia); this has many causes, including *haemoglobinopathies* (such as sickle cell anaemia), adverse reactions to drugs and immune reactions that have gone awry.

HAEMATINIC AGENTS

The use of haematinic agents is often only an adjunct to treatment of the underlying cause of the anaemia – for example, surgery for colon cancer (a common cause of iron deficiency) or antihelminthic drugs for patients with hookworm (a frequent cause of anaemia in parts of Africa and Asia; Ch. 56). Sometimes treatment consists of stopping an offending drug, for example a non-steroidal anti-inflammatory drug that is causing blood loss from the gastrointestinal tract (Ch. 27).

IRON

Iron is a transition metal with two important properties relevant to its biological role, namely its ability to exist in several oxidation states and to form stable coordination complexes.

The body of a 70-kg man contains about 4 g of iron, 65% of which circulates in the blood as haemoglobin. About one-half of the remainder is stored in the liver, spleen and bone marrow, chiefly as *ferritin* and *haemosiderin*. The iron in these molecules is available for haemoglobin synthesis. The rest, which is not available for haemoglobin synthesis, is present in myoglobin, cytochromes and various enzymes.

The distribution and turnover of iron in an average adult man are shown in Table 26.1 and Fig. 26.1. The corresponding values in a woman are approximately 45% less. Because most of the iron in the body is either part of – or destined to be part of – haemoglobin, the most obvious clinical result of iron deficiency is anaemia, and the only indication for therapy with iron is for treatment or prophylaxis of iron deficiency anaemia.

Haemoglobin is made up of four protein chain subunits (globins), each of which contains one haem moiety. Haem consists of a tetrapyrrole porphyrin ring containing ferrous (Fe^{2+}) iron. Each haem group can carry one oxygen molecule, which is bound reversibly to Fe^{2+} and to a histidine residue in the globin chain. This reversible binding is the basis of oxygen transport.

Table 26.1 The distribution of iron in the body of a healthy 70-kg man

Protein	Tissue	Iron content (mg)
Haemoglobin	Erythrocytes	2600
Myoglobin	Muscle	400
Enzymes (cytochromes, catalase, guanylyl cyclase, etc.)	Liver and other tissues	25
Transferrin	Plasma and extracellular fluid	8
Ferritin and haemosiderin	Liver	410
	Spleen	48
	Bone marrow	300

(Data from Jacobs, A., Worwood, M., 1982. Chapter 5. In: Hardisty, R.M., Weatherall, D.J. (Eds). Blood and Its Disorders. Blackwell Scientific, Oxford.)

IRON TURNOVER AND BALANCE

The normal daily requirement for iron is approximately 5 mg for men, and 15 mg for growing children and for menstruating women. A pregnant woman needs between 2 and 10 times this amount because of the demands of the fetus and increased requirements of the mother.[1] The average diet in Western Europe provides 15–20 mg of iron daily, mostly in meat. Iron in meat is generally present as haem, and about 20%–40% of haem iron is available for absorption.

▼ Humans are adapted to absorb haem iron. It is thought that one reason why modern humans have problems in maintaining iron balance (there are an estimated 500 million people with iron deficiency in the world) is that the change from hunting to grain cultivation 10,000 years ago led to cereals, which contain little utilisable iron, replacing meat in the diet. Non-haem iron in food is mainly in the ferric state, and this needs to be converted to ferrous iron for absorption. Iron salts have low solubility at the neutral pH of the small intestine; however, in the stomach, iron dissolves and binds to a mucoprotein carrier. In the presence of ascorbic acid, fructose and various amino acids, iron is detached from the carrier, forming soluble low molecular-weight complexes that enable it to remain in soluble form in the intestine. Ascorbic acid stimulates iron absorption partly by forming soluble iron–ascorbate chelates and partly by reducing ferric iron to the more soluble ferrous form. **Tetracycline** forms an insoluble iron chelate, impairing absorption of both substances.

The amount of iron in the diet and the various factors affecting its availability are thus important determinants in absorption, but the regulation of iron absorption is a function of the intestinal mucosa, influenced by the body's iron stores. Because there is no mechanism whereby iron excretion is regulated, the absorptive mechanism has a central role in iron balance as it is the sole mechanism by which body iron is controlled.

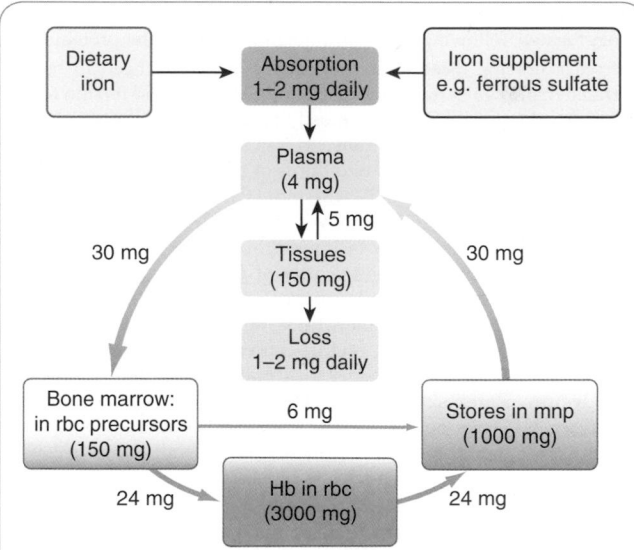

Fig. 26.1 Distribution and turnover of iron in the body. The quantities by the arrows indicate the usual amounts transferred each day. The transfer of 6 mg from red cell precursors to phagocytes represents aborted cells that fail to develop into functional red blood cells. *Hb*, haemoglobin; *mnp*, mononuclear phagocytes (mainly in liver, spleen and bone marrow); *rbc*, red blood cells.

[1]Each pregnancy 'costs' the mother 680 mg of iron, equivalent to 1300 mL of blood, owing to the demands of the fetus, plus requirements of the expanded blood volume and blood loss at delivery.

Iron absorption takes place in the duodenum and upper jejunum, and is a two-stage process involving uptake across the brush border into the mucosal cells, followed by transfer into the plasma. The second stage, which is rate limiting, is energy dependent. Haem iron in the diet is absorbed as intact haem, and the iron is released in the mucosal cell by the action of haem oxidase. Non-haem iron is absorbed in the ferrous state. Within the cell, ferrous iron is oxidised to ferric iron, which is bound to an intracellular carrier, a transferrin-like protein; the iron is then either held in storage in the mucosal cell as *ferritin* (if body stores of iron are high) or passed on to the plasma (if iron stores are low).

▼ Iron is carried in the plasma bound to *transferrin*, a β-globulin with two binding sites for ferric iron. The binding sites are normally only approximately 30% saturated. Plasma contains 4 mg of iron at any one time, but the daily turnover is about 30 mg (see Fig. 26.1). Most of the iron that enters the plasma is derived from mononuclear phagocytes, following the degradation of time-expired erythrocytes. Intestinal absorption and mobilisation of iron from storage depots contribute only small amounts. Most of the iron that leaves the plasma each day is used for haemoglobin synthesis by red cell precursors (erythroblasts). These have receptors that bind transferrin, releasing it again when its cargo of iron has been captured.

Iron is stored in two forms: soluble ferritin and insoluble *haemosiderin*. Ferritin is present in all cells, the mononuclear phagocytes of liver, spleen and bone marrow containing especially high concentrations. It is also present in plasma. The precursor of ferritin, *apoferritin*, is a protein of molecular weight 450,000, composed of 24 identical polypeptide subunits that enclose a cavity in which up to 4500 iron atoms can be stored. Apoferritin takes up ferrous iron, oxidises it and deposits the ferric iron in its core. In this form, it constitutes ferritin, the primary storage form of iron, from which the iron is most readily available. The lifespan of this iron-laden protein is only a few days. Haemosiderin is a degraded form of ferritin in which the iron cores of several ferritin molecules have aggregated, following partial disintegration of the outer protein shells.

Iron is not the most soluble of metals, hence its need to bind to transferrin (whilst transferring around the body) and ferritin for use inside cells (ferritin is found mostly inside cells but can exist in the plasma too, functioning to transport iron into cells). Ferritin in plasma contains very little iron, as two-thirds of the body's iron deposits are found within red blood cells, with more ferritin in the body than free unbound iron. The slow turnover of iron absorbed from the diet, transferred around the body by transferrin, then held in cellular storage by ferritin, means that the majority of total useful iron is held in erythrocytes, and their rapid turnover is the main source of liberated iron. Iron bound to plasma ferritin is, however, in equilibrium with the storage ferritin in cells, and its concentration in plasma (normal range 40–100 ng/mL) provides a clinically useful indicator of total body iron stores since values below 40 ng/mL signal mild iron deficiency despite normal haemoglobin, red cell morphology, serum iron concentration and transferrin saturation, with values below 20 and 10 ng/mL signalling moderate and severe anaemia, respectively.

The body has no means of actively excreting iron. Small amounts leave the body through shedding of mucosal cells containing ferritin, and even smaller amounts leave in the bile, sweat and urine. A total of about 1 mg is lost daily. Iron balance is therefore critically dependent on the active absorption mechanism in the intestinal mucosa. This absorption is influenced by the iron stores in the body, but the precise mechanism of this control is uncertain. Iron balance is summarised in Fig. 26.1. Since red cells contain approximately 0.6 mg iron per mL of blood, loss of only a few millilitres of blood per day substantially increases dietary iron requirement.

ADMINISTRATION OF IRON

Iron is usually given orally, e.g. as **ferrous sulfate**. Other salts for oral administration are **ferrous succinate**, **gluconate** or **fumarate**.

Parenteral (outside the alimentary canal) administration of iron (e.g. **iron-dextran**, **iron-sucrose**) may be necessary in individuals who are not able to absorb oral iron because of malabsorption syndromes, or as a result of surgical procedures or inflammatory conditions involving the gastrointestinal tract. It is also used for patients who do not tolerate oral preparations, and patients with chronic renal failure or with chemotherapy-induced anaemia who are receiving treatment with erythropoietin (see pp. 339–341). Iron-dextran can be given by deep intramuscular injection or slow intravenous infusion; iron-sucrose is given by slow intravenous infusion. A small initial dose is given because of the risk of anaphylactoid reaction.

Unwanted effects

The unwanted effects of oral iron administration are dose-related and include nausea, abdominal cramps and diarrhoea. Parenteral iron can cause anaphylactoid reactions (Ch. 58). Iron is an important nutrient for several pathogens and there is concern that excessive iron could worsen the clinical course of infection. Iron treatment is usually avoided during infection for this reason.

Acute iron toxicity, usually seen in young children who have swallowed attractively coloured iron tablets in mistake for sweets, can result in severe necrotising gastritis with vomiting, haemorrhage and diarrhoea, followed by circulatory collapse.

Clinical uses of iron salts

To treat iron deficiency anaemia, which can be caused by:
- *chronic blood loss* (e.g. with menorrhagia, hookworm, colon cancer);
- *increased demand* (e.g. in pregnancy and early infancy);
- *inadequate dietary intake* (uncommon in developed countries);
- *inadequate absorption* (e.g. following gastrectomy, or in diseases such as coeliac disease, where the intestinal mucosa is damaged by an immunologically based intolerance to the wheat protein gluten).

Iron overload

Chronic iron toxicity or iron overload occurs in chronic haemolytic anaemias requiring frequent blood transfusions, such as the *thalassaemias* (a large group of genetic disorders of globin chain synthesis) and *haemochromatosis* (a genetic iron storage disease with increased iron absorption, resulting in damage to liver, islets of Langerhans, joints and skin).[2]

The treatment of acute and chronic iron toxicity involves the use of iron chelators such as **desferrioxamine**. These drugs form a complex with ferric iron which, unlike unbound iron, is excreted in the urine. Desferrioxamine is not absorbed from the gut. For treating chronic iron overload (e.g. in thalassaemia), it must be given by slow subcutaneous infusion several times a week. For acute iron overdose, it

---

[2]'Bronze diabetes' – where chronic iron overload is treated by repeated bleeding, one of the few modern uses of this once near-universal 'remedy'; polycythaemia vera (caused by mutations in erythroid progenitors that increase their proliferation) is another.

is given intramuscularly or intravenously (as well as intragastrically to sequester unabsorbed iron). **Deferiprone** is an orally absorbed iron chelator, used as an alternative treatment for iron overload in patients with thalassaemia major who are unable to take desferrioxamine. Agranulocytosis and other blood dyscrasias are serious potential adverse effects. **Deferasirox** is similar, but can cause gastrointestinal bleeding.

Iron

- Iron is important for the synthesis of haemoglobin, myoglobin, cytochromes and other enzymes.
- Ferric iron (Fe^3+) must be converted to ferrous iron (Fe^2+) for absorption in the gastrointestinal tract.
- Absorption involves active transport into mucosal cells in the duodenum and jejunum (the upper ileum), from where it can be transported into the plasma and/or stored intracellularly as ferritin.
- Total body iron is controlled exclusively by absorption; in iron deficiency, more is transported into plasma than is stored as ferritin in jejunal mucosa.
- Iron loss occurs mainly by sloughing of ferritin-containing mucosal cells.
- Iron in plasma is bound to transferrin, and most is used for erythropoiesis. Some is stored as ferritin in other tissues. Iron from time-expired erythrocytes enters the plasma for reuse.
- The main therapeutic preparation is **ferrous sulfate**; **iron-sucrose** can be given as an intravenous infusion.
- Unwanted effects include gastrointestinal disturbances. Severe toxic effects occur if large doses are ingested; such acute poisoning can be treated with **desferrioxamine**, an iron chelator, as can chronic iron overload in diseases such as thalassaemia.

FOLIC ACID AND VITAMIN B$_{12}$

Vitamin B$_{12}$ and folic acid are essential constituents of the human diet, being necessary for DNA synthesis and consequently for cell proliferation. Their biochemical actions are interdependent (see key point box, p. 339), and treatment with folic acid corrects some, but not all, of the features of vitamin B$_{12}$ deficiency. Deficiency of either vitamin B$_{12}$ or folic acid affects tissues with a rapid cell turnover, particularly bone marrow, but vitamin B$_{12}$ deficiency also causes important neuronal disorders, which are not corrected (or may even be made worse) by treatment with folic acid. Deficiency of either vitamin causes *megaloblastic haematopoiesis*, in which there is disordered erythroblast differentiation and defective erythropoiesis in the bone marrow. Large abnormal erythrocyte precursors appear in the marrow, each with a high RNA:DNA ratio as a result of decreased DNA synthesis. The circulating abnormal erythrocytes ('macrocytes' – i.e. large red blood cells) are large fragile cells, often distorted in shape. Mild leukopenia and thrombocytopenia (i.e. low white blood cell and platelet counts) usually accompany the anaemia, and the nuclei of polymorphonuclear (PMN) leukocytes are structurally abnormal (hypersegmented – as young PMNs mature, their nuclei acquire 'lobes' in the form of discrete bulges, leading to hypersegmentation in post-mature cells. The nuclei of

megaloblasts – the precursors of macrocytic red cells in patients with B$_{12}$ or folate deficiency – are functionally asynchronous and feebly active, compared with the cells' low haemoglobin content). Neurological disorders caused by deficiency of vitamin B$_{12}$ include peripheral neuropathy and dementia, as well as *subacute combined degeneration*[3] of the spinal cord. Folic acid deficiency is caused by dietary deficiency, especially during increased demand (e.g. during pregnancy – particularly important because of the link between folate deficiency and neural tube defects in the baby (see Ch. 58) or because of chronic haemolysis in patients with haemoglobinopathies such as *sickle cell anaemia* – see p. 341). Vitamin B$_{12}$ deficiency, however, is usually due to decreased absorption (see p. 338).

FOLIC ACID

Some aspects of folate structure and metabolism are dealt with in Chapters 51 and 57, because several important antibacterial and anticancer drugs are antimetabolites that interfere with folate synthesis in microorganisms or tumour cells. Liver and green vegetables are rich sources of folate (also known as vitamin B$_9$). In healthy non-pregnant adults, the daily requirement is about 0.2 mg daily, but this is increased during pregnancy. Healthy fetal neural development in particular requires sufficient folate in the mother's diet, also leading to foetal neural development defects if insufficient.

Mechanism of action

Reduction of folic acid, catalysed by *dihydrofolate reductase* in two stages yields *dihydrofolate* (FH$_2$) and *tetrahydrofolate* (FH$_4$), co-factors which transfer methyl groups (1-carbon transfers) in several important metabolic pathways. FH$_4$ is essential for DNA synthesis because of its role as co-factor in the synthesis of purines and pyrimidines. It is also necessary for reactions involved in amino acid metabolism.

FH$_4$ is important for the conversion of deoxyuridylate monophosphate (DUMP) to deoxythymidylate monophosphate (DTMP). This reaction is rate limiting in mammalian DNA synthesis and is catalysed by thymidylate synthetase, with FH$_4$ acting as methyl donor.

Pharmacokinetic aspects

Therapeutically, folic acid is given orally and is absorbed in the ileum. Methyl-FH$_4$ is the form in which folate is usually carried in blood and which enters cells. It is functionally inactive until it is demethylated in a vitamin B$_{12}$-dependent reaction (see p. 338). Folate is taken up into hepatocytes and bone marrow cells by active transport. Within the cells, folic acid is reduced and formylated before being converted to the active polyglutamate form. **Folinic acid**, a synthetic FH$_4$, is converted much more rapidly to the polyglutamate form.

Unwanted effects

Unwanted effects do not occur even with large doses of folic acid – except possibly in the presence of vitamin B$_{12}$ deficiency, when it is possible that administration of folic acid may improve the anaemia while exacerbating the neurological lesion. It is therefore important to determine whether a megaloblastic anaemia is caused by folate or vitamin B$_{12}$ deficiency and treat accordingly.

---

[3]'Combined' because the lateral as well as the dorsal columns are involved, giving rise to motor as well as sensory symptoms.

Clinical uses of folic acid and vitamin B₁₂ (hydroxocobalamin)

Folic acid (vitamin B₉)
- Treatment of megaloblastic anaemia resulting from folate deficiency, which can be caused by:
  - *poor diet* (common in alcoholic individuals)
  - *malabsorption syndromes*
  - *drugs* (e.g. **phenytoin**).
- Treatment or prevention of toxicity from **methotrexate**, a folate antagonist (see Chs 27 and 57).
- Prophylactically in individuals at hazard from developing folate deficiency, for example:
  - *pregnant women* and *before conception* (especially if there is a risk of birth defects)
  - *premature infants*
  - patients with *severe chronic haemolytic anaemias*, including haemoglobinopathies (e.g. sickle cell anaemia).

Vitamin B₁₂ (hydroxocobalamin)
- Treatment of *pernicious anaemia* and other causes of vitamin B₁₂ deficiency.
- Prophylactically after surgical operations that remove the site of production of intrinsic factor (the stomach) or of vitamin B₁₂ absorption (the terminal ileum).

VITAMIN B₁₂

Vitamin B₁₂, also called cobalamin, corrects pernicious anaemia. The vitamin B₁₂ preparation used therapeutically is **hydroxocobalamin**, derived from cultured micro-organisms. The principal dietary sources are meat (particularly liver, where it is stored), eggs and dairy products. For activity, cobalamins must be converted to *methylcobalamin* (methyl-B₁₂) or *5′-deoxyadenosylcobalamin* (ado-B₁₂). The average European diet contains 5–25 µg of vitamin B₁₂ per day, and the daily requirement is 2–3 µg. Absorption requires *intrinsic factor* (a glycoprotein secreted by gastric parietal cells). Vitamin B₁₂, complexed with intrinsic factor, is absorbed by active transport in the terminal ileum. Healthy stomach secretes a large excess of intrinsic factor, but in patients with pernicious anaemia (an autoimmune disorder where the lining of the stomach atrophies), or following total gastrectomy, the supply of intrinsic factor is inadequate to maintain vitamin B₁₂ absorption in the long term. Surgical removal of the terminal ileum, for example, to treat Crohn's disease (see Ch. 31), can also impair B₁₂ absorption.

Vitamin B₁₂ is carried in the plasma by binding proteins called *transcobalamins*. It is stored in the liver, the total amount in the body being about 4 mg. This store is so large compared with the daily requirement, that if vitamin B₁₂ absorption stops suddenly – as after a total gastrectomy – it takes 2–4 years for evidence of deficiency to become manifest.

Mechanism of action

▼ Vitamin B₁₂ is required for two main biochemical reactions in humans.

The conversion of methyl-FH₄ to FH₄. The metabolic activities of vitamin B₁₂ and folic acid are linked in the synthesis of DNA. It is also through this pathway that folate/vitamin B₁₂ treatment can lower plasma homocysteine concentration. Because increased homocysteine concentrations may have undesirable vascular effects (Ch. 24, Table 24.1), this has potential therapeutic and public health implications. The reaction involves conversion of both methyl-FH₄ to FH₄ and homocysteine to methionine. The enzyme that accomplishes this (*homocysteine–methionine methyltransferase*) requires vitamin B₁₂ as co-factor and methyl-FH₄ as methyl donor. The methyl group from methyl-FH₄ is transferred first to B₁₂, and then to homocysteine to form methionine. Vitamin B₁₂ deficiency thus traps folate in the inactive methyl-FH₄ form, thereby depleting the folate polyglutamate coenzymes needed for DNA synthesis. Vitamin B₁₂-dependent methionine synthesis also affects the synthesis of folate polyglutamate coenzymes by an additional mechanism. The preferred substrate for polyglutamate synthesis is formyl-FH₄, and the conversion of FH₄ to formyl-FH₄ requires a formate donor such as methionine.

Isomerisation of methylmalonyl-CoA to succinyl-CoA. This isomerisation reaction is part of a route by which propionate is converted to succinate. Through this pathway, cholesterol, odd-chain fatty acids, some amino acids and thymine can be used for gluconeogenesis or for energy production via the tricarboxylic acid (TCA) cycle. Coenzyme B₁₂ (ado-B₁₂) is an essential co-factor, so methylmalonyl-CoA accumulates in vitamin B₁₂ deficiency. This distorts the pattern of fatty acid synthesis in neural tissue and may be the basis of neuropathy in vitamin B₁₂ deficiency.

Administration of vitamin B₁₂

When vitamin B₁₂ is used therapeutically (as **hydroxocobalamin**), it is usually given by injection[4] because, as explained above, vitamin B₁₂ deficiency commonly results from malabsorption. Patients with pernicious anaemia require life-long therapy, with maintenance injections every 3 months following a loading dose. Hydroxocobalamin does not cause unwanted effects.

HAEMATOPOIETIC GROWTH FACTORS

Every 60 seconds, a human being must generate about 120 million granulocytes and 150 million erythrocytes, as well as numerous mononuclear cells and platelets.[5] The cells responsible for this remarkable productivity are derived from a relatively small number of self-renewing, pluripotent stem cells laid down during embryogenesis. Maintenance of haematopoiesis necessitates a balance between self-renewal of the stem cells on the one hand, and differentiation into the various types of blood cell on the other. The factors involved in controlling this balance are the *haematopoietic growth factors*, which direct the division and maturation of the progeny of these cells down eight possible lines of development (Fig. 26.2). These cytokine growth factors are highly potent glycoproteins, acting at concentrations of 10^{-12} to 10^{-10} mol/L. They are present in plasma at very low concentrations under basal conditions, but on stimulation their concentrations can increase within hours by 1000-fold or more. *Erythropoietin* regulates the red cell line, and the

---

[4]At least in Anglo-Saxon countries; in France, very large doses of vitamin B₁₂ are given by mouth to achieve sufficient absorption for therapeutic efficacy despite the absence of intrinsic factor. Either method is a great improvement on eating the prodigious quantities of raw liver required by Minot and Murphy's 'liver diet' of 1925! – no matter how bad the taste of vitamin B₁₂, it's got to be better than that?
[5]That's your entire genome replicated faithfully for at least 200 million new blood cells every minute – our bodies are truly remarkable machines.

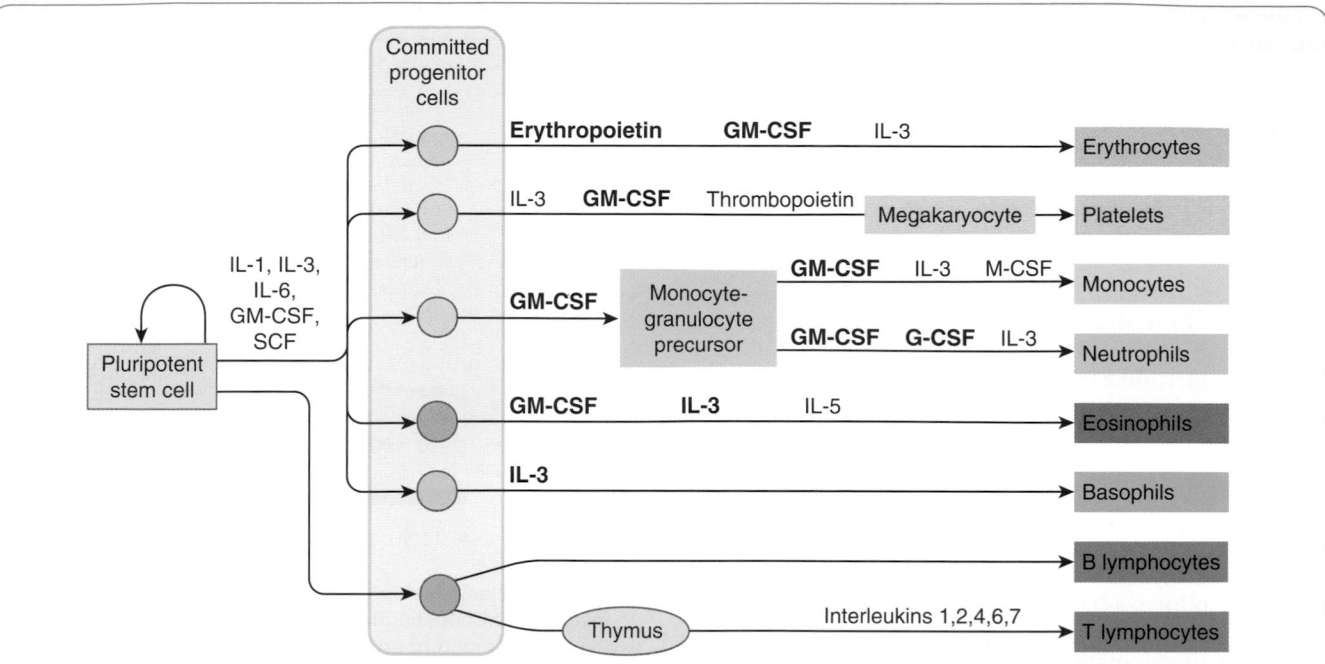

Fig. 26.2 **Haematopoietic growth factors in blood cell differentiation.** Various preparations of the factors shown in bold are in clinical use (see text). Most T cells generated in the thymus die by apoptosis; those that emerge are either CD4 or CD8 T cells. The colours used for the mature blood cells reflect how they appear in common staining preparations (and after which some are named). *CSF*, colony-stimulating factor; *G-CSF*, granulocyte CSF; *GM-CSF*, granulocyte–macrophage CSF; *IL-1*, interleukin-1; *IL-3*, interleukin-3 or multi-CSF; *M-CSF*, macrophage CSF; *SCF*, stem cell factor. (See also Ch. 7.)

Vitamin B$_{12}$ and folic acid

Both vitamin B$_{12}$ and folic acid are needed for DNA synthesis. Deficiencies particularly affect erythropoiesis, causing macrocytic megaloblastic anaemia.

Folic acid (vitamin B$_9$)

- There is active uptake of folic acid into cells and reduction to tetrahydrofolate (FH$_4$) by dihydrofolate reductase; extra glutamates are then added.
- Folate polyglutamate is a co-factor (a carrier of 1-carbon units) in the synthesis of purines and pyrimidines (especially thymidylate).

Vitamin B$_{12}$ (hydroxocobalamin)

- Vitamin B$_{12}$ needs intrinsic factor (a glycoprotein) secreted by gastric parietal cells for absorption in the terminal ileum.
- It is stored in the liver.
- It is required for:
  - conversion of methyl-FH$_4$ (inactive form of FH$_4$) to active formyl-FH$_4$, which, after polyglutamation, is a co-factor in the synthesis of purines and pyrimidines;
  - isomerisation of methylmalonyl-CoA to succinyl-CoA.
- Deficiency occurs most often in pernicious anaemia, which results from malabsorption caused by lack of intrinsic factor from the stomach. It causes neurological disease as well as anaemia.
- Vitamin B$_{12}$ is given by injection every 3 months to treat pernicious anaemia.

signal for its production is blood loss and/or low tissue oxygen tension. *CSFs* regulate the myeloid divisions of the white cell line, and the main stimulus for their production is infection (see also Ch. 7).

Recombinant erythropoietin (**epoietin**),[6] and recombinant granulocyte CSF (**filgrastim, lenograstim, pegfilgrastim**) are used clinically (see later); *thrombopoietin* has been manufactured in recombinant form but there are concerns about effects on tumour progression (it activates a cell surface protein that is an oncogene product) and it has been associated with severe immunologically mediated adverse effects. Some of the other haematopoietic growth factors (e.g. interleukin-3, interleukin-5 and various other cytokines) are covered in Chapter 7.

ERYTHROPOIETIN

Erythropoietin is a glycoprotein produced in juxtatubular cells in the kidney and also in macrophages; it stimulates committed erythroid progenitor cells to proliferate and generate erythrocytes (see Fig. 26.2). Recombinant human erythropoietins are made in cultured mammalian cells (because their pharmacokinetic properties depend critically on the degree of glycosylation, a post-translational modification that occurs in mammalian but not so predictably in bacterial cells) and used to treat anaemia caused by erythropoietin deficiency, for example in patients with chronic kidney disease, AIDS or cancer. Epoietin (recombinant human

---

[6]The first therapeutic agent to be produced by recombinant technology, by Amgen in 1989 – a huge commercial success, heralding the emergence of the biotechnology industry – albeit with some anxious moments (see Fig. 26.3).

erythropoietin) exists in several forms (alpha, beta, theta and zeta). It has a plasma half-life of about 5 hours, and is given by injection three times weekly. **Darbepoetin**, a hyperglycosylated form, has a longer half-life and can be administered less frequently, every 1–4 weeks; **methoxy polyethylene glycol-epoetin beta** is another preparation with long half-life. Epoietin and darbopoetin are given intravenously or subcutaneously, the response being greater after subcutaneous injection and faster after intravenous injection.

Epoietins are reaching the end of patent protection (e.g. the original **Procrit**) and the first 'biosimilar' products have been licensed (such as **Binocrit** and **Retacrit** in 2017 and 2018 respectively). Unlike the situation for small-molecule chemical entities where criteria for bioequivalence are relatively uncontroversial – Chapter 9 – biologically produced macromolecules may vary markedly with seemingly minor changes in manufacture, and have many opportunities to form immunologically distinct products during cell culture.

Unwanted effects

Transient influenza-like symptoms are common. Hypertension is also common and can cause encephalopathy with headache, disorientation and sometimes convulsions. Iron deficiency can be induced because more iron is required for the enhanced erythropoiesis. Blood viscosity increases as the haematocrit (i.e. the fraction of the blood that is occupied by red blood cells) rises, increasing the risk of thrombosis, especially during dialysis. There have been reports of a devastating chronic condition known as pure red cell aplasia (PRCA), connected with development of neutralising antibodies directed against erythropoietin which inactivate the endogenous hormone as well as the recombinant product (Berns, 2013). This has been a huge concern with indirect implications for quality control between batches of biological products and, indirectly, for the licensing of biosimilar products.

▼ Before 1998, only three cases of PRCA in association with epoietin treatment had been published. In that year, in response to concerns about transmitting bovine spongiform encephalopathy ('mad cow disease'), the formulation of the leading brand was changed, human serum albumin (used to stabilise the product) being replaced by polysorbate 80 and glycine. The incidence of PRCA increased abruptly, with approximately 250 documented cases by 2002, many of whom died or became completely dependent on blood transfusions. A large proportion had been treated with the new formulation. The mechanism whereby the manufacturing change led to the change in immunogenicity remains a matter of debate (Locatelli et al., 2007), but the packaging and storage were changed in 2003, since when the incidence of PRCA has declined (see Fig. 26.3). The moral is that immunogenicity is unpredictable and can be caused by seemingly minor changes in manufacture or storage (Kuhlmann & Marre, 2010).

Clinical use

Iron or folate deficiency must be corrected before starting treatment. Parenteral iron preparations are often needed (see p. 336). Haemoglobin must be monitored and maintained within the range 10–12 g/dL to avoid the unwanted effects described earlier. Erythrocyte-stimulating agents can be used but there are serious cardiovascular and thrombolytic adverse reactions that can occur, risking mortality. The clinical use of epoietin is given in the box later.

COLONY-STIMULATING FACTORS

CSFs are cytokines that stimulate the formation of maturing colonies of leukocytes, observable in tissue culture. They

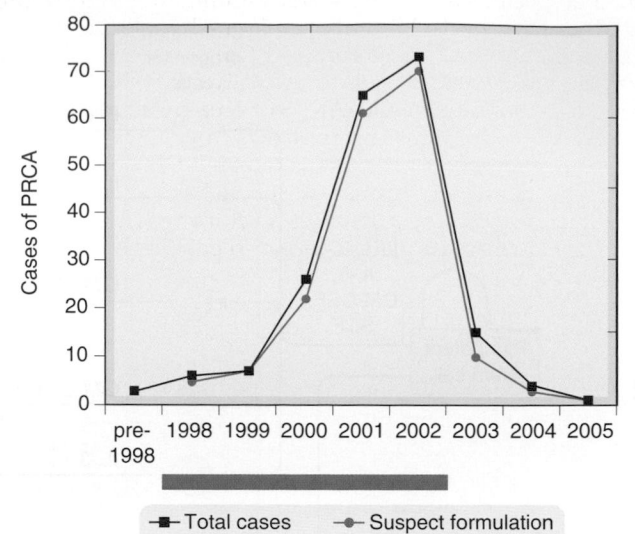

Fig. 26.3 Incidence of pure red cell aplasia (PRCA) in relation to introduction in 1998 of a changed formulation of the leading brand of epoietin. The incidence increased markedly and the suspect formulation *(blue)* accounted for almost all of the cases that were positive for anti-erythropoietin antibody *(red)*; the formulation and instructions for its administration and storage were changed again in 2003 with an abrupt subsequent decline in PRCA. The period when the suspect formulation was in use is indicated by the *blue rectangle*. (Redrawn from Kuhlmann & Marre, 2010.)

not only stimulate particular committed progenitor cells to proliferate (see Fig. 26.2) but also cause irreversible differentiation. The responding precursor cells have membrane receptors for specific CSFs and may express receptors for more than one factor, thus permitting collaborative interactions between factors.

Granulocyte CSF is produced mainly by monocytes, fibroblasts and endothelial cells, and controls primarily the development of neutrophils, increasing their proliferation and maturation, stimulating their release from bone marrow storage pools and enhancing their function. Recombinant forms (**filgrastim**, which is not glycosylated, and glycosylated **lenograstim**) are used therapeutically. **Pegfilgrastim** is a derivative of filgrastim conjugated with polyethylene glycol ('pegylated'), which has the effect of increasing its duration of action.

Thrombopoietin, made in liver and kidney, stimulates proliferation and maturation of megakaryocytes to form platelets. Recombinant thrombopoietin has been a tempting but horribly deceptive therapeutic target. Thrombocytopenia is a predictable and limiting toxicity of many chemotherapeutic regimens in oncology (Ch. 57), and a means to mitigate this would be a valuable prize. Recombinant thrombopoietin, seemingly the logical answer to this need, was manufactured and increased platelet counts in healthy volunteers and patients with mild chemotherapy-induced thrombocytopenia. But in early trials on healthy subjects, repeated dosing of a pegylated product caused the appearance of neutralising antibodies and consequently prolonged thrombocytopenia (Li et al., 2001), driving home the message from experience with erythropoietin (see Fig. 26.3) that subtle differences between biological products and natural mediators can lead to very serious immunologically mediated adverse effects. **Eltrombopag** (a small-molecule agonist administered orally) and **romiplostim** (a dimerised fusion protein analogue that binds to and activates thrombopoietin receptors working via the JAK/STAT pathway and administered by subcutaneous injection) are thrombopoietin agonists approved for treatment of patients with idiopathic thrombocytopaenic purpura (ITP) who have not responded to other treatments such as splenectomy; eltrombopag is also used to increase platelet counts in patients with aplastic anaemia.

Administration and unwanted effects

Filgrastim and lenograstim are given subcutaneously or by intravenous infusion. Pegfilgrastim is administered subcutaneously. Gastrointestinal effects, fever, bone pain, myalgia and rash are recognised adverse effects; less common effects include pulmonary infiltrates and enlargement of liver or spleen.

Haematopoietic growth factors

Erythropoietin

- Regulates red cell production.
- Is given intravenously, subcutaneously, intraperitoneally.
- Can cause transient flu-like symptoms, hypertension, iron deficiency and increased blood viscosity.
- Is available, as epoietin, to treat patients with anaemia caused by chronic renal failure.
- Granulocyte colony-stimulating factor.
- Stimulates neutrophil progenitors.
- Is available as **filgrastim**, **pegfilgrastim** or **lenograstim**; it is given parenterally.

Clinical uses of epoietin

- Anaemia of chronic *renal failure*.
- Anaemia during *chemotherapy* for cancer.
- Prevention of the anaemia that occurs in *premature infants* (unpreserved formulations are used because benzyl alcohol, used as a preservative, has been associated with a fatal toxic syndrome in neonates).
- To increase the yield of autologous blood before *blood donation*.
- Anaemia of *AIDS* (exacerbated by **zidovudine**).

Clinical uses of the colony-stimulating factors

Colony-stimulating factors are used in specialist centres:
- To reduce the severity/duration of neutropenia induced by cytotoxic drugs during:
  - intensive *chemotherapy* necessitating autologous *bone marrow rescue*
  - following *bone marrow transplant*.
- To harvest *progenitor cells*.
- To expand the number of harvested progenitor cells *ex vivo* before reinfusing them.
- For persistent neutropenia in *advanced HIV infection*.
- In aplastic anaemia.

HAEMOLYTIC ANAEMIA

Anaemia associated with increased red cell destruction can arise from genetic causes (e.g. sickle cell disease, thalassaemia, paroxysmal nocturnal haemoglobinuria) or a variety of non-genetic causes such as autoimmunity, infections and adverse drug reactions including haemolysis.

▼ *Sickle cell anaemia* is caused by a mutation in the gene that codes the β-globin chain of haemoglobin, resulting in a single amino acid substitution. The abnormal haemoglobin (haemoglobin S) can polymerise when deoxygenated, changing the physical properties of the red cells (which deform to a sickle shape, hence the name) and damaging cell membranes. This can block the microcirculation, causing painful crises, and haemolysis can reduce the availability of nitric oxide (Ch. 21) resulting in adverse cardiovascular effects, seen when NO depletion by extracellular haemoglobin causes acute hypertensive responses occurring generally during massive haemolysis (Schaer et al., 2013). Polymerisation, and the severity of the disease, are markedly reduced when other forms of haemoglobin (A and F) are present.
Paroxysmal nocturnal haemoglobinuria (PNH) is a rare and previously untreatable form of haemolytic anaemia caused by clonal expansion of haematopoietic stem cells with somatic mutations that prevent formation of glycophosphatidylinositol (GPI), which anchors many proteins to the cell surface, rendering the cell susceptible to complement-mediated haemolysis. In addition to anaemia, patients with PNH suffer from other features, including thrombosis, attacks of abdominal pain and pulmonary hypertension (Ch. 23).

DRUGS USED TO TREAT HAEMOLYTIC ANAEMIAS

Hydroxycarbamide (also known as **hydroxyurea**) is a cytotoxic drug that has been used for decades to lower the red cell and platelet counts in patients with *polycythaemia rubra vera* (a myeloproliferative disorder affecting especially the red cell lineage) or to treat chronic myeloid leukaemia. It is additionally used for sickle cell disease, and reduces the frequency of painful crises (Charache et al., 1995; Wang et al., 2011; Weatherall, 2011).

Mechanism of action

Hydroxycarbamide inhibits DNA synthesis by inhibiting *ribonucleotide reductase* and is S-phase specific (Ch. 6). It increases circulating haemoglobin F, while reducing haemoglobin S. Hydroxycarbamide metabolism gives rise to nitric oxide, which may contribute to its beneficial effect in sickle cell disease. Some of its beneficial effect in reducing painful crises could relate to anti-inflammatory effects secondary to its cytotoxic action.

Administration and unwanted effects

Hydroxycarbamide is administered by mouth once daily at a rather lower starting dose than is used for treating malignant disease; reduced doses are used in patients with impaired renal function. The blood count and haemoglobin F are monitored and the dose adjusted accordingly. Once stabilised, treatment may be continued indefinitely.

Myelosuppression, nausea and rashes are the commonest adverse effects. Animal studies demonstrated teratogenicity, and potential adverse effects on spermatogenesis. When used to treat malignant disease there is an increased risk of second malignancy, but this has not been observed when treating patients with sickle cell disease.

Eculizumab, licensed for the treatment of PNH, is a humanised monoclonal antibody that blocks the terminal

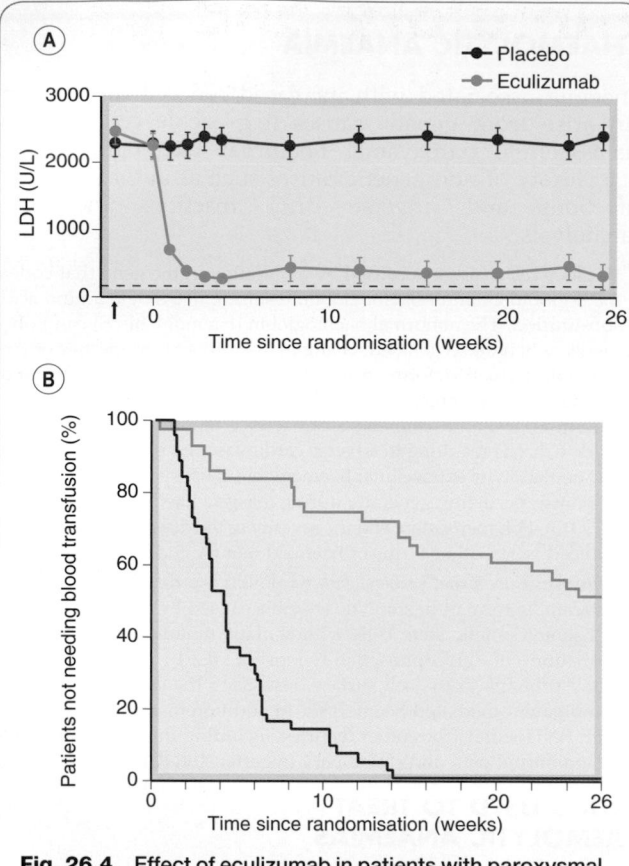

Fig. 26.4 Effect of eculizumab in patients with paroxysmal nocturnal haemoglobinuria (PNH). (A) Effect on plasma lactate dehydrogenase (LDH) activity, a measure of haemolysis. The horizontal dotted line shows the upper limit of normal. The arrow shows the baseline level at screening (n = 44 in placebo group, n = 43 in eculizumab group, *p* < 0.001). (B) Kaplan–Meier curves for the time to first transfusion during treatment in the same patients shown in (A) (*p* < 0.001). (Redrawn from Hillmen et al., 2006.)

complement protein C5 (Ch. 18). In a double-blind, randomised, controlled trial of 87 patients, treatment with eculizumab dramatically reduced haemolysis and transfusion requirement during 6 months of treatment (Fig. 26.4). Patients must be inoculated against meningococcal infection before treatment. It is administered by intravenous infusion weekly for 4 weeks and then approximately every 2 weeks. Serious adverse effects include infection, notably meningococcal infection, but are uncommon. The commonest adverse effects are headache and back pain.

In most forms of haemolytic anaemia, treatment is symptomatic (e.g. analgesia for painful crises in patients with sickle cell disease) and supportive (e.g. attention to fluid balance, oxygen therapy, blood transfusion when essential, treatment of iron overload, provision of adequate folate to support increased red cell turnover and, in some cases, antibiotics and immunisation). Acute haemolytic anaemia associated with autoantibodies may respond to treatment with glucocorticoids (Ch. 34).

REFERENCES AND FURTHER READING

General

Fishbane, S., 2009. Erythropoiesis-stimulating agent treatment with full anemia correction: a new perspective. Kidney Int. 75, 358–365.

Fishman, S.M., Christian, P., West, K.P., 2000. The role of vitamins in the prevention and control of anaemia. Public Health Nutr. 3, 125–150.

Kurzrock, R., 2005. Thrombopoietic factors in chronic bone marrow failure states: the platelet problem revisited. Clin. Cancer Res. 11, 1361–1367. (*Slow progress, see Li et al. below*)

Iron and iron deficiency

Andrews, N.C., 1999. Disorders of iron metabolism. N. Engl. J. Med. 341, 1986–1995.

Provan, D., Weatherall, D., 2000. Red cells, II: acquired anaemias and polycythaemia. Lancet 355, 1260–1268.

Toh, B.H., van Driel, I.R., Gleeson, P.A., 1997. Pernicious anaemia. N. Engl. J. Med. 337, 1441–1448. (*Immunopathogenesis of pernicious anaemia; excellent figures*)

EPO and pure red cell aplasia

Berns, J.S., 2013. Pure red cell aplasia due to anti-erythropoietin antibodies. http://www.uptodate.com/contents/pure-red-cell-aplasia-due-to-anti-erythropoietin-antibodies.

Kuhlmann, M., Marre, M., 2010. Lessons learned from biosimilar epoietins and insulins. Br. J. Diab. Vasc. Dis. 10, 90–97.

Locatelli, F., Del Vecchio, L., Pozzoni, P., 2007. Pure red-cell aplasia "epidemic" – mystery completely revealed? Perit. Dial. Int. 27 (Suppl. 2), S303–S307.

Colony-stimulating factors

Lieschke, G.J., Burges, A.W., 1992. Granulocyte colony-stimulating factor and granulocyte–macrophage colony-stimulating factor.

N. Engl. J. Med. 327, 1–35, 99–106. (*Worthwhile, comprehensive reviews*)

Mohle, R., Kanz, L., 2007. Hematopoietic growth factors for hematopoietic stem cell mobilization and expansion. Semin. Hematol. 44, 193–202.

Haemolytic anaemias

Charache, S., Terrin, M.L., Moore, R.D., et al., 1995. Effect of hydroxyurea on the frequency of painful crises in sickle-cell-anemia. N. Engl. J. Med. 332, 1317–1322. (*Important randomised, controlled trial evidence of efficacy and safety over mean follow-up of 21 months*)

Hillmen, P., Young, N.S., Schubert, J., et al., 2006. The complement inhibitor eculizumab in paroxysmal nocturnal hemoglobinuria. N. Engl. J. Med. 355, 1233–1243. (*Eculizumab is an effective therapy for PNH*)

Schaer, D.J., Buehler, P.W., Alayash, A.I., Belcher, J.D., Vercellotti, G.M., 2013. Hemolysis and free hemoglobin revisited: exploring hemoglobin and hemin scavengers as a novel class of therapeutic proteins. Blood 121, 1276–1284.

Wang, W.C., Ware, R.E., Miller, S.T., et al., 2011. for the BABY HUG investigators. Hydroxyurea in very young children with sickle-cell anaemia: a multicentre, randomised, controlled trial (BABY HUG). Lancet 377, 1663–1672. (*Landmark trial in infants*)

Weatherall, D.J., 2011. Hydroxycarbamide for sickle-cell anaemia in infancy. Lancet 377, 1628–1630. (*Good article on the background and mechanism of hydroycarbamide*)

Thrombopoietin and prolonged thrombocytopenia

Li, J., Yang, C., Xia, Y., et al., 2001. Thrombocytopenia caused by the development of antibodies to thrombopoietin. Blood 98, 3241–3248.

Anti-inflammatory and immunosuppressant drugs

27

OVERVIEW

This chapter deals with the main groups of anti-inflammatory and immunosuppressant drugs, together with their therapeutic uses in a range of different inflammatory and immune disorders. While generally associated with conditions such as rheumatoid arthritis, inflammation forms a significant component of many, if not most, of the diseases encountered in the clinic; consequently, anti-inflammatory drugs are extensively employed in virtually all branches of medicine. In England alone, 33.5 million prescriptions were written for these medicines in 2016 and since many are available from pharmacy counters they are widely used off-prescription by the general public.

INTRODUCTION

Anti-inflammatory drugs may be divided conveniently into seven major groups:

- Drugs that inhibit the cyclo-oxygenase (COX) enzyme – the *non-steroidal anti-inflammatory drugs* (NSAIDs) and the *coxibs*.
- Antirheumatoid drugs – the so-called *disease-modifying antirheumatic drugs* (DMARDs), together with some immunosuppressants.
- The glucocorticoids.
- Anticytokines and other biopharmaceutical agents.
- Antihistamines used for the treatment of allergic inflammation.
- Drugs specifically used to control gout.

In this chapter we first describe the therapeutic effects, mechanism of action and unwanted effects common to NSAIDs, and then deal in a little more detail with aspirin, paracetamol and drugs that are selective for COX-2. The antirheumatoid drugs comprise a rather varied group and include immunosuppressant drugs that are also used to treat other autoimmune diseases, and prevent rejection of organ transplants. The glucocorticoids are covered in Chapter 34, but are briefly discussed in this chapter. We then consider the biopharmaceutical 'revolution' which has changed the therapeutic landscape for patients with severe disease. Finally, we consider drugs that are used to control gout and the histamine H_1 receptor antagonists, which are used to treat acute allergic conditions.

CYCLO-OXYGENASE INHIBITORS

This group includes the 'traditional' (in the historical sense) NSAIDs[1] as well as the coxibs, which are more selective

[1]Here, we use the term NSAID to include the coxibs but this convention is not always followed in the literature.

for COX-2. NSAIDs, sometimes called the *aspirin-like drugs* or *antipyretic analgesics*, are among the most widely used of all medicines. There are now more than 50 different examples on the global market; common examples are listed in Table 27.1 and some significant NSAID structures are depicted in Fig. 27.1.

These drugs provide symptomatic relief from fever, pain and swelling in chronic joint disease such as occurs in osteo- and rheumatoid arthritis, as well as in more acute inflammatory conditions such as fractures, sprains, sports and other soft tissue injuries. They are also useful in the treatment of postoperative, dental and menstrual pain, as well as headaches and migraine. Several NSAIDs are available over the counter and are widely used to treat minor aches and pains and other ailments. There are also many different NSAID formulations available, including tablets, injections and gels. Virtually all these drugs, particularly the 'traditional' NSAIDs, can have significant unwanted effects, especially in the elderly. Newer agents generally provoke fewer adverse actions.

While there are differences between individual NSAIDs, their primary pharmacology is related to their shared ability to inhibit the fatty acid COX enzyme, thereby inhibiting the biosynthesis of prostaglandins and thromboxanes. As explained in Chapter 18, there are two common isoforms of this enzyme, COX-1 and COX-2 (although there may be further isoforms as yet uncharacterised). While they are closely related (>60% sequence identity) and catalyse the same reaction, there are important differences between the expression and role of these two isoforms. COX-1 is a constitutive enzyme expressed in most tissues, including blood platelets. It has a 'housekeeping' role in the body, being involved principally in tissue homeostasis. It is, for example, responsible for the production of prostaglandins involved in gastric cytoprotection (see Ch. 31), platelet aggregation (Ch. 25), renal blood flow autoregulation (Ch. 30) and the initiation of parturition (Ch. 36).

In contrast, COX-2 is induced in inflammatory cells when they are activated by (for example) the inflammatory cytokines – interleukin (IL)-1 and tumour necrosis factor (TNF)-α (see Ch. 19). Thus the COX-2 isoform is considered to be mainly responsible for the production of the prostanoid mediators of inflammation (Vane & Botting, 2001). There are, however, some significant exceptions. COX-2 is constitutively expressed in the kidney, generating prostacyclin, which plays a part in renal homeostasis (see Ch. 30), and in the central nervous system (CNS), where its function is not yet clear.

Though NSAIDs differ in toxicity and degree of patient acceptability and tolerance, their pharmacological actions are broadly similar, with certain important exceptions. **Aspirin** has other qualitatively different pharmacological actions and **paracetamol** is an interesting exception to the general NSAID stereotype (see later). Some notes on the relative selectivity of some NSAIDs and coxibs are provided in Table 27.1.

343

Table 27.1 Comparison of some common anti-inflammatory cyclo-oxygenase inhibitors

Type	Drug	Indication	COX selectivity	Comments
Propionates	Dexibruprofen	OA, MS, D, H&M	NT	Active enantiomer of ibuprofen
	Dexketoprofen	PO, D, H&M	NT	Isomer of ketoprofen
	Fenoprofen	RA, OA, MS, PO	Non-selective	Prodrug; activated in liver
	Felbinac	MS, OA	NT	Metabolite of fenbufen
	Flurbiprofen	RA, OA, MS, PO, D, H&M	Very COX-1 selective	—
	Ibuprofen	RA, OA, MS, PO, D, H&M	Weakly COX-1 selective	Suitable for children
	Ketoprofen	RA, OA, G, MS, PO, D	Weakly COX-1 selective	Suitable for mild disease
	Naproxen	RA, OA, G, MS, PO, D	Weakly COX-1 selective	Possibly CV safe?
	Tiaprofenic acid	RA, OA, MS	NT	—
Indoles and derivatives	Acemetacin	RD, OA, MS, PO	NT	Ester of indometacin
	Indometacin	RA, OA, G, MS, PO, D	Weakly COX-1 selective	Suitable for moderate to severe disease
	Sulindac	RA, OA, G, MS	Weakly COX-2 selective	Prodrug
Oxicams	Meloxicam	RA, OA, AS	Moderately COX-2 selective	Possibly fewer gastrointestinal effects
	Piroxicam	RA, OA, AS	Weakly COX-2 selective	—
	Tenoxicam	RA, OA, MS	NT	—
Sulfonyl and sulfonamide coxibs	Celecoxib	RA, OA, AS	Moderately COX-2 selective	Fewer gastrointestinal effects
	Etoricoxib	RA, OA, G, AS	Very COX-2 selective	—
	Parecoxib	PO	NT	Prodrug activated in liver
Phenylacetates	Aceclofenac	RA, OA, AS	NT	—
	Diclofenac	RA, OA, G, MS, PO, H&M	Weakly COX-2 selective	Moderate potency. Various salts
Fenamates	Mefenamic acid	RA, OA, PO, D	NT	Moderate activity
	Tolfenamic acid	H&M	NT	—
Miscellaneous	Ketorolac	PO	Highly COX-1 selective	Mainly ocular use
	Nabumetone	RA, OA	NT	Prodrug activated in liver
	Etodolac	RA, OA	Moderately COX-2 selective	Possibly fewer GI effects
Salicylates	Aspirin	Mainly CV usage	Weakly COX-1 selective	Component of many OTC preparations. Unsuitable for children.

The chemical classes of these NSAIDs are also shown because sometimes they are referred to in this manner.

AS, ankylosing spondylitis; *CV*, cardiovascular; *D*, dysmenorrhoea; *G*, acute gout; *GI*, gastrointestinal; *H&M*, headache and migraine; *MS*, musculoskeletal injuries and pain; *NT*, not tested; *OA*, osteoarthritis; *OTC*, over-the-counter; *PO*, postoperative pain; *RA*, rheumatoid arthritis.

(Data from British National Formulary 2017 and COX selectivity data, where tested, from Warner & Mitchell, 2004 and 2008.)

MECHANISM OF ACTION

In 1971, Vane and his colleagues demonstrated that the NSAIDs inhibit prostaglandin biosynthesis by a direct action on the COX enzyme and established the hypothesis that this single action explained the vast majority of their therapeutic actions and side effects. This has since been confirmed by numerous studies.

▼ COX enzymes are bifunctional, having two distinct catalytic activities. A *dioxygenase* step is followed by a second, *peroxidase*, reaction (see Ch. 18). Both COX-1 and COX-2 are haem-containing enzymes that exist as homodimers attached to intracellular membranes. Interestingly, only one monomer is catalytically active at one time. Binding of NSAIDs to one COX monomer can inhibit the catalytic activity of the entire dimeric complex. Structurally, COX-1 and COX-2 are similar; both contain a hydrophobic channel into which the arachidonic or other substrate fatty acids dock so that the oxygenation reaction can proceed. Most NSAIDs inhibit only the initial dioxygenation reaction. They are generally rapid 'competitive reversible' inhibitors of COX-1, but there are differences in their kinetics. Inhibition of COX-2 is more time-dependent and the inhibition is often irreversible. To block the enzymes, NSAIDs enter the hydrophobic channel, forming hydrogen bonds with an arginine residue at position 120, thus preventing substrate fatty acids from entering the catalytic domain. However, a single amino acid change (isoleucine to valine at position 523) in the structure of the entrance of this channel in COX-2 results in a 'bulge' in the channel that is not found in COX-1. This is important in understanding why some drugs, especially those with large sulfur-containing side groups, are more selective for the COX-2 isoform

Aspirin (Acetylsalicylic acid)

Salicylic acid

Ibuprofen

Naproxen

Indomethacin

Diclofenac

Paracetamol

Mefenamic acid

Celecoxib

Fig. 27.1 Significant structural features of some non-steroidal anti-inflammatory drugs (NSAIDs) and coxibs. Aspirin contains an acetyl group that is responsible for the inactivation of the cyclo-oxygenase (COX) enzyme. Salicylic acid is the end product when aspirin is de-acetylated but, oddly has anti-inflammatory activity in its own right. Paracetamol is a commonly used analgesic agent also of simple structure. Most 'classic' NSAIDs are carboxylic acids. Coxibs (celecoxib shown here as an example), however, often contain sulfonamide or sulfone groups. These are thought to be important in determining the selectivity of the molecule as they impede access to the hydrophobic channel in the COX-1 enzyme (see Fig. 27.2).

Therapeutic effects of cyclo-oxygenase (COX) inhibitors

These drugs inhibit COX enzymes, and therefore prostanoid synthesis, in inflammatory cells. Inhibition of the COX-2 isoform is probably crucial for their therapeutic actions which include:

- *An anti-inflammatory action*: the decrease in prostaglandin E_2 and prostacyclin reduces vasodilatation and, indirectly, oedema. Accumulation of inflammatory cells is not directly reduced.
- *An analgesic effect*: decreased prostaglandin generation means less sensitisation of nociceptive nerve endings to inflammatory mediators such as bradykinin and 5-hydroxytryptamine. Relief of headache is probably a result of decreased prostaglandin-mediated vasodilatation.
- *An antipyretic effect*: interleukin 1 releases prostaglandins in the central nervous system, where they elevate the hypothalamic set point for temperature control, thus causing fever. Non-steroidal anti-inflammatory drugs (NSAIDs) prevent this.

Important NSAIDs include **aspirin**, **ibuprofen**, **naproxen**, **indometacin**, **piroxicam** and **paracetamol**. Newer agents with more selective inhibition of COX-2 (and thus fewer adverse effects on the gastrointestinal tract) include **celecoxib** and **etoricoxib**.

(Fig. 27.2). Aspirin is, however, an anomaly. It enters the active site and acetylates a serine at position 530, irreversibly inactivating COX. This is the basis for aspirin's long-lasting effects on platelets. Interestingly, aspirin-inactivated COX-2 can still generate some hydroxyacids, but cannot produce the endoperoxide intermediate required for prostanoid synthesis.

PHARMACOLOGICAL ACTIONS

All the NSAIDs have actions very similar to those of aspirin, the archetypal NSAID which was introduced into clinical medicine in the 1890s. Their pharmacological profile is listed in the key points box.

Fig. 27.2 Schematic diagram comparing the binding sites of cyclo-oxygenase (COX)-1 and COX-2. The illustration shows the differences in non-steroidal anti-inflammatory (NSAID) binding sites in the two isoforms. Note that the COX-2 binding site is characterised by a 'side pocket' that can accommodate the realtively 'bulky' groups, such as the sulfonamide moiety of celecoxib, which would impede its access to the COX-1 site. Other NSAIDs, such as flurbiprofen (shown here), can enter the active site of either enzyme. (After Luong et al., 1996.)

Most traditional NSAIDs inhibit both COX-1 and COX-2, although their relative potency against the two isoforms differs. It is believed that the anti-inflammatory action (and probably most analgesic and antipyretic actions) of the NSAIDs are related to inhibition of COX-2, while their unwanted effects – particularly those affecting the gastrointestinal (GI) tract – are largely a result of their inhibition of COX-1. Compounds with a selective inhibitory action on COX-2 are now in clinical use, but while these drugs show fewer GI side effects, they are by no means as well tolerated as was once hoped. This is partly because many patients have already been exposed to less selective drugs and have already suffered some GI damage. Since COX-2 also seems to be important in healing and resolution, one can see how problems might still occur. There is also a concern about the cardiovascular effects of all NSAIDs when these are taken chronically.

THERAPEUTIC ACTIONS
ANTI-INFLAMMATORY EFFECTS

As described in Chapters 18 and 19, many mediators coordinate inflammatory and allergic reactions. The NSAIDs reduce those components in which prostaglandins, mainly derived from COX-2, play a significant part. These include not only the characteristic vasodilatation (because of reduced synthesis of vasodilator prostaglandins) but also the oedema of inflammation because vasodilatation facilitates and potentiates the action of mediators that increase the

permeability of postcapillary venules, such as histamine; Ch. 18).

▼ While NSAIDs suppress the signs and symptoms of inflammation, they have little or no action on underlying chronic disease itself. As a class, they are generally without direct effect on other aspects of inflammation, such as cytokine/chemokine release, leukocyte migration, lysosomal enzyme release and toxic oxygen radical production, which contribute to tissue damage in chronic inflammatory conditions such as rheumatoid arthritis, vasculitis and nephritis.

Other actions besides inhibition of COX may contribute to the anti-inflammatory effects of some NSAIDs. Reactive oxygen radicals produced by neutrophils and macrophages are implicated in tissue damage in some conditions, and some NSAIDs (e.g. **sulindac**) have oxygen radical-scavenging effects as well as COX inhibitory activity, so may decrease tissue damage. Aspirin also inhibits expression of the transcription factor NFκB (see Ch. 3), which has a key role in the transcription of the genes for inflammatory mediators.

ANTIPYRETIC EFFECTS

Neurons in the hypothalamus control the balance between heat production and heat loss, thereby regulating normal body temperature. Fever occurs when there is a disturbance of this hypothalamic 'thermostat', which raises body temperature. NSAIDs reset this thermostat. Once there has been a return to the normal 'set point', the temperature-regulating mechanisms (dilatation of superficial blood vessels, sweating, etc.) then operate to reduce temperature. Normal body temperature in healthy humans is not affected by NSAIDs.[2]

▼ The NSAIDs exert their antipyretic action largely through inhibition of prostaglandin production in the hypothalamus. During infection, bacterial endotoxins cause the release from macrophages of IL-1 (Ch. 18). In the hypothalamus this cytokine stimulates the generation of E-type prostaglandins that elevate the temperature set point. COX-2 may have a role here, because IL-1 induces this enzyme in the hypothalamic vascular endothelium. There is some evidence that prostaglandins are not the only mediators of fever, hence NSAIDs may have an additional antipyretic effect by mechanisms as yet unknown.

ANALGESIC EFFECTS

The NSAIDs are effective against mild or moderate pain, especially that arising from inflammation or tissue damage. Two sites of action have been identified.

Peripherally, NSAIDs decrease production of prostaglandins that sensitise nociceptors to inflammatory mediators such as bradykinin (see Chs 19 and 43) and they are therefore effective in arthritis, bursitis, pain of muscular and vascular origin, toothache, dysmenorrhoea, the pain of postpartum states and the pain of cancer metastases in bone. All conditions are associated with increased local prostaglandin synthesis probably as a result of COX-2 induction. Alone, or in combination with opioids, they decrease postoperative pain and in some cases can reduce the requirement for opioids by as much as one-third. Their ability to relieve headache may be related to the reduction in vasodilator prostaglandins acting on the cerebral vasculature.

In addition to these peripheral effects, there is a second, less well characterised central action in the spinal cord and possible elsewhere in the CNS. Peripheral inflammatory

---

[2]With possible exception of paracetamol, which has been used clinically to lower body temperature during surgery.

lesions increase COX-2 expression and prostaglandin release within the cord, facilitating transmission from afferent pain fibres to relay neurons in the dorsal horn (see Ch. 43).

UNWANTED EFFECTS

Overall, the burden of unwanted side effects amongst NSAIDs is high, probably reflecting the fact that they are used extensively, for extended periods of time, and often in the more vulnerable elderly population. When used for joint diseases (which usually necessitates fairly large doses and sustained treatment), there is a high incidence of side effects – particularly in the GI tract but also in the liver, kidney, spleen, blood and bone marrow.

Because prostaglandins are involved in gastric cytoprotection, platelet aggregation, renal vascular autoregulation and induction of labour, all NSAIDs share a broadly similar profile of mechanism-dependent side effects on these processes, although there may be other additional unwanted effects peculiar to individual members of the group. COX-2-selective drugs have less, but not negligible, GI toxicity.

Gastrointestinal disturbances

Adverse GI events are the commonest unwanted effects of the NSAIDs. They are believed to result mainly from inhibition of gastric COX-1, which synthesises prostaglandins that normally inhibit acid secretion and protect the mucosa (see Ch. 31, Fig. 31.2).

Mild symptoms of gastric discomfort ('dyspepsia') and nausea result from gastric mucosal damage, which in some cases progresses to manifest gastric bleeding and ulceration. It has been estimated that 34%–46% of users of NSAIDs will sustain some GI damage which, while it may be asymptomatic, can carry a risk of serious haemorrhage and/or perforation. These severe GI effects are said to result in the hospitalisation of over 100,000 people per year in the United States, some 15% of whom die from this iatrogenic disease (Fries, 1998). Damage is seen whether the drugs are given orally or systemically. However, in some cases (aspirin being a good example), local irritation of the gastric mucosa caused directly by the drug itself may compound the damage. Oral administration of 'replacement' prostaglandin analogues such as **misoprostol** (see Ch. 31) diminishes the gastric damage produced by these agents and is occasionally co-prescribed or combined in a single pill.

Based on extensive experimental evidence, it had been predicted that COX-2-selective agents would provide good anti-inflammatory and analgesic actions with less gastric damage. Two large prospective studies compared the GI side effects of two highly selective COX-2 inhibitors, **celecoxib** and **rofecoxib,** with those of standard comparator NSAIDs in patients with arthritis. The coxibs showed some benefit, although the results were not as clear-cut as had been hoped. The actual situation following therapy is complex because the degree to which the two COX isoforms are inhibited depends not only upon the intrinsic activity of the drug and the inhibitory kinetics as well as the pharmacokinetics. Warner and Mitchell (2008) have suggested that the degree to which NSAIDs inhibit COX-1 at the concentration at which they inhibit COX-2 by 80% is the best measure of 'selectivity'. Damage to the small intestine may also occur following NSAID treatment. It is not clear if a COX-dependent mechanism is involved.

Skin reactions

Rashes are common idiosyncratic unwanted effects of NSAIDs, particularly with **mefenamic acid** (10%–15% frequency) and **sulindac** (5%–10% frequency). They vary from mild erythematous, urticarial and photosensitivity reactions to more serious and potentially fatal diseases including *Stevens–Johnson syndrome* (a blistering rash that extends into the gut, see Ch. 58), and its more severe form, *toxic epidermal necrolysis*[3] (fortunately very rare). The mechanism is unclear.

Adverse renal effects

Therapeutic doses of NSAIDs in healthy individuals pose little threat to kidney function, but in susceptible patients they cause acute renal insufficiency, which is reversible on discontinuing the drug (see Ch. 58, Table 58.1). This occurs because of inhibition of the biosynthesis of those prostanoids (PGE_2 and PGI_2; prostacyclin) involved in the maintenance of renal blood flow, specifically in the PGE_2-mediated compensatory vasodilatation that occurs in response to the action of noradrenaline (norepinephrine) or angiotensin II (see Ch. 30). Neonates and the elderly are especially at risk, as are patients with heart, liver or kidney disease, or a reduced circulating blood volume.

Chronic NSAID consumption, especially NSAID abuse,[4] can cause analgesic nephropathy characterised by chronic nephritis and renal papillary necrosis (Ch. 30). **Phenacetin** (now withdrawn) was the main culprit; paracetamol, one of its major metabolites, is much less toxic. Regular use of prescribed doses of NSAIDs is less hazardous for the kidney than heavy and prolonged use of over-the-counter analgesics in a social context.

Cardiovascular side effects

Though aspirin is widely used clinically for its long-lasting antiplatelet action (see later) other NSAIDs generally lack this property and, as well as opposing the effects of some antihypertensive drugs, also raise blood pressure in patients not taking antihypertensive drugs, and therefore predispose to adverse cardiovascular events such as stroke and myocardial infarction. The hypertensive effect is dose- and time-dependent and rarely occurs with short-term (i.e. days) administration. It is now known that (with the exception of low-dose aspirin) these effects are common to most NSAIDs, especially following prolonged use. Patients with pre-existing cardiovascular risk are at particular risk. Some drugs (e.g. **naproxen**) appear to be better tolerated in this respect than others (see Ray et al., 2009).

▼ Astonishingly, given the fact that some of these drugs have been in use for half a century or more, this was only recognised as a serious issue during trials of the COX-2 inhibitor rofecoxib in 2000, after which continuing concern about the cardiovascular risk led to the addition of a 'warning label' in 2002. The results from a later long-term trial designed to assess the anticancer activity of rofecoxib confirmed a significantly increased the risk of cardiovascular events after 18 months of drug treatment. As a result, the drug was withdrawn in 2004.

[3]A horrible condition where skin peels away in sheets as if scalded.
[4]So called because the availability of NSAIDs (often in combination with other substances, such as caffeine) in over-the-counter proprietary medicines, has tempted some people to consume them in prodigious quantities, for every conceivable malady. Swiss workers manufacturing watches used to share analgesics in the same way as sweets or cigarettes!

The reasons for these adverse cardiovascular effects have been the subject of considerable debate and controversy. One attractive idea was that inhibition of prostacyclin (a potent vasodilator) production by COX-2 in vascular tissue could lead to a net hypertensive effect (see Grosser et al., 2006). This idea gained traction when it was shown that coxibs reduced the urinary output prostacyclin metabolites suggesting that COX-2 was the dominant isoform responsible for prostacyclin production in the vasculature. Others have argued that COX-1 is the main isoform in vascular tissue and that prostacyclin metabolites found in the urine predominately reflect intra-renal synthesis rather than overall vascular production (see Kirby et al., 2015). Prostaglandins are important in the regulation, by cells of the macula densa region, of renin release and hence blood pressure, so inhibition of COX-2 at this site may be the culprit. An alternative recent explanation is that renal COX-2 controls the methylarginine system suppressing the release of cardiotoxic asymmetrical dimethyl arginate (ADMA) by the constitutive nitric oxide synthase (NOS) enzyme (see Kirby et al., 2016 and Ch. 21). The problem has not yet been settled to everyone's satisfaction and a heated (and sometimes overheated) debate continues.

Other unwanted effects

Approximately 5% of patients exposed to NSAIDs experience aspirin-sensitive asthma. The exact mechanism is unknown, but inhibition of COX is implicated (see Ch. 29) and pre-existing viral infections may predispose. Aspirin is the worst offender, but there is cross-reaction with other NSAIDs, except possibly selective COX-2 inhibitors (see Ch. 29). Other, much less common, unwanted effects of NSAIDs include CNS effects, bone marrow disturbances and liver disorders, the last being more likely if there is already renal impairment.[5] Paracetamol overdose causes liver failure. All NSAIDs (except COX-2 inhibitors, including paracetamol in therapeutic doses) prevent platelet aggregation to some extent and therefore may prolong bleeding. Again, aspirin is the main problem in this regard.

SOME IMPORTANT NSAIDS AND COXIBS

Table 27.1 lists commonly used NSAIDs, and the clinical uses of the NSAIDs are summarised in the clinical box. We now look at some of the more significant drugs in a little more detail.

ASPIRIN

Aspirin (acetylsalicylic acid) was among the earliest drugs synthesised, and is still one of the most commonly consumed drugs worldwide.[6] It is also a common ingredient in many over-the-counter proprietary medicines (although increasingly less so). The drug itself is relatively insoluble, but its sodium and calcium salts dissolve readily in aqueous solutions.

While aspirin was originally an anti-inflammatory workhorse, it is seldom used for this purpose now, having been supplanted by other, better tolerated NSAIDs. Today, in addition to its widespread use as an over-the-counter remedy, its main clinical use is as a cardiovascular drug because of its ability to provide a prolonged suppression of platelet COX-1 and hence reduce aggregation (see Ch. 25).

---

[5]An odd side effect of the NSAID diclofenac came to light when a team of scientists investigated the curious decline in the vulture population of the Indian subcontinent. These birds feed on dead cattle some of which had been treated with diclofenac for veterinary reasons. Apparently, residual amounts of the drug in the carcasses proved uniquely toxic to this species.

[6]Indeed, many people do not seem to regard it as a 'drug' at all. Many studies of human platelet aggregation have been ruined by the failure of volunteers to declare their consumption of aspirin.

General unwanted effects of cyclo-oxygenase (COX) inhibitors

Unwanted effects, many stemming from inhibition of the constitutive housekeeping enzyme COX-1 isoform, are common, particularly in the elderly, and include the following:

- *Dyspepsia, nausea, vomiting* and *other GI effects*. Gastric and intestinal damage may occur with chronic use, with risk of haemorrhage, ulceration and perforation which can be life-threatening. The cause is suppression of gastroprotective prostaglandins in the gastric mucosa.
- *Adverse cardiovascular effects*. These can occur with many non-steroidal anti-inflammatory drugs (NSAIDs) and coxibs and may be related to inhibition of COX-2 in the kidney or elsewhere leading to hypertension.
- *Skin reactions*. Mechanism unknown.
- *Reversible renal insufficiency*. Seen mainly in individuals with compromised renal function when the compensatory prostaglandin I_2/E_2-mediated vasodilatation is inhibited.
- *Bronchospasm*. Seen in 'aspirin-sensitive' asthmatics. Uncommon with coxibs.
- *'Analgesic-associated nephropathy'*. This can occur following long-term high-dose regimes of NSAIDs and is often irreversible.
- *Liver disorders, bone marrow depression*. Relatively uncommon.

Clinical uses of non-steroidal anti-inflammatory drugs (NSAIDs)

NSAIDs are widely used but cause serious adverse effects (especially GI, renal, pulmonary and cardiovascular effects related to their main pharmacological actions, as well as idiosyncratic effects). Elderly patients and those with pre-existing disorders are at particular risk. The main uses are:

- *Antithrombotic*: e.g. **aspirin** (Ch. 25) for patients at high risk of arterial thrombosis (e.g. following myocardial infarction). Other NSAIDs that cause less profound inhibition of platelet thromboxane synthesis than does **aspirin**, *increase* the risk of thrombosis and should be avoided in high-risk individuals if possible.
- *Analgesia* (e.g. for headache, dysmenorrhoea, backache, bony metastases, postoperative pain):
  - short-term use: e.g. **aspirin**, **paracetamol**, **ibuprofen**;
  - chronic pain: more potent, longer-lasting drugs (e.g. **naproxen**, **piroxicam**) often combined with a low-potency opioid (e.g. **codeine**, Ch. 43);
  - to reduce the requirement for narcotic analgesics (the NSAID **ketorolac** is sometimes given postoperatively for this purpose).
- *Anti-inflammatory*: e.g. **ibuprofen**, **naproxen** for symptomatic relief in rheumatoid arthritis, gout, soft tissue disorders.
- *Antipyretic*: **paracetamol**.

▼ While inhibition of platelet function is a feature of most NSAIDs, the effect of aspirin is longer lasting. This is because it irreversibly acetylates COX enzymes, and while these proteins can be replaced in most cells, platelets, lacking a nucleus (and hence the cellular machinery for making new proteins), are not able to do so, and remain inactivated for their lifetime (approximately 10 days). Since a proportion of platelets is replaced each day from the bone marrow, this inhibition gradually abates but a small daily dose of aspirin (e.g. 75 mg/day) is all that is required to suppress platelet function to levels which benefit patients at risk for myocardial infarction and other cardiovascular problems (Ch. 25). The view that even patients not at risk would benefit from taking the drug prophylactically (primary prevention) was challenged in a meta-analysis (Baigent et al., 2009) suggesting that in the general population, the risk from gastrointestinal bleeding just outweighs the protective action. In cases where there is a previous history of cardiovascular episodes the case for prophylactic aspirin (secondary prevention) seems unassailable.

The use of aspirin has also been canvassed for other conditions. These include:

- Cancer – especially colonic and rectal cancer: aspirin (and some COX-2 inhibitors) may reduce the incidence of several types of cancer although one always has to be aware of the GI risk (see Patrignani & Patrono, 2016)
- Alzheimer's disease (Ch. 41): epidemiological evidence suggested that carefully selected doses of aspirin might be beneficial, at least in some groups (see Chang et al., 2016) although other studies have been less encouraging (see Waldstein et al., 2010).
- Radiation-induced diarrhoea.

Pharmacokinetic aspects

Aspirin, being a weak acid, is undissociated (i.e. not ionised) in the acid environment of the stomach, thus facilitating its passage across the mucosa. Most absorption, however, occurs in the ileum, because of the extensive surface area of the microvilli.

▼ Aspirin is rapidly (within 30 min) hydrolysed by esterases in plasma and tissues, particularly the liver, yielding *salicylate*. This compound itself has anti-inflammatory actions (indeed, it was the original anti-inflammatory from which aspirin was derived); the mechanism is not clearly understood, although it may depend upon inhibition of the NFκB system (Ch. 3) and only secondarily on COX inhibition. Oral salicylate is no longer used for treating inflammation, although it is a component of some topical preparations. Approximately 25% of the salicylate is oxidised; some is conjugated to give the glucuronide or sulfate before excretion, and about 25% is excreted unchanged, the rate of excretion being higher in alkaline urine (see Ch. 9).

The plasma half-life of aspirin will depend on the dose, but the duration of action is not directly related to the plasma half-life because of the irreversible nature of the action of the acetylation reaction by which it inhibits COX activity.

Unwanted effects

Salicylates (e.g. aspirin, **diflunisal** and **sulfasalazine**) may produce both local and systemic toxic effects. In addition to the general unwanted effects of NSAIDs outlined above., there are certain specific unwanted effects that occur with aspirin and other salicylates. *Reye's syndrome*, a rare disorder of children that is characterised by hepatic encephalopathy following an acute viral illness, carries a 20%–40% mortality. Since the withdrawal of aspirin for paediatric use, the incidence of Reye's syndrome has fallen dramatically. *Salicylism*, characterised by tinnitus (high pitched ringing in the ears), vertigo, decreased hearing and sometimes also nausea and vomiting, occurs with over-dosage of any salicylate.

Aspirin

Aspirin (acetylsalicylic acid) is the oldest non-steroidal anti-inflammatory drug. It acts by irreversibly inactivating cyclo-oxygenase (COX-) 1 and COX-2.

- In addition to its anti-inflammatory actions, aspirin strongly inhibits platelet aggregation, and its main clinical use now is in the therapy of cardiovascular disease.
- It is given orally and is rapidly absorbed; 75% is metabolised in the liver.
- Elimination of its metabolite salicylate follows first-order kinetics with low doses (half-life 4 h), and saturation kinetics with high doses (half-life over 15 h).

Unwanted effects:

- With therapeutic doses: GI symptoms, often including some gastric bleeding (usually slight and asymptomatic).
- With larger doses: dizziness, deafness and tinnitus ('salicylism'); compensatory respiratory alkalosis may occur.
- With toxic doses (e.g. from self-poisoning): uncompensated metabolic acidosis may occur, particularly in children.
- Aspirin has been linked with a rare but serious post-viral encephalitis (Reye's syndrome) in children and is not used for paediatric purposes.
- If given concomitantly with warfarin, aspirin can cause a potentially hazardous increase in the risk of bleeding.

▼ Acute salicylate poisoning (a medical emergency that occurs mainly in children and attempted suicides) causes major disturbance of acid–base and electrolyte balance. Salicylates uncouple oxidative phosphorylation (mainly in skeletal muscle), leading to hyperthermia, increased oxygen consumption and thus increased production of carbon dioxide. This stimulates respiration, which is also increased by a direct action of the drugs on the respiratory centre. The resulting hyperventilation causes a respiratory alkalosis that is normally compensated by renal mechanisms involving increased bicarbonate excretion. Larger doses actually cause a depression of the respiratory centre, less CO_2 is exhaled and therefore increases in the blood. Because this is superimposed on a reduction in plasma bicarbonate, an uncompensated respiratory acidosis will occur. This may be complicated by a metabolic acidosis, which results from the accumulation of metabolites of pyruvic, lactic and acetoacetic acids (an indirect consequence of uncoupled oxidative phosphorylation). Hyperthermia secondary to the increased metabolic rate is also likely to be present, and dehydration may follow repeated vomiting. In the CNS, initial stimulation with excitement is followed eventually by coma and respiratory depression. Bleeding can also occur, mainly as a result of depressed platelet aggregation.

Drug interactions

Aspirin may cause a potentially hazardous increase in the effect of warfarin, partly by displacing it from plasma protein binding sites (Ch. 11) thereby increasing its effective concentration and partly because its effect on platelets further interferes with haemostasis (see Ch. 25). Aspirin also antagonises the effect of some antihypertensive and uricosuric agents such as **probenecid** and **sulfinpyrazone**. Because low doses of aspirin may, on their own, reduce urate excretion (Ch. 30), it should not be used in gout.

PARACETAMOL

Paracetamol (called acetaminophen in the United States) is one of the most commonly used non-narcotic analgesic–antipyretic agents and is a component of many over-the-counter proprietary preparations. In some ways, the drug constitutes an anomaly: while it is an excellent analgesic (see Ch. 43) and antipyretic, its anti-inflammatory action is slight and seems to be restricted to a few special cases (e.g. inflammation following dental extraction; see Skjelbred et al., 1984). It is also substantially free of the gastric and platelet side effects of the other NSAIDs. For these reasons, paracetamol is sometimes not classified as an NSAID at all.

▼ The antipyretic and analgesic activities can be traced to inhibition of prostaglandin synthesis in the CNS. Paracetamol has been shown to inhibit prostaglandin biosynthesis in some experimental settings (e.g. in the CNS during fever) but not in others (see also Ch. 43). Various solutions to this puzzle have been suggested, including the possibility of a further paracetamol-sensitive COX isoform in the CNS. An alternative explanation is that it acts as a reducing agent to inhibit COX enzymes. Inhibition would be more effective in the particular oxidising milieu of the CNS (Ouellet & Percival, 2001).

Pharmacokinetic aspects

Paracetamol is well absorbed when given orally, with peak plasma concentrations reached in 30–60 min. The plasma half-life of therapeutic doses is 2–4 h, but with toxic doses it may be extended to 4–8 h. Paracetamol is inactivated in the liver, being conjugated to give the glucuronide or sulfate.

Unwanted effects

With therapeutic doses, side effects are few and uncommon, although allergic skin reactions sometimes occur. It is possible that regular intake of large doses over a long period may cause kidney damage. However, toxic doses (10–15 g) cause potentially fatal hepatotoxicity, and nephrotoxicity. This occurs when normal conjugation reactions are saturated and the drug is metabolised instead by mixed function oxidases. The resulting toxic metabolite, N-acetyl-p-benzoquinone imine (NABQI), is normally inactivated by conjugation with glutathione, but when this is depleted the toxic intermediate accumulates in the liver and the kidney tubules and causes necrosis. Chronic, but not acute, alcohol consumption can exacerbate paracetamol toxicity by inducing the liver microsomal enzymes producing the toxic metabolite but the situation is complex (see Prescott, 2000).

▼ The initial symptoms of acute paracetamol poisoning are nausea and vomiting, the hepatotoxicity being a delayed manifestation that occurs 24–48 h later. Further details of the toxic effects are given in Chapter 58. If the patient is seen sufficiently soon after ingestion, the liver damage can be prevented by administering agents that increase glutathione formation in the liver (**acetylcysteine** intravenously, or **methionine** orally). If more than 12 h have passed since the ingestion of a large dose, the antidotes, which themselves can cause adverse effects (nausea, allergic reactions), are less likely to be useful. Regrettably, ingestion of large amounts of paracetamol is a common method of suicide.

COXIBS

Several coxibs have been withdrawn following claims of cardiovascular and other toxicity, but three drugs are currently available for clinical use in the United Kingdom

Paracetamol

Paracetamol is a commonly used drug that is widely available over the counter. It has potent analgesic and antipyretic actions but much weaker anti-inflammatory effects than other non-steroidal anti-inflammatory drugs (NSAIDs). Its cyclo-oxygenase inhibitory action seems to be mainly restricted to the central nervous system (CNS) enzyme.

- It is given orally and metabolised in the liver (half-life 2–4 h).
- Toxic doses cause nausea and vomiting, then, after 24–48 h, potentially fatal liver damage by saturating normal conjugating enzymes, causing the drug to be converted by mixed function oxidases to N-acetyl-p-benzoquinone imine. If not inactivated by conjugation with glutathione, this compound reacts with cellular proteins causing tissue damage.
- Agents that increase glutathione (intravenous **acetylcysteine** or oral **methionine**) can prevent liver damage if given early.

and others may be available elsewhere. Coxibs are generally offered to patients for whom treatment with conventional NSAIDs would pose a high probability of serious GI side effects. However, these can still occur with coxibs, perhaps because COX-2 has been implicated in the healing of pre-existing ulcers, so inhibition could delay recovery from earlier lesions. As is the case with all NSAID treatment, cardiovascular risk should be assessed prior to long-term treatment.

Celecoxib and etoricoxib

Celecoxib and **etoricoxib** are used for symptomatic relief in the treatment of osteoarthritis and rheumatoid arthritis and some other conditions.

▼ Both are administered orally and have similar pharmacokinetic profiles, being well absorbed with peak plasma concentrations being achieved within 1–3 h. They are extensively (>99%) metabolised in the liver, and plasma protein binding is high (>90%). Common unwanted effects may include headache, dizziness, rashes and peripheral oedema caused by fluid retention. Because of the potential role of COX-2 in the healing of ulcers, patients with pre-existing disease should avoid the drugs.

Parecoxib

Parecoxib is a prodrug of **valdecoxib**. The latter drug has now been withdrawn, but parecoxib is licensed for the short-term treatment of postoperative pain. It is given by intravenous or intramuscular injection, and is rapidly and virtually completely (>95%) converted into the active valdecoxib by enzymatic hydrolysis in the liver.

▼ Maximum blood levels are achieved within approximately 30–60 min, depending on the route of administration. Plasma protein binding is high. The active metabolite, valdecoxib, is converted in the liver to various inactive metabolites, and has a plasma half-life of about 8 h. Skin reactions, some of them serious, have been reported with valdecoxib, and patients should be monitored carefully. The drug should also be given with caution to patients with impaired renal function, and renal failure has been reported in connection with this drug. Postoperative anaemia may also occur.

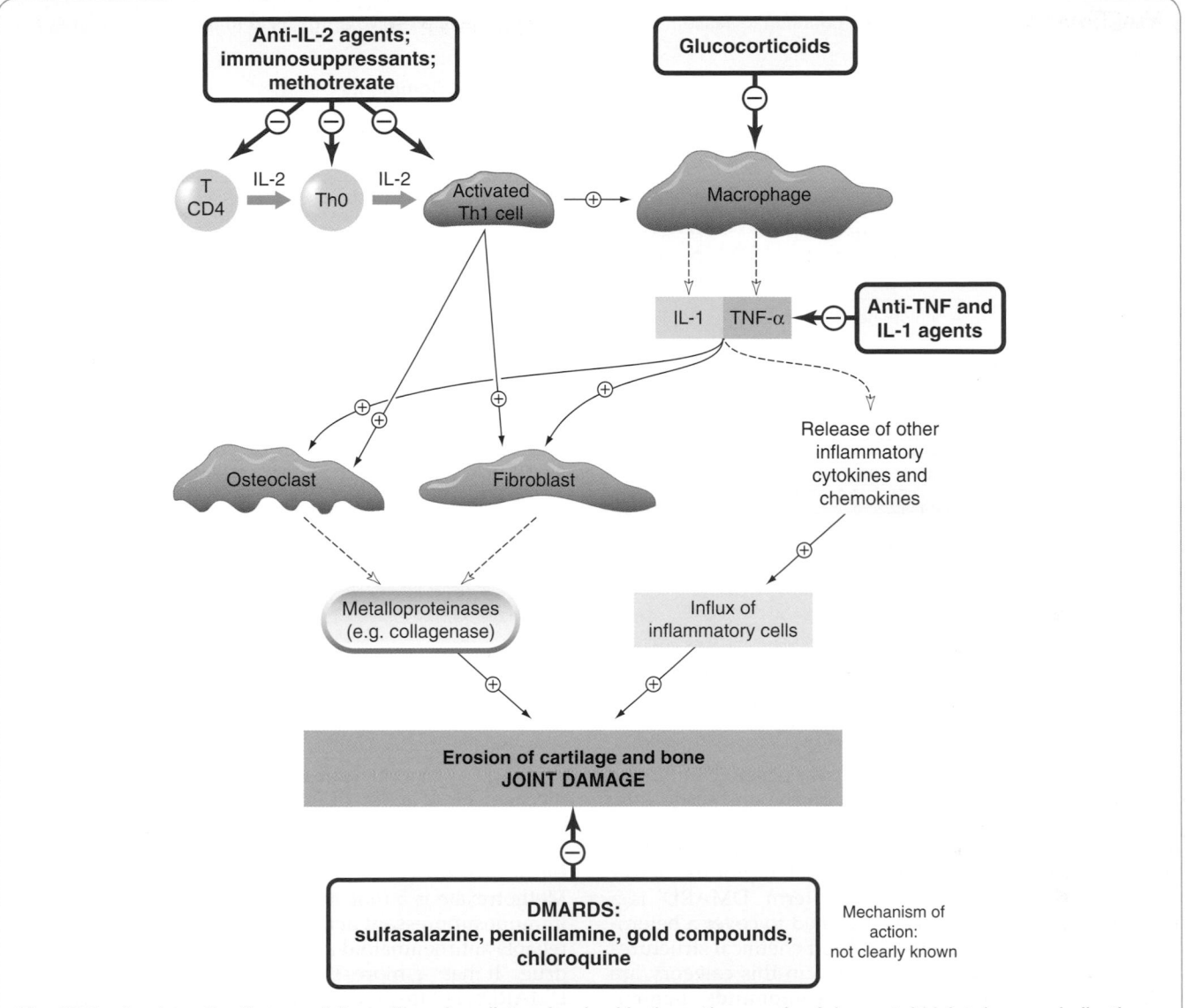

Fig. 27.3 A schematic diagram of the cells and mediators involved in the pathogenesis of rheumatoid joint damage, indicating the sites of action of antirheumatoid drugs. *DMARD*, disease-modifying antirheumatic drug. For details of the anti-TNF, IL-1 and IL-2 receptor agents, see Chapter 7 and Table 27.3.

ANTIRHEUMATOID DRUGS

Rheumatoid arthritis is one of the commonest chronic inflammatory conditions in developed countries, and a common cause of disability.[7] Affected joints become swollen, painful, deformed and immobile. One in three patients with rheumatoid arthritis is likely to become severely disabled. The disease also has cardiovascular and other systemic manifestations and carries an increased risk of mortality. The degenerative joint changes, which are driven by an autoimmune reaction, are characterised by inflammation, proliferation of the synovium and erosion of cartilage and bone. The primary

inflammatory cytokines, IL-1 and (especially) TNF-α, have a major role in the disease (Ch. 19). A simplified scheme showing the development of rheumatoid arthritis and the sites of action of therapeutic drugs, is given in Fig. 27.3. Davis and Matteson (2012) have reviewed the classification and treatment of this miserable and disabling affliction.

DISEASE-MODIFYING ANTIRHEUMATIC DRUGS

The drugs most frequently used in initial therapy are the 'disease-modifying antirheumatic drugs'[8] (DMARDs – especially **methotrexate**) and the NSAIDs. Unlike the NSAIDs, which only reduce the symptoms, DMARDs aim

---

[7]The term 'arthritis' simply refers to inflammatory joint disorders. Clinically, more than 50 distinguishable types are recognised. To the lay person though, arthritis usually denotes either *osteoarthritis* or *rheumatoid arthritis*. These are often confused although they are entirely separate entities.

[8]Historically classified as such because, unlike NSAIDs, they lowered the erythrocyte sedimentation rate (ESR) – a marker of acute inflammation linked to increased plasma fibrinogen. Today, other acute phase reactants such as C-reactive protein (CRP) are generally preferred by rheumatologists as biochemical markers of disease activity.

Table 27.2 Comparison of some common 'disease-modifying' and immunosuppressive drugs used in the treatment of the arthritides

Type	Drug	Indication	Comments
Gold complexes	Sodium aurothiomalate	Progressive RA	Many side effects. Long latency of action
Antimalarials	Chloroquine	Moderate RA, SLE	Used when other therapies fail
	Hydroxychloroquine sulfate	Moderate RA, SLE	Also useful for some skin disorders
Immunomodulators	Methotrexate	Moderate to severe RA, PS, JRA	A 'first-choice' drug. Also used in Crohn's disease and cancer treatment. Often used in combination with other drugs
	Azathioprine	RA, IBS	Used when other therapies fail. Also used in transplant rejection, IBS and eczema
	Ciclosporin	Severe RA, AD, PA	Used when other therapies fail, in some skin diseases and transplant rejection
	Cyclophosphamide	Severe RA	Used when other therapies fail
	Leflunomide	Moderate to severe RA, PA	Also used in psoriatic arthritis
NSAID	Sulfasalazine	RA, PA, JRA	A 'first-choice' drug. Also used in ulcerative colitis
Penicillin metabolite	Penicillamine	Severe RA	Many side effects. Long latency of action

AD, atopic dermatitis; *IBS*, inflammatory bowel disease; *JRA*, juvenile rheumatoid arthritis; *NSAID*, non-steroidal anti-inflammatory drug; *PA*, psoriatic arthritis; *PS*, psoriasis; *RA*, rheumatoid arthritis; *SLE*, systemic lupus erythematosus.
(Data from various sources, including the British National Formulary, 2017.)

to halt or reverse the underlying disease itself. Despite the fact that many of these claims err on the optimistic side, these drugs are nevertheless useful in the treatment of discrete groups of patients and Rau (2005) has argued for their continuing use despite the availability of the newer anticytokine agents (see later). The term 'DMARD' is a latex concept which has been stretched to cover a heterologous group of agents with different chemical structures and mechanisms of action. Included in this category are methotrexate, **sulfasalazine**, **gold compounds**, **penicillamine**, **chloroquine** and other antimalarials (Table 27.2) and various immunosuppressant drugs.

▼ The antirheumatoid action of most of these agents was discovered through a mixture of serendipity and clinical intuition. When they were introduced, nothing was known about their mechanism of action and decades of in vitro experiments have generally resulted in further bewilderment rather than understanding. When successful, DMARDs generally improve symptoms and reduce disease activity in rheumatoid arthritis, as measured by reduction in the number of swollen and tender joints, pain score, disability score, X-ray appearance and serum concentration of acute-phase proteins and of *rheumatoid factor* (an immunoglobulin IgM antibody against host IgG).

The DMARDs are sometimes referred to as *second-line drugs*, with the implication that they are only resorted to when other therapies (e.g. NSAIDs) failed, but DMARD therapy may be initiated as soon as a definite diagnosis has been reached. Their clinical effects are usually slow (months) in onset, and it is usual to provide NSAID 'cover' during this induction phase. If therapy is successful (and the success rate is variable), concomitant NSAID (or glucocorticoid) therapy can be reduced. Some DMARDs (e.g. methotrexate) have a place in the treatment of other chronic inflammatory diseases, whereas others (e.g. penicillamine) are not thought

to have a general anti-inflammatory action. Putative mechanisms of action of DMARDs have been reviewed by Cutolo (2002) and Chandrashekara (2013).

Methotrexate

Methotrexate is a folic acid antagonist with cytotoxic and immunosuppressant activity (Ch. 57). It has a useful and reliable antirheumatoid action and is a common first-choice drug. It has a more rapid onset of action than other DMARDs, but treatment must be closely monitored because of bone marrow depression, causing a drop in white cell and platelet counts (potentially fatal) and liver cirrhosis. It is, however, superior to most other DMARDs in terms of efficacy and patient tolerance, and is often given in conjunction with the anticytokine drugs.

Its mechanism of action is unrelated to its effect on folic acid (which is routinely co-administered to prevent blood disorders) but may well be connected with its ability to block adenosine uptake (see Ch. 17 and Chan & Cronstein, 2010).

Sulfasalazine

Sulfasalazine, another common first-choice DMARD in the United Kingdom, produces remission in active rheumatoid arthritis and is also used for chronic inflammatory bowel disease (see Ch. 31). It probably acts partly by inhibiting COX and lipoxygenase pathways or by scavenging toxic free radicals but it also reduces the release of IL-8 from colonic myofibroblasts, suggesting an additional immunosuppressive mechanism (Lodowska et al., 2015). The drug is a complex of a sulfonamide (sulfapyridine) and salicylate and is split into its component parts by bacteria in the colon. It is poorly absorbed after oral administration.

▼ Sulfasalazine is generally well tolerated but common side effects include GI disturbances, malaise and headache. Skin reactions and leukopenia can occur but are reversible on stopping the drug. The absorption of folic acid is sometimes impaired; this can be countered by giving folic acid supplements. A reversible decrease in sperm count has also been reported. As with other sulfonamides, bone marrow depression and anaphylactic-type reactions may occur in a few patients. Haematological monitoring may be necessary.

Penicillamine

Penicillamine is *dimethylcysteine*; it is produced by hydrolysis of penicillin and appears in the urine after treatment with that drug. The D-isomer is used in the therapy of rheumatoid disease. About 75% of patients with rheumatoid arthritis respond to penicillamine. Therapeutic effects are seen within weeks but do not reach a plateau for several months. Penicillamine is thought to modify rheumatoid disease partly by decreasing the immune response and IL-1 generation, and/or partly by preventing the maturation of newly synthesised collagen. However, the precise mechanism of action is still a matter of conjecture. The drug has a highly reactive thiol group and also has metal-chelating properties, which are put to good use in the treatment of *Wilson's disease* (pathological copper deposition causing neurodegeneration and liver disease) and heavy metal poisoning.

▼ Penicillamine is given orally, but only about half the dose is absorbed. It reaches peak plasma concentrations in 1–2 h and is excreted in the urine. Treatment is initiated with low doses and increased only gradually to minimise the unwanted effects, which occur in about 40% of patients and may necessitate cessation of therapy. Rashes and stomatitis are the most common unwanted effects but may resolve if the dosage is lowered. Anorexia, fever, nausea and vomiting, and disturbances of taste (the last related to the chelation of zinc) are seen, but often disappear with continued treatment. Proteinuria occurs in 20% of patients and should be monitored. Haematological monitoring is also required when treatment is initiated. Thrombocytopenia may require reduction in the dose. Leukopenia or aplastic anaemia are absolute contraindications, as are autoimmune conditions (e.g. thyroiditis, myasthenia gravis). Because penicillamine is a metal chelator, it should not be given with gold compounds (see later).

Gold

Gold is administered as an organic complex, **sodium aurothiomalate**. The anti-inflammatory effect develops slowly over 3–4 months. Pain and joint swelling subside, and the progression of bone and joint damage diminishes. The mechanism of action is not clear. Sodium aurothiomalate is given by deep intramuscular injection. Gold complexes gradually accumulate in synovial cells in joints as well as other tissues, such as liver cells, kidney tubules, the adrenal cortex and macrophages, and remain for some time after treatment is stopped. Excretion is mostly renal, but some is eliminated in the GI tract. The half-life is 7 days initially but increases with treatment, so the drug is usually given first at weekly, then at monthly intervals.

▼ Unwanted effects with aurothiomalate are seen in about one-third of patients treated, and serious toxic effects in about 1 patient in 10. Important unwanted effects include rashes (which can be severe), mouth ulcers, non-specific flu-like symptoms, proteinuria, thrombocytopenia and blood dyscrasias. Anaphylactic reactions can occur. If therapy is stopped when the early symptoms appear, the incidence of serious toxic effects is relatively low.

Antimalarial drugs

Hydroxychloroquine and chloroquine are 4-amino-quinoline drugs used mainly in the prevention and treatment of malaria (Ch. 55), but they are also used as DMARDs.

Chloroquine is usually reserved for cases where other treatments have failed. They are also used to treat another autoimmune disease, lupus erythematosus, but are contraindicated in patients with psoriatic arthropathy because they exacerbate the skin lesions. The related antimalarial, **mepacrine**, is also sometimes used for discoid (cutaneous) lupus. The antirheumatic effects do not appear until a month or more after the drug is started, and only about half the patients treated respond. The administration, pharmacokinetic aspects and unwanted effects of chloroquine are dealt with in Ch. 55; screening for ocular toxicity is particularly important.

IMMUNOSUPPRESSANT DRUGS

Immunosuppressants are used in the therapy of autoimmune disease and also to prevent and/or treat transplant rejection. Because they impair the immune response, they carry the hazard of a decreased response to infections and may facilitate the emergence of malignant cell lines. However, the relationship between these adverse effects and potency in preventing graft rejection varies with different drugs. The clinical use of immunosuppressants is summarised in the clinical box.

Clinical uses of immunosuppressant drugs

Immunosuppressant drugs are used by specialists, often in combination with glucorticoid and/or cytotoxic drugs:
- To slow the progress of rheumatoid and other arthritic diseases including psoriatic arthritis, ankylosing spondylitis, juvenile arthritis: *disease-modifying antirheumatic drugs* (DMARDs), e.g. **methotrexate**, **leflunomide**, **ciclosporin**; *cytokine modulators* (e.g. **adalimumab**, **etanercept**, **infliximab**) are used when the response to methotrexate or other DMARDs has been inadequate.
- To suppress rejection of transplanted organs, e.g. **ciclosporin**, **tacrolimus**, **sirolimus**.
- To suppress graft-versus-host disease following bone marrow transplantation, e.g. **ciclosporin**.
- In autoimmune disorders including idiopathic thrombocytopenic purpura, some forms of haemolytic anaemias and of glomerulonephritis and myasthenia gravis.
- In severe inflammatory bowel disease (e.g. **ciclosporin** in ulcerative colitis, **infliximab** in Crohn's disease).
- In severe skin disease (e.g. **pimecrolimus**, **tacrolimus** topically for atopic eczema uncontrolled by maximal topical glucocorticoids; **etanercept**, **infliximab** for very severe plaque psoriasis which has failed to respond to **methotrexate** or **ciclosporin**).

Most of these drugs act during the induction phase of the immunological response, reducing lymphocyte proliferation (see Ch. 7), although others also inhibit aspects of the effector phase. There are three main groups:

- drugs that inhibit IL-2 production or action (e.g. **ciclosporin**, **tacrolimus** and related drugs);

- drugs that inhibit cytokine gene expression (e.g. corticosteroids);
- drugs that inhibit purine or pyrimidine synthesis (e.g. **azathioprine**, **mycophenolate mofetil**, **leflunomide**).

Ciclosporin

Ciclosporin is a naturally occurring compound first identified in a fungus. It is a cyclic peptide of 11 amino acid residues (including some not found in animals) with potent immunosuppressive activity but no effect on the acute inflammatory reaction per se. Its unusual activity, which (unlike most earlier immunosuppressants) does not entail cytotoxicity, was discovered in 1972 and was crucial for the development of transplant surgery (for a detailed review, see Borel et al., 1996). The drug has numerous actions but those of relevance to immunosuppression are:

- decreased clonal proliferation of T cells, primarily by inhibiting IL-2 synthesis and possibly also by decreasing expression of IL-2 receptors;
- reduced induction and clonal proliferation of cytotoxic T cells from CD8+ precursor T cells;
- reduced function of the effector T cells responsible for cell-mediated responses (e.g. decreased delayed-type hypersensitivity);
- some reduction of T cell-dependent B-cell responses.

Immunosuppressants

- Clonal proliferation of T-helper cells can be decreased through inhibition of transcription of interleukin (IL)-2: **ciclosporin**, **tacrolimus**, **sirolimus** and **pimecrolimus** and glucocorticoids act in this way.
  - Ciclosporin-like drugs bind to cytosolic proteins (immunophilins) which inhibit calcineurin triggering changes in gene transcription.
  - They are given orally or intravenously; a common adverse effect is nephrotoxicity.
- For glucocorticoid actions, see separate box.
- Lymphocyte proliferation is also blocked by inhibitors of DNA synthesis such as:
  - **azathioprine**, through its active metabolite mercaptopurine;
  - **mycophenolate mofetil**, through inhibition of de novo purine synthesis;
  - **leflunomide**, through inhibition by a metabolite of pyrimidine synthesis.

The main action is a relatively selective inhibitory effect on IL-2 gene transcription, although a similar effect on interferon (IFN)-γ and IL-3 has also been reported. Normally, interaction of antigen with a T-helper (Th) cell receptor results in increased intracellular Ca^{2+} (Chs 2 and 7), which in turn stimulates *calcineurin*, a phosphatase. This activates various transcription factors that initiate IL-2 expression. Ciclosporin binds to *cyclophilin*, a cytosolic protein member of the immunophilin family (a group of proteins that act as intracellular receptors for such drugs). The drug–immunophilin complex binds to, and inhibits, calcineurin which acts in opposition to the many protein kinases involved in signal transduction (see Ch. 3),

thereby preventing activation of Th cells and production of IL-2 (Ch. 7).

Ciclosporin itself is poorly absorbed by mouth but can be given orally in a more readily absorbed formulation, or by intravenous infusion. After oral administration, peak plasma concentrations are usually attained in about 3–4 h. The plasma half-life is approximately 24 h. Metabolism occurs in the liver, and most of the metabolites are excreted in the bile. Ciclosporin accumulates in most tissues at concentrations three to four times that seen in the plasma. Some of the drug remains in lymphomyeloid tissue and remains in fat depots for some time after administration has stopped.

The commonest and most serious unwanted effect of ciclosporin is nephrotoxicity, which is thought to be unconnected with calcineurin inhibition. It may be a limiting factor in the use of the drug in some patients (see also Ch. 58). Hepatotoxicity and hypertension can also occur. Less important unwanted effects include anorexia, lethargy, hirsutism, tremor, paraesthesia (tingling sensation), gum hypertrophy (especially when co-prescribed with calcium antagonists for hypertension; Ch. 23) and GI disturbances. Ciclosporin has no depressant effects on the bone marrow.

Tacrolimus

Tacrolimus is a macrolide antibiotic of fungal origin with a very similar mechanism of action to ciclosporin, but higher potency. The main difference is that the internal receptor for this drug is not cyclophilin but a different immunophilin termed FKBP (FK-binding protein, so called because tacrolimus was initially termed FK506). The tacrolimus–FKBP complex inhibits calcineurin with the effects described previously. It is not used for arthritis but mainly in organ transplantation and severe atopic eczema. **Pimecrolimus** (used topically to treat atopic eczema) acts in a similar way. **Sirolimus** (used to prevent organ rejection after transplantation, and also in coating on cardiac stents to prevent restenosis; Ch. 22) also combines with an immunophilin, but activates a protein kinase to produce its immunosuppressant effect.

▼ Tacrolimus can be given orally, by intravenous injection or as an ointment for topical use in inflammatory disease of the skin. It is 99% metabolised by the liver and has a half-life of approximately 7 h. The unwanted effects of tacrolimus are similar to those of ciclosporin but are more severe. The incidence of nephrotoxicity and neurotoxicity is higher, but that of hirsutism is lower. GI disturbances and metabolic disturbances (hyperglycaemia) can occur. Thrombocytopenia and hyperlipidaemia have been reported but decrease when the dosage is reduced.

Azathioprine

Azathioprine interferes with purine synthesis and is cytotoxic. It is widely used for immunosuppression, particularly for control of autoimmune diseases such as rheumatoid arthritis and to prevent tissue rejection in transplant surgery. This drug is metabolised to mercaptopurine, an analogue that inhibits DNA synthesis (see Ch. 57). Because it inhibits clonal proliferation during the induction phase of the immune response (see Ch. 7) through a cytotoxic action on dividing cells, both cell-mediated and antibody-mediated immune reactions are depressed by this drug. As is the case with mercaptopurine itself, the main unwanted effect is depression of the bone marrow. Other toxic effects are nausea and vomiting, skin eruptions and a mild hepatotoxicity.

Cyclophosphamide

Cyclophosphamide is a potent immunosuppressant that is mainly used to treat cancer. Its mechanism of action is explained in Chapter 57. It has substantial toxicity and is therefore generally reserved for serious cases of rheumatoid arthritis in which all other therapies have failed.

Mycophenolate mofetil

Mycophenolate mofetil is a semisynthetic derivative of a fungal antibiotic, and is used for preventing organ rejection. In the body, it is converted to mycophenolic acid, which restrains proliferation of both T and B lymphocytes and reduces the production of cytotoxic T cells by inhibiting inosine monophosphate dehydrogenase. This enzyme is crucial for de novo purine biosynthesis in both T and B cells (other cells can generate purines through another pathway), so the drug has a fairly selective action.

▼ Mycophenolate mofetil is given orally and is well absorbed. Magnesium and aluminium hydroxides impair absorption, and colestyramine reduces plasma concentrations. The metabolite mycophenolic acid undergoes enterohepatic cycling and is eliminated by the kidney as the inactive glucuronide. Unwanted GI effects are common.

Leflunomide

Leflunomide, used mainly to treat rheumatoid arthritis and occasionally to prevent transplant rejection, has a relatively specific inhibitory effect on activated T cells. It is transformed to a metabolite that inhibits de novo synthesis of pyrimidines by inhibiting dihydro-orotate dehydrogenase. It is orally active and well absorbed from the GI tract. It has a long plasma half-life, and the active metabolite undergoes enterohepatic circulation. Unwanted effects include diarrhoea, alopecia, raised liver enzymes and indeed, a risk of hepatic failure. The long half-life increases the risk of cumulative toxicity.

Glucocorticoids

The therapeutic action of the glucocorticoids involves both their inhibitory effects on the immune response and their anti-inflammatory actions. These are described in Chapter 34, and their sites of action on cell-mediated immune reactions are indicated in Fig. 27.3. Glucocorticoids are immunosuppressant chiefly because, like ciclosporin, they restrain the clonal proliferation of Th cells, through decreasing transcription of the gene for IL-2. However, they also decrease the transcription of many other cytokine genes (including those for TNF-α, IFN-γ, IL-1 and many other interleukins) in both the induction and effector phases of the immune response. The synthesis and release of anti-inflammatory proteins (e.g. annexin 1, protease inhibitors) is also increased. These effects are mediated through inhibition of the action of transcription factors, such as activator protein-1 and NFκB as well as through the action of liganded glucocorticoid receptor in the cytosol of target cells (Ch. 3).

ANTICYTOKINE DRUGS AND OTHER BIOPHARMACEUTICALS

The *biopharmaceuticals* in this section represent the greatest technological and conceptual breakthrough in the treatment of severe chronic inflammation for decades (see Maini, 2005). These drugs are engineered recombinant antibodies and other proteins (see Ch. 5). As such, they are difficult and expensive to produce, and this limits their use. In the United Kingdom (in the National Health Service), they are generally restricted to patients who do not respond adequately to other DMARD therapy and they are administered under specialist supervision. Some are administered in combination with methotrexate, which apparently provides a synergistic anti-inflammatory action.

The characteristics and indications of some current biopharmaceuticals are shown in Table 27.3. The effect of two of these agents on rheumatoid arthritis is shown in Fig. 27.4. Many neutralise soluble cytokines. **Adalimumab, certolizumab pegol, golimumab, etanercept** and **infliximab** target TNF-α; **anakinra, secukinumab** and **canakinumab** target IL-1; **tocilizumab**, IL-6 and **ustekinumab**, ILs-12 and -23. **Abatacept, alemtuzumab, basiliximab, belatacept, daclizumab** and **natalizumab** target T cells, either disrupting activation, proliferation or emigration. **Rituximab** and **belimumab** target B cells. While they are not used for treating arthritis, basiliximab, belatacept and daclizumab are included in the table as they act to prevent the rejection of transplanted organs in a similar way – by suppressing T-cell proliferation.

There is some debate over the precise nature of the target of the anti-TNF agents. Some target both soluble and membrane-bound forms of TNF whereas others are more selective. Antibodies that target membrane-bound TNF (e.g. infliximab and adalimumab) may kill the host cell by complement-induced lysis. This produces a different quality of effect than simple sequestration of the soluble mediator (by, for example, etanercept). This fact is probably the reason why some of these drugs exhibit a slightly different pharmacological profile despite ostensibly acting through the same mechanism (see Arora et al., 2009, for further details).

▼ As proteins, none of these drugs can be given orally. Administration is usually by subcutaneous injection or intravenous infusion and their pharmacokinetic profiles vary enormously. Dosing regimes differ but (for example) anakinra is usually given daily, efalizumab and etanercept once or twice per week, adalimumab, certolizumab pegol, infliximab and rituximab every 2 weeks, and abatacept, belimumab, golimumab, natalizumab and tocilizumab every month. Sometimes a loading dose of these drugs is given as a preliminary to regular administration.

Usually, these biopharmaceuticals are only given to severely affected patients or to those in whom other therapies have failed. For reasons that are not entirely clear, a proportion of these patients (about 30%) do not respond and therapy is generally discontinued if no therapeutic benefit is evident within 2–4 weeks. Some studies suggest that if treatment is begun using drugs such as infliximab in combination with methotrexate this failure rate is reduced and a superior final therapeutic outcome achieved (van der Kooij et al., 2009).

Cytokines are crucial to the regulation of host defence systems (see Ch. 19), and leukocytes are key players in its successful functioning. One might predict, therefore, that anticytokine or antileukocyte therapy – like any treatment that interferes with immune function – may precipitate latent infections (e.g. tuberculosis or hepatitis B) or encourage opportunistic infections. Reports suggest that this is a problem with some of these agents (e.g. adalimumab, etanercept, infliximab, natalizumab and rituximab). The area has been reviewed by Bongartz et al. (2006). Another unexpected, but fortunately rare, effect seen with these drugs is the onset of psoriasis-like syndrome (Fiorino et al.,

Table 27.3 Some biopharmaceuticals used in the treatment of inflammatory disease

Target	Drug	Type	Mode of action	Indication
Soluble TNF	Adalimumab	Humanised mAb	Immunoneutralisation	RA (moderate–severe), PA, AS, PP, CD
	Certolizumab pegol	Pegylated ab fragment	Immunoneutralisation	RA[a] (moderate–severe)
	Golimumab	Humanised mAb	Immunoneutralisation	RA (moderate–severe), PA, PS
	Infliximab	Chimeric neutralising ab	Immunoneutralisation	RA[a] (moderate–severe), PA, AS, PP
	Etanercept	Fusion protein decoy receptor	Neutralisation	RA[a] (moderate–severe), PA, AS, PP
Soluble IL-1	Anakinra	Recombinant version of IL-1 ra	Neutralisation	RA[a] (moderate–severe)
	Secukinamab	Humanised mAb	Immunoneutralisation	AS, PA
	Canakinumab	Humanised mAb	Immunoneutralisation	G
Soluble IL-6	Tocilizumab	Humanised mAb	Immunoneutralisation	RA[a] (moderate–severe)
Soluble IL-12 and -23	Ustekinumab	Humanised mAb	Immunoneutralisation	PA, PP (severe)
T cells	Abatacept	Fusion protein	Prevents co-stimulation of T cells	RA[a] (moderate–severe)
	Alemtuzumab	Humanised mAb	Binds to CD 52 causing cell lysis	MS
	Basiliximab	Chimeric mAb	IL-2 receptor antagonists	Immunosuppression for transplantation surgery
	Belatacept	Fusion protein	Prevents activation of T cells	
	Daclizumab	Humanised mAb	IL-2 receptor antagonist	
	Natalizumab	Humanised mAb	VLA-4 on lymphocytes (neutralises)	Severe multiple sclerosis
B cells	Belimumab	Humanised mAb	Immunoneutralises B cell-activating factor	SLE
	Rituximab	Chimeric mAb	Causes B cells lysis	RA[a] (moderate–severe), some malignancies

[a]Used in conjunction with methotrexate.

ab, antibody; *AS*, ankylosing spondylitis; *CD*, Crohn's disease; *G*, severe gout; *IL*, interleukin; *mAb*, monoclonal antibody; *PA*, psoriatic arthritis; *PP*, plaque psoriasis (e.g. skin); *PS*, psoriasis; *RA*, rheumatoid arthritis; *SLE*, systemic lupus erythematosus; *TNF*, tumour necrosis factor.

(Data from various sources, including the British National Formulary, 2017.)

2009). Hypersensitivity, injection site reactions or mild GI symptoms may be seen with any of these drugs.

DRUGS USED IN GOUT

Gout is a metabolic disease in which urate crystals are deposited in tissues, usually because plasma urate concentration is raised. Sometimes this is linked to overindulgence in alcoholic beverages, especially beer, or purine-rich foods such as offal (urate is a product of purine metabolism). Increased cell turnover in haematological malignancies, particularly after treatment with cytotoxic drugs (see Ch. 57), or impaired excretion of uric acid by drugs such as ordinary therapeutic doses of aspirin (see earlier) are other causes. It is characterised by extremely painful intermittent attacks of acute arthritis produced by the deposition of the crystals in the synovial tissue of distal joints, such as the big toe, as well as the external ear – the common theme being that these tissues are generally relatively cool, favouring crystal deposition. An inflammatory response is evoked, involving activation of the kinin, complement and plasmin systems (see Chs 19 and 7, Fig. 7.1), generation of prostaglandins, lipoxygenase products such as leukotriene B4 (Ch. 18, Fig. 18.1), and local accumulation of neutrophil granulocytes. These engulf the crystals by phagocytosis, releasing tissue-damaging toxic oxygen metabolites and subsequently causing lysis of the cells with release of proteolytic enzymes. Urate crystals also induce the production of IL-1 and possibly other cytokines.

Drugs used to treat gout act in the following ways:

- by decreasing uric acid synthesis **allopurinol** (the main prophylactic drug) or **febuxostat**;
- by increasing uric acid excretion (*uricosuric agents*: **probenecid**, **sulfinpyrazone**; see Ch. 30);
- by inhibiting leukocyte migration into the joint (**colchicine**);
- as an 'IL-1 dependent' disease, biopharmaceuticals such as anakinra may be useful;
- by a general anti-inflammatory and analgesic effect (NSAIDs and occasionally glucocorticoids).

Their clinical uses are summarised in the clinical box (see later).

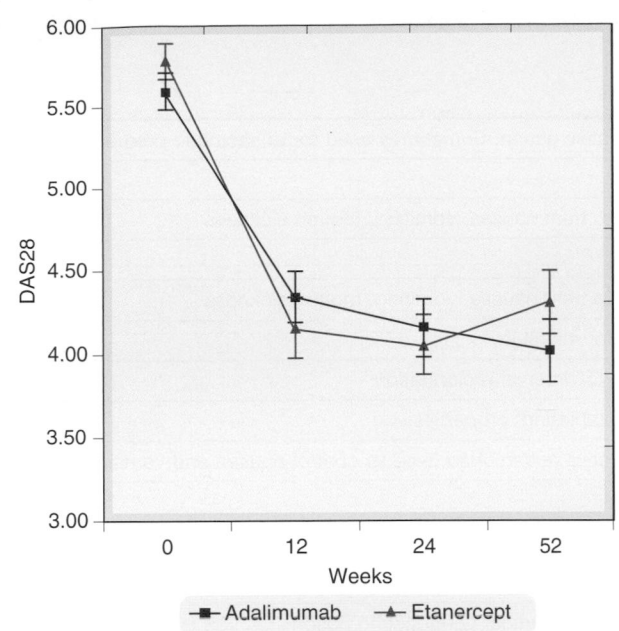

Fig. 27.4 **The effect of anticytokine biopharmaceuticals on rheumatoid arthritis.** In this figure, adalimumab (a humanised monoclonal antibody that neutralises tumour necrosis factor [TNF]) and etanercept (a fusion protein decoy receptor that binds to TNF) were used to treat patients with active rheumatoid arthritis. The Y-axis measures a composite disease activity scores obtained from clinical assessment of 28 joints (DAS28: the lower the score, the less swollen and painful the joints). (From Jobanputra et al., 2012.)

Fig. 27.5 Inhibition of uric acid synthesis by allopurinol. See text for details.

Drugs used in gout and hyperuricaemia

To treat acute gout:
- A non-steroidal anti-inflammatory drug (NSAID), e.g. **ibuprofen**, **naproxen**.
- **Colchicine** is useful if NSAIDs are contraindicated.
- A glucocorticoid, e.g. **hydrocortisone** (oral, intramuscular or intra-articular) is an alternative to an NSAID.
- For prophylaxis (must not be started until the patient is asymptomatic): **allopurinol**;
  a uricosuric drug (e.g. **probenecid**, **sulfinpyrazone**), for patients allergic to **allopurinol**
- **Rasburicase** by intravenous infusion for prevention and treatment of acute hyperuricaemia in patients with haematological malignancy at risk of rapid lysis.

Allopurinol
Allopurinol is an analogue of hypoxanthine that reduces the synthesis of uric acid by competitive inhibition of xanthine oxidase (Fig. 27.5). The drug is first converted by xanthine oxidase to alloxanthine, which persists in the tissue for a considerable time, and is an effective non-competitive inhibitor of the enzyme. Some inhibition of de novo purine synthesis also occurs.

Allopurinol reduces the concentration of the relatively insoluble urates and uric acid in tissues, plasma and urine, while increasing the concentration of their more soluble precursors, the xanthines and hypoxanthines. The deposition of urate crystals in tissues (tophi) is reversed, and the formation of renal urate stones is inhibited. Allopurinol is the drug of choice in the long-term treatment of gout, but it actually exacerbates inflammation and pain in an acute attack (see later). **Febuxostat** has a similar mechanism of action and pharmacology.

Allopurinol is given orally and is well absorbed. Its half-life is 2–3 h: its active metabolite alloxanthine (see Fig. 27.5) has a half-life of 18–30 h. Renal excretion is a balance between glomerular filtration and probenecid-sensitive tubular reabsorption.

Acute attacks of gout occur commonly during the early stages of therapy (possibly as a result of physicochemical changes in the surfaces of urate crystals as these start to re-dissolve), so treatment with allopurinol is never initiated during an acute attack and is usually initially combined with an NSAID. Unwanted effects are otherwise few. GI disturbances, allergic reactions (mainly rashes) and some blood problems can occur but usually disappear if the drug is stopped. Potentially fatal skin diseases such as toxic epidermal necrolysis and Stevens–Johnson syndrome are rare – but devastating.

▼ Allopurinol increases the effect of **mercaptopurine**, an antimetabolite used in cancer chemotherapy, which is inactivated by xanthine oxidase (Ch. 57), and also that of azathioprine (see Table 27.2), which is metabolised to mercaptopurine. Allopurinol also enhances the effect of another anticancer drug, cyclophosphamide (Ch. 57). The effect of **warfarin** is increased because its metabolism is inhibited.

Uricosuric agents
Uricosuric drugs increase uric acid excretion by a direct action on the renal tubule (see Ch. 30). They remain useful as prophylaxis for patients with severe recurrent gout who have severe adverse reactions to allopurinol. Common drugs include probenecid and sulfinpyrazone (which also has NSAID activity). **Benzbromarone** is also available on a

Table 27.4 Comparison of some commonly used systemic antihistamines (H₁ antagonists).

Type	Drug	Common anti-allergic use	Comments
'Sedating'	Alimemazine	U	Strong sedative action. Sometimes used for anaesthetic premedication
	Chlorphenamine	AE, H, U	—
	Cinnarizine	—	Also used to treat nausea, vomiting, motion sickness
	Clemastine	H, U	—
	Cyclizine	—	Also used to treat nausea, vomiting, motion sickness
	Cyproheptadine	H, U	Also used for migraine
	Hydroxyzine	U	May cause QT interval prolongation
	Ketotifen	H	Mast cell 'stabilising' properties.
	Promethazine	H, U, AE	Strong sedative action. Also used to control nausea and vomiting
'Non-sedating'	Acrivastine	H, U	—
	Bilastine	H, U	—
	Cetirizine	H, U	—
	Desloratadine	H, U	Metabolite of loratadine. Long-lasting action
	Fexofenadine	H, U	'Cardio-safe' metabolite of terfenadine
	Levocetirizine	H, U	Isomer of cetirizine
	Loratidine	H, U	—
	Mizolastine	H, U	May cause QT interval prolongation
	Rupatadine	H, U	Also antagonises PAF (see Ch. 18)

AE, allergic emergency (e.g. anaphylactic shock); *H,* hay fever; *PAF,* platelet activating factor; *S,* sedation; *U,* urticaria and/or pruritus.
(Data from various sources, including the British National Formulary, 2017.)

named patient basis for treatment of patients with renal impairment. Treatment with uricosuric drugs is initiated together with an NSAID, as in the case of allopurinol. However, aspirin and salicylates antagonise the action of uricosuric drugs and should not be used concurrently.

Although not strictly speaking in this group, **rasburicase**, a preparation containing the enzyme uric acid oxidase, is sometimes used for aggressive treatment of gout. It oxidises uric acid in the blood to allantoin, which is more soluble and thus more readily excreted.

Colchicine

Colchicine is an alkaloid extracted from the autumn crocus. It has a beneficial effect in gouty arthritis and can be used both to prevent and to relieve acute attacks. It prevents migration of neutrophils into the joint apparently by binding to tubulin, resulting in the depolymerisation of the microtubules and reduced cell motility. Colchicine-treated neutrophils exhibit erratic locomotion often likened to a 'drunken walk'. Colchicine may also prevent the production, by neutrophils that have phagocytosed urate crystals, of a putative inflammatory glycoprotein. Other mechanisms may also be important in bringing about its effects. At higher doses than are used to treat gout, colchicine inhibits mitosis, carrying a risk of serious bone marrow depression.

Colchicine is given orally, and is excreted partly in the GI tract and partly in the urine.

The acute unwanted effects of colchicine during therapy are largely GI and include nausea, vomiting and abdominal pain. Severe diarrhoea[9] may be a problem and with large doses, or prolonged treatment, its antimitotic action may cause serious side effects, including GI haemorrhage, kidney damage, bone marrow depression and peripheral neuropathy.

ANTAGONISTS OF HISTAMINE

Antihistamines were introduced by Bovet and his colleagues in the 1930s, before the discovery of the four histamine receptor subtypes described in Ch. 18. By convention, the generic term 'antihistamine' usually refers only to the H₁-receptor antagonists that are used for treating various inflammatory and allergic conditions, and it is these drugs that are discussed in this section

Details of some typical systemic H₁-receptor antagonists are shown in Table 27.4. In addition to these, there are several others that are primarily used topically (e.g. in nasal sprays or eye drops) in the treatment of hay fever and other allergic symptoms. These include **antazoline, azelastine, epinastine, olapatadine** and **emedastine**. In addition

---

[9]Because the therapeutic margin is so small, it used to be said by rheumatologists that 'patients must run before they can walk'!

to their H_1 antagonist activities, some antihistamines (e.g. **ketotifen**) may also have 'mast cell stabilising' and other anti-inflammatory properties unrelated to histamine antagonism (see Assanasen & Naclerio, 2002).

Pharmacological actions

Conventionally, the antihistamines are divided into 'first-generation' drugs, which cross the blood–brain barrier and often have sedating actions, and 'second-generation' drugs, which broadly speaking, do not. Some of the original second-generation agents (e.g. **terfenadine**) exhibited some cardiac toxicity (e.g. *torsade de pointes*, see Ch. 22). While the risk was extremely low, it was increased when the drug was taken with grapefruit juice or with agents that inhibit cytochrome P450 in the liver (see Chs 10 and 58). These drugs were therefore withdrawn and replaced by 'third-generation cardio-safe' drugs (often active metabolites of the original drugs, e.g. **fexofenadine**).

▼ Pharmacologically, most of the effects of the H_1-receptor antagonists follow from the actions of histamine outlined in Chapter 18. In vitro, for example, they decrease histamine-mediated contraction of the smooth muscle of the bronchi, the intestine and the uterus. They inhibit histamine-induced increases in vascular permeability and bronchospasm in the guinea pig in vivo, but are unfortunately of little value in allergic bronchospasm in humans. The clinical uses of H_1-receptor antagonists are summarised in the clinical box.

Clinical uses of histamine H_1-receptor antagonists

- Allergic reactions (see Ch. 7):
  - non-sedating drugs (e.g. **fexofenadine**, **cetirizine**) are used for allergic rhinitis (hay fever) and urticaria
  - topical preparations may be used for insect bites
  - injectable formulations are useful as an adjunct to **adrenaline** (**epinephrine**) for severe drug hypersensitivity reactions and emergency treatment of anaphylaxis.
- As antiemetics (see Ch. 31):
  - prevention of motion sickness (e.g. **cyclizine**, **cinnarizine**)
  - other causes of nausea, especially labyrinthine disorders.
  - For sedation (see Ch. 45, e.g. **promethazine**).

The CNS 'side effects' of some older H_1-receptor antagonists are sometimes more clinically useful than the peripheral H_1-antagonist effects (e.g. **chlorphenamine**; see Table 27.4). When used to treat allergies, the sedative effects are generally unwanted, but there are other occasions (e.g. in small children approaching bedtime) when they are more desirable. Even under these circumstances, other CNS effects, such as dizziness and fatigue, are unwelcome. Others are anti-emetic and are used to prevent motion sickness (e.g. **promethazine**; see Ch. 31).

Several H_1-receptor antagonists show weak blockade of α_1 adrenoceptors (e.g. promethazine). **Cyproheptadine** is a 5-HT antagonist as well as an H_1-receptor antagonist and **rupatadine** is also a platelet activating factor (PAF) antagonist.

Pharmacokinetic aspects

Most orally active H_1-receptor antagonists are well absorbed and remain effective for 3–6 h, although there are some prominent exceptions (e.g. **loratidine**, which is converted to a long-acting metabolite). Most appear to be widely distributed throughout the body, but some do not penetrate the blood–brain barrier, for example the non-sedating drugs mentioned above (see Table 27.4). They are mainly metabolised in the liver and excreted in the urine.

Many antihistamines have peripheral anti-muscarinic side effects. The commonest of these is dryness of the mouth, but blurred vision, constipation and retention of urine can also occur. Unwanted effects that are not mechanism-based are also seen; GI disturbances are fairly common, while allergic dermatitis can follow topical application.

POSSIBLE FUTURE DEVELOPMENTS IN ANTIINFLAMMATORY THERAPY

Undoubtedly the most exciting area of current development is in biopharmaceuticals (see Ch. 5). The success of the anti-TNF and other biological agents has been very gratifying and development of antibodies that neutralise inflammogens or block key leukocyte receptors or adhesion molecules is likely to continue. The main problem with this sector is their cost and lack of oral availability. This places a severe strain on health care budgets and often prevents them from being used as a first-line therapy. Hopefully, ways will be found to reduce the cost of production and development of these important medicines.

Clearly a low-cost alternative to a neutralising anti-TNF antibody would be a welcome development. *TNF-converting enzyme* (TACE; at least two forms) cleaves membrane-bound TNF thus releasing the soluble active form, and so might be an attractive target. A number of putative small-molecule inhibitors of this enzyme are effective in animal models but have not transferred well to the clinic (see Sharma et al., 2013 for a review) although there remains general optimism about this approach (see for example Ouvry et al., 2017).

The disconcerting realisation that all NSAIDs (and coxibs) have cardiovascular side effects has raised further questions about our existing therapeutic arsenal.[10] The area was reviewed by Atkinson et al. (2013). One of the few real innovations in the beleaguered NSAID area has been the design and synthesis of derivatised NSAIDs – conventional NSAIDs that have NO-donating, or other, 'protective' groups attached. The ability of these drugs to release NO following hydrolysis in plasma and tissue fluid reduces the risk of ulcerogenic events and may increase the anti-inflammatory activity. One of these drugs (e.g. **naproxcinod**, an NO-releasing derivative of naproxen) is undergoing clinical trials. Along similar lines, a novel group of NSAIDs that release H_2S – another gaseous mediator with protective properties – is being investigated (Wallace et al., 2015), while Kirby et al. (2016) have proposed that simple arginate salts of NSAIDs may lack the unwanted cardiovascular side effects of their parent drugs. The quest for a 'safe' NSAID continues.

---

[10]This does not, of course, apply to low-dose aspirin.

REFERENCES AND FURTHER READING

NSAIDs and coxibs

Baigent, C.L., Blackwell, L., Collins, R., et al., 2009. Aspirin in the primary and secondary prevention of vascular disease: collaborative meta-analysis of individual participant data from randomised trials. Lancet 373, 1849–1860. (*An important study of the use of aspirin in the prevention of cardiovascular disease*)

Baron, J.A., Sandler, R.S., Bresalier, R.S., et al., 2006. A randomized trial of rofecoxib for the chemoprevention of colorectal adenomas. Gastroenterology 131, 1674–1682. (*The increased risk of cardiovascular events observed during this trial indirectly led to the discovery that all NSAIDs and coxibs elevate blood pressure*)

Chang, C.W., Horng, J.T., Hsu, C.C., Chen, J.M., 2016. Mean daily dosage of aspirin and the risk of incident Alzheimer's dementia in patients with type 2 diabetes mellitus: a nationwide retrospective cohort study in Taiwan. J. Diabetes Res. 2016, 9027484.

Conaghan, P.G., 2012. A turbulent decade for NSAIDs: update on current concepts of classification, epidemiology, comparative efficacy, and toxicity. Rheumatol. Int. 32, 1491–1502. (*Excellent update on NSAIDs, coxibs and associated toxicity*)

FitzGerald, G.A., Patrono, C., 2001. The coxibs, selective inhibitors of cyclooxygenase-2. N. Engl. J. Med. 345, 433–442. (*Excellent coverage of the selective COX-2 inhibitors*)

Flower, R.J., 2003. The development of COX-2 inhibitors. Nat. Rev. Drug Discov. 2, 179–191. (*Reviews the work that led up to the development of the COX-2 inhibitors; several useful diagrams*)

Fries, J.F., 1998. Quality-of-life considerations with respect to arthritis and nonsteroidal anti-inflammatory drugs. Am. J. Med. 104, 14S–20S, discussion 21S–22S.

Grosser, T., Fries, S., FitzGerald, G.A., 2006. Biological basis for the cardiovascular consequences of COX-2 inhibition: therapeutic challenges and opportunities. J. Clin. Invest. 116, 4–15. (*Influential paper showing that prostacyclin – as assessed by its urinary metabolites - is reduced by Cox-2 inhibitors. This was attributed to a decrease in vascular production with obvious consequences for cardiovascular health*)

Henry, D., Lim, L.L., Garcia Rodriguez, L.A., et al., 1996. Variability in risk of gastrointestinal complications with individual non-steroidal anti-inflammatory drugs: results of a collaborative meta-analysis. BMJ 312, 1563–1566. (*Substantial analysis of the gastrointestinal effects of non-selective NSAIDs*)

Kirkby, N.S., Reed, D.M., Edin, M.L., et al., 2015. Inherited human group IVA cytosolic phospholipase A2 deficiency abolishes platelet, endothelial, and leucocyte eicosanoid generation. FASEB J. 29, 4568–4578. (*The authors took advantage of an extremely rare mutation in a human subject to demonstrate that most prostacyclin metabolites found in the urine arose from the kidney, not the vasculature. Read in conjunction with Grosser et al. above*)

Kirkby, N.S., Tesfai, A., Ahmetaj-Shala, B., et al., 2016. Ibuprofen arginate retains eNOS substrate activity and reverses endothelial dysfunction: implications for the COX-2/ADMA axis. FASEB J. 30, 4172–4179.

Luong, C., Miller, A., Barnett, J., et al., 1996. Flexibility of the NSAID binding site in the structure of human cyclooxygenase-2. Nat. Struct. Biol. 3, 927–933. (*An important research paper detailing the crystal structure of COX-2 and the relevance of this to NSAID and coxib action. Essential reading if you are seriously interested in this topic*)

Ouellet, M., Percival, M.D., 2001. Mechanism of acetaminophen inhibition of cyclooxygenase isoforms. Arch. Biochem. Biophys. 387, 273–280. (*Proposes a solution to the paracetamol mystery*)

Patrignani, P., Patrono, C., 2016. Aspirin and cancer. J. Am. Coll. Cardiol. 68, 967–976. (*Excellent review of this interesting topic. Recommended*)

Prescott, L.F., 2000. Paracetamol, alcohol and the liver. Br. J. Clin. Pharmacol. 49, 291–301.

Ray, W.A., Varas-Lorenzo, C., Chung, C.P., et al., 2009. Cardiovascular risks of non-steroidal anti-inflammatory drugs in patients after hospitalization for serious coronary heart disease. Circ. Cardiovasc. Qual. Outcomes 2, 155–163. (*This paper, together with an editorial on pages 146–147 of the same issue, present and comment on the findings from observational studies on the cardiovascular risk of a range of coxibs and NSAIDs*)

Skjelbred, P., Løkken, P., Skoglund, L.A., 1984. Post-operative administration of acetaminophen to reduce swelling and other inflammatory events. Curr. Ther. Res. 35, 377–385. (*A study showing that paracetamol can have anti-inflammatory properties under some circumstances*)

Waldstein, S.R., Wendell, C.R., Seliger, S.L., Ferrucci, L., Metter, E.J., Zonderman, A.B., 2010. Nonsteroidal anti-inflammatory drugs, aspirin, and cognitive function in the Baltimore longitudinal study of aging. J. Am. Geriatr. Soc. 58, 38–43.

Vane, J.R., 1971. Inhibition of prostaglandin synthesis as a mechanism of action for aspirin-like drugs. Nat. New Biol. 231, 232–239. (*The definitive, seminal article that proposed cyclo-oxygenase inhibition as a mechanism of action for the aspirin-like drugs*)

Vane, J.R., Botting, R.M. (Eds.), 2001. Therapeutic Roles of Selective COX-2 Inhibitors. William Harvey Press, London, p. 584. (*Outstanding multi-author book covering all aspects of the mechanisms of action, actions, adverse effects and clinical role of COX-2 inhibitors in a range of tissues; excellent coverage though a bit dated now*)

Wallace, J.L., 2000. How do NSAIDs cause ulcer disease? Baillière's Best Pract. Res. Clin. Gastroenterol. 14, 147–159. (*Proposes an interesting idea concerning the role of the two COX isoforms in gastric homeostasis*)

Warner, T.D., Mitchell, J.A., 2004. Cyclooxygenases: new forms, new inhibitors, and lessons from the clinic. FASEB J. 18, 790–804. (*Excellent review of COX-1/-2 inhibitors and the relative merits of coxibs and the physiological role of COX-2*)

Warner, T.D., Mitchell, J.A., 2008. COX-2 selectivity alone does not define the cardiovascular risks associated with non-steroidal anti-inflammatory drugs. Lancet 371, 270–273. (*Thoughtful article about cardiovascular risk of NSAIDs*)

Antirheumatoid drugs

Alldred, A., Emery, P., 2001. Leflunomide: a novel DMARD for the treatment of rheumatoid arthritis. Expert Opin. Pharmacother. 2, 125–137. (*Useful review and update of this DMARD*)

Bondeson, J., 1997. The mechanisms of action of disease-modifying antirheumatic drugs: a review with emphasis on macrophage signal transduction and the induction of proinflammatory cytokines. Gen. Pharmacol. 29, 127–150. (*Detailed review examining possible modes of action of these drugs*)

Borel, J.F., Baumann, G., Chapman, I., et al., 1996. In vivo pharmacological effects of ciclosporin and some analogues. Adv. Pharmacol. 35, 115–246. (*Borel was instrumental in the development of ciclosporin*)

Chan, E.S., Cronstein, B.N., 2010. Methotrexate – how does it really work? Nat. Rev. Rheumatol. 6, 175–178. (*An in-depth investigation of the actions of what is probably the most widely employed DMARD. Good diagrams*)

Chandrashekara, S., 2013. Pharmacokinetic consideration of synthetic DMARDs in rheumatoid arthritis. Expert Opin. Drug Metab. Toxicol. 9, 969–981.

Cutolo, M., 2002. Effects of DMARDs on IL-1Ra levels in rheumatoid arthritis: is there any evidence? Clin. Exp. Rheumatol. 20 (5 Suppl. 27), S26–S31. (*Reviews the actions of DMARDs on the generation and release of the endogenous IL-1 antagonist. An interesting slant on the mechanism of action of these drugs*)

Davis, J.M., 3rd, Matteson, E.L., 2012. My treatment approach to rheumatoid arthritis. Mayo Clin. Proc. 87, 659–673. (*Written from the viewpoint of a practical clinician, this review explains the latest guidance on classifying pathotypes of rheumatoid arthritis and adjusting the many different types of treatment to suit the patient*)

Lodowska, J., Gruchlik, A., Wolny, D., Wawszczyk, J., Dzierzewicz, Z., Weglarz, L., 2015. The Effect of sulfasalazine and 5-aminosalicylic acid on the secretion of interleukin 8 by human colon myofibroblasts. Acta Pol. Pharm. 72, 917–921.

Rau, R., 2005. Have traditional DMARDs had their day? Effectiveness of parenteral gold compared to biologic agents. Clin. Rheumatol. 24, 189–202. (*Argues for a continuing place of DMARDs in the clinic despite the introduction of the new biopharmaceuticals*)

Smolen, J.S., Kalden, J.R., Scott, D.L., et al., 1999. Efficacy and safety of leflunomide compared with placebo and sulphasalazine in active rheumatoid arthritis: a double-blind, randomised, multicentre trial. Lancet 353, 259–260. (*Gives details of the results of a clinical trial showing the efficacy of leflunomide*)

Anticytokine drugs and other biopharmaceuticals

Arora, T., Padaki, R., Liu, L., et al., 2009. Differences in binding and effector functions between classes of TNF antagonists. Cytokine 45, 124–131. (*A research paper detailing the significance of the membrane-bound versus soluble TNF neutralising actions of the drugs*)

Bongartz, T., Sutton, A.J., Sweeting, M.J., et al., 2006. Anti-TNF antibody therapy in rheumatoid arthritis and the risk of serious infections and malignancies: systematic review and meta-analysis of rare harmful effects in randomized controlled trials. JAMA 295, 2275–2285. (*The title is self-explanatory*)

Carterton, N.L., 2000. Cytokines in rheumatoid arthritis: trials and tribulations. Mol. Med. Today 6, 315–323. (*Good review of agents modulating the action of TNF-α and IL-1; simple, clear diagram of cellular action of these cytokines, and summaries of the clinical trials of the agents in tabular form*)

Choy, E.H.S., Panayi, G.S., 2001. Cytokine pathways and joint inflammation in rheumatoid arthritis. N. Engl. J. Med. 344, 907–916. (*Clear description of the pathogenesis of rheumatoid arthritis, emphasising the cells and mediators involved in joint damage; excellent diagrams of the interaction of inflammatory cells and of the mechanism of action of anticytokine agents*)

Feldmann, M., 2002. Development of anti-TNF therapy for rheumatoid arthritis. Nat. Rev. Immunol. 2, 364–371. (*Excellent review covering the role of cytokines in rheumatoid arthritis and the effects of anti-TNF therapy written by one of the pioneers of this type of therapy*)

Fiorino, G., Allez, M., Malesci, A., Danese, E., 2009. Review article: anti TNF-alpha induced psoriasis in patients with inflammatory bowel disease. Aliment. Pharmacol. Ther. 29, 921–927. (*Deals with this rare and unexpected side effect of anti-TNF therapy*)

Jobanputra, P., Maggs, F., Deeming, A., et al., 2012. A randomised efficacy and discontinuation study of etanercept versus adalimumab (RED SEA) for rheumatoid arthritis: a pragmatic, unblinded, non-inferiority study of first TNF inhibitor use: outcomes over 2 years. BMJ Open 2, 1–9.

van der Kooij, S.M., le Cessie, S., Goekoop-Ruiterman, Y.P., et al., 2009. Clinical and radiological efficacy of initial vs delayed treatment with infliximab plus methotrexate in patients with early rheumatoid arthritis. Ann. Rheum. Dis. 68, 1153–1158.

Maini, R.N., 2005. The 2005 International Symposium on Advances in Targeted Therapies: what have we learned in the 2000s and where are we going? Ann. Rheum. Dis. 64 (Suppl. 4), 106–108. (*An updated review dealing with the role of cytokines in the pathogenesis of rheumatoid arthritis and the results of clinical trials with anti-TNF and anti-IL-1 therapy written by one of the pioneers of this type of therapy*)

O'Dell, J.R., 1999. Anticytokine therapy – a new era in the treatment of rheumatoid arthritis. N. Engl. J. Med. 340, 310–312. (*Editorial with excellent coverage of the role of TNF-α in rheumatoid arthritis; summarises the differences between infliximab and etanercept*)

Antihistamines

Assanasen, P., Naclerio, R.M., 2002. Antiallergic anti-inflammatory effects of H_1-antihistamines in humans. Clin. Allergy Immunol. 17, 101–139. (*An interesting paper that reviews several alternative mechanisms whereby antihistamines may regulate inflammation*)

Leurs, R., Blandina, P., Tedford, C., Timmerm, N.H., 1998. Therapeutic potential of histamine H_3 receptor agonists and antagonists. Trends Pharmacol. Sci. 19, 177–183. (*Describes the available H_3 receptor agonists and antagonists, and their effects in a variety of pharmacological models, with discussion of possible therapeutic applications*)

Simons, F.E.R., Simons, K.J., 1994. Drug therapy: the pharmacology and use of H_1-receptor-antagonist drugs. N. Engl. J. Med. 23, 1663–1670. (*A bit dated now but contains effective coverage of the topic from the clinical viewpoint*)

New directions

Atkinson, T.J., Fudin, J., Jahn, H.L., Kubotera, N., Rennick, A.L., Rhorer, M., 2013. What's new in NSAID pharmacotherapy: oral agents to injectables. Pain Med. 14 (Suppl. 1), S11–S17.

Moss, M.L., Sklair-Tavron, L., Nudelman, R., 2008. Drug insight: tumor necrosis factor-converting enzyme as a pharmaceutical target for rheumatoid arthritis. Nat. Clin. Pract. Rheumatol. 4, 300–309. (*Accessible review dealing with this potentially important concept. Some good diagrams*)

Ouvry, G., Berton, Y., Bhurruth-Alcor, Y., et al., 2017. Identification of novel TACE inhibitors compatible with topical application. Bioorg. Med. Chem. Lett. 27, 1848–1853.

Sharma, M., Mohapatra, J., Acharya, A., et al., 2013. Blockade of tumor necrosis factor-alpha converting enzyme (TACE) enhances IL-1-beta and IFN-gamma via caspase-1 activation: a probable cause for loss of efficacy of TACE inhibitors in humans? Eur. J. Pharmacol. 701, 106–113. (*A discussion of the prospects and pitfalls of low molecular-weight TNF inhibitors*)

Wallace, J.L., de Nucci, G., Sulaieva, O., 2015. Toward more GI-friendly anti-inflammatory medications. Curr. Treat. Options Gastroenterol. 13, 377–385.

28 Skin

OVERVIEW

With a surface area of about 1.6–1.8 m² and a weight of about 4.5 kg in the average adult, skin qualifies as the largest and heaviest organ in the body. It is also an important target for drug therapy as well as cosmetic and other agents. Here, we look at the structure of human skin and briefly review some common skin disorders. We then discuss some of the many types of drugs that act upon, or through, this organ.

INTRODUCTION

Skin is a complex organ with many roles.[1] Firstly, it acts as a barrier. Being impermeable to water, it prevents the loss of moisture from the body as well as the ingress of water and many other substances into the body. It also cushions underlying tissues against thermal and mechanical damage and shields them from ultraviolet radiation and infection. Even if microorganisms survive in the slightly acidic environment of the skin's surface, they cannot easily cross the outer barrier of the skin. In the event that they do, they encounter specialised immunological surveillance systems comprising *Langerhans cells*, a type of dendritic cell, as well as mast cells and other immunocompetent cell types.[2]

A second function is thermoregulation. Approximately 10% of the total blood volume is contained within the dense capillary networks of the skin. Skin arterioles, controlled by the sympathetic nervous system, regulate blood flow and heat loss from the skin. Sweat glands (*eccrine glands*) in the skin secrete, under cholinergic control, an aqueous fluid which, upon evaporation, increases heat loss.

In the presence of sunlight, vitamin D_3 (cholecalciferol) is synthesised in the *stratum basale* and *stratum spinosum* of skin. Absence of this vitamin caused by inadequate exposure to the ultraviolet (UV B) component of sunlight can lead to deficiency symptoms (see Ch. 37). The dark-coloured pigment *melanin*, which protects skin against excessive and potentially damaging solar radiation and which gives skin its characteristic colour, is produced by melanocytes in the basal dermal layer. Melanin granule formation is stimulated by sunlight to match the prevailing light intensity.

---

[1]As the American humourist and songwriter Alan Sherman so succinctly put it, 'Skin's the thing that if you've got it outside/It keeps your insides in'.
[2]Dendritic cells were named as such by Paul Langerhans who discovered them when a medical student in 1868. Because of their shape, he mistook them for nerve cells, but they are actually phagocytic antigen-presenting immune cells of the monocyte/macrophage lineage.

Skin is also a profoundly sensory organ. It is densely innervated with neurons, including specific nerve endings that signal pain, heat and cold; specialised receptors that detect touch (*Meissner corpuscles*) and pressure (*Pacinian corpuscles*) as well as itch – a sensation unique to skin with an interesting pharmacology. The cell bodies of cutaneous sensory nerves reside in the dorsal root ganglia.

Being highly visible, skin and its specialised appendages, hair and nails, play an important part in social and sexual signalling. As such, it is an important target for cosmetic preparations, camouflaging agents, suntan lotions, anti-ageing compounds and more. Because unsightly skin can cause problems of social adjustment or even frank psychiatric illness, the distinction between a therapeutic agent and a cosmetic preparation can become blurred. In fact, the market for 'cosmeceuticals' as they are called is huge: in the United States alone over US$8 billion was spent on these compounds (many of which lack any proof of efficacy) in 2012 (Nolan et al., 2012).

Here we look briefly at some common conditions affecting the skin and at some of the drugs used to treat them (Table 28.1). In most cases, these drugs also have other uses and their mechanisms of action are described elsewhere in the book, so the appropriate cross-references are given in Table 28.1. Inflammation is a common feature of skin diseases, and anti-inflammatory drugs, discussed in detail in Chapter 27, are often used. In some other instances, the drugs themselves, or their particular utility, are almost unique to skin pharmacology, so they will be explained in a little more detail. Drugs used to treat skin infections and cancers are discussed in Chapters 52, 54 and 57.

Topical application of drugs onto the skin can be used as a route for systemic administration (see Ch. 9), and also to treat the underlying tissues. For example, non-steroidal anti-inflammatory drugs (NSAIDs) applied topically can reduce the inflammation of underlying joints and connective tissue with less unwanted effects than those seen after systemic administration (Klinge & Sawyer, 2013). However, we will not deal in depth with this topic here.

STRUCTURE OF SKIN

Skin comprises three main layers: the outermost layer, the *epidermis*, a middle layer, the *dermis*, and the innermost layer, the *subdermis*, sometimes called the *hypodermis* or *subcutis* (Fig. 28.1).

The epidermis consists largely of keratinocytes. There are four layers of cells: the *stratum basale* is the innermost layer and lies adjacent to the *dermoepidermal junction*. It comprises mainly dividing keratinocytes interspersed with melanocytes. The latter cells produce granules of melanin in *melanosomes*, which are transferred to the dividing keratinocytes. As the keratinocytes divide and mature

Table 28.1 Drug treatment of some common skin disorders

Disease	Class	Examples	Comments	Chapter
Acne	Antibacterials	Erythromycin, clindamycin, various antiseptic agents	For mild–moderate acne. Usually topical but sometimes systemic treatment is also used	52
	Retinoids	Isotretinoin, adapalene, tretinoin	For more severe disease. Often combined with anti-infective agents. Sometimes systemic treatment is also used	—
	Androgen antagonists	Co-cyprindiol	For moderate–severe disease	36
Alopecia	Anti-androgen, vasodilator	Finasteride, minoxidil	Generally in men only	36, 23
Hirsutism	Inhibitor of DNA/RNA synthesis	Eflornithine	Usually in women only	57
Infections	Antibacterials	Bacitracin, metronidazole, mupirocin, neomycin sulfate, polymixins, retapamulin, sulfadiazine, silver salts	Usually given topically but some drugs may be given orally.	52
	Antivirals	Aciclovir, penciclovir		53
	Antifungal	Amorolfine, clotrimazole, econazole, griseofulvin, ketaconazole, miconazole, terbinafine, tioconazole		54
	Antiparasite	Topical parasiticides e.g. benzyl benzoate, dimeticone, malathion, permethrin, tazarotene	—	55
Pruritus	Antihistamines, topical anaesthetics and related drugs	Crotamiton, diphenhydramine, doxepin	Antihistamines may be given topically or orally. Sometimes a 'sedating' antihistamine is useful	18
Eczema	Glucocorticoids	Mild–potent (i.e. hydrocortisone, betamethasone esters)	May be combined with antibacterial or antifungal agent if infection is present	27, 34
	Retinoids	Alitretinoin, acitretin	Given orally. Only used if glucocorticoid therapy has failed	—
	Calcineurin inhibitors	Picrolimus, tacrolimus	Often topical but sometimes systemic. Used for more severe disease	27
Psoriasis	Vitamin D analogues	Calcipotriol, calcitriol, tacalcitol	DMARDS and anticytokine drugs used for severe cases	5, 7, 27
	Retinoids	Acitretin, alitretinoin, tazarotene	Oral retinoids sometimes used	—
	Glucocorticoids	Moderate–potent (i.e. hydrocortisone butyrate, clobetasol propionate)	May be combined with antibacterial or antifungal agent if infection is present	27, 34, 52, 54
	Calcineurin inhibitors	Picrolimus, tacrolimus	Maybe given topically or systemically. Usually used for severe cases	27
Rosacea	Antibacterials or α_2 adrenergic agents	Doxycycline, erythromycin, metronidazole, tetracycline or brimonidine	Glucocorticoids are contraindicated	52
Urticaria	Antihistamines	Diphenhydramine, doxepin	Usually given orally. Sometimes a 'sedating' antihistamine is useful	18
Warts	Keratolytic agents and others	Formaldehyde, imiquimod, podophyllotoxin, salicylic acid, silver nitrate	Many of these substances are found in proprietary wart treatments	—

DMARDs, disease-modifying antirheumatic drugs.

Fig. 28.1 A simplified diagram showing the structure of the skin. The skin comprises three main layers coloured differently in the right-hand drawing: epidermis *(dark red/brown)*; dermis *(pink)*; and subdermis *(yellow)*. On the left is an enlarged diagram of the complex outer, epidermal, layer. Not shown are the apocrine glands within the hair follicles.

they progress towards the skin surface. In the next layer, they form the *stratum spinosum* ('spiny' layer), so-called because *desmosomes* (intercellular protein links) begin to appear on the cells. Gradually, these cells begin to flatten adopting a *squamous* (scaly) morphology. They lose their nuclei and the cytoplasm acquires a granular appearance. Lying immediately above this is a thin translucent layer of tissue called the *stratum lucidum*. The outermost layer of skin is the *stratum corneum*. By now, individual keratinocytes are no longer viable because they have fused together (corni-fied). Most tissues have 10–30 layers of these hardened sheets of tissue. The *corneocytes*, as they are now called, are surrounded with a hydrated proteinaceous envelope. Lipid bilayers occupy the extracellular space providing a hydrophilic waterproof layer. The water and lipid content of skin is critical to its function. If the moisture content of the hydrated layer falls, the skin loses its supple properties and cracks. The keratinocytes are normally replenished about every 45 days (Bergstresser & Taylor, 1977) and so healthy skin constantly sheds the outer layer of cornified cells. If this does not occur, patches of dry skin begin to appear.

Below the epidermis lies the dermis. This layer varies in thickness. In some tissues, it is very thick (e.g. the palms and the soles of the feet) and in others, very thin (e.g. the eyelids). Histologically, the dermis comprises a *papillary layer* and a deeper *reticular layer*. The main cell types are fibroblasts. These produce and secrete important structural elements of the skin such as glycoproteins, which contribute to the hydration of the tissue, and collagen and elastin that provide strength and elasticity. Other types of cells associated with the immune system are also present (see Ch. 7). The dermis is richly endowed with blood vessels and lymphatics and densely innervated.

Hair follicles, sebaceous glands and *sweat glands* are embedded in the dermis. Hair follicles are lined with specialised cells that produce keratin and associated melanocytes that produce pigment for the growing hair shaft. Associated with each hair follicle is an *erector pili* muscle that causes the hair shaft to become erect. Cold, fear and other strong emotional stimuli trigger this response giving the sensation of 'goose bumps'. Sebaceous glands associated with hair follicles coat the hair with waxy substances. The growth of hair and the activity of these glands is controlled by androgens.

There are two types of sweat glands: *apocrine* glands are associated with hair, especially in the armpits and perineum. They empty their proteinaceous secretion into the hair follicle. *Eccrine* glands, on the other hand, are distributed over much of the skin surface.

The innermost layer of skin is the hypodermis or cutis. This comprises connective tissue and adipose tissue, which may be particularly thick at some anatomical locations (e.g. the abdomen).

COMMON DISEASES OF THE SKIN

▼ Here we briefly review some common skin disorders, focusing on those for which specific drug treatment is available.

ACNE

▼ The most common form of the disease occurs during puberty, especially in boys but also (and sometimes devastatingly) in girls. Changes in circulating androgens stimulate the sebaceous glands associated with hair follicles, which become enlarged and blocked with sebum and debris. The confined material may become infected, causing an inflammatory reaction that compounds the problem. Normally acne disappears after puberty but some forms may persist or manifest in later life and require long-term treatment. If severe, acne can cause irreversible scarring and considerable psychological misery.

Skin

Skin is the largest and heaviest organ in the body. It is composed of three main components:

- *The epidermis*. This is the outermost layer and is comprised of four layers of keratinocytes with interspersed melanocytes. Keratinocytes divide in the basal layer and migrate upwards to the skin surface where they form cornified layers. Lipids in the extracellular spaces confer water-repellent properties.
- *The dermis*. The middle layer is of variable thickness. It consists of fibroblasts that produce structural components such as collagen and elastin as well as immunocompetent cells. Hair follicles and sweat glands are also embedded in this layer and it is densely innervated with nerves, blood vessels and lymphatics.
- *The subdermis* (*hypodermis* or *hypocutis*). This comprises connective tissue and varying amounts of adipose tissue.

Skin has four main functions:

- *A barrier*. Skin prevents the egress or ingress of water, other chemicals and microorganisms. It also acts as a mechanical and thermal barrier and a shock absorber.
- *Thermoregulation*. Vasodilatation of the rich capillary network of the skin, in combination with sweating, increases the loss of heat whilst vasoconstriction has the reverse effect.
- *Vitamin D synthesis*. In the presence of sunlight, vitamin D_3 is synthesised by cells in the epidermal layer.
- *A sensory organ*. Skin contains abundant sensory receptors for touch, heat, cold, pain and itch. Information arising from these dermal receptors is one of the chief ways in which we interact with the outside world.

ROSACEA

▼ The diagnostic feature of rosacea is the presence of a chronic hyperaemia of the facial skin. There is often a characteristic pattern with the erythema spreading across the nose, the cheeks and forehead. The erythema is caused by vasodilatation and dilated blood vessels close to the surface of the skin are usually visible. The affected skin may become dry and flaky; there may be a stinging or burning sensation, and a tendency to flush in response to various stimuli, including exertion, emotional stress, heat, sunlight and spicy foods.

There is a genetic basis for the disorder. It is more prevalent in women than men and may be exacerbated during the menopause. The disease cannot be cured and the symptoms can be very long lasting and difficult to control, with both drug and other therapies playing a role. There is a debate about the cause of rosacea. Infection may be a trigger but rosacea could be a disorder of the innate immune system in which antimicrobial peptides in the skin are indirectly responsible for the symptoms (see Antal et al., 2011; Yamasaki & Gallo, 2011). Antibiotics or α_2-agonist treatment are usually the first choices where clinical management demands drugs.

BALDNESS AND HIRSUTISM

▼ There are two main types of baldness, *male-pattern baldness* (*androgenic alopecia*) and *alopecia areata*. Androgenic alopecia is caused by rising androgen levels and so particularly affects men after puberty; it starts with bi-temporal recession and progresses. Androgens inhibit the growth of hair on the scalp but stimulate it elsewhere (e.g. the face, chest, back, etc.). Alopecia areata is a condition where hair falls out in patches that come and go. Eventually, these patches may coalesce, leading to total baldness. The disease seems to be of auto-immune origin.

Hirsutism is common in men (who seldom complain) but is less socially acceptable in women. Once again, rising androgen levels are the cause, stimulating the growth of hair on areas of the body where it does not normally occur in women (e.g. the face); this is commoner in some ethnic groups and seldom pathological but can be a symptom of androgenising endocrine tumours (such as *Sertoli–Leydig cell tumours*, which are rare functioning ovarian tumours).

ECZEMA

▼ This is a generic term and refers to a common condition where the skin becomes dry, itchy, flaky and inflamed. The distribution is distinctive, namely on flexor surfaces (e.g. wrists, elbows and behind the knees, in contrast to psoriasis). There are several potential causes. *Atopic eczema* (also called *atopic dermatitis*) is the most common inflammatory skin disease, affecting about a quarter of all children and about 5% of adults. It is often seen in patients who also suffer from asthma or seasonal rhinitis (hay fever), although the long-held notion that this type of eczema is *primarily* an immunological disorder has rather little support. It tends to run in families, indicating a genetic susceptibility. *Contact dermatitis* arises when the skin becomes 'sensitised' to a particular antigen. Nickel sensitivity is a classic example: contact with the metal either provokes the production of antibodies or modifies structural elements of the epidermis so that autoantibodies are produced. This is more often seen in women because it is a common component of (less-expensive) jewellery.[3] The pathophysiology is now believed to stem from disordered barrier function leading to epidermal water loss, and a vicious cycle of itching and scratching with release of inflammatory mediators. Penetration of allergens and interaction with IgE-bearing Langerhans cells can add a Th2-mediated immunological component. *Xerotic eczema* refers to eczema that is produced when the skin dries out. This is more common in the winter months, especially amongst older people.

PRURITUS

▼ Pruritus – itch – is a common symptom of skin diseases, but can also occur with systemic disorders, such as obstructive jaundice, or neurological disorders such as shingles (herpes zoster). Some drugs (e.g. opioids) also can cause itching. There is a complex relationship between the neural systems that detect and transduce pain and itch (see Greaves & Khalifa, 2004; Ikoma et al., 2006) and there may be a dedicated population of nociceptors that function as 'itch transducers'.

Skin diseases commonly causing itch include eczema, urticaria and psoriasis. These are largely caused by the release of inflammatory mediators in the skin from mast cells (e.g. histamine, leukotrienes, proteases and cytokines).

URTICARIA

▼ This term refers to a range of inflammatory changes in the skin characterised by the presence of raised wheals or bumps ('nettle rash'). They are normally surrounded by a red margin and are intensely itchy. There are many known causes, including exposure to the sun (*solar urticaria*[4]), heat or cold, insect bites or stings, foodstuffs or infection, as well as some drugs. Many cases are allergic in nature while others have no known cause. A bizarre manifestation of urticaria seen in some people is *dermographia* – literally 'skin writing'. This is an exaggerated form of the 'triple response' seen after injecting histamine into the skin (see Ch. 18) and in this case provoked by scratching or in some cases simply rubbing or stroking the skin.

---

[3]However, the number of men suffering from the condition is rising because of the popularity of skin piercing. If body art is your thing, insist on high-quality nickel-free jewellery.
[4]Not to be confused with *miliaria* (prickly heat), which is caused by blocked sweat glands.

Urticaria is associated with inflammatory changes in the dermis, including mast cell degranulation and the accompanying release of mediators. It may co-exist with a related condition, *angio-oedema*, which primarily affects the blood vessels of the subdermal layer. Urticaria can resolve relatively rapidly or can persist for weeks (*chronic urticaria*). The disorder can be difficult to manage and even glucocorticoids, which suppress most inflammatory responses, are usually ineffective.

PSORIASIS

▼ Aside from atopic dermatitis, psoriasis is the most common inflammatory skin disease affecting about 2%–3% of Europeans. It is an autoimmune condition and a genetic component and several susceptibility loci have been identified, most of which are connected with the operation of the immune system. Cytokines such as TNF, IL-17 and IL-23 are involved in the inflammatory mechanism and anti-cytokine biopharmaceuticals can be used to treat severe manifestations of the disease (see Ch. 7). Histologically, it manifests as inflammation accompanied by hyper-proliferation of keratinocytes. This leads to an accumulation of scaly dead skin at the sites of the disease. The most common form is *plaque psoriasis*. This presents as areas of scaly silvery-white skin surrounded by red margins. The distribution is usually quite characteristic, with plaques first appearing on the knees and elbows. The lesions may be painful and are sometimes itchy (in fact the word 'psoriasis' originates from Greek and literally means 'itchy skin', though in contrast to eczema, itch is by no means a predominant symptom).

Psoriasis can also affect the fingernails, giving a 'pitted' appearance, and/or the joints (typically but not exclusively the distal interphalangeal joints) or other connective tissue (*psoriatic arthritis*).

Psoriasis is generally a life-long condition but one that can appear and disappear for no apparent reason. Stress is said to be a precipitating factor, as is dry skin. Several drugs (e.g. β-adrenoceptor antagonists, NSAIDs and **lithium**) are purported to precipitate bouts of the disease (Basavaraj et al., 2010).

WARTS

▼ Warts are caused by infection with one of the many types of human papilloma virus (HPV). They are characterised by small raised lesions with an irregular shape. As infection of the epidermis by the virus causes *hyperkeratinisation*, they also have a 'rough' feel.

The many varieties of HPV are usually specific for particular tissues, so different strains give rise to different types of warts at diverse anatomical locations. The most common type is usually found on hands and feet (e.g. as *verrucas*). Other types of HPV specifically infect the anogenital region, giving *anogenital warts*.

Most warts are benign in nature and disappear spontaneously after a period of time (usually weeks–months). However, some types of HPV are linked to cancers such as cervical cancer. It is hoped that, in time, immunisation against HPV will reduce the incidence of this disease.

OTHER INFECTIONS

▼ In addition to acne and rosacea, there are a number of other important bacterial skin infections that can be treated with appropriate antibiotics, either topical or systemic. These include superficial skin infections such as *erysipelas* and *impetigo*, and *cellulitis*, which is a more deep-seated infection mainly involving the dermis and subdermis usually of the lower limbs.

Fungal infections of the skin are a common problem. *Tinea, candida* and other infections (see Ch. 54) affect skin at several sites (e.g. *tinea pedis* – 'athlete's foot'). These infections are easy to catch and can be difficult to eradicate completely.

The most common viral infections affecting the skin are *herpes simplex* (cold sores) and *herpes zoster* (shingles), which can be treated with antiviral drugs (see Ch. 53). The most common parasite infections of the skin are head lice (*Pediculus humanis capitus*), crab lice (*Pthirus pubis*) and scabies (*Sarcoptes scabiei*).

DRUGS ACTING ON SKIN

FORMULATION

Targeting drugs to the skin is both easy and difficult. Unlike most therapeutic situations, drugs can be applied directly to the diseased tissue in ointments, solutions, creams, pastes or dusting powders, etc. There is an important caveat, however: since skin is a highly effective barrier, it can prevent the entry of many medicinal agents and this can pose a problem. To reach its site of action (often the lower layer of the epidermis or the dermis), a drug has to pass through the epidermal layer with its highly enriched lipid and aqueous environment. The transdermal delivery of drugs is therefore a highly specialised topic (see Ch. 9). Generally speaking, absorption is facilitated if the molecule is predominately hydrophobic in nature: thus, for example, glucocorticoids are often derivatised with fatty acid esters to render them more easily absorbed. The use of a waterproof *occlusion dressing* to cover the skin after applying the drug improves absorption by keeping the epidermis fully hydrated.

The vehicle in which the drug is dissolved is also important. Creams and ointments – essentially stable oil/water emulsions – can be tailored to individual drugs. For example, **tacrolimus** formulated as an ointment can be used topically on the skin, whilst an oil-in-water is better for a water-soluble drug such as an NSAID. The appearance and odour of the formulated drug are also important. Most patients would rather take a tablet than apply creams that may be greasy, smelly or unsightly to large areas of skin (see Tan et al., 2012).

The physical condition of the skin is important in maintaining its barrier function and various agents can be used to protect the skin and promote repair. These include *emollients*, which re-hydrate the skin and *barrier creams* that help to prevent damage from irritants. Use of such agents is often indicated alongside treatment with drugs.

Many new ideas for formulating drugs for passage across the skin are under investigation, including the use of 'nanocarriers' and other sophisticated chemical measures (see Reis et al., 2017).

PRINCIPAL DRUGS USED IN SKIN DISORDERS

Many drugs in the dermatological arsenal are also used to treat other diseases and their mechanism of action is the same. The use of agents described below to treat specific skin disorders is shown in Table 28.1. We refer the reader to other chapters in the book where information about these agents may be found. Other drugs, such as analogues of vitamins A and D, are rather specific to skin pharmacology.

ANTIMICROBIAL AGENTS

Chapters 51–56 deal in depth with the mechanism of action of this group of drugs. Antibiotics can be applied topically in diseases such as impetigo and acne, or given systemically in the case of cellulitis or rosacea. Fungal infections of the skin are generally treated with topical fungicidal drugs but oral preparations of **ketoconazole** may be used under some circumstances. Herpes simplex infections may be

> **Drugs and the skin**
>
> *Formulation*. Because the skin comprises a unique combination of hydrophobic/hydrophilic structures, many drugs are not absorbed and special formulations may be necessary to promote penetration.
>
> Many drugs used for skin conditions are also used to treat disorders in other organs. The main groups are:
> - *Glucocorticoids*. Widely used to treat psoriasis, eczema and pruritus because of their anti-inflammatory properties. They are usually specially formulated to enhance topical penetration.
> - *Antimicrobial agents*. Used topically or systemically to treat skin infections (e.g. acne, impetigo, cellulitis and rosacea).
> - *Hormone antagonists*. Androgen antagonists are used topically or systemically to treat male-pattern baldness or hirsutism in women.
> - *Vitamin D derivatives*. Drugs such as **calcitriol**, **calcipotriol** and **tacalcitol** are used to treat psoriasis.
>
> Some drugs are used almost exclusively for skin disorders. These include:
> - *Retinoids*. These are derivatives of vitamin A and include **tretinoin**, **isotretinoin**, **alitretinoin**, **tazarotene** and **adapalene**. They are used to treat acne, eczema and psoriasis. They are usually given topically, but can be given systemically.

treated with topical or systemic **acyclovir** or **penciclovir** (see Ch. 53).

GLUCOCORTICOIDS AND OTHER ANTI-INFLAMMATORY AGENTS

As one might predict, antihistamines (Ch. 18) are useful when controlling mild pruritus, at least in some circumstances, e.g. eczema, insect bites and mild inflammation. Another topical drug which is useful in treating pruritus is **crotamiton**. This acts rapidly and has long-lasting effects. The mechanism of action is not known.

However, the main agents for treating inflammation of the skin are the glucocorticoids. These drugs are widely used to treat psoriasis, eczema and to suppress pruritus. Their general mechanism of action is described in Chapters 3, 27 and 34. Preparations used in dermatological practice are often formulated as fatty acid esters of the active drugs. This promotes their absorption through the highly hydrophobic layers of the skin but also alters their efficacy: for example, the potency of topical **hydrocortisone** on the skin is greatly enhanced by formulating it as a butyrate ester.

▼ Whilst schemes around the world vary, the convention is to classify these drugs by potency. For example:
- *Mild*, e.g. hydrocortisone;
- *Moderate*, e.g. **alclometasone dipropionate**, **clobetasone butyrate**, **fludroxycortide** and **fluocortolone**;
- *Potent*, e.g. **beclomethasone dipropionate**, **betamethasone** (various esters) **fluocinolone acetonide, fluocinonide, fluticasone propionate**, **mometasone fuorate** and **triamcinolone acetonide**;
- *Very potent*, e.g. **clobetasol propionate** and **diflucortolone valerate**.

The choice of glucocorticoid depends upon the severity of the disease and, because the thickness of skin varies from one location to the other, its anatomical site. They are sometimes used in combination with antibacterial or fungicidal drugs if they are to be used at the site of an infection.

The action of glucocorticoids on the skin is similar in mechanism to their effect elsewhere in the body. They are potent inhibitors of the release of inflammatory mediators from mast cells, of neutrophil activation and emigration, and immune cell activation (see Chs 7 and 27). Their topical application produces vasoconstriction in the skin causing a characteristic 'blanching' reaction.[5] The mechanism is unknown.

Unwanted effects. Generally speaking, short-term treatment with low potency steroid preparations is safe; some hydrocortisone formulations are available from pharmacies without prescription. There are potentially serious side effects associated with prolonged usage or with the more potent members of the class, however. These include:

- *Steroid 'rebound'*. If topical steroid therapy is suddenly discontinued, the underlying disease often returns in a more aggressive form. This is probably because the glucocorticoid receptor is down-regulated during topical treatment and can no longer respond to circulating glucocorticoids, which maintain an anti-inflammatory 'tone', when treatment is withdrawn. Gradually tapering the drug can avoid this problem.
- *Skin atrophy*. Catabolic effects of glucocorticoids (Ch. 34) can lead to atrophy of the skin, including stretch marks (striae) and small visible vessels (telangiectases), that is only partially reversible upon stopping treatment.
- *Systemic effects*. Systemic absorption can theoretically cause depression of the hypothalamic–pituitary–adrenal axis, as described in Ch. 34, but this does not seem to constitute a significant risk in normal clinical practice (Castela et al., 2012).
- *Spread of infection*. Because glucocorticoids suppress the immune system, there is a danger that they may encourage or reactivate infection. For this reason they are contraindicated in acne, where there is a co-existent infection.
- *'Steroid rosacea' (skin reddening and pimples)* is a recognised problem when treating facial skin with potent glucocorticoids.

For more serious cases of eczema or psoriasis or where glucocorticoids are ineffective, topical or systemic application of immunosuppressants such as **ciclosporin, pimecrolimus** or tacrolimus may be successful (Ch. 27). The use (often 'off label') of biopharmaceuticals such as **adalimumab** and **infliximab** and other 'cytokine modulators' by specialists in severe cases is increasing and looks very promising (see Williams, 2012; Noda et al., 2015).

DRUGS USED TO CONTROL HAIR GROWTH

Hair growth in both sexes is driven by androgens but so is male-pattern baldness. Because of this, androgen antagonists, or compounds that modulate androgen metabolism, can be used to treat both hirsutism in women and androgenic alopecia in men.

---

[5]This interesting observation was used by Cornell and Stoughton in 1985 as the basis for the first quantitative assay of glucocorticoid potency in man.

Co-cyprindol is mixture of an anti-androgen, **cyproterone acetate**, and a female sex hormone, **ethinylestrodiol**. Antagonising androgenic actions reduces sebum production by sebaceous glands and also hair growth (which is androgen-dependent), so it can be used for treating acne as well as hirsutism in women. Unwanted effects include venous thromboembolism and it is contraindicated in women with a family history of cardiovascular disease.

Finasteride inhibits the enzyme (5α-reductase) that converts testosterone to the more potent androgen, dihydrotestosterone (see Ch. 36). It is used topically (usually in combination with **minoxidil**) for the treatment of androgenic alopecia, as well as orally for prostatic hypertrophy. The treatment takes months to produce real changes. Unwanted effects resulting from its action on androgen metabolism include a reduction in libido, possibly impotence and tenderness of the breasts.

Eflornithine was originally developed as an antiprotozoal drug (see Ch. 55). It can be used topically to treat hirsutism because it irreversibly inhibits *ornithine decarboxylase* in hair follicles. This interrupts cell replication and the growth of new hair. Unwanted effects include skin reactions and acne.

Minoxidil is a vasodilator drug that was originally developed for treating hypertension (see Ch. 23). Applied topically, it is converted in hair follicles to a more potent metabolite, minoxidil sulfate (some preparations contain this salt). Perhaps because of its ability to increase blood supply to hair follicles, it stimulates growth of new hair and the progression of the new follicle through successive phases of the cell cycle (Ch. 6). Existing follicles, usually stalled in their resting (telogen) phase, must first be 'shed' to make way for new, rapidly growing follicles, so initial hair loss following treatment is a frequent, unwelcome – and rather alarming – action of the drug. Other unwanted effects

are few but some local irritation may occur. Hair loss recurs when topical application is discontinued.

RETINOIDS

Disturbances in vitamin A metabolism are known to result in skin pathology. The vitamin is normally acquired in ester form from dietary sources. It is converted to *retinol* in the gut and this seems to be a storage form of the vitamin.

Vitamin A has many biological roles. As *retinal*, it is an essential component of rhodopsin and hence crucial for normal vision. However, it can also undergo an irreversible oxidation to *retinoic acid*, which lacks any effects on the visual system, but has potent effects on skin homeostasis.

The retinoid drugs are derivatives of retinoic acid (Fig. 28.2). The principal examples are **acitretin, adapalene, alitretinoin, isotretinoin, tretinoin, tazarotene**. They are widely used (sometimes in combination with other drugs) for the treatment of acne, eczema and psoriasis. Topical application is the usual route of administration but oral therapy is sometimes used for severe cases.

Most workers believe that retinoids act by binding to RXR and RAR nuclear receptors (see Ch. 3 and Fig. 28.2) in their target cells, which include keratinocytes and the cells of sebaceous glands, although some have questioned this mechanism (Arechalde & Saurat, 2000). Retinoid binding proteins (RBP) on the surface of, and within, the cell aid in transport of the molecule to its receptor and facilitate its eventual catabolism (Napoli, 2017). The main dermatological actions of retinoids include modulation of epidermal cell growth and reduction in sebaceous gland activity and sebum production. They also have pleiotropic actions on the adaptive and innate immune system that produce a net anti-inflammatory effect (Fisher & Voorhees, 1996; Orfanos et al., 1997).

Fig. 28.2 The retinoid pathway. Vitamin A (retinol) is acquired largely through dietary sources and is reversibly converted to retinal (retinaldehyde). This may be combined with opsin to produce the visual pigment rhodopsin or irreversibly oxidised to retinoic acid. The latter species can interact with nuclear receptors (RXR and RAR; see Ch. 3) to produce changes in genes that modulate keratinocyte differentiation, reduce the size and output of sebaceous glands and exert a general anti-inflammatory action. The synthetic congeners acitretin, adapalene, alitretinoin, isotretinoin, tazarotene and tretinoin can act at the RXR and RAR, also producing potent actions in skin disorders such as acne and psoriasis.

Unwanted effects. After oral administration, retinoids may cause dry or flaky skin, stinging or burning sensations and joint pains, possibly because they can activate the TRPV1 receptor; (Yin et al., 2013). Retinoids are teratogenic (this is linked to the effects of retinoids on epidermal differentiation that underlie their efficacy) and can be used in women only in the presence of suitable contraception (see Chs 36 & 58).

VITAMIN D ANALOGUES

Vitamin D is actually a mixture of several related substances. Although classed as a 'vitamin' and therefore by implication an essential dietary factor, vitamin D_3 (cholecalciferol) is synthesised by the skin in the presence of sufficient sunlight (in fact, *phototherapy* is an important therapeutic modality in some skin disorders for this and other reasons). Other forms of the vitamin (e.g. D_2) can be obtained from the diet. The vitamin plays a crucial role in calcium and phosphate metabolism and bone formation (see Ch. 37). It also has complex regulatory actions on the immune system, reducing the activity of the adaptive system but increasing the activity of the innate immune system (Di Filippo et al., 2015; Trochoutsou et al., 2015).

The biologically active metabolite *calcitriol* (see Ch. 37) is synthesised in the body by a multi-step process that requires transformations in the liver and kidney (Fig. 37.4). At the molecular level, vitamin D and its analogues act though the VDR group of nuclear receptors (Ch. 3) in keratinocytes, fibroblasts, Langerhans cells and sebaceous gland cells, to modulate gene transcription. Amongst the effects seen after treatment are antiproliferative and pro-differentiation actions on keratinocytes, increased apoptosis of plaque keratinocytes (Tiberio et al., 2009) and the inhibition of T-cell activation (Tremezaygues & Reichrath, 2011).

The main analogues used are **calcitriol** itself, **calcipotriol** and **tacalcitol**. Their principal clinical use is treating psoriasis. Oral administration is possible but they are generally administered topically, sometimes in combination with a glucocorticoid.

Unwanted effects. There is always a concern about the possible effects of the drugs on bone and they should be avoided in patients who have problems related to calcium or bone metabolism. Topical application can lead to skin irritation.

AGENTS ACTING BY OTHER MECHANISMS

Many ancillary agents are used in dermatology, including topical antiseptics, emollients, soothing lotions and other substances. Amongst this group are '**coal tars**', which are poorly defined mixtures containing thousands of aromatic hydrocarbons generated during the conversion of coal to coke or gas and which contain chemicals that formed the basis for many early medicines. Coal tars have been used in dermatological practice for decades. Though their mechanism of action is unknown, they can bring about a useful therapeutic benefit in eczema, psoriasis and some other skin conditions, and are often the first agents to be tried. As one might expect, given their origin, coal tars contain carcinogenic substances but in clinical use, the risk appears to be slight (Roelofzen et al., 2010). Preparations containing coal tars are applied topically.

Amongst other drugs unique to skin pharmacology are **salicylic acid** and **podophyllotoxin**. Topical salicylic acid has a *keratolytic* effect in situations when excess skin is being produced (e.g. warts), causing epidermal layers to be shed. It is a common ingredient of numerous proprietary wart removers. Podophyllotoxin is a toxin extracted from plants of the podophyllum family. It is usually reserved for treating anogenital warts. It is applied topically and prevents the excess growth of skin, probably because it inhibits tubulin polymerisation and hence arrests the normal cell cycle.

Another agent used for anogenital warts is **imiquimod**. This drug is an immune modifier and is also used for the topical treatment some types of skin cancer (e.g. basal cell carcinoma). Its mechanism of action is not known but it may increase immune surveillance mechanisms. Unwanted effects include local skin reactions.

CONCLUDING REMARKS

Despite the plethora of preparations available to treat skin disorders, there is clearly still an unfilled therapeutic need in several areas (e.g. rosacea) and, as always, reducing the unwanted effects of existing drugs is a further worthwhile objective that would greatly enhance their clinical utility. Some of the most interesting ideas have arisen from reconsidering the design of the glucocorticoids, vitamin D analogues and especially the retinoids. All these drugs act predominantly through nuclear receptors and recent thinking suggests that differentiating the mechanisms of transrepression and transactivation of genes by these drugs may be an achievable goal. Clearly, the prospect of separating the calcaemic from the anti-inflammatory effects of vitamin D analogues (Tremezaygues & Reichrath, 2011) and improving the selectivity of retinoids (Orfanos et al., 1997) are very attractive therapeutic goals. Progress towards separating the useful from the unwanted effects of the glucocorticoids is already apparently yielding fruit (see Ch. 34 for a discussion of this).

It is perhaps surprising that 'itch' is still such a problem. Various new drug targets (e.g. NK_1-receptor antagonists, see Ch. 19) have been identified for treating chronic itch (reviewed in Benecke et al., 2013) but have not yet reached the market.

The search for new drugs to treat psoriasis and atopic dermatitis has largely focused upon the actions of biopharmaceuticals and the use of other immunomodulatory drugs (see Gniadecki & Calverley, 2002; Pastore et al., 2008; Noda et al., 2015).

REFERENCES AND FURTHER READING

Antal, A.S., Dombrowski, Y., Koglin, S., Ruzicka, T., Schauber, J., 2011. Impact of vitamin D3 on cutaneous immunity and antimicrobial peptide expression. Dermatoendocrinol. 3, 18–22. (*This paper explores the idea that, in addition to their protective role, antimicrobial peptides (cathelicidins) in the skin may actually cause some skin diseases such as* rosacea. *The paper also suggests that the inhibitory action of vitamin D analogues on cathelicidin production is a potential mechanism of action of these drugs*)

Arechalde, A., Saurat, J.H., 2000. Management of psoriasis: the position of retinoid drugs. Biodrugs 13, 327–333. (*Discusses the therapeutic action of retinoids, especially tazarotene, and concludes that the mechanism of action is not exclusively through binding to RXR and RAR receptors*)

Basavaraj, K.H., Ashok, N.M., Rashmi, R., Praveen, T.K., 2010. The role of drugs in the induction and/or exacerbation of psoriasis. Int. J. Dermatol. 49, 1351–1361. (*The title here is self-explanatory. Also explores the mechanisms by which drugs provoke the disease*)

Benecke, H., Lotts, T., Stander, S., 2013. Investigational drugs for pruritus. Expert Opin. Investig. Drugs 22, 1167–1179. (*Could be read in conjunction with the paper by Ikoma et al. – below*)

Bergstresser, P.R., Taylor, J.R., 1977. Epidermal 'turnover time' – a new examination. Br. J. Dermatol. 96, 503–509.

Castela, E., Archier, E., Devaux, S., et al., 2012. Topical corticosteroids in plaque psoriasis: a systematic review of risk of adrenal axis suppression and skin atrophy. J. Eur. Acad. Dermatol. Venereol. 26 (Suppl. 3), 47–51. (*This is a systemic literature review of the area and an analysis of data from many studies*)

Cornell, R.C., Stoughton, R.B., 1985. Correlation of the vasoconstriction assay and clinical activity in psoriasis. Arch. Dermatol. 121, 63–67.

Di Filippo, P., Scaparrotta, A., Rapino, D., et al., 2015. Vitamin D supplementation modulates the immune system and improves atopic dermatitis in children. Int. Arch. Allergy Immunol. 166, 91–96. (*The title is self-explanatory but this paper also explains how vitamin D alters the immune system. Easy to read*)

Fisher, G.J., Voorhees, J.J., 1996. Molecular mechanisms of retinoid actions in skin. FASEB J. 10, 1002–1013. (*Easy-to-read very readable review of retinoid action in the skin and a discussion of in vitro and in vivo models of retinoid action*)

Gniadecki, R., Calverley, M.J., 2002. Emerging drugs in psoriasis. Expert Opin. Emerg. Drugs 7, 69–90. (*Deals mainly with biological and anticytokine drugs as potential new therapies*)

Greaves, M.W., Khalifa, N., 2004. Itch: more than skin deep. Int. Arch. Allergy Immunol. 135, 166–172.

Ikoma, A., Steinhoff, M., Stander, S., Yosipovitch, G., Schmelz, M., 2006. The neurobiology of itch. Nat. Rev. Neurosci. 7, 535–547. (*A comprehensive review of the neural pathways and local mediators of pruritus and itch. Excellent diagrams. Highly recommended*)

James, K.A., Burkhart, C.N., Morrell, D.S., 2009. Emerging drugs for acne. Expert Opin. Emerg. Drugs 14, 649–659.

Klinge, S.A., Sawyer, G.A., 2013. Effectiveness and safety of topical versus oral nonsteroidal anti-inflammatory drugs: a comprehensive review. Phys. Sportsmed. 41, 64–74.

Naldi, L., Raho, G., 2009. Emerging drugs for psoriasis. Expert Opin. Emerg. Drugs 14, 145–163.

Napoli, J.L., 2017. Cellular retinoid binding-proteins, CRBP, CRABP, FABP5: Effects on retinoid metabolism, function and related diseases. Pharmacol. Ther. 173, 19–33. (*Interesting review about the role of intracellular binding proteins in retinoid action. Worth reading if you want to dig deeper into the subject*)

Noda, S., Krueger, J.G., Guttman-Yassky, E., 2015. The translational revolution and use of biologics in patients with inflammatory skin diseases. J. Allergy Clin. Immunol. 135, 324–336. (*Useful review of the use of biologics in skin diseases focusing on psoriasis and atopic dermatitis. Some useful diagrams. The immunology is somewhat high powered*)

Nolan, K.A., Marmur, E.S., 2012. Over-the-counter topical skincare products: a review of the literature. J. Drugs Dermatol. 11, 220–224.

Orfanos, C.E., Zouboulis, C.C., Almond-Roesler, B., Geilen, C.C., 1997. Current use and future potential role of retinoids in dermatology. Drugs 53, 358–388.

Pastore, S., Gubinelli, E., Leoni, L., Raskovic, D., Korkina, L., 2008. Biological drugs targeting the immune response in the therapy of psoriasis. Biologics 2, 687–697.

Reis, C.P., Rijo, P., Pereira, P., Antunes, A.F., 2017. Nanosystems for skin delivery: from drugs to cosmetics. Curr. Drug Metab. 18, 412–425.

Ritter, J.M., 2012. Drugs and the skin: psoriasis. Br. J. Clin. Pharmacol. 74, 393–395. (*Succinct and easily readable introduction to the treatment of psoriasis focusing on the role of cytokines in the disease mechanism and the utility of new biologicals. Good diagram. Highly recommended*)

Roelofzen, J.H., Aben, K.K., Oldenhof, U.T., et al., 2010. No increased risk of cancer after coal tar treatment in patients with psoriasis or eczema. J. Invest. Dermatol. 130, 953–961.

Schoepe, S., Schacke, H., May, E., Asadullah, K., 2006. Glucocorticoid therapy-induced skin atrophy. Exp. Dermatol. 15, 406–420. (*Good review of one of what is one of the main adverse effects of glucocorticoid therapy for skin disorders, together with a discussion of how this can be minimised*)

Tan, X., Feldman, S.R., Chang, J., Balkrishnan, R., 2012. Topical drug delivery systems in dermatology: a review of patient adherence issues. Expert Opin. Drug Deliv. 9, 1263–1271.

Tiberio, R., Bozzo, C., Pertusi, G., et al., 2009. Calcipotriol induces apoptosis in psoriatic keratinocytes. Clin. Exp. Dermatol. 34, 972–974.

Tremezaygues, L., Reichrath, J., 2011. Vitamin D analogs in the treatment of psoriasis: Where are we standing and where will we be going? Dermatoendocrinol. 3, 180–186. (*A very useful account of the biosynthesis and role of vitamin D and the action of its analogues in the regulation of skin inflammation. Recommended*)

Trochoutsou, A.I., Kloukina, V., Samitas, K., Xanthou, G., 2015. Vitamin-D in the immune system: genomic and non-genomic actions. Mini Rev. Med. Chem. 15, 953–963.

Williams, S.C., 2012. New biologic drugs get under the skin of psoriasis. Nat. Med. 18, 638. (*One-pager. Short account of the latest candidate biologicals used in the treatment of psoriasis*)

Yamasaki, K., Gallo, R.L., 2011. Rosacea as a disease of cathelicidins and skin innate immunity. J. Investig. Dermatol. Symp. Proc. 15, 12–15. (*Could be read in conjunction with the paper by Antal et al. – above*)

Yin, S., Luo, J., Qian, A., et al., 2013. Retinoids activate the irritant receptor TRPV1 and produce sensory hypersensitivity. J. Clin. Invest. 123, 3941–3951.

Respiratory system

29

OVERVIEW

Basic aspects of respiratory physiology (regulation of airway smooth muscle, pulmonary vasculature and glands) are considered as a basis for a discussion of pulmonary disease and its treatment. We devote most of the chapter to asthma, dealing first with pathogenesis and then the main drugs used in its treatment and prevention – inhaled bronchodilators and anti-inflammatory agents. We also discuss chronic obstructive pulmonary disease (COPD), as well as idiopathic pulmonary fibrosis. There are short sections on allergic emergencies, surfactants and the treatment of cough. Other important pulmonary diseases, such as bacterial infections (e.g. tuberculosis and acute pneumonias) and malignancies, are addressed in Chapters 52 and 57, respectively. Antihistamines, important in treatment of hay fever, are covered in Chapter 27 and pulmonary hypertension is discussed in Chapter 23.

THE PHYSIOLOGY OF RESPIRATION

CONTROL OF BREATHING

Respiration is controlled by spontaneous rhythmic discharges from the respiratory centre in the medulla, modulated by input from pontine and higher central nervous system (CNS) centres and vagal afferents from the lungs. Various chemical factors affect the respiratory centre, including the partial pressure of carbon dioxide in arterial blood (P_ACO_2) by an action on medullary chemoreceptors, and of oxygen (P_AO_2) by an action on the chemoreceptors in the carotid bodies.

Some voluntary control can be superimposed on the automatic regulation of breathing, implying connections between the cortex and the motor neurons innervating the muscles of respiration. Bulbar poliomyelitis and certain lesions in the brain stem result in loss of the automatic regulation of respiration without loss of voluntary regulation.[1]

REGULATION OF MUSCULATURE, BLOOD VESSELS AND GLANDS OF THE AIRWAYS

Irritant receptors and non-myelinated afferent nerve fibres respond to chemical irritants and cold air, and also to

---

[1]Referred to as *Ondine curse*. Ondine was a water nymph who fell in love with a mortal. When he was unfaithful to her, the king of the water nymphs put a curse on him – that he must stay awake in order to breathe. When exhaustion finally supervened and he fell asleep, he died. Such patients are treated with mechanical ventilation. In less extreme forms, patients whose respiratory centre is relatively insensitive hypoventilate and become hypoxic when they fall asleep, leading to multiple awakenings during the night.

inflammatory mediators. Efferent pathways controlling the airways include cholinergic parasympathetic nerves and non-noradrenergic non-cholinergic (NANC) inhibitory nerves (see Ch. 13). Inflammatory mediators (see Ch. 18) and other bronchoconstrictor mediators also have a role in diseased airways.

The tone of bronchial muscle influences airway resistance, which is also affected by the state of the mucosa and activity of the submucosal mucus-secreting glands in patients with asthma and bronchitis. Airway resistance can be measured indirectly by instruments that record the volume or flow of forced expiration. FEV_1 is the forced expiratory volume in 1 second. The peak expiratory flow rate (PEFR) is the maximal flow (expressed as L/min) after a full inhalation; this is simpler to measure at the bedside than FEV_1, which it follows closely.

EFFERENT PATHWAYS

Autonomic innervation

The autonomic innervation of human airways is reviewed by van der Velden and Hulsmann (1999).

Parasympathetic innervation. Parasympathetic innervation of bronchial smooth muscle predominates. Parasympathetic ganglia are embedded in the walls of the bronchi and bronchioles, and the postganglionic fibres innervate airway smooth muscle, vascular smooth muscle and glands. Five types of muscarinic (M) receptors are present (see Ch. 14, Table 14.2). M_3 receptors are pharmacologically the most important in airways disease. They are found on bronchial smooth muscle and gland cells, and mediate bronchoconstriction and mucus secretion. M_1 receptors are localised in ganglia and on postsynaptic cells, and facilitate nicotinic neurotransmission, whereas M_2 receptors are inhibitory autoreceptors mediating negative feedback on acetylcholine release by postganglionic cholinergic nerves. Stimulation of the vagus causes bronchoconstriction – mainly in the larger airways. The possible clinical relevance of the heterogeneity of muscarinic receptors in the airways is discussed later.

A distinct population of NANC nerves (see Ch. 13) also regulates the airways. Bronchodilators released by these nerves include *vasoactive intestinal polypeptide* (Table 13.2) and *nitric oxide* (NO; Ch. 21).

Sympathetic innervation. Sympathetic nerves innervate tracheobronchial blood vessels and glands, but not human airway smooth muscle. However, β adrenoceptors are abundantly expressed on human airway smooth muscle (as well as mast cells, epithelium, glands and alveoli) and β agonists relax bronchial smooth muscle, inhibit mediator release from mast cells and increase mucociliary clearance. In humans, β adrenoceptors in the airways are of the $β_2$ variety.

In addition to the autonomic innervation, non-myelinated sensory fibres, linked to irritant receptors in the lungs, release tachykinins such as *substance P*, *neurokinin A* and *neurokinin B* (see Ch. 19), producing *neurogenic inflammation*.

SENSORY RECEPTORS AND AFFERENT PATHWAYS

Slowly adapting *stretch receptors* control respiration via the respiratory centre. Unmyelinated sensory *C fibres* and rapidly adapting *irritant receptors* associated with myelinated vagal fibres are also important.

Physical or chemical stimuli, acting on irritant receptors on myelinated fibres in the upper airways and/or C-fibre receptors in the lower airways, cause coughing, broncho-constriction and mucus secretion. Such stimuli include cold air and irritants such as ammonia, sulfur dioxide, cigarette smoke and the experimental tool *capsaicin* (Ch. 43), as well as endogenous inflammatory mediators.

Regulation of airway muscle, blood vessels and glands

Afferent pathways
- Irritant receptors and C fibres respond to exogenous chemicals, inflammatory mediators and physical stimuli (e.g. cold air).

Efferent pathways
- Parasympathetic nerves cause bronchoconstriction and mucus secretion through M_3 receptors.
- Sympathetic nerves innervate blood vessels and glands, but not airway smooth muscle.
- β_2-Adrenoceptor agonists relax airway smooth muscle. This is pharmacologically important.
- Inhibitory non-noradrenergic non-cholinergic (NANC) nerves relax airway smooth muscle by releasing nitric oxide and vasoactive intestinal peptide.
- Excitation of sensory nerves causes neuroinflammation by releasing tachykinins: substance P and neurokinin A.

PULMONARY DISEASE AND ITS TREATMENT

Common symptoms of pulmonary disease include shortness of breath, wheeze, chest pain and cough with or without sputum production or haemoptysis (blood in the sputum). Ideally, treatment is of the underlying disease, but some-times symptomatic treatment, for example of cough, is all that is possible. The lung is an important target organ of many diseases addressed elsewhere in this book, including infections (Chs 52–56), malignancy (Ch. 57) and occupational and rheumatological diseases; drugs (e.g. **amiodarone**, **methotrexate**) can damage lung tissue and cause pulmonary fibrosis. Heart failure leads to pulmonary oedema (Ch. 23). Thromboembolic disease (Ch. 25) and pulmonary hyperten-sion (Ch. 23) affect the pulmonary circulation. In this present chapter, we concentrate on two important diseases of the airways: asthma and COPD.

BRONCHIAL ASTHMA

Asthma affects about 8% of the population; it is the commonest chronic disease in children in economically developed countries and is also common in adults. It is an inflammatory condition in which there is recurrent reversible airways obstruction in response to irritant stimuli that are too weak to affect non-asthmatic subjects. The obstruction usually causes wheeze and merits drug treatment,[2] although the natural history of asthma includes spontaneous remissions. Reversibility of airways obstruction in asthma contrasts with COPD, where the obstruction is either not reversible or at best incompletely reversible by bronchodilators.

CHARACTERISTICS OF ASTHMA

Asthmatic patients experience intermittent attacks of wheez-ing, shortness of breath – with difficulty especially in breathing out – and, sometimes, cough. As explained earlier, acute attacks are reversible, but the underlying pathological disorder can progress in older patients to a chronic state superficially resembling COPD.

Acute severe asthma (also known as *status asthmaticus*) is not easily reversed and causes hypoxaemia. Hospitalisa-tion is necessary, as the condition, which can be fatal, requires prompt and energetic treatment.

Asthma is characterised by:

- inflammation of the airways
- bronchial hyper-reactivity
- reversible airways obstruction

Bronchial hyper-reactivity (or hyper-responsiveness) is abnormal sensitivity to a wide range of stimuli, such as irritant chemicals, cold air and stimulant drugs, all of which can result in bronchoconstriction. In allergic asthma, these features may be initiated by sensitisation to allergen(s), but, once established, asthma attacks can be triggered by various stimuli such as viral infection, exercise (in which the stimulus may be cold air and/or drying of the airways) and atmospheric pollutants such as sulfur dioxide. Immu-nological desensitisation to allergens such as pollen or dust mites is popular in some countries but is not superior to conventional inhaled drug treatment.

PATHOGENESIS OF ASTHMA

The pathogenesis of asthma involves both genetic and environmental factors, and the asthmatic attack itself consists, in many subjects, of two main phases: an immediate and a late (or delayed) phase (Fig. 29.1).

Numerous cells and mediators play a part, and the full details of the complex events involved are still a matter of debate (Walter & Holtzman, 2005). The following simplified account is intended to provide a basis for understanding the rational use of drugs in the treatment of asthma.

Asthmatics have activated T cells, with a T-helper (Th)2 profile of cytokine production (see Ch. 19 and Table 19.2) in their bronchial mucosa. How these cells are activated is not fully understood, but allergens (Fig. 29.2) are one mechanism. The Th2 cytokines that are released do the following:

- Attract other inflammatory granulocytes, especially eosinophils, to the mucosal surface. Interleukin (IL)-5

---

[2]William Osler, 19th century doyen of American and British clinicians, wrote that 'the asthmatic pants into old age' – this at a time when the most effective drug that he could offer was to smoke stramonium cigarettes, a herbal remedy, the antimuscarinic effects of which were offset by direct irritation from the smoke. Its use persisted in English private schools into the 1950s, as one author can attest – much to the envy of his fellows!

and granulocyte–macrophage colony-stimulating factor prime eosinophils to produce cysteinyl leukotrienes (see Ch. 18), and to release granule proteins that damage the epithelium. This damage is one cause of bronchial hyper-responsiveness.

- Promote immunoglobulin (Ig)E synthesis and responsiveness in some asthmatics (IL-4 and IL-13 'switch' B cells to IgE synthesis and cause expression of IgE receptors on mast cells and eosinophils; they also enhance adhesion of eosinophils to endothelium).

Some asthmatics, in addition to these mechanisms, are also *atopic* – that is, they make allergen-specific IgE that binds to mast cells in the airways. Inhaled allergen cross-links IgE molecules on mast cells, triggering degranulation with

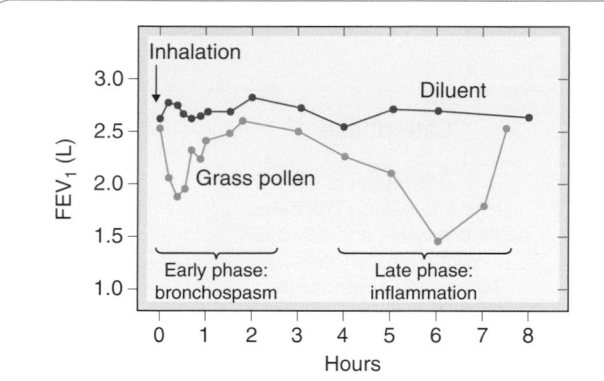

Fig. 29.1 Two phases of asthma demonstrated by the changes in forced expiratory volume in 1 second (FEV₁) after inhalation of grass pollen in an allergic subject. (From Cockcroft, D.W., 1983. Lancet ii, 253.)

release of histamine and leukotriene B₄, both of which are powerful bronchoconstrictors to which asthmatics are especially sensitive because of their airway hyper-responsiveness. This provides a mechanism for acute exacerbation of asthma in atopic individuals exposed to allergen. The effectiveness of **omalizumab** (an anti-IgE antibody; see p. 378) serves to emphasise the importance of IgE in the pathogenesis of asthma as well as in other allergic diseases. Noxious gases (e.g. sulfur dioxide, ozone) and airway dehydration can also cause mast cell degranulation.

Clinicians often refer to atopic or 'extrinsic' asthma and non-atopic or 'intrinsic' asthma; we prefer the terms allergic and non-allergic.

The immediate phase of an asthma attack

In allergic asthma the immediate phase (i.e. the initial response to allergen provocation) occurs abruptly and is mainly caused by spasm of the bronchial smooth muscle. Allergen interaction with mast cell-fixed IgE causes release of histamine, leukotriene B₄ and prostaglandin (PG)D₂ (Ch. 18).

Other mediators released include IL-4, IL-5, IL-13, macrophage inflammatory protein-1α and tumour necrosis factor (TNF)-α.

Various chemotaxins and chemokines (see Ch. 19) attract leukocytes – particularly eosinophils and mononuclear cells – setting the stage for the late phase (Fig. 29.3).

The late phase

The late phase or delayed response (see Figs 29.1 and 29.3) may be nocturnal. It is, in essence, a progressing inflammatory reaction, initiation of which occurred during the first phase, the influx of Th2 lymphocytes being of particular importance. The inflammatory cells include activated eosinophils. These release cysteinyl leukotrienes, interleukins IL-3, IL-5 and IL-8, and the toxic proteins *eosinophil cationic protein*, *major basic protein* and *eosinophil-derived neurotoxin*.

Fig. 29.2 The part played by T lymphocytes in allergic asthma. In genetically susceptible individuals, allergen *(green circle)* interacts with dendritic cells and CD4⁺ T cells, leading to the development of Th0 lymphocytes, which give rise to a clone of Th2 lymphocytes. These then (1) generate a cytokine environment that switches B cells/plasma cells to the production and release of immunoglobulin (Ig)E; (2) generate cytokines, such as interleukin (IL)-5, which promote differentiation and activation of eosinophils; and (3) generate cytokines (e.g. IL-4 and IL-13) that induce expression of IgE receptors. Glucocorticoids inhibit the action of the cytokines specified. *APC*, antigen-presenting dendritic cell; *B*, B cell; *P*, plasma cell; *Th*, T-helper cell.

Asthma

- Asthma is defined as recurrent reversible airway obstruction, with attacks of wheeze, shortness of breath and, often, nocturnal cough. Severe attacks cause hypoxaemia and are life-threatening.
- Essential features include:
  - airways inflammation, which causes
  - bronchial hyper-responsiveness, which in turn results in
  - recurrent reversible airway obstruction
- Pathogenesis involves exposure of genetically disposed individuals to allergens; activation of Th2 lymphocytes and cytokine generation promote:
  - differentiation and activation of eosinophils

- IgE production and release
- expression of IgE receptors on mast cells and eosinophils
- Important mediators include leukotriene B_4 and cysteinyl leukotrienes (C_4 and D_4); interleukins (IL)-4, IL-5, IL-13; and tissue-damaging eosinophil proteins.
- Antiasthmatic drugs include:
  - bronchodilators
  - anti-inflammatory agents
- Treatment is monitored by measuring forced expiratory volume in 1 second (FEV_1) or peak expiratory flow rate and, in acute severe disease, oxygen saturation and arterial blood gases.

Immediate phase

Late phase

Eliciting agent: allergen or non-specific stimulus

Infiltration of cytokine-releasing **Th2 cells,** and monocytes, and activation of inflammatory cells, particularly **eosinophils**

Mast cells, mononuclear cells

Mediators e.g. **cysLTs,** neuropeptides?, NO?, adenosine?

EMBP, ECP

Spasmogens **cysLTs,** H, PGD_2

Chemotaxins, chemokines

Epithelial damage

Bronchospasm

Airway inflammation

Airway hyper-reactivity

Reversed by β₂-adrenoceptor agonists, CysLT-receptor antagonists and theophylline

Bronchospasm, wheezing, coughing

Inhibited by glucocorticoids

Fig. 29.3 **Immediate and late phases of asthma, with the actions of the main drugs.** *CysLTs,* cysteinyl leukotrienes (leukotrienes C_4 and D_4); *ECP,* eosinophil cationic protein; *EMBP,* eosinophil major basic protein; *H,* histamine; *iNO,* induced nitric oxide. (For more detail of the Th2-derived cytokines and chemokines, see Ch. 17 and Ch. 6, Fig. 6.4.)

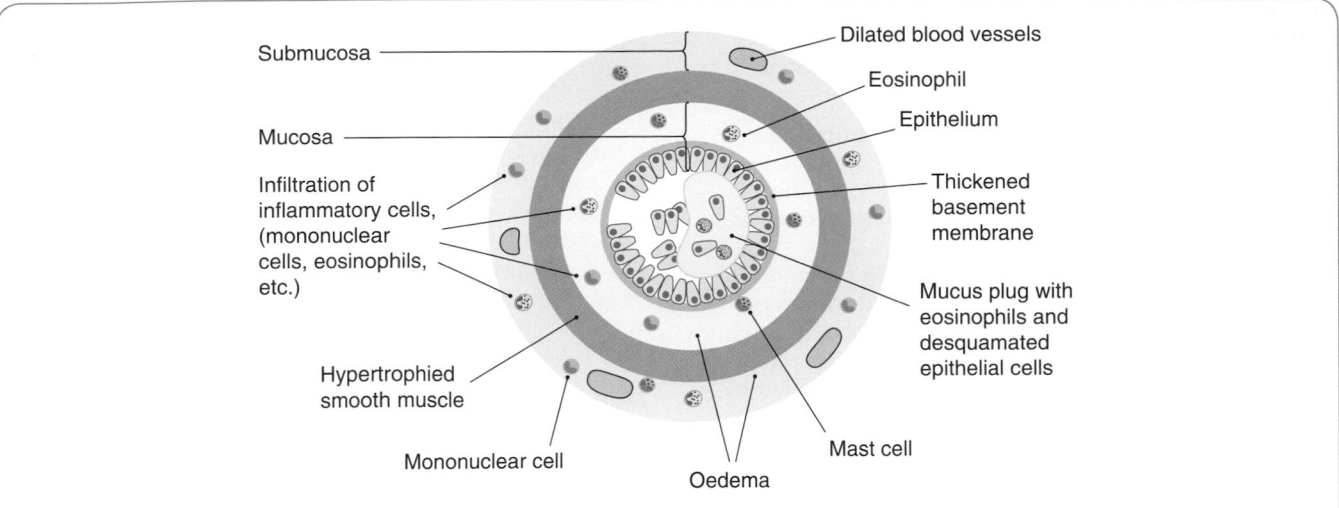

Fig. 29.4 Schematic diagram of a cross-section of a bronchiole, showing changes that occur with severe chronic asthma. The individual elements depicted are not, of course, drawn to scale.

These play an important part in the events of the late phase, the toxic proteins causing damage and loss of epithelium. Other putative mediators of the inflammatory process in the delayed phase are adenosine (acting on the A_1 receptor; see Ch. 17), induced NO (see Ch. 21) and neuropeptides (see Ch. 19).

Growth factors released from inflammatory cells act on smooth muscle cells, causing hypertrophy and hyperplasia, and the smooth muscle can itself release proinflammatory mediators and growth factors (Chs 6 and 19). Fig. 29.4 shows schematically the changes that take place in the bronchioles. Epithelial cell loss means that irritant receptors and C fibres are more accessible to irritant stimuli – an important mechanism of bronchial hyper-reactivity.

'Aspirin-sensitive' asthma

▼ Non-steroidal anti-inflammatory drugs (NSAIDs), especially **aspirin**, can precipitate asthma in sensitive individuals. Such aspirin-sensitive asthma (Ch. 27) is relatively uncommon (<10% of asthmatic subjects), and is often associated with nasal polyps. Individuals sensitive to one NSAID are usually also sensitive to other chemically unrelated cyclo-oxygenase (COX) inhibitors, sometimes including **paracetamol** (Ch. 27). Abnormal leukotriene production and sensitivity are implicated. Patients with aspirin-sensitive asthma produce more cysteinyl leukotriene and have greater airway hyper-responsiveness to inhaled cysteinyl leukotrienes than aspirin-tolerant asthmatics. Such airway hyper-responsiveness reflects elevated expression of cysteinyl leukotriene receptors on inflammatory cells, and this is down-regulated by aspirin desensitisation. In addition, aspirin and similar drugs directly activate eosinophils and mast cells in these patients through IgE-independent mechanisms.

DRUGS USED TO TREAT AND PREVENT ASTHMA

There are two categories of antiasthma drugs: *bronchodilators* and *anti-inflammatory agents*. Bronchodilators reverse the bronchospasm of the immediate phase; anti-inflammatory agents inhibit or prevent the inflammatory components of both phases (see Fig. 29.3). These two categories are not mutually exclusive: some drugs classified as bronchodilators also have some anti-inflammatory effect.

How best to use these drugs to treat asthma is complex. A guideline on the management of asthma (BTS/SIGN,

2016) specifies a stepwise approach for adults and children with chronic asthma. Very mild disease may be treated with short-acting bronchodilator (usually an inhaled short-acting β_2 agonist such as **salbutamol** or **terbutaline**, used as required), but if patients need this more than three times a week, a regular inhaled corticosteroid should be added. If the asthma remains uncontrolled, the next step is to add a long-acting bronchodilator (**salmeterol** or **formoterol**); and/or consider increased doses of inhaled corticosteroid. **Theophylline, tiotropium** (a long-acting muscarinic antagonist) or leukotriene antagonist (such as **montelukast)** are subsequent treatment options in patients who remain symptomatic. Addition of a regular oral corticosteroid (e.g. **prednisolone**) is recommended only in the small group of patients who do not achieve adequate control despite high-dose therapies with the other agents. Corticosteroids are the mainstay of therapy because they are the only asthma drugs that potently inhibit T-cell activation, and thus the inflammatory response, in the asthmatic airways. Omalizumab is an option in those with poorly controlled asthma despite treatment with oral corticosteroids. **Cromoglicate** (see p. 378) has only a weak effect and is now seldom used.

BRONCHODILATORS

The main drugs used as bronchodilators are β_2-adrenoceptor agonists; others include **theophylline**, cysteinyl leukotriene receptor antagonists and muscarinic receptor antagonists.

β-Adrenoceptor agonists

The β_2-adrenoceptor agonists are dealt with in Chapter 15. Their primary effect in asthma is to dilate the bronchi by a direct action on the β_2 adrenoceptors of smooth muscle. Being physiological antagonists of bronchoconstrictors (see Ch. 2), they relax bronchial muscle whatever spasmogen is involved. They also inhibit mediator release from mast cells and TNF-α release from monocytes, and increase mucus clearance by an action on cilia.

β_2-Adrenoceptor agonists are usually given by inhalation of aerosol, powder or nebulised solution (i.e. solution that has been converted into a cloud or mist of fine droplets), but some products may be given orally or by injection. A metered-dose inhaler is used for aerosol preparations.

Two categories of β₂-adrenoceptor agonists are used in asthma:

- Short-acting agents: **salbutamol** and **terbutaline**. These are given by inhalation; they act immediately, peaking within 30 min and the duration of action is 3–5 h; they are usually used on an 'as needed' basis to control symptoms.
- Longer-acting agents: e.g. **salmeterol** and **formoterol**. These are given by inhalation, and the duration of action is 8–12 h. They are not used 'as needed' but are given regularly, twice daily, as adjunctive therapy in patients whose asthma is inadequately controlled by glucocorticoids.

Antiasthma drugs: bronchodilators

- β₂-Adrenoceptor agonists (e.g. **salbutamol**) are first-line drugs (for details, see Ch. 14):
  - They act as physiological antagonists of the spasmogenic mediators but have little or no effect on the bronchial hyper-reactivity.
  - Salbutamol is given by inhalation; its effects start immediately and last 3–5 h, and it can also be given by intravenous infusion in status asthmaticus.
  - **Salmeterol** or **formoterol** are given regularly by inhalation; their duration of action is 8–12 h.
- **Theophylline** (often formulated as **aminophylline**):
  - is a methylxanthine;
  - inhibits phosphodiesterase and blocks adenosine receptors;
  - has a narrow therapeutic window: unwanted effects include cardiac dysrhythmia, seizures and GI disturbances;
  - is given intravenously (by slow infusion) for status asthmaticus, or orally (as a sustained-release preparation) as add-on therapy to inhaled corticosteroids and long-acting β₂ agonists (step 4);
  - is metabolised in the liver by P450; liver dysfunction and viral infections increase its plasma concentration and half-life (normally approximately 12 h);
  - interacts importantly with other drugs; some (e.g. specific antibiotics) increase the half-life of **theophylline**, others (e.g. anticonvulsants) decrease it.
- Cysteinyl leukotriene receptor antagonists (e.g. **montelukast**) are third-line drugs for asthma. They:
  - compete with cysteinyl leukotrienes at CysLT₁ receptors;
  - are used mainly as add-on therapy to inhaled corticosteroids and long-acting β₂ agonists (step 4).

Unwanted effects

The unwanted effects of β₂-adrenoceptor agonists result from systemic absorption and are given in Chapter 15. In the context of their use in asthma, the commonest adverse effect is *tremor*; other unwanted effects include *tachycardia* and *cardiac dysrhythmia*.

Clinical use of β₂-adrenoceptor agonists as bronchodilators

- Short-acting drugs (**salbutamol** or **terbutaline**, usually by inhalation) to prevent or treat wheeze in patients with reversible obstructive airways disease.
- Long-acting drugs (**salmeterol, formoterol**) to prevent bronchospasm (e.g. at night or with exercise) in patients requiring long-term bronchodilator therapy.

Methylxanthines (see Chs 17 and 49)

Theophylline (1,3-dimethylxanthine), which is also used as theophylline ethylenediamine (known as **aminophylline**), is the main therapeutic drug of this class, and has long been used as a bronchodilator.[3] Here we consider it in the context of respiratory disease, its only current therapeutic use.

Mechanism of action

The mechanism of theophylline is still unclear. The relaxant effect on smooth muscle has been attributed to inhibition of phosphodiesterase (PDE) isoenzymes, with resultant increase in cAMP and/or cGMP (see Ch. 4, Fig. 4.10). However, the concentrations necessary to inhibit the isolated enzymes exceed the therapeutic range of plasma concentrations.

Competitive antagonism of adenosine at adenosine A₁ and A₂ receptors (Ch. 17) may contribute, but the PDE inhibitor **enprofylline**, which is a potent bronchodilator, is not an adenosine antagonist.

Type IV PDE is implicated in inflammatory cells, and methylxanthines may have some anti-inflammatory effect. (**Roflumilast**, a type IV PDE inhibitor, is mentioned later in the context of COPD.)

Theophylline activates *histone deacetylase* (HDAC), which controls gene expression and may thereby reverse resistance to the anti-inflammatory effects of corticosteroids (Barnes, 2006).

Methylxanthines stimulate the CNS (Ch. 49) and respiratory stimulation may be beneficial in patients with COPD who suffer from reduced respiration and retention of CO₂. **Caffeine** has a special niche in treating hypoventilation of prematurity (see Ch. 49).

Unwanted effects

When theophylline is used in asthma, its other actions (CNS, cardiovascular, gastrointestinal [GI] and diuretic) result in unwanted side effects (e.g. insomnia, nervousness). The therapeutic plasma concentration range is 30–100 μmol/L, and adverse effects are common with concentrations greater than 110 μmol/L; thus there is a relatively narrow therapeutic window. Serious cardiovascular and CNS effects can occur when the plasma concentration exceeds 200 μmol/L. The most serious cardiovascular effect is *dysrhythmia* (especially during intravenous administration of aminophylline), which can be fatal. *Seizures* can occur with theophylline concentrations at

---

[3]Over 200 years ago, William Withering recommended 'coffee made very strong' as a remedy for asthma. Coffee contains caffeine, a related methylxanthine.

or slightly above the upper limit of the therapeutic range, and can be fatal in patients with impaired respiration due to severe asthma. Monitoring the concentration of theophylline in plasma is useful for optimising the dose.

Clinical use of theophylline

- In addition to steroids, in patients whose asthma does not respond adequately to β_2-adrenoceptor agonists.
- In addition to other bronchodilators and steroids in chronic obstructive pulmonary disease (COPD).
- Intravenously (as **aminophylline**, a combination of **theophylline** with **ethylenediamine** to increase its solubility in water) in acute severe asthma.

Pharmacokinetic aspects
Theophylline is given orally as a sustained-release preparation. Aminophylline can be given by slow intravenous injection of a loading dose followed by intravenous infusion.

Theophylline is well absorbed from the GI tract. It is metabolised by P450 enzymes in the liver; the mean elimination half-life is approximately 8 h in adults but there is wide inter-individual variation. The half-life is increased in liver disease, cardiac failure and viral infections, and is decreased in heavy cigarette smokers (as a result of enzyme induction leading to increased clearance). Unwanted drug interactions are clinically important: its plasma concentration is decreased by drugs that induce P450 enzymes (including **rifampicin**, **phenytoin** and **carbamazepine**). The concentration is increased by drugs that inhibit P450 enzymes, such as **erythromycin**, **clarithromycin**, **ciprofloxacin**, **diltiazem** and **fluconazole**. This is important in view of the narrow therapeutic window; antibiotics such as clarithromycin are often started when asthmatics are hospitalised because of a severe attack precipitated by a chest infection, and if the dose of theophylline is unaltered, severe toxicity can result.

Muscarinic receptor antagonists
Muscarinic receptor antagonists are dealt with in Chapter 14. **Ipratropium**, given by aerosol inhalation is the only short-acting muscarinic antagonist that is widely used clinically as a bronchodilator. Inhaled long-acting muscarinic antagonists, such as **tiotropium**, **aclidinium**, **umeclidinium**, and **glycopyrrolate**, are now available.

Ipratropium is a quaternary derivative of atropine. It does not discriminate between muscarinic receptor subtypes (see Ch. 14), and it is possible that its blockade of M_2 autoreceptors on the cholinergic nerves increases acetylcholine release and reduces the effectiveness of its antagonism at the M_3 receptors on smooth muscle. It is not particularly effective against allergen challenge, but it inhibits the augmentation of mucus secretion that occurs in asthma and may increase the mucociliary clearance of bronchial secretions. It has no effect on the late inflammatory phase of asthma.

Ipratropium is a quaternary nitrogen compound, and therefore highly polar and not well absorbed into the circulation (Ch. 9), limiting systemic effects. The maximum effect occurs approximately 30 min after inhalation and persists for 3–5 h. It has few unwanted effects and is, in general, safe and well tolerated. It can be used with β_2-adrenoceptor agonists, particularly in acute settings for symptomatic relief. See the clinical box later, for clinical uses.

Long-acting muscarinic antagonists are also quaternary ammonium compounds, designed to have greater selectivity towards the M_3 receptor, and to dissociate from the receptor very slowly, producing a sustained effect with regular daily dosing. They are often used together with long-acting β_2-adrenoceptor agonists in a combined inhaler for patients with COPD.

Clinical use of inhaled muscarinic receptor antagonists

- For asthma, as an adjunct to β_2-adrenoceptor agonists and steroids.
- For patients with chronic obstructive pulmonary disease (COPD), especially long-acting drugs (e.g. **tiotropium**).
- For bronchospasm precipitated by β_2-adrenoceptor antagonists.

Cysteinyl leukotriene receptor antagonists
Cysteinyl leukotrienes (LTC_4, LTD_4 and LTE_4) act on $CysLT_1$ and $CysLT_2$ receptors (see Ch. 18), both of which are expressed in respiratory mucosa and infiltrating inflammatory cells, but the functional significance of each is unclear. The 'lukast' drugs (**montelukast** and **zafirlukast**) antagonise only $CysLT_1$.

Lukasts inhibit exercise-induced asthma and decrease both early and late responses to inhaled allergen. They dilate the airways in mild asthma but are less effective than salbutamol, with which their action is additive. They reduce sputum eosinophilia, but there is no clear evidence that they modify the underlying inflammatory process in chronic asthma.

The lukasts are taken by mouth, in combination with an inhaled corticosteroid. They are generally well tolerated, adverse effects consisting mainly of headache and GI disturbances.

Histamine H_1-receptor antagonists
Although mast cell mediators, including histamine, play a part in the immediate phase of allergic asthma (see Fig. 29.3) and in some types of exercise-induced asthma, histamine H_1-receptor antagonists have no routine place in therapy, although they may be modestly effective in mild atopic asthma, especially when this is precipitated by acute histamine release in patients with concomitant allergy such as severe hay fever.

ANTI-INFLAMMATORY AGENTS

Glucocorticoids
Glucocorticoids (see Ch. 34) are the main drugs used for their anti-inflammatory action in asthma. They are not bronchodilators, but prevent the progression of chronic asthma and are effective in acute severe asthma (see clinical box, p. 378).[4]

---

[4]In 1900, Solis-Cohen reported that dried bovine adrenals had anti-asthma activity. He noted that the extract did not serve acutely 'to cut short the paroxysm' but was 'useful in averting recurrence of paroxysms'. Mistaken for the first report on the effect of adrenaline, his astute observation was probably the first on the efficacy of steroids in asthma.

Actions and mechanism

The basis of the anti-inflammatory action of glucocorticoids is discussed in Chapter 34. An important action, of relevance for asthma, is that they restrain clonal proliferation of Th cells by reducing the transcription of the gene for IL-2 and decrease formation of cytokines, in particular the Th2 cytokines that recruit and activate eosinophils and are responsible for promoting the production of IgE and the expression of IgE receptors. Glucocorticoids also inhibit the generation of the vasodilators PGE_2 and PGI_2, by inhibiting induction of COX-2 (Ch. 18, Fig. 18.3). By inducing *annexin 1*, (see Fig. 18.3) they could inhibit production of leukotrienes and platelet-activating factor, although there is currently no direct evidence that annexin 1 is involved in the therapeutic action of glucocorticoids in human asthma.

Corticosteroids inhibit the allergen-induced influx of eosinophils into the lung. Glucocorticoids up-regulate β_2 adrenoceptors, decrease microvascular permeability and indirectly reduce mediator release from eosinophils by inhibiting the production of cytokines (e.g. IL-5 and granulocyte–macrophage colony-stimulating factor) that activate eosinophils. Reduced synthesis of IL-3 (the cytokine that regulates mast cell production) may explain why long-term steroid treatment eventually reduces the number of mast cells in the respiratory mucosa, and hence suppresses the early-phase response to allergens and exercise.

Glucocorticoids are sometimes ineffective, even in high doses, for reasons that are incompletely understood. Many individual mechanisms could contribute to glucocorticoid resistance. The phenomenon has been linked to the number of glucocorticoid receptors, but in some situations other mechanisms are clearly in play – for example, reduced activity of *histone deacetylase* (HDAC) may be important in cigarette smokers.

The main compounds used are **beclometasone, budesonide, fluticasone, mometasone** and **ciclesonide**. These are given by inhalation with a metered-dose or dry-powder inhaler, the full effect on bronchial hyper-responsiveness being attained only after weeks or months of therapy. There are now several inhaler formulations where inhaled corticosteroids are combined together with long-acting β_2-adrenoceptor agonists (Cohen et al., 2016). Oral glucocorticoids (Ch. 34) are reserved for patients with the severest disease.

Unwanted effects

Serious unwanted effects are uncommon with inhaled steroids. Oropharyngeal candidiasis (thrush; Ch. 54) can occur (T lymphocytes are important in protection against fungal infection), as can sore throat and croaky voice, but use of 'spacing' devices, which decrease oropharyngeal deposition of the drug and increase airway deposition, reduces these problems. Regular high doses of inhaled glucocorticoids can produce some adrenal suppression, particularly in children, and necessitate carrying a 'steroid card' (Ch. 34). This is less likely with fluticasone, mometasone and ciclesonide, as these drugs are poorly absorbed from the GI tract and undergo almost complete presystemic metabolism. The unwanted effects of oral glucocorticoids are given in Fig. 34.7.

Cromoglicate and nedocromil

These two drugs, of similar chemical structure and properties, are now hardly used for the treatment of asthma. Although very safe, they have only weak anti-inflammatory

Clinical use of glucocorticoids in asthma

- Patients who require regular bronchodilators should be considered for glucocorticoid treatment (e.g. with low-dose inhaled **beclometasone**).
- More severely affected patients are treated with high-potency inhaled drugs (e.g. **fluticasone**).
- Patients with acute exacerbations of asthma may require intravenous **hydrocortisone** and oral **prednisolone**.
- A 'rescue course' of oral prednisolone may be needed at any stage of severity if the clinical condition is deteriorating rapidly.
- Prolonged treatment with oral prednisolone, in addition to inhaled bronchodilators and steroids, is needed by a few severely asthmatic patients.

effects and short duration of action. They are given by inhalation as aerosols or dry powders, and can also be used topically for allergic conjunctivitis or rhinitis. They are not bronchodilators, having no direct effects on smooth muscle, nor do they inhibit the actions of any of the known smooth muscle stimulants. Given prophylactically, they reduce both the immediate- and late-phase asthmatic responses and reduce bronchial hyper-reactivity.

Their mechanism of action is not fully understood. Cromoglicate is a 'mast cell stabiliser', preventing histamine release from mast cells. However, this is not the basis of its action in asthma, because compounds that are more potent than cromoglicate at inhibiting mast cell histamine release are ineffective against asthma.

Anti-IgE treatment

Omalizumab is a humanised monoclonal anti-IgE antibody. It is effective in patients with allergic asthma as well as in allergic rhinitis. It is of considerable theoretical interest (see review by Holgate et al., 2005), but it is expensive and its clinical role is principally for those patients with severe persistent confirmed allergic IgE-mediated asthma who have required continuous or frequent treatment with oral corticosteroids despite use of other standard therapies.

Inhibition of interleukin-5

Eosinophilic asthma is a recognised variant for which specific therapies (such as **mepolizumab** or **reslizumab**) targeted at human IL-5 are now available. IL-5 is the key cytokine involved in growth, differentiation and activation of eosinophils. Antibodies that inhibit IL-5 signalling result in reduced production and survival of eosinophils that mediate the allergic inflammatory process in patients with asthma.

Drugs in development

There are several novel agents targeted at mediators of eosinophilic airway inflammation (Bel & Ten Brinke, 2017). Examples of these cytokine targets and associated agents are IL-15 (**tralokinumab**), IL-4 (**dupilumab**) and thymic stromal lymphopoietin (**tezepelumab**). Inhibitors of prostaglandin D2 (see Fig. 29.3) are currently in clinical trials (**fevipiprant** and **timapiprant**).

Antiasthma drugs: glucocorticoids

Glucocorticoids (for details, see Ch. 34)

- These reduce the inflammatory component in chronic asthma and are life-saving in status asthmaticus (acute severe asthma).
- They do not prevent the immediate response to allergen or other challenges.
- The mechanism of action involves decreased formation of cytokines, particularly those generated by Th2 lymphocytes, decreased activation of eosinophils and other inflammatory cells.
- They are given by inhalation (e.g. **beclometasone**); systemic unwanted effects are uncommon at moderate doses, but oral thrush and voice problems can occur. Systemic effects can occur with high doses but are less likely with **mometasone** because of its presystemic metabolism. In deteriorating asthma, an oral glucocorticoid (e.g. **prednisolone**) or intravenous **hydrocortisone** is also given.

SEVERE ACUTE ASTHMA (STATUS ASTHMATICUS)

Severe acute asthma is a medical emergency requiring hospitalisation. Treatment includes oxygen (in high concentration, usually ≥60%), inhalation of nebulised salbutamol with ipratropium, and intravenous hydrocortisone followed by a course of oral prednisolone. Additional measures occasionally used include intravenous salbutamol or aminophylline, intravenous magnesium (considered to have bronchodilator effects), and antibiotics (if bacterial infection is present). Monitoring is by PEFR or FEV_1, and by measurement of arterial blood gases and oxygen saturation.

ALLERGIC EMERGENCIES

Anaphylaxis (Ch. 7) and *angio-oedema* are emergencies involving acute airways obstruction; **adrenaline** (epinephrine) is potentially life-saving. It is administered intramuscularly (or occasionally intravenously, as in anaphylaxis occurring in association with general anaesthesia). Patients at risk of acute anaphylaxis, for example, from food or insect sting allergy, may self-administer intramuscular adrenaline using a spring-loaded syringe. Oxygen, an antihistamine such as **chlorphenamine** and hydrocortisone are also indicated.

Angio-oedema is the intermittent occurrence of focal swelling of the skin or intra-abdominal organs caused by plasma leakage from capillaries. Most often, it is mild and 'idiopathic', but it can occur as part of acute allergic reactions, when it is generally accompanied by urticaria – 'hives' – caused by histamine release from mast cells. If the larynx is involved, it is life-threatening; swelling in the peritoneal cavity can be very painful and mimic a surgical emergency. It can be caused by drugs, especially *angiotensin-converting enzyme inhibitors* – perhaps because they block the inactivation of peptides such as bradykinin (Ch. 19) – and by aspirin and related drugs in patients who are aspirin sensitive (see Ch. 27). Hereditary angio-oedema is associated with lack of C1 esterase inhibitor – C1 esterase is an enzyme that degrades the complement component C1 (see Ch. 7).

Tranexamic acid (Ch. 25) or **danazol** (Ch. 36) may be used to prevent attacks in patients with hereditary angioneurotic oedema, and administration of partially purified C1 esterase inhibitor or fresh plasma, with antihistamines and glucocorticoids, can terminate acute attacks. **Icatibant**, a peptide bradykinin β_2 receptor antagonist (Ch. 19), is effective for acute attacks of hereditary angio-oedema. It is administered subcutaneously but can cause nausea, abdominal pain and nasal stuffiness.

CHRONIC OBSTRUCTIVE PULMONARY DISEASE

COPD is a major global health problem – current projections suggest that it will be the third commonest cause of death within 3 years (Adeloye et al., 2015). Cigarette smoking is the main cause, and is increasing in the developing world. Air pollution, also aetiologically important, is also increasing, and there is a huge unmet need for effective drugs. A resurgence of interest in new therapeutic approaches has yet to bear fruit but there are a number of promising avenues, in particular in defining subgroups of this rather heterogeneous disease that are responsive to particular therapeutic measures (McDonald, 2017).

Clinical features. The clinical picture starts with attacks of morning cough during the winter, and progresses to chronic cough with intermittent exacerbations, often initiated by an upper respiratory infection, when the sputum becomes purulent. There is progressive breathlessness. Some patients have a reversible component of airflow obstruction identifiable by an improved FEV_1 following a dose of bronchodilator. Pulmonary hypertension (Ch. 23) is a late complication, causing symptoms of heart failure (*cor pulmonale*). Exacerbations may be complicated by respiratory failure (i.e. reduced $P_{A}O_2$) requiring hospitalisation and intensive care. Tracheostomy and artificial ventilation, while prolonging survival, may serve only to return the patient to a miserable life.

Pathogenesis. There is fibrosis of small airways, resulting in obstruction, and/or destruction of alveoli and of elastin fibres in the lung parenchyma. The latter features are hallmarks of emphysema,[5] thought to be caused by proteases, including elastase, released during the inflammatory response. It is emphysema that causes respiratory failure, because it destroys the alveoli, impairing gas transfer. There is chronic inflammation (bronchitis), predominantly in small airways and lung parenchyma, characterised by increased numbers of macrophages, neutrophils and T lymphocytes. The inflammatory mediators have not been as clearly defined as in asthma. Lipid mediators, inflammatory peptides, reactive oxygen and nitrogen species, chemokines, cytokines and growth factors are all implicated (Barnes, 2004).

Principles of treatment. Stopping smoking (Ch. 49) slows the progress of COPD. Patients should be immunised against influenza and *Pneumococcus*, because superimposed infections with these organisms are potentially lethal. Glucocorticoids are less effective than in asthma. This contrast with asthma is puzzling, because in both diseases multiple inflammatory genes are activated, which might be expected to be turned off by glucocorticoids. Inflammatory gene activation results from acetylation of nuclear histones which opens up the chromatin structure, allowing gene

---

[5]Emphysema is a pathological condition sometimes associated with COPD, in which lung parenchyma is destroyed and replaced by air spaces that coalesce to form bullae – blister-like air-filled spaces in the lung tissue.

transcription and synthesis of inflammatory proteins to proceed. HDAC de-acetylates histones, and suppresses production of proinflammatory cytokines. Corticosteroids recruit HDAC to activated genes, switching off inflammatory gene transcription (Barnes et al., 2004). There is a link between the severity of COPD (but not of asthma) and reduced HDAC activity in lung tissue (Ito et al., 2005); furthermore, HDAC activity is inhibited by smoking-related oxidative stress, which may explain the relative lack of effectiveness of glucocorticoids in patients with COPD, as compared to those with asthma. Inhaled steroids do not influence the progressive decline in lung function in patients with COPD, but do improve the quality of life, probably as a result of a modest reduction in hospital admissions. This is counter-balanced by the increased risk of pneumonia associated with use of inhaled corticosteroids in patients with COPD.

Long-acting bronchodilators give modest benefit, but do not deal with the underlying inflammation. No currently licensed treatments reduce the progression of COPD or suppress the inflammation in small airways and lung parenchyma. Several new treatments that target the inflammatory process are in clinical development (Barnes, 2013). Some, such as chemokine antagonists, are directed against the influx of inflammatory cells into the airways and lung parenchyma, whereas others target inflammatory cytokines such as TNF-α. The PDE IV inhibitor **roflumilast** is licensed as an adjunct to bronchodilators for patients with severe COPD and frequent exacerbations. Other drugs that inhibit cell signalling (see Chs 3 and 6) include inhibitors of p38 mitogen-activated protein kinase, nuclear factor κβ and phosphoinositide-3 kinase-γ. More specific approaches include antioxidants, inhibitors of inducible NO synthase, and leukotriene β₄ antagonists. Other treatments have the potential to combat mucus hypersecretion, and there is a search for serine protease and matrix metalloprotease inhibitors to prevent lung destruction and the development of emphysema.

Specific aspects of treatment. Short- and long-acting inhaled bronchodilators can provide useful palliation in patients with a reversible component. The main short-acting drugs are ipratropium and salbutamol; long-acting drugs include muscarinic antagonists (e.g. **tiotropium**) which are often given together with β₂ agonists (such as **salmeterol** or **formoterol)** (Chs 14 and 15; Cohen et al, 2016). Theophylline (Ch. 17) can be given by mouth but is of uncertain benefit. Its respiratory stimulant effect may be useful for patients who tend to retain CO₂. Other respiratory stimulants (e.g. **doxapram**) are sometimes used briefly in acute respiratory failure (e.g. postoperatively) but have largely been replaced by non-invasive ventilation as well as mechanical ventilatory support (intermittent positive-pressure ventilation).

Long-term oxygen therapy administered at home prolongs life in patients with severe disease and hypoxaemia (at least if they refrain from smoking – an oxygen fire is not a pleasant way to go).

Acute exacerbations. Acute exacerbations of COPD are treated with inhaled O₂ in a concentration (initially, at least) of 24–28% O₂, that is, only just above atmospheric O₂ concentration (approximately 20%). The need for caution is because of the risk of precipitating CO₂ retention as a consequence of terminating the hypoxic drive to respiration. Blood gases and tissue oxygen saturation are monitored, and inspired O₂ subsequently adjusted accordingly. Antibiotics such as aminopenicillins, macrolides or tetracyclines are recommended if there is evidence of infection. Inhaled bronchodilators may provide some symptomatic improvement.

A systemically active glucocorticoid (intravenous hydrocortisone or oral prednisolone) is also administered routinely, although efficacy is modest.

IDIOPATHIC PULMONARY FIBROSIS

Idiopathic pulmonary fibrosis is a chronic debilitating inflammatory disorder that results in scarring of lung tissue and loss of elasticity. Lung expansion and gaseous exchange in the alveoli are impaired due to the fibrosis and consequent increased stiffness in pulmonary tissues. In the absence of a known aetiological agent, treatment is focused on the use of anti-fibrotic agents.

Pirfenidone is an immunosuppressant that reduces fibroblast proliferation and production of fibrosis-related mediators. The exact mechanism of pirfenidone is not known, but it appears to reduce fibrosis-related protein and cytokines, prevent accumulation of inflammatory cells, and inhibit expansion of extracellular matrix that is stimulated by cytokine growth factors such as transforming growth factor-β and platelet-derived growth factor (Borie et al., 2016). Clinical trials have demonstrated that pirfenidone can slow the decline in lung function and exercise capacity caused by pulmonary fibrosis.

Nintedanib is a small-molecule tyrosine kinase inhibitor that is thought to reduce inflammatory and fibrotic change in the lung. The drug acts through inhibition of signalling cascades from platelet-derived and fibroblast-derived growth factor receptors that are involved in the proliferation and differentiation of pulmonary fibroblasts and myoblasts (Borie et al., 2016). Clinical trials have demonstrated the efficacy of nintedanib in slowing the progressive loss of lung function that is seen in pulmonary fibrosis.

SURFACTANTS

Pulmonary surfactants act, not by binding to specific targets, but by lowering the surface tension of fluid lining the alveoli, allowing air to enter. They are effective in the prophylaxis and management of *respiratory distress syndrome* in newborn babies, especially premature babies in whom endogenous surfactant production is deficient. Examples include **beractant** and **poractant alpha**, which are derivatives of the physiological pulmonary surfactant protein. They are administered directly into the tracheobronchial tree via an endotracheal tube. (The mothers of premature infants are sometimes treated with glucocorticoids before birth in an attempt to accelerate maturation of the fetal lung and minimise incidence of this disorder.)

COUGH

Cough is a protective reflex that removes foreign material and secretions from the bronchi and bronchioles. It is a very common adverse effect of angiotensin-converting enzyme inhibitors, in which case the treatment is usually to substitute an alternative drug, often an angiotensin-receptor antagonist, less likely to cause this adverse effect (Ch. 23). It can be triggered by inflammation in the respiratory tract, for example, by undiagnosed asthma or chronic reflux with aspiration, or by neoplasia. In these cases, cough suppressant (antitussive) drugs are sometimes useful, for example for the dry painful cough associated with bronchial carcinoma, but are to be avoided in cases of chronic pulmonary infection, as they can cause undesirable thickening and retention of sputum, and in asthma because of the risk of respiratory depression.

DRUGS USED FOR COUGH

Opioid analgesics are the most effective antitussive drugs in clinical use (Ch. 43). They act by inhibiting an ill-defined 'cough centre' in the brain stem, and suppress cough in doses below those required for pain relief. Those used as cough suppressants have minimal analgesic actions and addictive properties. New opioid analogues that suppress cough by inhibiting release of excitatory neuropeptides through an action on μ receptors (see Table 43.2) on sensory nerves in the bronchi are being assessed.

Codeine (methylmorphine) is a weak opioid (see Ch. 43) with considerably less addiction liability than a strong opioid, and is a mild cough suppressant. It decreases secretions in the bronchioles, which thickens sputum, and inhibits ciliary activity. Constipation is common. **Dextromethorphan** (a drug with many actions, including μ-receptor and sigma-1-receptor agonist, non-selective serotonin-uptake inhibitor) and **pholcodine** (μ-receptor agonist with weak analgesic effects) have less adverse effects than codeine. Respiratory depression is a risk with all centrally acting cough suppressants. **Morphine** is used for palliative care in cases of lung cancer associated with distressing cough.

REFERENCES AND FURTHER READING

General
Barnes, P.J., 2011. Pathophysiology of allergic inflammation. Immunol. Rev. 242, SI31–SI50.
Bezemer, G.F.G., Sagar, S., van Bergenhenegouwen, J., et al., 2012. Dual role of toll-like receptors in asthma and chronic obstructive pulmonary disease. Pharmacol. Rev. 64, 337–358. (*Update on the role of TLRs in asthma and in COPD which discusses targeting these for airway diseases. TLR agonist, adjuvant and antagonist therapies could all be argued to be effective. Because of a possible dual role of TLRs in airway diseases with shared symptoms and risk factors but different immunological mechanisms, caution should be taken while designing pulmonary TLR-based therapies*)
Borie, R., Justet, A., Beltramo, G., et al., 2016. Pharmacological management of IPF. Respirology 21, 615–625.
Korkmaz, B., Horwitz, M.S., Jenne, D.E., Gauthier, F., 2010. Neutrophil elastase, proteinase 3, and cathepsin G as therapeutic targets in human diseases. Pharmacol. Rev. 62, 726–759. (*Describes the functions of these proteases, their role in human diseases and discusses identifying new therapeutics; also describes how non-human primate experimental models could assist*)
Melo, R.C.N., Liu, L., Xenakis, J.J., 2013. Eosinophil-derived cytokines in health and disease: unraveling novel mechanisms of selective secretion. Allergy 68, 274–284.
van der Velden, V.H.J., Hulsmann, A.R., 1999. Autonomic innervation of human airways: structure, function, and pathophysiology in asthma. Neuroimmunomodulation 6, 145–159. (*Review*)
Velasquez, R., Teran, L.M., 2011. Chemokines and their receptors in the allergic airway inflammatory process. Clin. Rev. Allergy Immunol. 41, 76–88.

Asthma
Berry, M., Hargadon, B., Morgan, A., et al., 2005. Alveolar nitric oxide in adults with asthma: evidence of distal lung inflammation in refractory asthma. Eur. Respir. J. 25, 986–991. (*Alveolar NO as a measure of distal airway inflammation*)
BTS/SIGN (British Thoracic Society/Scottish Intercollegiate Guideline Network), 2016. British Guideline on Management of Asthma. www.brit-thoracic.org.uk. (Accessed August 2017).
Pelaia, G., Cuda, G., Vatrella, A., et al., 2005. Mitogen-activated protein kinases and asthma. J. Cell. Physiol. 202, 642–653. (*Reviews involvement of mitogen-activated protein kinases in asthma pathogenesis, and discusses their possible role as molecular targets for antiasthma drugs*)
Wadsworth, S.J., Sandford, A.J., 2013. Personalised medicine and asthma diagnostics/management. Curr. Allergy Asthma Rep. 13, 118–129.
Walter, M.J., Holtzman, M.J., 2005. A centennial history of research on asthma pathogenesis. Am. J. Respir. Cell Mol. Biol. 32, 483–489.

Chronic obstructive pulmonary disease
Adeloye, D., Chua, S., Lee, C., et al., 2015. Global and regional estimates of COPD prevalence: Systematic review and meta-analysis. J. Glob. Health 5, 020415.
Barnes, P.J., 2004. Mediators of chronic obstructive pulmonary disease. Pharmacol. Rev. 56, 515–548. ('*The identification of inflammatory mediators and understanding their interactions is important for the development of anti-inflammatory treatments for this important disease*')

Barnes, P.J., 2013. New anti-inflammatory targets for chronic obstructive pulmonary disease. Nat. Rev. Drug Discov. 12, 543–559.
Barnes, P.J., Ito, K., Adcock, I.M., 2004. Corticosteroid resistance in chronic obstructive pulmonary disease: inactivation of histone deacetylase. Lancet 363, 731–733. (*Hypothesis that in patients with COPD, HDAC is impaired by cigarette smoking and oxidative stress, leading to reduced responsiveness to corticosteroids; see also Ito et al., 2005, below*)
Cohen, J.S., Miles, M.C., Donohue, J.F., Ohar, J.A., 2016. Dual therapy strategies for COPD: the scientific rationale for LAMA + LABA. Int. J. Chron. Obstruct. Pulmon. Dis. 11, 785–797. (*Good review of combination bronchodilator therapy in COPD*)
Ito, K., Ito, M., Elliott, W.M., et al., 2005. Decreased histone deacetylase activity in chronic obstructive pulmonary disease. N. Engl. J. Med. 352, 1967–1976. (*There is a link between the severity of COPD and the reduction in HDAC activity in the peripheral lung tissue; HDAC is a key molecule in the repression of production of proinflammatory cytokines in alveolar macrophages*)
McDonald, C.F., 2017. Eosinophil biology in COPD. N. Engl. J. Med. 377, 1680–1682.

Cough
Morice, A.H., Kastelik, J.A., Thompson, R., 2001. Cough challenge in the assessment of cough reflex. Br. J. Clin. Pharmacol. 52, 365–375.
Reynolds, S.M., Mackenzie, A.J., Spina, D., Page, C.P., 2004. The pharmacology of cough. Trends Pharmacol. Sci. 25, 569–576. (*Discusses the pathophysiological mechanisms of cough and implications for developing new antitussive drugs*)

Drugs and therapeutic aspects
Barnes, P.J., 2006. How corticosteroids control inflammation. Br. J. Pharmacol. 148, 245–254.
Bel, E.H., Ten Brinke, A., 2017. New anti-eosinophil drugs for asthma and COPD: targeting the trait! Chest 152 (6), 1276–1282.
Ben-Noun, L., 2000. Drug-induced respiratory disorders: incidence, prevention and management. Drug Saf. 23, 143–164. (*Diverse pulmonary adverse drug effects*)
Cazzola, M., Page, C.P., Calzetta, L., Matera, M.G., 2012. Pharmacology and therapeutics of bronchodilators. Pharmacol. Rev. 64, 450–504.
Conti, M., Beavo, J., 2007. Biochemistry and physiology of cyclic nucleotide phosphodiesterases: essential components in cyclic nucleotide signaling. Annu. Rev. Biochem. 76, 481–511.
Giri, S.N., 2003. Novel pharmacological approaches to manage interstitial lung fibrosis in the twenty first century. Annu. Rev. Pharmacol. Toxicol. 43, 73–95. (*Reviews approaches including maintaining intracellular nicotinamide adenine dinucleotide [NAD+] and ATP, blocking transforming growth factor-β and integrins, platelet-activating factor receptor antagonists and NO synthase inhibitors*)
Holgate, S.T., Djukanovic, R., Casale, T., Bousquet, J., 2005. Anti-immunoglobulin E treatment with omalizumab in allergic diseases: an update on anti-inflammatory activity and clinical efficacy. Clin. Exp. Allergy 35, 408–416. (*Reviews mechanism and clinical studies*)
Lewis, J.F., Veldhuizen, R., 2003. The role of exogenous surfactant in the treatment of acute lung injury. Annu. Rev. Physiol. 65, 613–642.

30 The kidney and urinary system

OVERVIEW

We set the scene with a brief outline of renal physiology based on the functional unit of the kidney – the nephron – before describing drugs that affect renal function. Emphasis is on diuretics – drugs that increase the excretion of Na⁺ ions and water, and reduce arterial blood pressure. We also mention drugs used to treat patients with renal failure and urinary tract disorders, several of which are also covered in other chapters.

INTRODUCTION

The main function of the kidneys is to maintain the constancy of the 'interior environment' by eliminating waste products and by regulating the volume, electrolyte content and pH of the extracellular fluid in the face of varying dietary intake and other environmental (e.g. climatic) demands. The kidneys receive approximately 20% of the cardiac output from which, in a young adult human, their glomeruli filter approximately 180 L of fluid per day, of which 99% is reabsorbed by the tubules. This results in a daily urine output of approximately 1.8 L (Table 30.1). The kidneys have important related endocrine functions including synthesis of erythropoietin (Ch. 25), renin (Ch. 23) and of the active form of vitamin D (Ch. 37), and are sites of action of mediators including vasopressin (Ch. 34) and angiotensin II (Ch. 23).

The kidneys are targets of the familiar range of pathological processes – infectious, structural, immunological, toxic (including drug toxicities) and so on – but the diverse diseases that result all converge via impairment of renal function (reduced glomerular filtration rate) to a common end stage of renal failure which (if the pathological process is reversible) may be acute and recoverable or (if not) chronic and irreversible other than by transplantation.

The main drugs that work by altering renal function – the diuretics – are crucial in treating cardiovascular disease, especially hypertension and heart failure (Ch 23), as well as management of patients with renal disease with an impaired ability to excrete salt and water. Immunosuppressant drugs (effective in several of the diseases that can cause renal failure, and crucial following renal transplantation) are covered in Chapter 27 and antibacterial drugs (used to treat renal and urinary tract infections) in Chapter 52. Several drugs that act on the autonomic nervous system influence the muscle of the bladder (the detrusor muscle) and its sphincter, and some of these are used therapeutically in attempts to improve symptoms of detrusor instability or urinary obstruction ('prostatism') (Chs 14, 15 and 36).

The kidneys are the main organ by which drugs and their metabolites are eliminated from the body (Ch. 10), so the dosing regimens of many drugs must be modified in patients with impaired renal function. A further challenge for clinical nephrologists is drug treatment of patients with renal failure who are being supported by an artificial form of dialysis that clears drugs differently from the kidneys. These are outside the scope of this book and interested readers are directed to the chapters by Golper, Udy and Lipman, and by Olyaei, Foster and Lermer in the Oxford Textbook of Clinical Nephrology (2015). Here we provide an introduction to renal physiology followed by coverage of drugs acting on the kidney, and short sections on drugs used in renal failure and drugs used in urinary tract disorders.

OUTLINE OF RENAL FUNCTION

The glomerular filtrate is similar in composition to plasma, apart from the absence of protein. As it passes through the renal tubule, about 99% of the filtered water, and much of the filtered Na⁺, is reabsorbed, and some substances are secreted into it from the blood.

Each kidney consists of an outer cortex, an inner medulla and the renal pelvis, which empties into the ureter. The functional unit is the nephron, of which there are approximately 1.4×10^6 in each kidney (approximately half this number in people with hypertension), with considerable variation between individuals. Nephron number declines with age, even in healthy people, accompanied by a predictable decline in renal function.

THE STRUCTURE AND FUNCTION OF THE NEPHRON

Each nephron consists of a *glomerulus, proximal tubule, loop of Henle, distal convoluted tubule* and *collecting duct* (Fig. 30.1). The glomerulus comprises a tuft of capillaries projecting into Bowman's capsule, a cup-like sack draining into the proximal tubule. Most nephrons lie largely or entirely in the cortex. The remaining 12%, called the *juxtamedullary nephrons,* have their glomeruli and convoluted tubules next to the junction of the medulla and cortex, and their loops of Henle pass deep into the medulla.

THE BLOOD SUPPLY TO THE NEPHRON

Nephrons possess the special characteristic of having two capillary beds in series with each other (see Fig. 30.1). The afferent arteriole of each cortical nephron branches to form the glomerulus; glomerular capillaries coalesce into the efferent arteriole which supplies a second capillary network in the cortex, around the convoluted tubules

Table 30.1 Reabsorption of fluid and solute in the kidney[a]

	Filtered/day	Excreted/day[b]	Percentage reabsorbed
Na^+ (mmol)	25,000	150	99+%
K^+ (mmol)	600	90	93+%
Cl^- (mmol)	18,000	150	99+%
HCO_3^- (mmol)	4900	0	100%
Total solute (mosmol)	54,000	700	87%
H_2O (L)	180	~1.5	99+%

[a]Typical values for a healthy young adult: renal blood flow, 1200 mL/min (20%–25% of cardiac output); renal plasma flow, 660 mL/min; glomerular filtration rate, 125 mL/min.
[b]These are typical figures for an individual eating a Western diet. The kidney excretes more or less of each of these substances to maintain the constancy of the internal milieu, so on a low-sodium diet (for instance in the Yanomami Indians of the upper Amazon basin), NaCl excretion may be reduced to below 10 mmol/day! At the other extreme, individuals living in some fishing communities in Japan eat (and therefore excrete) several hundred mmol/day.

and loops of Henle, before converging to form venules and then renal veins. By contrast, efferent arterioles of juxtamedullary nephrons lead to vessel loops (*vasa recta*) that pass deep into the medulla with the thin loops of Henle (see Fig. 30.1).

THE JUXTAGLOMERULAR APPARATUS

A conjunction of afferent arteriole, efferent arteriole and distal convoluted tubule near the glomerulus forms the juxtaglomerular apparatus (Fig. 30.2). At this site, there are specialised cells in both the afferent arteriole and the tubule. The latter, termed *macula densa* cells, respond to changes in the rate of flow and the composition of tubule fluid, and they control, probably by purinergic signalling (see Ch. 17), *renin* release from specialised granular renin-containing cells in the afferent arteriole (Ch. 23). These cells also release renin in response to decreased pressure in the afferent arteriole. Various chemical mediators also influence renin secretion, including β_2-adrenoceptor agonists, vasodilator prostaglandins and feedback inhibition from angiotensin II acting on AT_1 receptors (see Fig. 23.4). The role of the juxtaglomerular apparatus in the control of Na^+ balance is dealt with below.

GLOMERULAR FILTRATION

Fluid is driven from the capillaries into Bowman's capsule by hydrodynamic force opposed by the oncotic pressure of the plasma proteins, to which the glomerular capillaries are impermeable. All the low molecular-weight constituents

Fig. 30.1 **Simplified diagram of a juxtamedullary nephron and its blood supply.** The tubules and the blood vessels are shown separately for clarity. In the kidney, the peritubular capillary network surrounds the convoluted tubules, and the distal convoluted tubule passes close to the glomerulus, between the afferent and efferent arterioles. (This last is shown in more detail in Fig. 30.2.)

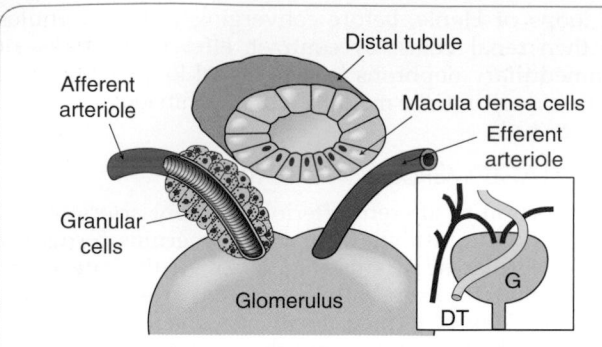

Fig. 30.2 The juxtaglomerular apparatus. The cutaway sections show the granular renin-containing cells around the afferent arteriole, and the macula densa cells in the distal convoluted tubule. The inset shows the general relationships between the structures. *DT*, distal tubule; *G*, glomerulus.

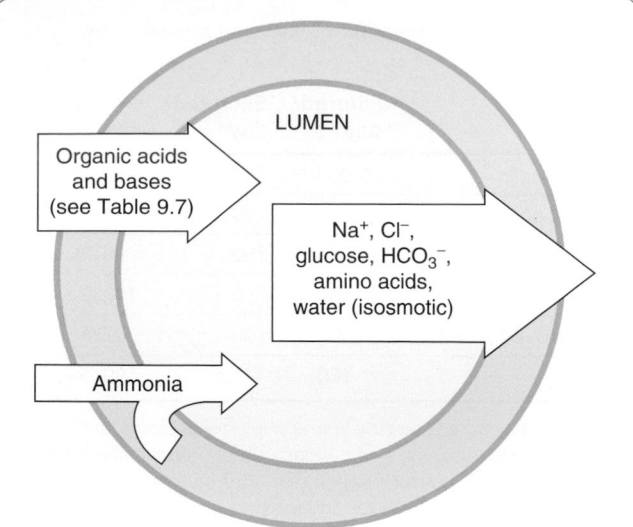

Fig. 30.3 Transport processes in the proximal convoluted tubule. The main driving force for the absorption of solutes and water from the lumen is the Na⁺-K⁺-ATPase in the basolateral membrane of the tubule cells. Many drugs are secreted into the proximal tubule (see Ch. 10). (Redrawn from Burg, 1985. Brenner, B.M., Rector, F.C. (eds). In: The Kidney, third ed., Philadelphia: WB Saunders, pp 145–175.)

of plasma appear in the filtrate, while albumin and larger proteins are retained in the blood.

TUBULAR FUNCTION

The apex (lumenal surface) of each tubular cell is surrounded by a tight junction, as in all epithelia. This is a specialised region of membrane that separates the intercellular space from the lumen. The movement of ions and water across the epithelium can occur *through* cells (the transcellular pathway) and *between* cells through the tight junctions (the paracellular pathway). A common theme is that energy is expended to pump Na⁺ out of the cell by Na⁺-K⁺-ATPase situated in the basolateral cell membrane and the resulting gradient of Na⁺ concentration drives the entry of Na⁺ from the lumen via various transporters that facilitate Na⁺ entry coupled with movement of other ions, either in the same direction as Na⁺, in which case they are called *symporters* or *co-transporters*, or in the opposite direction, in which case they are called *antiporters*. These transporters vary in different parts of the nephron, as described later.

THE PROXIMAL CONVOLUTED TUBULE

The epithelium of the proximal convoluted tubule is 'leaky', i.e. the tight junctions in the proximal tubule are not so 'tight' after all, being permeable to ions and water, and permitting passive flow in either direction. This prevents the build-up of large concentration gradients; thus, although approximately 60%–70% of Na⁺ reabsorption occurs in the proximal tubule, this transfer is accompanied by passive absorption of water so that fluid leaving the proximal tubule remains approximately isotonic to the glomerular filtrate.

Some of the transport processes in the proximal tubule are shown in Figs 30.3–30.5. The most important mechanism for Na⁺ entry into proximal tubular cells from the filtrate occurs by Na⁺/H⁺ exchange (see Fig. 30.5). Intracellular carbonic anhydrase is essential for production of H⁺ for secretion into the lumen. Na⁺ is reabsorbed from tubular fluid into the cytoplasm of proximal tubular cells in exchange for cytoplasmic H⁺. It is then transported out of the cells into the interstitium by a Na⁺-K⁺-ATPase (sodium pump) in the basolateral membrane. This is the main active transport mechanism of the nephron in terms of energy consumption. Reabsorbed Na⁺ then diffuses into blood vessels.

▼ Bicarbonate is normally completely reabsorbed in the proximal tubule. This is achieved by combination with protons, yielding carbonic acid, which dissociates to form carbon dioxide and water – a reaction catalysed by carbonic anhydrase present in the lumenal brush border of the proximal tubule cells (see Fig. 30.5A) – followed by passive reabsorption of the dissolved carbon dioxide.[1] The selective removal of sodium bicarbonate, with accompanying water, in the early proximal tubule causes a secondary rise in the concentration of chloride ions. Diffusion of chloride down its concentration gradient via the paracellular shunt (see Fig. 30.5A) leads, in turn, to a lumen-positive potential difference that favours reabsorption of sodium. The other mechanism involved in movement via the paracellular route is that sodium ions are secreted by Na⁺-K⁺-ATPase into the lateral intercellular space, somewhat raising its osmolality because of the 3 Na⁺:2 K⁺ stoichiometry of the transporter. This leads to osmotic movement of water across the tight junction (see Fig. 30.5A), in turn causing sodium and chloride ion reabsorption by convection (so-called solvent drag).

Many organic acids and bases are actively secreted into the tubule from the blood by specific transporters (see later, Fig. 30.3 and Ch. 10).

After passage through the proximal tubule, tubular fluid (now 30%–40% of the original volume of the filtrate) passes on to the loop of Henle.

THE LOOP OF HENLE, MEDULLARY COUNTER-CURRENT MULTIPLIER AND EXCHANGER

The loop of Henle consists of a descending and an ascending portion (see Figs 30.1 and 30.4), the ascending portion having both thick and thin segments. This part of the nephron

---

[1]The reaction is reversible, and the enzyme (as any catalyst) does not alter the equilibrium, just speeds up the rate with which it is attained. The concentrations inside the cell are such that carbon dioxide combines with water to produce carbonic acid: the same enzyme (carbonic anhydrase) catalyses this as well (see Fig. 30.5A).

Fig. 30.4 Schematic showing the absorption of sodium and chloride in the nephron and the main sites of action of drugs. Cells are depicted as a pink border round the yellow tubular lumen. Mechanisms of ion absorption at the apical margin of the tubule cell: *(1)* Na^+/H^+ exchange; *(2)* $Na^+/K^+/2Cl^-$ co-transport; *(3)* Na^+/Cl^- co-transport; *(4)* Na^+ entry through sodium channels. Sodium is pumped out of the cells into the interstitium by the Na^+-K^+-ATPase in the basolateral margin of the tubular cells (not shown). The numbers in the boxes give the concentration of ions as millimoles per litre of filtrate, and the percentage of filtered ions still remaining in the tubular fluid at the sites specified. *CT*, collecting tubule; *DT*, distal tubule; *PCT*, proximal convoluted tubule; *TAL*, thick ascending loop. (Data from Greger, 2000.)

enables the kidney to excrete urine that is either more or less concentrated than plasma, and hence to regulate the osmotic balance of the body as a whole. The loops of Henle of the juxtamedullary nephrons function as counter-current multipliers, and the vasa recta as counter-current exchangers. NaCl is actively reabsorbed in the thick ascending limb, causing hypertonicity of the interstitium. The descending limb is permeable to water, and this interstitial hypertonicity causes water to move out, so that the tubular fluid becomes progressively more concentrated as it approaches the bend.

▼ In juxtamedullary nephrons with long loops, there is extensive movement of water out of the tubule so that the fluid eventually reaching the tip of the loop has a high osmolality – normally approximately 1200 mosmol/kg, but up to 1500 mosmol/kg under conditions of dehydration – compared with plasma and extracellular fluid, which is approximately 300 mosmol/kg.[2] The hypertonic milieu of medulla, through which the collecting ducts of all nephrons pass on the way to the renal pelvis, is important in providing a mechanism by which the osmolarity of the urine is controlled.

The *ascending limb* has very low permeability to water, i.e. the tight junctions really are tight, enabling the build-up of a substantial concentration gradient across the wall of the tubule. It is here, in the thick ascending limb of the loop of Henle, that 20%–30% of filtered Na^+ is reabsorbed. There is active reabsorption of NaCl, unaccompanied by

water, reducing the osmolality of the tubular fluid and making the interstitial fluid of the medulla hypertonic. The osmotic gradient in the medullary interstitium is the key consequence of the counter-current multiplier system, the main principle being that small horizontal osmotic gradients stack up to produce a large vertical gradient. Urea contributes to the gradient because it is more slowly reabsorbed than water and may be added to fluid in the descending limb, so its concentration rises along the nephron until it reaches the collecting tubules, where it diffuses out into the interstitium. It is thus trapped in the inner medulla.

Ions move into cells of the thick ascending limb of the loop of Henle across the apical membrane by a $Na^+/K^+/2Cl^-$ co-transporter, driven by the Na^+ gradient produced by Na^+-K^+-ATPase in the basolateral membrane (see Fig. 30.5B). Most of the K^+ taken into the cell by the $Na^+/K^+/2Cl^-$ co-transporter returns to the lumen through apical potassium channels, but some K^+ is reabsorbed, along with Mg^{2+} and Ca^{2+}.

Reabsorption of salt from the thick ascending limb is not balanced by reabsorption of water, so tubular fluid is hypotonic with respect to plasma as it enters the distal convoluted tubule (see Fig. 30.4). The thick ascending limb is therefore sometimes referred to as the 'diluting segment'.

THE DISTAL TUBULE

In the early distal tubule, NaCl reabsorption, coupled with impermeability of the *zonula occludens* to water, further dilutes the tubular fluid. Transport is driven by Na^+-K^+-ATPase in the basolateral membrane. This lowers

---

[2]These figures are for humans; some other species, notably the desert rat, can do much better, with urine osmolalities up to 5000 mosmol/kg.

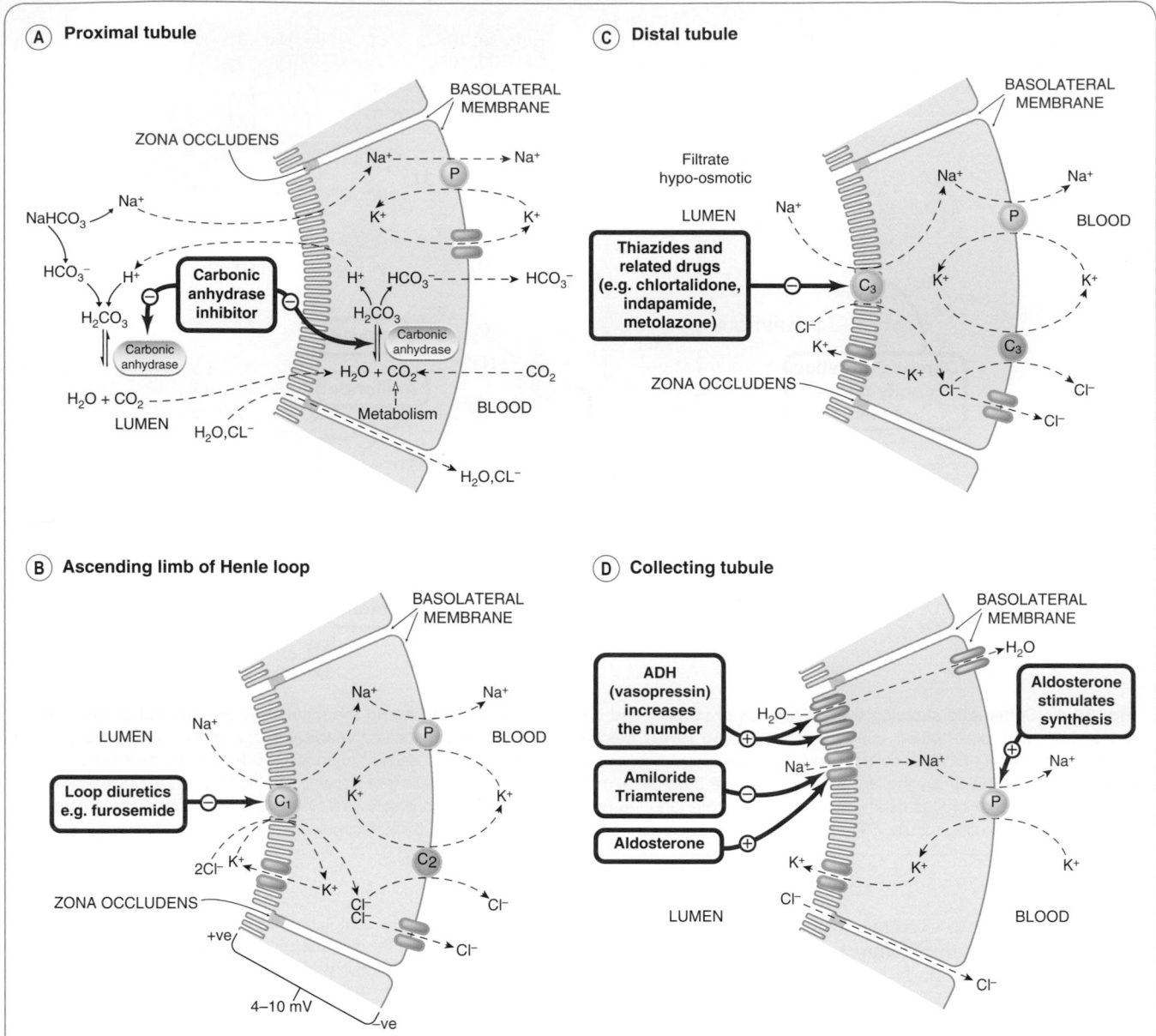

Fig. 30.5 **Drug effects on renal tubular ion transport.** The primary active transport mechanism is the Na^+/K^+ pump *(P)* in the basolateral membrane of cells in each location; the diagrams are simplified in that the pump exchanges three Na^+ for two K^+ ions. (A) Bicarbonate ion reabsorption in the proximal convoluted tubule, showing the action of carbonic anhydrase inhibitors. (B) Ion transport in the thick ascending limb of Henle loop, showing the site of action of loop diuretics, namely the $Na^+/K^+/2Cl^-$ co-transporter *(C₁)*. Chloride ions leave the cell both through basolateral chloride channels and by an electroneutral K^+/Cl^- co-transporter *(C₂)* which are also present in the distal tubule. (C) Salt transport in the distal convoluted tubule, showing the site of action of thiazide diuretics, namely the Na^+/Cl^- co-transporter *(C₃)*. (D) Actions of hormones and drugs on the collecting tubule. The cells are impermeable to water in the absence of antidiuretic hormone (ADH), and to Na^+ in the absence of aldosterone. Aldosterone acts on a nuclear receptor within the tubule cell and on membrane receptors. (Adapted from Greger, 2000.)

cytoplasmic Na^+ concentration, and consequently Na^+ enters the cell from the lumen down its concentration gradient, accompanied by Cl^-, by means of a Na^+/Cl^- co-transporter (see Fig. 30.5C).

The apical surfaces (lumen side) of distal tubular cells are permeable to Ca^{2+} via the TRPV5 channel. On the basolateral surface there is an active Na^+/Ca^{2+} transporter, and the basolateral ATP-dependent Na^+/K^+ pump produces the gradient for Ca^{2+} to be reabsorbed via a separate Na^+/Ca^{2+} basolateral antiporter. The excretion of Ca^{2+} is regulated

in this part of the nephron, by *parathormone (PTH)* and *calcitriol,* both of which increase Ca^{2+} reabsorption and phosphate excretion by increasing the synthesis of several of these transporters (see Ch. 37).

THE COLLECTING TUBULE AND COLLECTING DUCT

Distal convoluted tubules empty into collecting tubules, which coalesce to form collecting ducts (see Fig. 30.1). Collecting tubules include principal cells, which reabsorb Na^+ and secrete K^+ (see Fig. 30.5D), and two populations of intercalated cells, α and β, which secrete acid and base, respectively.

The tight junctions in this portion of the nephron are impermeable to water and cations. The movement of ions and water in this segment is under independent hormonal control: absorption of NaCl by *aldosterone* (Ch. 23), and absorption of water by *antidiuretic hormone* (ADH), also termed *vasopressin* (Ch. 34).

Aldosterone enhances Na^+ reabsorption and promotes K^+ excretion (see Fig. 30.5D). It promotes Na^+ reabsorption by:

- a rapid effect, up-regulating epithelial sodium channels in the collecting duct, increasing apical membrane permeability and hence reabsorption of sodium ions by an action on membrane aldosterone receptors.[3]
- delayed effects, via nuclear receptors (see Ch. 3), directing the synthesis of a specific protein mediator up-regulating and activating the basolateral Na^+/K^+ pump, which pumps three sodium ions out of the cell, into the interstitial fluid and two potassium ions into the cell from the interstitial fluid and stimulates synthesis of the epithelial sodium ion channel in addition to its rapid effect via the membrane receptor mentioned above.

ADH and nephrogenic diabetes insipidus. ADH is secreted by the posterior pituitary (Ch. 34) and acts on V_2 receptors in the basolateral membranes of cells in the collecting tubules and ducts, increasing expression of *aquaporin* (water channels; see Ch. 9) in the apical membranes (see Fig. 30.5D). This renders this part of the nephron permeable to water, allowing passive reabsorption of water as the collecting duct traverses the hyperosmotic region of the medulla, and hence the excretion of concentrated urine. Conversely, in the absence of ADH, collecting duct epithelium is impermeable to water, so hypotonic fluid that leaves the distal tubule remains hypotonic as it passes down the collecting ducts, leading to the excretion of dilute urine. Defective ADH secretion (Ch. 34) or action on the kidney results in *diabetes insipidus*, an uncommon disorder in which patients excrete large volumes of dilute urine.

Ethanol (Ch. 50) inhibits the secretion of ADH, causing a water diuresis (possibly familiar to some of our readers) as a kind of transient diabetes insipidus. **Nicotine** enhances ADH secretion (perhaps contributing to the appeal of an after-dinner cigar?).

Several drugs inhibit the action of ADH: **lithium** (used in psychiatric disorders; see Ch. 48, **demeclocycline** (a tetracycline used not as an antibiotic, but rather to treat inappropriate secretion of ADH from tumours or in other conditions), **colchicine** (Ch. 27) and *vinca alkaloids* (Ch. 57). Recently, more specific antagonists of ADH (e.g. **conivaptan, tolvaptan**) have been introduced for treatment of hyponatraemia. Any of these drugs, given in excess, can cause acquired forms of *nephrogenic* diabetes insipidus, caused by a failure of the renal collecting ducts to respond to ADH. Nephrogenic diabetes insipidus can also be caused by genetic disorders affecting the V_2 receptor or aquaporin.

---

[3]A mechanism distinct from regulation of gene transcription, which is the usual transduction mechanism for steroid hormones (Ch. 3).

Renal tubular function

- Protein-free glomerular filtrate enters via Bowman's capsule.
- Na^+-K^+-ATPase in the basolateral membrane is the main active transporter. It provides the Na^+-gradients (low cytoplasmic Na^+ concentrations) for passive transporters in the apical membranes which facilitate Na^+ entry (reabsorption) from the tubular fluid down a concentration gradient and in exchange for hydrogen ions (H^+).
- 60%–70% of the filtered Na^+ and >90% of HCO_3^- is absorbed in the proximal tubule.
- Carbonic anhydrase is key for $NaHCO_3$ reabsorption in the proximal tubule and also for distal tubular urine acidification.
- The thick ascending limb of Henle loop is impermeable to water; 20%–30% of the filtered NaCl is actively reabsorbed in this segment.
- Ions are reabsorbed from tubular fluid by a $Na^+/K^+/2Cl^-$ co-transporter in the apical membranes of the thick ascending limb.
- $Na^+/K^+/2Cl^-$ co-transport is inhibited by loop diuretics.
- Filtrate is diluted as it traverses the thick ascending limb as ions are reabsorbed, so that it is hypotonic when it leaves.
- The tubular counter-current multiplier actively generates a concentration gradient – small horizontal differences in solute concentration between tubular fluid and interstitium are multiplied vertically. The deeper in the medulla, the more concentrated is the interstitial fluid.
- Medullary hypertonicity is preserved passively by counter-current exchange in the vasa recta.
- Na^+/Cl^- co-transport (inhibited by thiazide diuretics) reabsorbs 5%–10% of filtered Na^+ in the distal tubule.
- K^+ is secreted into tubular fluid in the distal tubule and the collecting tubules and collecting ducts.
- In the absence of antidiuretic hormone (ADH), the collecting tubule and collecting duct have low permeability to salt and water. ADH increases water permeability.
- Na^+ is reabsorbed from the collecting duct through epithelial sodium channels.
- These epithelial Na^+ channels are activated by aldosterone and inhibited by **amiloride** and by **triamterene**. K^+ or H^+ is secreted into the tubule in exchange for Na^+ in this distal region.

ACID–BASE BALANCE

The kidneys (together with the lungs; Ch. 29) regulate the H^+ concentration of body fluids. Acid or alkaline urine can be excreted according to need, the usual requirement being to form acid urine to eliminate phosphoric and sulfuric acids generated during the metabolism of nucleic acids and of sulfur-containing amino acids consumed in the diet. Consequently, metabolic acidosis is a common accompaniment of renal failure. Altering urine pH to alter drug excretion is mentioned later.

POTASSIUM BALANCE

Extracellular K^+ concentration – critically important for excitable tissue function (see Ch. 4) – is tightly controlled through regulation of K^+ excretion by the kidney. Urinary K^+ excretion matches dietary intake, usually approximately 50–100 mmol in 24 h in Western countries. Many diuretics cause K^+ loss (see later).

Potassium ions are transported into collecting duct and collecting tubule cells from interstitial fluid by an Na^+-K^+-ATPase in the basolateral membrane which is under the control of aldosterone (see earlier, p. 387), and leak into the lumen through a K^+-selective ion channel. Na^+ passes from tubular fluid through sodium channels in the apical membrane down the electrochemical gradient created by the Na^+-K^+-ATPase; a lumen-negative potential difference across the cell results, increasing the driving force for K^+ secretion into the lumen. Thus K^+ secretion is coupled to Na^+ reabsorption.

Consequently, K^+ is lost when:

- more Na^+ reaches the collecting duct, as occurs with any diuretic acting proximal to the collecting duct;
- Na^+ reabsorption in the collecting duct is increased directly (e.g. in hyperaldosteronism).

Conversely, K^+ is retained when:

- Na^+ reabsorption in the collecting duct is decreased, for example by **amiloride** or **triamterene**, which block the sodium channel in this part of the nephron, or **spironolactone** or **eplerenone**, which antagonise aldosterone (see later).

EXCRETION OF ORGANIC MOLECULES

There are distinct mechanisms (see Ch. 10, Table 10.7) for secreting organic anions and cations into the proximal tubular lumen. Secreted anions include several important drugs, for example, *thiazides*, **furosemide**, **salicylate** (Ch. 27), and most *penicillins* and *cephalosporins* (Ch. 52). Similarly, several secreted organic cations are important drugs, for example, **triamterene**, **amiloride**, **atropine** (Ch. 14), **morphine** (Ch. 43) and **quinine** (Ch. 55). Both anion and cation transport mechanisms are, like other renal ion transport processes, indirectly powered by active transport of Na^+ and K^+, the energy being derived from Na^+-K^+-ATPase in the basolateral membrane.

Organic anions in the interstitial fluid are exchanged with cytoplasmic α-ketoglutarate by an antiport (i.e. an exchanger that couples uptake and release of α-ketoglutarate with, in the opposite direction, uptake and release of a different organic anion) in the basolateral membrane, and diffuse passively into the tubular lumen (see Fig. 30.3).

Organic cations diffuse into the cell from the interstitium and are then actively transported into the tubular lumen in exchange for H^+.

NATRIURETIC PEPTIDES

Endogenous A, B and C natriuretic peptides (ANP, BNP and CNP; see Chs 22 and 23) are involved in the regulation of Na^+ excretion. They are released from the heart in response to stretch (A and B), from endothelium (C) and from brain (B). They activate guanylyl cyclase (Ch. 3), and cause natriuresis both by renal haemodynamic effects (increasing glomerular capillary pressure by dilating afferent and constricting efferent arterioles) and by direct tubular

actions. The tubular actions include the inhibition of angiotensin II-stimulated Na^+ and water reabsorption in the proximal convoluted tubule, and of the action of ADH in promoting water reabsorption in the collecting tubule.

Within the kidney, the post-translational processing of ANP prohormone differs from that in other tissues, resulting in an additional four amino acids being added to the amino terminus of ANP to yield a related peptide, *urodilatin*, that promotes Na^+ excretion by acting on natriuretic peptide A receptors.

PROSTAGLANDINS AND RENAL FUNCTION

Prostaglandins (PGs; see Ch. 18) generated in the kidney influence its haemodynamic and excretory functions. The main renal prostaglandins in humans are vasodilator and natriuretic, namely PGE_2 in the medulla and PGI_2 (prostacyclin) in glomeruli. Factors that stimulate their synthesis include ischaemia, angiotensin II, ADH and bradykinin.

Prostaglandin biosynthesis is low under basal conditions. However, when vasoconstrictors (e.g. angiotensin II, noradrenaline) are released, local release of PGE_2 and PGI_2 compensates, preserving renal blood flow by their vasodilator action.

The influence of renal prostaglandins on salt balance and haemodynamics can be inferred from the effects of non-steroidal anti-inflammatory drugs (NSAIDs, which inhibit prostaglandin production by inhibiting cyclo-oxygenase; see Ch. 27). NSAIDs have little or no effect on renal function in healthy people, but predictably cause acute renal failure in clinical conditions in which renal blood flow depends on vasodilator prostaglandin biosynthesis. These include cirrhosis of the liver, heart failure, nephrotic syndrome, glomerulonephritis and extracellular volume contraction (see Ch. 58, Table 58.1). NSAIDs increase blood pressure in patients treated for hypertension by impairing PG-mediated vasodilatation and salt excretion. They exacerbate salt and water retention in patients with heart failure (see Ch. 23), partly by this same direct mechanism.[4]

DRUGS ACTING ON THE KIDNEY

DIURETICS

Diuretics increase the excretion of Na^+ and water. They decrease the reabsorption of Na^+ and an accompanying anion (usually Cl^-) from the filtrate, increased water loss being secondary to the increased excretion of NaCl (natriuresis). This can be achieved:

- by a direct action on the cells of the nephron
- indirectly, by modifying the content of the filtrate

Because a very large proportion of salt (NaCl) and water that passes into the tubule via the glomerulus is reabsorbed (see Table 30.1), even a small decrease in reabsorption can cause a marked increase in Na^+ excretion. A summary diagram of the mechanisms and sites of action of various

---

[1]Additionally, NSAIDs make many of the diuretics used to treat heart failure less effective by competing with them for the organic anion transport (OAT) mechanism mentioned above; loop diuretics and thiazides act from within the lumen by inhibiting exchange mechanisms – see later in this chapter – so blocking their secretion into the lumen reduces their effectiveness by reducing their concentrations at their sites of action.

diuretics is given in Fig. 30.4 and more detailed information on different classes of drugs in Fig. 30.5.

Most diuretics with a direct action on the nephron act from within the tubular lumen and reach their sites of action by being secreted into the proximal tubule (**spirono-lactone** is an exception).

DIURETICS ACTING DIRECTLY ON CELLS OF THE NEPHRON

The main therapeutically useful diuretics act on the:

- thick ascending loop of Henle
- early distal tubule
- collecting tubules and ducts

For a more detailed review of the actions and clinical uses of the diuretics, see Ellison and Subramanya (2015).

Loop diuretics

Loop diuretics (see Fig. 30.5B) are the most powerful diuretics (see Fig. 30.6 for a comparison with thiazides), capable of causing the excretion of 15%–25% of filtered Na^+. Their action is often described – in a phrase that conjures up a rather uncomfortable picture – as causing 'torrential urine flow'. The main example is **furosemide**; **bumetanide** and **torasemide** are alternative agents. These drugs act on the thick ascending limb, inhibiting the $Na^+/K^+/2Cl^-$ carrier in the lumenal membrane by combining with its Cl^- binding site.

Loop diuretics also have incompletely understood vascular actions. Intravenous administration of furosemide to patients with pulmonary oedema caused by acute heart failure (see Ch. 23) causes a therapeutically useful vasodilator effect independent of the onset of diuresis. Possible

mechanisms that have been invoked include decreased vascular responsiveness to vasoconstrictors such as angiotensin II and noradrenaline; increased formation of vasodilating prostaglandins (see earlier); decreased production of the endogenous ouabain-like natriuretic hormone (Na^+-K^+-ATPase inhibitor; see Ch. 22); and potassium-channel opening effects in resistance arteries (see Ellison & Subramanya, 2015).

Loop diuretics increase the delivery of Na^+ to the distal nephron, causing loss of H^+ and K^+. Because Cl^- but not HCO_3^- is lost in the urine, the plasma concentration of HCO_3^- increases as plasma volume is reduced – a form of metabolic alkalosis therefore referred to as 'contraction alkalosis'.

Loop diuretics increase excretion of Ca^{2+} and Mg^{2+} and decrease excretion of uric acid.

Pharmacokinetic aspects

Loop diuretics are absorbed from the gastrointestinal tract, and are usually given by mouth. They may also be given intravenously in urgent situations (e.g. acute pulmonary oedema) or when intestinal absorption is impaired, for example, as a result of reduced intestinal perfusion in patients with severe chronic congestive heart failure, who can become resistant to the action of orally administered diuretics. Given orally, they act within 1 h; given intravenously, they produce a peak effect within 30 min. Loop diuretics are strongly bound to plasma protein, and so do not pass directly into the glomerular filtrate. They reach their site of action – the lumenal membrane of the cells of the thick ascending limb – by being secreted in the proximal convoluted tubule by the organic acid transport mechanism; the fraction thus secreted is excreted in the urine.

In nephrotic syndrome,[5] loop diuretics become bound to albumin in the tubular fluid, and consequently are not available to act on the $Na^+/K^+/2Cl^-$ carrier – another cause of diuretic resistance.

The fraction of the diuretic not excreted in the urine is metabolised, mainly in liver – **bumetanide** by cytochrome P450 pathways and **furosemide** by glucuronide formation. The plasma half-life of both these drugs is approximately 90 min (longer in renal failure), and the duration of action 3–6 h. The clinical use of loop diuretics is given in the box.

Unwanted effects

Unwanted effects directly related to the renal action of loop diuretics are common.[6] Excessive Na^+ and water loss, especially in elderly patients, can cause hypovolaemia and hypotension. Potassium loss, resulting in low plasma K^+ (hypokalaemia), and metabolic alkalosis are common. Hypokalaemia increases the effects and toxicity of several drugs (e.g. **digoxin** and type III antidysrhythmic drugs, Ch. 22), so this is potentially a clinically important source of drug interaction. If necessary, hypokalaemia can be

Fig. 30.6 Dose–response curves for furosemide and hydrochlorothiazide, showing differences in potency and maximum effect 'ceiling'. Note that these doses are not used clinically. (Adapted from Timmerman, R.J. et al., 1964. Curr. Ther. Res 6, 88.)

---

[5]Several diseases that damage renal glomeruli impair their ability to retain plasma albumin, causing massive loss of albumin in the urine and a reduced concentration of albumin in the plasma, which can in turn cause peripheral oedema. This is referred to as nephrotic syndrome.
[6]Such unwanted effects are re-enacted in extreme form in Bartter syndrome type 1, a rare loss-of-function genetic disorder of the $Na^+/K^+/2Cl^-$ transporter, the features of which include polyhydramnios – caused by fetal polyuria – and, postnatally, renal salt loss, low blood pressure, hypokalaemic metabolic alkalosis and hypercalciuria.

Clinical uses of loop diuretics (e.g. furosemide)

- Loop diuretics are used (cautiously!), in conjunction with dietary salt restriction and often with other classes of diuretic, in the treatment of salt and water overload associated with:
  – *acute pulmonary oedema*
  – *chronic heart failure*
  – *cirrhosis of the liver complicated by ascites*
  – *nephrotic syndrome*
  – *renal failure*
- Treatment of *hypertension* complicated by renal impairment (thiazides are preferred if renal function is preserved).
- Treatment of *hypercalcaemia* after replacement of plasma volume with intravenous NaCl solution.

averted or treated by concomitant use of K⁺-sparing diuretics (see later), or supplementary potassium replacement. Hypomagnesaemia is less often recognised but can also be clinically important. Hyperuricaemia is common and can precipitate acute gout (see Ch. 27). Excessive diuresis leads to reduced renal perfusion and consequent impairment of renal function (an early warning of this is a rise in serum urea concentration).

Unwanted effects *unrelated to the renal actions* of the drugs are infrequent. Dose-related hearing loss (compounded by concomitant use of other ototoxic drugs such as aminoglycoside antibiotics) can result from impaired ion transport by the basolateral membrane of the stria vascularis in the inner ear. It occurs only at much higher doses than usually needed to produce diuresis. Adverse reactions unrelated to the main pharmacological effect (e.g. rashes, bone marrow depression) can occur.

Diuretics acting on the distal tubule

Diuretics acting on the distal tubule include thiazides (e.g. **bendroflumethiazide**, **hydrochlorothiazide**) and related drugs (e.g. **chlortalidone**, **indapamide** and **metolazone**; see Fig. 30.5C).

Thiazides are less powerful than loop diuretics, at least in terms of peak increase in rate of urine formation, and are preferred in treating uncomplicated hypertension (Ch. 23). They are better tolerated than loop diuretics, and in clinical trials have been shown to reduce risks of stroke and heart attack associated with hypertension. In the largest trial (ALLHAT, 2002), chlortalidone performed as well as newer antihypertensive drugs (an angiotensin-converting enzyme [ACE] inhibitor and a calcium antagonist, see Ch. 23). Thiazides bind the Cl⁻ site of the distal tubular Na⁺/Cl⁻ co-transport system, inhibiting its action and causing natriuresis with loss of sodium and chloride ions in the urine. The resulting contraction in blood volume stimulates renin secretion, leading to angiotensin formation and aldosterone secretion (Ch. 23, see Figs 23.4 and 23.9). This homeostatic mechanism limits the effect of the diuretic on blood pressure, resulting in an in vivo dose–hypotensive response relationship with only a gentle gradient during chronic dosing.

Effects of thiazides on Na⁺, K⁺, H⁺ and Mg²⁺ balance are qualitatively similar to those of loop diuretics, but smaller

in magnitude. In contrast to loop diuretics, however, thiazides reduce Ca²⁺ excretion, possibly advantageous in older patients at risk of osteoporosis and favouring thiazides over loop diuretics in this setting (Aung & Htay, 2011).

Although thiazides are milder than loop diuretics when used alone, co-administration with loop diuretics has a synergistic effect, because the loop diuretic delivers a greater fraction of the filtered load of Na⁺ to the site of action of the thiazide in the distal tubule.

Thiazide diuretics have a vasodilator action. When used in the treatment of hypertension (Ch. 23), the initial fall in blood pressure results from the decreased blood volume caused by diuresis, but vasodilatation contributes to the later phase.

Thiazide diuretics have a paradoxical effect in diabetes insipidus, where they *reduce* the volume of urine by interfering with the production of hypotonic fluid in the distal tubule, and hence reduce the ability of the kidney to excrete hypotonic urine (i.e. they reduce free water clearance).

Pharmacokinetic aspects

Thiazides and thiazide-related drugs are effective orally. All are excreted in the urine, mainly by tubular secretion, and they compete with uric acid for the organic anion transporter (OAT; see Ch. 9). Bendroflumethiazide has its maximum effect at about 4–6 h and duration is 8–12 h. Chlortalidone has a longer duration of action.

The clinical use of thiazide diuretics is given in the clinical box.

Clinical uses of thiazide diuretics (e.g. bendroflumethiazide)

- *Hypertension*.
- Mild *heart failure* (loop diuretics are usually preferred).
- Severe resistant *oedema* (**metolazone**, especially, is used, together with loop diuretics).
- To prevent recurrent stone formation in *idiopathic hypercalciuria*.
- *Nephrogenic diabetes insipidus*.

Unwanted effects

Apart from an increase in *urinary frequency*, the commonest unwanted effect of thiazides not obviously related to their main renal action is *erectile dysfunction*. This emerged in an analysis of reasons given by patients for withdrawing from blinded treatment in the Medical Research Council mild hypertension trial, where (to the surprise of the investigators) erectile dysfunction was substantially more common than in men allocated to a β-adrenoceptor antagonist or to placebo. Thiazide-associated erectile dysfunction is reversible; it is less common with the low doses used in current practice but remains a problem. *Potassium loss* can be important, as can loss of Mg²⁺. Excretion of uric acid is decreased, and hypochloraemic alkalosis can occur.

Impaired glucose tolerance (see Ch. 32), due to inhibition of insulin secretion, is thought to result from activation of K_ATP channels in pancreatic islet cells.[7] **Diazoxide**, a

---

[7]The chemically related sulfonylurea group of drugs used to treat diabetes mellitus (Ch. 32) act in the opposite way, by closing K_ATP channels and enhancing insulin secretion.

non-diuretic thiazide, also activates K_{ATP} channels, causing vasodilatation and impaired insulin secretion. **Indapamide** is said to lower blood pressure with less metabolic disturbance than related drugs, possibly because it is marketed at a lower equivalent dose.

Hyponatraemia is potentially serious, especially in the elderly. Hypokalaemia can be a cause of adverse drug interaction (see previously under Loop diuretics) and can precipitate encephalopathy in patients with severe liver disease.

Adverse reactions unrelated to the main pharmacology (e.g. rashes, blood dyscrasias) are not common but can be serious.

Aldosterone antagonists

Spironolactone and **eplerenone** (Weinberger, 2004) have limited diuretic action when used singly, because distal Na^+/K^+ exchange – the site on which they act – accounts for reabsorption of only 2% of filtered Na^+. They do, however, have marked antihypertensive effects (Ch. 23), prolong survival in selected patients with heart failure (Ch. 23) and can prevent hypokalaemia when combined with loop diuretics or with thiazides. They compete with aldosterone for its intracellular receptor (see Ch. 34), thereby inhibiting distal Na^+ retention and K^+ secretion (see Fig. 30.5D).

Pharmacokinetic aspects
Spironolactone is well absorbed from the gut. Its plasma half-life is only 10 min, but its active metabolite, **canrenone**, has a plasma half-life of 16 h. The action of spironolactone is largely attributable to canrenone. This, in addition to the slow turnover of membrane transporters, results in a slow onset of action, occurring over several days. Eplerenone has a shorter elimination half-life than canrenone and has no active metabolites. It is administered by mouth once daily.

Unwanted effects
Aldosterone antagonists predispose to hyperkalaemia, which is potentially fatal. Potassium supplements should not be co-prescribed other than in exceptional circumstances and then with close monitoring of plasma creatinine and electrolytes. Such monitoring is also needed if these drugs are used for patients with impaired renal function, especially if other drugs that can increase plasma potassium, such as *ACE inhibitors, angiotensin receptor antagonists* (sartans) (Ch. 23) or *β-adrenoceptor antagonists* (Ch. 15) are also prescribed – as they often are for patients with heart failure. Gastrointestinal upset is quite common. Actions of spironolactone/canrenone on progesterone and androgen receptors in tissues other than the kidney can cause gynaecomastia, menstrual disorders and testicular atrophy. Eplerenone has lower affinity for these receptors, and such oestrogen-like side effects are less common.

The clinical use of potassium-sparing diuretics is given in the clinical box.

Triamterene and amiloride

Like aldosterone antagonists, **triamterene** and **amiloride** have only limited diuretic efficacy, because they also act in the distal nephron, where only a small fraction of Na^+ reabsorption occurs. They act on the collecting tubules and collecting ducts, inhibiting Na^+ reabsorption by blocking

---

> ### Clinical uses of potassium-sparing diuretics (e.g. spironolactone, amiloride)
>
> - With K^+-losing (i.e. loop or thiazide) diuretics to prevent K^+ loss, where hypokalaemia is especially hazardous (e.g. patients requiring **digoxin** or **amiodarone**; see Ch. 22).
> - **Spironolactone** or **eplerenone** is used in:
>   - *heart failure*, to improve survival (see Ch. 22)
>   - *primary hyperaldosteronism* (Conn's syndrome)
>   - *resistant essential hypertension* (especially low-renin hypertension)
>   - *secondary hyperaldosteronism* caused by hepatic cirrhosis complicated by ascites

---

lumenal sodium channels (see Ch. 4), thereby indirectly decreasing K^+ excretion (see Fig. 30.5D).

They can be given with loop diuretics or thiazides in order to maintain potassium balance.

Pharmacokinetic aspects
Triamterene is well absorbed in the gastrointestinal tract. Its onset of action is within 2 h, and its duration of action 12–16 h. It is partly metabolised in the liver and partly excreted unchanged in the urine. Amiloride is less well absorbed and has a slower onset, with a peak action at 6 h and duration of about 24 h. Most of the drug is excreted unchanged in the urine.

Unwanted effects
The main unwanted effect, hyperkalaemia, is related to the pharmacological action of these drugs and can be dangerous, especially in patients with renal impairment or receiving other drugs that can increase plasma K^+ (see above). Gastrointestinal disturbances have been reported but are infrequent. Idiosyncratic reactions, for example, rashes, are uncommon.

Carbonic anhydrase inhibitors
Carbonic anhydrase inhibitors (see Fig. 30.5A) – for example, **acetazolamide** – increase excretion of bicarbonate with accompanying Na^+, K^+ and water, resulting in an increased flow of an alkaline urine and metabolic acidosis. These agents, although not now used as diuretics, are still used in the treatment of glaucoma to reduce the formation of aqueous humour (Ch. 14), in some types of infantile epilepsy (Ch. 46), and to accelerate acclimatisation to high altitude.

Urinary loss of bicarbonate depletes extracellular bicarbonate, and the diuretic effect of carbonic anhydrase inhibitors is consequently self-limiting. Acetazolamide is a sulfonamide and unwanted effects such as rashes, blood dyscrasias and interstitial nephritis can occur as with other sulfonamides (Ch. 52).

DIURETICS THAT ACT INDIRECTLY BY MODIFYING THE CONTENT OF THE FILTRATE
Osmotic diuretics
Osmotic diuretics are pharmacologically inert substances (e.g. **mannitol**) that are filtered in the glomerulus but not

reabsorbed (see Fig. 30.4).[8] Their main effect is exerted in those parts of the nephron that are freely permeable to water: the proximal tubule, descending limb of the loop and (in the presence of ADH; see earlier) the collecting tubules. Passive water reabsorption is reduced by the presence of non-reabsorbable solute within the tubule; consequently a larger volume of fluid remains within the proximal tubule. This has the secondary effect of reducing Na^+ reabsorption.

Therefore the main effect of osmotic diuretics is to increase the amount of water excreted, with a smaller increase in Na^+ excretion. They are sometimes used in acute renal failure, which can occur as a result of haemorrhage, injury or systemic infections. In acute renal failure, glomerular filtration rate is reduced, and absorption of NaCl and water in the proximal tubule becomes almost complete, so that more distal parts of the nephron virtually 'dry up', and urine flow ceases. Protein is deposited in the tubules and may impede the flow of fluid. Osmotic diuretics (e.g. **mannitol** given intravenously in a dose of 12–15 g) can limit these effects, at least if given in the earliest stages, albeit while increasing intravascular volume and risking left ventricular failure.

Osmotic diuretics are also used for the emergency treatment of acutely raised intracranial or intraocular pressure. Such treatment has nothing to do with the kidney, but relies on the increase in plasma osmolarity by solutes that do not enter the brain or eye, which results in efflux of water from these compartments.

Unwanted effects include transient expansion of the extracellular fluid volume (with a risk of precipitating left ventricular failure) and hyponatraemia. Headache, nausea and vomiting can occur.

DRUGS THAT ALTER THE pH OF THE URINE

It is possible, using pharmacological agents, to produce urinary pH values ranging from approximately 5 to 8.5.

Carbonic anhydrase inhibitors increase urinary pH by blocking bicarbonate reabsorption (see earlier). **Citrate** (given by mouth as a mixture of sodium and potassium salts) is metabolised via the Krebs cycle with generation of bicarbonate, which is excreted, alkalinising the urine. This may have some antibacterial effects, as well as improving dysuria (a common symptom of bladder infection, consisting of a burning sensation while passing urine). Additionally, some citrate is excreted in the urine as such and inhibits urinary stone formation. Alkalinisation is important in preventing certain weak acid drugs with limited aqueous solubility, such as *sulfonamides* (see Ch. 52), from crystallising in the urine; it also decreases the formation of uric acid and cystine stones by favouring the charged anionic form that is more water-soluble (Ch. 9).

Alkalinising the urine increases the excretion of drugs that are weak acids (e.g. salicylates and some barbiturates). Sodium bicarbonate is sometimes used to treat salicylate overdose (Ch. 10).

> **Diuretics**
>
> - Normally <1% of filtered Na^+ is excreted.
> - Diuretics increase the excretion of salt (NaCl or $NaHCO_3$) and water.
> - Loop diuretics, thiazides and K^+-sparing diuretics are the main therapeutic drugs.
> - Loop diuretics (e.g. **furosemide**) cause copious urine production. They inhibit the $Na^+/K^+/2Cl^-$ co-transporter in the thick ascending loop of Henle. They are used to treat heart failure and other diseases complicated by salt and water retention. Hypovolaemia and hypokalaemia are important unwanted effects.
> - Thiazides (e.g. **bendroflumethiazide**) have a smaller diuretic effect than loop diuretics. They inhibit the Na^+/Cl^- co-transporter in the distal convoluted tubule. They are used to treat hypertension, working partly through an indirect vasodilator action. Erectile dysfunction is an important adverse effect. Hypokalaemia and other metabolic effects (e.g. hyperuricaemia, hyperglycaemia) can occur, especially with high doses.
> - Potassium-sparing diuretics:
>   - act in the distal nephron and collecting tubules; they are weak diuretics but effective in some forms of hypertension and heart failure, and they can prevent hypokalaemia caused by loop diuretics or thiazides.
>   - canrenone, the active metabolite of **spironolactone** and **eplerenone** compete with aldosterone for its receptor.
>   - **amiloride** and **triamterene** act by blocking the sodium channels controlled by aldosterone's protein mediator.

Urinary pH can be decreased with **ammonium chloride**, but this is now rarely, if ever, used clinically.

DRUGS THAT ALTER THE EXCRETION OF ORGANIC MOLECULES

Uric acid metabolism and excretion are relevant in the treatment and prevention of gout (Ch. 27), and a few points about its excretion are made here. Normal plasma urate concentration is approximately 0.24 mmol/L, higher concentrations predisposing to gout (see Ch. 27)

Uric acid is derived from the catabolism of purines, and is present in plasma mainly as ionised urate. In humans, it passes freely into the glomerular filtrate, and most is then reabsorbed in the proximal tubule while a small amount is secreted into the tubule by the anion-secreting mechanism. The net result is excretion of approximately 8%–12% of filtered urate. The secretory mechanism is generally inhibited by low doses of drugs that affect uric acid transport (see later), whereas higher doses are needed to block reabsorption. Such drugs therefore tend to cause retention of uric acid at low doses, while promoting its excretion at higher doses. Drugs that increase the elimination of urate (*uricosuric agents*, e.g. **probenecid** and **sulfinpyrazone**) may be useful in such patients, although these have largely been supplanted by **allopurinol**, which inhibits urate synthesis (Ch. 27).

---

[8] In hyperglycaemia, glucose acts as an osmotic diuretic once plasma glucose exceeds the renal reabsorptive capacity (usually approximately 12 mmol/L), accounting for the cardinal symptom of polyuria in diabetes mellitus; see Chapter 32.

Probenecid inhibits the anion transporter responsible for the reabsorption of urate in the proximal tubule, increasing its excretion. It has the opposite effect on penicillin, inhibiting its secretion into the tubules and raising its plasma concentration. Given orally, probenecid is well absorbed in the gastrointestinal tract, maximal concentrations in the plasma occurring in about 3 h. Approximately 90% is bound to plasma albumin. Free drug passes into the glomerular filtrate but more is actively secreted into the proximal tubule, whence it may diffuse back because of its high lipid solubility (see also Ch. 10). Sulfinpyrazone acts similarly.

The main effect of uricosuric drugs is to block urate reabsorption and lower plasma urate concentration. Both probenecid and sulfinpyrazone inhibit the secretion as well as the reabsorption of urate and, if given in subtherapeutic doses, can actually increase plasma urate concentrations.

DRUGS USED IN RENAL FAILURE

Many drugs used in chronic renal failure (e.g. antihypertensives, vitamin D preparations and **epoetin**) are covered in other chapters. Electrolyte disorders are particularly important in renal failure, notably *hyperphosphataemia* and *hyperkalaemia*, and may require drug treatment.

HYPERPHOSPHATAEMIA

Phosphate metabolism is closely linked with that of calcium and is discussed in Chapter 37.

The antacid **aluminium hydroxide** (Ch. 31) binds phosphate in the gastrointestinal tract, reducing its absorption, but may increase plasma aluminium in dialysis patients.[9] Calcium-based phosphate-binding agents (e.g. calcium carbonate) are widely used to treat hyperphosphatemia. They are contraindicated in hypercalcaemia or hypercalciuria but until recently have been believed to be otherwise safe. However, calcium salts may predispose to tissue calcification (including of artery walls), and calcium-containing phosphate binders may actually contribute to the very high death rates from cardiovascular disease in dialysis patients.

An anion exchange resin, **sevelamer**, lowers plasma phosphate, and is less likely than calcium carbonate to cause arterial calcification (Tonelli et al., 2010). Sevelamer

is not absorbed from the gut and has an additional effect in lowering low-density lipoprotein cholesterol. It is given in gram doses by mouth three times a day with meals. Its adverse effects are gastrointestinal disturbance, and it is contraindicated in bowel obstruction.

HYPERKALAEMIA

Severe hyperkalaemia is life-threatening. Cardiac toxicity is counteracted directly by administering calcium gluconate intravenously (Table 22.1), and by measures that shift K^+ into the intracellular compartment, for example glucose plus insulin (Ch. 32). **Salbutamol**, administered intravenously or by inhalation, also causes cellular K^+ uptake and is used for this indication (e.g. Murdoch et al., 1991); it acts synergistically with insulin. Intravenous sodium bicarbonate is also often recommended, and moves potassium ions into cells in exchange for intracellular protons that emerge to buffer the extracellular fluid. Removal of excessive potassium from the body can be achieved by cation exchange resins such as **sodium** or **calcium polystyrene sulfonate** administered by mouth (in combination with **sorbitol** to prevent constipation) or as an enema. Dialysis is often needed.

DRUGS USED IN URINARY TRACT DISORDERS

Bed wetting (enuresis) is normal in very young children and persists in around 5% of children aged 10 years. Nocturnal enuresis in children aged 10 years or more may warrant treatment with **desmopressin** (an analogue of antidiuretic hormone, given by mouth or by nasal spray for the treatment of diabetes insipidus caused by ADH deficiency due to disease of the posterior pituitary gland Ch. 34), combined with restricting fluid intake in the evening.

Disordered micturition is also common in adults. Symptoms from benign prostatic hyperplasia may be improved by α_1-adrenoceptor antagonists, for example **doxazosin** or **tamsulosin** (Ch. 15), or by an inhibitor of androgen synthesis such as **finasteride** (Ch. 36).

Muscarinic receptor antagonists (Ch. 14) such as **oxybutinin** are used for neurogenic detrusor muscle instability ('overactive bladder'), but the dose is limited by their adverse effects. A selective β_3 agonist (**mirabegron**) is also licensed for this indication (Ch. 15), but can cause tachycardia and atrial fibrillation.

---

[9]Before Kerr identified the cause in Newcastle, the use of alum to purify municipal water supplies led to a horrible and untreatable neurodegenerative condition known as 'dialysis dementia', and also to a particularly painful and refractory form of bone disease.

REFERENCES AND FURTHER READING

Physiological aspects

Agre, P., 2004. Aquaporin water channels (Nobel lecture). Angew. Chem. Int. Ed. Engl. 43, 4278–4290.

Gamba, G., 2015. Molecular physiology and pathophysiology of electroneutral cation-chloride cotransporters. Physiol. Rev. 85, 423–493. (*Comprehensive review of this family: some of these cotransporters are targets for loop diuretics and thiazide-type diuretics, and inactivating mutations of three members of the family cause Bartter's, Gitelman's, and Anderman's diseases*)

Greger, R., 2000. Physiology of sodium transport. Am. J. Med. Sci. 319, 51–62. (*Outstanding article. Covers not only Na^+ transport but also, briefly, that of K^+, H^+, Cl^-, HCO_3^-, Ca^{2+}, Mg^{2+} and some organic substances in each of the main parts of the nephron. Discusses regulatory factors, pathophysiological aspects and pharmacological principles*)

Nigam, S.K., Bush, K.T., Martovetsky, G., 2016. The organic anion transporter (oat) family: a systems biology perspective. Physiol. Rev. 95, 83–123. (*The organic anion transporter (OAT) subfamily has received a great deal of attention because of its role in handling of common drugs including antibiotics, antivirals, diuretics, and nonsteroidal anti-inflammatory drugs in addition to toxins and nutrient vitamins and flavonoids*)

Drugs and therapeutic aspects

Diuretics

Aung, K., Htay, T., 2011. Thiazide diuretics and the risk of hip fracture. Cochrane Database Syst. Rev. (10), CD005185, doi:10.1002/14651858. CD005185.pub2.

Ellison, D.H., Subramanya, A.R., 2015. Clinical use of diuretics. In: Turner, N.N., Lameire, N., Goldsmith, D.J., Winearls, C.G.,

Himmelfarb, J.Remuzzi, G. (Eds.), Oxford Textbook of Clinical Nephrology, fourth ed. Oxford University Press, Oxford.

Shankar, S.S., Brater, D.C., 2003. Loop diuretics: from the Na–K–2Cl transporter to clinical use. Am. J. Physiol. Renal Physiol. 284, F11–F21. (*Reviews pharmacokinetics and pharmacodynamics of loop diuretics in health and in oedematous disorders*)

Weinberger, M.H., 2004. Eplerenone – a new selective aldosterone receptor antagonist. Drugs Today 40, 481–485. (*Review*)

Ca²⁺/PO₄⁻ (see also Diuretics section, above)

Tonelli, M., Pannu, N., Manns, B., 2010. Drug therapy: oral phosphate binders in patients with kidney failure. N. Engl. J. Med. 362, 1312–1324.

Vervloet, M., Cozzolino, M., 2017. Vascular calcification in chronic kidney disease: different bricks in the wall? Kidney Int. 91, 808–817. (*Complexity due to different kinds of vascular calcification in chronic kidney diosease patients, with different implications regarding vascular risk*)

Antihypertensives and renal protection

ALLHAT Officers and Coordinators for the ALLHAT Collaborative Research Group, 2002. Major outcomes in high-risk hypertensive patients randomized to angiotensin-converting enzyme inhibitor or calcium channel blocker vs diuretic: the Antihypertensive and Lipid-Lowering Treatment to Prevent Heart Attack Trial (ALLHAT). JAMA 288, 2981–2997. (*Massive trial; see also Appel, L.J. for editorial comment: 'The verdict from ALLHAT – thiazide diuretics are the preferred initial therapy for hypertension'. JAMA 288, 3039–3042*)

Nijenhuis, T., Vallon, V., van der Kemp, A.W., et al., 2005. Enhanced passive Ca²⁺ reabsorption and reduced Mg²⁺ channel abundance explains thiazide-induced hypocalciuria and hypomagnesemia. J. Clin. Invest. 115, 1651–1658. (*Micropuncture studies in mouse knock-outs showing that enhanced passive Ca²⁺ transport in the proximal tubule rather than active Ca²⁺ transport in distal convolution explains thiazide-induced hypocalciuria*)

Sodium and potassium ion disorders

Coca, S.G., Perazella, M.A., Buller, G.K., 2005. The cardiovascular implications of hypokalemia. Am. J. Kidney Dis. 45, 233–247. (*This review addresses the relative benefits of modulating potassium balance versus non-renal effects of aldosterone blockade*)

Murdoch, I.A., Dos Anjos, R., Haycock, G.B., 1991. Treatment of hyperkalaemia with intravenous salbutamol. Arch. Dis. Child. 66, 527–528. (*First description of this approach in children*)

Drug utilisation in kidney disease

Golper, T.A., Udy, A.A., Lipman, J., 2015. Drug dosing in acute kidney injury. In: Turner, N.N., Lameire, N., Goldsmith, D.J., Winearls, C.G., Himmelfarb, J.Remuzzi, G. (Eds.), Oxford Textbook of Clinical Nephrology, fourth ed. Oxford University Press, Oxford.

Olyaei, A.J., Foster, T.A., Lermer, E.V., 2015. Drug dosing in chronic kidney disease. In: Turner, N.N., Lameire, N., Goldsmith, D.J., Winearls, C.G., Himmelfarb, J.Remuzzi, G. (Eds.), Oxford Textbook of Clinical Nephrology, fourth ed. Oxford University Press, Oxford.

31

The gastrointestinal tract

OVERVIEW

In addition to its main function of digestion and absorption of food, the gastrointestinal (GI) tract is one of the major endocrine systems in the body. It also has its own integrative neuronal network, the enteric nervous system (see Ch. 13), which contains almost the same number of neurons as the spinal cord. It is the site of many common pathologies, ranging from simple dyspepsia to complex autoimmune conditions such as Crohn's disease, and medicines for treating GI disorders comprise some 8% of all prescriptions. In this chapter, we briefly review the physiological control of GI function and then discuss the pharmacological characteristics of drugs affecting gastric secretion and motility, and those used to treat intestinal inflammatory disease.

THE INNERVATION AND HORMONES OF THE GASTROINTESTINAL TRACT

The blood vessels and the glands (exocrine, endocrine and paracrine) of the GI tract are under both neuronal and hormonal control.

NEURONAL CONTROL

There are two principal intramural plexuses in the tract: the *myenteric plexus* (*Auerbach's plexus*) lies between the outer, longitudinal and the middle, circular muscle layers, and the *submucous plexus* (*Meissner's plexus*) lies on the lumenal side of the circular muscle layer. These plexuses are interconnected and their ganglion cells receive preganglionic parasympathetic fibres from the vagus. These are mostly cholinergic and excitatory, although a few are inhibitory. Incoming sympathetic fibres are largely postganglionic. In addition to innervating blood vessels, smooth muscle and some glandular cells directly, some sympathetic fibres terminate in these plexuses, where they inhibit acetylcholine secretion (see Ch. 13).

The neurons within the plexuses constitute the *enteric nervous system* and secrete not only acetylcholine and noradrenaline (norepinephrine), but also 5-hydroxytryptamine (5-HT), purines, nitric oxide and a variety of pharmacologically active peptides (see Chs 13–21). The enteric plexus also contains sensory neurons, which respond to mechanical and chemical stimuli.

HORMONAL CONTROL

The hormones of the GI tract include both endocrine and paracrine secretions. The endocrine secretions (i.e. substances released into the bloodstream) are mainly peptides synthesised by endocrine cells in the mucosa. Important examples include *gastrin* and *cholecystokinin*. The paracrine secretions include many regulatory peptides released from special cells found throughout the wall of the tract. These hormones act on nearby cells, and in the stomach the most important of these is *histamine*. Some of these paracrine factors also function as neurotransmitters.

Orally administered drugs are, of course, absorbed during their passage through the GI tract (Ch. 9). Other functions of the GI tract that are important from the viewpoint of pharmacological intervention are:

* gastric secretion
* vomiting (emesis) and nausea
* gut motility and defecation
* the formation and excretion of bile

GASTRIC SECRETION

The stomach secretes about 2.5 L of gastric juice daily. The principal exocrine components are proenzymes such as *prorennin* and *pepsinogen* elaborated by the *chief* or *peptic* cells, and *hydrochloric acid* (HCl) and *intrinsic factor* (see Ch. 26) secreted by the *parietal* or *oxyntic* cells. The production of acid is important for promoting proteolytic digestion of foodstuffs, iron absorption and killing pathogens. Mucus-secreting cells also abound in the gastric mucosa. Bicarbonate ions are secreted and trapped in the mucus, creating a gel-like protective barrier that maintains the mucosal surface at a pH of 6–7 in the face of a much more acidic environment (pH 1–2) in the lumen. Alcohol and bile can disrupt this protective layer. Locally produced 'cytoprotective' prostaglandins stimulate the secretion of both mucus and bicarbonate.

Disturbances in these secretory and protective mechanisms are thought to be involved in the pathogenesis of *peptic ulcer*, and indeed in other types of gastric damage such as *gastro-oesophageal reflux disease* (GORD[1]) and injury caused by non-steroidal anti-inflammatory drugs (NSAIDs).

THE REGULATION OF ACID SECERETION BY PARIETAL CELLS

Disturbances of acid secretion are important in the pathogenesis of peptic ulcer and constitute a particular target for drug action. The secretion of the parietal cells is an isotonic solution of HCl (150 mmol/L) with a pH less than 1, the concentration of hydrogen ions being more than a million times higher than that in the plasma. To produce this, Cl⁻ is actively transported into *canaliculi* in the cells

---

[1]Or GERD in the United States, to reflect the different spelling of *esophageal*.

Fig. 31.1 A schematic illustration of the secretion of hydrochloric acid by the gastric parietal cell. Secretion involves a proton pump (P), which is an H^+-K^+-ATPase, a symport carrier (C) for K^+ and Cl^-, and an antiport (A), which exchanges Cl^- and HCO_3^-. An additional Na^+/H^+ antiport situated at the interface with the plasma may also have a role (not shown).

that communicate with the lumen of the gastric glands and thus with the stomach itself. This is accompanied by K^+ secretion, which is then exchanged for H^+ from within the cell by a K^+-H^+-ATPase (the 'proton pump', Fig. 31.1). Within the cell, carbonic anhydrase catalyses the combination of carbon dioxide and water to give carbonic acid, which dissociates into H^+ and bicarbonate ions. The latter exchanges across the basal membrane of the parietal cell for Cl^-. The principal mediators that directly – or indirectly – control parietal cell acid output are:

- histamine (a stimulatory local hormone)
- gastrin (a stimulatory peptide hormone)
- acetylcholine (a stimulatory neurotransmitter)
- prostaglandins E_2 and I_2 (local hormones that inhibit acid secretion)
- somatostatin (an inhibitory peptide hormone)

HISTAMINE

Histamine is discussed in Chapter 18, and only those aspects of its pharmacology relevant to gastric secretion will be dealt with here. Neuroendocrine cells abound in the stomach and the dominant type are the *ECL cells* (enterochromaffin-like cells). These are histamine-containing cells similar to mast cells, which lie close to the parietal cells. They sustain a steady basal release of histamine, which is further increased by gastrin and acetylcholine. Histamine acts in a paracrine fashion on parietal cell H_2 receptors, increasing intracellular cAMP. These cells are responsive to histamine concentrations that are below the threshold required for vascular H_2 receptor activation.

GASTRIN

Gastrin is a polypeptide of 34 residues but also exists in shorter forms. It is synthesised by *G cells* in the gastric antrum and secreted into the portal blood, acting as a circulating hormone. Its main action is stimulation of acid secretion by ECL cells through its action at gastrin/cholecystokinin (CCK)$_2$ receptors,[2] which elevate intracellular Ca^{2+}. Gastrin receptors also occur on the parietal cells but their significance in the control of physiological secretion is controversial. CCK$_2$ receptors are blocked by the experimental drugs such as **netazepide** and **proglumide** (Fig. 31.2), but none of these agents have progressed into licensed clinical use.

Gastrin also stimulates histamine synthesis by ECL cells and indirectly increases pepsinogen secretion, stimulates blood flow and increases gastric motility. Release of gastrin is controlled by both neuronal transmitters and blood-borne mediators, as well as by the chemistry of the stomach contents. Amino acids and small peptides directly stimulate the gastrin-secreting cells, as do milk and solutions of calcium salts, explaining why it is inappropriate to use calcium-containing salts as antacids.

ACETYLCHOLINE

Acetylcholine, released (together with a battery of other neurotransmitters and peptides), from postganglionic cholinergic neurons, stimulates specific muscarinic M_3 receptors on the surface of the parietal cells (see Ch. 14), thereby elevating intracellular Ca^{2+} and stimulating acid secretion. It also has complex effects on other cell types; by inhibiting somatostatin release from *D cells*, it potentiates its action on parietal cell acid secretion.

PROSTAGLANDINS

Most cells of the GI tract produce prostaglandins (PGs; see Ch. 18), the most important being PGE$_2$ and I$_2$. Prostaglandins exert 'cytoprotective' effects on many aspects of gastric function including increasing bicarbonate secretion (EP$_{1/2}$ receptors), increasing the release of protective mucin (EP$_4$ receptor), reducing gastric acid output, probably by acting on EP$_{2/3}$ receptors on ECL cells and preventing the vasoconstriction (and thus damage to the mucosa) that follows injury or insult. The latter is probably an action mediated through EP$_{2/4}$ receptors. **Misoprostol** (see later) is a synthetic prostaglandin that probably exploits many of these effects to bring about its therapeutic action.

SOMATOSTATIN

This peptide hormone is released from *D cells* at several locations within the stomach. By acting at its somatostatin (SST)$_2$ receptor, it exerts paracrine inhibitory actions on gastrin release from G cells, histamine release from ECL cells, as well as directly on parietal cell acid output.

THE COORDINATION OF FACTORS REGULATING ACID SECRETION

The regulation of the parietal cell is complex and many local hormones probably play a role in the fine-tuning of the secretory response. The generally accepted model today is that the *gastrin–ECL–parietal cell axis* is the dominant

---

[2]These two peptides share the same, biologically active, C-terminal pentapeptide sequence.

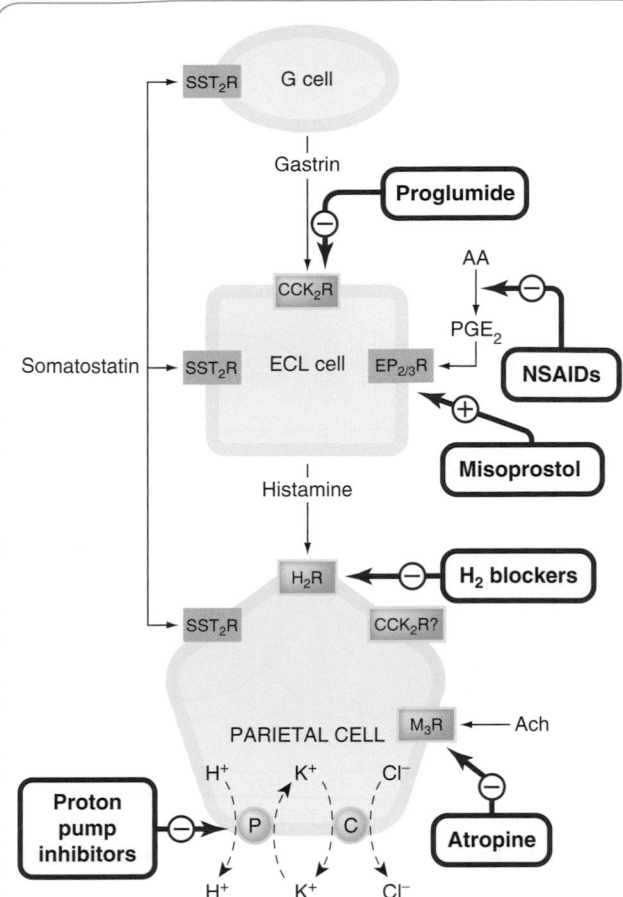

Fig. 31.2 Schematic diagram showing the regulation of the acid-secreting gastric parietal cell, illustrating the site of action of drugs influencing acid secretion. The initial step in controlling physiological secretion is the release of gastrin from G cells. This acts through its gastrin/cholecystokinin (CCK$_2$) receptor on mast cell-like histamine-secreting enterochromaffin (ECL) cells to release histamine and may also have a secondary direct effect on parietal cells themselves, although this is not entirely clear. Histamine acts on parietal cell H$_2$ receptors to elevate cAMP that activates the secretion of acid by the proton pump. Direct vagal stimulation also provokes acid secretion and released acetylcholine directly stimulates M$_3$ receptors on parietal cells. The influence of somatostatin on G cells, ECL cells and parietal cells is inhibitory. Local (or therapeutically administered) prostaglandins exert inhibitory effects predominately on ECL cell function. Receptors depicted in *red* have inhibitory effects on cell secretion, whilst those in *blue* stimulate cell secretion. *AA*, arachidonic acid; *ACh*, acetylcholine; *C*, symport carrier for K$^+$ and Cl$^-$; *CCK$_2$*, gastrin/cholecystokinin receptor; *NSAIDs*, non-steroidal anti-inflammatory drugs; *P*, proton pump (H$^+$-K$^+$-ATPase); *PGE$_2$*, prostaglandin E$_2$.

cells to elevate cAMP and to activate the secretion of protons as described.

Direct vagal stimulation can also provoke acid secretion (the basis for 'stress ulcers') through a release of acetylcholine, which directly stimulates M$_3$ receptors on parietal cells. Somatostatin probably exerts a tonic inhibitory influence on G cells, ECL and parietal cells, and local (or therapeutically administered) prostaglandins, acting through EP$_{2/3}$ receptors, exert inhibitory effects predominantly on ECL cell function.

This control system is clearly complex, but prolonged exposure of tissues to excess acid secretion is dangerous and must be tightly regulated (see Schubert & Peura, 2008).

Secretion of gastric acid, mucus and bicarbonate

The control of the gastrointestinal tract is through nervous and humoral mechanisms.

- Acid is secreted from gastric parietal cells by a proton pump (K$^+$-H$^+$-ATPase).
- The three endogenous secretagogues for acid are histamine, acetylcholine and gastrin.
- Prostaglandins E$_2$ and I$_2$ inhibit acid, stimulate mucus and bicarbonate secretion, and dilate mucosal blood vessels.
- Somatostatin inhibits all phases of parietal cell activation.

The genesis of peptic ulcers involves:
- infection of the gastric mucosa with *Helicobacter pylori*;
- an imbalance between the mucosal-damaging, (acid, pepsin) and the mucosal-protecting, agents (mucus, bicarbonate, prostaglandins E$_2$ and I$_2$, and nitric oxide).

DRUGS USED TO INHIBIT OR NEUTRALISE GASTRIC ACID SECRETION

The principal clinical indications for reducing acid secretion are *peptic ulceration* (both duodenal and gastric), *GORD* (in which gastric secretion causes damage to the oesophagus) and the *Zollinger–Ellison syndrome* (a rare hypersecretory condition caused by a gastrin-producing tumour). If untreated, GORD can cause a dysplasia of the oesophageal epithelium which may progress to a potentially dangerous pre-cancerous condition called *Barrett oesophagus*.

The reasons why peptic ulcers develop are not fully understood, although infection of the stomach mucosa with *Helicobacter pylori*[3] – a Gram-negative bacillus that causes chronic gastritis – is now generally considered to be a major cause (especially of duodenal ulcer) and forms the usual basis for therapy. Treatment of *H. pylori* infection is discussed later.

Many non-specific NSAIDs (see Ch. 27) cause gastric bleeding and erosions by inhibiting cyclo-oxygenase I, the enzyme responsible for synthesis of protective prostaglandins. More selective cyclo-oxygenase II inhibitors such as **celecoxib** appear to cause less stomach damage (but see Ch. 27 for a discussion of this issue).

mechanism for controlling acid secretion. According to this idea (see Fig. 31.2), which is supported by the majority of transgenic 'knock-out' mouse studies, the initial step in controlling physiological secretion is the release of gastrin from G cells. This acts through its CCK$_2$ receptor on ECL cells to release histamine and may also have a secondary direct effect on parietal cells themselves, although this has been disputed. Histamine acts on H$_2$ receptors on parietal

---

[3]*H. pylori* infection in the stomach has also been classified as a class 1 (definite) carcinogen for gastric cancer.

Therapy of peptic ulcer and reflux oesophagitis aims to decrease the secretion of gastric acid with H₂ receptor antagonists or proton pump inhibitors, and/or to neutralise secreted acid with antacids (see Huang & Hunt, 2001). These treatments are often coupled with measures to eradicate *H. pylori* (see Blaser, 1998; Horn, 2000).

HISTAMINE H₂ RECEPTOR ANTAGONISTS

The discovery and development of histamine H₂-blocking drugs by Black and his colleagues in 1972 was a major breakthrough in the treatment of gastric ulcers – a condition that could hitherto only be treated by (sometimes rather heroic) surgery.[4] Indeed, the ability to distinguish between histamine receptor subtypes using pharmacological agents was, in itself, a major intellectual achievement. H₂ receptor antagonists competitively inhibit histamine actions at all H₂ receptors, but their main clinical use is as inhibitors of gastric acid secretion. They can inhibit histamine- and gastrin-stimulated acid secretion; pepsin secretion also falls with the reduction in volume of gastric juice. These agents not only decrease both basal and food-stimulated acid secretion by 90% or more, but numerous clinical trials indicate that they also promote healing of gastric and duodenal ulcers. However, relapses are likely to follow cessation of treatment.

The main drugs used are **cimetidine**, **ranitidine** (sometimes in combination with **bismuth**), **nizatidine** and **famotidine**. There is little difference between them. The effect of cimetidine on gastric secretion in human subjects is shown in Fig. 31.3. The clinical use of H₂ receptor antagonists is explained in the clinical box.

Clinical use of agents affecting gastric acidity

- Histamine H₂ receptor antagonists (e.g. **ranitidine**):
  - *peptic ulcer*
  - *reflux oesophagitis*
- Proton pump inhibitors (e.g. **omeprazole**, **lansoprazole**):
  - *peptic ulcer*
  - *reflux oesophagitis*
  - as one component of therapy for *Helicobacter pylori* infection
  - *Zollinger–Ellison* syndrome (a rare condition caused by gastrin-secreting tumours)
- Antacids (e.g. magnesium trisilicate, aluminium hydroxide, alginates):
  - *dyspepsia*
  - symptomatic relief in *peptic ulcer* or (**alginate**) *oesophageal reflux*
- **Bismuth chelate:**
  - as one component of therapy for *H. pylori* infection

Pharmacokinetic aspects and unwanted effects

The drugs are generally given orally and are well absorbed, although preparations for intramuscular and intravenous use are also available (except famotidine). Dosage regimens

Fig. 31.3 **The effect of cimetidine on betazole-stimulated gastric acid and pepsin secretion in humans.** Either cimetidine or a placebo was given orally 60 min prior to a subcutaneous injection (1.5 mg/kg) of betazole, a relatively specific histamine H₂-receptor agonist that stimulates gastric acid secretion. (Modified from Binder & Donaldson, 1978.)

vary depending on the condition under treatment. Low-dosage over-the-counter formulations of cimetidine, ranitidine and famotidine are available from pharmacies for short-term use, without prescription.

Unwanted effects are rare. Diarrhoea, dizziness, muscle pains, alopecia, transient rashes, confusion in the elderly and hypergastrinaemia have been reported. Cimetidine sometimes causes gynaecomastia in men and, rarely, a decrease in sexual function. This is probably caused by a modest affinity for androgen receptors. Cimetidine (but not other H₂ receptor antagonists) also inhibits cytochrome P450, and can retard the metabolism (and thus potentiate the action) of a range of drugs including oral anticoagulants and tricyclic antidepressants.

PROTON PUMP INHIBITORS

The first proton pump inhibitor was **omeprazole**, which irreversibly inhibits the H⁺-K⁺-ATPase (the proton pump), the terminal step in the acid secretory pathway (see Figs 31.1 and 31.2). Both basal and stimulated gastric acid secretion (Fig. 31.4) is reduced. The drug comprises a racemic mixture of two enantiomers. As a weak base, it accumulates in the acid environment of the canaliculi of the stimulated parietal cell where it is converted into an achiral form and is then able to react with, and inactivate, the ATPase. This preferential accumulation means that it has a specific effect

---

[4]This era has been referred to as the 'BC' – before cimetidine – era of gastroenterology (Schubert & Peura, 2008)! It is an indication of the clinical importance of the development of this drug.

Fig. 31.4 The inhibitory action of omeprazole on acid secretion from isolated human gastric glands stimulated by 50 μmol/L histamine. Acid secretion was measured by the accumulation of a radiolabelled weak base, aminopyrine (AP), in the secretory channels. The data represent the mean and standard error of measurements from eight patients. (Adapted from Lindberg, P. et al., 1987. Trends Pharmacol. Sci. 8, 399–402.)

on these cells. Other proton pump inhibitors (all of which have a similar mode of activation and pharmacology) include **esomeprazole** (the [S] isomer of omeprazole), **lansoprazole**, **pantoprazole** and **rabeprazole**. The clinical indication for these drugs is given in the clinical box (see earlier).

Pharmacokinetic aspects and unwanted effects

Oral administration is the most common route of administration, although some injectable preparations are available. Omeprazole is given orally, but as it degrades rapidly at low pH, it is administered as capsules containing enteric-coated granules. Following absorption in the small intestine, it passes from the blood into the parietal cells and then into the canaliculi where it exerts its effects. Increased doses give disproportionately higher increases in plasma concentration (possibly because its inhibitory effect on acid secretion improves its own bioavailability). Although its half-life is about 1 h, a single daily dose affects acid secretion for 2–3 days, partly because of the accumulation in the canaliculi and partly because it inhibits the H^+-K^+-ATPase irreversibly. With daily dosage, there is an increasing antisecretory effect for up to 5 days, after which a plateau is reached.

Unwanted effects of this class of drugs are uncommon. They may include headache, diarrhoea (both sometimes severe) and rashes. Acid-suppression with proton pump inhibitors is associated with increased risk of *Clostridium difficile* diarrhoea, particularly in patients who are immunosuppressed or have been receiving antibiotics. Dizziness, somnolence, mental confusion, impotence, gynaecomastia, and pain in muscles and joints have been reported. Proton pump inhibitors should be used with caution in patients with liver disease, or in women who are pregnant or breastfeeding. The use of these drugs may 'mask' the symptoms of gastric cancer.

ANTACIDS

Antacids are the simplest way to treat the symptoms of excessive gastric acid secretion. They directly neutralise

acid and this also has the effect of inhibiting the activity of peptic enzymes, which practically ceases at pH 5. Given in sufficient quantity for long enough, they can produce healing of duodenal ulcers, but are less effective for gastric ulcers.

Most antacids in common use are salts of magnesium and aluminium. Magnesium salts cause diarrhoea and aluminium salts, constipation – so mixtures of these two can, happily, be used to preserve normal bowel function. Preparations of these substances (e.g. **magnesium trisilicate** mixtures and some proprietary aluminium preparations) containing high concentrations of sodium should not be given to patients on a sodium-restricted diet. Numerous antacid preparations are available; a few of the more significant are given later.

Magnesium hydroxide is an insoluble powder that forms magnesium chloride in the stomach. It does not produce systemic alkalosis, because Mg^{2+} is poorly absorbed from the gut. Another salt, magnesium trisilicate, is an insoluble powder that reacts slowly with the gastric juice, forming magnesium chloride and colloidal silica. This agent has a prolonged antacid effect, and it also adsorbs pepsin. **Magnesium carbonate** is also used.

Aluminium hydroxide gel forms aluminium chloride in the stomach; when this reaches the intestine, the chloride is released and is reabsorbed. Aluminium hydroxide raises the pH of the gastric juice to about 4, and also adsorbs pepsin. Its action is gradual, and its effect continues for several hours.[5] Colloidal aluminium hydroxide combines with phosphates in the GI tract and the increased excretion of phosphate in the faeces that occurs results in decreased excretion of phosphate via the kidney. This effect has been used in treating patients with chronic renal failure (see Ch. 30). Other preparations such as **hydrotalcite** contain mixtures of both aluminium and magnesium salts.

Alginates or **simeticone** are sometimes combined with antacids. Alginates are believed to increase the viscosity and adherence of mucus to the oesophageal mucosa, forming a protective barrier, whereas simeticone is an anti-foaming agent, intended to relieve bloating and flatulence.

TREATMENT OF *HELICOBACTER PYLORI* INFECTION

H. pylori infection has been implicated as a causative factor in the production of gastric and, more particularly, duodenal ulcers, as well as a risk factor for gastric cancer. Indeed, some would argue that infectious gastroduodenitis is actually the chief clinical entity associated with ulcers, and gastric cancer its prominent sequela. Certainly, eradication of *H. pylori* infection promotes rapid and long-term healing of ulcers, and it is routine practice to test for the organism in patients presenting with suggestive symptoms. If the test is positive, then the organism can generally be eradicated with a 1- or 2-week regimen of 'triple therapy', comprising a proton pump inhibitor in combination with the antibacterials **amoxicillin** and **metronidazole** or **clarithromycin** (see Ch. 52); other combinations are also used. Bismuth-containing preparations (see later) are sometimes added.

---

[5]There was a suggestion – no longer widely believed – that aluminium could trigger Alzheimer's disease. In fact, aluminium is not absorbed to any significant extent following oral administration of aluminium hydroxide, although when introduced by other routes (e.g. during renal dialysis with aluminium-contaminated solutions) it is extremely toxic.

While elimination of the bacillus can produce long-term remission of ulcers, reinfection with the organism can occur.

DRUGS THAT PROTECT THE MUCOSA

Some agents, termed *cytoprotective*, are said to enhance endogenous mucosal protection mechanisms and/or to provide a physical barrier over the surface of the ulcer.

Bismuth chelate
Bismuth chelate (tripotassium dicitratobismuthate) is sometimes used in combination regimens to treat *H. pylori*. It has toxic effects on the bacillus, and may also prevent its adherence to the mucosa or inhibit its bacterial proteolytic enzymes. It is also believed to have other mucosa-protecting actions, by mechanisms that are unclear, and is widely used as an over-the-counter remedy for mild GI symptoms. Very little is absorbed, but if renal excretion is impaired, the raised plasma concentrations of bismuth can result in encephalopathy.

Unwanted effects include nausea and vomiting, and blackening of the tongue and faeces.

Sucralfate
Sucralfate is a complex of aluminium hydroxide and sulfated sucrose, which releases aluminium in the presence of acid. The residual complex carries a strong negative charge and binds to cationic groups in proteins, glycoproteins, etc. It can form complex gels with mucus, an action that is thought to decrease the degradation of mucus by pepsin and to limit the diffusion of H^+ ions. Sucralfate can also inhibit the action of pepsin and stimulate secretion of mucus, bicarbonate and prostaglandins from the gastric mucosa. All these actions contribute to its mucosa-protecting action.

Sucralfate is given orally and about 30% is still present in the stomach 3 h after administration. In the acid environment, the polymerised product forms a tenacious paste, which can sometimes produce an obstructive lump (known as a *bezoar*[6]) that gets stuck in the stomach. It reduces the absorption of a number of other drugs, including fluoroquinolone antibiotics, **theophylline**, **tetracycline**, **digoxin** and **amitriptyline**. Because it requires an acid environment for activation, antacids given concurrently or prior to its administration will reduce its efficacy.

Unwanted effects are few, the most common being constipation. Less common effects apart from bezoar formation, include dry mouth, nausea, vomiting, headache and rashes.

Misoprostol
Prostaglandins of the E and I series have a generally homeostatic protective action in the GI tract, and a deficiency in endogenous production (after ingestion of an NSAID, for example) may contribute to ulcer formation. **Misoprostol** is a stable analogue of prostaglandin E_1. It is given orally and is used to promote the healing of ulcers or to prevent the gastric damage that can occur with chronic use of NSAIDs. It exerts a direct action on the ECL cell (and possibly parietal cell also; see Fig. 31.2), inhibiting the basal secretion of gastric acid as well as the stimulation of production seen in response to food, pentagastrin and caffeine. It also increases mucosal blood flow and augments the secretion of mucus and bicarbonate.

Unwanted effects include diarrhoea and abdominal cramps; uterine contractions can also occur, so the drug should not be given during pregnancy (unless deliberately to induce a therapeutic abortion; see Ch. 36). Prostaglandins and NSAIDs are discussed more fully in Chapters 7 and 27.

VOMITING

Nausea and vomiting are unwanted side effects of many clinically used drugs, notably those used for cancer chemotherapy but also opioids, general anaesthetics and digoxin. They also occur in motion sickness,[7] during early pregnancy and in numerous disease states (e.g. migraine) as well as bacterial and viral infections.

THE REFLEX MECHANISM OF VOMITING
Vomiting is a defensive response intended to rid the organism of toxic or irritating material. Poisonous compounds, bacterial toxins, many cytotoxic drugs (as well as mechanical distension) trigger the release, from enterochromaffin cells in the lining of the GI tract, of mediators such as 5-HT. These transmitters trigger signals in vagal afferent fibres. The physical act of vomiting is co-ordinated centrally by the *vomiting* (or *emetic*) *centre* in the medulla; Fig. 31.5. Actually, this is not a discrete anatomical location but a network of neural pathways that integrate signals arriving from other locations. One of these, in the *area postrema* is known as the *chemoreceptor trigger zone* (CTZ). The CTZ receives inputs from the labyrinth in the inner ear through the *vestibular nuclei* (which explains the mechanism of motion sickness) and vagal afferents arising from the GI tract. Toxic chemicals in the bloodstream can also be detected directly by the CTZ because the blood–brain barrier is relatively permeable in this area. The CTZ is therefore a primary site of action of many emetic and antiemetic drugs (Table 31.1).

The vomiting centre also receives signals directly from vagal afferents, as well as those relayed through the CTZ. In addition, it receives input from higher cortical centres, explaining why unpleasant or repulsive sights or smells, or strong emotional stimuli, can sometimes induce nausea and vomiting.

The main neurotransmitters involved in this neurocircuitry are acetylcholine, histamine, 5-HT, dopamine and substance P and receptors for these transmitters have been demonstrated in the relevant areas (see Chs 13–17). It has been hypothesised that enkephalins (see Ch. 43) are also implicated in the mediation of vomiting, acting possibly at δ (CTZ) or μ (vomiting centre) opioid receptors. Substance P (see Ch. 19) acting at neurokinin-1 receptors in the CTZ, and endocannabinoids (Ch. 20), may also be involved.

The neurobiology of nausea is much less well understood. Nausea and vomiting may occur together or separately and may subserve different physiological functions (see

---

[6]From the Persian word meaning 'a cure for poisoning'. It refers to the belief that a concoction made from lumps of impacted rubbish retrieved from the stomach of goats would protect against poisoning by one's enemies.

[7]In fact, the word *nausea* is derived from the Greek word meaning 'boat', with the obvious implication of associated motion sickness. *Vomiting* is derived from a Latin word and a *vomitorium* was the 'fast exit' passageway in ancient theatres. It has a certain resonance, as we think you will agree!

Fig. 31.5 Schematic diagram of the factors involved in the control of vomiting, with the probable sites of action of antiemetic drugs. There are three important centres located in the medulla. The chemoreceptor trigger zone (CTZ), the vomiting centre and the vestibular nuclei. The vomiting centre receives inputs from the CTZ, the gastrointestinal (GI) tract (through vagal afferent connections) and higher cortical centres and coordinates the physical act of emesis. Vagal afferents arising from the GI tract also feed into the CTZ directly as does input from the vestibular nuclei, which in turn, receive inputs from the labyrinth. (Based partly on a diagram from Rojas & Slusher, 2012.)

Andrews & Horn, 2006). From the pharmacologist's viewpoint, it is easier to control vomiting than nausea, and many effective antiemetics (e.g. 5-HT$_3$ antagonists) are much less successful in this regard.

ANTIEMETIC DRUGS

Several antiemetic agents are available, and these are generally used for specific conditions, although there may be some overlap. Such drugs are of particular importance as an adjunct to cancer chemotherapy, where the nausea and vomiting produced by many cytotoxic drugs (see Ch. 57) can be almost unendurable.[8] In using drugs to treat the morning sickness of pregnancy, the problem of potential damage to the fetus has always to be borne in mind. In general, all drugs should be avoided during the first 3

months of pregnancy, if possible. Details of the main categories of antiemetics are given later, and their main clinical uses are summarised in the box. The clinical box and Table 31.1 give an overview of their likely sites of action and their clinical utility.

RECEPTOR ANTAGONISTS

Many H$_1$ (see Ch. 27), muscarinic (see Ch. 14), 5-HT$_3$ (see Ch. 16), dopamine (see Ch. 47) and neurokinin NK$_1$ receptor antagonists exhibit clinically useful antiemetic activity.

H$_1$ receptor antagonists

Cinnarizine, cyclizine and **promethazine** are the most commonly employed; they are effective against nausea and vomiting arising from many causes, including motion sickness and the presence of irritants in the stomach. None is very effective against substances that act directly on the CTZ. Promethazine is used for morning sickness of pregnancy (on the rare occasions when this is so severe that drug treatment is justified), and has been used by NASA to treat space motion sickness. Drowsiness and sedation,

---

[8]It was reported that a young, medically qualified patient being treated by combination chemotherapy for sarcoma stated that 'the severity of vomiting at times made the thought of death seem like a welcome relief'.

Table 31.1 Sites of action of common antiemetic drugs

Class	Drugs	Site of action	Comments
Antihistamines	Cinnarizine, cyclizine, promethazine	H_1 receptors in the CNS (causing sedation) and possibly anticholinergic actions in the vestibular apparatus	Widely effective regardless of cause of emesis
Antimuscarinics	Hyoscine	Anticholinergic actions in the vestibular apparatus and possibly elsewhere	Mainly motion sickness
Cannabinoids	Nabilone	Probably CB_1 receptors in the GI tract	CINV in patients where other drugs have been ineffective
Dopamine antagonists	Phenothiazines: prochlorphenazine, perphenazine, trifluorphenazine, chlorpromazine	D_2 receptors in CTZ	CINV, PONV, RS
	Related drugs: droperidol, haloperidol	D_2 receptors in GI tract	CINV, PONV, RS
	Metoclopramide	D_2 receptors in the CTZ and GI tract	PONV, CINV
Glucocorticoids	Dexamethasone	Probably multiple sites of action, including the GI tract	PONV, CINV; typically used in combination with other drugs
5-HT$_3$ antagonists	Granisteron, ondansetron, palonosetron	5-HT$_3$ receptors in CTZ and GI tract	PONV, CINV
Neurokinin-1 antagonists	Aprepitant, fosaprepitant	NK_1 receptors in CTZ, vomiting centre and possibly the GI tract	CINV; given in combination with another drug

5-HT, 5-hydroxytryptamine; *CINV*, cytotoxic drug-induced vomiting; *CNS*, central nervous system; *CTZ*, chemoreceptor trigger zone; *GI*, gastrointestinal; *PONV*, postoperative nausea and vomiting; *RS*, radiation sickness.

The reflex mechanism of vomiting

Emetic stimuli include:
- chemicals or drugs in the blood or intestine;
- neuronal input from the gastrointestinal (GI) tract, labyrinth and central nervous system (CNS).

Pathways and mediators include:
- impulses from the chemoreceptor trigger zone and various other CNS centres relayed to the vomiting centre;
- chemical transmitters such as histamine, acetylcholine, dopamine, 5-hydroxytryptamine (5-HT) and substance P, acting on H_1, muscarinic, D_2, 5-HT$_3$ and NK_1 receptors, respectively.

Antiemetic drugs include:
- H_1 receptor antagonists (e.g. **cinnarizine**);
- muscarinic antagonists (e.g. **hyoscine**);
- 5-HT$_3$ receptor antagonists (e.g. **ondansetron**);
- D_2 receptor antagonists (e.g. **metoclopramide**);
- cannabinoids (e.g. **nabilone**);
- neurokinin-1 antagonists (e.g. **aprepitant**, **fosaprepitant**).

Main side effects of principal antiemetics include:
- drowsiness and antiparasympathetic effects (**hyoscine, nabilone > cinnarizine**);
- dystonic reactions (**metoclopramide**);
- general CNS disturbances (**nabilone**);
- headache, GI tract upsets (**ondansetron**).

Clinical use of antiemetic drugs

- Histamine H_1 receptor antagonists (see also clinical box in Ch. 27):
  - **Cyclizine**: motion sickness, vestibular disorders, nausea and vomiting associated with surgery and postoperative narcotic analgesic use.
  - **Cinnarizine**: motion sickness, vestibular disorders (e.g. Menière's disease).
  - **Promethazine**: severe morning sickness of pregnancy, motion sickness, vestibular disorders.
- Muscarinic receptor antagonists:
  - **Hyoscine**: motion sickness.
- Dopamine D_2 receptor antagonists:
  - Phenothiazines (e.g. **prochlorperazine**): vomiting caused by migraine, vestibular disorders, radiation, viral gastroenteritis, severe morning sickness of pregnancy.
  - **Metoclopramide**: vomiting caused by migraine, radiation, gastrointestinal disorders, cytotoxic drugs, prevention of nausea and vomiting in the postoperative period.
  - **Domperidone** is less liable to cause central nervous system side effects in patients with Parkinson's disease as it penetrates the blood–brain barrier poorly.
- 5-Hydroxytryptamine (5-HT)$_3$ receptor antagonists (e.g. **ondansetron**): cytotoxic drugs or radiation, postoperative vomiting.
- Cannabinoids (e.g. **nabilone**): cytotoxic drugs (see Ch. 20).
- NK_1 receptor antagonists (e.g. **fosaprepitant**): cytotoxic drugs.

while possibly contributing to their clinical efficacy, are the chief unwanted effects.

Betahistine has complicated effects on histamine action, antagonising H_3 receptors but having a weak agonist activity on H_1 receptors. It is used to control the nausea and vertigo associated with *Menière's disease*.[9]

Muscarinic receptor antagonists

Hyoscine (scopolamine) is employed principally for prophylaxis and treatment of motion sickness, and may be administered orally or as a transdermal patch. Dry mouth and blurred vision are the most common unwanted effects. Drowsiness also occurs, but the drug has less sedative action than the antihistamines because of poor central nervous system penetration.

5-HT$_3$ receptor antagonists

Granisetron, **ondansetron** and **palonosetron** (see Ch. 16) are of particular value in preventing and treating the vomiting and, to a lesser extent the nausea, commonly encountered postoperatively as well as that caused by radiation therapy or administration of cytotoxic drugs such as **cisplatin**. The primary site of action of these drugs is the CTZ. They may be given orally or by injection (sometimes helpful if nausea is already present). Unwanted effects such as headache and GI upsets are relatively uncommon.

Dopamine antagonists

Antipsychotic phenothiazines (see Ch. 47), such as **chlorpromazine**, **perphenazine**, **prochlorperazine** and **trifluoperazine**, are effective antiemetics commonly used for treating the more severe nausea and vomiting associated with cancer, radiation therapy, cytotoxic drugs, opioids, anaesthetics and other drugs. They can be administered orally, intravenously or by suppository. They act mainly as antagonists of the dopamine D_2 receptors in the CTZ (see Fig. 31.5) but they also block histamine and muscarinic receptors.

Unwanted effects are common and include sedation (especially chlorpromazine), hypotension and extrapyramidal symptoms including dystonias and tardive dyskinesia (Ch. 47).

Other antipsychotic drugs, such as **haloperidol**, the related compound **droperidol** and **levomepromazine** (Ch. 47), also act as D_2 antagonists in the CTZ and can be used for acute chemotherapy-induced emesis.

Metoclopramide and domperidone

Metoclopramide is a D_2 receptor antagonist (see Fig. 31.5), closely related to the phenothiazine group, that acts centrally on the CTZ and also has a peripheral action on the GI tract itself, increasing the motility of the oesophagus, stomach and intestine. This not only adds to the antiemetic effect, but explains its use in the treatment of gastro-oesophageal reflux and hepatic and biliary disorders. As metoclopramide also blocks dopamine receptors elsewhere in the central nervous system, it produces a number of unwanted effects including disorders of movement (more common in children and young adults), fatigue, motor restlessness, spasmodic

torticollis (involuntary twisting of the neck) and oculogyric crises (involuntary upward eye movements). It stimulates prolactin release (see Chs 34 and 36) causing galactorrhoea and disorders of menstruation.

Domperidone is a similar drug used to treat vomiting due to cytotoxic therapy as well as GI symptoms. Unlike metoclopramide, it does not readily penetrate the blood–brain barrier and is consequently less prone to producing central side effects. However, domperidone is associated with a small increased risk of serious cardiac adverse effects (particularly at higher doses and in older patients), and its use is now restricted.

Both drugs are given orally, have plasma half-lives of 4–5 h and are excreted in the urine.

NK$_1$ receptor antagonists

Substance P causes vomiting when injected intravenously and is released by GI vagal afferent nerves as well as in the vomiting centre itself. **Aprepitant** blocks substance P (NK$_1$) receptors (see Ch. 19) in the CTZ and vomiting centre. Aprepitant is given orally, and is effective in controlling the late phase of emesis caused by cytotoxic drugs, with few significant unwanted effects. **Fosaprepitant** is a prodrug of aprepitant, which is administered intravenously.

OTHER ANTIEMETIC DRUGS

Anecdotal evidence originally suggested the possibility of using cannabinoids (see Ch. 20) as antiemetics (see Pertwee, 2001). The synthetic cannabinol **nabilone** has been found to decrease vomiting caused by agents that stimulate the CTZ, and is sometimes effective where other drugs have failed. The antiemetic effect is antagonised by **naloxone**, which implies that opioid receptors may be important in the mechanism of action. Nabilone is given orally; it is well absorbed from the GI tract and is metabolised in many tissues. Its plasma half-life is approximately 120 min, and its metabolites are excreted in the urine and faeces.

Unwanted effects are common, especially drowsiness, dizziness and dry mouth. Mood changes and postural hypotension are also fairly frequent. Some patients experience hallucinations and psychotic reactions, resembling the effect of other cannabinoids (see Ch. 20).

High-dose glucocorticoids (particularly **dexamethasone**; see Chs 27 and 34) can also control emesis, especially when this is caused by cytotoxic drugs. The mechanism of action is not clear. Dexamethasone is typically deployed in combination with metoclopramide or ondansetron in patients receiving cytotoxics, or in postoperative nausea and vomiting.

THE MOTILITY OF THE GI TRACT

Drugs that alter the motility of the GI tract include:

- purgatives, which accelerate the passage of food through the intestine;
- agents that increase the motility of the GI smooth muscle without causing purgation;
- antidiarrhoeal drugs, which decrease motility;
- antispasmodic drugs, which decrease smooth muscle tone.

---

[9]A disabling condition named after the eponymous French physician who discovered that the nausea and vertigo that characterise this condition were associated with a disorder of the inner ear.

Clinical uses of drugs that affect the motility of the GI tract are summarised in the clinical box below.

> ### Drugs and GI tract motility
>
>
> - Purgatives include:
>   - bulk laxatives (e.g. **ispaghula husk**, first choice for slow action);
>   - osmotic laxatives (e.g. **lactulose**);
>   - faecal softeners (e.g. **docusate**);
>   - stimulant purgatives (e.g. **senna**).
> - Drugs used to treat diarrhoea:
>   - oral rehydration with isotonic solutions of NaCl plus glucose and starch-based cereal (important in infants);
>   - antimotility agents, e.g. **loperamide** (unwanted effects: drowsiness and nausea).

PURGATIVES

The transit of food through the intestine may be hastened by several different types of drugs, including laxatives, faecal softeners and stimulant purgatives. The latter agents may be used to relieve constipation or to clear the bowel prior to surgery or examination.

BULK AND OSMOTIC LAXATIVES

The *bulk laxatives* include **methylcellulose** and certain plant extracts such as **sterculia**, **agar**, **bran** and **ispaghula husk**. These agents are polysaccharide polymers that are not digested in the upper part of the GI tract. They form a bulky hydrated mass in the gut lumen promoting peristalsis and improving faecal consistency. They may take several days to work but have no serious unwanted effects.

The *osmotic laxatives* consist of poorly absorbed solutes – the saline purgatives – and **lactulose**. The main salts in use are magnesium sulfate and magnesium hydroxide. By producing an osmotic load, these agents trap increased volumes of fluid in the lumen of the bowel, accelerating the transfer of the gut contents through the small intestine. This results in an abnormally large volume entering the colon, causing distension and purgation within about an hour. Abdominal cramps can occur. The amount of magnesium absorbed after an oral dose is usually too small to have adverse systemic effects, but these salts should be avoided in small children and in patients with poor renal function, in whom they can cause heart block, neuromuscular block or central nervous system depression. While isotonic or hypotonic solutions of saline purgatives cause purgation, hypertonic solutions can cause vomiting. Sometimes, other sodium salts of phosphate and citrate are given rectally, by suppository, to relieve constipation.

Lactulose is a semisynthetic disaccharide of fructose and galactose. It is poorly absorbed and produces an effect similar to that of the other osmotic laxatives. It takes 2–3 days to act. Unwanted effects, seen with high doses, include flatulence, cramps, diarrhoea and electrolyte disturbance. Tolerance can develop. Another agent, **macrogol**, which consists of inert ethylene glycol polymers, acts in the same way, and is sometimes formulated together with electrolyte ions to ensure that the laxative effect does not cause marked changes in sodium, potassium and water balance.

FAECAL SOFTENERS

Docusate sodium is a surface-active compound that acts in the GI tract in a manner similar to a detergent and produces softer faeces. It is also a weak stimulant laxative. Other agents that achieve the same effect include **arachis oil**, which is given as an enema, and **liquid paraffin**, although this is now seldom used.

STIMULANT LAXATIVES

The stimulant laxative drugs act mainly by increasing electrolyte and hence water secretion by the mucosa, and by increasing peristalsis – possibly by stimulating enteric nerves. Abdominal cramping may be experienced as a side effect with almost any of these drugs.

Bisacodyl may be given by mouth but is often given by suppository. In the latter case, it stimulates the rectal mucosa, inducing defecation in 15–30 min. Glycerol suppositories act in the same manner. **Sodium picosulfate** and docusate sodium have similar actions. The former is given orally and is often used in preparation for intestinal surgery or colonoscopy.

Senna and **dantron** are **anthraquinone** laxatives. The active principle (after hydrolysis of glycosidic linkages in the case of the plant extract, senna) directly stimulates the myenteric plexus, resulting in increased peristalsis and thus defecation. Dantron is similar. As this drug is a skin irritant and may be carcinogenic, it is generally used only in the terminally ill.

Laxatives of any type should not be used when there is obstruction of the bowel. Overuse can lead to an atonic colon where the natural propulsive activity is diminished. In these circumstances, the only way to achieve defecation is to take further amounts of laxatives, so a sort of dependency arises.

DRUGS THAT INCREASE GASTROINTESTINAL MOTILITY

Domperidone is primarily used as an antiemetic (as described previously), but it also increases GI motility (although the mechanism is unknown).

Metoclopramide (also an antiemetic) stimulates gastric motility, causing a marked acceleration of gastric emptying. It is useful in gastro-oesophageal reflux and in disorders of gastric emptying, but is ineffective in paralytic ileus.

Prucalopride is a selective 5-HT$_4$ receptor agonist that has marked prokinetic properties on the gut. It is generally only used when other types of laxative treatment have failed.

Lubiprostone is a chloride channel-2 activator that acts on cells in the apical membrane of the small intestine to promote chloride and fluid secretion into the lumen, with associated improvements in gut motility and softer stool. It has regulatory approval for treatment of constipation due to opioids, in irritable bowel syndrome, and in patients who have failed to respond to non-drug treatment of constipation.

Naloxegol is a μ opioid-receptor antagonist that is similar to naloxone, but with the addition of a pegylated portion to prevent penetration into the central nervous system. Naloxegol counteracts the reduced GI motility and hypertonicity that is seen in opioid-induced constipation, but without exerting any adverse effect on the analgesic properties of opioid agonists centrally. **Methylnaltrexone** is a peripheral opioid-receptor antagonist that is licensed for opioid-induced constipation, and there are a number of related compounds (examples include **naldemedine** and **axelopran**) in development (Nelson & Camilleri, 2016).

ANTIDIARRHOEAL AGENTS

There are numerous causes of diarrhoea, including underlying disease, infection, toxins and even anxiety. It may also arise as a side effect of drug or radiation therapy. The consequences range from mild discomfort and inconvenience to a medical emergency requiring hospitalisation, parenteral fluid and electrolyte replacement therapy. Globally, acute diarrhoeal disease is one of the principal causes of death in malnourished infants, especially in developing countries where medical care is less accessible and 1–2 million children die each year for want of simple counter-measures.

During an episode of diarrhoea, there is an increase in the motility of the GI tract, accompanied by an increased secretion, coupled with a decreased absorption, of fluid. This leads to a loss of electrolytes (particularly Na$^+$) and water. Cholera toxins and some other bacterial toxins produce a profound increase in electrolyte and fluid secretion by irreversibly activating the G proteins that couple the surface receptors of the mucosal cells to adenylyl cyclase (see Ch. 3).

There are three approaches to the treatment of severe acute diarrhoea:

- maintenance of fluid and electrolyte balance;
- use of anti-infective agents;
- use of spasmolytic or other antidiarrhoeal agents.

The maintenance of fluid and electrolyte balance by means of oral rehydration is the first priority. Wider application of this cheap and simple remedy could save the lives of many infants in the developing world. Indeed, many patients require no other treatment.

In the ileum, as in the nephron, there is co-transport of Na$^+$ and glucose across the epithelial cell. The presence of glucose (and some amino acids) therefore enhances Na$^+$ absorption and thus water uptake. Preparations of sodium chloride and glucose for oral rehydration are available in powder form, ready to be dissolved in water before use.

Many GI infections are viral in origin. Those that are bacterial generally resolve fairly rapidly, so the use of anti-infective agents is usually neither necessary nor useful. Other cases may require more aggressive therapy, however. *Campylobacter* spp. is the commonest cause of bacterial gastroenteritis in the United Kingdom, and severe infections may require **ciprofloxacin**. The most common bacterial organisms encountered by travellers include *Escherichia coli*, *Salmonella* and *Shigella*, as well as protozoa such as *Giardia* and *Cryptosporidium* spp. Drug treatment (Chs 52 and 55) may be necessary in these and other more serious infections.

TRAVELLERS' DIARRHOEA

Millions of people cross international borders each year. Many travel hopefully, but many return with GI symptoms such as diarrhoea, having encountered enterotoxin-producing *E. coli* (the most common cause) or other organisms. Most infections are mild and self-limiting, requiring only oral replacement of fluid and salt, as detailed previously. General principles for the drug treatment of travellers' diarrhoea are detailed by Gorbach (1987).[10] Up-to-date

information on the condition, including the prevalence of infectious organisms around the globe as well as recommended treatment guidelines, is issued in the United Kingdom by the National Travel Health Network and Centre (see web links in the reference list).

ANTIMOTILITY AND SPASMOLYTIC AGENTS

The main pharmacological agents that decrease motility are opioids (Ch. 43) and muscarinic receptor antagonists (Ch. 14). Agents in this latter group are seldom employed as primary therapy for diarrhoea because of their actions on other systems, but small doses of **atropine** are sometimes used, combined with **diphenoxylate**. The action of **morphine**, the archetypal opiate, on the alimentary tract is complex; it increases the tone and rhythmic contractions of the intestine but diminishes propulsive activity. The pyloric, ileocolic and anal sphincters are contracted, and the tone of the large intestine is markedly increased. Its overall effect is constipating.

The main opioids used for the symptomatic relief of diarrhoea are **codeine** (a morphine congener), diphenoxylate and **loperamide** (both **pethidine** congeners that do not readily penetrate the blood–brain barrier and are used only for their actions in the gut). All may have unwanted effects, including constipation, abdominal cramps, drowsiness and dizziness. Complete loss of intestinal motility (paralytic ileus) can also occur. They should not be used in young (<4 years of age) children.

Loperamide is the drug of first choice for pharmacotherapy of travellers' diarrhoea and is a component of several proprietary antidiarrhoeal medicines. It has a relatively selective action on the GI tract and undergoes significant enterohepatic cycling. It reduces the frequency of abdominal cramps, decreases the passage of faeces and shortens the duration of the illness.

Diphenoxylate also lacks morphine-like activity in the central nervous system, although large doses (25-fold higher) produce typical opioid effects. Preparations of diphenoxylate usually contain atropine as well. Codeine and loperamide have antisecretory actions in addition to their effects on intestinal motility.

'Endogenous opioids', enkephalins (Ch. 43), also play a role in regulation of intestinal secretion. **Racecadotril** is a prodrug of **thiorphan**, an inhibitor of enkephalinase. By preventing the breakdown of enkephalins, this drug reduces the excessive intestinal secretion seen during episodes of diarrhoea. It is used in combination with rehydration therapy.

Cannabinoid receptor agonists also reduce gut motility in animals, most probably by decreasing acetylcholine release from enteric nerves. There have been anecdotal reports of a beneficial effect of cannabis against dysentery and cholera.

Drugs that reduce GI motility are also useful in irritable bowel syndrome and diverticular disease. Muscarinic receptor antagonists (Ch. 14) used for this purpose include atropine, hyoscine, **propantheline** and **dicycloverine**. The last named is thought to have some additional direct relaxant action on smooth muscle. All produce antimuscarinic side effects such as dry mouth, blurred vision and urinary retention. **Mebeverine**, a derivative of reserpine, has a direct relaxant action on GI smooth muscle. Unwanted effects are few.

ADSORBENTS

Adsorbent agents are used in the symptomatic treatment of some types of diarrhoea, although properly controlled

---

[10]Who flippantly (although accurately) observed that 'travel broadens the mind and loosens the bowels'.

trials proving efficacy have not been carried out. The main preparations used contain kaolin, pectin, chalk, charcoal, methylcellulose and activated attapulgite (magnesium aluminium silicate). It has been suggested that these agents may act by adsorbing microorganisms or toxins, by altering the intestinal flora or by coating and protecting the intestinal mucosa, but there is no hard evidence for this. Kaolin is sometimes given as a mixture with morphine (e.g. kaolin and morphine mixture BP).

DRUGS FOR CHRONIC BOWEL DISEASE

This category comprises *irritable bowel syndrome* (IBS) and *inflammatory bowel disease* (IBD). IBS is characterised by bouts of diarrhoea, constipation or abdominal pain. The aetiology of the disease is uncertain, but psychological factors may play a part. Treatment is symptomatic, with a high-residue diet plus loperamide or a laxative if needed.

Eluxadoline is a mixed μ and κ opioid-receptor agonist and δ-receptor antagonist that has recently been licensed for treatment of IBS with diarrhoea. The drug acts on opioids receptors in enteric neurons that regulate motility and visceral sensation in the GI tract, resulting in slowing of intestinal transit and improved stool consistency. Eluxadoline has low oral bioavailability and is considered to have limited potential for adverse effects on opioid receptors in the central nervous system (see Corsetti & Whorwell, 2016).

Linaclotide has recently received regulatory approval for symptomatic treatment of moderate to severe IBS with constipation in adults. It is a synthetic peptide that is structurally related to endogenous guanylin peptides. Linaclotide is an agonist at the guanylate cyclase-C receptor on the luminal surface of intestinal epithelium, and increases the concentration of cyclic guanosine monophosphate in the intestinal cells. This results in greater secretion of chloride and bicarbonate ions and intestinal fluid, as well as more rapid intestinal transit. Clinical trials have demonstrated improvements in bowel movements and reduction in abdominal discomfort, although diarrhoea is a recognised adverse effect (see Corsetti & Whorwell, 2016).

Ulcerative colitis and *Crohn's disease* are forms of IBD, affecting the colon or ileum. They are autoimmune inflammatory disorders, which can be severe and progressive, requiring long-term drug treatment with anti-inflammatory and immunosuppressant drugs (see Ch. 27), and occasionally surgical resection. The following agents are commonly used.

GLUCOCORTICOIDS

Glucocorticoids are potent anti-inflammatory agents and are dealt with in Chapters 27 and 34. The drugs of choice are generally **prednisolone** or **budesonide** (although others can be used). They are administered orally or locally into the bowel by suppository or enema.

AMINOSALICYLATES

While glucocorticoids are useful for the acute attacks of IBDs, they are not the ideal for the long-term treatment because of their side effects. Maintenance of remission in both ulcerative colitis and Crohn's disease is generally achieved with aminosalicylates, although they are less useful in the latter condition.

Sulfasalazine consists of the sulfonamide sulfapyridine linked to 5-aminosalicylic acid (5-ASA). The latter forms the active moiety when it is released in the colon. Its mechanism of action is obscure. It may reduce inflammation by scavenging free radicals, by inhibiting prostaglandin and leukotriene production, and/or by decreasing neutrophil chemotaxis and superoxide generation. Its unwanted effects include diarrhoea, salicylate sensitivity and interstitial nephritis. 5-ASA is not absorbed, but the sulfapyridine moiety, which seems to be therapeutically inert in this instance, is absorbed, and its unwanted effects are those associated with the sulfonamides (see Ch. 52).

Newer compounds in this class, which presumably share a similar mechanism of action, include **mesalazine** (5-ASA itself), **olsalazine** (a 5-ASA dimer linked by a bond that is hydrolysed by colonic bacteria) and **balsalazide** (a prodrug from which 5-ASA is also released following hydrolysis of a diazo linkage).

OTHER DRUGS

Methotrexate and the immunosuppressants **ciclosporin**, **tacrolimus**, **azathioprine** and **6-mercaptopurine** (see Ch. 27) are also sometimes used in patients with severe IBD. The biopharmaceuticals **infliximab**, **adalimumab** and **golimumab**, monoclonal antibodies directed against tumour necrosis factor (TNF)-α (see Ch. 27), have also been used with success. These drugs are expensive, and their principal indication is for moderate and severe Crohn's disease that is unresponsive to glucocorticoids or immunomodulators.

Newer biopharmaceuticals agents have been developed towards alternative targets in the inflammatory pathway. **Vedolizumab** is a humanised monoclonal antibody with specific binding properties for α4β7 integrin on T-helper lymphocytes that migrate to the gut. The inhibition of α4β7 integrin stops the interaction of these lymphocytes with mucosal addressin cell adhesion molecule-1 on gut epithelial cells, thus reducing the inflammatory effects in the bowel tissue that arise from trans-migration of T lymphocytes. In contrast, **ustekinumab** is targeted at the p40 protein subunit of interleukin (IL)-12 and IL-23, and prevents these cytokines from binding to IL-12Rβ1 receptors on immune cells. Vedolizumab and ustekinumab are indicated in those with moderately to severely active Crohn's disease, who have not responded to or cannot tolerate conventional treatment and other biopharmaceuticals.

The antiallergy drug sodium **cromoglicate** (see Ch. 29) is sometimes used for treating GI symptoms associated with food allergies.

DRUGS AFFECTING THE BILIARY SYSTEM

The commonest pathological condition of the biliary tract is *cholesterol cholelithiasis* – the formation of gallstones with high cholesterol content. Surgery is generally the preferred option, but there are orally active drugs that dissolve non-calcified 'radiolucent' cholesterol gallstones. The principal agent is **ursodeoxycholic acid**, a minor constituent of human bile (but the main bile acid in the bear, hence *urso*-). Diarrhoea is the main unwanted effect.

Biliary colic, the pain produced by the passage of gallstones through the bile duct, can be very intense, and immediate relief may be required. Morphine relieves the pain effectively, but it may have an undesirable local effect because it constricts the sphincter of Oddi and raises the pressure in the bile duct. **Buprenorphine** may be preferable. Pethidine has similar actions, although it relaxes other smooth muscle, for example, that of the ureter. Atropine is commonly employed to relieve biliary spasm because it has antispasmodic action and may be used in conjunction with morphine. **Glyceryl trinitrate** (see Ch. 22) can produce a marked fall of intrabiliary pressure and may be used to relieve biliary spasm.

FUTURE DIRECTIONS

The quest for novel antisecretory drugs is an ongoing task. Amongst the newer agents that have undergone evaluation are gastrin/cholecystokinin-2 receptor antagonists (with little success) and potassium competitive acid-blocking drugs (Inatomi et al., 2016). The latter agents work because potassium ions are exchanged for protons by the proton pump (see Fig. 31.1) and so potassium antagonists with rapid onset of action and sustained effect would represent a promising modality for inhibiting the secretion of acid. Unfortunately, the agents produced so far have not been conclusively proven to be superior to proton pump inhibitors, and currently, the two available agents (**revaprazan**, **vonoprazan**) are licensed only in a few Asian countries (Inatomi et al., 2016).

REFERENCES AND FURTHER READING

Innervation and hormones of the gastrointestinal tract

Hansen, M.B., 2003. The enteric nervous system II: gastrointestinal functions. Pharmacol. Toxicol. 92, 249–257. (*Small review on the role of the enteric nervous system in the control of gastrointestinal motility, secretory activity, blood flow and immune status; easy to read*)

Sanger, G.J., 2004. Neurokinin NK_1 and NK_3 receptors as targets for drugs to treat gastrointestinal motility disorders and pain. Br. J. Pharmacol. 141, 1303–1312. (*Useful review that deals with the present and potential future uses of neurokinin antagonists in gastrointestinal physiology and pathology*)

Spiller, R., 2002. Serotonergic modulating drugs for functional gastrointestinal diseases. Br. J. Clin. Pharmacol. 54, 11–20. (*An excellent and 'easily digestible' article describing the latest thinking on the use of 5-hydroxytryptamine agonists and antagonists in gastrointestinal function; useful diagrams*)

Gastric secretion

Binder, H.J., Donaldson, R.M., Jr., 1978. Effect of cimetidine on intrinsic factor and pepsin secretion in man. Gastroenterology 74, 371–375.

Chen, D., Friis-Hansen, L., Håkanson, R., Zhao, C.M., 2005. Genetic dissection of the signaling pathways that control gastric acid secretion. Inflammopharmacology 13, 201–207. (*Describes experiments using receptor 'knock-outs' to analyse the mechanisms that control gastric acid production*)

Cui, G., Waldum, H.L., 2007. Physiological and clinical significance of enterochromaffin-like cell activation in the regulation of gastric acid secretion. World J. Gastroenterol. 13, 493–496. (*Short review on the central role of ECL cells in the regulation of gastric acid secretion. Easy to read*)

Horn, J., 2000. The proton-pump inhibitors: similarities and differences. Clin. Ther. 22, 266–280, discussion 265. (*Excellent overview*)

Huang, J.Q., Hunt, R.H., 2001. Pharmacological and pharmacodynamic essentials of H(2)-receptor antagonists and proton pump inhibitors for the practising physician. Best Pract. Res. Clin. Gastroenterol. 15, 355–370.

Inatomi, N., Matsukawa, J., Sakurai, Y., Otake, K., 2016. Potassium-competitive acid blockers: advanced therapeutic option for acid-related diseases. Pharmacol. Ther. 168, 12–22. (*A good account of the shortcomings of current anti-secretory drugs and developments in the field*)

Linberg, P., Brandstrom, A., Wallmark, B., 1987. Structure-activity relationships of omeprazole analogues and their mechanism of action. Trends Pharmacol. Sci. 8, 399–402.

Schubert, M.L., Peura, D.A., 2008. Control of gastric acid secretion in health and disease. Gastroenterology 134, 1842–1860. (*Excellent review of the physiology and pharmacology of gastric acid secretion. Authoritative and well illustrated*)

Drugs in GI disorders

Black, J.W., Duncan, W.A.M., Durant, C.J., et al., 1972. Definition and antagonism of histamine H_2-receptors. Nature 236, 385–390. (*Seminal paper outlining the pharmacological approach to inhibition of acid secretion through antagonism at an alternative histamine receptor*)

Blaser, M.J., 1998. *Helicobacter pylori* and gastric diseases. BMJ 316, 1507–1510. (*Succinct review, emphasis on future developments*)

Klotz, U., 2000. The role of aminosalicylates at the beginning of the new millennium in the treatment of chronic inflammatory bowel disease. Eur. J. Clin. Pharmacol. 56, 353–362.

Mossner, J., Caca, K., 2005. Developments in the inhibition of gastric acid secretion. Eur. J. Clin. Invest. 35, 469–475. (*Useful overview of several new directions in gastrointestinal drug development*)

Pertwee, R.G., 2001. Cannabinoids and the gastrointestinal tract. Gut 48, 859–867.

Nausea and vomiting

Andrews, P.L., Horn, C.C., 2006. Signals for nausea and emesis: implications for models of upper gastrointestinal diseases. Auton. Neurosci. 125, 100–115.

Hesketh, P.J., 2001. Potential role of the NK_1 receptor antagonists in chemotherapy-induced nausea and vomiting. Support. Care Cancer 9, 350–354.

Hornby, P.J., 2001. Central neurocircuitry associated with emesis. Am. J. Med. 111, 106S–112S. (*Comprehensive review of central control of vomiting*)

Rojas, C., Slusher, B.S., 2012. Pharmacological mechanisms of 5-HT(3) and tachykinin NK(1) receptor antagonism to prevent chemotherapy-induced nausea and vomiting. Eur. J. Pharmacol. 684, 1–7.

Tramèr, M.R., Moore, R., Reynolds, D.J., McQuay, H.J., 1997. A quantitative systematic review of ondansetron in treatment of established postoperative nausea and vomiting. Br. Med. J. 314, 1088–1092.

Yates, B.J., Miller, A.D., Lucot, J.B., 1998. Physiological basis and pharmacology of motion sickness: an update. Brain Res. Bull. 5, 395–406. (*Good account of the mechanisms underlying motion sickness and its treatment*)

Motility of the gastrointestinal tract

Corsetti, M., Whorwell, P., 2016. Novel pharmacological therapies for irritable bowel syndrome. Expert Rev. Gastroenterol. Hepatol. 10, 807–815. (*Good review article covering current treatments*)

De Las Casas, C., Adachi, J., Dupont, H., 1999. Travellers' diarrhoea. Aliment. Pharmacol. Ther. 13, 1373–1378. (*Review article*)

Gorbach, S.L., 1987. Bacterial diarrhoea and its treatment. Lancet 1378–1382.

Nelson, A.D., Camilleri, M., 2016. Opioid-induced constipation: advances and clinical guidance. Ther. Adv. Chronic Dis. 7, 121–134.

The biliary system

Bateson, M.C., 1997. Bile acid research and applications. Lancet 349, 5–6.

Useful Web resources

www.nathnac.org. (*This is the site for the UK Health Protection Agency's National Travel Health Network and Centre. There are two components to the site, one for lay people and one for health professionals. Click on the latter and enter 'Travellers' diarrhoea' as a search term to retrieve current information and advice*)

32 The control of blood glucose and drug treatment of diabetes mellitus

OVERVIEW

In this chapter we describe the endocrine control of blood glucose by pancreatic hormones, especially *insulin* but also *glucagon* and *somatostatin*, and the gut hormones (*incretins*) *glucagon-like peptide-1* (GLP-1) and *gastric inhibitory peptide* (GIP, which is also known as glucose-dependent insulinotropic peptide). This underpins coverage of diabetes mellitus and its treatment with insulin preparations (including insulin analogues), and other hypoglycaemic agents – metformin, sulfonylureas, α-glucosidase inhibitors, long-acting incretin mimetics such as exenatide, gliptins, which potentiate incretins by blocking their degradation, and renal tubular sodium–glucose co-transport inhibitors.

INTRODUCTION

Insulin is the main hormone controlling intermediary metabolism. Its most striking acute effect is to lower blood glucose. Reduced (or absent) secretion of insulin causes *diabetes mellitus*. It is often coupled with reduced sensitivity to its action, 'insulin resistance', which is closely related to obesity. Diabetes mellitus, recognised since ancient times, is named for the production of sugary urine in copious volumes (due to the osmotic diuretic action of the high urine glucose concentration). Diabetes is rapidly increasing to epidemic proportions (in step with obesity, Ch. 33), and its consequences are dire – especially accelerated atherosclerosis (myocardial and cerebral infarction, gangrene or limb amputation), kidney failure, neuropathy and blindness.

In this chapter, we first describe the control of blood sugar. The second part of the chapter is devoted to the different kinds of diabetes mellitus and the role of drugs in their treatment. Diabetes, along with obesity (Ch. 33), hypertension (Ch. 23), dyslipidaemia (Ch. 24), and fatty infiltration of the liver, comprise a 'metabolic syndrome', a common pathological cluster and a rapidly growing problem that is associated with many life-threatening conditions. Drugs that act on some of the many mechanisms that become deranged in metabolic syndrome, including several directed at controlling blood sugar, have been developed, but clinical success has so far been modest.

CONTROL OF BLOOD GLUCOSE

Glucose is the obligatory source of energy for the adult brain, and physiological control of blood glucose reflects the need to maintain adequate fuel supplies in the face of intermittent food intake and variable metabolic demands. More fuel is made available by feeding than is required immediately, and excess calories are stored as glycogen or fat. During fasting, these energy stores need to be mobilised in a regulated manner. The most important regulatory hormone is *insulin*, the actions of which are described below. Increased blood glucose stimulates insulin secretion (Fig. 32.1), whereas reduced blood glucose reduces insulin secretion. The effect of glucose on insulin secretion depends on whether the glucose load is administered intravenously or by mouth. Glucose administered by mouth is more effective in stimulating insulin secretion because it stimulates release from the gut of *incretin* hormones which promote insulin secretion (see Fig. 32.1). Glucose is less effective in stimulating insulin secretion in patients with diabetes (Fig. 32.2). *Hypoglycaemia*, caused by excessive exogenous insulin, not only reduces endogenous insulin secretion but also elicits secretion of an array of 'counter-regulatory' hormones, including *glucagon*, *adrenaline* (Ch. 15), *glucocorticoids* (Ch. 34) and *growth hormone* (Ch. 34), all of which increase blood glucose. Their main effects on glucose uptake and carbohydrate metabolism are summarised and contrasted with those of insulin in Table 32.1.

The kidneys also have an important role in glucose regulation. Substantial amounts of glucose (approximately 900 mmol or 160 g) are filtered each day from the plasma into the renal tubules (Abdul-Ghani et al., 2015). However, in those with normal glucose homeostasis, very little or no glucose is excreted in the urine because renal tubular sodium–glucose co-transporters (SGLT) reclaim all the filtered glucose. The co-transporters are large transmembrane proteins (670 amino acids) that actively transport glucose against the concentration gradient through a mechanism that involves coupling with sodium transport (Abdul-Ghani et al., 2011). There are two SGLT variants in the kidney – SGLT2 (located in the early convoluted segment of the proximal tubule) has low affinity but high capacity, and is responsible for reclaiming about 90% of the filtered renal glucose, whilst the remaining 10% is reclaimed by high affinity, low capacity SGLT1 (located further on in the distal straight segment of the proximal tubule; DeFronzo et al., 2012). SGLT1 is also found in the heart, lungs and gastrointestinal (GI) tract, whereas SGLT2 is principally located in the kidney so selective inhibitors of SGLT2 can promote glucose excretion without influencing glucose transport in other organs.

The evolutionary role of SGLT in the kidney has been attributed to the benefits of retaining glucose in times when starvation or food shortages were commonplace. However, when the renal capacity for glucose re-absorption is exceeded in diabetes, glucose spills over into the urine (glycosuria) and causes an osmotic diuresis (polyuria) which, in turn, results in dehydration, thirst and increased drinking (polydipsia). The chronically elevated glucose concentrations

Table 32.1 The effect of hormones on blood glucose

Hormone	Main actions	Main stimuli for secretion	Main effect
Main regulatory hormone			
Insulin	↑ Glucose uptake ↑ Glycogen synthesis ↓ Glycogenolysis ↓ Gluconeogenesis	Acute rise in blood glucose Incretins (GIP and GLP-1)	↓ Blood glucose
Main counter-regulatory hormones			
Glucagon	↑ Glycogenolysis ↑ Glyconeogenesis		
Adrenaline (epinephrine)	↑ Glycogenolysis	Hypoglycaemia (i.e. blood glucose <3 mmol/L), (e.g. with exercise, stress, high-protein meals), etc.	↑ Blood glucose
Glucocorticoids	↓ Glucose uptake ↑ Gluconeogenesis ↓ Glucose uptake and utilisation		
Growth hormone	↓ Glucose uptake		

GIP, gastric inhibitory peptide; *GLP-1*, glucagon-like peptide-1.

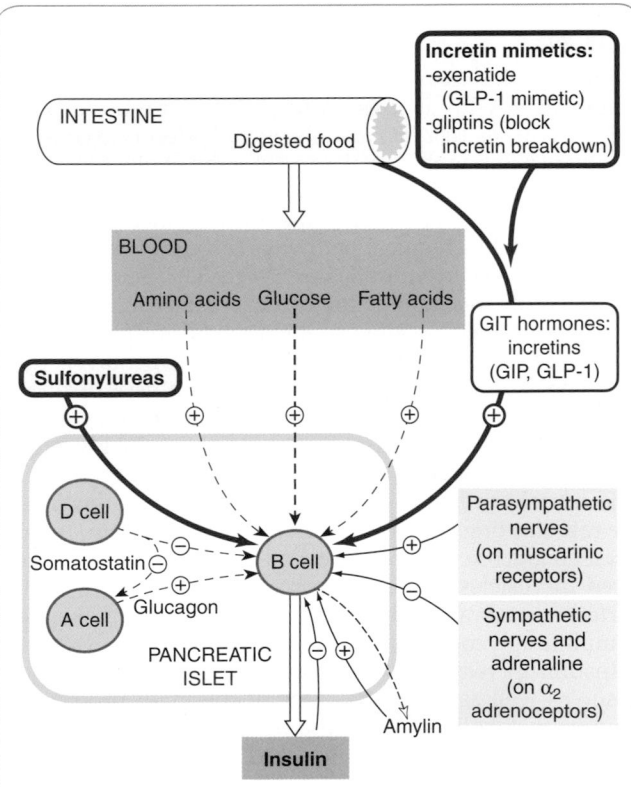

Fig. 32.1 Factors regulating insulin secretion. Blood glucose is the most important factor. Drugs used to stimulate insulin secretion are shown in *red-bordered boxes*. Glucagon potentiates insulin release but opposes some of its peripheral actions and increases blood glucose. *GIP*, gastric inhibitory peptide; *GIT*, gastrointestinal tract; *GLP-1*, glucagon-like peptide-1.

Fig. 32.2 Schematic diagram of the two-phase release of insulin in response to a constant glucose infusion. The first phase is missing in type 2 (non insulin-dependent) diabetes mellitus, and both are missing in type 1 (insulin-dependent) diabetes mellitus. The first phase is also produced by amino acids, sulfonylureas, glucagon and gastrointestinal tract hormones. (Data from Pfeifer, M.A., Halter, J.B., Porte, D. Jr., 1981. Am. J. Med. 70, 579–588.)

in patients with diabetes leads to up-regulation of SGLT2 expression and greater re-absorption of glucose, thus reducing glycosuria at the expense of worsening hyperglycaemia (DeFronzo et al., 2012). Because SGLT2 is a co-transporter that reabsorbs sodium ions with glucose, its increased expression also causes salt retention and hypertension.

PANCREATIC ISLET HORMONES

The islets of Langerhans, the endocrine part of the pancreas, contain four main types of peptide-secreting cells: β (or B) cells secrete *insulin*, α (or A) cells secrete *glucagon*, δ (or D) cells secrete *somatostatin*, PP cells secrete *pancreatic polypeptide* (PP) plus one minor player, ε (or E) cells. These are present in the developing pancreas and secrete *ghrelin*, a peptide hormone that releases growth hormone and is implicated in appetite control (Ch. 32).

▼ PP is a 36-amino acid peptide closely related to neuropeptide Y (Ch. 13) and peptide YY (Ch. 33). It is released by eating a meal and is implicated in control of food intake (Ch. 33): PP acts on G protein-coupled receptors and also inhibits secretion of exocrine pancreatic secretions and contraction of intestinal and biliary smooth muscle.

The core of each islet contains mainly the predominant β cells surrounded by a mantle of α cells interspersed with δ cells or PP cells (see Fig. 32.1). In addition to insulin, β cells secrete a peptide known as *islet amyloid polypeptide* or *amylin*, which delays gastric emptying and opposes insulin by stimulating glycogen breakdown in striated muscle, and C-peptide (see p. 412). Glucagon opposes insulin, increasing blood glucose and stimulating protein breakdown in muscle. Somatostatin inhibits secretion of insulin and of glucagon. It is widely distributed outside the pancreas and is also released from the hypothalamus, inhibiting the release of growth hormone from the pituitary gland (Ch. 34).

INSULIN

Insulin was the first protein for which the amino acid sequence was determined (by Sanger's group in Cambridge in 1955). It consists of two peptide chains (of 21 and 30 amino acid residues) linked by two disulfide bonds.

SYNTHESIS AND SECRETION

Like other peptide hormones (see Ch. 19), insulin is synthesised as a precursor (preproinsulin) in the rough endoplasmic reticulum. Preproinsulin is transported to the Golgi apparatus, where it undergoes proteolytic cleavage to proinsulin and then to insulin plus a fragment of uncertain function called C-peptide.[1] Insulin and C-peptide are stored in granules in β cells, and are normally co-secreted by exocytosis in equimolar amounts together with smaller and variable amounts of proinsulin.

The main factor controlling the synthesis and secretion of insulin is the blood glucose concentration (see Fig. 32.1). β cells respond both to the absolute glucose concentration and to the rate of change of blood glucose. Other physiological stimuli to insulin release include amino acids (particularly arginine and leucine), fatty acids, the parasympathetic nervous system and *incretins* (especially *GLP-1* and *GIP*, see p. 413). Pharmacologically, sulfonylurea drugs (see p. 416) act by releasing insulin.

There is a steady basal release of insulin and an increase in blood glucose stimulates an additional response. This response has two phases: an initial rapid phase reflecting release of stored hormone, and a slower, delayed phase reflecting continued release of stored hormone and new synthesis (see Fig. 32.2). The response is abnormal in diabetes mellitus, as discussed later.

ATP-sensitive potassium channels (K_{ATP}; Ch. 4) determine the resting membrane potential in β cells. Glucose enters β cells via a surface membrane transporter called Glut-2, and its subsequent metabolism via glucokinase (which is the rate-limiting glycolytic enzyme in β cells) links insulin secretion to extracellular glucose. The consequent rise in ATP within β cells blocks K_{ATP} channels, causing membrane depolarisation. Depolarisation opens voltage-dependent calcium channels, leading to Ca^{2+} influx. This triggers insulin secretion in the presence of amplifying messengers, including diacylglycerol, non-esterified arachidonic acid (which

facilitates further Ca^{2+} entry) and 12-lipoxygenase products of arachidonic acid (mainly *12-S-hydroxyeicosatetraenoic acid* or *12-S*-HETE; see Ch. 18). Phospholipases are commonly activated by Ca^{2+}, but free arachidonic acid is liberated in β cells by an ATP-sensitive Ca^{2+}-insensitive (ASCI) phospholipase A_2. Consequently, in β cells, Ca^{2+} entry and arachidonic acid production are both driven by ATP, linking cellular energy status to insulin secretion.

Insulin release is inhibited by the sympathetic nervous system (see Fig. 32.1). Adrenaline (epinephrine) increases blood glucose by inhibiting insulin release (via α_2 adrenoceptors) and by promoting glycogenolysis via β_2 adrenoceptors in striated muscle and liver. Several peptides, including somatostatin, galanin (an endogenous K_{ATP} activator) and amylin, also inhibit insulin release.

About one-fifth of the insulin stored in the pancreas of the human adult is secreted daily. The plasma insulin concentration after an overnight fast is 20–50 pmol/L. Plasma insulin concentration is reduced in patients with type 1 (insulin-dependent) diabetes mellitus (see p. 413), and markedly increased in patients with *insulinomas* (uncommon functioning tumours of β cells), as is C-peptide, with which it is co-released.[2] It is also raised in obesity and other normoglycaemic insulin-resistant states.

ACTIONS

Insulin is the main hormone controlling intermediary metabolism, with actions on liver, fat and muscle (Table 32.2). It is an *anabolic hormone*: its overall effect is to conserve fuel by facilitating the uptake and storage of glucose, amino acids and fats after a meal. Acutely, it reduces blood glucose. Consequently, a fall in plasma insulin increases blood glucose. The biochemical pathways through which insulin exerts its effects are summarised in Fig. 32.3, and molecular aspects of its mechanism are discussed below.

Insulin influences glucose metabolism in most tissues, especially the liver, where it inhibits glycogenolysis (glycogen breakdown) and gluconeogenesis (synthesis of glucose from non-carbohydrate sources) while stimulating glycogen synthesis. It also increases glucose utilisation by glycolysis, but the overall effect is to increase hepatic glycogen stores.

In muscle, unlike liver, uptake of glucose is slow and is the rate-limiting step in carbohydrate metabolism. Insulin causes a glucose transporter called Glut-4, which is sequestered in vesicles, to be expressed within minutes on the surface membrane. This facilitates glucose uptake, and stimulates glycogen synthesis and glycolysis.

Insulin increases glucose uptake by Glut-4 in adipose tissue as well as in muscle. One of the main products of glucose metabolism in adipose tissue is glycerol, which is esterified with fatty acids to form triglycerides, thereby affecting fat metabolism (see Table 32.2).

Insulin increases synthesis of fatty acid and triglyceride in adipose tissue and in liver. It inhibits lipolysis, partly via dephosphorylation – and hence inactivation – of lipases (see Table 32.2). It also inhibits the lipolytic actions of

---

[1]Not to be confused with C-reactive peptide, which is an acute-phase reactant used clinically as a marker of inflammation (Ch. 7).

[2]Insulin for injection does not contain C-peptide, which therefore provides a means of distinguishing endogenous from exogenous insulin. This is used to differentiate insulinoma (an insulin-secreting tumour causing high circulating insulin with high C-peptide) from surreptitious injection of insulin (high insulin with low C-peptide). Deliberate induction of hypoglycaemia by self-injection with insulin is a well-recognised, if unusual, manifestation of psychiatric disorder, especially in health professionals – it has also been used in murder.

Table 32.2 Effects of insulin on carbohydrate, fat and protein metabolism

Type of metabolism	Liver cells	Fat cells	Muscle
Carbohydrate metabolism	↓ Gluconeogenesis ↓ Glycogenolysis ↑ Glycolysis ↑ Glycogenesis	↑ Glucose uptake ↑ Glycerol synthesis	↑ Glucose uptake ↑ Glycolysis ↑ Glycogenesis
Fat metabolism	↑ Lipogenesis ↓ Lipolysis	↑ Synthesis of triglycerides ↑ Fatty acid synthesis ↓ Lipolysis	
Protein metabolism	↓ Protein breakdown	–	↑ Amino acid uptake ↑ Protein synthesis

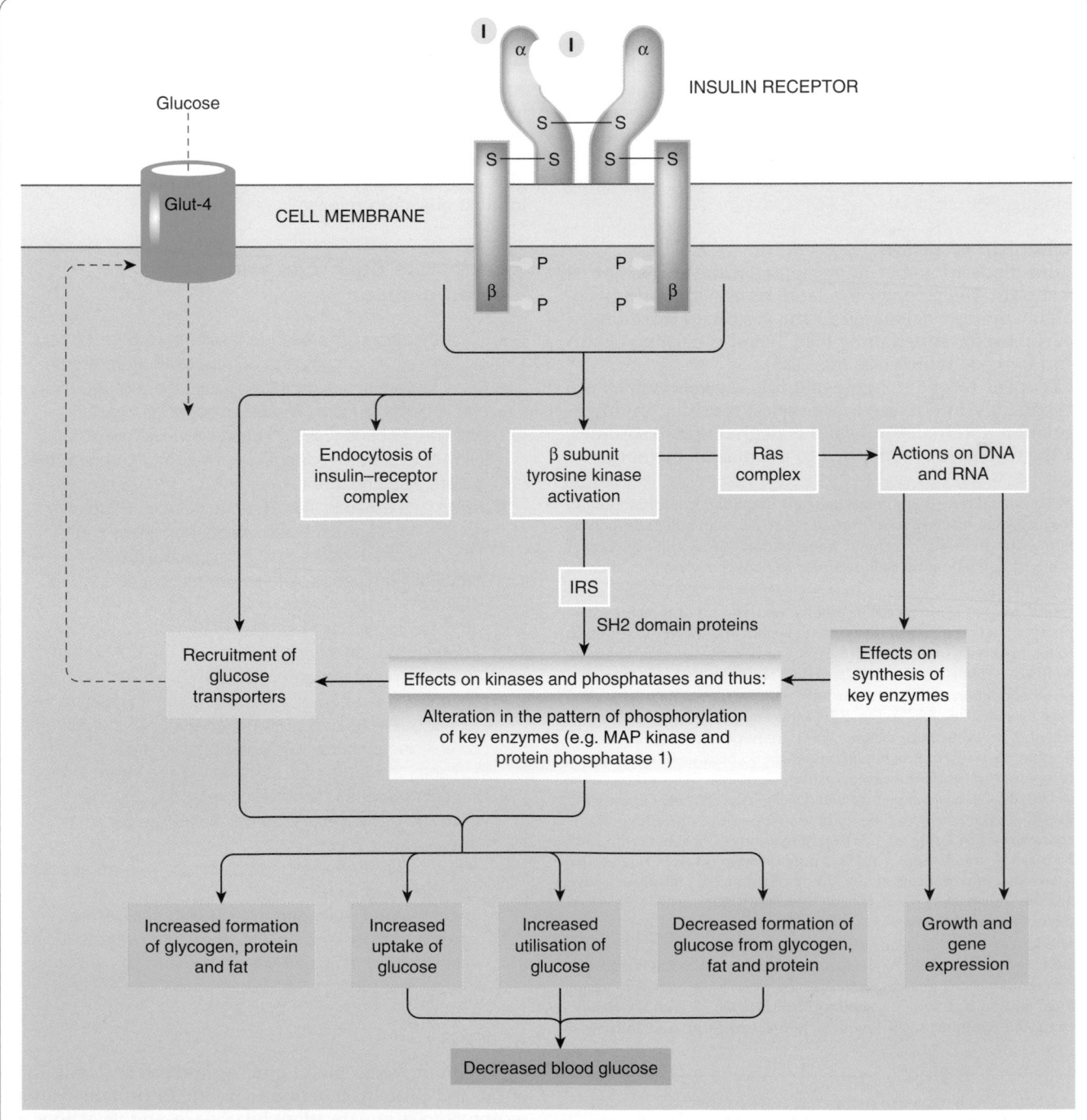

Fig. 32.3 Insulin signalling pathways. *I*, insulin; *Glut-4*, an insulin-sensitive glucose transporter present in muscle and fat cells; *IRS*, insulin receptor substrate (several forms: 1–4).

adrenaline, growth hormone and glucagon by opposing their actions on adenylyl cyclase.

Insulin stimulates uptake of amino acids into muscle and increases protein synthesis. It also decreases protein catabolism and inhibits oxidation of amino acids in the liver.

Other metabolic effects of insulin include transport into cells of K^+, Ca^{2+}, nucleosides and inorganic phosphate.[3]

Long-term effects of insulin

In addition to rapid effects on metabolism, exerted via altered activity of enzymes and transport proteins, insulin has long-term actions via altered enzyme synthesis. It is an important anabolic hormone during fetal development. It stimulates cell proliferation (mitogenic action) and is implicated in somatic and visceral growth and development.

Mitogenic actions of insulin are of great concern in the development of insulin analogues; **insulin glargine** (one widely used analogue; see p. 415) is six- to eight-fold more mitogenic than human insulin, and cultured breast cancer cells proliferate in response to near-therapeutic concentrations of this analogue in vitro, but it is not known if there is any clinically significant parallel in vivo. Mammary tumours developed in rats given one long-acting insulin analogue.

Mechanism of action

Insulin binds to a specific receptor on the surface of its target cells. The receptor is a large transmembrane glycoprotein complex belonging to the tyrosine kinase-linked type 3 receptor superfamily (Ch. 3) and consisting of two α and two β subunits (see Fig. 32.3).

Occupied receptors aggregate into clusters, which are subsequently internalised in vesicles, resulting in down-regulation. Internalised insulin is degraded in lysosomes, but the receptors are recycled to the plasma membrane.

▼ The signal transduction mechanisms that link receptor binding to the biological effects of insulin are complex. Receptor autophosphorylation – the first step in signal transduction – is a consequence of dimerisation, allowing each receptor to phosphorylate the other, as explained in Chapter 3.

Insulin receptor substrate (IRS) proteins undergo rapid tyrosine phosphorylation specifically in response to insulin and insulin-like growth factor-1 but not to other growth factors. The best-characterised substrate is IRS-1, which contains 22 tyrosine residues that are potential phosphorylation sites. It interacts with proteins that contain a so-called SH2 domain (see Ch. 3, Fig. 3.15), thereby passing on the insulin signal. Knock-out mice lacking IRS-1 are hyporesponsive to insulin (insulin-resistant) but do not become diabetic, because of robust β-cell compensation with increased insulin secretion. By contrast, mice lacking IRS-2 fail to compensate and develop overt diabetes, implicating the IRS-2 gene as a candidate for human type 2 diabetes (IRS proteins are reviewed by Lavin et al., 2016). Activation of phosphatidylinositol 3-kinase by interaction of its SH2 domain with phosphorylated IRS has several important effects, including recruitment of insulin-sensitive glucose transporters (Glut-4) from the Golgi apparatus to the plasma membrane in muscle and fat cells.

The longer-term actions of insulin entail effects on DNA and RNA, mediated partly at least by the Ras signalling complex. Ras is a protein that regulates cell growth and cycles between an active GTP-bound form and an inactive GDP-bound form (see Chs 3 and 57). Insulin shifts the equilibrium in favour of the active form, and initiates a phosphorylation cascade that results in activation of mitogen-activated protein kinase (MAP-kinase), which in turn activates several nuclear transcription factors, leading to the expression of genes that are involved with cell growth and with intermediary metabolism.

Insulin for treatment of diabetes mellitus is considered below.

GLUCAGON
SYNTHESIS AND SECRETION

Glucagon is a single-chain polypeptide of 21 amino acid residues synthesised mainly in the α cell of the islets, but also in the upper GI tract. It has considerable structural homology with other GI tract hormones, including secretin, vasoactive intestinal peptide and GIP (see Ch. 31).

Amino acids (especially L-arginine) stimulate glucagon secretion, as does ingestion of a high-protein meal, but diurnal variation in plasma glucagon concentrations is less than for insulin. Glucagon secretion is stimulated by low and inhibited by high concentrations of glucose and fatty acids in the plasma. Sympathetic nerve activity and circulating adrenaline stimulate glucagon release via β adrenoceptors. Parasympathetic nerve activity also increases secretion, whereas somatostatin, released from δ cells adjacent to the glucagon-secreting α cells in the periphery of the islets, inhibits glucagon release.

Endocrine pancreas and blood glucose

- Islets of Langerhans secrete insulin from β (or B) cells, glucagon from α cells and somatostatin from δ cells.
- Many factors stimulate insulin secretion, but the main one is blood glucose. Incretins, especially gastric inhibitory peptide (GIP) and glucagon-like peptide-1 (GLP-1) secreted, respectively, by K and L cells in the gut are also important.
- Insulin has essential metabolic actions as a fuel-storage hormone and also affects cell growth and differentiation. It decreases blood glucose by:
  - increasing glucose uptake into muscle and fat via Glut-4
  - increasing glycogen synthesis
  - decreasing gluconeogenesis
  - decreasing glycogen breakdown.
- Glucagon is a fuel-mobilising hormone, stimulating gluconeogenesis and glycogenolysis, also lipolysis and proteolysis. It increases blood sugar and also increases the force of contraction of the heart.
- Diabetes mellitus is a chronic metabolic disorder in which there is hyperglycaemia. There are two main types:
  - type 1 (insulin-dependent) diabetes, with an absolute deficiency of insulin;
  - type 2 (non insulin-dependent) diabetes, with a relative deficiency of insulin associated with reduced sensitivity to its action (insulin resistance).

ACTIONS

Glucagon increases blood glucose and causes breakdown of fat and protein. It acts on specific G protein–coupled receptors to stimulate adenylyl cyclase, and its actions are

---

[3]The action on K^+ is exploited in the emergency treatment of hyperkalaemia by intravenous glucose with insulin (see Ch. 30).

somewhat similar to β-adrenoceptor–mediated actions of adrenaline. Unlike adrenaline, however, its metabolic effects are more pronounced than its cardiovascular actions. Glucagon is proportionately more active on liver, while the metabolic actions of adrenaline are more pronounced on muscle and fat. Glucagon stimulates glycogen breakdown and gluconeogenesis, and inhibits glycogen synthesis and glucose oxidation. Its metabolic actions on target tissues are thus the opposite of those of insulin. Glucagon increases the rate and force of contraction of the heart, although less markedly than adrenaline.

Clinical uses of glucagon are summarised in the clinical box.

Clinical uses of glucagon

- **Glucagon** can be given intramuscularly or subcutaneously as well as intravenously.
- Treatment of *hypoglycaemia* in unconscious patients (who cannot drink); unlike intravenous glucose, it can be administered by non-medical personnel (e.g. spouses or ambulance crew). It is useful if obtaining intravenous access is difficult.
- Treatment of *acute cardiac failure* precipitated by β-adrenoceptor antagonists.

SOMATOSTATIN

Somatostatin is secreted by the δ cells of the islets. It is also generated in the hypothalamus, where it inhibits the release of growth hormone (see Ch. 33). In the islet, it inhibits release of insulin and of glucagon. **Octreotide** is a long-acting analogue of somatostatin. It inhibits release of a number of hormones, and is used clinically to relieve symptoms from several uncommon gastroenteropancreatic endocrine tumours, and for treatment of acromegaly[4] (the endocrine disorder caused by a functioning tumour of cells that secrete growth hormone from the anterior pituitary; see Ch. 34).

AMYLIN (ISLET AMYLOID POLYPEPTIDE)

▼ The term *amyloid* refers to amorphous protein deposits in different tissues that occur in a variety of diseases, including several neurodegenerative conditions (see Ch. 41). Amyloid deposits occur in the pancreas of patients with diabetes mellitus, although it is not known if this is functionally important. The major component of pancreatic amyloid is a 37-amino acid residue peptide known as islet amyloid polypeptide or amylin. This is stored with insulin in secretory granules in β cells and is co-secreted with insulin. Amylin delays gastric emptying. Supraphysiological concentrations stimulate the breakdown of glycogen to lactate in striated muscle. Amylin also inhibits insulin secretion (see Fig. 32.1). It is structurally related to calcitonin (see Ch. 37) and has weak calcitonin-like actions on calcium metabolism and osteoclast activity. It is also about 50% identical with calcitonin gene-related peptide (CGRP; see Ch. 19), and large intravenous doses cause vasodilatation, presumably by an action on CGRP receptors.

Pramlintide, an amylin analogue with three proline substitutions that reduce its tendency to aggregate into insoluble fibrils, is approved in the United States to treat patients with type 1 diabetes and for type 2 diabetics who use mealtime insulin but have not achieved satisfactory glucose control. It is injected subcutaneously before each major meal as an adjunct to insulin, and reduces insulin requirements. Pramlintide reduces the speed of gastric emptying and decreases the postprandial rise in glucagon. Unwanted effects include hypoglycaemia and nausea – it is contraindicated in patients with loss of gastric motility (gastroparesis), a complication of diabetic autonomic neuropathy (Younk et al., 2011).

INCRETINS

La Barre suggested in the 1930s that crude secretin contained two active principles: 'excretin', which stimulates the exocrine pancreas, and 'incretin', which stimulates insulin release. He proposed that incretin presented possibilities for the treatment of diabetes. 'Excretin' did not catch on (perhaps not helped by an unfortunate association with other bodily functions – at least to an Anglo-Saxon ear), but 'incretin' has gone from strength to strength, and some 80 years later several incretin-based drugs are now licensed for clinical use (see later). Incretin action proved to be due to peptide hormones released from the gut, mainly *GIP* and *GLP-1*. These are both members of the glucagon peptide superfamily (Ch. 19). GIP is a 42-amino acid peptide stored in and secreted by enteroendocrine K cells in the duodenum and proximal jejunum. GLP-1 is secreted by L cells which are more widely distributed in the gut, including in the ileum and colon as well as more proximally. Two forms of GLP-1 are secreted after a meal: GLP-1(7-37) and GLP-1(7-36) amide; these are similarly potent. Most of the circulating activity is due to GLP-1(7-36) amide. Release of GIP and GLP-1 by ingested food provides an early stimulus to insulin secretion before absorbed glucose or other products of digestion reach the islet cells in the portal blood (see Fig. 32.1). As well as stimulating insulin secretion, both these hormones inhibit pancreatic glucagon secretion and slow the rate of absorption of digested food by reducing gastric emptying. They are also implicated in control of food intake via appetite and satiety (see Ch. 33). The actions of GIP and GLP-1 are terminated rapidly by dipeptidyl peptidase-4 (DPP-4). This enzyme is a membrane glycoprotein with rather wide substrate specificity – it has been implicated in suppression of malignancy and in atherogenesis (e.g. Waumans et al., 2015), but inhibitors are licensed to treat diabetes (see later, p. 418).

DIABETES MELLITUS

Diabetes mellitus is a chronic metabolic disorder characterised by a high blood glucose concentration – hyperglycaemia (fasting plasma glucose >7.0 mmol/L, or plasma glucose >11.1 mmol/L, 2 h after a meal) – caused by insulin deficiency, often combined with insulin resistance. There are two main types of diabetes mellitus:

1. **Type 1 diabetes** (previously known as insulin-dependent diabetes mellitus – IDDM – or juvenile-onset diabetes), in which there is an absolute deficiency of insulin.
2. **Type 2 diabetes** (previously known as non insulin-dependent diabetes mellitus – NIDDM – or maturity-onset diabetes), in which there is a relative deficiency of insulin associated with reduced sensitivity to its action (insulin resistance).

---

[4]Octreotide is used either short term before surgery on the pituitary tumour, or while waiting for radiotherapy of the tumour to take effect, or if other treatments have been ineffective.

Hyperglycaemia occurs because of uncontrolled hepatic glucose output and reduced uptake of glucose by skeletal muscle with reduced glycogen synthesis. Insulin deficiency causes muscle wasting through increased breakdown and reduced synthesis of proteins. Diabetic ketoacidosis is an acute emergency that is predominantly seen in patients with type 1 diabetes. It develops in the absence of insulin because of accelerated breakdown of fat to acetyl-CoA, which, in the absence of aerobic carbohydrate metabolism, is converted to acetoacetate and β-hydroxybutyrate (which cause acidosis) and acetone (a ketone).

Various complications develop as a consequence of the metabolic derangements in diabetes, often over several years. Many of these are the result of disease of blood vessels, either large (macrovascular disease) or small (microangiopathy). Dysfunction of vascular endothelium (see Ch. 23) is an early and critical event in the development of vascular complications. Oxygen-derived free radicals, protein kinase C and non-enzymic products of glucose and albumin called *advanced glycation end products* (AGE) have been implicated. Macrovascular disease consists of accelerated atheroma (Ch. 24) and its thrombotic complications (Ch. 25), which are commoner and more severe in diabetic patients. Microangiopathy is a distinctive feature of diabetes mellitus and particularly affects the retina, kidney and peripheral nerves. Diabetes mellitus is the commonest cause of chronic renal failure, a huge and rapidly increasing problem, and a major burden to society as well as to individual patients. Co-existent hypertension promotes progressive renal damage, and treatment of hypertension slows the progression of diabetic nephropathy and reduces the risk of myocardial infarction. Angiotensin-converting enzyme inhibitors or angiotensin receptor antagonists (Ch. 23) are more effective in preventing diabetic nephropathy than other antihypertensive drugs, perhaps because they prevent fibroproliferative actions of angiotensin II and aldosterone.

Diabetic neuropathy[5] is associated with accumulation of osmotically active metabolites of glucose, produced by the action of aldose reductase, but *aldose reductase inhibitors* have been disappointing as therapeutic drugs (see Farmer et al., 2012, for a review).

Type 1 diabetes can occur at any age, but patients are usually young (children or adolescents) and not obese when they first develop symptoms. There is an inherited predisposition, with a 10- to 15-fold increased incidence in first-degree relatives of an index case, and strong associations with particular histocompatibility antigens (HLA types). Identical twins are less than fully concordant, so environmental factors such as viral infection (e.g. with coxsackie virus or echovirus) are believed to be necessary for genetically predisposed individuals to express the disease. Viral infection may damage pancreatic β cells and expose antigens that initiate a self-perpetuating autoimmune process. The patient becomes overtly diabetic only when more than 90% of the β cells have been destroyed. This natural history provides a tantalising prospect of intervening in the pre-diabetic stage, and a variety of strategies have been mooted,

including immunosuppression, early insulin therapy, antioxidants, nicotinamide and many others; so far these have disappointed, but this remains a very active field.

Type 2 diabetes is accompanied both by insulin resistance (which precedes overt disease) and by impaired insulin secretion, each of which are important in its pathogenesis. Such patients are often obese and usually present in adult life, the incidence rising progressively with age as β-cell function declines. Treatment is initially dietary, although oral hypoglycaemic drugs usually become necessary, and most patients ultimately benefit from exogenous insulin. Prospective studies have demonstrated a relentless deterioration in diabetic control[6] with increasing age and duration of disease.

Insulin secretion (basal, and in response to a meal) in a type 1 and a type 2 diabetic patient is contrasted schematically with that in a healthy control in Fig. 32.2.

There are many other less common forms of diabetes mellitus in addition to the two main ones described earlier (for example, syndromes associated with autoantibodies directed against insulin receptors which cause severe insulin resistance, functional α-cell tumours, 'glucagonomas', and many other rarities), and hyperglycaemia can also be a clinically important adverse effect of several drugs, including glucocorticoids (Ch. 34), high doses of thiazide diuretics (Ch. 30) and several of the protease inhibitors used to treat HIV infection (Ch. 53).

DRUGS USED IN THE TREATMENT OF DIABETES

The main groups of drugs used are:

Agents given by injection
- Insulin, in various forms and formulations (used in type 1 and type 2 diabetes)
- Incretin mimetics (e.g. **exenatide, liraglutide**)

Oral agents (used in type 2 diabetes)
- Biguanides (e.g. **metformin**)
- Sulfonylureas (e.g. **tolbutamide, glibenclamide, glipizide**) and related drugs (e.g. **repaglinide, nateglinide**)
- Thiazolidinediones (e.g. **pioglitazone**)
- Gliptins (e.g. **sitagliptin**)
- Glucose transport inhibitors (e.g. **empagliflozin**)

INSULIN TREATMENT

The effects of insulin and its mechanism of action are described earlier. Here we describe pharmacokinetic aspects and adverse effects, both of which are central to its therapeutic use. Insulin for clinical use was once either porcine or bovine but is now almost entirely human (made in expression systems by recombinant DNA technology, Ch. 5). Animal insulins are liable to elicit an immune response; this is less of an issue with recombinant human insulins. Although recombinant insulin is more consistent in quality than insulins extracted from pancreases of freshly slaughtered animals, doses are still quantified in terms of units of activity (Ch. 8), with which doctors and patients are familiar, rather than of mass.

[5]Neuropathy ('disease of the nerves') causes dysfunction of peripheral nerve fibres, which can be motor, sensory or autonomic. Diabetic neuropathy often causes numbness in a 'stocking' distribution caused by damage to sensory fibres, and postural hypotension and erectile dysfunction due to autonomic neuropathy.

[6]Diabetic control is not easily estimated by determination of blood glucose, because this is so variable. Instead, glycated haemoglobin (haemoglobin A$_{1C}$) is measured. This provides an integrated measure of control over the lifespan of the red cell: approximately 120 days. In healthy individuals, 4%–6% (20–42 mmol/mol) of haemoglobin is glycated; levels above 6.5% (48 mmol/mol) are indicative of diabetes.

Pharmacokinetic aspects and insulin preparations

Insulin is destroyed in the GI tract, and is ordinarily given by injection – usually subcutaneously, but intravenously or occasionally intramuscularly in emergencies. Intraperitoneal insulin can be used in rare instances in patients with diabetes, through a continuous infusion pump, or through ambulatory peritoneal dialysis for those with end stage renal failure. Other potential approaches include incorporation of insulin into biodegradable polymer microspheres as a slow-release formulation, and its encapsulation with a lectin in a glucose-permeable membrane.[7] Once absorbed, insulin has an elimination half-life of approximately 10 min. It is inactivated enzymically in the liver and kidney, and 10% is excreted in the urine. Renal impairment reduces insulin requirement.

One of the main problems in using insulin is to avoid wide fluctuations in plasma concentration and thus in blood glucose. Different formulations vary in the timing of their peak effect and duration of action. *Soluble insulin* produces a rapid and short-lived effect. Longer-acting preparations are made by precipitating insulin with protamine or zinc, thus forming finely divided amorphous solid or relatively insoluble crystals, which are injected as a suspension from which insulin is slowly absorbed. These preparations include *isophane insulin* and amorphous or crystalline *insulin zinc suspensions*. Mixtures of different forms in fixed proportions are available.

More recently, modifications of insulin molecules have focused on two different areas – one being the production of molecules with a more rapid onset of action to cover mealtimes, and the other being even longer-acting formulations. Development of rapid-acting analogues is based on amino acid substitutions that promote formation of insulin monomers for faster absorption, whilst reducing the aggregation of insulin dimers and hexamers (Atkin et al., 2015). Example of these analogues include insulin aspart, insulin lispro and insulin glulisine, which involve different amino acid switches at positions such as B28 or B29 in the insulin molecule. These analogues act more rapidly (onset of action <15 min and typically reaching peak concentrations within 40–70 min after injection) but for a shorter time than natural insulin, enabling patients to inject themselves immediately before the start of a meal rather than 30 min before eating with human insulin.

Basal or longer-acting insulin analogues are designed with the opposite intention, namely to provide a constant basal insulin supply and mimic physiological postabsorptive basal insulin secretion. **Insulin glargine**, which is a clear solution, forms a microprecipitate at the physiological pH of subcutaneous tissue, and absorption from the subcutaneous site of injection is prolonged. In contrast, subcutaneous injection of **insulin detemir** causes the molecules to bind together more avidly, thus slowing the absorption into the circulation (Atkin et al., 2015). **Insulin degludec** is formed by the addition of a fatty-diacid side chain to human insulin, and the resulting molecules join up to form a depot of long multihexamers after subcutaneous injection. Monomers of insulin degludec slowly dissociate from this depot, thus giving a protracted duration of action >40 h.

Various dosage regimens are used. Some type 1 patients inject a combination of short- and intermediate-acting insulins twice daily, before breakfast and before the evening meal. Improved control of blood glucose can be achieved with multiple daily injections of rapid-acting insulin analogues given with meals, and a basal insulin analogue injected once daily (often at night). Insulin pumps are used in hospital to control blood glucose acutely and are also available in a portable form that delivers continuous subcutaneous infusion for outpatients. The most sophisticated forms of pump regulate the dose by means of a sensor that continuously measures blood glucose, but these are not yet used routinely – this seemingly logical approach is limited by the complexity of insulin's effects on intermediary metabolism (see Table 32.2, Fig. 32.3) which are imperfectly captured by existing continuous glucose monitoring technology, and by risks of infection.

Unwanted effects

The main undesirable effect of insulin is hypoglycaemia. This is common and, if very severe, can cause brain damage or sudden cardiac death. In the Diabetes Control and Complications Trial mentioned before, intensive insulin therapy resulted in a three-fold increase in severe hypoglycaemic episodes compared with usual care. The treatment of hypoglycaemia is to take a sweet drink or snack or, if the patient is unconscious, to give intravenous glucose or intramuscular glucagon (see clinical box, p. 413). Rebound hyperglycaemia ('Somogyi effect') can follow insulin-induced hypoglycaemia, because of the release of counter-regulatory hormones (e.g. adrenaline, glucagon and glucocorticoids). This can cause hyperglycaemia before breakfast following an unrecognised hypoglycaemic attack during sleep in the early hours of the morning. It is essential to appreciate this possibility to avoid the mistake of increasing (rather than reducing) the evening dose of insulin in this situation.

Allergy to human insulin is unusual but can occur. It may take the form of local or systemic reactions. Insulin resistance as a consequence of antibody formation is rare. Theoretical concerns regarding mitogenic effects of insulin analogues are mentioned earlier (p. 412).

Biguanides

Metformin (present in French lilac, *Galega officinalis*, which was used to treat diabetes in traditional medicine for centuries) is the only biguanide used clinically to treat type 2 diabetes, for which it is now a drug of first choice.[8]

Actions and mechanism

The molecular target or targets through which biguanides act remain unclear, but their biochemical actions are well understood, and include:

- reduced hepatic glucose production (gluconeogenesis) which is markedly increased in type 2 diabetes;
- increased glucose uptake and utilisation in skeletal muscle (i.e. reduced insulin resistance);
- reduced carbohydrate absorption from the intestine;
- increased fatty acid oxidation;
- reduced circulating low-density and very low-density lipoprotein (LDL and VLDL, respectively, see Ch. 24).

[7]This could, in theory, provide variable release of insulin controlled by the prevailing glucose concentration, because glucose and glycated insulin compete for binding sites on the lectin.

[8]Metformin had a very slow start. It was first synthesised in 1922, one of a large series of biguanides with many different pharmacological actions, which proved largely unsuitable for clinical use. Its glucose-lowering effect was noted early on, but was eclipsed by the discovery of insulin. It did not receive FDA approval until 1995.

Clinical uses of insulin and other hypoglycaemic drugs for injection

- Patients with *type 1 diabetes* require long-term **insulin**:
  - an intermediate-acting preparation (e.g. **isophane insulin**) or a long-acting analogue (e.g. **glargine**) is often combined with soluble insulin or a short-acting analogue (e.g. **lispro**) taken before meals.
- **Soluble insulin** is used (intravenously) in treatment of hyperglycaemic emergencies (e.g. *diabetic ketoacidosis*).
- Approximately one-third of patients with *type 2 diabetes* ultimately require **insulin**.
- Short-term treatment of patients with type 2 diabetes or impaired glucose tolerance during intercurrent events (e.g. *operations, infections, myocardial infarction*).
- During pregnancy, for *gestational diabetes* not controlled by diet alone.
- Emergency treatment of *hyperkalaemia*: **insulin** is given with glucose to lower extracellular K^+ via redistribution into cells.
- Glucagon-like peptide-1 **(GLP-1) agonist** for type 2 diabetes in addition to oral agents to improve control and lose weight.

Reduced hepatic gluconeogenesis is especially important. Metformin decreases hepatic glucose production directly or indirectly by inhibiting the mitochondrial respiratory chain complex I (reviewed by Viollet et al., 2012). The resulting increase in AMP activates AMP-activated protein kinase (AMPK) which is a master regulator of energy homeostasis in eukaryotes (Myers et al., 2017). Activation of AMPK in the duodenum triggers release of GLP-1 which stimulates a gut–brain–liver vagal network that regulates hepatic glucose production (Duca et al., 2015). Chronic administration of metformin alters recirculation of bile acids and composition of the gut microbiome in type 2 leading to increased GLP-1 secretion in diabetes patients (Napolitano et al., 2014).

Metformin has a half-life of about 3 h and is excreted unchanged in the urine.

Unwanted effects

Metformin, while preventing hyperglycaemia, does *not* cause hypoglycaemia, and the commonest unwanted effects are dose-related GI disturbances (e.g. anorexia, diarrhoea, nausea), which are usually, but not always, transient. Lactic acidosis is a rare but potentially fatal toxic effect, and metformin should not be given routinely to patients with renal or hepatic disease, hypoxic pulmonary disease or shock. Such patients are predisposed to lactic acidosis because of reduced drug elimination or reduced tissue oxygenation. It should be avoided in other situations that predispose to lactic acidosis including alcohol intoxication, and some forms of mitochondrial myopathy that are associated with diabetes. Long-term use may interfere with absorption of vitamin B_{12}.

Clinical use

Metformin is used to treat patients with type 2 diabetes. It does not stimulate appetite (rather the reverse; see earlier!) and is the drug of first choice in the majority of type 2 patients who are obese, provided they have unimpaired renal and hepatic function. It can be combined with other glucose-lowering agents if blood glucose is inadequately controlled. Potential uses outside type 2 diabetes include other syndromes with accompanying insulin resistance including polycystic ovary syndrome, non-alcoholic fatty liver disease, gestational diabetes and some forms of premature puberty.

Sulfonylureas

The sulfonylureas were developed following the chance observation that a sulfonamide derivative (which was being used to treat typhoid) caused hypoglycaemia. Numerous sulfonylureas are available. The first used therapeutically were **tolbutamide** and **chlorpropamide**. Chlorpropamide has a long duration of action and a substantial fraction is excreted in the urine. Consequently, it can cause severe hypoglycaemia, especially in elderly patients in whom renal function declines inevitably but insidiously (Ch. 30). It causes flushing after alcohol because of a disulfiram-like effect (Ch. 50), and has an action like that of antidiuretic hormone on the distal nephron, giving rise to hyponatraemia and water intoxication. Williams (1994) comments that 'time honoured but idiosyncratic chlorpropamide should now be laid to rest' – a sentiment with which we concur. Tolbutamide, however, remains useful. So-called second-generation sulfonylureas (e.g. **glibenclamide**, **glipizide**; Table 32.3) are more potent, but their maximum hypo-glycaemic effect is no greater and control of blood glucose no better than with tolbutamide. These drugs all contain the sulfonylurea moiety and act in the same way, but different substitutions result in differences in pharmacokinetics and hence in duration of action (see Table 32.3).

Mechanism of action

The principal action of sulfonylureas is on β cells (see Fig. 32.1), stimulating insulin secretion and thus reducing plasma glucose. High-affinity binding sites for sulfonylureas are present on the K_{ATP} channels (Ch. 4) in the surface membranes of β cells, and the binding of various sulfonylureas parallels their potency in stimulating insulin release. Block by sulfonylurea drugs of K_{ATP} channel activation causes depolarisation of β cells, Ca^{2+} entry and insulin secretion. (Compare this with the physiological control of insulin secretion, see Fig. 32.1.)

Pharmacokinetic aspects

Sulfonylureas are well absorbed after oral administration, and most reach peak plasma concentrations within 2–4 h. The duration of action varies (see Table 32.3). All bind strongly to plasma albumin and are implicated in interactions with other drugs (e.g. salicylates and sulfonamides) that compete for these binding sites (see Ch. 9). Most sulfonylureas (or their active metabolites) are excreted in the urine, so their action is increased and prolonged in the elderly and in patients with renal disease.

Most sulfonylureas cross the placenta and enter breast milk and their use is contraindicated in pregnancy and in breastfeeding.

Table 32.3 Oral hypoglycaemic sulfonylurea drugs

Drug	Relative potency[a]	Duration of action and (half-life) (hours)	Pharmacokinetic aspects[b]	General comments
Tolbutamide	1	6–12 (4)	Some converted in liver to weakly active hydroxytolbutamide; some carboxylated to inactive compound Renal excretion	A safe drug; least likely to cause hypoglycaemia May decrease iodide uptake by thyroid Contraindicated in liver failure
Glibenclamide[c]	150	18–24 (10)	Some is oxidised in the liver to moderately active products and is excreted in urine; 50% is excreted unchanged in the faeces	May cause hypoglycaemia The active metabolite accumulates in renal failure
Glipizide	100	16–24 (7)	Peak plasma levels in 1 h Most is metabolised in the liver to inactive products, which are excreted in urine; 12% is excreted in faeces	May cause hypoglycaemia Has diuretic action Only inactive products accumulate in renal failure

[a]Relative to tolbutamide.
[b]All are highly protein bound (90%–95%).
[c]Termed glyburide in the United States.

Unwanted effects

The sulfonylureas are usually well tolerated. Unwanted effects are specified in Table 32.3. The commonest adverse effect is hypoglycaemia, which can be severe and prolonged, the highest incidence occurring with long-acting chlorpropamide and glibenclamide and the lowest with tolbutamide. Long-acting sulfonylureas are best avoided in the elderly and in patients with even mild renal impairment because of the risk of hypoglycaemia. Sulfonylureas stimulate appetite and often cause weight gain. This is a major concern in obese diabetic patients. About 3% of patients experience GI upsets. Allergic rashes can occur, and bone marrow toxicity (Ch. 58), although rare, can be severe.

During and for a few days after acute myocardial infarction in diabetic patients, insulin must be substituted for sulfonylurea treatment. Such substitution is associated with a substantial reduction in short-term mortality, although it remains unclear if this is due to a beneficial effect specific to insulin or to avoiding a detrimental effect of sulfonylurea drugs in this setting, or both. Another vexing question is whether prolonged therapy with oral hypoglycaemic drugs has adverse cardiovascular effects. Blockade of K_{ATP} in heart and vascular tissue could theoretically have adverse effects, and an observational study recorded an increased risk of death and cardiovascular disease during follow-up for up to 8 years in newly diagnosed type 2 diabetic patients treated with sulfonylureas compared with those treated with metformin (Evans et al., 2006).

Drug interactions

Several drugs augment the hypoglycaemic effect of sulfonylureas. Non-steroidal anti-inflammatory drugs, warfarin, some uricosuric drugs (e.g. **sulfinpyrazone**), alcohol, monoamine oxidase inhibitors, some antibacterial drugs (including sulfonamides, **trimethoprim** and **chloramphenicol**) and some imidazole antifungal drugs have all been reported to produce severe hypoglycaemia when given

with a sulfonylurea. The probable basis of most of these interactions is competition for metabolising enzymes, but interference with plasma protein binding or with transport mechanisms facilitating excretion may play some part.

Agents that decrease the action of sulfonylureas on blood glucose include high doses of thiazide diuretics (Chs 22 and 30) and glucocorticoids (pharmacodynamic interactions).

Clinical use

Sulfonylureas are used to treat type 2 diabetes in its early stages, but because they require functional β cells, they are not useful in type 1 or late-stage type 2 diabetes. They can be combined with metformin.

OTHER DRUGS THAT STIMULATE INSULIN SECRETION

Several drugs that act, like the sulfonylureas, by blocking the sulfonylurea receptor on K_{ATP} channels in pancreatic β cells but lack the sulfonylurea moiety have been developed. These include **repaglinide** and **nateglinide** which, though much less potent than most sulfonylureas, have rapid onset and offset kinetics leading to short duration of action and a low risk of hypoglycaemia.[9] These drugs are administered shortly before a meal to reduce the postprandial rise in blood glucose in type 2 diabetic patients inadequately controlled with diet and exercise. They may cause less weight gain than conventional sulfonylureas. Later in the course of the disease, they can be combined with metformin or other oral hypoglycaemic agents. Unlike glibenclamide, these drugs are relatively selective for K_{ATP} channels on β cells versus K_{ATP} channels in vascular smooth muscle.

Thiazolidinediones (glitazones): pioglitazone

The thiazolidinediones (or *glitazones*) were developed following the chance observation that a **clofibrate** analogue,

---

[9]It is ironic that these aggressively marketed drugs share many of the properties of tolbutamide, the oldest, least expensive and least fashionable of the sulfonylureas.

ciglitazone, which was being screened for effects on lipids, unexpectedly lowered blood glucose. Ciglitazone caused liver toxicity, and this class of drugs (despite considerable commercial success) has been dogged by adverse effects (especially cardiovascular), regulatory withdrawals and controversy. No clinical trials of these agents have demonstrated a beneficial effect on mortality, and they were licensed on the basis of statistically significant effects on haemoglobin A1c (a surrogate marker of longer-term diabetes status) of uncertain clinical significance. **Pioglitazone** is the only drug of this class that remains in clinical use, its predecessors, rosiglitazone and troglitazone, having faced regulatory action because of increased risk of heart attacks and liver damage, respectively – at the time, a *cause célèbre*, and very expensive for the companies involved.

Effects

The effect of thiazolidinediones on blood glucose is slow in onset, the maximum effect being achieved only after 1–2 months of treatment. They act by enhancing the effectiveness of endogenous insulin, thereby reducing hepatic glucose output, and increasing glucose uptake into muscle.

They reduce the amount of exogenous insulin needed to maintain a given level of blood glucose by approximately 30%. Reduced blood glucose concentration is accompanied by reduced insulin and free fatty acid concentrations. Weight gain of 1–4 kg is common, usually stabilising in 6–12 months. Some of this is attributable to fluid retention: there is an increase in plasma volume of up to 500 mL, with a concomitant reduction in haemoglobin concentration caused by haemodilution; there is also an increase in extravascular fluid, and increased deposition of subcutaneous (as opposed to visceral) fat.

Mechanism of action

Thiazolidinediones bind to a nuclear receptor called the *peroxisome proliferator-activated receptor-γ* (PPARγ), which is complexed with retinoid X receptor (RXR; see Ch. 3).[10] It remains something of a mystery that glucose homeostasis should be so responsive to drugs that bind to receptors found mainly in fat cells; it has been suggested that the explanation may lie in resetting of the glucose–fatty acid (Randle) cycle by the reduction in circulating free fatty acids.

Unwanted effects

Clinical trial data have demonstrated significantly increased risk of a range of adverse events with pioglitazone, including heart failure, bone fracture, oedema, and weight gain. (Liao et al., 2017), and glitazones are now far less frequently used.

Clinical use

Pioglitazone is additive with other oral hypoglycaemic drugs in terms of effect on blood glucose, and a combination tablet with metformin is marketed.

α-Glucosidase inhibitors

Acarbose, an inhibitor of intestinal α-glucosidase, is used in type 2 diabetes inadequately controlled by diet with or without other agents. It delays carbohydrate absorption, reducing the postprandial increase in blood glucose. The commonest adverse effects are related to its main action and consist of flatulence, loose stools or diarrhoea, and abdominal pain and bloating. Like metformin, it may be particularly helpful in obese type 2 patients, and it can be co-administered with metformin.

Incretin mimetics and related drugs

Exenatide is a synthetic version of *exendin-4*, a peptide found in the saliva of the Gila monster (a lizard that presumably evolved this as means to disable its prey by rendering them hypoglycaemic).

GLP-1 agonists lower blood glucose after a meal by increasing insulin secretion, suppressing glucagon secretion and slowing gastric emptying (see earlier). They reduce food intake (by an effect on satiety, see Ch. 33) and are associated with modest weight loss. They reduce hepatic fat accumulation.

GLP-1 agonists are administered by subcutaneous injection, either once daily (exenatide, **liraglutide, lixisenatide**) or once weekly (extended release exenatide, **albiglutide, dulaglutide**). Pancreatitis is rare but potentially severe.

GLP-1 agonists are used in patients with type 2 diabetes in combination with other drugs (metformin with or without a sulfonylurea, pioglitazone, insulin).

Gliptins

Gliptins (e.g. **sitagliptin, vildagliptin, saxagliptin, linagliptin**) are synthetic drugs that competitively inhibit dipeptidyl peptidase-4 (DPP-4), thereby lowering blood glucose by potentiating endogenous incretins (GLP-1 and GIP, see p. 413) which stimulate insulin secretion. They do not cause weight loss or weight gain.

They are absorbed from the gut and administered once (or, in the case of vildagliptin, twice) daily by mouth. They are eliminated partly by renal excretion and are also metabolised by hepatic CYP enzymes. They are usually well tolerated with a range of mild GI adverse effects; liver disease, heart failure (particularly with saxagliptin or alogliptin) and pancreatitis (incidence approximately 0.1%–1%) are less common but potentially serious. There is also concern that they may act as tumour promoters (see Ch. 58). Gliptins are used for type 2 diabetes in addition to other oral hypoglycaemic drugs (see clinical box on uses of oral hypoglycaemic drugs, p. 420).

Evidence of cardiovascular efficacy or effect on mortality is inconsistent, with liraglutide the only agent to produce a demonstrable reduction in major adverse cardiac events (Paneni & Luscher, 2017), whereas neither sitagliptin nor exenatide have shown such benefits in large-scale clinical trials.

Glucose transport inhibitors

Several SGLT2 inhibitors are licensed for use in type 2 diabetes. Examples include **canagliflozin, dapagliflozin**, and **empagliflozin**.

Mechanism of action

The SGLT2 inhibitors act by promoting glucose excretion into the urine, thereby reducing the concentration of circulating glucose. The resulting glycosuria is associated with an osmotic diuresis and salt excretion

---

[10]Compare with fibrates (to which thiazolidinediones are structurally related), which bind to PPARα (see Ch. 24).

Effects

Clinical studies have found elevated amounts of glucose in the urine over sustained periods, and an associated increase in urinary volume. As the efficacy of SGLT2 inhibitors rely on adequate renal function and urine output, these agents have limited or no effect in patients with chronic kidney disease. Clinical trials have confirmed improvements in fasting and post-prandial glucose concentrations, and significant reduction in glycosylated haemoglobin (Storgaard et al., 2016). The osmotic diuretic effect and the caloric loss (from glucose in the urine) also leads to reduction in systolic blood pressure and body weight (Abdul-Ghani et al., 2015). A clinical trial of empaglifozen (EMPA-REG OUTCOME) reported substantial reductions in cardiovascular endpoints, to which these haemodynamic effects probably contributed substantially (Paneni & Luscher, 2017).

Pharmacokinetic aspects

SGLT2 inhibitors are rapidly absorbed, with time to peak plasma concentrations of less than 2 h. They are highly bound to plasma proteins (>80%).

Unwanted effects

A significant increase in the risk of urinary tract and fungal infections such as candidal vaginitis or balanitis has been reported with SGLT2 inhibition, presumably due to the glycosuria (Storgaard et al., 2016). Natriuresis with diuresis can lead to increased urinary volume, hypotension and dehydration, and is accentuated with concomitant use of thiazide diuretics.

Safety signals that are currently under regulatory evaluation include potential serious adverse events such as increased susceptibility to diabetic ketoacidosis, and lower limb amputations.

Clinical use

SGLT2 inhibitors are licensed for use in type 2 diabetes, either alone (when metformin is inappropriate) or in combination with insulin or other oral glucose lowering therapies. Typically, this would involve SGLT2 use in dual or triple therapy where sulfonylureas are not tolerated or have not been sufficiently efficacious. A potential advantage of SGLT2 inhibition in those with inadequate diabetes control is that the amount of glucose excreted in the urine will be proportionately greater in patients whose plasma glucose concentrations are high.

The SGLT2 inhibitors are also considered to have a relatively low risk of hypoglycaemia, and are therefore a recommended option in patients who are susceptible to hypoglycaemia.

TREATMENT OF DIABETES MELLITUS

Insulin is essential for the treatment of type 1 diabetes, and a valuable component of the treatment of many patients with type 2 disease.

▼ For many years it was assumed, as an act of faith, that normalising plasma glucose would reduce the risk of diabetic complications. The Diabetes Control and Complications Trial (American Diabetes Association, 1993) showed that this faith was well placed: type 1 diabetic patients were randomly allocated to intensive or conventional management. Mean fasting blood glucose concentration was 2.8 mmol/L lower in the intensively treated group, who had a substantial reduction in the occurrence and progression of retinopathy, nephropathy and neuropathy over a period of 4–9 years. Benefits, including reduced atheromatous as well as microvascular disease, were long-lasting and outweighed adverse effects, which included a three-fold increase in severe hypoglycaemic attacks and modest excess weight gain.

The UK Prospective Diabetes Study showed that *lowering blood pressure* markedly improves outcome in type 2 diabetes. Normalisation of blood glucose was not achieved even in intensively treated patients. Better metabolic control did improve outcome, but (in contrast to lowering blood pressure) the magnitude of the benefit was disappointing and statistically significant only for microvascular complications. In long-term follow-up, patients from this study who had been allocated to intensive treatment continued to have better outcomes than patients treated with diet alone (despite diabetic control becoming similar in the two groups after the blinded treatment period had finished), suggesting that early diabetic control (within the first 12 years from diagnosis) is important (Holman et al., 2008). By contrast, studies of intensive control later in the course of the disease have been disappointing with harm from hypoglycaemia outweighing any benefit.

Realistic goals in type 2 diabetic patients are usually less ambitious than in younger type 1 patients. Dietary restriction leading to weight loss in overweight and obese patients is the cornerstone (albeit one with a tendency to crumble), combined with increased exercise. Oral agents are used to control symptoms from hyperglycaemia, as well as to limit microvascular complications, and are introduced early. Dietary measures and statins to prevent atheromatous disease (Ch. 24) are crucial. Details of dietary management and treatment for specific diabetic complications are beyond the scope of this book. Glitazones and drugs that mimic or potentiate incretins reduce glycated haemoglobin (typically by 0.5–1 percentage points) but their effects (if any) on clinical outcomes such as diabetic complications have not been consistently demonstrated. There is some evidence that **pioglitazone**, **liraglutide** and **empagliflozin** can improve cardiovascular outcomes in type 2 diabetic patients (Paneni & Lüscher, 2017) – possibly due to cardiovascular actions distinct from their metabolic effects.

Drugs used in diabetes mellitus

Insulin and other injectable drugs

- Human **insulin** is made by recombinant DNA technology. For routine use, it is given subcutaneously (by intravenous infusion in emergencies).
- Different formulations of **insulin** differ in their duration of action:
  - fast- and short-acting **soluble insulin**: peak action after subcutaneous dose 2–4 h and duration 6–8 h; it is the only formulation that can be given intravenously
  - intermediate-acting insulin (e.g. **isophane insulin**)
  - long-acting forms (e.g. **insulin zinc suspension**)
- The main unwanted effect is hypoglycaemia.
- Altering the amino acid sequence (insulin analogues, e.g. **lispro** and **glargine**) can usefully alter **insulin** kinetics.
- **Insulins** are used for all type 1 diabetic patients and approximately one-third of patients with type 2 diabetes.
- **Exenatide** and **liraglutide** are injectable glucagon-like peptide-1 (GLP-1) agonists used as add-on treatment in certain inadequately controlled type 2 diabetic patients. Unlike **insulin** they cause weight loss.

Oral hypoglycaemic drugs

- These are used in type 2 diabetes.
- Biguanides (e.g. **metformin**):
  - have complex peripheral actions in the presence of residual insulin, increasing glucose uptake in striated muscle and inhibiting hepatic glucose output and intestinal glucose absorption
  - cause anorexia and encourage weight loss
  - can be combined with sulfonylureas
- Sulfonylureas and other drugs that stimulate insulin secretion (e.g. **tolbutamide**, **glibenclamide**, **nateglinide**):

- can cause hypoglycaemia (which stimulates appetite and leads to weight gain)
- are effective only if β cells are functional
- block ATP-sensitive potassium channels in β cells
- are well tolerated but promote weight gain and are associated with more cardiovascular disease than is **metformin**
- Thiazolidinediones have been associated with serious cardiac toxicity.
  Pioglitazone is the only one still widely marketed; it:
  - increases insulin sensitivity and lowers blood glucose in type 2 diabetes
  - can cause weight gain and oedema
  - increases osteoporotic fractures
  - is a peroxisome proliferator-activated receptor-γ (a nuclear receptor) agonist
- Gliptins (e.g. **sitagliptin**):
  - potentiate endogenous incretins by blocking dipeptidyl peptidase-4 (DPP-4)
  - are added to other orally active drugs to improve control in patients with type 2 diabetes
  - are weight-neutral; they are usually well tolerated but pancreatitis is a concern
- Sodium–glucose co-transporter (SGLT)2 inhibitors (e.g. empagliflozin)
  - Promote urinary excretion of glucose
  - Have potentially beneficial effects on weight, blood pressure and cardiovascular outcome
  - Increase the risk of dehydration and urinary tract infections
- α-Glucosidase inhibitor, **acarbose**:
  - reduces carbohydrate absorption
  - causes flatulence and diarrhoea

Clinical uses of oral hypoglycaemic drugs

- *Type 2 diabetes mellitus*, to reduce symptoms from hyperglycaemia (e.g. thirst, excessive urination). ('Tight' control of blood glucose has only a small effect on vascular complications in this setting.)
- **Metformin** is preferred, especially for obese patients unless contraindicated by factors that predispose to lactic acidosis (renal or liver failure, poorly compensated heart failure, hypoxaemia).
- **Acarbose** (α-glucosidase inhibitor) reduces carbohydrate absorption; it causes flatulence and diarrhoea.
- Drugs that act on the sulfonylurea receptor (e.g. **tolbutamide**, **glibenclamide**) are well tolerated but often promote weight gain. They are associated with increased cardiovascular risk compared with **metformin**.
- **Pioglitazone** improves control (reduces haemoglobin A_{1c}) but increases weight, causes heart failure, fluid

retention and increases risk of fractures. Glucagon-like peptide (GLP)-1 agonists (e.g. **exenatide, lixisenatide,** or **liraglutide**) are injected once daily or (**extended release exenatide**) once weekly in obese patients inadequately controlled on two hypoglycaemic drugs. These agents are associated with the potential for weight loss or prevention of weight gain in overweight or obese patients.
- Dipeptidyl peptidase-4 (DPP-4) inhibitors (gliptins, e.g. **sitagliptin**) improve control, are well tolerated and weight-neutral, but outcome evidence is inconsistent. Pancreatitis and heart failure are possible adverse effects of concern.
- Sodium–glucose co-transporter (SGLT)2 inhibitors improve control, but long-term outcomes and safety data are still emerging.

REFERENCES AND FURTHER READING

References

Abdul-Ghani, M.A., Norton, L., DeFronzo, R.A., 2011. Role of sodium-glucose cotransporter 2 (SGLT 2) inhibitors in the treatment of type 2 diabetes. Endocr. Rev. 32 (4), 515–531.

Abdul-Ghani, M.A., Norton, L., DeFronzo, R.A., 2015. Renal sodium-glucose cotransporter inhibition in the management of type 2 diabetes mellitus. Am. J. Physiol. Renal Physiol. 309 (11), F889–F900.

American Diabetes Association, 1993. Implications of the diabetes control and complications trial. Diabetes 42, 1555–1558. (*Landmark clinical trial*)

Atkin, S., Javed, Z., Fulcher, G., 2015. Insulin degludec and insulin aspart: novel insulins for the management of diabetes mellitus. Ther. Adv. Chronic. Dis. 6 (6), 375–388. (*Excellent summary of development and pharmacokinetics of insulin analogues*)

DeFronzo, R.A., Davidson, J.A., Del Prato, S., 2012. The role of the kidneys in glucose homeostasis: a new path towards normalizing glycaemia. Diabetes Obes. Metab. 14 (1), 5–14. (*Good review article discussing glucose homeostasis and the kidney*)

Duca, F.A., Cote, C.D., Rasmussen, B.A., et al., 2015. Metformin activates a duodenal Ampk-dependent pathway to lower hepatic glucose production in rats. Nat. Med. 21, 506–511.

Evans, J.M.M., Ogston, S.A., Emslie-Smith, A., Morris, A.D., 2006. Risk of mortality and adverse cardiovascular outcomes in type 2 diabetes: a comparison of patients treated with sulfonylureas and metformin. Diabetologia 49, 930–936. (*Observational cohort study in 5700 newly treated type 2 patients, 1000 deaths in up to 8 years follow-up. Sulfonylurea use was associated with increased risk of death and of cardiovascular disease. Not proof but pretty suggestive!*)

Holman, R.R., Sanjoy, K.P., Bethel, M.A., et al., 2008. 10-year follow-up of intensive glucose control in type 2 diabetes. N. Engl. J. Med. 359, 1577–1589.

Liao, H.W., Saver, J.L., Wu, Y.L., Chen, T.H., Lee, M., Ovbiagele, B., 2017. Pioglitazone and cardiovascular outcomes in patients with insulin resistance, pre-diabetes and type 2 diabetes: a systematic review and meta-analysis. BMJ open. 7 (1), e013927.

Myers, R.W., Guan, H.P., Ehrhart, J., et al., 2017. Systemic pan-AMPK activator MK-8722 improves glucose homeostasis but induces cardiac hypertrophy. Science 357, 507–511.

Napolitano, A., Miller, S., Nicholls, A.W., et al., 2014. Novel gut-based pharmacology of metformin in patients with type 2 diabetes mellitus. PLoS ONE 9, e100778.

Paneni, F., Luscher, T.F., 2017. Cardiovascular protection in the treatment of type 2 diabetes: a review of clinical trial results across drug classes. Science 120, S17–S27. (*Good summary of cardiovascular outcomes in trials of different classes of hypoglycaemic agents*)

Storgaard, H., Gluud, L.L., Bennett, C., et al., 2016. Benefits and harms of sodium-glucose co-transporter 2 inhibitors in patients with type 2 diabetes: a systematic review and meta-analysis. PLoS ONE 11 (11).

Viollet, B., Guigas, B., Garcia, N.S., Leclerc, J., Foretz, M., Andreelli, F., 2012. Cellular and molecular mechanisms of metformin: an overview. Clin. Sci. 122, 253–270. (*Reviews mechanisms as a setting for novel therapeutic uses, for example in non-alcoholic fatty liver disease*)

Waumans, Y., Baerts, L., Kehoe, K., Lambeir, A.M., De Meester, I., 2015. The dipeptidyl peptidase family, prolyl oligopeptidase, and prolyl carboxypeptidase in the immune system and inflammatory disease, including atherosclerosis. Front. Immunol. 6, 387.

Williams, G., 1994. Management of non-insulin dependent diabetes mellitus. Lancet 343, 95–100.

Yu, D.M.T., Yao, T.W., Chowdhary, S., 2010. The dipeptidyl peptidase IV family in cancer and cell biology. FEBS J. 277, 1126–1144. (*Discusses current understanding of this unique family of enzymes*)

Further reading

Physiological and pathophysiological aspects

Lavin, D.P., White, M.F., Brazil, D.P., 2016. IRS proteins and diabetic complications. Diabetologia 59, 2280–2291. (*Reviews the role of IRS proteins in linking cell surface receptors to intracellular signalling cascades and potential mechanisms that lead to development and progression of diabetic complications'*)

Withers, D.J., Gutierrez, J.S., Towery, H., et al., 1998. Disruption of IRS-2 causes type 2 diabetes in mice. Nature 391, 900–904. (*Dysfunction of IRS-2 may 'contribute to the pathophysiology of human type 2 diabetes'; see also accompanying commentary by Avruch, J., A signal for β-cell failure, pp. 846–847*)

Zimmet, P., Alberti, K.G.M.M., Shaw, J., 2001. Global and societal implications of the diabetes epidemic. Nature 414, 782–787. (*Changes in human behaviour have resulted in a dramatic increase in type 2 diabetes worldwide*)

Insulins

Owens, D.R., Zinman, B., Bolli, G.B., 2001. Insulins today and beyond. Lancet 358, 739–746. (*Reviews the physiology of glucose homeostasis, genetically engineered 'designer' insulins and developments in insulin delivery and glucose sensing*)

Oral hypoglycaemic drugs

Gale, E.A.M., 2001. Lessons from the glitazones: a story of drug development. Lancet 357, 1870–1875. (*Fighting stuff: 'Troglitazone was voluntarily withdrawn in Europe, but went on to generate sales of over $2 billion in the USA and caused 90 cases of liver failure before being withdrawn. Rosiglitazone and pioglitazone reached the USA for use alone or in combination with other drugs whereas in Europe the same dossiers were used to apply for a limited licence as second-line agents. How should we use them? How did they achieve blockbuster status without any clear evidence of advantage over existing therapy?'*)

Guan, Y., Hao, C., Cha, D.R., et al., 2005. Thiazolidinediones expand body fluid volume through PPARγ stimulation of ENaC-mediated renal salt absorption. Nat. Med. 11, 861–865. (*Mechanism of fluid retention caused by thiazolidinediones and suggestion that amiloride may provide a specific therapy for this*)

Other drugs for diabetes, and therapeutic aspects

Brenner, B.M., Cooper, M.E., de Zeeuw, D., et al., 2001. Effects of losartan on renal and cardiovascular outcomes in patients with type 2 diabetes and nephropathy. N. Engl. J. Med. 345, 861–869. (*Significant renal benefits from the AT_1 antagonist; see also two adjacent articles: Lewis, E.J., et al., pp. 851–860, and Parving, H.-H., et al., pp. 870–878, and an editorial on prevention of renal disease caused by type 2 diabetes by Hostetter, T.H., pp. 910–911*)

Farmer, K.L., Li, C.Y., Dobrowsky, R.T., 2012. Diabetic neuropathy: should a chaperone accompany our therapeutic approach? Pharmacol. Rev. 64, 880–900. (*Currently no satisfactory therapy*)

Younk, L.M., Mikeladze, M., Davis, S.N., 2011. Pramlintide and the treatment of diabetes: a review of the data since its introduction. Expert Opin. Pharmacother. 12, 1439–1451. (*'Pramlintide significantly reduces hemoglobin A(1c) and body weight in patients with type 1 and type 2 diabetes mellitus. Newer research is focusing on weight loss effects of pramlintide and pramlintide plus metreleptin in nondiabetic obese individuals'*)

33 Obesity

OVERVIEW

Obesity is a growing health issue around the world and is reaching epidemic proportions in some nations. The problem is not restricted to the inhabitants of the affluent countries, to the adult population or to any one socioeconomic class. Body fat represents stored energy and obesity occurs when the homeostatic mechanisms controlling energy balance become disordered or overwhelmed. In this chapter we first outline the endogenous regulation of appetite and body mass, and then consider the main health implications of obesity and its pathophysiology. We conclude with a discussion of the drugs currently licensed for the treatment of obesity and glance at possible future pharmacological treatments for this condition.

INTRODUCTION

Survival requires a continuous provision of energy to maintain homeostasis, even when the supply of food is intermittent. Evolution has furnished a mechanism for storing excess energy latent in foodstuffs in adipose tissue as energy-dense triglycerides, such that these can be easily mobilised when food is scarce. This mechanism, controlled by the so-called *thrifty genes*, was an obvious asset to our hunter–gatherer ancestors, but in many societies a combination of sedentary lifestyle, genetic susceptibility, cultural influences and unrestricted access to an ample supply of calorie-dense foods has led to a global epidemic of obesity, or 'globesity' as it is sometimes called. Obesity is one component of a cluster of disorders described in other chapters, which often coexist in the same individual, comprising what is now described as 'metabolic syndrome' (formerly 'metabolic X syndrome'), and which constitutes a rapidly growing public health problem.

DEFINITION OF OBESITY

'Obesity' may be defined as an illness where health (and hence life expectancy) is adversely affected by excess body fat.[1] But at what point does an individual become 'obese'? The generally accepted (WHO) benchmark is the body mass index (BMI). The BMI is expressed as W/h^2, where W = body weight (in kg), h = height (in metres). Although it is not a perfect index (e.g. it does not distinguish between fat and lean mass), the BMI is generally well correlated with other measurements of body fat, and it is widely utilised as a convenient index. While there are problems in defining a 'healthy' weight for a particular population,

the WHO classifies adults with a BMI of ≥25 as being overweight and those with a BMI of ≥30 as obese. Childhood obesity is more difficult to assess.

Since the BMI obviously depends on the overall energy balance, another operational definition of obesity would be that it is a multifactorial disorder of energy balance in which calorie intake over the long term exceeds energy output.

OBESITY AS A HEALTH PROBLEM

Obesity is a growing and costly global health problem. The WHO in 2016 estimated that worldwide obesity has doubled since 1980 and there were more than 1.9 billion overweight adults, approximately one-third of whom – amounting to more than 13% of the world's population – were obese according to the criteria outlined earlier. National obesity levels vary enormously, being less than 4% in Japan and parts of Africa, but a staggering 40% or more in parts of Polynesia. Adult obesity levels in the United States, Europe and the United Kingdom (among others) have increased three-fold since 1980, with figures of 34% being quoted for the United States by WHO (2016) and about 25% for many other industrialised nations including the United Kingdom. The disease is not confined to adults: some 42 million children or infants under 5 years old are estimated to be overweight. In the United States, the number of overweight children has doubled and the number of overweight adolescents has trebled since 1980, although there are now signs of it stabilising at around 17% (data from the US Center for Disease Control and Prevention, 2015). Ironically, obesity often coexists with malnutrition in many developing countries. All socioeconomic classes are affected. In the poorest countries, it is the top socioeconomic classes in whom obesity is prevalent, but in the affluent West it is usually the reverse.

Overall, more people die in the world from being overweight and obese than being underweight, and the financial burden on the healthcare system is huge. An influential report (McKinsey Global Institute, 2014) estimated the global economic burden was estimated at US$2.1 trillion in 2014, 2.9% of the global GDP – more than the cost incurred by armed violence, war and terrorism taken altogether.

▼ While obesity itself is rarely fatal, it often coexists with metabolic and other disorders (particularly hypertension, hypercholesterolaemia and type 2 diabetes), together comprising the *metabolic syndrome*. This carries a high risk of cardiovascular conditions, strokes, cancers (particularly hormone-dependent), respiratory disorders (particularly sleep apnoea) and digestive problems, as well as osteoarthritis. One commentator (Kopelman, 2000) has remarked that obesity 'is beginning to replace under-nutrition and infectious diseases as the most significant contributor to ill health'. Increasingly, social stigma is suffered by obese individuals, leading to a sense of psychological isolation.

---

[1] 'Persons who are naturally very fat are apt to die earlier than those who are slender' observed Hippocrates.

The risk of developing type 2 diabetes (which represents 85% of all cases of the disease) rises sharply with increasing BMI. The WHO reports that some 90% of those diagnosed with the disease are obese. In a study of the disease in women, the risk of developing diabetes was closely correlated with BMI, increasing five-fold when the BMI was 25 kg/m^2, to 93-fold when the BMI was 35 kg/m^2 or above (Colditz et al., 1995). Cardiovascular disease is also increased in the obese individual, and the increased thoracic and abdominal adipose tissue reduces lung volume and makes respiration difficult. Obese subjects also have an increased risk of colon, breast, prostate, gall bladder, ovarian and uterine cancer. Numerous other disorders are associated with excess body weight, including osteoarthritis, hyperuricaemia and male hypogonadism. 'Gross' obesity (BMI ≥40 kg/m^2) is associated with a 12-fold increase in mortality in the group aged 25–35 years compared with those in this age group with a BMI of 20–25 kg/m^2.

HOMEOSTATIC MECHANISMS CONTROLLING ENERGY BALANCE

A common view, and one that is implicitly encouraged by authors of numerous self-help books as well as the enormously lucrative dieting industry, is that obesity is simply the result of bad diet or willful overeating (hyperphagia). In truth, however, the situation is more complex. On its own, dieting seldom provides a lasting solution: the failure rate is high (probably 90%), and most dieters eventually return to their original starting weight. This suggests the operation of some intrinsic homeostatic system to maintain a particular set weight. This mechanism is normally exceptionally precise, and is capable of regulating energy balance to within 0.17% per decade (Weigle, 1994), a truly astonishing feat, considering the day-to-day variations in food intake.

When exposed to the same dietary choices, some individuals will become obese whereas others will not. Studies of obesity in monozygotic and dizygotic twins have established a strong genetic influence on the susceptibility to the condition, and studies of rare mutations in mice (and more recently in humans) have led to the discovery and elucidation of the neuroendocrine pathways that match food intake with energy expenditure. These, in turn, have led to the concept that disorders of these control systems are largely responsible for the onset and maintenance of obesity.

THE ROLE OF GUT AND OTHER HORMONES IN BODY WEIGHT REGULATION

At the beginning of the 20th century it was observed that patients with damage to the hypothalamus tended to gain weight. In the 1940s it was also shown that discrete lesions in the hypothalamus of rodents caused them to become obese or exhibit unusual feeding behaviour. On the basis of early (1953) observations in rats, Kennedy proposed that a hormone released from adipose tissue acted on the hypothalamus to regulate body fat and food intake. These seminal findings set the stage for future discoveries in this area.

It was also observed that mice became obese as a result of mutations in certain genes. At least five of these have now been characterised, including the *Ob* (obesity), *Tub* (tubby), *Fat* and *Db* (diabetes) genes. Mice that are homozygous for mutant forms of these genes – *Ob/Ob* mice and *Db/Db* mice – eat excessively, have low energy expenditure, become grossly fat and have numerous metabolic and other abnormalities. Weight gain in an *Ob/Ob* mouse is suppressed if its circulation is linked to that of a normal mouse, implying that the obesity is caused by lack of a blood-borne factor.

An important conceptual breakthrough came in 1994, when Friedman and his colleagues (see Zhang et al., 1994) cloned the *Ob* gene and identified its protein product as the polypeptide *leptin*.[2] When recombinant leptin was administered systemically to *Ob/Ob* mice, it strikingly reduced food intake and body weight. It had a similar effect when injected directly into the lateral or the third ventricle, implying that it acted on the regions of the brain that control food intake and energy balance. Recombinant leptin has similar effects in humans (Fig. 33.1).

Leptin mRNA is expressed in adipocytes; its synthesis is increased by glucocorticoids, insulin and oestrogens, and is reduced by β-adrenoceptor agonists. In normal human subjects, the release of leptin is pulsatile and varies according to the state of the fat stores and the BMI. Insulin (see Ch. 32) may also stimulate leptin release although the relationship between these two hormones is complex.

In addition to leptin and insulin, several other mediators originating mainly from the gastrointestinal (GI) tract as well as in the hypothalamus, play a crucial role in determining food intake, meal size and the feeling of satisfaction produced ('satiety').[3] Peptide hormones secreted by cells in the wall of the small intestine in response to the arrival of food (see Ch. 31) are important in this connection. Table 33.1 and Fig. 33.2 summarise the chief characteristics of these mediators.

The majority of these peptides are released either during, or in anticipation of, eating and most are inhibitory in nature, producing either satiety or satiation. Two exceptions are the gastric hormone, ghrelin, which promotes hunger, and leptin itself, which is controlled by the amount of adipose tissue and is thus more involved with the longer-term energy status of the individual. The main targets for these hormones are receptors on vagal afferent fibres or within the hypothalamus (or elsewhere in the central nervous system [CNS]). Here, they modulate the release of other neurotransmitters that exert a fine regulation over eating behaviour, energy expenditure and body weight. Other actions of these peptide hormones include the release of insulin by the *incretins* (see Ch. 32), which include glucagon-like peptide-1 (GLP-1) and gastric inhibitory peptide (GIP).

Another factor, *nesfatin 1*, has recently attracted attention as a potentially important regulator of feeding behaviour and energy homeostasis (see Ramesh et al., 2017). This is an 82-amino acid peptide produced from a precursor molecule *nucleobindin 2*. Unlike many of the hormones already discussed, nesfatin 1 may be produced by many peripheral and central tissues. It acts centrally to produce an anorexigenic effect by modulating the neuropeptides in the hypothalamic circuits described later. It may also have additional actions on the pancreas as well as GI function and even the cardiovascular system.

NEUROLOGICAL CIRCUITS THAT CONTROL BODY WEIGHT AND EATING BEHAVIOUR
CONTROL OF FOOD INTAKE

The manner in which all these hormonal signals are processed and integrated with other viscerosensory, gustatory or

[2]The word is derived from the Greek *leptos*, meaning thin.
[3]The terminology can be confusing. 'Hunger' obviously refers to the desire to eat; 'satiation' is the feeling that you have eaten enough in the course of a meal. 'Satiety' refers to the feeling after a meal that you don't yet need another.

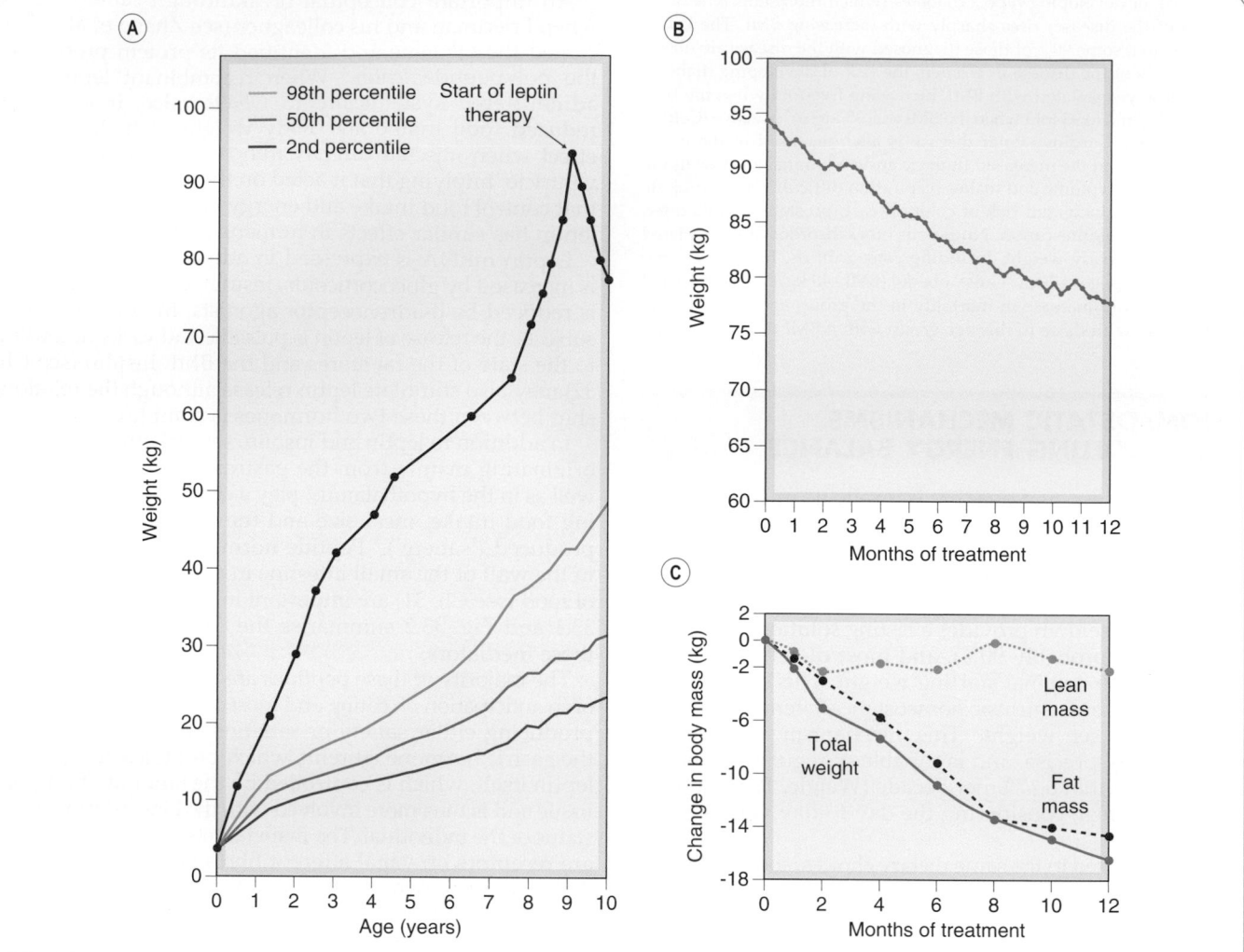

Fig. 33.1 The effect of recombinant leptin on body weight in a 9-year-old severely obese child with endogenous leptin deficiency because of a frame shift mutation in the leptin gene. Although of normal birth weight, the child began gaining weight at 4 months and was constantly demanding food. Prior to treatment, the child weighed 94.4 kg. Weight loss began after 2 weeks' treatment, and her eating pattern returned to normal. She had lost 15.6 kg of body fat after 1 year of treatment. (Data and figure adapted from Farooqi et al., 1999.)

Table 33.1 Some peripheral hormones that regulate eating behaviour

Hormone	Source	Stimulus to release	Target	Effect
CCK	GI tract	During feeding or just before	Vagal afferents	Limits size of meal
Amylin, insulin, glucagon	Pancreas	During feeding or just before	Vagal afferents	Limits size of meal
PYY3–36	Ileum, colon	After feeding	Brain stem, hypothalamus	Postpones need for next meal
GLP-1	Stomach	After feeding	Brain stem, hypothalamus	Postpones need for next meal
Oxyntomodulin	Stomach	After feeding	Brain stem, hypothalamus	Postpones need for next meal
Leptin	Adipose tissue	Adiposity 'status'	Brain stem, arcuate nucleus	Longer-term regulation of food intake
Ghrelin	Stomach	Hunger, feeding	Vagus, hypothalamus	Increases food intake by increasing size and number of meals
Nesfatin 1	Hypothalamus, pancreas, adipose tissue and GI tract	Food intake	Orexigenic NPY neurones.	Decreases appetite

424

CCK, cholecystokinin; *GI,* gastrointestinal; *GLP-1,* glucagon-like peptide-1; *NPY,* neuropeptide Y; *PYY3–36,* peptide YY.

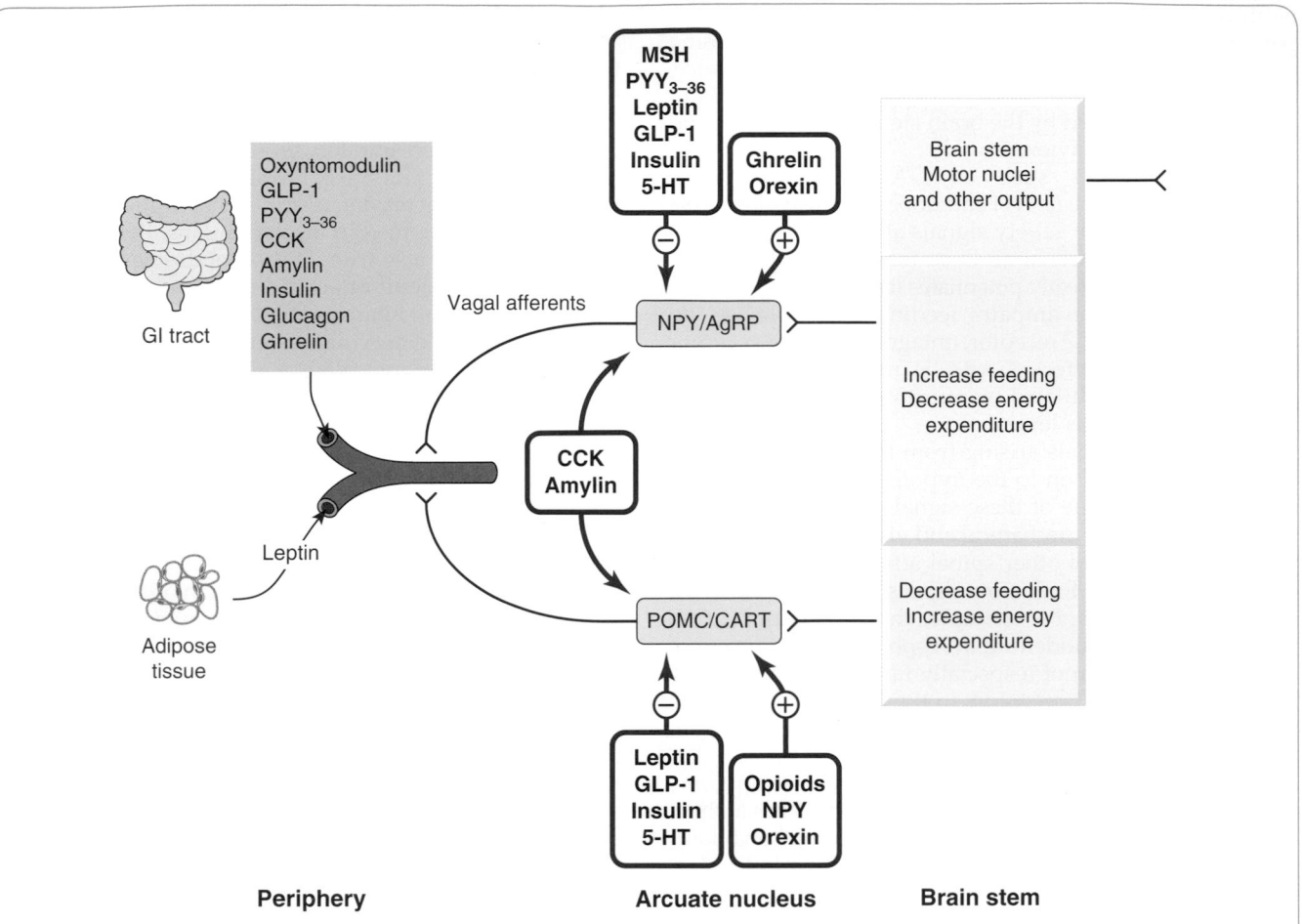

Fig. 33.2 A simplified representation of the role of peripheral hormones and other mediators in the regulation of energy balance and fat stores. The primary level of hypothalamic control is vested in two groups of neurons, with opposing actions, in the arcuate nucleus (ARC). In one group, the peptides neuropeptide Y (NPY) and agouti-related peptide (AgRP) are co-localised; the other contains the polypeptides prepro-opiomelanocortin (POMC) and cocaine- and amphetamine-related transcript (CART), which release α melanocyte-stimulating hormone (MSH). Blood-borne hormones arising from the GI tract or adipose tissue are sensed by receptors on vagal and other afferents and are relayed through the nucleus tractus solitarius to modify the activity of these neuronal circuits. The influence of hormones on each neuronal group is indicated. Some (e.g. leptin) arise from the peripheral blood and influence the ARC neurons directly or indirectly through neuronal signals; while others (e.g. 5-hydroxytryptamine [5-HT], orexin) originate within the central nervous system itself. Activation of the NPY/AgRP group by, for example, a fall in leptin or an increase in ghrelin levels results in increased food intake and decreased energy expenditure. In the POMC/CART group of neurons, increased leptin or other hormone levels triggered by overfeeding produces a predominately inhibitory effect on feeding behaviour. Several other hormones such as cholecystokinin (CCK) and amylin also alter the properties of the ARC neurons although the mechanism is not clear. The recently discovered factor, nesfatin 1, is not shown. *GLP-1*, glucagon-like peptide-1; *PYY_{3-36}*, peptide YY. (Modified from Adan et al., 2008.)

olfactory information within the CNS is complex. Many sites are involved in different aspects of the process and some 50 hormones and neurotransmitters are implicated. The account we present here is therefore necessarily an oversimplification: the Further Reading list should be consulted for a more complete picture.

As early lesioning studies predicted, the hypothalamus is the main brain centre that regulates appetite, feeding behaviour and energy status, although other sites in the brain such as the nucleus accumbens (NAc), the amygdala and, especially, the nucleus tractus solitarius (NTS) in the medulla, are also crucial. Within the hypothalamus, the arcuate nucleus (ARC), situated in the floor of the third ventricle, is a key site. It receives afferent signals originating from the GI tract and contains receptors for leptin and other significant hormones. It also has extensive reciprocal connections with other parts of the hypothalamus involved

in monitoring energy status, in particular the paraventricular nuclei and the ventromedial hypothalamus. Fig. 33.2 summarises in a simplified fashion some of the interactions that occur in the ARC.

Within the ARC are two groups of functionally distinct neurons that exert opposite effects on appetite. One group, termed *anorexigenic* (appetite-suppressing), secrete pro-opiomelanocortin (POMC)-derived peptides (such as α melanocyte-stimulating hormone; α-MSH) or cocaine- and amphetamine-regulated transcript (CART[4])-derived peptides. The other group, termed *orexigenic* (appetite-promoting)

---

[4]So called because the administration of cocaine or amphetamine stimulates the transcription of this gene. Its expression in the hypothalamus is related to nutritional status implicating it in the control of appetite. Its receptor is unknown but it probably modulates the action of NPY and leptin.

neurons, secrete neuropeptide Y (NPY) or agouti-related peptide (AgRP). As these groups of neurons have opposing actions, energy homeostasis depends, in the first instance, on the balance between these actions, the final effects of which are transduced by the brain stem motor system and change feeding behaviour.

Neurotransmitters such as GABA, noradrenaline, 5-hydroxytryptamine (5-HT) and dopamine also play a role in the modulation of satiety signals alongside the peptide transmitters. Noradrenaline is co-localised with NPY in some neurons and greatly potentiates its hyperphagic action. Deficit of dopamine impairs feeding behaviour, as do agonists at the 5-HT$_{2C}$ receptor; antagonists at this receptor have the reverse effect. GABA is released from AgRP neurons and is modulated by nutritional status as well as by hormones such as leptin.

Many neural signals arising from the GI tract are integrated, and relayed on to the hypothalamus, by the NTS in the medulla. Some of these signals, including those of gustatory, olfactory, mechanical and viscerosensory signals, arise from vagal and other spinal afferents originating in the GI tract or liver. Endocrine signals have more complex signalling pathways. For example, cholecystokinin (CCK) is secreted by the duodenum in response to the process of eating and digestion of (especially fatty) foodstuffs. CCK acts locally on CCK$_A$ receptors in the GI tract to stimulate vagal afferents and also acts on CCK$_B$ receptors in the brain to function as a satiety factor.

Ghrelin, the only hormone known to increase appetite, stimulates growth hormone release (Ch. 34) and has a direct action on neurons in the ARC to modify feeding behaviour. Blood ghrelin levels normally fall after eating but not in obese individuals (English et al., 2002). Interestingly, polymorphisms in the ghrelin gene may be important in the pathogenesis of the *Prader–Willi syndrome*, a rare genetic childhood disorder that predisposes to life-threatening obesity.

Leptin also targets these neurons in the ARC. Falling leptin levels activate the orexigenic neurons, resulting in increased food intake and synthesis and storage of fat (anabolism), as well as decreased energy expenditure. Conversely, rising leptin levels activate the second group of neurons, producing the opposite anorexigenic and catabolic effect.

Inputs from other parts of the CNS also influence feeding behaviour. Of importance to us is the input from the NAc. This centre seems to regulate those aspects of eating that are driven by pleasure or reward – the so-called 'hedonic' aspects of eating (see also Ch. 50). The endocannabinoid system (Ch. 20) is important in this response. The hypothalamus contains large amounts of 2-arachidonyl glycerol and anandamide as well as the CB$_1$ receptor. Administration of endogenous or exogenous (e.g. Δ9-THC) cannabinoids provokes a powerful feeding response.[5] This system in turn may be modulated by 'stress' and other factors in the environment.

Many other hormones such as prolactin, androgens and oestrogens can modulate the activity of the hypothalamic control centres, and the situation is complex. The reader is referred to Cornejo et al. (2016) for a summary of recent thinking in this area.

CONTROL OF ENERGY EXPENDITURE

Balancing food intake is the energy expenditure required to maintain metabolism, physical activity and thermogenesis (heat production). The metabolic aspects include, among other things, cardiorespiratory work and the energy required by a multitude of enzymes. Physical activity increases all these, as well as increasing energy consumption by skeletal muscles. Exposure to cold also stimulates thermogenesis, and the reverse is also true. The, often dramatic (20%–40% increase), thermogenic effect of feeding itself may provide a partial protection against developing obesity.

The sympathetic nervous system (sometimes in concert with thyroid hormone) plays a significant part in energy regulation in cardiovascular and skeletal muscle function during physical activity, as well as the thermogenic response of adipose tissue and the response to cold. Both 'white' and (especially) 'brown' fat cells (the colour is caused by the high density of mitochondria) play a major role in thermogenesis. Brown fat, which is densely innervated by the sympathetic nervous system, is abundant in rodents and human infants, although in human adults these cells are generally to be found more interspersed amongst white fat cells. Because of their abundant mitochondria, they are remarkable heat generators. The basis for this, as determined in mice, is the presence of *mitochondrial uncoupling proteins* (UCP). Three isoforms, UCP-1, -2 and -3, are known and have different distributions, although all are found in brown fat. These proteins 'uncouple' oxidative phosphorylation, so that mitochondria dissipate most energy as heat rather than producing ATP. As one might anticipate, exposure to cold or leptin administration increases both the activity and (after prolonged stimulation) the amount of UCP-1 in brown fat. Noradrenaline, acting on β adrenoceptors (mainly β$_3$) in brown fat, increases the activity of the peroxisome proliferator-activated receptor-γ (PPARγ) transcription factor, which, in turn, activates the gene for UCP-1. The expression of β$_3$ adrenoceptors is decreased in genetically obese mice.

THE PATHOPHYSIOLOGY OF HUMAN OBESITY

In most adults, body fat and body weight remain more or less constant over many years, even decades, in the face of very large variations in food intake and energy expenditure amounting to about a million calories per year. The steady-state body weight and BMI of an individual, as explained, depends upon the integration of multiple interacting regulatory pathways. How, then, does obesity occur? Why is it so difficult for the obese to lose weight and maintain the lower weight?

The main determinant is manifestly a disturbance of the homeostatic mechanisms that control energy balance, and genetic factors that underlie this disturbance. Other factors, such as food availability and lack of physical activity, also contribute. Additionally, of course, there are overlaying social, cultural and psychological aspects. We discuss here the physiological and genetic mechanisms; the role of social, cultural and psychological aspects we will leave (with a profound sigh of relief) to the psychosociologists!

FOOD INTAKE AND OBESITY

As Spiegelman and Flier (1996) point out, 'one need not be a rocket scientist to notice that increased food intake

---

[5]This effect is responsible for the 'munchies', a common side effect of smoking cannabis.

Energy balance

Energy balance depends on food intake, energy storage in fat and energy expenditure. In most individuals the process is tightly regulated by a homeostatic system that integrates inputs from a number of internal sensors and external factors. Important components of the system include the following:

- Hormones that signal the status of fat stores (e.g. leptin). Increasing fat storage promotes leptin release from adipocytes.
- Hormones released from the gut during feeding that convey sensations of hunger (e.g. ghrelin), satiety (e.g. cholecystokinin [CCK]) or satiation (e.g. peptide YY [PYY_{3-36}]).
- This hormonal information together with neural, gustatory, olfactory and viscerosensory input is integrated in the hypothalamus. The arcuate nucleus is a key site.
- Two groups of opposing neurons in the arcuate nucleus sense hormonal and other signals. Those secreting pro-opiomelanocortin (POMC)/ cocaine- and amphetamine-regulated transcript (CART) products promote feeding while those secreting neuropeptide Y (NPY)/ agouti-related peptide (AgRP) inhibit feeding. Many other central nervous system neurotransmitters (e.g. endocannabinoids) are involved.

The net output from this process is relayed to other sites in the brain stem motor nuclei that control feeding behaviour.

tends to be associated with obesity'. A typical obese subject will usually gain 20 kg over a decade or so. This means that there has been a daily excess of energy input over energy requirement of 30–40 kcal initially (i.e. 1.5%–2%), increasing gradually to maintain the increased body weight.

The type of food eaten, as well as the quantity, can disturb energy homeostasis. Fat is an energy-dense foodstuff, and it may be that the satiety mechanisms regulating appetite, which react rapidly to carbohydrate and protein, react too slowly to stop an individual consuming excess fat.

However, when obese individuals reduce their calorie intake as part of a diet regime, they shift into negative energy balance. When they lose weight, the resting metabolic rate decreases, and there is a concomitant reduction in energy expenditure. Thus an individual who was previously obese and is now of normal weight generally needs fewer calories to maintain that weight than an individual who has never been obese. The decrease in energy expenditure appears to be largely caused by an alteration in the conversion efficiency of chemical energy to mechanical work in the skeletal muscles. This adaptation to the caloric reduction contributes to the difficulty of maintaining weight loss by diet.

PHYSICAL EXERCISE AND OBESITY

It used to be said that the only exercise effective in combating obesity was pushing one's chair back from the table. It is now recognised that physical activity – i.e. increased energy expenditure – has a much more positive role in reducing

fat storage and adjusting energy balance in the obese, particularly if associated with modification of the diet. A serendipitous natural population study provides an example. Many years ago, a tribe of Pima Indians split into two groups. One group in Mexico continued to live simply at subsistence level, eating frugally and spending most of the week in hard physical labour. They are generally lean and have a low incidence of type 2 diabetes. The other group settled in the United States – an environment with easy access to calorie-rich food and less need for hard physical work. They are, on average, 57 lb (26 kg) heavier than the Mexican group and have a high incidence of early-onset type 2 diabetes.

OBESITY AS A DISORDER OF THE HOMEOSTATIC CONTROL OF ENERGY BALANCE

Because the homeostatic control of energy balance is complex, it is not easy to determine exactly what goes wrong in obesity.[6] When the leptin story unfolded, it was thought that alterations in leptin kinetics might provide a simple explanation. There is a considerable inter-individual variation in sensitivity to leptin, and some individuals seem to produce insufficient amounts of this hormone. Paradoxically, however, plasma leptin is often higher in obese than non-obese subjects, not lower as might be expected. The reason for this is that resistance to leptin, rather than insufficient hormone, is more prevalent in obesity. Such resistance could be caused by defects in leptin carriage in the circulation, transport into the CNS, in leptin receptors in the hypothalamus (as occurs in obese *Db/Db* mice) or in postreceptor signalling.

Mediators other than leptin are also implicated. For example, tumour necrosis factor (TNF)-α, a cytokine that can relay information from fat tissue to brain, is increased in the adipose tissue of insulin-resistant obese individuals. Reduced insulin sensitivity of muscle and fat also occurs, as well as decreased β₃-adrenoceptor function in brown adipose tissue; alternatively, the uncoupling protein UCP-2 in adipocytes, may be dysfunctional.

A further suggestion is that alterations in the function of specific nuclear receptors, such as PPARα, β and γ, may play a role in obesity. These receptors regulate gene expression of enzymes associated with lipid and glucose homeostasis, and they also promote the formation of adipose tissue. PPARγ is expressed preferentially in fat cells and synergises with another transcription factor, C/EBPα, to convert precursor cells to fat cells (see Spiegelman & Flier, 1996). The gene for UCP in white fat cells also has regulatory sites that respond to PPARα and C/EBPα. **Pioglitazone**, used to treat type 2 diabetes (see Ch. 32), activates PPARγ and causes weight gain. The pathophysiology of obesity could involve disturbance(s) in any of the multitude of other factors involved in energy balance.

GENETIC FACTORS AND OBESITY

Analyses of large-scale studies of over 100,000 human monozygotic and dizygotic twin pairs indicated that 50%–90% of the variance of BMI can be attributed to genetic

---

[6]Even the type of gut flora has come under scrutiny as a potential determining factor in obesity (see review by Duranti et al., 2017). The notion that this could be supplemented with 'probiotics' to modify the risk is attracting attention. 'Holy shit!' was the title of one magazine article on the subject (*The Economist*, 12 November 2009).

factors, and suggested a relatively minor role for environmental influences (Barsh et al., 2000). The updated Human Obesity Gene Map (Rankinen et al., 2006) identified >250 *quantitative trait loci*[7] that contribute to obesity in humans. The prevailing view is that *susceptibility* to obesity is largely determined genetically, while environmental factors regulate the *expression* of the disease.

Obesity is conventionally classified as being *monogenic*, *syndromic* or *common (polygenic)*, depending upon the genetic background to the disease. As the name implies, monogenic obesity arises through the action of a single gene. The discovery that spontaneous mutations arising in single genes (e.g. the *Ob/Ob* genotype) produced obese phenotypes in mice led to a search for equivalent genes in humans. A review (Pérusse et al., 2005) identified over 170 human obesity cases that could be traced to single gene mutations in 10 different genes. Mutations in the POMC gene, the gene for FTO gene (fat mass- and obesity-associated gene), the leptin gene itself or the gene for its receptor are sometimes the culprits. Melanocortin MC_4 receptor mutations are the most common (1%–6%) in obese patients but there are many other potential candidates (e.g. see Barsh et al., 2000).

Polygenic (common) obesity comprises most of the cases of the disease. Here, obesity is usually the result of contributions of many genes, each of which has a small effect on the overall phenotype. Other genes that may influence obesity include the neurotransmitter receptors involved in the central processing of appetite/energy expenditure (e.g. the CB_1, D_2, $5\text{-}HT_{2C}$ receptors), the β_3 adrenoceptor and the glucocorticoid receptor. Decreased function of the β_3 adrenoceptor gene could be associated with impairment of lipolysis in white fat or with thermogenesis in brown fat. A mutation of this gene has been found to be associated with abdominal obesity, insulin resistance and early-onset type 2 diabetes in some subjects and a markedly increased propensity to gain weight in a separate group of morbidly obese subjects. Alterations in the function of the glucocorticoid receptor could be associated with obesity through the permissive effect of glucocorticoids on several aspects of fat metabolism and energy balance. The significance of polymorphisms in the ghrelin gene has already been mentioned.

In syndromic obesity, the obesity is associated with a distinctive clinical picture. Prader–Willi syndrome is the most common (at 1 in 15,000–25,000 live births) and is associated with defects in gene expression on chromosome 15q. The clinical picture is multifaceted and obesity is only one component.

Recently, the interpretation of genetic data in obesity has become even more complicated with the recognition of the importance of epigenetic modification of the genome. The subject cannot be discussed here but is well reviewed by Lopomo et al. (2016). Clearly it will be a while before we have a clear appreciation of all these issues.

PHARMACOLOGICAL APPROACHES TO THE PROBLEM OF OBESITY

The first weapons in the fight against obesity are diet and exercise. Unfortunately, these often fail or show only

Obesity

- Obesity is a multifactorial disorder of energy balance, in which long-term calorie intake exceeds energy output.
- A subject with a body mass index (BMI) (W/h²) of 20–25 kg/m² is considered as having a healthy body weight, one with a BMI of 25–30 kg/m² as overweight, and one with a BMI >30 kg/m² as obese.
- Obesity is a growing problem in most rich nations; the incidence – at present approximately >30% in the United States and >20% in Europe – is increasing.
- A BMI >30 kg/m² significantly increases the risk of type 2 diabetes, hypercholesterolaemia, hypertension, ischaemic heart disease, gallstones and some cancers.
- The causes of obesity include:
  - dietary, exercise, social, financial and cultural factors;
  - genetic susceptibility;
  - deficiencies in the synthesis or action of leptin or other gut hormone signals;
  - defects in the hypothalamic neuronal systems responding to any of these signals;
  - defects in the systems controlling energy expenditure (e.g. reduced sympathetic activity), decreased metabolic expenditure of energy or decreased thermogenesis caused by a reduction in β_3 adrenoceptor-mediated tone and/or dysfunction of the proteins that uncouple oxidative phosphorylation.

short-term efficacy, leaving surgical techniques (such as gastric stapling or bypass) or drug therapy as a viable alternative. *Bariatric* (weight loss) surgery is much more effective than currently licensed drugs, and is believed to work chiefly, not by mechanically limiting gastric capacity, but by its effects on gut hormone responses to feeding, acting, for example, to produce earlier satiety. This may be construed as indirect evidence for the utility of pharmacological measures designed to interrupt these messengers.

The attempt to control body weight with drugs has had a long and regrettably, a largely undistinguished[8] history. Many types of 'anorectic' (appetite suppressant) agents have been tested in the past, including the uncoupling agent **dinitrophenol** (DNP), **amphetamine** and derivatives such as **dexfenfluramine** and **fenfluramine**. All have been withdrawn from clinical use because of serious adverse effects. DNP, an industrial chemical, is advertised online for slimmers and body-builders as a weight loss and 'fat-burning agent', and has caused deaths among those who use it for this purpose. It blocks mitochondrial ATP production, diverting energy metabolism to generate heat instead

---

[7]In other words, a stretch of DNA which correlates with the development of obesity and which is likely therefore to contain – or be linked to – a relevant gene.

[8]As the showman Bynum said: 'There's a sucker born every minute … and one born to take him' … thyroxine (to increase metabolic rate, Ch. 35), swallowing parasites (intestinal worms compete for ingested food), amphetamines (Ch. 59), drugs that cause malabsorption, hence leaking fat per rectum (see later in this chapter) … really!

Fig. 33.3 The effect of treatment with the centrally acting appetite suppressant, sibutramine, alone or in combination with lifestyle modification. In this study, 224 obese patients were given sibutramine alone, lifestyle modification counselling alone or sibutramine together with a 'brief' or more extensive programme of lifestyle counselling. The Y axis shows the weight loss in kg (± standard error) over time (X axis). It is evident that sibutramine is far more effective as a weight-loss therapy when combined with lifestyle changes. This is a common experience when treating obesity. Note: Sibutramine has been withdrawn because of adverse cardiovascular side effects. (Redrawn from Wadden et al., 2005.)

of ATP and increasing the overall metabolic rate, which can cause life-threatening hyperthermia.[9]

CENTRALLY ACTING APPETITE SUPPRESSANTS

There have been many attempts to use centrally acting drugs to control appetite and this is an area which is still being actively exploited by drug hunters. **Sibutramine** (now withdrawn in most countries because of clinical trial evidence demonstrating increased cardiovascular risk) inhibits the reuptake of 5-HT and noradrenaline at the hypothalamic sites that regulate food intake.[10] Its main effects are to reduce food intake and cause dose-dependent weight loss (Fig. 33.3). It enhanced satiety and was reported to produce a reduction in waist circumference, a decrease in plasma triglycerides and very-low-density lipoproteins, but an increase in high-density lipoproteins. Like many similar drug regimes, sibutramine was much more effective when combined with lifestyle modification (Wadden et al., 2005).

However, other serotoninergic drugs have shown promise. **Lorcaserin**, a 5-HT$_{2C}$ receptor agonist (see Chs 16 and 38), was approved in the United States in 2012 for uses as an appetite suppressant in certain patients. It acts by increasing

POMC levels in the hypothalamus. In clinical trials it enhanced weight loss through dieting, but patients regained weight after stopping the drug. **Qsymia**, a mixture of an old appetite suppressant drug, **phentermine** and an anticonvulsant, **topiramate** was approved in the United States in 2012 despite some reservations about cardiovascular and other side effects. The drug stimulates the synaptic release of serotonin as well as noradrenaline and dopamine (and increases GABA action).

Other centrally acting drugs that are used in some countries for treating obesity include **Contrave**, a mixture of the opioid-receptor antagonist **naltrexone** and the noradrenaline–dopamine uptake–reuptake inhibitor, **bupropion**. The cannabinoid pathway was the target of the CB$_1$ receptor antagonist **rimonabant** which was originally developed to promote smoking cessation (see Ch. 20). This drug was introduced as an appetite suppressant following some encouraging clinical trials but was eventually withdrawn in the United States in 2008 because of adverse effects on mood seen in some patients. A similar fate overtook another promising CB$_1$ antagonist, **taranabant**.

ORLISTAT

The only drug currently (2017) licensed in the United Kingdom for the treatment of obesity is the lipase inhibitor **orlistat**, used with concomitant dietary and other therapy (e.g. exercise).

In the intestine, orlistat reacts with serine residues at the active sites of gastric and pancreatic lipases, irreversibly inhibiting these enzymes and thereby preventing the breakdown of dietary fat to fatty acids and glycerol. It therefore decreases absorption (and correspondingly causes faecal excretion) of some 30% of dietary fat. Given in conjunction with a low-calorie diet in obese individuals, it produces a modest but consistent loss of weight compared with placebo-treated control subjects. In a meta-analysis of 11 long-term placebo-controlled trials encompassing more than 6000 patients, orlistat was found to produce a 2.9% greater reduction in body weight than in the control group, and 12% more patients lost 10% or more of their body weight compared with the controls (Padwal et al., 2003).

Orlistat is also reported to be effective in patients suffering from type 2 diabetes and other complications of obesity. It reduces leptin levels and blood pressure, protects against weight loss-induced changes in biliary secretion, delays gastric emptying and gastric secretion and improves several important metabolic parameters without interfering with the release or action of thyroid or other important hormones (Curran & Scott, 2004). It does not induce changes in energy expenditure.

PHARMACOKINETIC ASPECTS AND UNWANTED EFFECTS

Virtually all (97%) of orlistat is excreted in the faeces (83% unchanged), with only negligible amounts of the drug or its metabolites being absorbed.

Abdominal cramps, flatus with discharge and faecal incontinence can occur, as can intestinal borborygmi (rumbling) and oily spotting. Surprisingly, in view of the possibility of these antisocial effects occurring, the drug is well tolerated. Supplementary therapy with fat-soluble vitamins may be needed. The absorption of contraceptive pills and **ciclosporin** (see Ch. 27) may be decreased. The former is not usually clinically significant but the latter is potentially more serious. Given its good safety record,

---

[9]DNP is reported to have been given to Russian soldiers in the Second World War, to keep them warm.

[10]Many antidepressant drugs act by the same mechanism (see Ch. 48), and also cause weight loss by reducing appetite. However, sibutramine does not have antidepressant properties. Furthermore, depressed patients are often obese, and antidepressant drugs are used to treat both conditions (see Appolinario et al., 2004).

orlistat has recently been licensed for inclusion in some over-the-counter medicines for weight loss.

Clinical uses of anti-obesity drugs

- The main treatment of obesity is a suitable diet and increased exercise.
- **Orlistat**, which causes fat malabsorption, is used together with dietary restriction in obese individuals, and also in overweight patients who have additional cardiovascular risk factors (e.g. diabetes mellitus, hypertension).
  - Orlistat therapy should be stopped after 12 weeks if the patient has not been able to lose at least 5% of their body weight from the time of drug initiation.
- Many centrally acting appetite suppressants (e.g. fenfluramine, sibutramine) have been withdrawn because of addiction, pulmonary hypertension or other serious adverse effects.
- Gastrointestinal ('bariatric') surgery for obesity influences incretin secretion, and is effective in severe obesity.

NEW APPROACHES TO OBESITY THERAPY

As might be imagined, the quest for further effective anti-obesity agents is the subject of prodigious efforts by the pharmaceutical industry.

Rare cases of leptin deficiency in patients have been successfully treated by long-term treatment with the hormone, but this is unlikely to be of more than limited use in the future. Many other approaches are being piloted (see Kang & Park, 2012). Some aim to exploit the action or production of neuroendocrine satiety signals such as CCK to produce appetite suppression. Many of these GI satiety hormones produce such effects when given systemically to humans or rodents, although these are not always useful; for example, CCK reduces meal size but increases meal frequency (West et al., 1984). Glucagon-like peptides such as **liraglutide**, which is used for treating type 2 diabetes (Ch. 32), also has anorexic actions (Astrup et al., 2009) and is approved in the United States for obesity treatment (by injection only). Other peptides trialled include amylin, oxyntomodulin and leptin analogues and NPY antagonists. Even vaccination against ghrelin or somatostatin has been mooted as a therapeutic strategy (Bhat et al., 2017).

Other strategies aim to alter the CNS levels of neurotransmitters such as NPY or melanocortins, which transduce hormonal signals regulating appetite (Halford, 2006). The tractability of the MC_4 receptor itself as a drug target, coupled with the observation that defects in MC_4 signalling are prevalent in obesity, has attracted much interest from the pharmaceutical industry.

Given the importance of the sympathetic nervous system in the control of energy regulation, one might predict that β_3-adrenoceptor agonists might be useful therapeutics. Disappointingly, whilst having been extensively researched (see Arch, 2008), they have so far failed to yield an acceptable therapeutic lead. In contrast, the serotonergic system remains squarely in the frame for the development of further anti-obesity agents (Oh et al., 2016).

Kang and Park (2012) highlight the value of combination therapies targeting complex pathways involved in appetite regulation. Most drug therapies are much more effective when used in conjunction with lifestyle and other behavioural modification. The importance of this joint approach is reviewed by Vetter et al. (2010).

In summary, at the time of writing, it is disappointing to report that the number of drugs licensed for use in obesity, at least in the United Kingdom, seems to be inversely proportional to the growing magnitude of the associated health problem. In some other countries, such as the United States, the situation is slightly better (Daneschvar et al., 2016) although there has been some debate about how useful this latest group of drugs will really prove to be (Kim, 2016). All in all, it is depressing that despite all the groundbreaking work on the neuroendocrine control of feeding and body weight, so few really novel drugs have found their way on to the market. The lack of sustained success with pharmacological therapies has led to the emergence of bariatric surgery as a more promising long-term option for reducing complications such as hypertension and diabetes mellitus in patients with severe obesity.

REFERENCES AND FURTHER READING

Body weight regulation and obesity

Adan, R.A., Vanderschuren, L.J., la Fleur, S.E., 2008. Anti-obesity drugs and neural circuits of feeding. Trends Pharmacol. Sci. 29, 208–217. (*Very accessible overview of the area. Recommended*)

Ahima, R.S., Osei, S., 2001. Molecular regulation of eating behaviour: new insights and prospects for future strategies. Trends Mol. Med. 7, 205–213. (*Praiseworthy short review; excellent figures and useful tables of the mediators involved in stimulation and inhibition of feeding behaviour*)

Barsh, G.S., Farooqi, I.S., O'Rahilly, S., 2000. Genetics of body-weight regulation. Nature 404, 644–651.

Colditz, G.A., Willett, W.C., Rotnitzky, A., Manson, J.E., 1995. Weight gain as a risk factor for clinical diabetes mellitus in women. Ann. Intern. Med. 122, 481–486.

Cornejo, M.P., Hentges, S.T., Maliqueo, M., Coirini, H., Becu-Villalobos, D., Elías, C.F., 2016. Neuroendocrine regulation of metabolism. J. Neuroendocrinol. 28, 1–12. (*A readable account of the latest developments in the field of neuroendocrine control of apetite and feeding. Covers some material not included here. Recommended*)

Duranti, S., Ferrario, C., van Sinderen, D., Ventura, M., Turroni, F., 2017. Obesity and microbiota: an example of an intricate relationship. Genes Nutr. 12 (18). (*Review role of gut bacteria in obesity*)

English, P.J., Ghatei, M.A., Malik, I.A., et al., 2002. Food fails to suppress ghrelin levels in obese humans. J. Clin. Endocrinol. Metab. 87, 2984–2987.

Farooqi, I.S., Jebb, S.A., Langmack, G., et al., 1999. Effects of recombinant leptin therapy in a child with congenital leptin deficiency. N. Engl. J. Med. 341, 879–884. (*A classic clinical paper on the role of leptin in the control of feeding behaviour and weight gain*)

Kennedy, G.C., 1953. The role of depot fat in the hypothalamic control of food intake in the rat. Proc. R. Soc. Lond. B. Biol Sci 140, 578–592. (*The paper that put forward the proposal, based on experiments on rats, that there was a hypothalamus-based homeostatic mechanism for controlling body fat*)

Kopelman, P.G., 2000. Obesity as a medical problem. Nature 404, 635–643.

Pérusse, C., Rankinen, T., Zuberi, A., et al., 2005. The human obesity gene map: the 2004 update. Obes. Res. 13, 381–490. (*Detailed review of the genes, markers and chromosomal regions that have been shown to be associated with human obesity*)

Lopomo, A., Burgio, E., Migliore, L., 2016. Epigenetics of obesity. Prog. Mol. Biol. Transl. Sci. 140, 151–184.

McKinsey Global Institute, 2014. Overcoming obesity: an initial economic analysis, p. 120.

Ramesh, N., Gawli, K., Pasupulleti, V., Unniappan, S., 2017. Metabolic and cardiovascular actions of nesfatin-1: implications in health and disease. Curr. Pharm. Des. 23, 1453–1464.

Rankinen, T., Zuberi, A., Chagnon, Y.C., et al., 2006. The human obesity gene map: the 2005 update. Obesity (Silver Spring) 14, 529–644.

Schwartz, M.W., Woods, S.C., Porte, D.J., et al., 2000. Central nervous control of food intake. Nature 404, 661–671. (*Outlines a model that delineates the roles of hormones and neuropeptides in the control of food intake. Outstanding diagrams. Note that there are several other excellent articles in this* Nature Insight *supplement on obesity*)

Spiegelman, B.M., Flier, J.S., 1996. Adipogenesis and obesity: rounding out the big picture. Cell 87, 377–389.

Spiegelman, B.M., Flier, J.S., 2001. Obesity regulation and energy balance. Cell 104, 531–543. (*Excellent review of the CNS control of energy intake/body weight, monogenic obesities, leptin physiology, central neural circuits, the melanocortin pathway, the role of insulin and adaptive thermogenesis*)

Weigle, D.S., 1994. Appetite and the regulation of body composition. FASEB J. 8, 302–310.

Zhang, Y., Proenca, R., Maffei, M., et al., 1994. Positional cloning of the mouse obese gene and its human homologue. Nature 372, 425–432.

Drugs in obesity

Appolinario, J.C., Bueno, J.R., Coutinho, W., 2004. Psychotropic drugs in the treatment of obesity: what promise? CNS Drugs 18, 629–651.

Arch, J.R., 2008. The discovery of drugs for obesity, the metabolic effects of leptin and variable receptor pharmacology: perspectives from beta$_3$-adrenoceptor agonists. Naunyn Schmiedebergs Arch. Pharmacol. 378, 225–240. (*A comprehensive review that focuses on the quest for anti-obesity drugs that act through the β_3 adrenoceptor. Useful comments and insights into the field as a whole*)

Astrup, A., Rossner, S., Van Gaal, L., et al.; NN8022-1807 Study Group, 2009. Effects of liraglutide in the treatment of obesity: a randomised, double-blind, placebo-controlled study. Lancet 374, 1606–1616.

Bhat, S.P., Sharma, A., 2017. Current drug targets in obesity pharmacotherapy - A review. Curr. Drug Targets 18, 983–993. (*Useful review of diverse agents being trialed as potential anti-obesity agents. Includes hormone and other agents*)

Chiesi, M., Huppertz, C., Hofbauer, K.G., 2001. Pharmacotherapy of obesity: targets and perspectives. Trends Pharmacol. Sci. 22, 247–254. (*Commendable, succinct review; table of the potential targets, and useful, simple figures of the central and peripheral pathways of energy regulation and of the regulation of thermogenesis*)

Collins, P., Williams, G., 2001. Drug treatment of obesity: from past failures to future successes? Br. J. Clin. Pharmacol. 51, 13–25. (*Overview – from a clinical perspective – of currently available anti-obesity drugs and potential future drugs; well written*)

Crowley, V.E.F., Yeo, G.S.H., O'Rahilly, S., 2002. Obesity therapy: altering the energy intake-and-expenditure balance sheet. Nat. Rev. Drug Discov. 1, 276–286. (*Review stressing that pharmacological approaches to obesity therapy necessitate altering the balance between energy intake and expenditure and/or altering the partitioning of nutrients between lean tissue and fat*)

Curran, M.P., Scott, L.J., 2004. Orlistat: a review of its use in the management of patients with obesity. Drugs 64, 2845–2864.

Daneschvar, H.L., Aronson, M.D., Smetana, G.W., 2016. FDA-approved anti-obesity drugs in the United States. Am. J. Med. 129 (879), e871–e876. (*A brief review of five drugs recently approved by the FDA for the treatment of obesity. Covers most of the pharmacology of these drugs. Useful*)

Di Marzo, V., Matias, I., 2005. Endocannabinoid control of food intake and energy balance. Nat. Neurosci. 8, 585–589. (*A discussion of the putative role of endocannabinoids in this complex physiological mechanism; also considers therapeutic applications arising from this area*)

Halford, J.C., 2006. Obesity drugs in clinical development. Curr. Opin. Invest. Drugs 7, 312–318.

Kang, J.G., Park, C.Y., 2012. Anti-obesity drugs: a review about their effects and safety. Diabetes Metab. J. 36, 13–25. (*A brief and easy-to-read review dealing with prospective new drug therapies for obesity*)

Kaplan, L.M., 2005. Pharmacological therapies for obesity. Gastroenterol. Clin. North Am. 34, 91–104.

Kim, S., 2016. Drugs to treat obesity: do they work? Postgrad. Med. J. 92, 401–406. (*A rather critical look at some recent drug candidates which point out that the average weight loss is only some 3%-10% of the starting weight*)

Oh, C.M., Park, S., Kim, H., 2016. Serotonin as a new therapeutic target for diabetes mellitus and obesity. Diabetes Metab. J. 40, 89–98. (*Mainly deals with the potential regulatory role of 5-HT in the peripheral regulation of tissue metabolism and its potential for exploitation for future anti-obesity agents*)

Padwal, R., Li, S.K., Lau, D.C., 2003. Long-term pharmacotherapy for overweight and obesity: a systematic review and meta-analysis of randomized controlled trials. Int. J. Obes. Relat. Metab. Disord. 27, 1437–1446.

Wadden, T.A., Berkowitz, R.I., Womble, G., et al., 2005. Randomized trial of lifestyle modification and pharmacotherapy for obesity. N. Engl. J. Med. 353, 2111–2120.

Vetter, M.L., Faulconbridge, L.F., Webb, V.L., Wadden, T.A., 2010. Behavioral and pharmacologic therapies for obesity. Nat. Rev. Endocrinol. 6, 578–588. (*This review stresses the importance of lifestyle changes in combination with drug therapy to combat obesity*)

West, D.B., Fey, D., Woods, S.C., 1984. Cholecystokinin persistently suppresses meal size but not food intake in free-feeding rats. Am. J. Physiol. 246, R776–R787.

Wilding, J.P.H. (Ed.), 2008. Pharmacotherapy of obesity. In: Parnham, M.J., Bruinvels, J. (Eds.), Milestones in Drug Therapy. Birkhäuser, Basle. (*This book covers a wide variety of topics connected with obesity and its therapy. The contributors are experts in the field*)

Useful web resource

www.who.int. (*This is the World Health Organization Web page that carries data about the prevalence of 'globesity' and its distribution around the world; click on the 'Health Topics' link and navigate to 'Obesity' in the alphabetical list of topics for further information*)

www.cdc.gov. (*This is the web page for the US Center for Disease Control and Prevention. There is a link here to a list of health topics from which you can select 'Obesity'*)

34 The pituitary and the adrenal cortex

OVERVIEW

The pituitary gland and the adrenal cortex release hormones that regulate salt and water balance, energy expenditure, growth, sexual behaviour, immune function and many other vital mechanisms. The commander-in-chief of this impressive hormonal campaign is the hypothalamus and the functioning unit is known as the *hypothalamo–pituitary–adrenal* **(HPA) axis. In the first part of this chapter we review the control of pituitary function by hypothalamic hormones, and the physiological roles and clinical utilities of both anterior and posterior pituitary hormones. The second part of the chapter focuses on adrenal hormones and, in particular, the anti-inflammatory effect of glucocorticoids. This should be read in conjunction with the relevant sections of Chapters 3 and 27.**

THE PITUITARY GLAND

The pituitary gland comprises three histologically distinct structures which arise from two separate embryological precursors (Fig. 34.1). The *anterior pituitary* and the *intermediate lobe* are derived from the endoderm of the buccal cavity, while the *posterior pituitary* is derived from neural ectoderm. The anterior and posterior lobes receive independent neuronal input from the hypothalamus, with which they have an intimate functional relationship.

THE ANTERIOR PITUITARY GLAND

The anterior pituitary gland (*adenohypophysis*) secretes a number of hormones crucial for normal physiological function. Within this tissue are specialised cells such as *corticotrophs*, *lactotrophs* (*mammotrophs*), *somatotrophs*, *thyrotrophs* and *gonadotrophs*, which secrete hormones that regulate different endocrine organs of the body (Table 34.1). Interspersed among these are other cell types, including *folliculostellate cells*, which exert a nurturing and regulatory influence on the hormone-secreting endocrine cells.

Secretion from the anterior pituitary is largely regulated by the release from the hypothalamus of, what are generally known as, 'releasing factors' – in effect, local hormones – that reach the pituitary through the bloodstream.[1] The blood supply to the hypothalamus divides to form a meshwork of capillaries, the *primary plexus*, which drains into the *hypophyseal portal vessels*. These pass through the pituitary

stalk to feed a *secondary plexus* of capillaries in the anterior pituitary. Peptidergic neurons in the hypothalamus secrete a variety of releasing or inhibitory hormones directly into the capillaries of the primary capillary plexus (see Table 34.1 and Fig. 34.1). Most of these regulate the secretion of hormones from the anterior lobe, although the *melanocyte-stimulating hormones* (MSHs) are secreted mainly from the intermediate lobe.

The release of stimulatory hormones is regulated by negative feedback pathways between the hormones of the hypothalamus, the anterior pituitary and the peripheral endocrine glands. Hormones secreted from the peripheral glands exert regulatory actions on both the hypothalamus and the anterior pituitary, constituting the *long negative feedback* pathways. Anterior pituitary hormones acting directly on the hypothalamus comprise the *short negative feedback* pathway.

The peptidergic neurons in the hypothalamus are themselves influenced by other centres within the central nervous system (CNS) and mediated through neural pathways that release dopamine, noradrenaline, 5-hydroxytryptamine and the opioid peptides (which are particularly abundant in the hypothalamus). Hypothalamic control of the anterior pituitary is also exerted through the *tuberohypophyseal dopaminergic pathway* (see Ch. 40), the neurons of which lie in close apposition to the primary capillary plexus. Dopamine secreted directly into the hypophyseal portal circulation reaches the anterior pituitary via the bloodstream, inhibiting the secretion of prolactin (see Ch. 36).

HYPOTHALAMIC HORMONES

The secretion of anterior pituitary hormones, then, is primarily regulated by the peptide 'releasing factors' that originate from the hypothalamus. The most significant are described in more detail later. Somatostatin and gonadotrophin-releasing hormone are used therapeutically, the others have mainly diagnostic utilities or are useful research tools. Some of these peptides also function as neurotransmitters or neuromodulators elsewhere in the CNS (Ch. 40).

SOMATOSTATIN

Somatostatin is a peptide of 14 amino acid residues. It inhibits the release of growth hormone and thyroid-stimulating hormone (TSH, thyrotrophin) from the anterior pituitary (Fig. 34.2), and insulin and glucagon from the pancreas. It also decreases the release of most gastrointestinal (GI) hormones, and reduces gastric acid and pancreatic secretion.

Octreotide is a long-acting analogue of somatostatin. It is used for the treatment of *carcinoid* and other hormone-secreting tumours (Ch. 16). It also has a place in the therapy of *acromegaly* (a condition in which there is oversecretion of growth hormone in an adult). It also constricts splanchnic blood vessels, and is used to treat bleeding *oesophageal*

---

[1]The term 'factor' was originally coined at a time when their structure and function were not known. These are blood-borne messengers, and as such are clearly hormones but the nomenclature, though irrational, lingers on.

Fig. 34.1 Schematic diagram of vascular and neuronal relationships between the hypothalamus, the posterior pituitary and the anterior pituitary. The main portal vessels to the anterior pituitary lie in the pituitary stalk and arise from the primary plexus in the hypothalamus, but some (the short portal vessels) arise from the vascular bed in the posterior pituitary (not shown).

Fig. 34.2 Control of growth hormone secretion and its actions. Drugs are shown in *red-bordered boxes*. *GHRF*, growth hormone-releasing factor; *IGF-1*, insulin-like growth factor-1.

varices. Octreotide is generally given subcutaneously. The peak action is at 2 h, and the suppressant effect lasts for up to 8 h.

Unwanted effects include pain at the injection site and GI disturbances. Gallstones and postprandial hyperglycaemia

have also been reported and acute hepatitis or pancreatitis has occurred in a few cases.

Lanreotide and **pasireotide** have similar effects. Lanreotide is also used in the treatment of thyroid tumours, while pasireotide, which is a particularly potent analogue, is used in the treatment of *Cushing's syndrome* when surgery is inappropriate or has been ineffective.

GONADOTROPHIN-RELEASING HORMONE

Gonadotrophin- (or luteinising hormone [LH]-) releasing hormone (GnRH, previously known as LHRH) is a decapeptide that releases both *follicle-stimulating hormone* and *luteinising hormone* from gonadotrophs. **Gonadorelin**[2] and its analogues (**buserelin**, **goserelin**, **leuprorelin**, **nafarelin** and **triptorelin**) are used mainly in the treatment of infertility and some hormone-dependent tumours (see Ch. 36).

GROWTH HORMONE-RELEASING FACTOR (SOMATORELIN)

Growth hormone-releasing factor (GHRF) is a peptide with 44 amino acid residues. The main action of GHRF is summarised in Fig. 34.2.

▼ An analogue, **sermorelin** (discontinued in some countries), has been used as a diagnostic test for growth hormone secretion. Given intravenously, subcutaneously or intranasally, it causes secretion of growth hormone within minutes and peak concentrations in 1 h. The action is selective for the somatotrophs in the anterior pituitary, and no other pituitary hormones are affected. Unwanted effects are rare.

THYROTROPHIN-RELEASING HORMONE

Thyrotrophin-releasing hormone (TRH) from the hypothalamus releases TSH from the thyrotrophs.

▼ **Protirelin** (now discontinued in the United Kingdom) is a synthetic TRH that has been used for the diagnosis of thyroid disorders (see Ch. 35). Given intravenously in normal subjects, it causes an increase in plasma TSH concentration, whereas in patients with hyperthyroidism there is a blunted response because the raised blood thyroxine concentration has a negative feedback effect on the anterior pituitary. The opposite occurs with hypothyroidism, where there is an intrinsic defect in the thyroid itself.

CORTICOTROPHIN-RELEASING FACTOR

Corticotrophin-releasing factor (CRF) is a peptide that releases **adrenocorticotrophic hormone** (ACTH, corticotrophin) and β-endorphin from corticotrophs in the anterior pituitary gland. CRF acts synergistically with *antidiuretic hormone* (ADH; arginine-vasopressin, see Ch. 30), and both its action and release are inhibited by glucocorticoids (see Fig. 34.4). Synthetic preparations have been used to test the ability of the pituitary to secrete ACTH, and to assess whether ACTH deficiency is caused by a pituitary or a hypothalamic defect. It has also been used to evaluate hypothalamic pituitary function after therapy for Cushing's syndrome (see Fig. 34.7).

ANTERIOR PITUITARY HORMONES

The main hormones of the anterior pituitary are listed in Table 34.1. The gonadotrophins are dealt with in Chapter 36 and TSH in Chapter 35. The actions of the remainder are summarised below.

---

[2]In this context, the suffix '-relin' denotes peptides that stimulate hormone release.

Table 34.1 Hormones secreted by the hypothalamus and the anterior pituitary and some related drugs

Hypothalamic factor/hormone[a]	Effect on anterior pituitary	Main effects of anterior pituitary hormone
CRF	Releases ACTH (corticotrophin) *Analogue:* tetracosactide	Stimulates secretion of adrenal cortical hormones (mainly glucocorticoids); maintains integrity of adrenal cortex.
TRH *Analogue:* protirelin	Releases TSH (thyrotrophin)	Stimulates synthesis and secretion of thyroid hormones; maintains integrity of thyroid gland.
GHRF (somatorelin) *Analogue:* sermorelin	Releases GH (somatotrophin) *Analogue:* somatropin	Regulates growth, partly directly, but also by releasing somatomedins from the liver and elsewhere; increases protein synthesis, increases blood glucose, stimulates lipolysis.
Growth hormone release-inhibiting factor (somatostatin) *Analogues:* octreotide, lanreotide, paseriotide	Inhibits the release of GH	Prevents effects of GHRF. Blocks TSH release.
GnRH *Analogues:* 'gonadorelin analogues' – buserelin, goserelin, leuprorelin, naferelin, triptorelin	Releases FSH (see Ch. 36)	Stimulates the growth of the ovum and the Graafian follicle (female) and gametogenesis (male); with LH, stimulates the secretion of oestrogen throughout the menstrual cycle and progesterone in the second half.
	Release of LH or interstitial cell-stimulating hormone (see Ch. 36)	Stimulation of ovulation and the development of the corpus luteum; with FSH, stimulation of secretion of oestrogen and progesterone in the menstrual cycle; in male, regulation of testosterone secretion.
PRF	Releases prolactin	Together with other hormones, prolactin promotes development of mammary tissue during pregnancy and stimulates milk production in the postpartum period.
Prolactin release-inhibiting factor (probably dopamine)	Inhibits the release of prolactin	Prevents effects of PRF.
MSH-releasing factor	Releases α-, β- and γ-MSH	Promotes formation of melanin, which causes darkening of skin; MSH has anti-inflammatory actions and also regulates appetite/feeding.
MSH release-inhibiting factor	Inhibits the release of α-, β- and γ-MSH	Prevents effects of MSH.

[a]These hormones are often spelled without the 'h' (e.g. corticotropin, thyrotropin, etc.) in contemporary texts. We have retained the original nomenclature in this edition.
ACTH, adrenocorticotrophic hormone; *CRF*, corticotrophin-releasing factor; *FSH*, follicle stimulating hormone; *GH*, growth hormone; *GHRF*, growth hormone-releasing factor; *GnRH*, gonadotrophin (or luteinising hormone)-releasing hormone; *LH*, luteinising hormone; *MSH*, melanocyte-stimulating hormone; *PRF*, prolactin-releasing factor; *TRH*, thyrotrophin-releasing hormone; *TSH*, thyroid-stimulating hormone.

GROWTH HORMONE (SOMATOTROPHIN)

Growth hormone is secreted by the somatotroph cells and is the most abundant pituitary hormone. Secretion is high in the newborn, decreasing at 4 years to an intermediate level, which is then maintained until after puberty, after which there is a further decline. Recombinant human growth hormone, **somatropin**, is available for treating growth defects and other developmental problems.

Regulation of secretion

Secretion of growth hormone is regulated by the action of hypothalamic GHRF and modulated by somatostatin, as described above and outlined in Fig. 34.2. A different peptide releaser of growth hormone ('ghrelin') is released from the stomach and pancreas and is implicated in the control of appetite and of body weight (Ch. 33). One of the mediators of growth hormone action, insulin-like growth factor (IGF)-1,

which is released from the liver, has an inhibitory effect on growth hormone secretion by stimulating somatostatin release from the hypothalamus.

As with other anterior pituitary secretions, growth hormone release is pulsatile, and its plasma concentration may fluctuate 10- to 100-fold. These surges occur repeatedly during the day and night, and reflect the dynamics of hypothalamic control. Deep sleep is a potent stimulus to growth hormone secretion, particularly in children.

Actions

The main effect of growth hormone (and its analogues) is to stimulate normal growth. To do so, it acts in conjunction with other hormones secreted from the thyroid, the gonads and the adrenal cortex. It stimulates hepatic production of the IGFs – also termed *somatomedins* – which mediate most of its anabolic actions. IGF-1 (the principal mediator) mediates many of these anabolic effects, stimulating the uptake of amino acids and increasing protein synthesis by skeletal muscle (and therefore muscle bulk) as well as by the cartilage at the epiphyses of long bones (thus influencing bone growth). Receptors for IGF-1 exist on many other cell types, including liver cells and fat cells.

Disorders of production and clinical use

Deficiency of growth hormone (or failure of its action) results in *pituitary dwarfism*. In this condition, which may result from lack of GHRF or a lack of IGF generation or action, the normal proportions of the body are maintained even though overall stature is reduced. Growth hormone is used therapeutically in these patients (often children) as well as those suffering from the short stature caused by chronic renal insufficiency or associated with the chromosomal disorder known as *Turner's syndrome*.

Humans are insensitive to growth hormone of other species, so human growth hormone (hGH) must be used clinically. Human cadavers were the original source, but this led to the spread of *Creutzfeldt–Jakob disease*, a prion-mediated neurodegenerative disorder (Ch. 41). hGH is now prepared by recombinant DNA technology (somatropin), which avoids this risk. Satisfactory linear growth can be achieved by giving somatropin subcutaneously, six to seven times per week, and therapy is most successful when started early.

hGH is also used illicitly by athletes (see Ch. 59) to increase muscle mass. The large doses used have serious side effects, causing abnormal bone growth and cardiomegaly. It has also been tested as a means of combating the bodily changes in senescence; clinical trials have shown increases in body mass, but no functional improvement. Human recombinant IGF-1 (**mecasermin**) is also available for the treatment of growth failure in children who lack adequate amounts of this hormone.

An excessive production of growth hormone in children results in *gigantism*. An excessive production in adults, which is usually the result of a benign pituitary tumour, results in *acromegaly*, in which there is enlargement mainly of the jaw and of the hands and feet. The dopamine agonist **bromocriptine** and octreotide may mitigate the condition. Another useful agent is **pegvisomant**, a modified analogue of growth hormone prepared by recombinant technology that is a highly selective antagonist of growth hormone actions.

PROLACTIN

Prolactin is secreted from the anterior pituitary gland by lactotroph (mammotroph) cells. These are abundant in the gland and increase in number during pregnancy, probably under the influence of oestrogen.

REGULATION OF SECRETION

Prolactin secretion is under tonic inhibitory control by dopamine (acting on D_2 receptors on the lactotrophs) released from the hypothalamus (Fig. 34.3 and see Table 34.1). The main stimulus for release is suckling; in rats, both the smell and the sounds of hungry pups are also effective triggers. Neural reflexes from the breast may stimulate the secretion from the hypothalamus of prolactin-releasing factor(s), possible candidates for which include TRH and **oxytocin**. Oestrogens increase both prolactin secretion and the proliferation of lactotrophs through the release, from a subset of lactotrophs, of the neuropeptide *galanin*. Dopamine antagonists (used mainly as antipsychotic

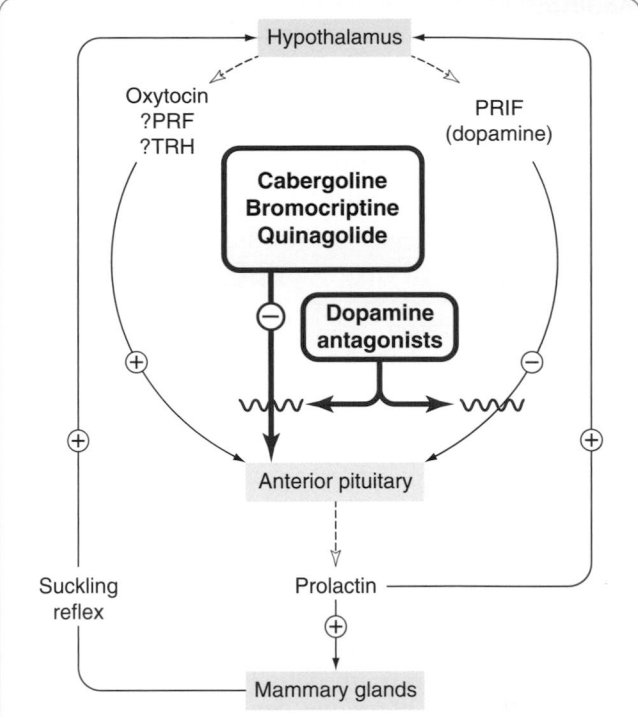

Fig. 34.3 **Control of prolactin secretion.** Drugs are shown in *red-bordered boxes*. *PRF*, prolactin-releasing factor(s); *PRIF*, prolactin release-inhibiting factor(s); *TRH*, thyrotrophin-releasing hormone.

drugs; see Ch. 47) are potent stimulants of prolactin release, whereas agonists such as bromocriptine (Chs 40 and 47) suppress prolactin release. Bromocriptine is also used in Parkinson's disease (Ch. 41).

Actions

The prolactin receptor is a single transmembrane domain receptor of the kinase-linked type (Ch. 3) related to the cytokine receptors. Several different isoforms and splice variants are known. These are found not only in the mammary gland but are widely distributed throughout the body, including the brain, ovary, heart, lungs and immune system. The main function of prolactin in women is the control of milk production. At parturition the prolactin concentration rises and lactation is initiated. Maintenance of lactation depends on suckling (see earlier), which causes a 10- to 100-fold increase in blood prolactin levels within 30 min.

Together with other hormones, prolactin is responsible for the proliferation and differentiation of mammary tissue during pregnancy. It also inhibits gonadotrophin release and/or the response of the ovaries to these trophic hormones. This is one of the reasons why ovulation does not usually occur during breastfeeding.

▼ According to one rather appealing hypothesis, the high postpartum concentration of prolactin reflects its biological function as a 'parental' hormone. Certainly, broodiness and nest-building activity can be induced in birds, mice and rabbits by prolactin injections. Prolactin also exerts other, apparently unrelated, actions, including stimulating mitogenesis in lymphocytes. There is some evidence that it may play a part in regulating immune responses.

Modification of prolactin secretion

Prolactin itself is not used clinically. **Bromocriptine**, a dopamine receptor agonist, is used to decrease excessive prolactin secretion (*hyperprolactinaemia*). It is well absorbed orally, and peak concentrations occur after 2 h. Unwanted reactions include nausea and vomiting. Dizziness, constipation and postural hypotension may also occur. **Cabergoline** and **quinagolide** are similar.

Clinical uses of bromocriptine

- To prevent lactation.
- To treat galactorrhoea (i.e. non-puerperal lactation in either sex), owing to excessive prolactin secretion.
- To treat prolactin-secreting pituitary tumours (prolactinomas).
- In the treatment of Parkinson's disease (Ch. 41) and of acromegaly.

ADRENOCORTICOTROPHIC HORMONE

Adrenocorticotrophic hormone (ACTH, corticotrophin) is the anterior pituitary secretion that controls the synthesis and release of the glucocorticoids of the adrenal cortex (see Table 34.1). It is a 39-residue peptide derived from the precursor pro-opiomelanocortin (POMC) by sequential proteolytic processing. It acts on the MC_2 member of the family of melanocortin receptors (see later). Failure of ACTH action because of defects in its receptor or intracellular signalling pathways can lead to severe glucocorticoid deficiency (Chan et al., 2008). Details of the regulation of ACTH secretion are shown in Fig. 34.4.

▼ This hormone occupies (together with cortisone) an important place in the history of inflammation therapy because of the work of Hench and his colleagues in the 1940s, who first observed that both substances had anti-inflammatory effects in patients with rheumatoid disease. The effect of ACTH was thought to be secondary to stimulation of the adrenal cortex but, interestingly, the hormone also has anti-inflammatory actions in its own right, through activation of macrophage (melanocortin) MC_3 receptors (Getting et al., 2002).

ACTH itself is not often used in therapy today, because its action is less predictable than that of the corticosteroids and it may provoke antibody formation. **Tetracosactide (tetracosactrin)**, a synthetic polypeptide that consists of the first 24 N-terminal residues of human ACTH, suffers from some of the same drawbacks but is now widely used for assessing the competency of the adrenal cortex. The drug is given intramuscularly or intravenously, and the concentration of hydrocortisone in the plasma is measured by radioimmunoassay.

Actions

Acting through MC_2 receptors, tetracosactide and ACTH have two actions on the adrenal cortex:

- Stimulation of the synthesis and release of glucocorticoids. This action occurs within minutes of injection, and the ensuing biological actions are predominately those of the released steroids.
- A trophic action on adrenal cortical cells, and regulation of the levels of key mitochondrial steroidogenic enzymes. The loss of this effect accounts for the adrenal atrophy that results from chronic glucocorticoid administration, which suppresses ACTH secretion.

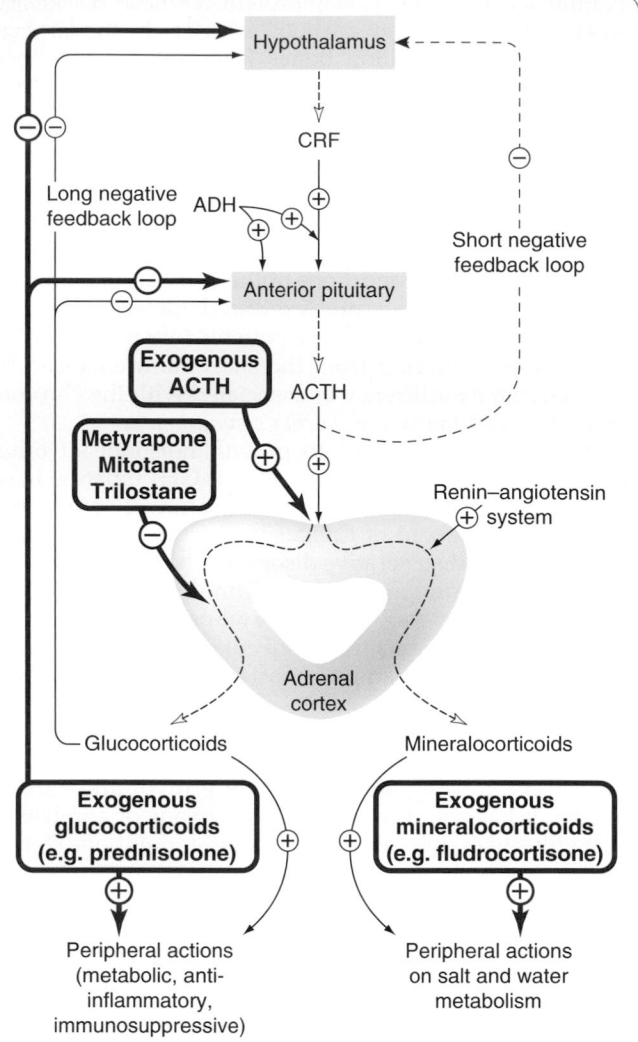

Fig. 34.4 Regulation of synthesis and secretion of adrenal corticosteroids. The long negative feedback loop is more physiologically significant than the short loop *(dashed lines)*. Adrenocorticotrophic hormone (ACTH, corticotrophin) has only a minimal effect on mineralocorticoid production. Drugs are shown in *red-bordered boxes*. *ADH*, antidiuretic hormone (vasopressin); *CRF*, corticotrophin-releasing factor.

MELANOCYTE-STIMULATING HORMONE (MSH)

α-, β- and γ-MSH are peptide hormones with structural similarity to ACTH and are derived from the same precursor. Together, these peptides are referred to as *melanocortins*, because their first recognised action was to stimulate the production of melanin by specialised skin cells called *melanocytes*. As such, they play an important part in determining hair colouration, skin colour and reaction to ultraviolet light.

MSH acts on melanocortin receptors, of which five (MC_{1-5}) have been cloned. These are G protein–coupled receptors (GPCRs) that activate cAMP synthesis. Melanin formation is controlled by the MC_1 receptor. Excessive α-MSH production can provoke abnormal proliferation of melanocytes and may predispose to melanoma.

▼ Melanocortins exhibit numerous other biological effects. For example, α-MSH inhibits the release of interleukin (IL)-1β and tumour necrosis factor (TNF)-α, reduces neutrophil infiltration, and exhibits anti-inflammatory and antipyretic activity. Levels of α-MSH are increased in synovial fluid of patients with rheumatoid arthritis. These immunomodulatory effects are transduced by MC_1 and MC_3 receptors. Agonists at these receptors with potential anti-inflammatory activity are being sought. Central injection of α-MSH also causes changes in animal behaviour, such as increased grooming and sexual activity as well as reduced feeding through actions on MC_4 receptors, and agonists of MC_4 are under investigation as potential treatments for obesity and for erectile impotence.

Intracerebroventricular or intravenous injection of γ-MSH increases blood pressure, heart rate and cerebral blood flow. These effects are also likely to be mediated by the MC_4 receptor.

Two naturally occurring ligands for melanocortin receptors (*agouti-signalling protein* and *agouti-related peptide*, together called the *agouti*) have been discovered in human tissues. These are proteins that competitively antagonise the effect of MSH at melanocortin receptors.

The anterior pituitary gland and hypothalamus

- The anterior pituitary gland secretes hormones that regulate:
  - the release of *glucocorticoids* from the adrenal cortex
  - the release of *thyroid hormones*
  - the release of sex hormones: *ovulation* in the female and *spermatogenesis* in the male
  - *growth*
  - *mammary gland* structure and function
- Each anterior pituitary hormone is itself regulated by a specific hypothalamic releasing factor. Feedback mechanisms govern the release of these factors. Clinically useful drugs of this type include:
  - *growth hormone-releasing factor* (**sermorelin**) and analogues of growth hormone (**somatrophin**)
  - *thyrotrophin-releasing factor* (**protirelin**) and thyroid-stimulating hormone (thyrotrophin; used to test thyroid function)
  - **octreotide** and **lanreotide**, analogues of **somatostatin**, which inhibit growth hormone release
  - *corticotrophin-releasing factor*, used in diagnosis
  - *gonadotrophin-releasing factor*, **gonadorelin** and *analogues*. Used to treat infertility and some carcinomas

POSTERIOR PITUITARY GLAND

The posterior pituitary gland (neurohypophysis) consists largely of the terminals of nerve cells originating from the *supraoptic* and *paraventricular nuclei* of the hypothalamus. Their axons form the *hypothalamic–hypophyseal tract*, and the fibres terminate in dilated nerve endings in close association with capillaries in the posterior pituitary gland (see Fig. 34.1). Peptides, synthesised in the hypothalamic nuclei, pass down these axons into the posterior pituitary, where they are stored and eventually secreted into the bloodstream.

The two main hormones of the posterior pituitary are **oxytocin** (which contracts the smooth muscle of the uterus;

Adrenocorticotrophic hormone and the adrenal steroids

- Adrenocorticotrophic hormone (ACTH; **tetracosactrin**, **tetracosactide**) stimulates synthesis and release of glucocorticoids (e.g. **hydrocortisone**), as well as some androgens, from the adrenal cortex.
- Corticotrophin-releasing factor (CRF) from the hypothalamus regulates ACTH release, and is regulated in turn by neural factors and negative feedback effects of plasma glucocorticoids.
- Mineralocorticoid (e.g. aldosterone) release from the adrenal cortex is controlled by the renin–angiotensin system.

for details see Ch. 36) and **vasopressin** (ADH; see Chs 23 and 30). They are highly homologous cyclic nonapeptides. Several analogues have been synthesised that vary in their antidiuretic, vasopressor and oxytocic (uterine stimulant) properties.

VASOPRESSIN

Regulation of secretion and physiological role
Vasopressin released from the posterior pituitary has a crucial role in the control of the water content of the body through its action on the cells of the distal part of the nephron and the collecting tubules in the kidney (see Ch. 30). The hypothalamic nuclei that control fluid balance lie close to the nuclei that synthesise and secrete vasopressin.

One of the main stimuli for vasopressin release is an increase in plasma osmolarity (which produces a sensation of thirst). A decrease in circulating blood volume (*hypovolaemia*) is another, and here the stimuli arise from stretch receptors in the cardiovascular system or from angiotensin release. *Diabetes insipidus* is a condition in which large volumes of dilute urine are produced because vasopressin secretion is reduced or absent, or because of a reduced sensitivity of the kidney to the hormone.

Vasopressin receptors
There are three classes of receptor: V_{1A}, V_{1B} and V_2. All are GPCRs. V_2 receptors stimulate adenylyl cyclase, which mediates the main physiological actions of vasopressin in the kidney, whereas the V_{1A} and V_{1B} receptors are coupled to the phospholipase C/inositol trisphosphate system.

The receptor for oxytocin (OT receptor) is also a GPCR, which primarily signals through phospholipase C stimulation but has a secondary action on adenylyl cyclase. Vasopressin is a partial agonist at OT, but its effects are limited by the distribution of the receptor, which, as might be inferred from its classic action on the pregnant uterus, is high in the myometrium, endometrium, mammary gland and ovary. The central actions of oxytocin (and vasopressin) have also attracted the attention of sociobiologists as they are important in 'pair bonding' and the other psychosocial interactions.[3]

---

[3]Oxytocin is released during childbirth, lactation and orgasm and has been shown to promote trust and other prosocial behaviour. This has earned it the nickname of the 'love hormone' (or even more nauseatingly, the 'cuddle hormone') in the popular press and internet discussion groups.

Actions
Renal actions

Vasopressin binds to V_2 receptors in the basolateral membrane of the cells of the distal tubule and collecting ducts of the nephron. Its main effect in the collecting duct is to increase the rate of insertion of water channels (*aquaporins*) into the lumenal membrane, thus increasing the permeability of the membrane to water (see Ch. 30). It also activates urea transporters and transiently increases Na^+ absorption, particularly in the distal tubule.

Several drugs affect the action of vasopressin. Non-steroidal anti-inflammatory drugs and **carbamazepine** increase, and **lithium**, **colchicine** and **vinca alkaloids** decrease, vasopressin effects. The effects of the last two agents are secondary to their action on the microtubules required for translocation of water channels. The V_2 receptor antagonists **tolvaptan and demeclocycline** (actually a tetracycline antibiotic) counteract the action of vasopressin in renal tubules and can be used to treat patients with water retention combined with urinary salt loss (and thus *hyponatraemia*) caused by excessive secretion of the hormone. This *syndrome of inappropriate ADH secretion* ('SIADH') is associated with lung or other malignancies or head injury. Specific V_2 receptor antagonists are also being investigated in the treatment of heart failure (Ch. 23).

Other non-renal actions

Vasopressin causes contraction of smooth muscle, particularly in the cardiovascular system, by acting on V_{1A} receptors (see Ch. 23). The affinity of vasopressin for these receptors is lower than that for V_2 receptors, and smooth muscle effects are seen only with doses larger than those affecting the kidney. Vasopressin also stimulates blood platelet aggregation and mobilisation of coagulation factors. When released into the pituitary portal circulation it promotes the release of ACTH from the anterior pituitary by an action on V_{1B} receptors (see Fig. 34.4). In the CNS, vasopressin, like oxytocin, is believed to have a role in modulating emotional and social behaviour.

Pharmacokinetic aspects

Vasopressin, and various peptide analogues, are used clinically either for the treatment of diabetes insipidus or as vasoconstrictors. Several analogues have been developed to (a) increase their duration of action and (b) shift the relative potency between the V_1 and V_2 receptors.

The main substances used are:

- *vasopressin itself*: short duration of action, weak selectivity for V_2 receptors, given by subcutaneous or intramuscular injection, or by intravenous infusion;
- *desmopressin*: increased duration of action, V_2-selective and therefore fewer pressor effects, can be given by several routes including nasal spray;
- *terlipressin*: increased duration of action, low but protracted vasopressor action (and minimal antidiuretic properties), used to reduce bleeding (e.g. from oesophageal varices) and maintain blood pressure;
- *felypressin*: a short-acting vasoconstrictor that is injected with local anaesthetics such as prilocaine to prolong their action (see Ch. 44).

Vasopressin itself is rapidly eliminated, with a plasma half-life less than 10 min and a short duration of action. Tissue peptidases metabolise the hormone and 33% is removed by the kidney. Desmopressin is less subject to degradation by peptidases, and its plasma half-life is 75 min.

Unwanted effects

There are few unwanted effects and these are mainly cardiovascular in nature: intravenous vasopressin may cause spasm of the coronary arteries with resultant angina, but this risk can be minimised if the antidiuretic peptides are administered intranasally.

The posterior pituitary gland

- The posterior pituitary gland secretes:
  - oxytocin (see Ch. 36)
  - antidiuretic hormone (**vasopressin**), which acts on V_2 receptors in the distal kidney tubule to increase water reabsorption and, in higher concentrations, on V_{1A} receptors to cause vasoconstriction. It also stimulates adrenocorticotrophic hormone secretion.
- Substances available for clinical use are **vasopressin** and the analogues **desmopressin**, **felypressin** and **terlipressin**.

Clinical uses of antidiuretic hormone (vasopressin) and analogues

- Diabetes insipidus: **felypressin, desmopressin**.
- Initial treatment of bleeding oesophageal varices: **vasopressin, terlipressin, felypressin**. (**Octreotide** – a somatostatin analogue – is also used, but direct injection of sclerosant via an endoscope is the main treatment.)
- Prophylaxis against bleeding in haemophilia (e.g. before tooth extraction): **vasopressin, desmopressin** (by increasing the concentration of factor VIII).
- **Felypressin** is used as a vasoconstrictor with local anaesthetics (see Ch. 44).
- **Desmopressin** is used for persistent nocturnal enuresis in older children and adults.

THE ADRENAL CORTEX

The adrenal glands consist of two parts: the inner *medulla*, which secretes catecholamines (see Ch. 15), and the outer *cortex*, which secretes adrenal steroids. The cortex comprises three concentric zones: the *zona glomerulosa* (the outermost layer), which elaborates mineralocorticoids, the *zona fasciculata*, which elaborates glucocorticoids, and the innermost *zona reticularis*, which produces androgen precursors. The principal adrenal steroids are those with glucocorticoid and mineralocorticoid activities.[4] Androgen secretion (see Ch. 36) by the cortex is not considered further in this chapter.

---

[4]So named because early experimenters noticed that separate fractions of adrenal gland extracts caused changes in either blood glucose or salt and water retention.

Table 34.2 Comparison of the main corticosteroid agents used for systemic therapy (using hydrocortisone as a standard)

Compound	Relative affinity for GR	Approximate relative potency in clinical use		Duration of action after oral dose[a]	Comments
		Anti-inflammatory	Sodium retaining		
Hydrocortisone (cortisol)	1	1	1	Short	Drug of choice for replacement therapy.
Cortisone	0 (Prodrug)	0.8	0.8	Short	Inactive until converted to hydrocortisone; not used as anti-inflammatory because of mineralocorticoid effects.
Deflazacort	0 (Prodrug)	3	Minimal	Short	Converted by plasma esterases into active metabolite. Similar utility to prednisolone.
Prednisolone	2.2	4	0.8	Intermediate	Drug of choice for systemic anti-inflammatory and immunosuppressive effects.
Prednisone	0 (Prodrug)	4	0.8	Intermediate	Inactive until converted to prednisolone.
Methylprednisolone	11.9	5	Minimal	Intermediate	Anti-inflammatory and immunosuppressive.
Triamcinolone	1.9	5	None	Intermediate	Relatively more toxic than others.
Dexamethasone	7.1	27	Minimal	Long	Anti-inflammatory and immunosuppressive, used especially where water retention is undesirable (e.g. cerebral oedema); drug of choice for suppression of ACTH production.
Betamethasone	5.4	27	Negligible	Long	Anti-inflammatory and immunosuppressive, used especially when water retention is undesirable.
Fludrocortisone	3.5	15	150	Short	Drug of choice for mineralocorticoid effects.
Aldosterone	0.38	None	500	N/A	Endogenous mineralocorticoid.

[a]Duration of action (half-lives in hours): short, 8–12; intermediate, 12–36; long, 36–72. Some drugs are inactive until converted to active compounds in vivo and therefore have negligible affinity for the glucocorticoid receptor.

GR, glucocorticoid receptor.

(Data for relative affinity obtained from Baxter & Rousseau, 1979.)

The mineralocorticoids regulate water and electrolyte balance, and the main endogenous hormone is *aldosterone*. The glucocorticoids have widespread actions on carbohydrate and protein metabolism, as well as potent regulatory effects on host defence mechanisms (Chs 7 and 27). The adrenal gland secretes a mixture of glucocorticoids; in humans the main hormone is *hydrocortisone* (also, confusingly, known as *cortisol*), and in rodents it is *corticosterone*. The mineralocorticoid and glucocorticoid actions are not completely separated in naturally occurring steroids and some glucocorticoids have quite substantial effects on water and electrolyte balance. In fact, both hydrocortisone and aldosterone are equiactive on mineralocorticoid receptors but, in mineralocorticoid-sensitive tissues such as the kidney, the action of *11β-hydroxysteroid dehydrogenase Type 2* converts hydrocortisone to the inactive metabolite cortisone,[5] thereby preventing the tissue from responding to hydrocortisone. Interestingly, there is increasing evidence that some glucocorticoid synthesis can take place locally at extra-adrenal sites such as thymus and skin (see Talaber et al., 2015; Hannen et al., 2017) providing a fresh perspective on the local control of inflammatory processes.

With the exception of *replacement therapy*, glucocorticoids are most commonly employed for their anti-inflammatory and immunosuppressive properties (see Ch. 27). In this therapeutic context, their metabolic and other actions are seen as unwanted side effects. Synthetic steroids have been developed in which exhibit a partial separation of the glucocorticoid from the mineralocorticoid actions (Table 34.2), but it has not yet been possible completely to separate the anti-inflammatory from the other actions of the glucocorticoids.

▼ The adrenal gland is essential to life, and animals deprived of these glands are able to survive only under rigorously controlled conditions. In humans, a deficiency in corticosteroid production, termed *Addison's disease*, is characterised by muscular weakness, low blood pressure, depression, anorexia, loss of weight and hypoglycaemia. Addison's disease may have an autoimmune aetiology, or it may be secondary to destruction of the gland by chronic inflammatory conditions such as tuberculosis.

When corticosteroids are produced in excess, the clinical picture depends on which molecular species predominates. Excessive *glucocorticoid* activity results in *Cushing's syndrome*, the manifestations of which are outlined in Fig. 34.7. This can be caused by hypersecretion from the adrenal glands or by prolonged therapeutic use of

---

[5]Oddly, it was cortisone that Hench originally demonstrated to have potent anti-inflammatory activity in his classic studies of 1949. The reason for this apparent anomaly is the presence in some tissues of the enzyme *11β-hydroxysteroid dehydrogenase Type 1* which can reduce cortisone to cortisol (i.e. hydrocortisone), thus restoring its biological activity.

glucocorticoids. An excessive production of *mineralocorticoids* results in retention of Na^+ and loss of K^+. This may be caused by hyperactivity or tumours of the adrenals (*primary hyperaldosteronism*, or *Conn's syndrome*, an uncommon but important cause of hypertension; see Ch. 23), or by excessive activation of the renin–angiotensin system such as occurs in some forms of kidney disease, cirrhosis of the liver or congestive cardiac failure (*secondary hyperaldosteronism*).

GLUCOCORTICOIDS

Synthesis and release

Glucocorticoids are not stored in the adrenal gland but are synthesised under the influence of circulating ACTH secreted from the anterior pituitary gland (see Fig. 34.4) and released in a pulsatile fashion into the blood. While glucocorticoids are continuously released, there is a well-defined circadian rhythm in the secretion in healthy humans, with the net blood concentration being highest early in the morning, gradually diminishing throughout the day and reaching a low point in the evening or night. ACTH secretion itself (also pulsatile in nature) is regulated by CRF released from the hypothalamus, and by vasopressin released from the posterior pituitary gland. The release of both ACTH and CRF, in turn, is reflexly inhibited by the ensuing rising concentrations of glucocorticoids in the blood.

Opioid peptides also exercise a tonic inhibitory control on the secretion of CRF, and psychological factors, excessive heat or cold, injury or infections can also affect the release of both vasopressin and CRF. This is the principal mechanism whereby the HPA axis is activated in response to perceived threats in the external environment.

The biosynthetic precursor of glucocorticoids is cholesterol (Fig. 34.5). The initial conversion of cholesterol to *pregnenolone* is the rate-limiting step and is regulated by ACTH. Some biosynthetic reactions can be inhibited by drugs and these have a utility in treating Cushing's disease or adrenocortical carcinoma. **Metyrapone** prevents the β-hydroxylation at C11, and thus the formation of hydrocortisone and corticosterone. Synthesis is blocked at the 11-deoxycorticosteroid stage, leaving intermediates that have no effects on the hypothalamus and pituitary, so there is a marked increase in ACTH in the blood. Metyrapone can therefore be used to test ACTH production, and may also be used to treat patients with Cushing's syndrome. **Trilostane** (previously used to treat Cushing's syndrome and primary hyperaldosteronism but now largely restricted to veterinary indications) blocks an earlier enzyme in the pathway – the *3β-dehydrogenase*. **Aminoglutethimide** inhibits the initial step in the biosynthetic pathway and has the same overall effect as metyrapone.

Trilostane and aminoglutethimide are not currently used in the United Kingdom but **ketoconazole**, an antifungal agent (Ch. 54), also inhibits steroidogenesis and may be of value in the specialised treatment of Cushing's syndrome. **Mitotane** suppresses glucocorticoid synthesis by a direct (and unknown) mechanism on the adrenal gland. It is chiefly used to treat adrenocortical carcinomas.

Mechanism of glucocorticoid action

The glucocorticoid effects relevant to this discussion are initiated by interaction of the drugs with specific intracellular glucocorticoid receptors[6] belonging to the nuclear receptor superfamily (although there may be other binding proteins or sites; see Norman et al., 2004). This superfamily also includes the receptors for mineralocorticoids, the sex steroids, thyroid hormones, vitamin D_3 and retinoic acid (see Ch. 3). The actual mechanism of transcriptional control is complex, with at least four mechanisms operating within the nucleus. These are summarised diagrammatically in Fig. 34.6.

When the nuclear actions of glucocorticoid receptors were first discovered it was thought that this mechanism could account for all the actions of the hormones, but a surprising discovery overturned this idea. Reichardt et al. (1998), using transgenic mice in which the glucocorticoid receptor was unable to dimerise (and therefore unable to function in the nucleus), found that glucocorticoids were still able to exert a great many biological actions. This suggested that in addition to controlling gene expression within the nucleus, the liganded receptor itself could initiate important signal transduction events while still in the cytosolic compartment (there may even be a subpopulation of receptors that reside there permanently). One such effect seems to be interaction of the receptor with the regulatory complex, NF-κB (see Fig. 34.6 and Ch. 3) and other important interactions may involve protein kinases/phosphatase signalling systems. Some of these cytosolic actions are very rapid. For example, the liganded glucocorticoid receptor-induced phosphorylation by PKC and subsequent release of the protein *annexin A1*, which has potent inhibitory effects on leukocyte trafficking and other anti-inflammatory actions, occurs in minutes and cannot be accounted for by changes in protein synthesis and there are many other examples (see Buttgereit & Scheffold, 2002).

In recent years, our understanding of the glucocorticoid field has been further enriched by the discovery of numerous isoforms and splice variants of glucocorticoid receptor (GR), some of which are expressed in a tissue-specific manner (see Oakley & Cidlowsky, 2013). This opens up a real possibility of highly selective glucocorticoid drugs in the future.

> ## Mechanism of action of the glucocorticoids
>
> - Glucocorticoids bind intracellular receptors that then dimerise, migrate to the nucleus and interact with DNA to modify gene transcription, inducing synthesis of some proteins and inhibiting synthesis of others.
> - Many acute glucocorticoid actions are mediated by signalling systems triggered by the liganded receptor in the cytosol. Some are very rapid.
> - There may be different populations of receptors including membrane bound receptors which may also transduce rapid actions.
> - Tissue and spice variants of the glucocorticoid receptor are found to be distributed in a tissue-specific fashion.

Actions

General metabolic and systemic effects

The main metabolic effects are on carbohydrate and protein metabolism. The glucocorticoids cause both a decrease in the uptake and utilisation of glucose and an increase in gluconeogenesis, resulting in a tendency to hyperglycaemia

---

[6]Reader beware! The glucocorticoid receptor is also referred to as the *Type II corticosteroid receptor*. The Type I corticosteroid receptor being what we more usually call the mineralocorticoid receptor (MR).

Fig. 34.5 **Biosynthesis of corticosteroids, mineralocorticoids and sex hormones.** All steroid hormones are synthesised from cholesterol. The biosynthetic pathway involves successive steps of hydroxylation and dehydrogenation and these are targets for drugs. Intermediates are shown in *green boxes*; interconversions occur between the pathways. *Blue boxes* indicate circulating hormones. Drugs are shown in *red-bordered boxes* adjacent to their sites of action. Glucocorticoids are produced by cells of the zona fasciculata, and their synthesis is stimulated by adrenocorticotrophic hormone (ACTH); aldosterone is produced by cells of the zona glomerulosa, and its synthesis is stimulated by angiotensin II (angio II). Metyrapone inhibits glucocorticoid synthesis, aminoglutethimide and trilostane block synthesis of all three types of adrenal steroid (see text for details). Carbenoxolone inhibits the interconversion of hydrocortisone and cortisone in the kidney. Not shown is mitotane, which suppresses adrenal hormone synthesis through an unknown mechanism. Enzymes: *17-α-OH*, 17-α-hydroxylase; *3-β-dehyd*, 3-β-dehydrogenase; *21-β-OH*, 21-β-hydroxylase; *11-β-OH*, 11-β-hydroxylase; *11-β-dehyd*, 11-β-hydroxysteroid dehydrogenase.

(see Ch. 32). There is a concomitant increase in glycogen storage, which may be a result of insulin secretion in response to the increase in blood sugar. Overall, there is decreased protein synthesis and increased protein breakdown, particularly in muscle, and this can lead to tissue wasting. Catecholamines and some other hormones cause lipase activation through a cAMP-dependent kinase, the synthesis of which requires the 'permissive' presence of glucocorticoids and are several other examples of this type of hormone action have been observed. Large doses of glucocorticoids given over a long period result in the redistribution of body fat characteristic of Cushing's syndrome (Fig. 34.7).

Glucocorticoids tend to produce a negative calcium balance by decreasing Ca^{2+} absorption in the GI tract and increasing its excretion by the kidney. Together with increased breakdown of bone matrix protein this may cause osteoporosis. In higher, non-physiological concentrations, the glucocorticoids have some mineralocorticoid actions, causing Na^+ retention and K^+ loss – possibly by swamping the protective 11β-hydroxysteroid dehydrogenase and acting at mineralocorticoid receptors.

Fig. 34.6 **Molecular mechanism of action of glucocorticoids.** The schematic figure shows four possible ways by which the liganded glucocorticoid receptor can control gene expression following translocation into the nucleus. (A) Basic transactivation mechanism. Here, the transcriptional machinery (TM) is presumed to be operating at a low level. The liganded glucocorticoid receptor (GR) dimer binds to one or more 'positive' glucocorticoid response elements (GREs) within the promoter sequence *(shaded zone)* and upregulates transcription. (B) Basic transrepression mechanism. The TM is constitutively driven by transcription factors (TF). In binding to the 'negative' GRE (nGRE), the receptor complex displaces these factors and expression falls. (C) Fos/Jun mechanism. Transcription is driven at a high level by Fos/Jun transcription factors binding to their AP-1 regulatory site. This effect is reduced in the presence of the GR. (D) Nuclear factor (NF)-κβ mechanism. The TFs P65 and P50 bind to the NF-κβ site, promoting gene expression. This is prevented by the presence of the GR, which binds the TFs, preventing their action (this may occur in the cytoplasm also). (For further details of the structure of the glucocorticoid receptor, see Ch. 3.) (Redrawn from Oakley & Cidlowski, 2001.)

Negative feedback effects on the anterior pituitary and hypothalamus
Both endogenous and exogenous glucocorticoids have a negative feedback effect on the secretion of CRF and ACTH (see Fig. 34.4), thus inhibiting the secretion of endogenous glucocorticoids and potentially causing atrophy of the adrenal cortex. If therapy is prolonged, it may take many months to return to normal function once the drugs are stopped.

Anti-inflammatory and immunosuppressive effects
Endogenous glucocorticoids maintain a low-level anti-inflammatory tone, and are secreted in increased amounts in response to inflammatory stimuli. Consequently, adrenalectomised animals and humans with adrenal insufficiency show a heightened response to even mild insults

and injuries. On this basis, it has been suggested that a failure of appropriate glucocorticoid secretion in response to injury or infection may underlie certain chronic inflammatory human pathologies.

Exogenous glucocorticoids are the anti-inflammatory drugs *par excellence*, and when given therapeutically, suppress the operation of both the innate and adaptive immune system. They reverse virtually all types of inflammatory reaction, whether caused by invading pathogens, by chemical or physical stimuli, or by inappropriately deployed immune responses such as are seen in hypersensitivity or autoimmune disease. When used prophylactically to suppress graft rejection, glucocorticoids are more efficient in suppressing the initiation and generation of the immune response than they are in preventing the operation of an established response where clonal proliferation has already occurred.

Euphoria
(though sometimes
depression or psychotic
symptoms, and emotional
lability)

Buffalo hump

(Hypertension)

Thinning
of skin

Thin arms
and legs:
muscle wasting

(Benign intracranial
hypertension)

(Cataracts)

Moon face, with red
(plethoric) cheeks

Increased
abdominal fat

(Avascular necrosis
of femoral head)

Easy bruising

Poor wound
healing

Also:
Osteoporosis
Tendency to hyperglycaemia
Negative nitrogen balance
Increased appetite
Increased susceptibility to infection
Obesity

Fig. 34.7 Cushing's syndrome. This is caused by excessive exposure to endogenous glucocorticoids, by disease (e.g. an adrenocorticotrophic hormone-secreting tumour) or by prolonged administration of glucocorticoid drugs (*iatrogenic Cushing's syndrome*). *Italicised* effects are particularly common. Less frequent effects, related to dose and duration of therapy, are shown in *parentheses*. (Redrawn from Baxter & Rousseau, 1979)

Given that glucocorticoids modify the expression of so many genes (approximately 1% of the total genome is affected), and that the extent and direction of regulation varies between tissues and even at different times during disease, you will not be surprised to learn that their anti-inflammatory effects are complex.

Actions on *inflammatory* cells include:

- decreased egress of neutrophils from blood vessels and reduced activation of neutrophils, macrophages and mast cells secondary to decreased transcription of the genes for cell adhesion factors and cytokines;
- decreased overall activation of T-helper (Th) cells, reduced clonal proliferation of T cells, and a 'switch' from the Th1 to the Th2 immune response (see Ch. 7);
- decreased fibroblast function, less production of collagen and glycosaminoglycans, and, under some circumstances, reduced healing and repair.

Actions on the mediators of inflammatory and immune responses (Chs 18 and 19) include:

- decreased production of prostanoids through reduced expression of cyclo-oxygenase II and suppression of substrate arachidonic acid release;
- decreased generation of many cytokines, including IL-1, IL-2, IL-3, IL-4, IL-5, IL-6, IL-8, TNF-α, cell adhesion factors and granulocyte–macrophage

colony-stimulating factor. These are largely secondary to inhibition of gene transcription;
- reduction in the concentration of complement components in the plasma;
- decreased generation of nitric oxide by the inducible nitric oxide synthase 2 (NOS2) isoform;
- decreased release of histamine and other mediators from basophils and mast cells;
- decreased immunoglobulin G (IgG) production;
- increased synthesis of anti-inflammatory factors such as IL-10, IL-1-soluble receptor and annexin 1.

Endogenous anti-inflammatory glucocorticoids circulate constantly in the blood and are increased during inflammatory episodes – or even by the anticipation of a stressful event. It is suggested (see Munck et al., 1984), that the anti-inflammatory and immunosuppressive actions of endogenous glucocorticoids play a crucial counter-regulatory role, in that they prevent excessive activation of inflammation and other powerful defence reactions that might, if unchecked, threaten homeostasis. Certainly, this view is borne out by experimental work. While these drugs are of great value in treating conditions characterised by hypersensitivity and unwanted inflammation, they carry the hazard that they are able to suppress the same defence reactions that protect us from infection and other insults.

Unwanted effects

Low-dose glucocorticoid replacement therapy is usually without problems but serious unwanted effects occur with large doses or prolonged administration of glucocorticoids. The major effects are as follows:

- *Suppression of the response to infection or injury*: opportunistic infection can be potentially very serious unless quickly treated with antimicrobial agents along with an increase in the dose of steroid. Oral thrush (candidiasis, a fungal infection; see Ch. 54) frequently occurs when glucocorticoids are taken by inhalation, because of suppression of local anti-infective mechanisms. Wound healing is impaired, and peptic ulceration may also occur.
- *Cushing's syndrome* (see Fig. 34.7).
- *Osteoporosis*, with the attendant hazard of fractures, is one of the main limitations to long-term glucocorticoid therapy. These drugs influence bone density both by regulation of calcium and phosphate metabolism and through effects on collagen turnover. They reduce osteoblast function (which deposits bone matrix) and increase the activity of osteoclasts (which digest bone matrix). An effect on the blood supply to bone can result in avascular necrosis of the head of the femur (see Ch. 37).
- *Hyperglycaemia* produced by exogenous glucocorticoids may develop into frank diabetes.
- *Muscle wasting* and proximal muscle weakness.
- In children, *inhibition of growth*[7] if treatment is continued for more than 6 months.
- *CNS effects*: euphoria and psychosis with short-term administration, depression with chronic treatment.

[7]However, some of the diseases for which glucocorticoids are indicated themselves retard growth. In a classical trial, glucocorticoid treatment *increased* growth in adolescents with inflammatory bowel disease as the disease resolved (Whittington et al., 1977).

- *Other effects*: glaucoma (in genetically predisposed persons), raised intracranial pressure and an increased incidence of cataracts.

Sudden withdrawal of the drugs after prolonged therapy may result in acute adrenal insufficiency because of suppression of the patient's capacity to synthesise corticosteroids.[8] Careful procedures for phased withdrawal should be followed. Recovery of full adrenal function usually takes about 8 weeks, although it can take 18 months or more after prolonged high-dose treatment.

Pharmacokinetic aspects

There are many glucocorticoid drugs in therapeutic use. Although **cortisol** (**hydrocortisone**), the endogenous hormone, is often used, synthetic derivatives are even more common. These have different physicochemical properties as well as varying potencies and have been optimised for administration by oral, systemic or intra-articular routes or for topical application such as by aerosol directly into the respiratory tract or nose or as eye drops. They may be formulated as creams or ointments for application to the skin (see Ch. 28); or as foam enemas for the GI tract (Ch. 31). Topical administration diminishes the likelihood of systemic toxic effects unless large quantities are used. When prolonged use of systemic glucocorticoids is necessary, therapy on alternate days may decrease suppression of the HPA axis and other unwanted effects.

Endogenous glucocorticoids are transported in the plasma bound to *corticosteroid-binding globulin* (CBG) and to albumin. About 77% of plasma hydrocortisone is bound to CBG, but many synthetic glucocorticoids are not bound at all. Albumin has a lower affinity for hydrocortisone but binds both natural and synthetic steroids. Both CBG-bound and albumin-bound steroids are biologically inactive. Hydrocortisone has a plasma half-life of 90 min, although many of its biological effects have a latency of 2–8 h.

As small lipophilic molecules, glucocorticoids probably enter their target cells by simple diffusion. Biological inactivation, which occurs in liver cells and elsewhere, is initiated by reduction of the C4–C5 double bond. Cortisone and **prednisone** are inactive until converted in vivo by the 11β dehydrogenase type 1 to hydrocortisone and **prednisolone**, respectively.

The clinical uses of systemic glucocorticoids are summarised in the clinical box. Dexamethasone has a special use: it is used to test HPA axis function. In the dexamethasone suppression test a relatively low dose of dexamethasone is given, usually at night. This would be expected to suppress the hypothalamus and pituitary, resulting in a reduced ACTH secretion and hydrocortisone output in the plasma about 9 h later. Failure of suppression implies hypersecretion of ACTH or of glucocorticoids (Cushing's syndrome).

MINERALOCORTICOIDS

The main endogenous mineralocorticoid is aldosterone. Its chief action is to increase Na^+ reabsorption by the distal tubules in the kidney, with a concomitant increase in excretion of K^+ and H^+ (see Ch. 30). An excessive secretion of mineralocorticoids, as in *Conn's syndrome*, causes marked Na^+ and water retention, with increased extracellular fluid

Actions of glucocorticoids

Common drugs used systemically include **hydrocortisone**, **prednisolone** and **dexamethasone**.

Metabolic actions

- *Carbohydrates*: decreased uptake and utilisation of glucose accompanied by increased gluconeogenesis; this causes a tendency to hyperglycaemia.
- *Proteins*: increased catabolism, reduced anabolism.
- *Lipids*: a permissive effect on lipolytic hormones and a redistribution of fat, as observed in Cushing's syndrome.

Regulatory actions

- *Hypothalamus and anterior pituitary gland*: a negative feedback action resulting in reduced release of ACTH and therefore endogenous glucocorticoids.
- *Cardiovascular system*: reduced vasodilatation, decreased fluid exudation.
- *Musculoskeletal*: decreased osteoblast and increased osteoclast activity.
- *Inflammation and immunity*:
  - in acute inflammation: decreased influx and activity of leukocytes;
  - in chronic inflammation: decreased activity of mononuclear cells, decreased angiogenesis, less fibrosis;
  - in lymphoid tissues: decreased clonal expansion of T and B cells, and decreased action of cytokine-secreting T cells. Switch from Th1 to Th2 response;
  - decreased production and action of many pro-inflammatory cytokines, including interleukins, tumour necrosis factor-α and granulocyte–macrophage colony-stimulating factor;
  - reduced generation of eicosanoids;
  - decreased generation of IgG;
  - decrease in complement components in the blood;
  - increased release of *anti-inflammatory* factors such as interleukin (IL)-10, IL-1ra and annexin 1.
- Overall effects: reduction in the activity of the innate and acquired immune systems, but also diminution in the protective aspects of the inflammatory response and sometimes decreased healing.

volume and sometimes hypokalaemia, alkalosis and hypertension. Decreased secretion, as in some patients with Addison's disease, causes Na^+ loss and a marked decrease in extracellular fluid volume. There is a concomitant decrease in the excretion of K^+, resulting in hyperkalaemia.

Regulation of aldosterone synthesis and release

The regulation of the synthesis and release of aldosterone depends mainly on the electrolyte composition of the plasma and on the activity of the angiotensin II system (see Fig. 34.4; Chs 23 and 30). Low plasma Na^+ or high plasma K^+ concentrations directly stimulate aldosterone release from the zona glomerulosa cells of the adrenal. Depletion of Na^+ also activates the renin–angiotensin system (see Ch. 23, Fig. 23.4). One of the effects of angiotensin II is to increase the synthesis and release of aldosterone (see Ch. 30, Fig. 30.5).

---

[8]Patients on long-term glucocorticoid therapy are advised to carry a card stating, 'I am a patient on STEROID TREATMENT which must not be stopped abruptly'.

Pharmacokinetics and unwanted actions of the glucocorticoids

- Administration can be oral, topical or parenteral. Most naturally occurring glucocorticoids are transported in the blood by corticosteroid-binding globulin or albumen and enter cells by diffusion. They are metabolised in the liver.
- Unwanted effects are seen mainly after prolonged systemic use as anti-inflammatory or immunosuppressive agents but not usually following replacement therapy. The most important of these are:
  - suppression of response to infection
  - suppression of endogenous glucocorticoid synthesis
  - metabolic actions (see earlier)
  - osteoporosis
  - iatrogenic Cushing's syndrome (see Fig. 34.7)

Clinical uses of glucocorticoids

- Replacement therapy for patients with adrenal failure (*Addison's disease*).
- Anti-inflammatory/immunosuppressive therapy (see also Ch. 27):
  - in *asthma* (Ch. 29)
  - topically in various inflammatory conditions of skin, eye, ear or nose (e.g. *eczema*, *allergic conjunctivitis* or *rhinitis*; see Ch. 28)
  - *hypersensitivity states* (e.g. severe allergic reactions)
  - in miscellaneous diseases with autoimmune and inflammatory components (e.g. *rheumatoid arthritis* and other 'connective tissue' diseases, *inflammatory bowel diseases*, some forms of *haemolytic anaemia*, *idiopathic thrombocytopenic purpura*)
  - to prevent graft-versus-host disease following organ or bone marrow transplantation
- In neoplastic disease (Ch. 57):
  - in combination with cytotoxic drugs in treatment of specific malignancies (e.g. *Hodgkin's disease*, *acute lymphocytic leukaemia*)
  - to reduce cerebral oedema in patients with metastatic or primary *brain tumours* (**dexamethasone**).

Mechanism of action

Like other steroid hormones, aldosterone acts through specific intracellular receptors of the nuclear receptor family. Unlike the glucocorticoid receptor, which is present in most cells, the *mineralocorticoid receptor* (also called the *corticosteroid receptor Type I*) is restricted to a few tissues, such as the kidney and the transporting epithelia of the colon and bladder. Cells containing mineralocorticoid receptors also contain the 11β-hydroxysteroid dehydrogenase type 2 enzyme, which converts hydrocortisone (cortisol) into inactive cortisone, but does not inactivate aldosterone. This ensures that the cells are appropriately affected only by the mineralocorticoid hormone itself. Interestingly, this

enzyme is inhibited by **carbenoxolone**, a compound derived from liquorice (and previously used to treat gastric ulcers; see Ch. 31). If this inhibition is marked, cortisol accumulates and acts on the mineralocorticoid receptor, producing an effect similar to Conn's syndrome (*primary hyperaldosteronism*) except that the circulating aldosterone concentration is not raised.

As with the glucocorticoids, the interaction of aldosterone with its receptor initiates transcription and translation of specific proteins, resulting in an increase in the number of sodium channels in the apical membrane of the renal tubular cell, and subsequently an increase in the number of Na^+-K^+-ATPase molecules in the basolateral membrane (see Fig. 30.5), causing increased K^+ excretion (see Ch. 30). In addition to the genomic effects, there is evidence for a rapid *non-genomic* effect of aldosterone on Na^+ influx, through an action on the Na^+-H^+ exchanger in the apical membrane.

Clinical use of mineralocorticoids and antagonists
The main clinical use of mineralocorticoids is replacement therapy of patients with Addison's disease. The most commonly used drug is **fludrocortisone** (see Table 34.2 and Fig. 34.4), which can be taken orally to supplement the necessary glucocorticoid replacement. **Spironolactone** is a competitive antagonist of aldosterone, and it also prevents the mineralocorticoid effects of other adrenal steroids on the renal tubule (Ch. 30). Side effects include gynaecomastia and impotence, because spironolactone also has some blocking action on androgen and progesterone receptors. It is used to treat primary or secondary hyperaldosteronism and, in conjunction with other drugs, for the treatment of resistant hypertension and of heart failure (Ch. 23) and oedema (Ch. 30). **Eplerenone** has a similar indication and mechanism of action, although fewer side effects as it has lower affinity for sex hormone receptors (Ch. 23).

Mineralocorticoids

Fludrocortisone is given orally to produce a mineralocorticoid effect. This drug:
- increases Na^+ reabsorption in distal tubules and increases K^+ and H^+ efflux into the tubules;
- acts on intracellular receptors that modulate DNA transcription, causing synthesis of Na^+ channel and other proteins that mediate the effect of the drug;
- may be used together with a glucocorticoid in replacement therapy regimes.

NEW DIRECTIONS IN GLUCOCORTICOID THERAPY

Glucocorticoids are highly effective in controlling inflammation, but their utility is constrained by their potentially harmful side effects. The ideal solution would be a glucocorticoid possessing the anti-inflammatory but not the unwanted metabolic or other effects.

Following the discovery of cortisol, the pharmaceutical industry pursued this ambitious goal by testing straightforward structural analogues of cortisol. While this yielded many new active and interesting compounds (several of which are in clinical use today), none achieved a true 'separation' of the glucocorticoid actions. There have been recently been fresh attempts to accomplish this. The development of structural analogues at novel sites on the steroid template (e.g. Uings et al., 2013) has met with more success, and structural details of the receptor revealed by X-ray crystallography has enabled the design of non-steroidal receptor ligands (see, for example, Biggadike et al., 2009; He et al., 2014). Another approach has been to add other functional groups on to the steroid molecule, which alters the conformation of the liganded receptor. Fiorucci et al. (2002) attached a nitric oxide donating group to prednisolone, finding augmented efficacy and reduced unwanted effects. The compound is reported to be useful in the treatment of inflammatory bowel disease (see Schacke et al., 2007). The design of 'soft' glucocorticoids which are rapidly metabolised to inactive species thereby limiting their capacity for producing side effects is also being investigated (see Dobricic et al., 2017).

Many investigators in this area have been influenced by the 'dissociated steroids' or 'transrepression hypothesis': this is the notion, based upon some experimental observations, that the anti-inflammatory effects of glucocorticoids are generally caused by the *down*-regulation (*transrepression*) of genes such as those coding for cytokines, whilst the unwanted effects are usually caused by *up*-regulation (*transactivation*) of metabolic and other genes (e.g. tyrosine amino transferase and phosphoenol pyruvate carboxykinase).

Because transactivation and transrepression utilise different molecular pathways (see Fig. 34.6) which depend upon different conformational states of the GR, researchers have sought **S**elective **G**lucocorticoid **R**eceptor **A**gonists (SEGRAs) that promote one set of actions without the other. The application of this idea has been reviewed by Schacke et al. (2007) and the development of compounds for treating skin and ocular conditions has been reported (Schacke et al., 2009; Spinelli et al., 2014). However, some anti-inflammatory effects of glucocorticoids do not fit neatly into this scheme (Vandevyver et al., 2013); its shortcomings have been reviewed by Clark and Belvisi (2012).

Another approach focuses upon the histone deacetylase enzymes that facilitate the transcriptional regulation of genes following nuclear receptor binding to hormone response elements (Hayashi et al., 2004). There may be a specific isoform of this enzyme that deals with gene up-regulation, and if this could be inhibited, it would lessen the possibility of those unwanted effects. Barnes (2011) has reviewed this approach, particularly as it relates to the therapy of asthma. A more general review of the whole area, with particular relevance to the treatment of rheumatic diseases, has been provided by Strehl et al. (2011). Other molecular tactics that show promise include the use of GILZ (**G**lucocorticoid-**I**nduced **L**eucine **Z**ipper protein) as a therapeutic agent (Beaulieu & Morand, 2011) or exploitation of the cytosolic, non-genomic actions of these drugs (Jiang et al., 2014)

The quest for the glucocorticoid magic bullet continues.

REFERENCES AND FURTHER READING

The hypothalamus and pituitary

Chan, L.F., Clark, A.J., Metherell, L.A., 2008. Familial glucocorticoid deficiency: advances in the molecular understanding of ACTH action. Horm. Res. 69, 75–82. (*This paper and the one by the same group below (Clark et al.) discuss research into the role of the ACTH signalling system in familial glucocorticoid deficiency. An expert piece of scientific detective work. The second paper is more accessible*)

Chini, B., Manning, M., Guillon, G., 2008. Affinity and efficacy of selective agonists and antagonists for vasopressin and oxytocin receptors: an 'easy guide' to receptor pharmacology. Prog. Brain Res. 170, 513–517. (*The title is self-explanatory! Also deals with the prospects for new drugs in this area*)

Clark, A.J., Metherell, L.A., Cheetham, M.E., Huebner, A., 2005. Inherited ACTH insensitivity illuminates the mechanisms of ACTH action. Trends Endocrinol. Metab. 16, 451–457. (*See also Chan et al. above*)

Drolet, G., Rivest, S., 2001. Corticotropin-releasing hormone and its receptors; an evaluation at the transcription level *in vivo*. Peptides 22, 761–767.

Freeman, M.E., Kanyicska, B., Lerant, A., Nagy, G., 2000. Prolactin: structure, function and regulation of secretion. Physiol. Res. 80, 1524–1585. (*Comprehensive review of prolactin and its receptors*)

Getting, S.J., Christian, H.C., Flower, R.J., Perretti, M., 2002. Activation of melanocortin type 3 receptor as a molecular mechanism for adrenocorticotropic hormone efficacy in gouty arthritis. Arthritis Rheum. 46, 2765–2775. (*Original paper that demonstrates that ACTH has intrinsic anti-inflammatory actions that are independent of adrenal stimulation*)

Guillemin, R., 2005. Hypothalamic hormones a.k.a. hypothalamic releasing factors. J. Endocrinol. 184, 11–28. (*This little review focuses on the history of research in this field and covers the discovery and characterisation of the principal releasing factors. Something to read if you are drawn to this area*)

Lamberts, S.W.J., van der Lely, A.J., de Herder, W.W., Hofland, L.J., 1996. Octreotide. N. Engl. J. Med. 334, 246–254. (*A review covering somatostatin receptors, somatostatin analogues and treatment of tumours expressing somatostatin receptors with octreotide*)

Schneider, F., Tomek, W., Grundker, C., 2006. Gonadotropin-releasing hormone (GnRH) and its natural analogues: a review. Theriogenology 66, 691–709. (*Focuses mainly on the use of such agents in veterinary medicine*)

Thibonnier, M., Coles, P., Thibonnier, A., et al., 2001. The basic and clinical pharmacology of nonpeptide vasopressin receptor antagonists. Annu. Rev. Pharmacol. 41, 175–202. (*Authoritative account of ADH receptors and the search for new antagonists*)

Wikberg, J.E.S., Muceniece, R., Mandrika, I., et al., 2000. New aspects on the melanocortins and their receptors. Pharmacol. Res. 42, 393–420. (*Detailed review of the varied biological roles of melanocortins and their receptors*)

Glucocorticoids

Barnes, P.J., 2011. Glucocorticosteroids: current and future directions. Br. J. Pharmacol. 163 (1), 29–43. (*Useful and accessible review focusing on general mechanisms with especial reference to asthma*)

Beaulieu, E., Morand, E.F., 2011. Role of GILZ in immune regulation, glucocorticoid actions and rheumatoid arthritis. Nat. Rev. Rheumatol. 7, 340–348. (*Details the role of glucocorticoid-induced leucine zipper protein in GC action and speculates that it could be used as a stand-alone therapeutic agent with some advantages over GC treament*)

Buttgereit, F., Scheffold, A., 2002. Rapid glucocorticoid effects on immune cells. Steroids 67, 529–534. (*A short paper which details some of the effects of GCs on cells which can't be accounted for by genomic mechanisms*)

Baxter, J.D., Rousseau, G.G. (Eds.), 1979. Glucocorticoid Hormone Action. Monographs on Endocrinology. Springer-Verlag, Berlin, p. 12. (*Another very useful source of information although it is somewhat dated now*)

Biggadike, K., Bledsoe, R.K., Coe, D.M., et al., 2009. Design and x-ray crystal structures of high-potency nonsteroidal glucocorticoid agonists exploiting a novel binding site on the receptor. Proc. Natl. Acad. Sci. U. S. A. 106, 18114–18119. (*Explores the design of new non-steroid drugs that bind to the glucocorticoid receptor*)

Buckingham, J.C., 1998. Stress and the hypothalamo–pituitary–immune axis. Int. J. Tissue React. 20, 23–34. (*Excellent review of the complexities of the effect of stress on HPA axis function*)

Clark, A.R., Belvisi, M.G., 2012. Maps and legends: the quest for dissociated ligands of the glucocorticoid receptor. Pharmacol. Ther. 134, 54–67. (*Very readable account of the 'transrepression' hypothesis and its shortcomings*)

D'Acquisto, F., Perretti, M., Flower, R.J., 2008. Annexin-A1: a pivotal regulator of the innate and adaptive immune systems. Br. J. Pharmacol. 155, 152–169. (*Reviews the role of the glucocorticoid-regulated protein annexin-A1 in mediating anti-inflammatory actions of glucocorticoid drugs*)

Dobricic, V., Jacevic, V., Vucicevic, J., Nikolic, K., Vladimirov, S., Cudina, O., 2017. Evaluation of biological activity and computer-aided design of new soft glucocorticoids. Arch. Pharm. (Weinheim) 350 (5).

Fiorucci, S., Antonelli, E., Distrutti, E., et al., 2002. NCX-1015, a nitric-oxide derivative of prednisolone, enhances regulatory T cells in the lamina propria and protects against 2,4,6-trinitrobenzene sulfonic acid-induced colitis in mice. Proc. Natl. Acad. Sci. U. S. A. 99, 15770–15775.

Hannen, R., Udeh-Momoh, C., Upton, J., et al., 2017. Dysfunctional skin-derived glucocorticoid synthesis is a pathogenic mechanism of psoriasis. J. Invest. Dermatol. (*One of two recent papers (see Talaber et al. below) that overturn the idea that GCs can only be synthesised in the adrenal cortex*)

Hayashi, R., Wada, H., Ito, K., Adcock, I.M., 2004. Effects of glucocorticoids on gene transcription. Eur. J. Pharmacol. 500, 51–62. (*Good basic review of glucocorticoid action; easy to read*)

He, Y., Yi, W., Suino-Powell, K., et al., 2014. Structures and mechanism for the design of highly potent glucocorticoids. Cell Res. 24, 713–726.

Jiang, C.L., Liu, L., Tasker, J.G., 2014. Why do we need nongenomic glucocorticoid mechanisms? Front. Neuroendocrinol. 35, 72–75. (*Another short, but thought-provoking, paper on the potential role of non-genomic GC actions in the physiological response to stress*)

Kirwan, J., Power, L., 2007. Glucocorticoids: action and new therapeutic insights in rheumatoid arthritis. Curr. Opin. Rheumatol. 19, 233–237. (*Written mainly from the viewpoint of a practising rheumatologist, this review offers interesting insights into the use of these drugs to modify severe chronic arthritic disease*)

Munck, A., Guyre, P.M., Holbrook, N.J., 1984. Physiological functions of glucocorticoids in stress and their relation to pharmacological actions. Endocr. Rev. 5, 25–44. (*Seminal review suggesting that the anti-inflammatory/immunosuppressive actions of the glucocorticoids have a physiological function; required reading if you want to understand glucocorticoid physiology and pharmacology*)

Norman, A.W., Mizwicki, M.T., Norman, D.P., 2004. Steroid-hormone rapid actions, membrane receptors and a conformational ensemble model. Nat. Rev. Drug Discov. 3, 27–41. (*Fairly advanced reading but contains many useful tables and excellent diagrams; well worth the effort if this subject interests you*)

Oakley, R.H., Cidlowski, J.A., 2001. The glucocorticoid receptor: expression, function and regulation of glucocorticoid responsiveness. In: Goulding, N.J., Flower, R.J. (Eds.), Milestones in Drug Therapy: Glucocorticoids. Birkhäuser Verlag, Basle, pp. 55–80. (*The book is a useful source of information on all aspects of glucocorticoid biology and pharmacology, containing chapters by some of the leaders in the field*)

Oakley, R.H., Cidlowski, J.A., 2013. The biology of the glucocorticoid receptor: new signaling mechanisms in health and disease. J. Allergy Clin. Immunol. 132, 1033–1044. (*A fascinating account of the role of splice variants and GR isoforms in glucocorticoid action*)

Spinelli, S.L., Xi, X., McMillan, D.H., et al., 2014. Mapracorat, a selective glucocorticoid receptor agonist, upregulates RelB, an anti-inflammatory nuclear factor-kappaB protein, in human ocular cells. Exp. Eye Res. 127, 290–298.

Reichardt, H.M., Kaestner, K.H., Tuckermann, J., et al., 1998. DNA binding of the glucocorticoid receptor is not essential for survival. Cell 93, 531–541. (*An account of the work that changed the way we think about glucocorticoid receptor actions*)

Schacke, H., Berger, M., Rehwinkel, H., Asadullah, K., 2007. Selective glucocorticoid receptor agonists (SEGRAs): novel ligands with an improved therapeutic index. Mol. Cell. Endocrinol. 275, 109–117. (*This paper and the next describe the ideas behind the 'SEGRA' concept and the drugs that have been produced as a result*)

Schacke, H., Zollner, T.M., Docke, W.D., et al., 2009. Characterization of ZK 245186, a novel, selective glucocorticoid receptor agonist for the topical treatment of inflammatory skin diseases. Br. J. Pharmacol. 158, 1088–1103.

Song, I.H., Gold, R., Straub, R.H., et al., 2005. New glucocorticoids on the horizon: repress, don't activate! J. Rheumatol. 32, 1199–1207. (*Good summary of the various approaches taken to circumvent glucocorticoid side effects*)

Strehl, C., Spies, C.M., Buttgereit, F., 2011. Pharmacodynamics of glucocorticoids. Clin. Exp. Rheumatol. 29, S13–S18. (*General review of glucocorticoid mechanisms with especial reference to the treatment of rheumatic disorders*)

Tak, P.P., Firestein, G.S., 2001. NF-kappaB: a key role in inflammatory diseases. J. Clin. Invest. 107, 7–11. (*Succinct and very readable account of the role of nuclear factor (NF)κβ in inflammation*)

Talaber, G., Jondal, M., Okret, S., 2015. Local glucocorticoid production in the thymus. Steroids 103, 58–63. (*One of two recent papers [see Hannen et al. above] that overturn the idea that GCs can only be synthesised in the adrenal cortex*)

Uings, I.J., Needham, D., Matthews, J., et al., 2013. Discovery of GW870086: a potent anti-inflammatory steroid with a unique pharmacological profile. Br. J. Pharmacol. 169, 1389–1403.

Vandevyver, S., Dejager, L., Tuckermann, J., Libert, C., 2013. New insights into the anti-inflammatory mechanisms of glucocorticoids: an emerging role for glucocorticoid-receptor-mediated transactivation. Endocrinology 154, 993–1007.

Mineralocorticoids

Bastl, C., Hayslett, J.P., 1992. The cellular action of aldosterone in target epithelia. Kidney Int. 42, 250–264. (*A detailed review covering the aldosterone receptor and regulation of gene expression, aldosterone action on electrogenic and electroneutral Na+ transport, and on K+ and H+ secretion*)

Jaisser, F., Farman, N., 2016. Emerging roles of the mineralocorticoid receptor in pathology: toward new paradigms in clinical pharmacology. Pharmacol. Rev. 68, 49–75. (*This review is an extremely comprehensive account of mineralocorticoid action and whilst it concentrates on the role of the MR in pathology, it also contains a great deal of basic information on the physiology and pharmacology of the MR*)

35 The thyroid

OVERVIEW

Diseases of the thyroid gland are common, and in this chapter we deal with drug therapy used to mitigate these disorders. We set the scene by briefly outlining the structure, regulation and physiology of the thyroid, and highlight the most common abnormalities of thyroid function. We then consider the drugs that can be used to replace thyroid hormones when these are deficient or cease to function adequately, or which decrease thyroid function when this is excessive.

SYNTHESIS, STORAGE AND SECRETION OF THYROID HORMONES

The thyroid gland secretes three main hormones: in this chapter we focus on two of these, *thyroxine* (T_4) and *tri-iodothyronine* (T_3). The third hormone secreted by this gland is *calcitonin*, which is involved in the control of plasma $[Ca^{2+}]$. It is used to treat osteoporosis and other metabolic bone diseases. It is dealt with in Ch 37. The term 'thyroid hormones' will be used here solely to refer to T_4 and T_3.

Both T_3 and T_4 circulate in the blood tightly bound (>99%) to plasma proteins, mainly *thyroxine binding globulin* (TBG). The majority (~85%) of the secreted thyroid hormone is T_4. This is converted into the (three- to five-fold) more active species, T_3, in a tissue-specific manner. Both hormones are critically important for normal growth and development and for controlling energy metabolism.

The functional unit of the thyroid is the follicle or acinus. Each follicle consists of a single layer of epithelial cells surrounding a cavity, the *follicle lumen*, which is filled with a thick colloid containing *thyroglobulin*. Thyroglobulin is a large glycoprotein, each molecule of which contains about 115 tyrosine residues. It is synthesised, glycosylated and then secreted into the lumen of the follicle, where iodination of the tyrosine residues occurs. Surrounding the follicles is a dense capillary network and the blood flow through the gland is very high in comparison with other tissues. The main steps in the synthesis, storage and secretion of thyroid hormone (Fig. 35.1) are:

- uptake of plasma iodide by the follicle cells;
- oxidation of iodide and iodination of tyrosine residues of thyroglobulin;
- secretion of thyroid hormone.

UPTAKE OF PLASMA IODIDE BY THE FOLLICLE CELLS

Iodide uptake must occur against a concentration gradient (normally about 25:1) so it is an energy-dependent process. Iodide is captured from the blood and moved to the lumen by two transporters: the Na^+/I^- symporter (NIS) located at the basolateral surface of the thyrocytes (the energy being provided by Na^+/K^+-ATPase), and *pendrin*[1] (PDS), an I^-/Cl^- porter in the apical membranes (Nilsson, 2001). Uptake is very rapid: labelled iodide (^{125}I) is found in the lumen within 40 s of intravenous injection. Numerous mutations have been discovered in the NIS and PDS genes and these contribute to thyroid disease in some patients.

OXIDATION OF IODIDE AND IODINATION OF TYROSINE RESIDUES

The oxidation of iodide and its incorporation into thyroglobulin (termed the *organification* of iodide) is catalysed by *thyroperoxidase*, an enzyme situated at the inner surface of the cell at the interface with the colloid. The reaction requires the presence of hydrogen peroxide (H_2O_2) as an oxidising agent. Iodination occurs after the tyrosine has been incorporated into thyroglobulin. The process is shown in Fig. 35.2.

Tyrosine residues are iodinated first at position 3 on the ring, forming monoiodotyrosine (MIT) and then, in some molecules, at position 5 as well, forming di-iodotyrosine (DIT). While still incorporated into thyroglobulin, these molecules are then coupled in pairs, either MIT with DIT to form T_3, or two DIT molecules to form T_4 (Figs 35.2 and 35.3). The mechanism for coupling is believed to involve a peroxidase system similar to the iodination reaction. About one-fifth of the tyrosine residues in thyroglobulin are iodinated in this way.

The iodinated thyroglobulin of the thyroid forms a large store of thyroid hormone within the gland, with a relatively slow turnover. This is in contrast to some other endocrine secretions (e.g. the hormones of the adrenal cortex), which are not stored but synthesised and released as required.

SECRETION OF THYROID HORMONE

The thyroglobulin molecule is taken up into the follicle cell by endocytosis. The endocytotic vesicles then fuse with lysosomes, and proteolytic enzymes act on thyroglobulin, releasing T_4 and T_3 to be secreted into the plasma. The surplus MIT and DIT, which are released at the same time, are scavenged by the cell and the iodide is removed enzymatically and reused.

REGULATION OF THYROID FUNCTION

Thyrotropin-releasing hormone (TRH), released from the hypothalamus in response to various stimuli, releases

---

[1]So called because it is implicated in the pathophysiology of *Pendred syndrome*, named after the eponymous English physician who first described this autosomal recessive form of familial goitre in association with sensorineural deafness.

Fig. 35.1 **Diagram of thyroid hormone synthesis and secretion, with the sites of action of some drugs used in the treatment of thyroid disorders.** Iodide in the blood is transported by the carriers Na^+/I^- symporter (NIS) and pendrin (PDS) through the follicular cell and into the colloid-rich lumen, where it is incorporated into tyrosines in thyroglobulin under the influence of the thyroperoxidase enzyme and monoiodotyrosine units are produced and coupled to produce the hormones (see text for details). Thyroid-stimulating hormone (thyrotropin; TSH) stimulates the endocytosis of thyroglobulin and the hormones are subsequently cleaved from the globulin by lysosomal enzymes and exported into the blood. *DIT*, di-iodotyrosine; *L*, lysosome; *MIT*, monoiodotyrosine; *P*, pseudopod; *T*, tyrosine; T_3, tri-iodothyronine; T_4, thyroxine; *TG*, thyroglobulin.

Fig. 35.2 **Iodination of tyrosyl residues by the thyroperoxidase–H_2O_2 complex.** This probably involves two sites on the enzyme, one of which removes an electron from iodide to give the free radical I•; another removes an electron from tyrosine to give the tyrosyl radical *(shown by orange dot)*. Monoiodotyrosine results from the addition of the two radicals.

Fig. 35.3 **The structures of thyroxine T_3 and T_4.** The position of the iodine residues are indicated in *orange*. T_4 is converted, in a tissue-specific manner, to the more active species T_3 by mono de-iodination at position 5 of the ring. The basic tyrosine unit is shaded in *yellow*.

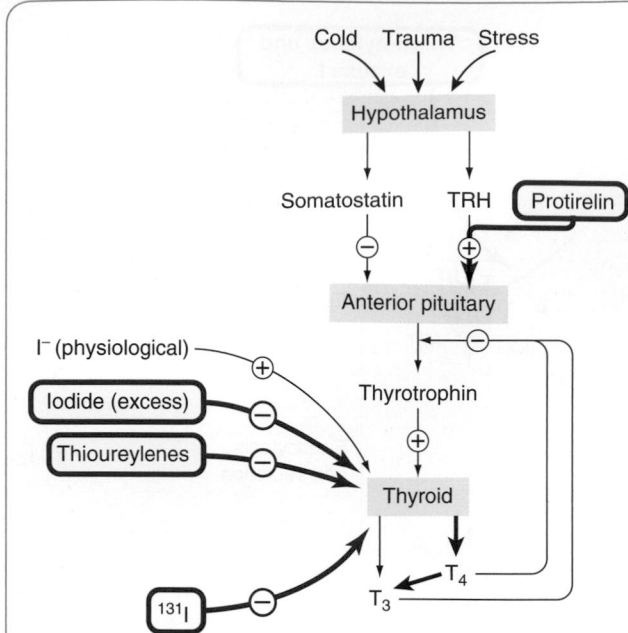

Fig. 35.4 Regulation of thyroid hormone secretion. Iodide (I⁻) is essential for thyroid hormone synthesis, but excess of endogenous or exogenous iodide (30 times the daily requirement of iodine) may be used to inhibit the increased thyroid hormone production of thyrotoxicosis. Protirelin, as well as recombinant human thyrotropin-releasing hormone (rhTRH) is sometimes used to stimulate the system for diagnostic purposes. Larger amounts of iodine (as the ^{131}I isotope) are used for ablation of thyroid tissue (see text for details). T_3, tri-iodothyronine; T_4, thyroxine.

Fig. 35.5 The effect of equimolar doses of tri-iodothyronine (T_3) and thyroxine (T_4) on basal metabolic rate (BMR) in a hypothyroid subject. Note that this figure is meant only to illustrate overall differences in effect; thyroxine is not given clinically in a single bolus dose as here, but in regular daily doses so that the effect builds up to a plateau. The apparent differences in potency really represent differences in kinetics, reflecting the prohormone role of T_4. (Modified from Blackburn et al., 1954.)

thyroid-stimulating hormone (TSH; thyrotrophin) from the anterior pituitary (Fig. 35.4), as does the synthetic tripeptide **protirelin** (pyroglutamyl-histidyl-proline amide), which is used in this way for diagnostic purposes. TSH acts on receptors on the membrane of thyroid follicle cells through a mechanism that involves cAMP and phosphatidylinositol 3-kinase. It has a trophic action on thyroid cells and controls all aspects of thyroid hormone synthesis, mainly by stimulating transcription of the iodide transporter genes, thereby increasing the uptake of iodide by follicle cells. This, in turn, controls all aspects of thyroid hormone synthesis including:

• the synthesis and secretion of thyroglobulin;
• the generation of H_2O_2 and the iodination of tyrosine;
• the endocytosis and proteolysis of thyroglobulin;
• the actual secretion of T_3 and T_4;
• the blood flow through the gland.

The production of TSH is also regulated by a negative feedback effect of thyroid hormones on the anterior pituitary gland and the hypothalamus; T_3 is more active than T_4 in this respect. The peptide **somatostatin** also reduces basal TSH release. The control of the secretion of TSH thus depends on a balance between the actions of T_3/T_4 and TRH (and probably also somatostatin) on the pituitary and most likely on the hypothalamus also. However, the relationship between T_3/T_4 concentration and TSH secretion is not linear. Small changes in thyroid hormones can produce very large changes in TSH secretion whilst large changes

in TSH produce only small alterations in T_3/T_4. It is important to recognise this, as measurement of TSH is a key diagnostic tool when assessing thyroid function in patients.

The other main factor influencing thyroid function is the plasma iodide concentration. About 100 nmol of T_4 is synthesised daily, necessitating uptake by the gland of approximately 500 nmol of iodide each day (equivalent to about 70 μg of iodine). A reduced iodine intake, with reduced plasma iodide concentration, will result in a decrease of hormone production and an increase in TSH secretion. An increased plasma iodide has the opposite effect, although this may be modified by other factors. The overall feedback mechanism responds to changes of iodide slowly over fairly long periods of days or weeks, because there is a large reserve capacity for the binding and uptake of iodide in the thyroid. The size and vascularity of the thyroid are reduced by an increase in plasma iodide and this is exploited therapeutically in preparing hyperthyroid patients for surgery to the gland. Diets deficient in iodine eventually result in a continuous excessive compensatory secretion of TSH, and eventually in an increase in vascularity and (sometimes gross) hypertrophy of the gland.[2]

ACTIONS OF THE THYROID HORMONES

The physiological actions of the thyroid hormones fall into two main categories: those affecting metabolism and those affecting growth and development. Both T_3 and T_4 are extensively plasma bound and only the free concentrations of the hormones are active.

EFFECTS ON METABOLISM

The thyroid hormones produce a general increase in the metabolism of carbohydrates, fats and proteins, and regulate these processes in most tissues, T_3 being three to five times more active than T_4 in this respect (Fig. 35.5). Although

---

[2]'Derbyshire neck' was the name given to this condition in a part of the United Kingdom where sources of dietary iodine were once scarce.

the thyroid hormones directly control the activity of some of the enzymes of carbohydrate metabolism, most effects are brought about in conjunction with other hormones, such as insulin, glucagon, the glucocorticoids and the catecholamines. There is an increase in oxygen consumption and heat production, which is manifested as an increase in the measured basal metabolic rate. This reflects the action of these hormones on tissues such as heart, kidney, liver and muscle, although not on others, such as the gonads, brain or spleen. This calorigenic action is important as part of the response to a cold environment. Administration of thyroid hormone results in augmented cardiac rate and output, and increased tendency to dysrhythmias such as atrial fibrillation.

EFFECTS ON GROWTH AND DEVELOPMENT

The thyroid hormones have a critical effect on growth, partly by a direct action on cells, but also indirectly by influencing growth hormone production and potentiating its effects on its target tissues. The hormones are important for a normal response to *parathormone* (Ch. 37) and calcitonin as well as for skeletal development; they are also essential for normal growth and maturation of the central nervous system.

MECHANISM OF ACTION

While there is some evidence for non-genomic actions (see Bassett et al., 2003), thyroid hormones act mainly through a specific nuclear receptor, TR (Ch. 3). Two distinct genes, TRα and TRβ, code for several receptor isoforms that have distinct functions. T_4 may be regarded as a prohormone, because when it enters the cell, it is converted to T_3, which then binds with high affinity to TR. This interaction is likely to take place in the nucleus, where TR isoforms generally act as a constitutive repressor of target genes. When T_3 is bound, these receptors change conformation, the co-repressor complex is released and a co-activator complex is recruited, which then activates transcription, resulting in generation of mRNA and protein synthesis. Some rare cases of thyroid hormone resistance linked to TRβ mutations, have been reported (Lai et al., 2015).

TRANSPORT AND METABOLISM OF THYROID HORMONES

Plasma concentrations of these hormones can be measured by radioimmunoassay, and are approximately 1×10^{-7} mol/L (T_4) and 2×10^{-9} mol/L (T_3). Both are eventually metabolised in their target tissues by deiodination, deamination, decarboxylation and conjugation with glucuronic and sulfuric acids. The liver is a major site of metabolism and the free and conjugated forms are excreted partly in the bile and partly in the urine. The half-life of T_3 is a few hours, whereas that of T_4 varies between 3–4 days in hyperthyroidism, and 9–10 days in hypothyroidism[3]. Abnormalities in the metabolism of these hormones may occur naturally or be induced by drugs or heavy metals, and this may give rise to a variety of (uncommon) clinical conditions such as the 'low T_3 syndrome'.

ABNORMALITIES OF THYROID FUNCTION

Thyroid disorders are among the most common endocrine diseases in all age groups, including children. Subclinical thyroid disease is prevalent in the middle-aged and elderly. Thyroid disorders are accompanied by many extra-thyroidal symptoms, particularly in the heart, gastrointestinal system and skin. One (rare) cause of organ dysfunction is thyroid cancer. Many other thyroid disorders have an autoimmune basis – in fact, autoimmune thyroid disease is the commonest autoimmune disease. The reason for this is not clear, although it may be linked to a breakdown in immune tolerance to the TSH receptor, although other factors cannot be ruled out (Lee et al., 2015). It may be linked to other autoimmune conditions such as rheumatoid arthritis.

There are two main types of autoimmune thyroid disorder, *Graves' disease*[4] and *Hashimoto's disease*. Both are associated with the production of thyroid autoantibodies and immune damage to the gland itself.[5] Oddly perhaps, they result in different clinical pictures with Graves' disease leading to thyrotoxicosis while Hashimoto's thyroiditis leads to hypoactive thyroid. Regardless of causation, thyroid dysfunction is often associated with typical gross enlargement of the gland, known as *goitre*. Like other autoimmune diseases, such thyroid disorders are more common in women than men and occur with increased frequency during pregnancy (Cignini et al., 2012).

HYPERTHYROIDISM (THYROTOXICOSIS)

In thyrotoxicosis there is excessive secretion and activity of the thyroid hormones, resulting in a high metabolic rate, an increase in skin temperature and sweating, and heat intolerance. Nervousness, tremor, tachycardia and increased appetite associated with loss of weight occur. There are several types of hyperthyroidism, but only two are common: *exophthalmic* or *diffuse toxic goitre* (Graves' disease) and *toxic nodular goitre*.

Diffuse toxic goitre is an organ-specific autoimmune disease caused by autoantibodies to the TSH receptor which activate it, increasing T_4 secretion. Constitutively active mutations of the TRH receptor may also be involved. As is indicated by the name, patients with exophthalmic goitre have protrusion of the eyeballs. The pathogenesis of this condition is not fully understood, but it is thought to be caused by the presence of TSH receptor-like proteins in orbital tissues. There is also an enhanced sensitivity to catecholamines. Toxic nodular goitre is caused by a benign tumour, and may develop in patients with long-standing simple goitre. This condition does not usually have concomitant exophthalmos. The antidysrhythmic drug **amiodarone** (Ch. 22) is rich in iodine and can cause either hyperthyroidism or hypothyroidism. Some iodine-containing radiocontrast agents, such as **iopanoic acid** and its congeners, used as imaging agents to visualise the gall bladder,

---

[3]Correcting hypothyroidism by administration of T_4 therefore takes 2–3 weeks to reach equilibrium.

[4]After a Dublin physician who connected 'violent and long continued palpitations in females' with enlargement of the thyroid gland. Their complaints of fluttering hearts and lumps in their throats had previously been attributed to hysteria.
[5]John F Kennedy Jr suffered from Graves' disease. He inherited a propensity for autoimmune diseases from his father JFK, who himself suffered from the autoimmune *Addison's disease*, in which adrenal glands are the main organs affected. JFK's sister Eunice also suffered from Addison's disease.

may also interfere with thyroid function. The chronic use of psychotropic agents may precipitate a variety of thyroid abnormalities (Bou Khalil & Richa, 2011).

SIMPLE, NON-TOXIC GOITRE

A dietary deficiency of iodine, if prolonged, causes a rise in plasma TRH and eventually an increase in the size of the gland. This condition is known as simple or non-toxic goitre. Another cause is ingestion of *goitrogens* (e.g. from cassava root). The enlarged thyroid usually manages to produce normal amounts of thyroid hormone, although if the iodine deficiency is very severe, hypothyroidism may supervene.

HYPOTHYROIDISM

A decreased activity of the thyroid results in hypothyroidism, and in severe cases *myxoedema*. Once again, this disease is usually of immunological in origin, and the manifestations include low metabolic rate, slow speech, deep hoarse voice, lethargy, bradycardia, sensitivity to cold and mental impairment. Patients also develop a characteristic thickening of the skin (caused by the subcutaneous deposition of glycosaminoglycans), which gives myxoedema its name. In Hashimoto's thyroiditis, there is an immune reaction against thyroglobulin or some other component of thyroid tissue, which can lead to both hypothyroidism and myxoedema. Genetic factors play an important role. Destruction of glandular tissue whilst treating thyroid tumours with radioiodine is another cause of hypothyroidism. Some drugs (e.g. cholecystographic agents or anti-epileptic drugs) as well as environmental 'endocrine disruptors'[6] may interfere with the normal production of thyroid hormones.

Thyroid deficiency during development, affecting 1 in 3000–4000 births, causes congenital hypothyroidism, characterised by gross retardation of growth and mental deficiency.[7]

DRUGS USED IN DISEASES OF THE THYROID

HYPERTHYROIDISM

Hyperthyroidism may be treated pharmacologically or surgically. In general, surgery is now used only when there are mechanical problems resulting from compression of the trachea by the thyroid. Under such circumstances it is usual to remove only part of the organ. Although the condition of hyperthyroidism can be controlled with antithyroid drugs, these drugs do not alter the underlying autoimmune mechanisms or improve the exophthalmos associated with Graves' disease.

RADIOIODINE

Radioiodine is a first-line treatment for hyperthyroidism (particularly in the United States). The isotope used is ^{131}I (usually as the sodium salt), and the dose generally 5–15 mCi. Given orally, it is taken up and processed by the thyroid in the same way as the stable form of iodide, eventually becoming incorporated into thyroglobulin. The

isotope emits both β and γ radiation. The γ rays pass through the tissue without causing damage, but the β particles have a very short range; they are absorbed by the tissue and exert a powerful cytotoxic action that is restricted to the cells of the thyroid follicles, resulting in significant destruction of the tissue. ^{131}I has a half-life of 8 days, so by 2 months its radioactivity has effectively disappeared. It is given as one single dose, but its cytotoxic effect on the gland is delayed for 1–2 months and does not reach its maximum for a further 2 months.

Hypothyroidism will eventually occur after treatment with radioiodine, particularly in patients with Graves' disease, but is easily managed by replacement therapy with T_4. Radioiodine is best avoided in children or pregnant patients (because of potential damage to the fetus). There is theoretically an increased risk of thyroid cancer but this has not been seen following therapeutic treatment.

The uptake of ^{131}I and other isotopes of iodine is also used diagnostically as a test of thyroid function. A tracer dose of the isotope is given orally or intravenously and the amount accumulated by the thyroid is measured by a γ-scintillation counter placed over the gland. ^{131}I is also used for the treatment of thyroid cancer.

> ### The thyroid
>
> - Thyroid hormones, tri-iodothyronine (T_3) and thyroxine (T_4), are synthesised by iodination of tyrosine residues on thyroglobulin within the lumen of the thyroid follicle.
> - Hormone synthesis and secretion are regulated by thyroid-stimulating hormone (thyrotropin) and influenced by plasma iodide.
> - There is a large pool of T_4 in the body; it has a low turnover rate and is found mainly in the circulation.
> - There is a small pool of T_3 in the body; it has a fast turnover rate and is found mainly intracellularly.
> - Within target cells, the T_4 is converted to T_3, which interacts with a nuclear receptor to regulate gene transcription.
> - T_3 and T_4 actions:
>   - stimulation of metabolism, causing increased oxygen consumption and increased metabolic rate;
>   - regulation of growth and development.
> - Abnormalities of thyroid function include:
>   - hyperthyroidism (thyrotoxicosis): either diffuse toxic goitre or toxic nodular goitre;
>   - hypothyroidism: in adults this causes myxoedema, in infants, gross retardation of growth and mental deficiency;
>   - simple non-toxic goitre caused by dietary iodine deficiency, usually with normal thyroid function.

THIOUREYLENES

This group of drugs comprises **carbimazole** and **propylthiouracil**. Chemically, they are related to thiourea, and the thiocarbamide (S–C–N) group is essential for antithyroid activity.

Mechanism of action

Thioureylenes decrease the output of thyroid hormones from the gland, and cause a gradual reduction in the signs

---

[6]These are man-made chemicals such as pesticides or herbicides (e.g. polychlorinated biphenyls) that persist in the environment and are ingested in foodstuffs. The endocrine system is particularly sensitive to these, especially during development.
[7]An older term for this condition, *cretinism*, has been dropped.

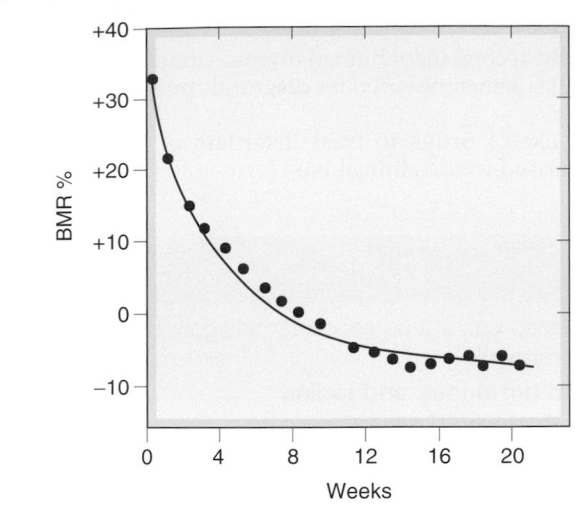

Fig. 35.6 Time course of fall of basal metabolic rate (BMR) during treatment with an antithyroid drug, **carbimazole.** The curve is exponential, corresponding to a daily decrease in BMR of 3.4%. (Modified from Furth et al., 1963.)

and symptoms of thyrotoxicosis, with the basal metabolic rate and pulse rate returning to normal over a period of 3–4 weeks. Their mode of action is not completely understood, but there is evidence that they reduce the iodination of tyrosyl residues in thyroglobulin (see Figs 35.1 and 35.2) by inhibiting the thyroperoxidase-catalysed oxidation reactions, possibly by acting as substrates thus competitively inhibiting the interaction with tyrosine. Propylthiouracil has the additional effect of reducing the deiodination of T_4 to T_3 in peripheral tissues.

Pharmacokinetic aspects

Thioureylenes are given orally. Carbimazole is rapidly converted to an active metabolite. An average dose of carbimazole produces more than 90% inhibition of thyroid incorporation of iodine within 12 h. The full clinical response to this and other antithyroid drugs, however, may take several weeks (Fig. 35.6), partly because T_4 has a long half-life, and also because the thyroid may have large stores of hormone, which need to be depleted before the drug's action can be fully manifest. Propylthiouracil is thought to act somewhat more rapidly because of its additional effect as an inhibitor of the peripheral conversion of T_4 to T_3.

Both drugs may be used during pregnancy but both can cross the placenta and may affect the fetal thyroid gland. They also appear in breast milk, but this effect is less pronounced with propylthiouracil, because it is more strongly bound to plasma protein. After degradation, the metabolites of these drugs are excreted in the urine. The thioureylenes may be concentrated in the thyroid.

Unwanted effects

The most dangerous unwanted effects of thioureylene drugs are neutropenia and agranulocytosis (see Ch. 26). These are relatively rare, having an incidence of 0.1%–1.2%, and are reversible on cessation of treatment. Patients must be warned to report symptoms (especially sore throat) immediately and have a blood count. Rashes (2%–25%) and other

symptoms including headaches, nausea, jaundice and arthralgia, are common. Rare cases of fetal abnormalities have been reported with carbimazole.

IODINE/IODIDE

Iodine is converted in vivo to iodide (I⁻), which temporarily inhibits the release of thyroid hormones. When high doses of iodine are given to thyrotoxic patients, the symptoms subside within 1–2 days. There is inhibition of the secretion of thyroid hormones and, over a period of 10–14 days, a marked reduction in vascularity of the gland, which becomes smaller and firmer. Iodine is often given orally in a solution with potassium iodide ('*Lugol iodine*'). With continuous administration, its effect reaches maximum within 10–15 days and then decreases. The mechanism of action is not entirely clear; it may inhibit iodination of thyroglobulin, possibly by reducing the H_2O_2 generation that is necessary for this process.

The main uses of iodine/iodide are for the preparation of hyperthyroid subjects for surgical resection of the gland, and as part of the treatment of severe thyrotoxic crisis (*thyroid storm*). It is also used following exposure to accidental leakage of radioactive iodine from nuclear reactors, to reduce uptake of the radioactive isotope in the thyroid. Allergic reactions can occur; these include angio-oedema, rashes and drug fever. Lacrimation, conjunctivitis, pain in the salivary glands and a cold-like syndrome are dose-related adverse effects connected to the concentration of iodide by transport mechanisms in tears and saliva.

OTHER DRUGS USED

The β-adrenoceptor antagonists, for example, **propranolol** and **nadolol** (Ch. 15), are not antithyroid agents as such, but they are useful for decreasing many of the signs and symptoms of hyperthyroidism – the tachycardia, dysrhythmias, tremor and agitation. They are used during the preparation of thyrotoxic patients for surgery, as well as in most hyperthyroid patients during the initial treatment period while the thioureylenes or radioiodine take effect, or as part of the treatment of acute hyperthyroid crisis. Eye drops containing **guanethidine**, a noradrenergic-blocking agent (Ch. 15), are used to mitigate the exophthalmos of hyperthyroidism (which is not relieved by antithyroid drugs); it acts by relaxing the sympathetically innervated smooth muscle that causes eyelid retraction. Glucocorticoids (e.g. **prednisolone** or **hydrocortisone**) or surgical decompression may be needed to mitigate severe exophthalmia in Graves' disease.

HYPOTHYROIDISM

There are no drugs that specifically augment the synthesis or release of thyroid hormones. The only effective treatment for hypothyroidism, unless it is caused by iodine deficiency (which is treated with iodide), is to administer the thyroid hormones themselves as replacement therapy. Synthetic T_4 (official name: **levothyroxine**) and T_3 (official name: **liothyronine**), identical to the natural hormones, are given orally. Levothyroxine, as the sodium salt in doses of 50–100 µg/day, is the usual first-line drug of choice. Liothyronine has a faster onset but a shorter duration of action, and is generally reserved for acute emergencies such as the rare condition of myxoedema coma, where these properties are an advantage.

Unwanted effects may occur with overdose, and in addition to the signs and symptoms of hyperthyroidism there is a risk of precipitating angina pectoris, cardiac dysrhythmias or even cardiac failure. The effects of less severe overdose are more insidious; the patient feels well but bone resorption is increased, leading to osteoporosis (Ch. 37).

The use of drugs to treat thyroid cancer is a specialist subject and will not be covered here. Bikas et al. (2016)

review the latest generation of drugs to be used for this purpose.

Finally, recombinant human thyroid-stimulating hormone (rhTSH) is sometimes used for diagnostic purposes following surgery.

The use of drugs to treat disorders of the thyroid is summarised in the clinical box.

Clinical use of drugs acting on the thyroid

Radioiodine (^{131}I)
- Hyperthyroidism (Graves' disease, multinodular toxic goitre).
- Relapse of hyperthyroidism after failed medical or surgical treatment.

Carbimazole or propylthiouracil
- Hyperthyroidism (diffuse toxic goitre); at least 1 year of treatment is needed.
- Preliminary to surgery for toxic goitre.
- Part of the treatment of thyroid storm (very severe hyperthyroidism); **propylthiouracil** is preferred,

combined with a β-adrenoceptor antagonist (e.g. **propranolol**).

Thyroid hormones and iodine
- **Levothyroxine** (T_4) is the standard replacement therapy for hypothyroidism.
- **Liothyronine** (T_3), administered by slow intravenous injection, is used for myxoedema coma.
- Iodine dissolved in aqueous potassium iodide (**'Lugol iodine'**) is used short term to control thyrotoxicosis preoperatively. It reduces the vascularity of the gland.

REFERENCES AND FURTHER READING

Bassett, J.H.D., Harvey, C.B., Williams, G.R., 2003. Mechanisms of thyroid hormone receptor-specific nuclear and extranuclear actions. Mol. Cell. Endocrinol. 213, 1–11. (*An excellent and comprehensive review dealing with the actions of thyroid hormones through the nuclear receptor mechanism as well as other actions through G protein-coupled receptors and other pathways*)

Bikas, A., Vachhani, S., Jensen, K., Vasko, V., Burman, K.D., 2016. Targeted therapies in thyroid cancer: an extensive review of the literature. Expert Rev. Clin. Pharmacol. 1–15. (*This reference reviews the properties of some of the latest generation of drugs to be used in thyroid carcinoma, such as the tyrosine kinase inhibitors*)

Blackburn, C.M., McConahey, W.M., Keating, F.R., Jr., Albert, A., 1954. Calorigenic effects of single intravenous doses of L-triiodothyronine and L-thyroxine in myxedematous persons. J. Clin. Invest. 33, 819–824.

Bou Khalil, R., Richa, S., 2011. Thyroid adverse effects of psychotropic drugs: a review. Clin. Neuropharmacol. 34, 248–255. (*Many patients taking psychotropic drugs present with thyroid problems. This review deals with the role played by antipsychotic drugs in this phenomenon*)

Cignini, P., Cafa, E.V., Giorlandino, C., Capriglione, S., Spata, A., Dugo, N., 2012. Thyroid physiology and common diseases in pregnancy: review of literature. J. Prenat. Med. 6, 64–71. (*Makes the point that increased rates of thyroid abnormalities are seen in pregnancy and that many go undiagnosed. Also deals with clinical management of these cases*)

Furth, E.D., Becker, D.V., Schwartz, M.S., 1963. Significance of rate of response of basal metabolic rate and serum cholesterol in hyperthyroid patients receiving neomercazole and other antithyroid agents. J. Clin. Endocrinol. Metab. 23, 1130–1140.

Hadj Kacem, H., Rebai, A., Kaffel, N., et al., 2003. PDS is a new susceptibility gene to autoimmune thyroid diseases: association and linkage study. J. Clin. Endocrinol. Metab. 88, 2274–2280. (*Interesting article on the PDS transporter protein and its contribution to disease susceptibility*)

Kahaly, G.J., Dillmann, W.H., 2005. Thyroid hormone action in the heart. Endocr. Rev. 26, 704–728. (*A very interesting review focusing on the cardiac actions of thyroid hormones; much historical detail*)

Kelly, G.S., 2000. Peripheral metabolism of thyroid hormones: a review. Altern. Med. Rev. 5, 306–333. (*This review focuses on the role of peripheral metabolism in thyroid hormone action*)

Kojic, K.L., Kojic, S.L., Wiseman, S.M., 2012. Differentiated thyroid cancers: a comprehensive review of novel targeted therapies. Exp. Rev. Anticancer Ther. 12, 345–357. (*A review dealing with the pharmacotherapy of the most common type of thyroid cancer, differentiated thyroid carcinoma*)

Lai, S., Zhang, S., Wang, L., et al., 2015. A rare mutation in patients with resistance to thyroid hormone and review of therapeutic strategies. Am. J. Med. Sci. 350, 167–174. (*Worth reading if you are interested in this rare disorder*)

Lee, H.J., Li, C.W., Hammerstad, S.S., Stefan, M., Tomer, Y., 2015. Immunogenetics of autoimmune thyroid diseases: a comprehensive review. J. Autoimmun. 64, 82–90. (*An immunological view of disorders such as Graves' and Hashimoto's disease. Interesting but moderately complex*)

Mastorakos, G., Karoutsou, E.I., Mizamtsidi, M., Creatsas, G., 2007. The menace of endocrine disruptors on thyroid hormone physiology and their impact on intrauterine development. Endocrine 3, 219–237. (*A review of endocrine disrupters and their effects on the thyroid. Not mainstream reading but an interesting topic*)

McAninch, E.A., Bianco, A.C., 2016. The history and future of treatment of hypothyroidism. Ann. Intern. Med. 164, 50–56. (*Very comprehensive history of the diagnosis and treatment of hypothyroidism. Good review if you want to go into this subject in more detail*)

Nilsson, M., 2001. Iodide handling by the thyroid epithelial cell. Exp. Clin. Endocrinol. Diabetes 109, 13–17. (*Useful and readable review of iodide handling by the thyroid gland*)

Roberts, C.G., Ladenson, P.W., 2004. Hypothyroidism. Lancet 363, 793–803. (*Authoritative and accessible review dealing with this thyroid pathology*)

Sheehan, M.T., 2016. Biochemical testing of the thyroid: TSH is the best and, oftentimes, only test needed - A review for primary care. Clin. Med. Res. 14, 83–92. (*This review was written primarily for primary care physicians who have to test thyroid function in their patients. However, it contains a small review on the physiology and endocrinology of the thyroid as well as a lot of information about abnormal thyroid tests. Easy to read and recommended*)

Surks, M.I., Ortiz, E., Daniels, G.H., et al., 2004. Subclinical thyroid disease: scientific review and guidelines for diagnosis and management. JAMA 291, 228–238. (*Discusses and reviews the treatment of subclinical thyroid disease in detail; primarily of interest to clinical students*)

Yen, P.M., 2001. Physiological and molecular basis of thyroid hormone action. Physiol. Rev. 81, 1097–1142. (*Comprehensive review of thyroid hormone–receptor interaction and the effects of thyroid hormone on target tissues*)

Zhang, J., Lazar, M., 2000. The mechanism of action of thyroid hormones. Annu. Rev. Physiol. 62, 439–466. (*Detailed review of the molecular aspects of thyroid hormone–receptor interaction*)

36

The reproductive system

OVERVIEW

In this chapter, we describe the endocrine control of the female and male reproductive systems as the basis for understanding drug actions in sex hormone replacement, contraception, treatment of infertility, management of labour and treatment of erectile dysfunction.

INTRODUCTION

Drugs that affect reproduction (both by preventing conception and more recently for treating infertility) transformed society in the latter half of the last century. In this chapter, we briefly summarise salient points in reproductive endocrinology as a basis for understanding the numerous important drugs that work on the male and female reproductive systems. Such drugs are used for contraception, to treat infertility, as sex hormone replacement and in obstetric practice to influence labour. They are also used to influence lifestyle (Ch. 59). The principle of negative feedback is stressed and is central to understanding how hormones interact to control reproduction[1] – many drugs, including agents used to prevent or assist conception, work by influencing negative feedback mechanisms. The chapter concludes with a short section on erectile dysfunction.

ENDOCRINE CONTROL OF REPRODUCTION

Hormonal control of the reproductive systems in men and women involves sex steroids from the gonads, hypothalamic mediators including the decapeptide gonadotrophin-releasing hormone (GnRH), and glycoprotein gonadotrophins from the anterior pituitary gland (Ch. 34). Kisspeptin, a protein that is a G protein–coupled receptor ligand for a receptor known as GPR54, initiates secretion of GnRH at puberty. GnRH is released from the hypothalamus to act on the anterior pituitary triggering the release of luteinising hormone (LH), and follicle-stimulating hormone (FSH). These gonadotrophic hormones control sexual maturation and gametogenesis. Kisspeptin has been linked with sexual bonding. Neurokinin B (NKB, Ch. 19) is also implicated in

controlling the secretion of GnRH in humans, with possible roles in pregnancy, sexual maturation and the menopause. It is present, together with kisspeptin and dynorphin, in the arcuate nucleus of the hypothalamus where these mediators are implicated in generating pulsatile release of GnRH. NKB is implicated in menopausal flushing and NK3 receptor block has reduced such flushing (Prague et al., 2017).

Anti-Müllerian hormone (AMH) is a glycoprotein which controls sexual development in the fetus and follicle formation in adult women (Behringer, 1994). It is activated at a specific time in the male fetus and inhibits the development of the female reproductive tract (Müllerian ducts) in the male embryo. AMH is also produced in adult women, regulating follicle formation in the ovaries. It is produced by granulosa cells, which surround the eggs, and is a biomarker of ovarian reserve and in disorders such as polycystic ovary syndrome.

NEUROHORMONAL CONTROL OF THE FEMALE REPRODUCTIVE SYSTEM

Increased secretion of hypothalamic and anterior pituitary hormones occurs in girls at puberty and stimulates secretion of oestrogen from the ovaries. This causes maturation of the reproductive organs and development of secondary sexual characteristics, and also accelerated growth followed by closure of the epiphyses of the long bones. Sex steroids, *oestrogens* and *progesterone*, are thereafter involved in the menstrual cycle, and in pregnancy. A simplified outline is given in Figs 36.1 and 36.2.

The menstrual cycle begins with menstruation, which lasts for 3–6 days, during which the superficial layer of uterine endometrium is shed. The endometrium regenerates during the follicular phase of the cycle after menstrual flow has stopped. A releasing factor, GnRH, is secreted from peptidergic neurons in the hypothalamus which discharge in a pulsatile fashion, approximately one burst per hour. GnRH stimulates the anterior pituitary to release gonadotrophic hormones (see Fig. 36.1) – FSH and LH. These act on the ovaries to promote development of small groups of follicles, each of which contains an ovum. One follicle develops faster than the others and forms the Graafian follicle (see Figs 36.1 and 36.2E), which secretes oestrogens, and the rest degenerate. The ripening Graafian follicle consists of thecal and granulosa cells surrounding a fluid-filled core, within which lies an ovum. Oestrogens are responsible for the proliferative phase of endometrial regeneration, which occurs from day 5 or 6 until mid-cycle (see Fig. 36.2B and F). During this phase, the endometrium increases in thickness and vascularity, and at the peak of oestrogen secretion there is a prolific cervical secretion of mucus of pH 8–9, rich in protein and carbohydrate, which facilitates entry of spermatozoa. Oestrogen has a negative feedback effect on the anterior pituitary, decreasing gonadotrophin

---

[1]Recognition that negative feedback is central to endocrine control was a profound insight, made in 1930 by Dorothy Price, a laboratory assistant in the University of Chicago experimenting on effects of testosterone in rats. She referred to it as 'reciprocal influence' and it helps in understanding how many reproductive hormones seem, confusingly, to cause both an effect and its opposite if given in different doses or over different time courses.

Fig. 36.1 Hormonal control of the female reproductive system. The Graafian follicle (GF) is shown developing on the *left*, then involuting to form the corpus luteum (CL) on the right, after the ovum (●) has been released. *FSH*, follicle-stimulating hormone; *GnRH*, gonadotrophin-releasing hormone; *LH*, luteinising hormone.

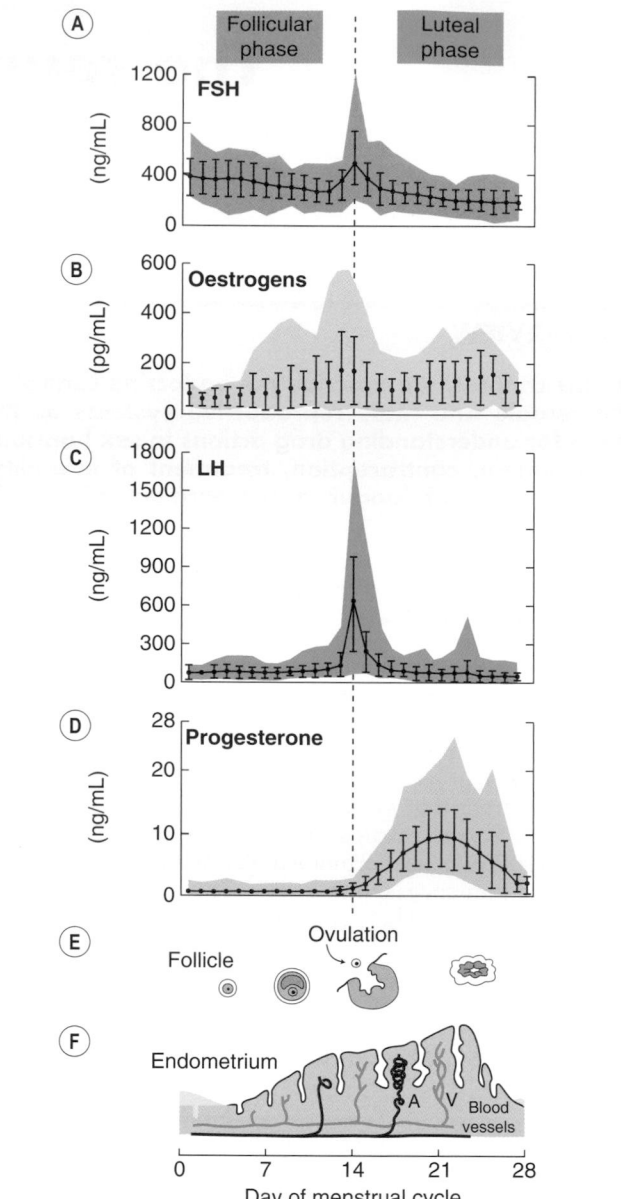

Fig. 36.2 Plasma concentrations of ovarian hormones and gonadotrophins in women during normal menstrual cycles. Values are the mean ± standard deviation of 40 women. The *shaded areas* indicate the entire range of observations. Day 1 is the onset of menstruation. Mean plasma hormone concentrations (A–D) are shown in relation to day of menstrual cycle. (E and F) show diagrammatically the changes in the ovarian follicle and the endometrium during the cycle. Ovulation on day 14 of the menstrual cycle occurs with the mid-cycle peak of luteinising hormone (LH), represented by the *vertical dashed line*. A, arterioles; *FSH*, follicle-stimulating hormone; *V*, venules. (After van de Wiele, R. L., Dyrenfurth, I. 1974. Pharmacol. Rev. 25, 189–217.)

release during chronic administration of oestrogen as oral contraception (see pp. 463–464). In contrast, the spike of endogenous oestrogen secretion just before mid-cycle sensitises LH-releasing cells of the pituitary to the action of the GnRH and causes the mid-cycle surge of LH secretion (see Fig. 36.2C). This, in turn, causes rapid swelling and rupture of the Graafian follicle, resulting in ovulation. If fertilisation occurs, the fertilised ovum passes down the fallopian tubes to the uterus, starting to divide as it goes.

Stimulated by LH, cells of the ruptured follicle proliferate and develop into the *corpus luteum*, which secretes progesterone. Progesterone acts, in turn, on oestrogen-primed endometrium, stimulating the secretory phase of the cycle, which renders the endometrium suitable for the implantation of a fertilised ovum. During this phase, cervical mucus becomes more viscous, less alkaline, less copious and in general less welcoming for sperm. Progesterone exerts negative feedback on the hypothalamus and pituitary, decreasing the release of LH. It also has a thermogenic effect, causing a rise in body temperature of about 0.5°C at ovulation, which is maintained until the end of the cycle.

If implantation of a fertilised ovum does not occur, progesterone secretion stops, triggering menstruation. If implantation does occur the corpus luteum continues to secrete progesterone which, by its effect on the hypothalamus and anterior pituitary, prevents further ovulation. The chorion (an antecedent of the placenta) secretes human chorionic gonadotrophin (HCG), which maintains the lining of the uterus during pregnancy. For reasons that are not

physiologically obvious, HCG has an additional pharmacological action, exploited therapeutically in treating infertility (see p. 463), of stimulating ovulation. As pregnancy proceeds, the placenta develops further hormonal functions and secretes a variety of hormones, including gonadotrophins, progesterone and oestrogens. Progesterone secreted

Fig. 36.3 The biosynthetic pathway for the androgens and oestrogens, with sites of drug action. (See also Fig. 34.5.) Finasteride is used in benign prostatic hyperplasia, and anastrozole to treat breast cancer in postmenopausal women.

during pregnancy controls the development of the secretory alveoli in the mammary gland, while oestrogen stimulates the lactiferous ducts. After parturition oestrogen, along with prolactin (see Ch. 34), is responsible for stimulating and maintaining lactation, whereas supraphysiological doses of oestrogen suppress lactation.

Oestrogens, progestogens (progesterone-like drugs), androgens and the gonadotrophins are described below – see Fig. 36.3 for biosynthetic pathways.

Hormonal control of the female reproductive system

- The menstrual cycle starts with menstruation.
- Gonadotrophin-releasing hormone, released from the hypothalamus, acts on the anterior pituitary to release follicle-stimulating hormone (FSH) and luteinising hormone (LH).
- FSH and LH stimulate follicle development in the ovary. FSH is the main hormone stimulating oestrogen release. LH stimulates ovulation at mid-cycle and is the main hormone controlling subsequent progesterone secretion from the corpus luteum.
- Oestrogen controls the proliferative phase of the endometrium and has negative feedback effects on the anterior pituitary. Progesterone controls the later secretory phase, and has negative feedback effects on both the hypothalamus and anterior pituitary.
- If a fertilised ovum is implanted, the corpus luteum continues to secrete progesterone.
- After implantation, human chorionic gonadotrophin (HCG) from the chorion becomes important, and later in pregnancy progesterone, HCG and other hormones are secreted by the placenta.

Fig. 36.4 Hormonal control of the male reproductive system. *FSH*, follicle-stimulating hormone; *GnRH*, gonadotrophin-releasing hormone; *ICSH*, interstitial cell-stimulating hormone.

NEUROHORMONAL CONTROL OF THE MALE REPRODUCTIVE SYSTEM

As in women, hypothalamic, anterior pituitary and gonadal hormones control the male reproductive system.

A simplified outline is given in Fig. 36.4. GnRH controls the secretion of gonadotrophins by the anterior pituitary. This secretion is not cyclical as in menstruating women, although it is pulsatile in both sexes, as with other anterior pituitary hormones (see Ch. 34). FSH is responsible for the integrity of the seminiferous tubules, and after puberty is important in gametogenesis through an action on Sertoli cells, which nourish and support developing spermatozoa. LH, which in the male is also called *interstitial cell-stimulating hormone* (ICSH), stimulates the interstitial cells (Leydig cells) to secrete androgens – in particular *testosterone.* LH/ICSH secretion begins at puberty, and the consequent secretion of testosterone causes maturation of the reproductive organs and development of secondary sexual characteristics. Thereafter, the primary function of testosterone is the maintenance of spermatogenesis and hence fertility – an action mediated by Sertoli cells. Testosterone is also important in the maturation of spermatozoa as they pass through the epididymis and vas deferens. A further action is a feedback effect on the anterior pituitary, modulating its sensitivity to GnRH and thus influencing secretion of LH/ICSH. Testosterone has marked anabolic effects, causing development of the musculature and increased bone growth which results in the pubertal growth spurt, followed by closure of the epiphyses of the long bones.

Secretion of testosterone is mainly controlled by LH/ICSH, but FSH also plays a part, possibly by releasing a factor similar to GnRH from the Sertoli cells which are its primary target. The interstitial cells that synthesise testosterone also have receptors for prolactin, which may influence testosterone production by increasing the number of receptors for LH/ICSH.

BEHAVIOURAL EFFECTS OF SEX HORMONES

As well as controlling the menstrual cycle, sex steroids affect sexual behaviour. Two types of control are recognised: *organisational* and *activational*.

Organisational control refers to the fact that sexual differentiation of the brain can be permanently altered by the presence or absence of sex steroids at key stages in development. In rats, administration of androgens to females within a few days of birth results in long-term virilisation of behaviour. Conversely, neonatal castration of male rats causes them to develop behaviourally as females. Brain development in the absence of sex steroids follows female lines, but is switched to the male pattern by exposure of the hypothalamus to androgen at a key stage of development. Similar but less complete behavioural virilisation of female offspring has been demonstrated following androgen administration in non-human primates, and probably also occurs in humans if pregnant women are exposed to excessive androgen.

The *activational* effect of sex steroids refers to their ability to modify sexual behaviour after brain development is complete. In general, oestrogens and androgens increase sexual activity in the appropriate sex. **Oxytocin**, which is important during parturition (see pp. 465–466), also has roles in mating and parenting behaviours, its action in the central nervous system being regulated by oestrogen (see Ch. 34).

DRUGS AFFECTING REPRODUCTIVE FUNCTION

OESTROGENS

Oestrogens are synthesised by the ovary and placenta, and in small amounts by the testis and adrenal cortex. The starting substance for synthesis of oestrogen and other steroids is cholesterol. The immediate precursors to the oestrogens are androgenic substances – androstenedione or testosterone (see Fig. 36.3). There are three main endogenous oestrogens in humans: *oestradiol, oestrone* and *oestriol* (see Fig. 36.3). Oestradiol is the most potent and is

the principal oestrogen secreted by the ovary. At the beginning of the menstrual cycle, the plasma concentration is 0.2 nmol/L, rising to ~2.2 nmol/L in mid-cycle.

Actions

Oestrogen acts in concert with progesterone, and induces synthesis of progesterone receptors in uterus, vagina, anterior pituitary and hypothalamus. Conversely, progesterone decreases oestrogen receptor expression in the reproductive tract. *Prolactin* (see Ch. 34) also influences oestrogen action by increasing the numbers of oestrogen receptors in the mammary gland, but has no effect on oestrogen receptor expression in the uterus.

Effects of exogenous oestrogen in females depend on the state of sexual maturity when the oestrogen is administered:

- *In primary hypogonadism:* oestrogen stimulates development of secondary sexual characteristics and accelerates growth.
- *In adults with primary amenorrhoea:* oestrogen, given cyclically with a progestogen, induces an artificial cycle.
- *In sexually mature women:* oestrogen (with a progestogen) is contraceptive.
- *At or after the menopause:* oestrogen replacement prevents menopausal symptoms and bone loss.

Oestrogens have several metabolic actions, including mineralocorticoid (retention of salt and water) and mild anabolic actions. They increase plasma concentrations of high-density lipoproteins, a potentially beneficial effect (Ch. 24) that may contribute to the relatively low risk of atheromatous disease in premenopausal women compared with men of the same age. However, oestrogens also increase the coagulability of blood, and increase the risk of thromboembolism.

Mechanism of action

Oestrogen binds to nuclear receptors, as do other steroid hormones (Ch. 3). There are at least two types of oestrogen receptor, termed ERα and ERβ. Binding is followed by interaction of the resultant complexes with nuclear sites and subsequent genomic effects. In addition to these 'classic' intracellular receptors, some oestrogen effects, in particular its rapid vascular actions, are initiated by interaction with membrane receptors, including a G protein–coupled oestrogen receptor (GPER), which was cloned from vascular endothelial cells and plays a part in regulating vascular tone and cell growth as well as lipid and glucose homeostasis (Barton & Prossnitz, 2015). Acute vasodilatation caused by 17-β-oestradiol is mediated by nitric oxide, and a plant-derived (phyto-) oestrogen called genistein (which is selective for ERβ, as well as having quite distinct effects due to inhibition of protein kinase C) is as potent as 17-β-oestradiol in this regard (Walker et al., 2001). Oestrogen receptor modulators (receptor-selective oestrogen agonists or antagonists) are mentioned later.

Preparations

Many preparations (oral, transdermal, intramuscular, implantable and topical) of oestrogens are available for a wide range of indications. These include natural (e.g. **oestradiol**, **oestriol**) and synthetic (e.g. **mestranol**, **ethinylestradiol**, **diethylstilbestrol**) oestrogens. Oestrogens are presented either as single agents or combined with progestogen.

Pharmacokinetic aspects

Natural and synthetic oestrogens are well absorbed in the gastrointestinal (GI) tract, but after absorption the natural oestrogens are rapidly metabolised in the liver, whereas synthetic oestrogens are degraded less rapidly. There is variable enterohepatic cycling. Most oestrogens are readily absorbed from skin and mucous membranes. They may be given as intravaginal creams or pessaries for local effect. In the plasma, natural oestrogens are bound to albumin and to a sex steroid-binding globulin. Natural oestrogens are excreted in the urine as glucuronides and sulfates.

Unwanted effects

Unwanted effects of oestrogens range from the common and tiresome to the life-threatening but rare: breast tenderness, nausea, vomiting, anorexia, retention of salt and water with resultant oedema, and increased risk of thromboembolism. More details of the unwanted effects of oral contraceptives are given later.

Used intermittently for postmenopausal replacement therapy, oestrogens cause menstruation-like bleeding. Oestrogen causes endometrial hyperplasia unless given cyclically with a progestogen. When administered to males, oestrogens result in feminisation.

There is current concern regarding environmental effects of oestrogens, including various pesticides that act on oestrogen receptors as well as oestrogens excreted in urine. Either of these sources of oestrogen can pollute groundwater and damage aquatic wildlife as well as posing risks to human health (Adeel et al., 2017; McLachlan, 2016).

Oestrogen administration to pregnant women can cause genital abnormalities in their offspring: carcinoma of the vagina was more common in young women whose mothers were given diethylstilbestrol in early pregnancy in a misguided attempt to prevent miscarriage (see Ch. 58).

The clinical uses of oestrogens and antioestrogens are summarised in the box (p. 460). In addition, see the section later on postmenopausal hormone replacement therapy (HRT).

OESTROGEN RECEPTOR MODULATORS

Raloxifene, a 'selective [o]estrogen receptor modulator' (SERM), has anti-oestrogenic effects on breast and uterus but oestrogenic effects on bone, lipid metabolism and blood coagulation. It is used for prevention and treatment of postmenopausal osteoporosis (Ch. 37) and reduces the incidence of oestrogen receptor-positive breast cancer similarly to **tamoxifen** but with fewer adverse events (Barrett-Connor et al., 2006; Vogel et al., 2006). The US FDA has supported its use to reduce the risk of invasive breast cancer in postmenopausal women with osteoporosis and in postmenopausal women at high risk for invasive breast cancer. Unlike oestrogen, it does not prevent menopausal flushes.

Tamoxifen has an antioestrogenic action on mammary tissue but oestrogenic actions on plasma lipids, endometrium and bone. It produces mild oestrogen-like adverse effects consistent with partial agonist activity. The tamoxifen–oestrogen receptor complex does not readily dissociate, so there is interference with the recycling of receptors.

Tamoxifen upregulates transforming growth factor-β (TGF-β), a cytokine that retards the progression of malignancy, and that also has a role in controlling the balance between bone-producing osteoblasts and bone-resorbing osteoclasts (Ch. 37).

The use of tamoxifen to treat and prevent breast cancer is discussed further in Chapter 57.

ANTIOESTROGENS

Antioestrogens compete with natural oestrogens for receptors in target organs; in addition to SERMs (raloxifene, tamoxifen), which are partial agonists in some tissues and antagonists in others, there are drugs that are pure oestrogen receptor antagonists.

Clomiphene inhibits oestrogen binding in the anterior pituitary, so preventing negative feedback and acutely increasing secretion of GnRH and gonadotrophins. This stimulates and enlarges the ovaries, increases oestrogen secretion and induces ovulation. It is used in treating infertility caused by lack of ovulation. Twins are common, but multiple pregnancy is unusual.

See the clinical box on oestrogens and antioestrogens for a summary of clinical uses.

PROGESTOGENS

The natural progestational hormone (progestogen) is *progesterone* (see Figs 36.2 and 36.3). This is secreted by the corpus luteum in the second part of the menstrual cycle, and by the placenta during pregnancy. Small amounts are also secreted by the testis and adrenal cortex.

Progestogens act, as do other steroid hormones, on nuclear receptors. The density of progesterone receptors is controlled by oestrogens (see p. 458).

Preparations

There are two main groups of progestogens:

1. The naturally occurring hormone and its derivatives (e.g. **hydroxyprogesterone**, **medroxyprogesterone**, **dydrogesterone**). Progesterone itself is virtually inactive orally, because of presystemic hepatic metabolism. Other derivatives are available for oral administration, intramuscular injection or administration via the vagina or rectum.
2. Testosterone derivatives (e.g. **norethisterone**, **norgestrel** and **ethynodiol**) can be given orally. The first two have some androgenic activity and are metabolised to give oestrogenic products. Newer progestogens used in contraception include **desogestrel** and **gestodene**; they may have fewer adverse effects on lipids than ethynodiol and may be considered for women who experience side effects such as acne, depression or breakthrough bleeding with the older drugs. However, these newer drugs have been associated with higher risks of venous thromboembolic disease (see later).

Actions

The pharmacological actions of the progestogens are in essence the same as the physiological actions of progesterone described previously. Specific effects relevant to contraception are detailed later.

Pharmacokinetic aspects

Injected progesterone is bound to albumin, not to the sex steroid-binding globulin. Some is stored in adipose tissue. It is metabolised in the liver, and the products, pregnanolone

Clinical uses of progestogens are summarised in the next box.

ANTIPROGESTOGENS

Mifepristone is a partial agonist at progesterone receptors. It sensitises the uterus to the action of prostaglandins. It is given orally and has a plasma half-life of 21 h. Mifepristone is used, in combination with a prostaglandin (e.g. **gemeprost**; see p. 466), as a medical alternative to surgical termination of pregnancy (see clinical box).

Oestrogens and antioestrogens

- The endogenous oestrogens are oestradiol (the most potent), oestrone and oestriol; there are numerous exogenous synthetic forms (e.g. **ethinylestradiol**).
- Mechanism of action involves interaction with nuclear receptors (ERα or ERβ) in target tissues, resulting in modification of gene transcription. Some of the rapid vascular and metabolic effects of oestrogens are mediated by a G protein–coupled [o]estrogen receptor (GPER).
- Their pharmacological effects depend on the sexual maturity of the recipient:
  - before puberty, they stimulate development of secondary sexual characteristics;
  - given cyclically in the female adult, they induce an artificial menstrual cycle and are used for contraception;
  - given at or after the menopause, they prevent menopausal symptoms and protect against osteoporosis, but increase thromboembolism.
- Antioestrogens are competitive antagonists or partial agonists. **Tamoxifen** is used in oestrogen-dependent breast cancer. **Clomiphene** induces ovulation by inhibiting the negative feedback effects on the hypothalamus and anterior pituitary.
- Selective modulators of the oestrogen receptor are oestrogen agonists in some tissues but antagonists in others. **Raloxifene** (one such drug) is used to treat and prevent osteoporosis.

Clinical uses of oestrogens and antioestrogens

Oestrogens
- Replacement therapy:
  - primary ovarian failure (e.g. Turner's syndrome);
  - secondary ovarian failure (menopause) for flushing, vaginal dryness and to preserve bone mass.
- Contraception.
- Prostate and breast cancer (these uses have largely been superseded by other hormonal manipulations; see Ch. 57).

Antioestrogens
- To treat oestrogen-sensitive breast cancer (**tamoxifen**).
- To induce ovulation (**clomiphene**) in treating infertility.

and pregnanediol, are conjugated with glucuronic acid and excreted in the urine.

Unwanted effects
Unwanted effects of progestogens include weak androgenic actions. Other unwanted effects include acne, fluid retention, weight change, depression, change in libido, breast discomfort, premenstrual symptoms, irregular menstrual cycles and breakthrough bleeding. There is an increased incidence of thromboembolism.

Progestogens and antiprogestogens

- The endogenous hormone is progesterone. Examples of synthetic drugs are the progesterone derivative **medroxyprogesterone** and the testosterone derivative **norethisterone**.
- Mechanism of action involves intracellular receptor/altered gene expression. Oestrogen stimulates synthesis of progesterone receptors, whereas progesterone inhibits synthesis of oestrogen receptors.
- Main therapeutic uses are in oral contraception and oestrogen replacement regimens, and to treat endometriosis.
- The antiprogestogen **mifepristone**, in combination with prostaglandin analogues, is an effective medical alternative to surgical termination of early pregnancy.

Clinical uses of progestogens and antiprogestogens

Progestogens
- Contraception:
  - with **oestrogen** in *combined oral contraceptive pill*;
  - as *progesterone-only contraceptive pill*;
  - as *injectable* or *implantable* progesterone-only contraception;
  - as part of an *intrauterine* contraceptive system.
- Combined with **oestrogen** for *oestrogen replacement therapy* in women with an intact uterus, to prevent endometrial hyperplasia and carcinoma.
- For *endometriosis*.
- In *endometrial carcinoma*; use in breast and renal cancer has declined.
- Poorly validated uses have included various menstrual disorders.

Antiprogestogens
- Medical termination of pregnancy: **mifepristone** (partial agonist) combined with a prostaglandin (e.g. **gemeprost**).

POSTMENOPAUSAL HORMONE REPLACEMENT THERAPY (HRT)

At the menopause, whether natural or surgically induced, ovarian function decreases and oestrogen levels fall. There is a long history of disagreement regarding the pros and cons of HRT in this context, with the prevailing wisdom undergoing several revisions over the years (see Davis et al., 2005). HRT normally involves the cyclic or continuous administration of low doses of one or more oestrogens, with or without a progestogen. Short-term HRT has some clear-cut benefits:

- improvement of symptoms caused by reduced oestrogen, for example, hot flushes and vaginal dryness;
- prevention and treatment of osteoporosis, but other drugs are usually preferable for this (Ch. 37).

Oestrogen replacement does not reduce the risk of coronary heart disease, despite earlier hopes, nor is there evidence that it reduces age-related decline in cognitive function. Drawbacks include:

- cyclical withdrawal bleeding;
- adverse effects related to progestogen (see later);
- increased risk of endometrial cancer if oestrogen is given unopposed by progestogen;
- increased risk of breast cancer, related to the duration of HRT use and disappearing within 5 years of stopping;
- increased risk of venous thromboembolism (risk approximately doubled in women using combined HRT for 5 years).

The web links in the reference list provide best estimates of risks of cancer (breast, endometrium, ovary), venous thromboembolism, stroke and coronary artery disease in relation to age and duration of HRT use.

Oestrogens used in HRT can be given orally (conjugated oestrogens, oestradiol, oestriol), vaginally (oestriol), by transdermal patch (oestradiol) or by subcutaneous implant (oestradiol). **Tibolone** is marketed for the short-term treatment of symptoms of oestrogen deficiency and for postmenopausal prophylaxis of osteoporosis in women at high risk of fracture when other prophylaxis is contraindicated or not tolerated. It has oestrogenic, progestogenic and weak androgenic activity, and can be used continuously without cyclical progesterone (avoiding the inconvenience of withdrawal bleeding).

ANDROGENS

Testosterone is the main natural androgen. It is synthesised mainly by the interstitial cells of the testis, and in smaller amounts by the ovaries and adrenal cortex. Adrenal androgen production is influenced by adrenocorticotrophic hormone (ACTH, corticotrophin). As for other steroid hormones, cholesterol is the starting substance. Dehydroepiandrosterone and androstenedione are important intermediates. They are released from the gonads and the adrenal cortex, and converted to testosterone in the liver (see Fig. 36.3).

Actions

In general, the effects of exogenous androgens are the same as those of testosterone, and depend on the age and sex of the recipient. If prepubertal boys are given androgens, they do not reach their full predicted height because of premature closure of the epiphyses of the long bones. In boys at the age of puberty, there is rapid development of secondary sexual characteristics (i.e. growth of facial, axillary and pubic hair, deepening of the voice), maturation of the reproductive organs and a marked increase in muscular strength. There is a growth spurt with an acceleration in the usual increase in height that occurs year on year in younger children, followed by fusion of the bony epiphyses and cessation of linear growth. In adults, the anabolic effects can be accompanied by retention of salt and water. The skin thickens and may darken, and sebaceous glands become more active, predisposing to acne. Body weight and muscle mass increase, partly due to water retention. Androgens cause a feeling of well-being and an increase in physical vigour, and may increase libido. Whether they are responsible for sexual behaviour as such is controversial, as is their contribution to aggressive behaviour. Paradoxically, testosterone administration inhibits spermatogenesis, so reducing male fertility.

Mechanism of action

In most target cells, testosterone works through an active metabolite, dihydrotestosterone, to which it is converted locally by a 5α-reductase enzyme. In contrast, testosterone itself causes virilisation of the genital tract in the male embryo and regulates LH/ICSH production in anterior pituitary cells. Testosterone and dihydrotestosterone modify gene transcription by interacting with nuclear receptors.

Preparations

Testosterone itself can be given by subcutaneous implantation or by transdermal patches (male replacement dose approximately 2.5 mg/day). Various esters (e.g. enanthate and propionate) are given by intramuscular depot injection. Testosterone undecanoate and mesterolone can be given orally.

Pharmacokinetic aspects

If given orally, testosterone is rapidly metabolised in the liver. Virtually all testosterone in the circulation is bound to plasma protein – mainly to the sex steroid-binding globulin. Approximately 90% of endogenous testosterone is eliminated as metabolites. The elimination half-life of the free hormone is short (10–20 min). It is converted in the liver to androstenedione (see Fig. 36.3), which has weak androgenic activity. Synthetic androgens are less rapidly metabolised, and some are excreted in the urine unchanged.

Unwanted effects

Unwanted effects of androgens include decreased gonadotrophin release during continued use, with resultant male infertility,[2] and salt and water retention leading to oedema. Adenocarcinoma of the liver has been reported. Androgens impair growth in children (via premature fusion of epiphyses), cause acne and lead to masculinisation in girls. Adverse effects of testosterone replacement and monitoring for these are reviewed by Rhoden and Morgentaler (2004).

The clinical uses of androgens are given in the clinical box.

ANABOLIC STEROIDS

Androgens can be modified chemically to alter the balance of anabolic and other effects. 'Anabolic steroids' (e.g. **nandrolone**) increase protein synthesis and muscle development disproportionately, but clinical use (e.g. in debilitating or muscle wasting disease) has been disappointing. They

---

[2]Large doses of androgens also adversely affect female fertility, but physiological concentrations of androgen are now believed to be important for female fertility (Prizant et al., 2014)

Androgens and the hormonal control of the male reproductive system

- Gonadotrophin-releasing hormone from the hypothalamus acts on the anterior pituitary to release both follicle-stimulating hormone, which stimulates gametogenesis, and luteinising hormone (also called interstitial cell-stimulating hormone), which stimulates androgen secretion.
- The endogenous hormone is testosterone; intramuscular depot injections of testosterone esters are used for replacement therapy.
- Mechanism of action is via intracellular receptors.
- Effects depend on age/sex, and include development of male secondary sexual characteristics in prepubertal boys and masculinisation in women.

Clinical uses of androgens and anti-androgens

- Androgens (**testosterone** preparations) as hormone replacement in:
  - male hypogonadism due to pituitary or testicular disease (e.g. 50–100 mg per day as gel applied to the skin)
- Anti-androgens (e.g. **flutamide**, **cyproterone**) are used as part of the treatment of prostatic cancer.
- 5α-Reductase inhibitors (e.g. **finasteride**) are used in benign prostatic hyperplasia.

are used in the therapy of aplastic anaemia and (notoriously) abused by some athletes (Ch. 59), as is testosterone itself. Unwanted effects are described above, under Androgens. In addition, cholestatic jaundice, liver tumours and increased risk of coronary heart disease are recognised adverse effects of high-dose anabolic steroids.

ANTI-ANDROGENS

Both oestrogens and progestogens have anti-androgen activity, oestrogens mainly by inhibiting gonadotrophin secretion and progestogens by competing at androgen receptors in target organs. **Cyproterone** is a derivative of progesterone and has weak progestational activity. It is a partial agonist at androgen receptors, competing with dihydrotestosterone for receptors in androgen-sensitive target tissues. Through its effect in the hypothalamus, it depresses the synthesis of gonadotrophins. It is used as an adjunct in the treatment of prostatic cancer during initiation of GnRH agonist treatment (see later). It is also used in the therapy of precocious puberty in males, and of masculinisation and acne in women. It also has a central nervous system effect, decreasing libido, and has been used to treat hypersexuality in male sexual offenders.[3]

Flutamide is a non-steroidal anti-androgen used with GnRH agonists in the treatment of prostate cancer.

Drugs can have anti-androgen action by inhibiting synthetic enzymes. **Finasteride** inhibits the enzyme (5α-reductase) that converts testosterone to dihydro-testosterone (see Fig. 36.3). This active metabolite has greater affinity than testosterone for androgen receptors in the prostate gland. Finasteride is well absorbed after oral administration, has a half-life of about 7 h, and is excreted in the urine and faeces. It is used to treat benign prostatic hyperplasia, although α₁-adrenoceptor antagonists, for example, **terazosin** or **tamsulosin** (Chs 15 and 30), are more effective (working by the entirely different mechanism of relaxing smooth muscle in the capsule of the prostate gland and opposing α₁-adrenoceptor-mediated prostatic growth). Surgery is another option.

GONADOTROPHIN-RELEASING HORMONE: AGONISTS AND ANTAGONISTS

GnRH (previously known as luteinising hormone-releasing hormone, LHRH) is a decapeptide that controls the secretion of FSH and LH by the anterior pituitary. Secretion of GnRH is controlled by neural input from other parts of the brain, and through negative feedback by the sex steroids (Figs 36.1 and 36.5). Exogenous androgens, oestrogens and progestogens all inhibit GnRH secretion, but only progestogens exert this effect at doses that do not have marked hormonal actions on peripheral tissues, presumably because progesterone receptors in the reproductive tract are sparse unless they have been induced by previous exposure to oestrogen. **Danazol** (see later) is a synthetic steroid that inhibits release of GnRH and, consequently, of gonadotrophins (FSH and LH). **Clomifene** is an oestrogen antagonist that stimulates gonadotrophin release by inhibiting the negative feedback effects of endogenous oestrogen; it is used to treat infertility (see clinical box, p. 460, and Fig. 36.5).

Synthetic GnRH is termed **gonadorelin**. Numerous analogues of GnRH, both agonists and antagonists, have

Fig. 36.5 Regulation of gonadotrophin (follicle-stimulating hormone, FSH; luteinising hormone, LH) release from the anterior pituitary. *GnRHR*, gonadotrophin-releasing hormone receptor.

---

[3]Very different doses are used for these different conditions, for example, 2 mg/day for acne, 100 mg/day for hypersexuality and 300 mg/day for prostatic cancer.

been synthesised. **Buserelin, leuprorelin, goserelin** and **nafarelin** are agonists, the last being 200 times more potent than endogenous GnRH.

Pharmacokinetics and clinical use

GnRH agonists, given by subcutaneous infusion in pulses to mimic physiological secretion of GnRH, stimulate gonadotrophin release (see Fig. 36.5) and induce ovulation. They are absorbed intact following nasal administration (Ch. 9). Continuous use, by nasal spray or as depot preparations, stimulates gonadotrophin release transiently, but then paradoxically inhibits gonadotrophin release (see Fig. 36.5) because of down-regulation (desensitisation) of GnRH receptors in the pituitary. GnRH analogues are given in this fashion to cause gonadal suppression in various sex hormone-dependent conditions, including prostate and breast cancers, endometriosis (endometrial tissue outside the uterine cavity) and large uterine fibroids. Continuous, non-pulsatile administration inhibits spermatogenesis and ovulation. GnRH agonists are used by specialists in infertility treatment, not to stimulate ovulation (which is achieved using gonadotrophin preparations) but to suppress the pituitary before administration of FSH or HCG.

Unwanted effects of GnRH analogues

Unwanted effects of GnRH agonists in women, for example, flushing, vaginal dryness and bone loss, result from hypo-oestrogenism. The initial stimulation of gonadotrophin secretion on starting treatment can transiently worsen pain from bone metastases in men with prostate cancer, so treatment is started only after the patient has received an androgen receptor antagonist such as **flutamide** (see earlier and Ch. 57).

DANAZOL

Actions and pharmacokinetics

Danazol inhibits gonadotrophin secretion (especially the mid-cycle surge), and consequently reduces oestrogen synthesis in the ovary (see Fig. 36.5). In men, it reduces androgen synthesis and spermatogenesis. It has androgenic activity. It is orally active and metabolised in the liver.

Danazol is used in sex hormone-dependent conditions including endometriosis, breast dysplasia (benign breast lumps) and gynaecomastia. An additional special use is to reduce attacks of swelling in hereditary angio-oedema (Ch. 29).

Unwanted effects are common, and include GI disturbances, weight gain, fluid retention, dizziness, menopausal symptoms, muscle cramps and headache. Danazol is virilising in women.

GONADOTROPHINS AND ANALOGUES

Gonadotrophins (FSH, LH and HCG) are glycoproteins produced and secreted by the anterior pituitary (FSH and LH, see Ch. 34) or chorion and placenta (HCG). Large amounts of gonadotrophins are present in the urine of women following the menopause, in whom oestrogen no longer exerts feedback inhibition on the pituitary, which consequently secretes large amounts of FSH and LH.[4]

Preparations

Gonadotrophins are extracted from urine of pregnant (HCG) or postmenopausal women (human menopausal gonadotrophin, which contains a mixture of FSH and LH). Recombinant FSH (**follitropin**) and LH (**lutropin**) are also available.

Pharmacokinetics and clinical use

Gonadotrophin preparations are given by injection. They are used to treat infertility caused by lack of ovulation as a result of hypopituitarism, or following failure of treatment with **clomiphene**; they are also used by specialists to induce ovulation to enable eggs to be collected for in vitro fertilisation. For this use, gonadotrophin is usually administered after secretion of endogenous FSH and LH has been suppressed (see p. 463). Gonadotrophins are also sometimes used in men with infertility caused by a low sperm count as a result of hypogonadotrophic hypogonadism (a disorder that is sometimes accompanied by lifelong anosmia, i.e. lack of sense of smell). (Gonadotrophins do not, of course, work for patients whose low sperm count is the result of primary testicular failure.) HCG has been used to stimulate testosterone synthesis in boys with delayed puberty, but testosterone is usually preferred.

> ## Gonadotrophin-releasing hormone and gonadotrophins
>
> - Gonadotrophin-releasing hormone is a decapeptide; **gonadorelin** is the synthetic form. **Nafarelin** is a potent analogue.
> - Given in pulsatile fashion, they stimulate gonadotrophin release; given continuously, they inhibit it.
> - The gonadotrophins, follicle-stimulating hormone and luteinising hormone, are glycoproteins.
> - Preparations of gonadotrophins (e.g. chorionic gonadotrophin) are used to treat infertility caused by failure of ovulation.
> - **Danazol** is a modified progestogen that inhibits gonadotrophin production by actions on the hypothalamus and anterior pituitary.

DRUGS USED FOR CONTRACEPTION

ORAL CONTRACEPTIVES

There are two main types of oral contraceptives:

1. Combinations of an oestrogen with a progestogen (the combined pill).
2. Progestogen alone (the progestogen-only pill).

THE COMBINED PILL

The combined oral contraceptive pill is extremely effective, at least in the absence of intercurrent illness and of treatment with potentially interacting drugs (see p. 464). The oestrogen in most combined preparations (second-generation pills)[5] is **ethinylestradiol**, although a few preparations contain

---

[4]This forms the basis for the standard blood test, estimation of plasma LH/FSH concentrations, to confirm whether a woman is postmenopausal.

[5]The first-generation pills, containing more than 50 µg of oestrogen, were shown in the 1970s to be associated with an increased risk of deep vein thrombosis and pulmonary embolism.

mestranol instead. The progestogen may be **norethisterone**, **levonorgestrel**, **ethynodiol**, or – in 'third-generation' pills – **desogestrel** or **gestodene**, which are more potent, have less androgenic action and cause less change in lipoprotein metabolism, but which probably cause a greater risk of thromboembolism than do second-generation preparations. The oestrogen content is generally 20–50 μg of ethinylestradiol or its equivalent, and a preparation is chosen with the lowest oestrogen and progestogen content that is well tolerated and gives good cycle control. This combined pill is taken for 21 consecutive days followed by 7 pill-free days, which causes a withdrawal bleed. Normal cycles of menstruation usually commence fairly soon after discontinuing treatment, and permanent loss of fertility (which may be a result of early menopause rather than a long-term consequence of the contraceptive pill) is rare.
The mode of action is as follows:

- Oestrogen inhibits secretion of FSH via negative feedback on the anterior pituitary, and thus suppresses development of the ovarian follicle.
- Progestogen inhibits secretion of LH and thus prevents ovulation; it also makes the cervical mucus less suitable for the passage of sperm.
- Oestrogen and progestogen act in concert to alter the endometrium in such a way as to discourage implantation.

They may also interfere with the coordinated contractions of the cervix, uterus and fallopian tubes that facilitate fertilisation and implantation.

Hundreds of millions of women worldwide have used this method since the 1960s, and in general the combined pill constitutes a safe and effective method of contraception. There are distinct health benefits from taking the pill (see below), and serious adverse effects are rare. However, minor unwanted effects constitute drawbacks to its use, and several important questions need to be considered.

Common adverse effects
The common adverse effects are:

- weight gain, owing to fluid retention or an anabolic effect, or both;
- mild nausea, flushing, dizziness, depression or irritability;
- skin changes (e.g. acne and/or an increase in pigmentation);
- amenorrhoea of variable duration on cessation of taking the pill.

Questions that need to be considered
Is there an increased risk of cardiovascular disease (venous thromboembolism, myocardial infarction, stroke)?
With second-generation pills (oestrogen content less than 50 μg), the risk of thromboembolism is small (incidence approximately 15 per 100,000 users per year, compared with 5 per 100,000 non-pregnant non-users per year or 60 episodes of thromboembolism per 100,000 pregnancies). The risk is greatest in subgroups with additional factors, such as smoking (which increases risk substantially) and long-continued use of the pill, especially in women over 35 years of age. The incidence of thromboembolic disease is approximately 25 per 100,000 users per year in users of preparations containing **desogestrel** or **gestodene**, which is still a small absolute risk compared with the risk of thromboembolism in an

unwanted pregnancy. In general, provided risk factors, e.g. smoking, hypertension and obesity, have been identified, combined oral contraceptives are safe for most women for most of their reproductive lives.

Is cancer risk affected?
Ovarian and endometrial cancer risk is *reduced*.

Is blood pressure increased?
A marked increase in arterial blood pressure occurs in a small percentage of women shortly after starting the combined oral contraceptive pill. This is associated with increased circulating angiotensinogen, and disappears when treatment is stopped. Blood pressure is therefore monitored when oral contraceptive treatment is started, and an alternative contraceptive substituted if necessary.

Beneficial effects
Besides avoiding unwanted pregnancy, other desirable effects of the combined contraceptive pill include decreased menstrual symptoms such as irregular periods and intermenstrual bleeding. Iron deficiency anaemia and premenstrual tension are reduced, as are benign breast disease, uterine fibroids and functional cysts of the ovaries.

THE PROGESTOGEN-ONLY PILL

The drugs used in progestogen-only pills include **norethisterone**, **levonorgestrel** or **ethynodiol**. The pill is taken daily without interruption. The mode of action is primarily on the cervical mucus, which is made inhospitable to sperm. The progestogen probably also hinders implantation through its effect on the endometrium (see Fig. 36.2) and on the motility and secretions of the fallopian tubes (see p. 456).

Potential beneficial and unwanted effects
Progestogen-only contraceptives offer a suitable alternative to the combined pill for some women in whom oestrogen is contraindicated, and are suitable for women whose blood pressure increases unacceptably during treatment with oestrogen. However, their contraceptive effect is less reliable than that of the combination pill, and missing a dose may result in conception. Disturbances of menstruation (especially irregular bleeding) are common. Only a small proportion of women use this form of contraception, so long-term safety data are less reliable than for the combined pill.

PHARMACOKINETICS OF ORAL CONTRACEPTIVES: DRUG INTERACTIONS

Combined and progestogen-only oral contraceptives are metabolised by hepatic cytochrome P450 enzymes. Because the minimum effective dose of oestrogen is used (to avoid excess risk of thromboembolism), any increase in its clearance may result in contraceptive failure, and indeed enzyme-inducing drugs can have this effect, not only for combined but also for progesterone-only pills. Such drugs include **rifampicin** and **rifabutin**, as well as **carbamazepine**, **phenytoin** and others, including the herbal preparation St John's Wort (Ch. 48).

OTHER DRUG REGIMENS USED FOR CONTRACEPTION
POSTCOITAL (EMERGENCY) CONTRACEPTION

Oral administration of **levonorgestrel**, alone or combined with oestrogen, is effective if taken within 72 h of

Oral contraceptives

The combined pill

- The combined pill contains an oestrogen and a progestogen. It is taken for 21 consecutive days out of 28.
- Mode of action: the oestrogen inhibits follicle-stimulating hormone release and therefore follicle development; the progestogen inhibits luteinising hormone release and therefore ovulation, and makes cervical mucus inhospitable for sperm; together, they render the endometrium unsuitable for implantation.
- Drawbacks: weight gain, nausea, mood changes and skin pigmentation can occur.
- Serious unwanted effects are rare. A small proportion of women develop reversible hypertension; there is a small increase in diagnosis of breast cancer, possibly attributable to earlier diagnosis, and of cervical cancer. There is an increased risk of thromboembolism with third-generation pills, especially in women with additional risk factors (e.g. smoking) and with prolonged use.
- There are several beneficial effects, not least the avoidance of unwanted pregnancy, which itself carries risks to health.

The progestogen-only pill

- The progestogen-only pill is taken continuously. It differs from the combined pill in that the contraceptive effect is less reliable and is mainly a result of the alteration of cervical mucus. Irregular bleeding is common.

unprotected intercourse and repeated 12 h later. Nausea and vomiting are common (and the pills may then be lost: replacement tablets can be taken with an antiemetic such as **domperidone**). Insertion of an intrauterine device is more effective than hormonal methods, and works up to 5 days after intercourse.

LONG-ACTING PROGESTOGEN-ONLY CONTRACEPTION

Medroxyprogesterone can be given intramuscularly as a contraceptive. This is effective and safe. However, menstrual irregularities are common, and infertility may persist for many months after the final dose.

Levonorgestrel implanted subcutaneously in non-biodegradable capsules is used by approximately 3 million women worldwide. This route of administration avoids first-pass metabolism. The capsules release their progestogen content slowly over 5 years. Irregular bleeding and headache are common.

A levonorgestrel-impregnated intrauterine system provides prolonged, reliable contraception and, in contrast to standard copper containing devices, *reduces* menstrual bleeding.

THE UTERUS

The physiological and pharmacological responses of the uterus vary at different stages of the menstrual cycle and during pregnancy.

THE MOTILITY OF THE UTERUS

Uterine muscle contracts rhythmically both in vitro and in vivo, contractions originating in the muscle itself. Myometrial cells in the fundus act as pacemakers and give rise to conducted action potentials. The electrophysiological activity of these pacemaker cells is regulated by the sex hormones.

The non-pregnant human uterus contracts spontaneously but weakly during the first part of the cycle, and more strongly during the luteal phase and during menstruation. Uterine movements are depressed in early pregnancy because oestrogen, potentiated by progesterone, hyperpolarises myometrial cells. This suppresses spontaneous contractions. Towards the end of gestation, however, contractions recommence; these increase in force and frequency, and become fully coordinated during parturition. The nerve supply to the uterus includes both excitatory and inhibitory sympathetic components: adrenaline, acting on β_2 adrenoceptors, inhibits uterine contraction, whereas noradrenaline, acting on α adrenoceptors, stimulates contraction.

DRUGS THAT STIMULATE THE UTERUS

Drugs that stimulate the pregnant uterus and are important in obstetrics include **oxytocin**, **ergometrine** and prostaglandins.

OXYTOCIN

The neurohypophyseal hormone oxytocin (an octapeptide) regulates myometrial activity, causing uterine contraction (Ch. 34). Oxytocin release is stimulated by cervical dilatation, and by suckling; its role in parturition is incompletely understood but the fact that an antagonist (**atosiban**, see later) is effective in delaying the onset of labour implicates it in the physiology of parturition.

Oestrogen induces oxytocin receptor synthesis and, consequently, the uterus at term is highly sensitive to this hormone. Given by slow intravenous infusion to induce labour, oxytocin causes regular coordinated contractions that travel from fundus to cervix. Both amplitude and frequency of these contractions are related to dose, the uterus relaxing completely between contractions during low-dose infusion. Larger doses further increase the frequency of the contractions, and there is incomplete relaxation between them. Still higher doses cause sustained contractions that interfere with blood flow through the placenta and cause fetal distress or death.

Oxytocin contracts myoepithelial cells in the mammary gland, which causes 'milk let-down' – the expression of milk from the alveoli and ducts. It also has a vasodilator action. A weak antidiuretic action can result in water retention, which can be problematic in patients with cardiac or renal disease, or with pre-eclampsia.[6] Oxytocin and oxytocin receptors are also found in the brain, particularly in the limbic system, and are believed to play a role in mating and parenting behaviour.

The clinical use of synthetic oxytocin is given in the box on p. 467.

Oxytocin can be given by intravenous injection or intramuscularly, but is most often given by intravenous infusion. It is inactivated in the liver and kidneys, and by circulating placental oxytocinase.

---

[6]Eclampsia is a pathological condition (involving, among other things, high blood pressure, swelling and seizures) that occurs in pregnant women – it is usually preceded by milder changes ('pre-eclampsia').

Unwanted effects of oxytocin include dose-related hypotension, due to vasodilatation, with associated reflex tachycardia. Its antidiuretic hormone-like effect on water excretion by the kidney causes water retention and, unless water intake is curtailed, consequent hyponatraemia.

ERGOMETRINE

Ergot (*Claviceps purpurea*) is a fungus that grows on rye and contains a surprising variety of pharmacologically active substances (see Ch. 16). Ergot poisoning, which was once common, was often associated with abortion. In 1935, **ergometrine** was isolated and recognised as the oxytocic principle in ergot.

Ergometrine contracts the human uterus. This action depends partly on the contractile state of the organ. On a contracted uterus (the normal state following delivery), ergometrine has relatively little effect. However, if the uterus is inappropriately relaxed, ergometrine initiates strong contraction and reduces bleeding from the placental bed (the raw surface from which the placenta has detached). Ergometrine also has a moderate vasoconstrictor action.

The mechanism of action of ergometrine on smooth muscle is not understood. It is possible that it acts partly on α adrenoceptors, like the related alkaloid ergotamine (see Ch. 15), and partly on 5-hydroxytryptamine receptors.

The clinical use of ergometrine is given in the box on p. 467.

Ergometrine can be given orally, intramuscularly or intravenously. It has a very rapid onset of action and its effect lasts for 3–6 h.

Ergometrine can produce vomiting, probably by an effect on dopamine D_2 receptors in the chemoreceptor trigger zone (see Ch. 31, Fig. 31.5). Vasoconstriction with an increase in blood pressure associated with nausea, blurred vision and headache can occur, as can vasospasm of the coronary arteries, resulting in angina.

PROSTAGLANDINS

Prostaglandins are discussed in detail in Chapter 18. The endometrium and myometrium have substantial prostaglandin-synthesising capacity, particularly in the second, proliferative phase of the menstrual cycle. Prostaglandin $(PG)F_{2\alpha}$ is generated in large amounts, and has been implicated in the ischaemic necrosis of the endometrium that precedes menstruation (although it has relatively little vasoconstrictor action on many human blood vessels, in contrast to some other mammalian species). Vasodilator prostaglandins, PGE_2 and PGI_2 (prostacyclin), are also generated by the uterus.

In addition to their vasoactive properties, the E and F prostaglandins contract uterine smooth muscle, whose sensitivity to these prostaglandins increases during gestation. Their role in parturition is not fully understood, but as cyclo-oxygenase inhibitors can delay labour (see later), they probably play some part in this.

Prostaglandins also play a part in two of the main disorders of menstruation: dysmenorrhoea (painful menstruation) and menorrhagia (excessive blood loss). Dysmenorrhoea is associated with increased production of PGE_2 and $PGF_{2\alpha}$; non-steroidal anti-inflammatory drugs, which inhibit prostaglandin biosynthesis (see Ch. 27), are used to treat dysmenorrhoea. Menorrhagia, in the absence of other uterine pathology, may be caused by a combination of increased vasodilatation and reduced haemostasis. Increased generation by the uterus of PGI_2 (which inhibits platelet aggregation) could impair haemostasis as well as causing vasodilatation. Non-steroidal anti-inflammatory drugs (e.g. **mefenamic acid**) are used to treat menorrhagia as well as dysmenorrhoea.

Prostaglandin preparations

Prostaglandins of the E and F series promote coordinated contractions of the body of the pregnant uterus, while relaxing the cervix. E and F prostaglandins reliably cause abortion in early and middle pregnancy, unlike oxytocin which generally does not cause expulsion of the uterine contents at this stage. The prostaglandins used in obstetrics are **dinoprostone** (PGE_2), **carboprost** (15-methyl $PGF_{2\alpha}$) and **gemeprost** or **misoprostol** (PGE_1 analogues). Dinoprostone can be given intravaginally as a gel or as tablets. Carboprost is given by deep intramuscular injection. Gemeprost or misoprostol are given intravaginally.

Unwanted effects

Unwanted effects include uterine pain, nausea and vomiting, and diarrhoea. Dinoprost can cause hypotension. When combined with mifepristone, a progestogen antagonist that sensitises the uterus to prostaglandins, lower doses of the prostaglandins (e.g. misoprostol) can be used to terminate pregnancy and side effects are reduced.

The clinical box shows the clinical uses of prostaglandins (also Ch. 18).

> ### Drugs acting on the uterus
>
> - At parturition, **oxytocin** causes regular coordinated uterine contractions, each followed by relaxation; **ergometrine**, an ergot alkaloid, causes uterine contractions with an increase in basal tone. **Atosiban**, an antagonist of oxytocin, delays labour.
> - Prostaglandin (PG) analogues, for example, **dinoprostone** (PGE_2) and **dinoprost** ($PGF_{2\alpha}$), contract the pregnant uterus but relax the cervix. Cyclo-oxygenase inhibitors inhibit PG synthesis and delay labour. They also alleviate symptoms of dysmenorrhoea and menorrhagia.
> - The β_2-adrenoceptor agonists (e.g. **ritodrine**) inhibit spontaneous and oxytocin-induced contractions of the pregnant uterus.

DRUGS THAT INHIBIT UTERINE CONTRACTION

Selective β_2-adrenoceptor agonists, such as **ritodrine** or **salbutamol**, inhibit spontaneous or oxytocin-induced contractions of the pregnant uterus. These uterine relaxants are used in selected patients to prevent premature labour occurring between 22 and 33 weeks of gestation in otherwise uncomplicated pregnancies. They can delay delivery by 48 h, time that can be used to administer glucocorticoid therapy to the mother so as to mature the lungs of the baby and reduce neonatal respiratory distress. It has been difficult to demonstrate that any of the drugs used to delay labour improve the outcome for the baby. Risks to the mother, especially pulmonary oedema, increase after 48 h, and myometrial response is reduced, so prolonged treatment is avoided. Cyclo-oxygenase inhibitors (e.g. **indometacin**) inhibit labour, but their use could cause problems in the baby, including renal dysfunction and delayed closure of the ductus arteriosus, both of which are influenced by endogenous prostaglandins.

An oxytocin receptor antagonist, **atosiban**, provides an alternative to a β_2-adrenoceptor agonist. It is given as an intravenous bolus followed by an intravenous infusion for not more than 48 h. Adverse effects include vasodilatation, nausea, vomiting and hyperglycaemia.

Clinical uses of drugs acting on the uterus

Myometrial stimulants (oxytocics)

- **Oxytocin** is used to *induce or augment labour* when the uterine muscle is not functioning adequately. It can also be used to treat *postpartum haemorrhage*.
- **Ergometrine** is used to treat *postpartum haemorrhage*. **Carboprost** can be used if patients do not respond to **ergometrine**.
- A preparation containing both **oxytocin** and **ergometrine** is used for the management of the third stage of labour; the two agents together can also be used, before surgery, to control bleeding due to incomplete abortion.
- **Gemeprost** (intravaginally) or **misoprostol** (following mifepristone) are used to terminate pregnancy.

Myometrial relaxants

- The β-adrenoceptor agonists (e.g. **ritodrine**) are used to delay *preterm labour*.
- **Atosiban** (oxytocin antagonist) also delays preterm labour.

ERECTILE DYSFUNCTION

Erectile function depends on complex interactions between physiological and psychological factors. Erection is caused by vasorelaxation in the arteries and arterioles supplying the erectile tissue. This increases penile blood flow; the consequent increase in sinusoidal filling compresses the venules, occluding venous outflow and causing erection. During sexual intercourse, reflex contraction of the ischio-cavernosus muscles compresses the base of the corpora cavernosa, and the intracavernosal pressure can reach several hundred millimetres of mercury during this phase of rigid erection. Innervation of the penis includes autonomic and somatic nerves. Nitric oxide is probably the main mediator of erection and is released both from nitrergic nerves and from endothelium (Ch. 21, Fig. 21.6).

Erectile function is adversely affected by several thera-peutic drugs (including many antipsychotic, antidepressant and antihypertensive agents), and psychiatric and vascular disease (especially in association with endothelial dysfunc-tion) can themselves cause erectile dysfunction, which is common in middle-aged and older men, even if they have no psychiatric or cardiovascular problems.[7] There are several organic causes, including hypogonadism (see clinical box,

p. 462), hyperprolactinaemia (see Ch. 34), arterial disease and various causes of neuropathy (most commonly diabetes), but often no organic cause is identified.

Over the centuries, there has been a huge trade in parts of various creatures that have the misfortune to bear some fancied resemblance to human genitalia, in the pathetic belief that consuming these will restore virility or act as an aphrodisiac (i.e. a drug that stimulates libido). Alcohol (Ch. 50) 'provokes the desire but takes away the perfor-mance', and cannabis (Ch. 20) can also release inhibitions and probably does the same. **Yohimbine** (an α_2-adrenoceptor antagonist; Ch. 15) may have some positive effect in this regard, but trials have proved inconclusive. **Apomorphine** (a dopamine agonist; Ch. 39) causes erections in humans as well as in rodents when injected subcutaneously, but it is a powerful emetic, a disadvantage in this context. The picture picked up somewhat when it was found that injecting vasodilator drugs directly into the corpora cavernosa causes penile erection. **Papaverine** (Ch. 23), if necessary with the addition of **phentolamine**, was used in this way. The route of administration is not acceptable to most men, but diabetics in particular are often not needle-shy, and this approach was a real boon to many such patients. PGE_1 (**alprostadil**) is often combined with other vasodilators when given intracavernosally. It can also be given transurethrally as an alternative (albeit still a somewhat unromantic one) to injection. Adverse effects of all these drugs include priapism (prolonged and painful erection with risk of permanent tissue damage), which is no joke. Treatment consists of aspiration of blood and, if necessary, cautious intracaver-nosal administration of a vasoconstrictor such as **phenyle-phrine**. Intracavernosal and transurethral preparations are still available to treat erectile failure, but orally active phosphodiesterase inhibitors are now generally the drugs of choice.

PHOSPHODIESTERASE TYPE V INHIBITORS

Sildenafil, the first selective phosphodiesterase type V inhibitor (see also Chs 21 and 23), was found accidentally to influence erectile function.[8] **Tadalafil** and **vardenafil** are similar. Tadalafil is longer acting than sildenafil. In contrast to intracavernosal vasodilators, phosphodiesterase type V inhibitors do not cause erection independent of sexual desire, but enhance the erectile response to sexual stimula-tion. They have transformed the treatment of erectile dysfunction.

Mechanism of action

Phosphodiesterase V is the isoform that inactivates cGMP. Nitrergic nerves release nitric oxide (or a related nitrosothiol) which diffuses into smooth muscle cells, where it activates guanylyl cyclase. The resulting increase in cytoplasmic cGMP mediates vasodilatation via activation of protein kinase G (Ch. 4, Fig. 4.10). Consequently, inhibition of phosphodiesterase V potentiates the effect on penile vascular smooth muscle of endothelium-derived nitric oxide and of nitrergic nerves that are activated by sexual stimulation (Fig. 36.6). Other vascular beds are also affected, suggesting other possible uses, notably in pulmonary hypertension (Ch. 23).

---

[7]In randomised controlled trials, an appreciable proportion of men who discontinued treatment because of erectile dysfunction had been receiving placebo.

[8]Sildenafil was originally intended to treat angina, but bulging bedclothes were noticed in early clinical trials, providing the opportunity for the drug to be developed for a less crowded and more profitable indication than angina.

Fig. 36.6 Mechanism of phosphodiesterase V (PDE V) inhibitors on penile erection, and of the interaction of PDE V inhibitors with organic nitrates. The *large grey rectangle* denotes a vascular smooth muscle cell in the corpora cavernosa. Sexual stimulation releases nitric oxide (NO) from nitrergic nerves and this activates guanylyl cyclase, increasing cGMP production and hence activating protein kinase G (PKG), causing vasodilatation and penile erection. cGMP is inactivated by PDE V, so PDE V inhibitors (e.g. sildenafil) potentiate NO and promote penile erection. NO from organic nitrates such as glyceryl trinitrate (GTN) is also potentiated leading to generalised vasodilatation and hypotension.

Pharmacokinetic aspects and drug interactions

Peak plasma concentrations of sildenafil occur approximately 30–120 min after an oral dose and are delayed by eating, so it is taken an hour or more before sexual activity. It is given as a single dose as needed. It is metabolised by CYP3A4, which is induced by **carbamazepine**, **rifampicin** and **barbiturates**, and inhibited by **cimetidine**, macrolide antibiotics, antifungal imidazolines and some antiviral drugs (such as **ritonavir**). These drugs can interact with sildenafil. Tadalafil has a longer half-life than sildenafil, so can be taken longer before sexual activity. A clinically important pharmacodynamic interaction of all phosphodiesterase V inhibitors occurs with all organic nitrates, which work through increasing cGMP (Ch. 21) and are therefore markedly potentiated by sildenafil (see Fig. 36.6). Consequently, concurrent nitrate use, including use of **nicorandil**, contraindicates the concurrent use of any phosphodiesterase type V inhibitor.[9]

Unwanted effects

Many of the unwanted effects of phosphodiesterase type V inhibitors are caused by vasodilatation in other vascular beds; these effects include hypotension, flushing and headache. Visual disturbances have occasionally been reported and are of concern because sildenafil has some action on phosphodiesterase VI, which is present in the retina and important in vision (a cGMP-dependent process too). The manufacturers advise that sildenafil should not be used in patients with hereditary retinal degenerative diseases (such as retinitis pigmentosa) because of the theoretical risk posed by this. Vardenafil is more selective for the type V isozyme than is sildenafil (reviewed by Doggrell, 2005), but is also contraindicated in patients with hereditary retinal disorders.

---

[9]This is important not only for sufferers from angina who take nitrates such as glyceryl trinitrate or isosorbide mononitrate therapeutically or prophylactically and are at risk of hypotension because of coronary artery disease, but also asymptomatic individuals who take amyl nitrate recreationally ('poppers') because of its effect on pelvic blood vessels.

REFERENCES AND FURTHER READING

Sex hormones and their control

Adeel, M., Song, X., Wang, Y., Dennis Francis, D., Yang, Y., 2017. Environmental impact of estrogens on human, animal and plant life: a critical review. Environ. Int. 99, 107–119. (*Review of environmental issues*)

Barrett-Connor, E., Mosca, L., Collins, P., et al., 2006. Effects of raloxifene on cardiovascular events and breast cancer in postmenopausal women. N. Engl. J. Med. 355, 125–137. (*Reduced breast cancer*)

Barton, M., Prossnitz, E.R., 2015. Emerging roles of GPER in diabetes and atherosclerosis. Trends Endocrinol. Metab. 26, 185–192. (*Evidence for a central role of GPER in a wide range of vascular and metabolic processes*)

Behringer, R.R., 1994. The in vivo roles of Müllerian-inhibiting substance. Curr. Top. Dev. Biol. 29, 171–187. (*Known as Anti-Müllerian hormone, AMH*)

Chen, Z., Yuhanna, I.S., Galcheva-Gargova, Z., et al., 1999. Estrogen receptor-alpha mediates the nongenomic activation of endothelial nitric oxide synthase by estrogen. J. Clin. Invest. 103, 401–406. (*Acute vasodilator action of oestrogen may involve membrane ER rather than the classic intracellular receptor pathway*)

Gruber, C.J., Tschugguel, W., Schneeberger, C., Huber, J.C., 2002. Production and actions of estrogens. N. Engl. J. Med. 346, 340–352. (*Review focusing on the new biochemical aspects of the action of oestrogen – including phyto-oestrogens and selective oestrogen receptor modulators – as well as physiological and clinical aspects*)

McLachlan, J.A., 2016. Environmental signaling: from environmental estrogens to endocrine-disrupting chemicals and beyond. Andrology 4, 684–694. (*Review, including epigenetic mechanisms of inter-generational adverse effects*)

Prizant, H., Gleicher, N., Sen, A., 2014. Androgen actions in the ovary: balance is key. J. Endocrinol. 222, R141–R151. (*Androgens play an important role in female fertility*)

Rhoden, E.L., Morgentaler, A., 2004. Risks of testosterone-replacement therapy and recommendations for monitoring. N. Engl. J. Med. 350, 482–492. (*Review*)

Vogel, V., Constantino, J., Wickerman, L., et al., 2006. Effects of tamoxifen vs. raloxifene on the risk of developing invasive breast cancer and other disease outcomes. JAMA 295, 2727–2741. (*Raloxifene had similar efficacy as tamoxifen with fewer thrombotic events*)

Walker, H.A., Dean, T.S., Sanders, T.A.B., et al., 2001. The phytoestrogen genistein produces acute nitric oxide-dependent dilation of human forearm vasculature with similar potency to 17 beta-estradiol. Circulation 103, 258–262.

Contraceptives

Djerassi, C., 2001. This Man's Pill: Reflections on the 50th Birthday of the Pill. Oxford University Press, New York. (*Scientific and autobiographical memoir by polymath steroid chemist who worked on 'the pill' at its inception under Syntex in Mexico, and has continued thinking about human reproduction in a broad biological and biosocial sense ever since*)

Postmenopausal aspects

Davis, S.R., Dinatale, I., Rivera-Woll, L., Davison, S., 2005. Postmenopausal hormone therapy: from monkey glands to transdermal patches. J. Endocrinol. 185, 207–222. (*Reviews the history of knowledge of the menopause and the development of hormonal therapy for climacteric complaints, and summarises current evidence for specific benefits and risks of hormone treatment*)

Hulley, S., Grady, D., Bush, T., et al., 1998. Randomized trial of estrogen plus progestin for secondary prevention of coronary heart disease in postmenopausal women. JAMA 280, 605–613. (*Study showing that incidence of fatal myocardial infarction was similar in the two groups, despite favourable changes in low- and high-density-lipoprotein cholesterol in the HRT group. Venous thromboembolism was increased by a factor of 2.89 in the active group*)

Prague, J.K., Roberts, R.E., Comninos, A.N., 2017. Neurokinin 3 receptor antagonism as a novel treatment for menopausal hot flushes: a phase 2, randomised, double-blind, placebo-controlled trial. Lancet 389, 1809–1820. (*A neurokinin 3 receptor antagonist relieved hot flush symptoms without the need for oestrogen exposure*)

The uterus

Norwitz, E.R., Robinson, J.N., Challis, J.R., 1999. The control of labor. N. Engl. J. Med. 341, 660–666. (*Review*)

Thornton, S., Vatish, M., Slater, D., 2001. Oxytocin antagonists: clinical and scientific considerations. Exp. Physiol. 86, 297–302. (*Reviews rationale for uterine relaxants in preterm labour; evidence for administering atosiban; and the role of oxytocin, vasopressin and their receptors in the onset of labour*)

Erectile dysfunction

Doggrell, S.A., 2005. Comparison of clinical trials with sildenafil, vardenafil and tadalafil in erectile dysfunction. Expert Opin. Pharmacother. 6, 75–84. (*Vardenafil is similarly effective to sildenafil. Its only advantage is that it does not inhibit phosphodiesterase VI to alter colour perception, a rare side effect that sometimes occurs with sildenafil. Tadalafil has a longer duration of action*)

Useful Web resource

https://www.gov.uk/drug-safety-update/hormone-replacement-therapy-updated-advice. (*Risks of cancer [breast, endometrium, ovary], venous thromboembolism, stroke and coronary artery disease in relation to age and duration of HRT use*)

37 Bone metabolism

OVERVIEW

In this chapter we consider first the cellular and biochemical processes involved in bone remodelling, and the various mediators that regulate these processes. We then describe the drugs used to treat disorders of bone, including new agents.

INTRODUCTION

The human skeleton undergoes a continuous process of remodelling throughout life – some bone being resorbed and new bone being laid down continuously – resulting in the complete skeleton being replaced every 10 years. Structural deterioration and decreased bone mass (osteoporosis) occur with advancing age and constitute a worldwide health problem. Other conditions that lead to treatable pathological changes in bone include nutritional deficiencies and malignancy. There have recently been significant advances in the understanding of bone biology, which have led in turn to several valuable new drugs.

BONE STRUCTURE AND COMPOSITION

The human skeleton consists of 80% cortical bone and 20% trabecular bone. Cortical bone is the dense, compact outer part and trabecular bone, the inner meshwork. The former predominates in the shafts of long bones, the latter in the vertebrae, the epiphyses of long bones and the iliac crest. Trabecular bone, having a large surface area, is metabolically more active and more affected by factors that lead to bone loss (see later).

The main minerals in bone are calcium and phosphates. More than 99% of the calcium in the body is in the skeleton, mostly as crystalline hydroxyapatite but some as non-crystalline phosphates and carbonates; together, these make up half the bone mass.

The main bone cells are *osteoblasts*, *osteoclasts* and *osteocytes*.

- Osteoblasts are bone-forming cells derived from precursor cells in the bone marrow and the periosteum: they secrete important components (particularly collagen) of the extracellular matrix of bone – which is known as *osteoid*. They also have a role in the activation of osteoclasts (Figs 37.1 and 37.2).
- Osteoclasts are multinucleated bone-resorbing cells derived from precursor cells of the macrophage/monocyte lineage.
- Osteocytes are derived from osteoblasts which, during the formation of new bone, become embedded in the bony matrix and differentiate into osteocytes. These cells form a connected cellular network that, along with nerve fibres located in bone, influences the response to mechanical loading. Osteocytes sense mechanical strain, and respond by triggering bone remodelling (see later) and secreting *sclerostin*, a glycoprotein that binds to receptors on osteoblasts to inhibit bone formation (McClung, 2017).
- Other important cells in bone include monocytes/macrophages, lymphocytes and vascular endothelial cells; these secrete cytokines and other mediators implicated in bone remodelling.

Osteoid is the organic matrix of bone and its principal component is collagen. Other components such as *proteoglycans*, *osteocalcin* and various phosphoproteins are also important; one of these, *osteonectin*, binds to both calcium and collagen and thus links these two major constituents of bone matrix.

Calcium phosphate crystals are deposited as hydroxyapatite $[Ca_{10}(PO_4)_6(OH)_2]$ in the osteoid, converting it into hard bone matrix.

In addition to its structural function, bone plays a major role in calcium homeostasis.

BONE REMODELLING

There has been substantial progress in our understanding of bone remodelling (see reviews by Harslof & Langdahl, 2016; Tabatabaei-Malazy, 2017.)

The process of remodelling involves:

- activity of osteoblasts and osteoclasts (see Fig. 37.1);
- actions of various cytokines (see Figs 37.1 and 37.2);
- turnover of bone minerals – particularly calcium and phosphate;
- actions of several hormones: parathyroid hormone (PTH), the vitamin D family, oestrogens, growth hormone, steroids, calcitonin and various cytokines.

Diet, drugs and physical factors (exercise, loading) also affect remodelling. Bone loss – of 0.5%–1% per year – starts aged 35–40 years in both sexes, and accelerates by as much as 10-fold during the menopause in women or with castration in men, and then gradually settles at 1%–3% per year. The loss during the menopause is due to increased osteoclast activity and affects mainly trabecular bone; the later loss in both sexes with increasing age is due to decreased osteoblast numbers and affects mainly cortical bone.

THE ACTION OF CELLS AND CYTOKINES

A cycle of remodelling starts with recruitment of osteoclast precursors followed by cytokine-induced differentiation of these to mature multinucleated osteoclasts (see Fig. 37.1).

Fig. 37.1 **The bone-remodelling cycle and the action of hormones, cytokines and drugs.** *Quiescent trabecular bone:* Cytokines such as insulin-like growth factor (IGF) and transforming growth factor (TGF)-β, shown as dots, are embedded in the bone matrix. *Bone resorption* and *bone formation* are illustrated. Embedded bisphosphonates (BPs), are ingested by osteoclasts (OCs) when bone is resorbed (not shown). *IL,* interleukin; *OB,* osteoblasts; *PTH,* parathyroid hormone.

Fig. 37.2 **Schematic diagram of the role of the osteoblast and cytokines in the differentiation and activation of the osteoclast and the action of drugs thereon.** The osteoblast is stimulated to express a surface ligand, the RANK ligand (RANKL). RANKL interacts with a receptor on the osteoclast – an osteoclast differentiation and activation receptor termed RANK (receptor activator of nuclear factor κB), which causes differentiation and activation of the osteoclast progenitors to form mature osteoclasts. Bisphosphonates inhibit bone resorption by osteoclasts. Anti-RANKL antibodies (e.g. denosumab) bind RANKL and prevent the RANK–RANKL interaction. Sclerostin inhibits proliferation of osteoblasts and stimulates RANKL secretion. Drugs used clinically are in *red-bordered boxes.* *IL,* interleukin; *M-CSF,* macrophage colony-stimulating factor; *OPG,* osteoprotegerin; *PTH,* parathyroid hormone.

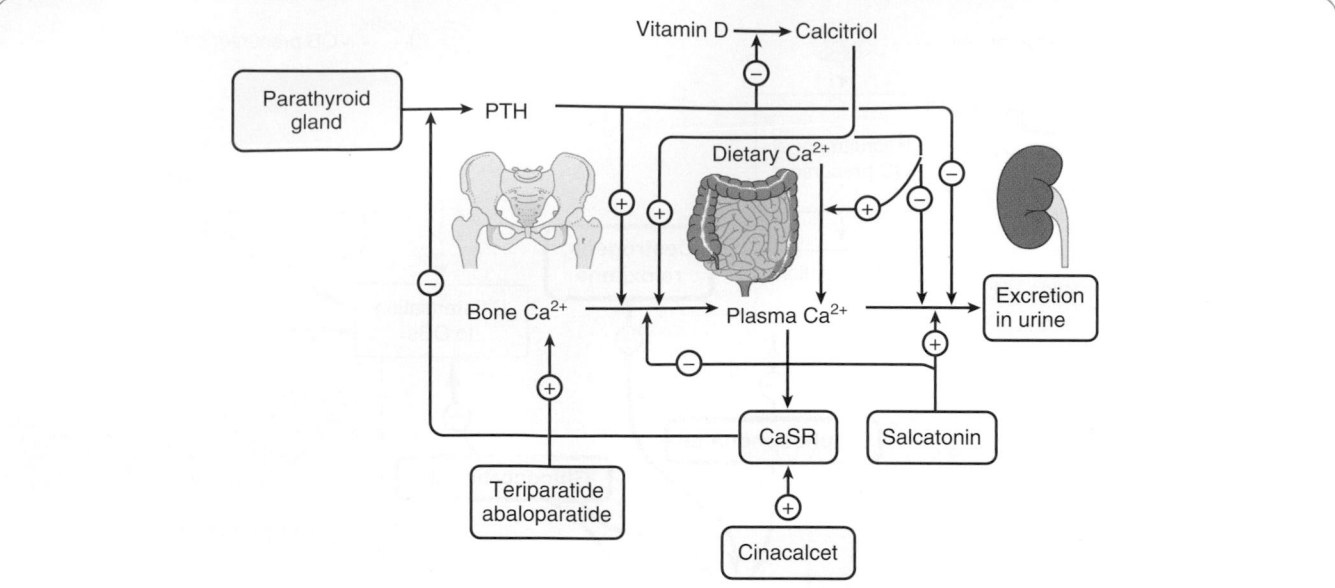

Fig. 37.3 The main factors involved in maintaining the concentration of Ca²⁺ in the plasma and the action of drugs. The calcium receptor on the parathyroid cell is a G protein–coupled receptor. Endogenous calcitonin, secreted by the thyroid, inhibits Ca²⁺ mobilisation from bone and decreases its reabsorption in the kidney, thus reducing blood Ca²⁺. *CaSR*, calcium-sensing receptor; *PTH*, parathyroid hormone.

The osteoclasts adhere to an area of trabecular bone, developing a ruffled border at the attachment site. They move along the bone, digging a pit by secreting hydrogen ions and proteolytic enzymes, mainly *cathepsin K*. This process gradually liberates cytokines such as insulin-like growth factor (IGF)-1 and transforming growth factor (TGF)-β, which have been embedded in the osteoid (see Fig. 37.1); these in turn recruit and activate successive teams of osteoblasts that have been stimulated to develop from precursor cells and are awaiting the call to duty (see Fig. 37.1). The osteoblasts invade the site, synthesising and secreting osteoid and secreting IGF-1 and TGF-β (which become embedded in the osteoid; see earlier). Some osteoblasts become embedded in the osteoid, forming osteocytes; others interact with and activate osteoclast precursors – and we are back to the beginning of the cycle.

Cytokines other than IGF-1 and TGF-β involved in bone remodelling include other members of the TGF-β family, including *bone morphogenic proteins* (BMPs), several interleukins, various hormones and members of the tumour necrosis factor (TNF) family. A member of this last family – a ligand for a receptor on the osteoclast precursor cell – is of particular importance. The receptor is termed (wait for it – biological terminology has fallen over its own feet here) *RANK*, which stands for *receptor activator of nuclear factor kappa B* (NF-κB), NF-κB being the principal transcription factor involved in osteoclast differentiation and activation. And the ligand is termed, unsurprisingly, RANK ligand (RANKL).

▼ Osteoblasts synthesise and release *osteoprotegerin* (OPG) which is identical with RANK and functions as a decoy receptor. In a sibling-undermining process by osteoblast and osteoclast precursor cells, OPG can bind to RANKL[1] (generated by the very same cells as OPG) and inhibit RANKL's binding to the functional receptor, RANK, on

the osteoclast precursor cell (see Fig. 37.2). The ratio of RANKL to OPG is critical in the formation and activity of osteoclasts and the RANK, RANKL, OPG system is fundamental to bone remodelling (reviewed by Boyce & Xing, 2008; Wright et al., 2009). **Denusomab** is an antibody directed against RANKL that is used clinically to treat osteoporosis.

THE TURNOVER OF BONE MINERALS

The main bone minerals are calcium and phosphates.

CALCIUM METABOLISM

The daily turnover of bone minerals during remodelling involves about 700 mg of calcium. Calcium has numerous roles in physiological functioning. Intracellular Ca²⁺ is part of the signal transduction mechanism of many cells (see Ch. 4), so the concentration of Ca²⁺ in the extracellular fluid and the plasma, normally about 2.5 mmol/L, needs to be controlled with great precision. The plasma Ca²⁺ concentration is regulated by interactions between PTH and various forms of vitamin D (Figs 37.3 and 37.4); calcitonin also plays a part.

Calcium absorption in the intestine involves a Ca²⁺-binding protein, the synthesis of which is regulated by calcitriol (see Fig. 37.3). It is probable that the overall calcium content of the body is regulated largely by this absorption mechanism, because urinary Ca²⁺ excretion normally remains more or less constant. However, with high blood Ca²⁺ concentrations urinary excretion increases, and with low blood concentrations urinary excretion can be reduced by PTH and calcitriol, both of which enhance Ca²⁺ reabsorption in the renal tubules (see Fig. 37.3).

PHOSPHATE METABOLISM

Phosphates are important constituents of bone, and are also critically important in the structure and function of all the cells of the body. They are constituents of nucleic acids, provide energy in the form of ATP, and control

---

[1]RANKL is also sometimes confusingly termed *OPG ligand*.

Fig. 37.4 Summary of the actions of the vitamin D endocrine system and the action of drugs. Exogenous ergocalciferol, vitamin (vit) D_2 (formed in plants by ultraviolet [UV] light), is converted to the corresponding D_2 metabolites in liver and kidney, as is the D_2 analogue dihydrotachysterol (not shown). Calcifediol and calcitriol are metabolites of vitamin D_3 and constitute the 'hormones' 25-hydroxy-vitamin D_3 and 1,25-dihydroxy-vitamin D_3, respectively. Alfacalcidol (1α-hydroxycholecalciferol) is 25-hydroxylated to calcitriol in the liver. *OB*, osteoblast.

– through phosphorylation – the activity of many functional proteins. They also have roles as intracellular buffers and in the excretion of hydrogen ions in the kidney.

Phosphate absorption is an energy-requiring process regulated by *calcitriol*. Phosphate deposition in bone, as hydroxyapatite, depends on the plasma concentration of PTH, which, with calcitriol, mobilises both Ca^{2+} and phosphate from the bone matrix. Phosphate is excreted by the kidney; here PTH inhibits reabsorption and thus increases excretion.

HORMONES INVOLVED IN BONE METABOLISM AND REMODELLING

The main hormones involved in bone metabolism and remodelling are PTH, members of the vitamin D family, oestrogens and calcitonin. Glucocorticoids and thyroid hormone also affect bone.

PARATHYROID HORMONE

PTH, which consists of a single-chain polypeptide of 84 amino acids, is an important physiological regulator of

Bone remodelling

- Bone is continuously remodelled throughout life. The events of the remodelling cycle are as follows:
  - osteoclasts, having been activated by osteoblasts, resorb bone by digging pits in trabecular bone. Into these pits the bone-forming osteoblasts secrete osteoid (bone matrix), which consists mainly of collagen but also contains osteocalcin, osteonectin, phosphoproteins and the cytokines insulin growth factor (IGF) and transforming growth factor (TGF)-β;
  - the osteoid is then mineralised, i.e. complex calcium phosphate crystals (hydroxyapatites) are deposited.
- Bone metabolism and mineralisation involve the action of parathyroid hormone, the vitamin D family, and various cytokines (e.g. IGF, the TGF-β family and interleukins). Declining physiological levels of oestrogens and therapeutic levels of glucocorticoids can result in bone resorption not balanced by bone formation – leading to osteoporosis.

Ca^{2+} metabolism. It acts on PTH type 1 receptor,[2] G protein-coupled receptors present in various tissues, especially bone – where it is expressed on osteoblast cell membranes and kidney to maintain the plasma Ca^{2+} concentration via activation of adenylyl cyclase and phospholipase C. A closely related molecule, known as parathyroid hormone-related peptide (PTHrP) bears the same N-terminal end as PTH, and can activate PTH receptors in broadly similar ways (Harslof & Langdahl, 2016). When PTH activates the osteoblast PTH type 1 receptor, osteoblasts express RANKL, which binds to RANK on osteoclasts, activating them and increasing the resorption rate.

PTH mobilises Ca^{2+} from bone, promotes its reabsorption by the kidney and stimulates the synthesis of calcitriol, which in turn increases Ca^{2+} absorption from the intestine and synergises with PTH in mobilising bone Ca^{2+} (see Figs 37.3 and 37.4). PTH promotes phosphate excretion, and thus its net effect is to increase the concentration of Ca^{2+} in the plasma and lower that of phosphate.

PTH receptors exist in two conformations (R0 and RG). Shorter duration of activation (and anabolic effect) is seen with ligands that have greater affinity for the RG conformation, whereas ligands that bind to the R0 state have a more prolonged duration of action that leads to bone resorption. Sustained levels of PTH mobilise Ca^{2+} from bone and reduce renal Ca^{2+} excretion. In contrast, low intermittent therapeutic doses of PTH stimulate osteoblast activity and enhance bone formation.

Parathyroid hormone is synthesised in the cells of the parathyroid glands and stored in vesicles. The principal factor controlling secretion is the concentration of ionised calcium in the plasma, low plasma Ca^{2+} stimulating secretion, high plasma Ca^{2+} decreasing it by binding to and activating a Ca^{2+}-sensing G protein–coupled surface receptor (CaSR, see Ch. 3 and Fig. 37.3). (For reviews, see Stewart, 2004; Deal, 2009.) **Cinacalcet** increases the sensitivity of CaSR to plasma Ca^{2+}, thereby reducing PTH secretion.

Teriparatide and **abaloparatide** are clinically licensed shorter-chain synthetic analogues of PTH and PTHrP, respectively.

VITAMIN D

Vitamin D (calciferol) consists of a group of lipophilic precursors that are converted in the body into biologically active metabolites that function as true hormones, circulating in the blood and regulating the activities of various cell types (see Reichel et al., 1989). Their main action, mediated by nuclear receptors of the steroid receptor superfamily (see Ch. 3), is the maintenance of plasma Ca^{2+} by increasing Ca^{2+} absorption in the intestine, mobilising Ca^{2+} from bone and decreasing its renal excretion (see Fig. 37.3). In humans, there are two important forms of vitamin D, termed D$_2$ and D$_3$:

1. Dietary *ergocalciferol* (D$_2$), derived from ergosterol in plants.
2. *Cholecalciferol* (D$_3$), generated in the skin from 7-dehydrocholesterol by the action of ultraviolet irradiation during sun exposure, or formed from cholesterol in the wall of the intestine.

Cholecalciferol is converted to *calcifediol* (25-hydroxy-vitamin D$_3$) in the liver, and this is converted to a series of other metabolites of varying activity in the kidney, the most potent of which is *calcitriol* (1,25-dihydroxy-vitamin D$_3$); see Fig. 37.4.

The synthesis of calcitriol from calcifediol is regulated by PTH, and is also influenced by the phosphate concentration in the plasma and by the calcitriol concentration itself through a negative feedback mechanism (see Fig. 37.4). Receptors for calcitriol are ubiquitous, and calcitriol is important in the functioning of many cell types.

The main actions of calcitriol are to stimulate absorption of Ca^{2+} and phosphate in the intestine, and to mobilise Ca^{2+} from bone, but it also increases Ca^{2+} reabsorption in the kidney tubules (see Fig. 37.3). It promotes maturation of osteoclasts and stimulates their activity (see Figs 37.1 and 37.3). It decreases collagen synthesis by osteoblasts. However, the effect on bone is complex and not confined to mobilising Ca^{2+}, because in clinical vitamin D deficiency (see p. 477), in which the mineralisation of bone is impaired, administration of vitamin D restores bone formation. One explanation may lie in the fact that calcitriol stimulates synthesis of *osteocalcin*, the Ca^{2+}-binding protein of bone matrix.

OESTROGENS

Oestrogens have an important role in maintaining bone integrity in adult women, acting on osteoblasts and osteoclasts. Oestrogen inhibits the cytokines that recruit osteoclasts and opposes the bone-resorbing, Ca^{2+}-mobilising action of PTH. It increases osteoblast proliferation, augments production of TGF-β and BMPs, and inhibits apoptosis. Withdrawal of oestrogen, as happens physiologically at the menopause, frequently leads to osteoporosis.

CALCITONIN

Calcitonin is a peptide hormone secreted by 'C' cells found in the thyroid follicles (see Ch. 35).

The main action of calcitonin is on bone; it inhibits bone resorption by binding to an inhibitory receptor on osteoclasts. In the kidney, it decreases the reabsorption of Ca^{2+} and phosphate in the proximal tubules. Its overall effect is to decrease the plasma Ca^{2+} concentration (see Fig. 37.3).

Secretion is determined mainly by the plasma Ca^{2+} concentration. A calcitonin analogue, **salcatonin**, is used clinically (see later).

OTHER HORMONES

Physiological concentrations of glucocorticoids are required for osteoblast differentiation. Higher concentrations inhibit bone formation by inhibiting osteoblast differentiation and activity, and may stimulate osteoclast action – leading to osteoporosis, which is a feature of Cushing's syndrome (Fig. 34.7) and an important adverse effect of glucocorticoid administration (Ch. 34).

Thyroxine stimulates osteoclast action, reducing bone density and liberating Ca^{2+}. Osteoporosis occurs in association with thyrotoxicosis, and it is important not to use excessive thyroxine for treating hypothyroidism (see Ch. 35).

---

[2]The type 1 receptor is the main one; the PTH type 2 receptor is also a transmembrane-spanning G protein–coupled receptor expressed in a number of tissues including central nervous system, pancreas, testis and placenta. Its functions are less well understood.

474

DISORDERS OF BONE

The reduction of bone mass with distortion of the micro-architecture is termed *osteoporosis*; a reduction in the mineral

Parathyroid hormone, vitamin D and bone mineral homeostasis

- The vitamin D family give rise to true hormones; precursors are converted to calcifediol in the liver, then to the main hormone, calcitriol, in the kidney.
- Calcitriol increases plasma Ca^{2+} by mobilising it from bone, increasing its absorption in the intestine and decreasing its excretion by the kidney.
- Parathyroid hormone (PTH) acts mainly on the PTH type 1 receptor on osteoblasts and in the kidney. Intermittent stimulation of PTH receptors with synthetic PTH analogues stimulates bone formation.
- Calcitonin (secreted from the thyroid) reduces Ca^{2+} resorption from bone by inhibiting osteoclast activity.

content is termed *osteopenia*. Dual-energy X-ray absorptiometry (DXA) and quantitative computed tomography are the standard methods for assessing osteoporosis severity and monitoring the effect of treatment (Riggs et al., 2012). Osteoporotic bone fractures easily after minimal trauma. The commonest causes of osteoporosis are postmenopausal deficiency of oestrogen and age-related deterioration in bone homeostasis. It is estimated that 50% of women and 20% of men over the age of 50 will have a fracture due to osteoporosis. With increasing life expectancy, osteoporosis has increased to epidemic proportions and is an important public health problem, affecting about 75 million people in the United States, Japan and Europe. Other predisposing factors include catabolic hormones that favour protein breakdown such as excessive thyroxine or glucocorticoid administration. Other preventable or treatable diseases of bone include *osteomalacia* and *rickets* (the juvenile form of osteomalacia), in which there are defects in bone mineralisation due to vitamin D deficiency, either due to dietary deficiency of vitamin D and lack of sunlight, or to renal disease resulting in reduced synthesis of the active calcitriol hormone (Ch. 30) and *Paget's disease*, in which there is distortion of the processes of bone resorption and remodelling as a consequence of mutation in the gene that codes for a ubiquitin-binding protein[3] called sequestosome 1 (Rea et al., 2013), which is a scaffold protein in the RANK/NF-κB signalling pathway (see p. 472).

DRUGS USED IN BONE DISORDERS

Two types of agent are currently used for treatment of osteoporosis:

1. *Antiresorptive drugs* that decrease bone loss, e.g. bisphosphonates, calcitonin, selective [o]estrogen receptor modulators (SERMs), **denusomab**, calcium.
2. *Anabolic agents* that increase bone formation, e.g. PTH, **teriparatide**.

---

[3]Ubiquitin (Ch. 6) is a small regulatory protein present in almost all cells of the body ('ubiquitous'). It directs proteins to compartments in the cell, including the proteasome which destroys and recycles proteins. Ubiquitin-binding proteins interact with ubiquitinated targets and regulate diverse biological processes, including endocytosis, signal transduction, transcription and DNA repair.

Rickets and osteomalacia are treated with vitamin D preparations.

Paget's disease is common but only a small percentage of patients are symptomatic; if medical treatment is needed for symptoms such as bone pain, intermittent courses of bisphosphonates such as risedronate, **pamidronate** or **zoledronate** (see later) can provide benefit that lasts for a number of years, and are much more convenient than frequent injections of **salcatonin**, previously the only effective medical treatment.

BISPHOSPHONATES

Bisphosphonates (Fig. 37.5) are enzyme-resistant analogues of pyrophosphate, a normal constituent of tissue fluids that accumulates in bone and has a role in regulating bone resorption. Bisphosphonates inhibit bone resorption by an action mainly on the osteoclasts. They form tight complexes with calcium in the bone matrix, and are released slowly as bone is resorbed by the osteoclasts, which are thus exposed to high local bisphosphonate concentrations.

Mechanism of action

Bisphosphonates reduce the rate of bone turnover. They can be grouped into two classes:

1. Simple compounds that are very similar to pyrophosphate (e.g. **etidronate, clodronate**). These are incorporated into ATP analogues that accumulate within the osteoclasts and promote their apoptosis.
2. Potent amino-bisphosphonates (e.g. **pamidronate, alendronate, risedronate, ibandronate, zoledronate**). These prevent bone resorption by interfering with the anchoring of cell surface proteins to the osteoclast membrane by prenylation, thereby preventing osteoclast attachment to bone (see Strewler, 2005).

Fig. 37.5 Structure of bisphosphonates. Replacement of the oxygen atom in pyrophosphate renders the compounds enzyme-resistant. Addition of an N-containing side chain alters the mechanism of action (see text) and greatly increases potency.

Pharmacokinetic aspects

Bisphosphonates are given orally on an empty stomach with plenty of water in a sitting or standing position at least 30 min before breakfast because of their propensity to cause severe oesophageal problems or, in the case of pamidronate, ibandronate and of zoledronate, intravenously. They are poorly absorbed from the gut. About 50% of absorbed drug accumulates at sites of bone mineralisation, where it remains adsorbed onto hydroxyapatite crystals, potentially for months or years, until the bone is resorbed. The free drug is excreted unchanged by the kidney.

Absorption is impaired by food, particularly milk, so the drugs must be taken on an empty stomach.

Unwanted effects include gastrointestinal (GI) disturbances including peptic ulcers and oesophagitis (sometimes with erosions or stricture formation). Bone pain occurs occasionally. Atypical femoral fractures are described during long-term treatment, especially of osteoporosis, and the need for continued use should be re-evaluated periodically (e.g. after 5 years). Given intravenously, some bisphosphonates (in particular zoledronate) can lead to osteonecrosis (literally 'death of bone') of the jaw, especially in patients with malignant disease; a dental check is needed before treatment (followed by any indicated remedial work). After zoledronate infusion supplemental calcium and vitamin D are administered for at least 10 days.

Clinical use

Alendronate, ibandronate and risedronate are given orally for prophylaxis and treatment of osteoporosis. Etidronate is an alternative. Clodronate is used in patients with malignant disease involving bone and pamidronate is given by intravenous infusion to treat hypercalcaemia of malignancy or to treat Paget's disease. Ibandronate is given intravenously every 3–4 weeks in patients with breast cancer metastatic to bone, or every 3 months to treat postmenopausal osteoporosis. Zoledronate, which is given as an intravenous infusion, is used for advanced malignancy involving bone, for Paget's disease and for selected cases of osteoporosis (postmenopausal or in men) when it is administered once a year or even less frequently (see clinical box below).

Bisphosphonates

- Orally active, stable analogues of pyrophosphate, which are incorporated into remodelling bone and remain there for months to years.
- Released when osteoclast-mediated bone resorption occurs, exposing osteoclasts to their effects.
- First-generation compounds (e.g. **etidronate**) act by promoting apoptosis of osteoclasts.
- Second-generation compounds (e.g. **risedronate**) with N-containing side chains are much more potent, and prevent osteoclast action by inhibiting prenylation reactions required for membrane anchoring of functional proteins.
- Used long term for prevention and treatment of osteoporosis, and for symptomatic Paget's disease.
- Main unwanted effect is gastrointestinal (especially oesophageal) disturbance; a rare but serious adverse effect of the most potent drugs (notably **zoledronate**) is osteonecrosis of the jaw.

Clinical uses of bisphosphonates

- *Osteoporosis*:
  - 'primary' prevention of fractures in high-risk individuals (e.g. with established osteoporosis, several risk factors for osteoporosis, chronic treatment with systemic glucocorticoids);
  - 'secondary' prevention after an osteoporotic fracture;
  - **alendronate** by mouth, given daily or once weekly in addition to calcium with vitamin D_3. **Risedronate** or **etidronate** are alternatives; **zoledronate** is given annually or even less often by intravenous infusion; it is the most potent bisphosphonate and more likely to cause osteonecrosis of the jaw – dental check and remedial dental work are prerequisites of treatment.
- *Malignant disease* involving bone (e.g. metastatic breast cancer, multiple myeloma):
  - to reduce bone damage, pain and hypercalcaemia (e.g. **clodronate**, **ibandronate**, **zoledronate**).
- *Paget's disease* of bone (e.g. **risedronate**, **pamidronate**) administered intermittently as required in patients who are symptomatic.

OESTROGENS AND RELATED COMPOUNDS

The decline in endogenous oestrogen is a major factor in postmenopausal osteoporosis, and there is evidence that giving oestrogen as hormone replacement therapy (HRT; see Ch. 36) can ameliorate this. But HRT has actions on many systems, and newer agents (e.g. **raloxifene**, see Ch. 36) have been developed that exhibit agonist actions on some tissues and antagonist actions on others. These are termed *selective oestrogen receptor modulators* (SERMs).

RALOXIFENE

Raloxifene is a SERM that stimulates osteoblasts and inhibits osteoclasts. It also has agonist actions on the cardiovascular system, and antagonist activity on mammary tissue and the uterus.

It is well absorbed in the GI tract, and undergoes extensive first-pass metabolism in the liver, yielding the glucuronide, which undergoes enterohepatic recycling. Overall bioavailability is only about 2%. Despite the low plasma concentration, raloxifene is concentrated in tissues, and is converted to an active metabolite in liver, lungs, bone, spleen, uterus and kidney. Its half-life averages 32 h. It is excreted mainly in the faeces.

Unwanted effects include hot flushes, leg cramps, flu-like symptoms and peripheral oedema. Less common are thrombophlebitis and thromboembolism. Other rarer adverse effects are thrombocytopenia, GI disturbances, rashes, raised blood pressure and arterial thromboembolism. Raloxifene is not recommended for primary prevention of osteoporotic fractures, but is one alternative to a bisphosphonate for secondary prevention in postmenopausal women who cannot tolerate a bisphosphonate.

PARATHYROID HORMONE AND TERIPARATIDE

PTH and fragments of PTH given in small doses paradoxically *stimulate* osteoblast activity and *enhance* bone formation, and are used treat osteoporosis, especially in those who are receiving systemic corticosteroids. The main compound currently used is **teriparatide** – the peptide fragment (1–34) of recombinant PTH. A closely related molecule, abaloparatide (consisting of the 34 amino acids in human PTH-related peptide), has recently been licensed in the United States for postmenopausal women with osteoporosis who are at high risk of fracture, or unable to take other available therapies. It is thought that the greater affinity of abaloparatide for the RG conformation of the PTH-1 receptor will result in increased bone formation without provoking bone resorption (Harslof & Langdahl, 2016).

Teriparatide reverses osteoporosis by stimulating new bone formation. It increases bone mass, structural integrity and bone strength by increasing the number of osteoblasts and by activating those osteoblasts already in bone. It also reduces osteoblast apoptosis.

Teriparatide is given subcutaneously once daily. It is well tolerated, and serious adverse effects are few. Nausea, dizziness, headache and arthralgias can occur. Mild hypercalcaemia, transient orthostatic hypotension and leg cramps have been reported. Owing to concerns regarding long-term efficacy and safety, the maximal treatment duration of teriparatide should be limited to 24 months, and must not be repeated.

VITAMIN D PREPARATIONS

Vitamin D preparations are used in the treatment of vitamin D deficiencies, bone problems associated with renal failure ('renal osteodystrophy') and hypoparathyroidism – acute hypoparathyroidism is treated with intravenous calcium and injectable vitamin D preparations.

The main vitamin D preparation used clinically is **ergocalciferol**. Other preparations are **alfacalcidol** and **calcitriol**. All can be given orally and are well absorbed unless there is obstructive liver disease (vitamin D is fat soluble, and bile salts are necessary for absorption). **Paricalcitol,** a synthetic vitamin D analogue with less potential to cause hypercalcaemia, is used to treat and prevent the secondary hyperparathyroidism that occurs in patients with chronic renal failure because of associated hyperphosphataemia (Salusky, 2005).

Given orally, vitamin D is bound to a specific α-globulin in the blood and exogenous vitamin D persists in fat for many months after dosing. The main route of elimination is in the faeces.

The clinical uses of vitamin D preparations are given in the box.

Excessive intake of vitamin D causes hypercalcaemia. If hypercalcaemia persists, especially in the presence of elevated phosphate concentrations, calcium salts are deposited in the kidney and urine, causing renal failure and kidney stones.

Clinical uses of vitamin D

- Deficiency states: prevention and treatment of *rickets*, *osteomalacia* and vitamin D deficiency owing to *malabsorption* and *liver disease* (**ergocalciferol**).
- Hypocalcaemia caused by *hypoparathyroidism* (**ergocalciferol**).
- *Osteodystrophy* of *chronic renal failure*, which is the consequence of decreased calcitriol generation (**calcitriol** or **alphacalcidol**).
Plasma Ca^{2+} levels should be monitored during therapy with vitamin D.

BIOPHARMACEUTICALS

Denosumab is a recombinant human monoclonal antibody that inhibits RANKL, the primary signal for bone resorption (see p. 472), and is particularly useful when bisphosphonates are not appropriate. It is licensed for use in men and postmenopausal women with osteoporosis who are at high risk of fracture. Denusomab can be used for prevention of skeleton-related adverse events in patients with bone metastases from solid tumours, as well as to treat bone loss in patients who are receiving hormone ablation therapy for breast or prostate cancer. Calcium and vitamin D deficiencies need to be corrected and necessary dental work needs to be undertaken before treatment with denosumab to reduce the risk of osteonecrosis of the jaw (as with potent bisphosphonates, see clinical box, p. 476). It is administered as subcutaneous injections (60 mg) every 6 months for women with postmenopausal osteoporosis or men with prostate cancer at increased risk of osteoporosis because of hormone ablation, or more frequently (monthly) in patients with bone metastases. Adverse effects include altered bowel habit (diarrhoea or constipation), dyspnoea, hypocalcaemia, hypophosphataemia, infection (including respiratory, ear, cellulitis) or rash as well as (rarely) osteonecrosis of the jaw.

CALCITONIN

The main preparation available for clinical use (see the clinical box) is **salcatonin** (synthetic salmon calcitonin). Synthetic human calcitonin is also available. Calcitonin is given by subcutaneous or intramuscular injection, and there may be a local inflammatory action at the injection site. It can also be given intranasally, which is more convenient but less effective. Its plasma half-life is 4–12 min, but its action lasts for several hours.

Unwanted effects include nausea and vomiting. Facial flushing may occur, as may a tingling sensation in the hands and an unpleasant taste in the mouth.

Clinical uses of calcitonin/salcatonin

These agents are now less used.
- *Hypercalcaemia* (e.g. associated with neoplasia).
- *Paget's disease* of bone (to relieve pain and reduce neurological complications) – but it is much less convenient than an injected high-potency bisphosphonate.
- Postmenopausal and corticosteroid-induced *osteoporosis* (with other agents).

CALCIUM SALTS

Calcium salts used therapeutically include **calcium gluconate** and **calcium lactate**, given orally. Calcium gluconate is also used for intravenous injection in emergency treatment of hyperkalaemia (Ch. 30); intramuscular injection is not used because it causes local necrosis.

Calcium carbonate, an antacid and phosphate binder (Ch. 30), is usually very little absorbed from the gut (an advantage since an effect within the stomach or intestine is the desired outcome for a drug intended to buffer gastric acid and to reduce ileal phosphate absorption), but there is concern that low-level systemic absorption has the potential to cause arterial calcification in patients with renal failure, especially if complicated by hyperphosphataemia (the product of calcium and phosphate ion concentrations is sometimes used clinically to estimate the risk of tissue deposition of insoluble calcium phosphate).

Unwanted effects: oral calcium salts can cause GI disturbance. Intravenous administration in emergency treatment of hyperkalaemia requires care, especially in patients receiving cardiac glycosides, the toxicity of which is influenced by extracellular calcium ion concentration (see Ch. 22).

The clinical uses of calcium salts are given in the clinical box.

> ### Clinical uses of calcium salts
>
>
> - Dietary deficiency.
> - Hypocalcaemia caused by *hypoparathyroidism* or *malabsorption* (intravenous for acute tetany).
> - Calcium carbonate is an antacid; it is poorly absorbed and binds phosphate in the gut. It is used to treat *hyperphosphataemia* (Ch. 30).
> - Prevention and treatment of *osteoporosis* (often with oestrogen or selective oestrogen receptor modulators (SERMs) in women, bisphosphonate, vitamin D).
> - Cardiac dysrhythmias caused by severe *hyperkalaemia* (intravenous; see Ch. 30).

CALCIMIMETIC COMPOUNDS

Calcimimetics enhance the sensitivity of the parathyroid Ca^{2+}-sensing receptor to the concentration of blood Ca^{2+}, with a consequent decrease in secretion of PTH and reduction in serum Ca^{2+} concentration. There are two types of calcimimetics:

1. Type I are agonists, and include various inorganic and organic cations; Sr^{2+} is an example.
2. Type II are allosteric activators (see Ch. 3) that activate the receptor indirectly. Examples include **cinacalcet**, which is an oral preparation used for the treatment of hyperparathyroidism (see Fig. 37.3; Peacock et al., 2005), and **etelcalcetide,** a recently licensed injectable formulation that has a longer elimination half-life than cinacalcet (Hamano et al., 2017).

POTENTIAL NEW THERAPIES

Romosozumab is a monoclonal antibody that increases bone formation and reduces bone resorption through inhibition of sclerostin which is produced by osteoclasts (McClung, 2017). Although romosozumab appears to be more efficacious than alendronate in preventing fractures, there are safety concerns that have slowed progress towards licensing.

REFERENCES AND FURTHER READING

Bone disorders and bone remodelling

Boyce, B.F., Xing, L., 2008. Functions of RANKL/RANK/OPG in bone modeling and remodeling. Arch. Biochem. Biophys. 473, 139–146. (*Good review of the role of the RANK/RANKL/OPG in osteoclast formation and the transcription factors involved*)

Deal, C., 2009. Potential new drug targets for osteoporosis. Nat. Clin. Pract. Rheumatol. 5, 174–180. (*Outstanding review; good diagrams*)

Deftos, L.J., 2005. Treatment of Paget's disease – taming the wild osteoclast. N. Engl. J. Med. 353, 872–875. (*Editorial covering the use of OPG and zoledronic acid for Paget's disease. See also article by Cundy et al. in the same issue, pp. 918–923*)

Imai, Y., Youn, M.Y., Inoue, K., 2013. Nuclear receptors in bone physiology and diseases. Physiol. Rev. 93, 481–523. (*Reviews roles of various nuclear receptor-mediated signalling pathways in bone physiology and disease*)

Khosla, S., Westendorf, J.J., Oursler, M.J., 2008. Building bone to reverse osteoporosis and repair fractures. J. Clin. Invest. 118, 421–428. (*Good review; covers the role of Wnt signalling and sclerostin secretion*)

McClung, M.R., 2017. Clinical utility of anti-sclerostin antibodies. Bone 96, 3–7. (*Describes new advances in the understanding of drugs targeted at sclerostin*)

Rea, S.L., Walsh, J.P., Layfield, R., Ratajczak, T., Xu, J., 2013. New insights into the role of sequestosome 1/p62 mutant proteins in the pathogenesis of Paget's disease of bone. Endocrine Rev. 34, 501–524. (*Outlines recent advances in understanding of the multiple pathophysiological roles of SQSTM1/p62 protein, with particular emphasis on their relationship to Paget's disease of bone*)

Reichel, H., Koeftler, H.P., Norman, A.W., 1989. The role of the vitamin D endocrine system in health and disease. N. Engl. J. Med. 320, 980–991. (*Classic*)

Reid, J., 2008. Anti-resorptive therapies for osteoporosis. Semin. Cell Dev. Biol. 19, 5473–5478. (*Excellent review of the actions of current and novel anti-resorptive drugs*)

Riggs, B.L., Khosla, S., Melton, L.J., 2012. Better tools for assessing osteoporosis. J. Clin. Invest. 122, 4323–4324. (*Describes the current gold standard methods of dual-energy X-ray absorptiometry (DXA) and quantitative computed tomography*)

Stewart, J.F., 2004. Translational implications of the parathyroid calcium receptor. N. Engl. J. Med. 351, 324–326. (*Succinct article with useful diagrams*)

Wright, H.L., McCarthy, H.S., Middleton, J., Marshall, M.J., 2009. RANK, RANKL and osteoprotegerin in bone biology and disease. Curr. Rev. Musculoskelet. Med. 2, 56–64. (*Synopsis of the structures of RANK, RANKL and OPG, and the intracellular RANK/RANKL signalling pathways with a review of diseases linked to their malfunction*)

Drugs used to treat bone disorders

Clemett, D., Spenser, C.M., 2000. Raloxifene: a review of its use in postmenopausal osteoporosis. Drugs 60, 379–411. (*Comprehensive review covering the mechanism of action, pharmacology, pharmacokinetic aspects, therapeutic use and adverse effects of raloxifene*)

Cummings, S.R., San Martin, J., McClung, M.R., et al., 2009. Denosumab for prevention of fractures in postmenopausal women with osteoporosis. N. Engl. J. Med. 361, 818–820. (*'Freedom Trial' with 239 collaborators. Denosumab was effective in reducing fracture risk in women with osteoporosis*)

Hamano, N., Komaba, H., Fukagawa, M., 2017. Etelcalcetide for the treatment of secondary hyperparathyroidism. Expert Opin. Pharmacother. 18, 529–534.

Harslof, T., Langdahl, B.L., 2016. New horizons in osteoporosis therapies. Curr. Opin. Pharmacol. 28, 38–42. (Comprehensive review of the mechanisms and targets of new treatments for osteoporosis)

Khosla, S., 2009. Increasing options for the treatment of osteoporosis. N. Engl. J. Med. 361, 818–820. (*Editorial*)

Nemeth, E.F., Heaton, W.H., Miller, M., et al., 2004. Pharmacodynamics of the type II calcimimetic compound cinacalcet HCl. J. Pharmacol. Exp. Ther. 398, 627–635. (*Detailed study of pharmacokinetic aspects and the pharmacological action of cinacalcet hydrochloride*)

Peacock, M., Bilezikian, J.P., Klassen, P.S., et al., 2005. Cinacalcet hydrochloride maintains long-term normocalcaemia in patients with primary hyperparathyroidism. J. Clin. Endocrinol. Metab. 90, 135–141.

Reginster, J.Y., Deroisy, R., Neuprez, A., et al., 2009. Strontium ranelate: new data on fracture prevention and mechanisms of action. Curr. Osteoporos. Rep. 7, 96–102. (*Stresses that in 5-year studies this drug has* proved efficacious in both decreasing bone reabsorption and stimulating bone formation, and has a positive risk–benefit ratio)

Rogers, M.J., 2003. New insights into the mechanisms of action of the bisphosphonates. Curr. Pharm. Des. 9, 2643–2658. (*Covers the different mechanisms of action of the simple bisphosphonates and the nitrogen-containing bisphosphonates*)

Salusky, I.B., 2005. Are new vitamin D analogues in renal bone disease superior to calcitriol? Pediatr. Nephrol. 20, 393–398.

Strewler, G.J., 2005. Decimal point – osteoporosis therapy at the 10-year mark. N. Engl. J. Med. 350, 1172–1174. (*Crisp article concentrating mainly on bisphosphonates*)

Tabatabaei-Malazy, O., Salari, P., Khashayar, P., LarijanI, B., 2017. New horizons in treatment of osteoporosis. Daru 25, 2. (*Comprehensive overview of recent developments in drug therapy*)

38 Chemical transmission and drug action in the central nervous system

OVERVIEW

Brain function is the single most important aspect of physiology that defines the difference between humans and other species. Disorders of brain function, whether primary or secondary to malfunction of other systems, are a major concern of human society, and a field in which pharmacological intervention plays a key role. In this chapter we introduce some basic principles of neuropharmacology that underlie much of the material in the other chapters describing drug action on the central nervous system.

INTRODUCTION

There are two reasons why understanding the action of drugs on the central nervous system (CNS) presents a particularly challenging problem. The first is that centrally acting drugs are of special significance to humankind. Not only are they of major therapeutic importance,[1] but they are also the drugs that humans most commonly administer to themselves for non-medical reasons (e.g. alcohol, tea and coffee, nicotine, cannabis, MDMA [ecstasy], opioids, cocaine, amphetamines and so on). The second reason is that the CNS is functionally far more complex than any other system in the body (also uniquely protected by a blood–brain barrier), and this makes the understanding of drug effects very much more difficult. The relationship between the behaviour of individual cells and that of the organ as a whole is far less direct in the brain than in other organs. Currently, the links between a drug's action at the biochemical and cellular level and its effects on brain function remain largely mysterious. Functional brain imaging is beginning to reveal relationships between brain activity in specific regions and mental function, and this tool is being used increasingly to probe drug effects. Despite sustained progress in understanding the cellular and biochemical effects produced by centrally acting drugs, and the increasing use of brain imaging to study brain function and drug effects, the gulf between our understanding of drug action at the cellular level and at the functional and behavioural level remains, for the most part, very wide.

In some instances, our understanding of brain function and how drugs alter it is more advanced. Thus, the relationship between dopaminergic pathways in the extrapyramidal system and the effects of drugs in alleviating or exacerbating the symptoms of Parkinson's disease (see Ch. 41) is clear cut. Many CNS drugs are used to treat psychiatric disorders

that are defined according to their symptomatology rather than on the basis of causative factors or clinical signs and investigations. What is called 'schizophrenia' or 'depression' on the basis of particular symptoms is likely to consist of several distinct disorders caused by different mechanisms and responding to drugs in different ways. Furthermore, in disorders such as schizophrenia and depression, disease-induced cognitive deficits may contribute to the behavioural symptoms and in chronic pain the affective state (mood) of the sufferer may be changed and exacerbate the painful condition. Much effort is going into pinning down the biological basis of psychiatric disorders – a necessary step to improve the design of better drugs for clinical use – but the task is daunting and progress is slow.

In this chapter we outline the general principles governing the action of drugs on the CNS. Most neuroactive drugs work by interfering with the chemical signals that underlie brain function, and the next two chapters discuss the major CNS transmitter systems and the ways in which drugs affect them. In Chapter 41, we focus on neurodegenerative diseases, and the remaining chapters in this section deal with the main classes of neuroactive drugs that are currently in use.

Background information will be found in neurobiology and neuropharmacology textbooks such as Iversen et al. (2009), Kandel et al. (2013) and Nestler et al. (2015).

CHEMICAL SIGNALLING IN THE NERVOUS SYSTEM

The brain (like every other organ in the body!) is basically a chemical machine; it controls the main functions of a higher animal across timescales ranging from milliseconds (e.g. returning a 100 mph tennis serve) to years (e.g. remembering how to ride a bicycle).[2] The chemical signalling mechanisms cover a correspondingly wide dynamic range, as summarised, in a very general way, in Fig. 38.1. Currently, we understand much about drug effects on events at the fast end of the spectrum – synaptic transmission and neuromodulation – but much less about long-term adaptive processes, although it is quite evident that the latter are of great importance for the neurological and psychiatric disorders that are susceptible to drug treatment.

The original concept of neurotransmission envisaged a substance released by one neuron and acting rapidly, briefly and at short range on the membrane of an adjacent (post-synaptic) neuron, causing excitation or inhibition. The principles outlined in Chapter 13 apply to the central as well as the peripheral nervous system. It is now clear that

---

[1]In England and Wales in 2015, over 200 million prescriptions (about 20% of all prescriptions), costing £1.93 billion, were for CNS drugs as defined by the *British National Formulary*. This amounted to over three prescriptions per person across the whole population.

[2]Memory of drug names and the basic facts of pharmacology seems to come somewhere in the middle of this range (skewed towards the short end).

Timescale	Process	Chemical mediators	Molecular mechanisms
ms	Impulse conduction	None	Voltage-gated ion channels (Ch. 4)
	Transmitter release	$[Ca^{2+}]_i$	Exocytosis (Ch. 4)
	Fast synaptic transmission	Fast transmitters (e.g. glutamate, GABA, ACh)	Ligand-gated ion channels (Ch. 3)
s	Slow synaptic transmission	Slow transmitters (e.g. monoamines, peptides, ACh)	G protein-coupled receptors (Ch. 3) linked to ion channels, $[Ca^{2+}]_i$, second messengers Soluble guanylyl cyclase (Ch. 21)
min	Neuromodulation	Slow transmitters + others (e.g. NO, arachidonic acid metabolites)	
	Synaptic plasticity		
h	Delayed pharmacological effects	Many neuroactive drugs (e.g. antidepressants, Ch. 48)	Receptor up-/down-regulation ? Altered gene expression
	Pharmacological tolerance	Many neuroactive drugs (Ch. 50) (e.g. opioids, benzodiazepines)	
day	Structural remodelling	Chemokines Cytokines Growth factors ? Adhesion molecules ? Steroids	Kinase-linked receptors controlling gene expression
month/year	Degeneration, regeneration and repair (very limited in CNS)		

Fig. 38.1 **Chemical signalling in the nervous system.** Knowledge of the mediators and mechanisms becomes sparser as we move from the rapid events of synaptic transmission to the slower ones involving remodelling and alterations of gene expression. *ACh*, acetylcholine; *CNS*, central nervous system; *NO*, nitric oxide.

chemical mediators within the brain can produce slow and long-lasting effects; that they can act rather diffusely, at a considerable distance from their site of release (e.g. GABA acting at extrasynaptic GABA_A receptors, see Ch. 39); and that they can also produce other diverse effects, for example, on transmitter synthesis, on the expression of neurotransmitter receptors and on neuronal morphology, in addition to affecting the ionic conductance of the postsynaptic cell membrane. The term *neuromodulator* is often used to denote a mediator, the actions of which do not conform to the original neurotransmitter concept. The term is not clearly defined, and it covers not only the diffusely acting neuropeptide mediators, but also mediators such as nitric oxide (NO, Ch. 21) and arachidonic acid metabolites (Ch. 18), which are not stored and released like conventional neurotransmitters, and may come from non-neuronal cells, particularly glia, as well as neurons. In general, *neuromodulation* relates to synaptic plasticity, including short-term physiological events such as the regulation of presynaptic transmitter release or postsynaptic excitability. Longer-term *neurotrophic* effects are involved in regulating the growth and morphology of neurons, as well as their functional properties. Table 38.1 summarises the types of chemical mediator that operate in the CNS.

Glial cells, particularly astrocytes, which are the main non-neuronal cells in the CNS and outnumber neurons by 10 to 1, also play an important signalling role. Once thought of mainly as housekeeping cells, whose function was merely to look after the fastidious neurons, they are increasingly seen as 'inexcitable neurons' with a major communications role (see Matsas & Tsacopolous, 2013; Vasile et al., 2017), albeit on a slower timescale than that of neuronal communication. These cells express a range of receptors and transporters, and also release a wide variety of mediators, including glutamate, D-serine, ATP, lipid mediators and growth factors. They respond to chemical signals from neurons, and also from neighbouring astrocytes and microglial cells (the CNS equivalent of macrophages, which function much like inflammatory cells in peripheral tissues). Electrical coupling between astrocytes causes them often to respond in concert in a particular brain region, thus controlling the chemical environment in which the neurons operate. Although they do not conduct action potentials, and do not send signals to other parts of the body, astrocytes are otherwise very similar to neurons and play a crucial communication role within the brain. This is a rapidly expanding area of research and drug development. It is an area to watch closely.

Table 38.1 Types of chemical mediators in the central nervous system

Mediator type[a]	Examples	Targets	Main functional role
Conventional small-molecule mediators	Glutamate, GABA, acetylcholine, dopamine, 5-hydroxytryptamine, etc.	Ligand-gated ion channels G protein–coupled receptors	Fast and slow synaptic neurotransmission Neuromodulation
Neuropeptides	Substance P, neuropeptide Y, endorphins, orexins, corticotrophin-releasing factor, etc.	G protein–coupled receptors	Neuromodulation
Lipid mediators	Prostaglandins, endocannabinoids	G protein–coupled receptors	Neuromodulation
'Gaseous' mediators	Nitric oxide, carbon monoxide, hydrogen sulfide, etc	Guanylyl cyclase	Neuromodulation
Neurotrophins, cytokines	Nerve growth factor, brain-derived neurotrophic factor, interleukin-1	Kinase-linked receptors	Neuronal growth, survival and functional plasticity
Steroids	Androgens, oestrogens	Nuclear and membrane receptors	Functional plasticity

[a]Most central nervous system pharmacology has been centred on small-molecule mediators and, less commonly, neuropeptides. Other mediator types are now being targeted for therapeutic purposes.

Chemical transmission in the central nervous system

- The basic processes of synaptic transmission in the central nervous system are essentially similar to those operating in the periphery (Ch. 13).
- Glial cells, particularly astrocytes, participate actively in chemical signalling, functioning essentially as 'inexcitable neurons'.
- The terms *neurotransmitter*, *neuromodulator* and *neurotrophic factor* refer to chemical mediators that operate over different timescales. In general:
  - *neurotransmitters* are released by presynaptic terminals and produce rapid excitatory or inhibitory responses in postsynaptic neurons;
  - fast neurotransmitters (e.g. glutamate, GABA) operate through ligand-gated ion channels
  - slow neurotransmitters and neuromodulators (e.g. dopamine, neuropeptides, prostanoids) operate mainly through G protein–coupled receptors;
  - *neuromodulators* are released by neurons and by astrocytes, and produce slower pre- or postsynaptic responses;
  - *neurotrophic factors* are released mainly by non-neuronal cells and act on tyrosine kinase-linked receptors that regulate gene expression and control neuronal growth and phenotypic characteristics.
- The same agent (e.g. glutamate, 5-hydroxytryptamine, acetylcholine) may act through both ligand-gated channels and G protein–coupled receptors, and function as both neurotransmitter and neuromodulator.
- Many chemical mediators, including glutamate, nitric oxide and arachidonic acid metabolites, are produced by glia as well as neurons.
- Many mediators (e.g. cytokines, chemokines, growth factors and steroids) control long-term changes in the brain (e.g. synaptic plasticity and remodelling), mainly by affecting gene transcription.

TARGETS FOR DRUG ACTION

▼ To recapitulate what was discussed in Chapters 2 and 3, neuroactive drugs act primarily on one of four types of target proteins, namely ion channels, receptors, enzymes and transport proteins. Of the four main receptor families – ionotropic receptors, G protein–coupled receptors, kinase-linked receptors and nuclear receptors – current neuroactive drugs target mainly the first two.

In the last three decades, knowledge about these targets in the CNS has accumulated rapidly, particularly as follows:

- As well as 40 or more small-molecule and peptide mediators, the importance of other 'non-classical' mediators – NO, eicosanoids, growth factors, etc. – has become apparent.
- Considerable molecular diversity of known receptor molecules and ion channels (see Ch. 3) has been revealed.
- Receptors and channels are each expressed in several subtypes, and many possess sites for allosteric modulation and exist in multiple heteromeric complexes, all of which add to the diversity of potential drug targets. In most cases, we are only beginning to discover what this diversity means at a functional level. The molecular diversity of such targets raises the possibility of developing drugs with improved selectivity of action, e.g. interacting with one kind of GABA$_A$ receptor without affecting others (see Ch. 45). The potential of these new approaches in terms of improved drugs for neurological and psychiatric diseases is large but as yet unrealised.

Our knowledge of the neurobiology of epilepsy, schizophrenia and depressive illnesses is advancing and hopefully this will result in new strategies for treating these disabling conditions. The pathophysiology and genetic causes of neurodegeneration are beginning to be understood (see Ch. 41) ushering in long-awaited gene therapies for CNS disorders. In this regard, **nusinersen**, an antisense oligonucleotide that corrects the genetic defect that causes spinal muscular atrophy, has recently been approved for clinical use.

DRUG ACTION IN THE CENTRAL NERVOUS SYSTEM

As already emphasised, the molecular and cellular mechanisms underlying drug action in the CNS and in the periphery have much in common. Understanding how drugs affect brain function is, however, problematic. One difficulty is the complexity of neuronal interconnections in the brain – the wiring diagram. Fig. 38.2 illustrates in a schematic way the kind of interconnections that typically exist for, say, a noradrenergic neuron in the *locus coeruleus* (see Ch. 40), shown as **neuron 1** in the diagram, releasing **transmitter** *a* at its terminals. Release of *a* affects **neuron 2** (which releases **transmitter** *b*), and also affects neuron 1 by direct feedback and, indirectly, by affecting presynaptic inputs impinging on neuron 1. The firing pattern of neuron 2 also affects the system, partly through interneuronal connections (**neuron 3**, releasing **transmitter** *c*). Even at this grossly oversimplified level, the effects on the system of blocking or enhancing the release or actions of one or other of the transmitters are difficult to predict, and will depend greatly on the relative strength of the various excitatory and inhibitory synaptic connections, and on external inputs (*x* and *y* in the diagram). Added to this complexity is the influence of glial cells, mentioned previously.

A further important complicating factor is that a range of secondary, adaptive responses is generally set in train by any drug-induced perturbation of the system. Typically, an increase in transmitter release, or interference with transmitter reuptake, is countered by inhibition of transmitter synthesis, enhanced transporter expression or decreased receptor expression. These changes, which involve altered gene expression, generally take time (hours, days or weeks) to develop and are not evident in acute pharmacological experiments.

In the clinical situation, the effects of psychotropic drugs often take weeks to develop, so it is likely that they reflect adaptive responses and slowly developing changes in perception rather than the immediate pharmacodynamic effects of the drug. This is well documented for antipsychotic and antidepressant drugs (Chs 47 and 48). The development of dependence on opioids, benzodiazepines and psychostimulants is similarly gradual in onset (Ch. 50). Thus one has to take into account not only the primary interaction of the drug with its target, but also the longer-term secondary response of the brain to this primary effect; it is often this secondary response, rather than the primary effect, which leads to clinical benefit.

BLOOD–BRAIN BARRIER

▼ A key factor in CNS pharmacology is the blood–brain barrier (see Ch. 9), penetration of which requires molecules to traverse the vascular endothelial cells rather than going between them. Inflammation can disrupt the integrity of the blood–brain barrier, allowing previously impermeable drugs such as **penicillin** to cross. In general, only small non-polar molecules can diffuse passively across cell membranes. Some neuroactive drugs penetrate the blood–brain barrier in this way, but many do so via transporters, which either facilitate entry into the brain or diminish it by pumping the compound from the endothelial cell interior back into the bloodstream. Drugs that gain entry in this way include **levodopa** (Ch. 41), **valproate** (Ch. 46) and various sedative histamine antagonists (Ch. 18). Active extrusion of drugs from the brain occurs via P-glycoprotein, an ATP-driven drug efflux transporter, and related transporter proteins (see Ch. 9). Many antibacterial and anticancer drugs are excluded from the brain while some CNS-acting drugs – including certain opioid, antidepressant, antipsychotic and anti-epileptic drugs – are actively extruded from the brain (see Linnet & Ejsing, 2008). Variation in the activity of efflux transporters between individuals is an important consideration (Chs 9 and 12).

Drug action in the central nervous system

- The basic types of drug target (ion channels, receptors, enzymes and transporter proteins) described in Chapter 3 apply in the central nervous system, as elsewhere.
- Most of these targets occur in several different molecular isoforms, giving rise to subtle differences in function and pharmacology.
- Many of the currently available neuroactive drugs are relatively non-specific, affecting several different targets, the principal ones being receptors, ion channels and transporters.
- The relationship between the pharmacological profile and the therapeutic effect of neuroactive drugs is often unclear.
- Slowly developing secondary responses to the primary interaction of the drug with its target are often important (e.g. the delayed efficacy of antidepressant drugs, and tolerance and dependence with opioids).

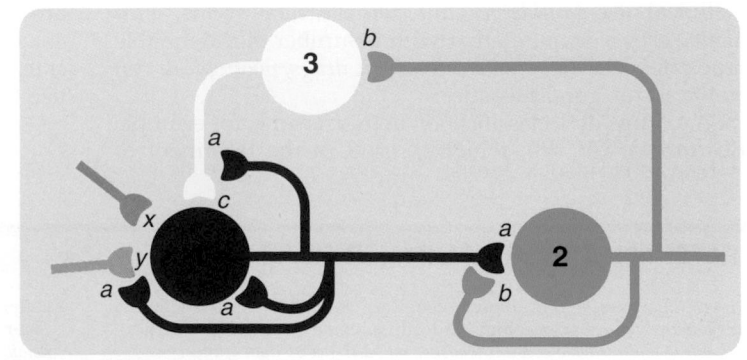

Fig. 38.2 Simplified scheme of neuronal interconnections in the central nervous system. Neurons *1*, *2* and *3* are shown releasing transmitters *a*, *b* and *c*, respectively, which may be excitatory or inhibitory. Boutons of neuron *1* terminate on neuron *2*, but also on neuron *1* itself, and on presynaptic terminals of other neurons that make synaptic connections with neuron *1*. Neuron *2* also feeds back on neuron *1* via interneuron *3*. Transmitters (*x and y*) released by other neurons are also shown impinging on neuron *1*. Even with such a simple network, the effects of drug-induced interference with specific transmitter systems can be difficult to predict.

Table 38.2 General classification of drugs acting on the central nervous system

Class	Definition	Examples	See chapter
General anaesthetic agents	Drugs used to produce surgical anaesthesia	Isoflurane, desflurane, propofol, etomidate	42
Analgesic drugs	Drugs used clinically for controlling pain	Opiates Neuropathic pain – carbamazepine, gabapentin, amitriptyline, duloxetine	43
Anxiolytics and sedatives	Drugs that reduce anxiety and cause sleep	Benzodiazepines (e.g. diazepam, chlordiazepoxide, flurazepam, clonazepam)	45
Anti-epileptic drugs Synonym: anticonvulsants	Drugs used to reduce seizures	Carbamazepine, valproate, lamotrigine	46
Antipsychotic drugs Synonym: antischizophrenic drugs	Drugs used to relieve the symptoms of schizophrenic illness	Clozapine, haloperidol, risperidone	47
Antidepressant drugs	Drugs that alleviate the symptoms of depressive illness	Selective serotonin reuptake inhibitors, tricyclic antidepressants, monoamine oxidase inhibitors	48
Psychomotor stimulants Synonym: psychostimulants	Drugs that cause wakefulness and euphoria	Amphetamine, cocaine, methylphenidate, caffeine	49
Psychotomimetic drugs Synonym: hallucinogens	Drugs that cause disturbance of perception (particularly visual hallucinations) and of behaviour in ways that cannot be simply characterised as sedative or stimulant effects	Lysergic acid diethylamide, mescaline, MDMA (ecstasy)	49
Cognition enhancers Synonym: nootropic drugs	Drugs that improve memory and cognitive performance	Acetylcholinesterase inhibitors: donepezil, galantamine, rivastigmine	41
		NMDA receptor antagonists: memantine Others: piracetam, modafinil	39

NMDA, N-methyl-D-aspartate.

THE CLASSIFICATION OF PSYCHOTROPIC DRUGS

Psychotropic drugs are defined as those that affect mood and behaviour. Because these indices of brain function are difficult to define and measure, there is no consistent basis for classifying psychotropic drugs. Instead, we find a confusing mêlée of terms relating to chemical structure (*benzodiazepines, butyrophenones*, etc.), biochemical target (*monoamine oxidase inhibitors, serotonin reuptake inhibitors*, etc.), behavioural effect (*hallucinogens, psychomotor stimulants*) or clinical use (*antidepressants, antipsychotic agents, anti-epileptic drugs*, etc.), together with a number of indefinable rogue categories (*atypical antipsychotic drugs, nootropic drugs*) thrown in for good measure.

Some drugs defy classification in this scheme, for example **lithium** (see Ch. 48), which is used in the treatment of manic depressive psychosis, and **ketamine** (see Ch. 42), which is classed as a dissociative anaesthetic but produces psychotropic effects rather similar to those produced by phencyclidine (PCP, Ch. 49).

Table 38.2 provides a general classification of centrally acting drugs. In practice, the use of drugs in psychiatric illness frequently cuts across specific therapeutic categories. For example, it is common for antipsychotic drugs to be used as 'tranquillisers' to pacify extremely anxious or unruly patients, or to treat bipolar depression (Ch. 48). Antidepressant drugs are often used to treat anxiety (Ch. 45) and neuropathic pain (Ch. 43), and certain psychostimulants are of proven efficacy for treating hyperactive children (Ch. 49). Here we will adhere to the conventional pharmacological categories, but it needs to be emphasised that in clinical use these distinctions are often disregarded.

REFERENCES AND FURTHER READING

Iversen, L.L., Iversen, S.D., Bloom, F.E., Roth, R.H., 2009. Introduction to Neuropsychopharmacology. Oxford University Press, New York. (*Excellent and readable account focusing on basic rather than clinical aspects*)

Kandel, E., Schwartz, J.H., Jessell, T.M., 2013. Principles of Neural Science, fifth ed. Elsevier, New York. (*Excellent and detailed standard text on neurobiology – little emphasis on pharmacology*)

Linnet, K., Ejsing, T.B., 2008. A review on the impact of P-glycoprotein on the penetration of drugs into the brain. Focus on psychotropic drugs. Eur. Neuropsychopharmacol. 18, 157–169. (*Review of how P-glycoprotein can limit the brain concentration of antidepressant and antipsychotic drugs*)

Matsas, R., Tsacopolous, M., 2013. The functional roles of glial cells in health and disease: dialogue between glia and neurons. Adv. Exp. Biol. Med. 468. (*This volume contains a number of chapters on the emerging view of glial cell function*)

Nestler, E.J., Hyman, S.E., Holzman, M., Malenka, R.C., 2015. Molecular Neuropharmacology, third ed. McGraw-Hill, New York. (*Good textbook*)

Vasile, F., Dossi, E., Rouach, N., 2017. Human astrocytes: structure and function in the healthy brain. Brain Struct. Funct. 222, 2017–2029. (*Informative review*)

39

Amino acid transmitters

OVERVIEW

In this chapter we discuss the major neurotransmitters in the central nervous system (CNS), namely the excitatory transmitter, glutamate, and the inhibitory transmitters, GABA and glycine. It is an area in which scientific interest has been intense in recent years. Unravelling the complexities of amino acid receptors and signalling mechanisms has thrown considerable light on their role in brain function and their likely involvement in CNS disease. Drugs that target specific receptors and transporters have been developed, but translating this knowledge into drugs for therapeutic use is only now beginning to happen. Here, we present the pharmacological principles and include recent references for those seeking more detail.

EXCITATORY AMINO ACIDS

EXCITATORY AMINO ACIDS AS CNS TRANSMITTERS

L-Glutamate is the principal and ubiquitous excitatory transmitter in the central nervous system.

▼ The realisation of glutamate's importance came slowly (see Watkins & Jane, 2006). By the 1950s, work on the peripheral nervous system had highlighted the transmitter roles of acetylcholine and catecholamines and, as the brain also contained these substances, there seemed little reason to look further. The presence of **γ-aminobutyric acid** (GABA; see p. 493) in the brain, and its powerful inhibitory effect on neurons, were discovered in the 1950s, and its transmitter role was postulated. At the same time, work by Curtis's group in Canberra showed that glutamate and various other acidic amino acids produced a strong excitatory effect, but it seemed inconceivable that such workaday metabolites could actually be transmitters. Through the 1960s, GABA and excitatory amino acids (EAAs) were thought, even by their discoverers, to be mere pharmacological curiosities. In the 1970s, the humblest amino acid, glycine, was established as an inhibitory transmitter in the spinal cord, giving the lie to the idea that transmitters had to be exotic molecules, too beautiful for any role but to sink into the arms of a receptor. Once glycine had been accepted, the rest quickly followed. A major advance was the discovery of EAA antagonists, based on the work of Watkins in Bristol, which enabled the physiological role of glutamate to be established unequivocally, and also led to the realisation that EAA receptors are heterogeneous.

To do justice to the wealth of discovery in this field in the past 25 years is beyond the range of this book; for more detail see Traynelis et al. (2010) and Nicoletti et al. (2011). Here we concentrate on pharmacological aspects. With regard to novel drug development, many promising new compounds interacting with EAAs commenced development for the treatment of a wide range of neurological and psychiatric disorders but have failed because of lack of efficacy or adverse effects, and only a few drugs[1] have made it into clinical use. The field has yet to make a major impact on therapeutics. The major problem has been that EAA-mediated neurotransmission is ubiquitous in the brain and so agonist and antagonist drugs exert effects at many sites, giving rise not only to therapeutically beneficial effects, but also to other, unwanted, harmful effects.

METABOLISM AND RELEASE OF EXCITATORY AMINO ACIDS

Glutamate is widely and fairly uniformly distributed in the CNS, where its concentration is much higher than in other tissues. It has an important metabolic role, the metabolic and neurotransmitter pools being linked by transaminase enzymes that catalyse the interconversion of glutamate and α-ketoglutarate (Fig. 39.1). Glutamate in the CNS comes mainly from either glucose, via the Krebs cycle, or glutamine, which is synthesised by glial cells and taken up by the neurons; very little comes from the periphery. The interconnection between the pathways for the synthesis of EAAs and inhibitory amino acids (GABA and glycine), shown in Fig. 39.1, makes it difficult to use experimental manipulations of transmitter synthesis to study the functional role of individual amino acids, because disturbance of any one step will affect both excitatory and inhibitory mediators.

In common with other fast neurotransmitters, glutamate is stored in synaptic vesicles and released by Ca^{2+}-dependent exocytosis; specific transporter proteins account for its uptake by neurons and other cells, and for its accumulation by synaptic vesicles (see Ch. 13). Released glutamate is taken up into nerve terminals and neighbouring astrocytes (Fig. 39.2) by $Na^+/H^+/K^+$ dependent transporters (cf. monoamine transporters – Chs 13 and 14), and transported into synaptic vesicles, by a different transporter driven by the proton gradient across the vesicle membrane. Several EAA transporters have been cloned and characterised in detail (see Jensen et al., 2015). Glutamate transport can, under some circumstances (e.g. depolarisation by increased extracellular $[K^+]$), operate in reverse and constitute a source of glutamate release, a process that may occur under pathological conditions such as brain ischaemia (see Ch. 41). Glutamate taken up by astrocytes is converted to glutamine and recycled, via transporters, back to the neurons, which convert the glutamine back to glutamate (see Fig. 39.2). Glutamine, which lacks the pharmacological activity of glutamate, thus serves as a pool of inactive transmitter under the regulatory control of the astrocytes, which act as ball boys, returning

---

[1]**Perampanel**, a non-competitive AMPA receptor antagonist, has been approved for the treatment of epilepsy (Ch. 46). **Memantine**, an NMDA antagonist, licensed for the treatment of moderate to severe Alzheimer's disease (Ch. 41), has been used for some time, as has the dissociative anaesthetic **ketamine**, an NMDA channel blocker (Ch. 42).

Fig. 39.1 **Metabolism of transmitter amino acids in the brain.** Transmitter substances are marked with *green boxes*. *GABA-T*, GABA transaminase; *GAD*, glutamic acid decarboxylase.

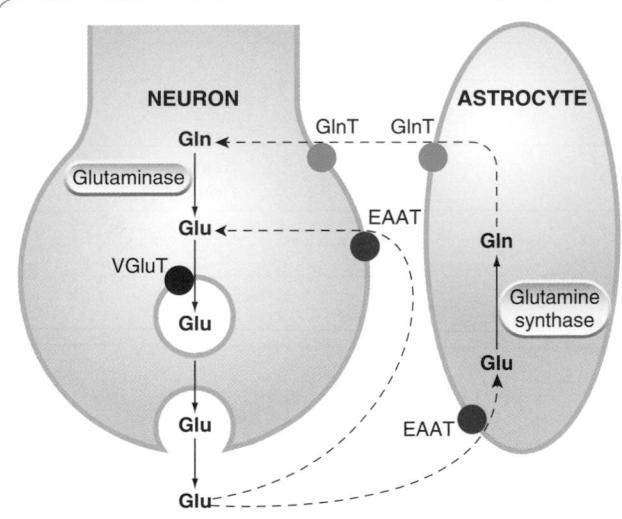

Fig. 39.2 **Transport of glutamate (Glu) and glutamine (Gln) by neurons and astrocytes.** Released glutamate is captured partly by neurons and partly by astrocytes, which convert most of it to glutamine. *EAAT*, excitatory amino acid transporter; *GlnT*, glutamine transporter; *VGluT*, vesicular glutamate transporter.

the ammunition in harmless form in order to rearm the neurons.

There may be value in developing enhancers and inhibitors of glutamate uptake for the treatment of CNS disorders in which the level of extracellular glutamate may be abnormal, e.g. neurodegeneration (see Ch. 41), schizophrenia (see Ch. 47) and depression (see Ch. 48). In contrast to the

situation with monoamine synthesis and transport (Chs 15 and 40), few drugs (none in clinical use) are known that interfere specifically with glutamate metabolism.

GLUTAMATE

GLUTAMATE RECEPTOR SUBTYPES

Glutamate and related EAAs, such as aspartate and homocysteate, activate both ionotropic (ligand-gated cation channels) and metabotropic (G protein–coupled) receptors (see Ch. 3 for a general description of ionotropic and metabotropic receptors).

IONOTROPIC GLUTAMATE RECEPTORS

On the basis of studies with selective agonists and antagonists (Fig. 39.3 and Table 39.1), three main subtypes of ionotropic receptors for glutamate can be distinguished: **NMDA**, **AMPA** and **kainate**[2] receptors, named originally according to their specific agonists. These ligand-gated channels comprise four subunits, each with the 'pore loop' structure shown in Fig. 3.5 (Ch. 3). There are some 16 different receptor subunits and their nomenclature has, until recently, been somewhat confusing.[3] Here, in this brief, general description, we use the International Union of Basic and Clinical Pharmacology (IUPHAR) recommended terminology because it simplifies the subject considerably, but beware confusion when reading older papers. NMDA receptors are heteromers assembled from seven types of subunit (GluN1, GluN2A, GluN2B, GluN2C, GluN2D, GluN3A, GluN3B). The subunits comprising AMPA receptors (GluA1–4) and kainate receptors (GluK1–5) are closely related to, but distinct from, GluN subunits. AMPA and kainite receptors can be homomeric or heteromeric. Receptors comprising different subunits can have different pharmacological and physiological characteristics, e.g. AMPA receptors lacking the GluA2 subunit have much higher permeability to Ca^{2+} than the others, which has important functional consequences (see Ch. 4). AMPA receptor subunits are also subject to other kinds of variation, namely alternative splicing, giving rise to the engagingly named *flip* and *flop* variants, RNA editing at the single amino acid level, and associated auxiliary subunits, all of which contribute yet more functional diversity to this diverse family.

AMPA receptors, and in certain brain regions kainate receptors, serve to mediate fast excitatory synaptic transmission in the CNS – absolutely essential for our brains to function. NMDA receptors (which often coexist with AMPA receptors) contribute a slow component to the excitatory synaptic potential (Fig. 39.4B), the magnitude of which varies in different pathways. NMDA, kainate and AMPA receptors are also expressed on nerve terminals where they can enhance or reduce transmitter release.[4] AMPA receptors

---

[2] In the past, AMPA and kainate receptors were often lumped together as AMPA/kainate or non-NMDA receptors, but they each have distinct subunit compositions and should not be grouped together.
[3] An international committee has sought to bring order to the area but, despite the logic of their recommendations, how generally accepted they will be remains to be seen (see Collingridge et al., 2009 and <www.guidetopharmacology.org>). Scientists can get very stuck in their ways.
[4] In the CNS, presynaptic ligand-gated ion channels such as kainate and NMDA receptors as well as nicotinic and P2X receptors (see Ch. 40) control neurotransmitter release. An explanation of how this control can be either facilitatory or inhibitory is given in Khakh and Henderson (2000).

Fig. 39.3 **Structures of agonists acting on glutamate, GABA and glycine receptors.** The receptor specificity of these compounds is shown in Tables 39.1 and 39.2. *AMPA,* (S)-α-amino-3-hydroxy-5-methylisoxazole-4-propionic acid; *L-AP4,* L-2-amino-4-phosphonopentanoic acid; *NMDA,* N-methyl-D-aspartic acid.

Table 39.1 **Properties of ionotropic glutamate receptors**

	NMDA		AMPA	Kainate
Subunit composition	Tetramers consisting of GluN1–3 subunits		Tetramers consisting of GluA1–4 subunits (variants splicing and RNA editing)	Tetramers consisting of GluK1–5 subunits
	Receptor site	*Modulatory site (glycine)*		
Endogenous agonist(s)	Glutamate Aspartate	Glycine D-Serine	Glutamate	Glutamate
Other agonist(s)[a]	NMDA	D-Cycloserine	AMPA	Kainate Domoate[b]
Antagonist(s)[a]	AP5, CPP	7-Chloro-kynurenic acid, HA-966	NBQX	NBQX ACET
Other modulators	Polyamines (e.g. spermine, spermidine) Mg^{2+}, Zn^{2+}		Cyclothiazide Perampanel Piracetam CX-516	—
Channel blockers	Dizocilpine (MK801) Phencyclidine, ketamine Remacemide Memantine Mg^{2+}		—	—
Effector mechanism	Ligand-gated cation channel (slow kinetics, high Ca^{2+} permeability)		Ligand-gated cation channel (fast kinetics; channels possessing GluA2 subunits show low Ca^{2+} permeability)	Ligand-gated cation channel (fast kinetics, low Ca^{2+} permeability)
Location	Postsynaptic (some presynaptic, also glial) Wide distribution		Postsynaptic (also glial)	Pre- and postsynaptic
Function	Slow epsp Synaptic plasticity (long-term potentiation, long-term depression) Excitotoxicity		Fast epsp Wide distribution	Fast epsp Presynaptic inhibition Limited distribution

[a]Structures of experimental compounds can be found in Brauner-Osborne et al. (2002).
[b]A neurotoxin from mussels (see Ch. 41).
ACET, -(S)-1-(2-amino-2-carboxyethyl)-3-(2-carboxy-5-phenylthiophene-3-yl-methyl)-5-methylpyrimidine-2,4-dione; *AP5,* 2-amino-5-phosphonopentanoic acid; *CPP,* 3-(2-carboxypiperazin-4-yl)-propyl-1-phosphonic acid; *CX-516,* 1-(quinoxalin-6-ylcarbonyl)-piperidine; *epsp,* excitatory postsynaptic potential; *NBQX,* 2,3-dihydro-6-nitro-7-sulfamoyl-benzoquinoxaline; *NMDA,* N-methyl-D-aspartic acid. (Other structures are shown in Fig. 39.3.)

Fig. 39.4 Effects of excitatory amino acid receptor antagonists on synaptic transmission. (A) AP5 (*N*-methyl-D-aspartic acid [NMDA] antagonist) prevents long-term potentiation (LTP) in the rat hippocampus without affecting the fast excitatory postsynaptic potential (epsp). Top records show the extracellularly recorded fast epsp (*downward deflection*) before, and 50 min after, a conditioning train of stimuli (100 Hz for 2 s). The presence of LTP in the control preparation is indicated by the increase in epsp amplitude. In the presence of AP5 (50 μmol/L), the normal epsp is unchanged, but LTP does not occur. Lower trace shows epsp amplitude as a function of time. The conditioning train produces a short-lasting increase in epsp amplitude, which still occurs in the presence of AP5, but the long-lasting effect is prevented. (B) Block of fast and slow components of epsp by CNQX (6-cyano-7-nitroquinoxaline-2,3-dione; AMPA receptor antagonist) and AP5 (NMDA receptor antagonist). The epsp (*upward deflection*) in a hippocampal neuron recorded with intracellular electrode is partly blocked by CNQX (5 μmol/L), leaving behind a slow component, which is blocked by AP5 (50 μmol/L). (Panel [A] from Malinow, R., Madison, D., Tsien, R.W., 1988. Nature 335, 821; panel [B] from Andreasen, M., Lambert, J. D., Jensen, M. S., 1989. J. Physiol. 414, 317–336.)

Fig. 39.5 Main sites of drug action on *N*-methyl-D-aspartic acid (NMDA) and GABA_A receptors. Both receptors are multimeric ligand-gated ion channels. Drugs can act as agonists or antagonists at the neurotransmitter receptor site or at modulatory sites associated with the receptor. They can also act to block the ion channel at one or more distinct sites. In the case of the GABA_A receptor, the mechanism by which 'channel modulators' (e.g. ethanol, anaesthetic agents, neurosteroids) facilitate channel opening is uncertain; they may affect both ligand-binding and channel sites. The location of the different binding sites shown in the figure is largely imaginary, although study of mutated receptors is revealing where they actually reside. Examples of the different drug classes are given in Tables 39.1 and 39.3.

occur on astrocytes as well as on neurons, and these cells play an important role in communication in the brain.

Binding studies show that ionotropic glutamate receptors are most abundant in the cortex, basal ganglia and sensory pathways. NMDA and AMPA receptors are generally co-localised, but kainate receptors have a much more restricted distribution. Expression of the many different receptor subtypes in the brain also shows distinct regional differences, but we have hardly begun to understand the significance of this extreme organisational complexity.

Special features of NMDA receptors

NMDA receptors and their associated channels have been studied in more detail than the other types and show special pharmacological properties, summarised in Fig. 39.5, that are postulated to play a role in pathophysiological mechanisms.

- They are highly permeable to Ca^{2+}, as well as to other cations, so activation of NMDA receptors is particularly effective in promoting Ca^{2+} entry.
- They are readily blocked by Mg^{2+}, and this block shows marked voltage dependence. It occurs at

Fig. 39.6 Facilitation of *N*-methyl-D-aspartic acid (NMDA) by glycine. Recordings from mouse brain neurons in culture (whole-cell patch clamp technique). Downward deflections represent inward current through excitatory amino acid-activated ion channels. (A) NMDA (10 μmol/L) or glycine (1 μmol/L) applied separately had little or no effect, but together produced a response. (B) The response to glutamate (Glu,10 μmol/L) was strongly potentiated by glycine (Gly, 1 μmol/L). (C and D) Responses of AMPA and kainate receptors to quisqualate (Quis) and kainate (Kai) were unaffected by glycine. (From Johnson, J.W., Ascher, P., 1987. Glycine potentiates the NMDA response in cultured mouse brain neurons. Nature 325, 529–531.)

physiological Mg^{2+} concentrations when the cell is normally polarised, but disappears if the cell is depolarised.

- Activation of NMDA receptors requires glycine as well as glutamate (Fig. 39.6). The binding site for glycine is distinct from the glutamate binding site, i.e. glycine is an allosteric modulator (see Ch. 2), and both have to be occupied for the channel to open. This discovery by Johnson and Ascher caused a stir, because glycine had hitherto been recognised as an inhibitory transmitter (see p. 497), so to find it facilitating excitation ran counter to the prevailing doctrine. The concentration of glycine required depends on the subunit composition of the NMDA receptor: for some NMDA receptor subtypes, physiological variation of the glycine concentration may serve as a regulatory mechanism, whereas others are fully activated at all physiological glycine concentrations. Competitive antagonists at the glycine site (see Table 39.1) indirectly inhibit the action of glutamate. **D-serine**, somewhat surprisingly,[5] may also function as an endogenous activator of the glycine site on the NMDA receptor.
- Some endogenous polyamines (e.g. **spermine**, **spermidine**) act at an allosteric site distinct from that of glycine to facilitate channel opening. The experimental drugs **ifenprodil** and **eliprodil** block their action.
- Other allosteric sites have been identified on the NMDA receptor and positive and negative allosteric modulators with novel patterns of GluN2 subunit

selectivity have been discovered (Zhu & Paoletti, 2015).
- **Aspartate** and **homocysteate** activate NMDA receptors and may be endogenous activators in certain brain regions.
- Some well-known anaesthetic and psychotomimetic agents, such as **ketamine** (Ch. 42) and **phencyclidine** (Ch. 49), are selective blocking agents for NMDA-operated channels. The experimental compound **dizocilpine** shares this property.

METABOTROPIC GLUTAMATE RECEPTORS

There are eight different metabotropic glutamate receptors (mGlu[1-8]) which are unusual in showing no sequence homology with other G protein–coupled receptors (Ferraguti & Shigemoto, 2006). They function as homo- and heterodimers[6] (see Ch. 3) cross-linked by a disulfide bridge across the extracellular domain of each protein (see Goudet et al., 2009). They are members of class C G protein–coupled receptors, possessing a large extracellular N-terminus domain that forms a Venus fly trap-like structure into which glutamate binds. They can be divided into three groups on the basis of their sequence homology, G protein coupling and pharmacology (Table 39.2). Alternatively, spliced receptor variants have been reported.

mGlu receptors are widely distributed throughout the CNS (see Ferraguti & Shigemoto, 2006) on neurons, where they regulate cell excitability and synaptic transmission, and on glia. Neuronal group 1 mGlu receptors are located postsynaptically and are largely excitatory. By raising intracellular $[Ca^{2+}]$, they modify responses through

---

[5]Surprising, because it is the 'wrong' enantiomer for amino acids of higher organisms. Nevertheless, vertebrates possess specific enzymes and transporters for this D-amino acid, which is abundant in the brain.

[6]It has been suggested that mGlu receptors may form heterodimers with non mGlu receptors such as the 5-HT[2A] receptor (González-Maeso et al., 2008).

Table 39.2 Metabotropic glutamate receptors

	Group 1	Group 2	Group 3
Members	mGlu$_1$, mGlu$_5$	mGlu$_2$, mGlu$_3$	mGlu$_4$, mGlu$_6$,[a] mGlu$_7$, mGlu$_8$
G protein coupling	G$_q$	G$_i$/G$_o$	G$_i$/G$_o$
Agonist	DHPG CHPG[b]	Eglumegad[c]	L-AP4 (S)-3,4-DCPG[d]
Antagonist	LY367385[e] S-4-CPG	LY341495	CPPG
Neuronal location	Somatodendritic	Somatodendritic and nerve terminals	Nerve terminals

[a]mGlu$_6$ is found only in the retina.
[b]mGlu$_5$ selective.
[c]Formerly known as LY354740.
[d]mGlu$_8$ selective.
[e]mGlu$_1$ selective.
CHPG, (RS)-2-chloro-5-hydroxyphenylglycine; CPPG, (RS)-α-cyclopropyl-4-phosphonophenylglycine; DHPG, 3,5-dihydroxyphenylglycine; L-AP4, 2-amino-4-phosphonobutyrate; (S)-3,4-DCPG, (S)-3,4-dicarboxyphenylglycine; S-4-CPG, (S)-4-carboxyphenylglycine.

ionotropic glutamate receptors (Fig. 39.7). Group 2 and 3 mGlu receptors are mostly presynaptic receptors and their activation tends to reduce synaptic transmission and neuronal excitability. They can be autoreceptors, involved in reducing glutamate release or heteroreceptors, e.g. when present on GABA-containing terminals.

SYNAPTIC PLASTICITY AND LONG-TERM POTENTIATION

▼ As well as participating in synaptic transmission, glutamate receptors play a role in long-term adaptive and pathological changes in the brain, and are of particular interest as potential drug targets.

In this context, two aspects of glutamate receptor function are of particular pathophysiological importance, namely *synaptic plasticity*, discussed here, and *excitotoxicity* (discussed in Ch. 41).

Synaptic plasticity is a general term used to describe long-term changes in synaptic connectivity and efficacy, either following physiological alterations in neuronal activity (as in learning and memory), or resulting from pathological disturbances (as in epilepsy, chronic pain or drug dependence). Synaptic plasticity underlies much of what we call 'brain function', allowing it to be influenced by past experience. Needless to say, no single mechanism is responsible; however, one significant and much-studied component is *long-term potentiation* (LTP), a phenomenon in which AMPA and NMDA receptors play a central role.

LTP (see Bear et al., 2015; Bliss & Cooke, 2011) is a prolonged (hours in vitro, days or weeks in vivo) enhancement of synaptic transmission that occurs at various CNS synapses following a short (conditioning) burst of high-frequency presynaptic stimulation. Its counterpart is *long-term depression* (LTD), which is produced at some synapses by a longer train of stimuli at lower frequency (see Massey & Bashir, 2007; Bliss & Cooke, 2011). These phenomena have been studied at various synapses in the CNS, most especially in the hippocampus, which plays a central role in learning and memory (see Fig. 39.4). It

has been argued that 'learning', in the synaptic sense, can occur if synaptic strength is enhanced following simultaneous activity in both pre- and postsynaptic neurons. LTP shows this characteristic; it does not occur if presynaptic activity fails to excite the postsynaptic neuron, or if the latter is activated independently, for instance by a different presynaptic input. The mechanisms underlying both LTP and LTD differ somewhat at different synapses in the brain (see Bear et al., 2015). Here only a brief, generic view of the underlying events is given. LTP initiation may involve both presynaptic and postsynaptic components, and results from enhanced activation of postsynaptic AMPA receptors at glutamatergic synapses and (probably) to enhanced glutamate release (although the argument rumbles on about whether increased transmitter release does or does not occur in LTP; see Nicoll, 2017). The response of postsynaptic AMPA receptors to glutamate is increased due to phosphorylation of the AMPA receptor subunits by kinases such as Ca^{2+}/calmodulin-dependent protein kinase (CaMKII) and protein kinase C (PKC), thus enhancing their conductance, as well as to increased expression and trafficking of AMPA receptors to synaptic sites. LTD, on the other hand, results from modest Ca^{2+} entry into the cell activating phosphatases that reduce AMPA receptor phosphorylation and enhance AMPA receptor internalisation (see Connor & Wang, 2016).

LTP is reduced by agents that block the synthesis or effects of nitric oxide or arachidonic acid. These mediators (see Chs 18 and 21) may act as retrograde messengers through which events in the postsynaptic cell are able to influence the presynaptic nerve terminal. Endogenous cannabinoids released by the postsynaptic cell, may also act as retrograde messengers to enhance glutamate release (see Chs 20 and 40).

Two special properties of the NMDA receptor underlie its involvement in LTP, namely voltage-dependent channel block by Mg^{2+} and its high Ca^{2+} permeability. At normal membrane potentials, the NMDA channel is blocked by Mg^{2+}; a sustained postsynaptic depolarisation produced by glutamate acting repeatedly on AMPA receptors, however, removes the Mg^{2+} block, and NMDA receptor activation then allows Ca^{2+} to enter the cell. Activation of group 1 mGlu receptors also contributes to the increase in [Ca^{2+}]$_i$. This rise in [Ca^{2+}]$_i$ in the postsynaptic cell activates protein kinases, phospholipases and nitric oxide synthase, which act jointly with other cellular processes to facilitate transmission via AMPA receptors. Initially, during the induction phase of LTP, phosphorylation of AMPA receptors increases their responsiveness to glutamate. Later, during the maintenance phase, more AMPA receptors are recruited to the membrane of postsynaptic dendritic spines as a result of altered receptor trafficking; later still, various other mediators and signalling pathways are activated, causing structural changes and leading to a permanent increase in the number of synaptic contacts.

The general descriptions of LTP and LTD given earlier are intended to provide the uninitiated reader with an overview of the topic. There are subtle differences in their forms and in the mechanisms underlying them at different synapses in the CNS. How LTP and LTD, in all of their guises, relate to different forms of memory is slowly being worked out (see Kessels & Malinow, 2009; Connor & Wang, 2016). Thus there is hope that drugs capable of modifying LTP and LTD may improve learning and memory.

DRUGS ACTING ON GLUTAMATE RECEPTORS
ANTAGONISTS AND NEGATIVE MODULATORS

Inotropic glutamate receptor antagonists

The main types and examples of ionotropic glutamate antagonists are shown in Table 39.1. They are selective for the main receptor types but generally not for specific subtypes. Many of these compounds, although very useful as experimental tools in vitro, are unable to penetrate the blood–brain barrier, so they are not effective when given systemically.

NMDA receptors, as discussed before, require glycine as well as NMDA to activate them, so blocking the glycine site is an alternative way to produce antagonism. **Kynurenic**

Fig. 39.7 Mechanisms of long-term potentiation. (A) With infrequent synaptic activity, glutamate (G) activates mainly AMPA receptors. There is insufficient glutamate to activate metabotropic receptors, and *N*-methyl-D-aspartic acid NMDA receptor channels are blocked by Mg^{2+}. (B) After a conditioning train of stimuli, enough glutamate is released to activate metabotropic receptors, and NMDA channels are unblocked by the sustained depolarisation. The resulting increase in $[Ca^{2+}]_i$ activates various enzymes, including the following:

- Ca^{2+}/calmodulin-dependent protein kinase (CaMKII) and protein kinase C (PKC) phosphorylate various proteins, including AMPA receptors (causing them to be trafficked to areas of synaptic contact on dendritic spines and facilitation of transmitter action) and other signal transduction molecules controlling gene transcription (not shown) in the postsynaptic cell.
- Nitric oxide synthase (NOS); release of nitric oxide (NO) facilitates glutamate release (retrograde signalling, otherwise known as NO turning back).
- Phospholipase A_2 (not shown) catalyses the formation of arachidonic acid (Ch. 18), a retrograde messenger that increases presynaptic glutamate release.
- A phospholipase (NAPE-PLD, not shown) that catalyses production of the endocannabinoids (Ch. 20) that act as retrograde messengers to enhance glutamate release.
- Brain-derived neurotrophic factor (BDNF) released from nerve terminals and postsynaptic structures (not shown) plays a multimodal role in the early and later stages of LTP. *Arg,* Arginine; *IP₃,* inositol (1,4,5) trisphosphate; *NO,* nitric oxide; *PI,* phosphatidylinositol.

acid and the more potent analogue **7-chloro-kynurenic acid** act in this way. Another site of block is the channel itself, where substances such as ketamine, phencyclidine and **memantine** act. These agents are lipid soluble and thus able to cross the blood–brain barrier.

The potential therapeutic interest in ionotropic glutamate receptor antagonists lies mainly in the reduction of brain damage following strokes and head injury (Ch. 41), as well as in the treatment of epilepsy (Ch. 46) and Alzheimer's disease (Ch. 41). They have also been considered for indications such as drug dependence (Ch. 50), schizophrenia (Ch. 47) and depression (Ch. 48). Trials with NMDA antagonists and channel blockers have so far proved disappointing, and a serious drawback of these agents is their tendency to cause hallucinatory and other disturbances (also a feature of phencyclidine; Ch. 49). Only two NMDA receptor antagonists,

ketamine (anaesthesia, analgesia and depression; see Chs 42, 43 and 48) and **memantine** (Alzheimer's disease; Ch. 41), are in clinical use. Ketamine is also used for its psychoactive properties (see Ch. 49) inducing feelings akin to an 'out-of-body' experience (going 'through the K-hole'). It is possible that antagonists selective for NMDA receptors containing the GluN2B subunit, which is highly Ca^{2+} permeable, may be effective for treating neurodegeneration and have fewer CNS side effects. The non-competitive AMPA receptor antagonist **perampanel** has been introduced as an anti-epileptic drug (see Ch. 46). The prospects for kainate receptor antagonists appear promising – antagonists for GluK1 have shown potential for the treatment of pain, migraine, epilepsy, stroke and anxiety (see Jane et al., 2009).

Overall, the promise foreseen for ionotropic glutamate receptor antagonists in the clinic has been less successful than was hoped. The problem may be that glutamate is such a ubiquitous and multifunctional mediator – involved, it seems, in almost every aspect of brain function – that attempting to improve a specific malfunction by flooding the brain with a compound that affects the glutamate system in some way is just too crude a strategy. The new hope is that subunit selective negative allosteric modulators may have fewer side effects than previous generations of orthosteric antagonists.

Metabotropic glutamate receptor antagonists

While antagonists that discriminate between the different groups of mGlu receptors are available (see Table 39.2), it has proven more difficult to develop selective antagonists for the subtypes within the groups. mGlu receptors, like many G protein–coupled receptors, possess allosteric modulatory sites, which can be either inhibitory or facilitatory (see Ch. 3). Antagonists or negative allosteric modulators acting at group 1 mGlu receptors have potential for the treatment of fragile X syndrome,[7] various pain states, Parkinson's disease (including the control of **levodopa**-induced dyskinesias, see Ch. 41), neuroprotection, epilepsy and drug abuse; whereas antagonists or negative allosteric modulators of group 2 mGlu receptors have potential as cognition enhancers (see Nicoletti et al., 2011).

AGONISTS AND POSITIVE MODULATORS

Ionotropic glutamate receptors

Various agonists at ionotropic glutamate receptors that are used experimentally are shown in Table 39.1. From the clinical perspective, interest centres on the theory that positive AMPA receptor modulators may improve memory and cognitive performance. Early examples include **cyclothiazide**, **piracetam** (approved for use in certain forms of epilepsy, see Ch. 46) and CX-516 (**Ampalex**). These positive allosteric modulators, known as *ampakines*, can act in subtly different ways to increase response amplitude, slow deactivation and attenuate desensitisation of AMPA receptor-mediated currents. They therefore increase AMPA-mediated synaptic responses and enhance LTP as well as up-regulating the production of nerve growth factors such as *brain-derived neurotrophic factor* (BDNF). Originally, ampakines were

thought to have therapeutic potential as cognition enhancers (nootropics or 'smart drugs') and for the treatment of schizophrenia, depression, attention deficit hyperactivity disorder (ADHD) and Parkinson's disease (see Lynch, 2006) but so far clinical trials have been disappointing. A more recently developed ampakine, CX1739, is in clinical trial for the treatment of drug-induced respiratory depression. Inhibition of the glycine transporter GlyT1 leads to an elevation of extracellular glycine levels throughout the brain and, through potentiation of NMDA receptor-mediated responses, could be beneficial in the treatment of various neurological disorders (see Harvey & Yee, 2013).

Metabotropic glutamate receptors

Developing selective agonists of mGlu receptors has proven to be quite difficult; recently, selective positive allosteric modulators have been developed (see Nicoletti et al., 2011). Group 2 and 3 mGlu receptors are located presynaptically on nerve terminals and agonists at these receptors decrease glutamate release. Group 2 mGlu agonists and positive allosteric modulators were therefore thought to have therapeutic potential to decrease neuronal cell death in stroke and in the treatment of epilepsy, but to date clinical trials have been disappointing. Agonists and positive allosteric modulators may be useful in treating anxiety as well as in controlling the positive symptoms of schizophrenia. Group 3 mGlu receptor positive allosteric modulators may be useful in treating anxiety and Parkinson's disease.

γ-AMINOBUTYRIC ACID (GABA)

GABA is the main inhibitory transmitter in the brain. In the spinal cord and brain stem, glycine is also important (see p. 497).

SYNTHESIS, STORAGE AND FUNCTION

GABA occurs in brain tissue but not in other mammalian tissues, except in trace amounts. It is particularly abundant (about 10 µmol/g tissue) in the nigrostriatal system, but occurs at lower concentrations (2–5 µmol/g) throughout the grey matter.

GABA is formed from glutamate (see Fig. 39.1) by the action of glutamic acid decarboxylase (GAD), an enzyme found only in GABA-synthesising neurons in the brain.[8] Immunohistochemical labelling of GAD is used to map the GABA pathways in the brain. GABAergic neurons and astrocytes take up GABA via specific transporters, thus removing GABA after it has been released. GAT1 is the predominant GABA transporter in the brain and is located primarily on GABAergic nerve terminals where it recycles GABA. GAT3 is located predominantly on astrocytes around the GABAergic synapse. GABA transport is inhibited by **guvacine**, **nipecotic acid** and **tiagabine**. Tiagabine is used to treat epilepsy (Ch. 46). In astrocytes GABA can be destroyed by a transamination reaction in which the amino group is transferred to α-oxoglutaric acid (to yield glutamate), with the production of succinic semialdehyde and

---

[7]Fragile X syndrome is caused by mutation of a single gene on the X chromosome. It affects about 1:4000 children of either sex, causing mental retardation, autism and motor disturbances.

[8]It has been suggested that GABA can also be synthesised in the brain from putrescine by the action of diamine oxidase and aldehyde dehydrogenase.

Excitatory amino acids

- Glutamate is the main fast excitatory transmitters in the central nervous system.
- Glutamate is formed mainly from the Krebs cycle intermediate α-ketoglutarate by the action of GABA transaminase.
- There are three main ionotropic glutamate receptors and eight metabotropic receptors.
- *N*-methyl-D-aspartic acid (NMDA), (*S*)-α-amino-3-hydroxy-5-methylisoxazole-4-propionic acid (AMPA) and kainate receptors are ionotropic receptors regulating cation channels.
- The channels controlled by NMDA receptors are highly permeable to Ca^{2+} and are blocked by Mg^{2+}.
- AMPA and kainate receptors are involved in fast excitatory transmission; NMDA receptors mediate slower excitatory responses and, through their effect in controlling Ca^{2+} entry, play a more complex role in controlling synaptic plasticity (e.g. long-term potentiation).
- Competitive NMDA receptor antagonists include **AP5** (2-amino-5-phosphonopentanoic acid) and **CPP** (3-(2-carboxypirazin-4-yl)-propyl-1-phosphonic acid); the NMDA-operated ion channel is blocked by **ketamine** and **phencyclidine**.
- **NBQX** (2,3-dihydro-6-nitro-7-sulfamoyl-benzoquinoxaline) is an AMPA and kainate receptor antagonist.
- NMDA receptors require low concentrations of glycine as a co-agonist, in addition to glutamate; **7-chlorokynurenic acid** blocks this action of glycine.
- NMDA receptor activation is increased by endogenous polyamines, such as **spermine**, acting on a modulatory site that is blocked by **ifenprodil**.
- The entry of excessive amounts of Ca^{2+} produced by NMDA receptor activation can result in cell death – excitotoxicity (see Ch. 41).
- Metabotropic glutamate receptors ($mGlu_{1–8}$) are dimeric G protein–coupled receptors. $mGlu_1$ and $mGlu_5$ receptors couple through G_q to inositol trisphosphate formation and intracellular Ca^{2+} release. They play a part in glutamate-mediated synaptic plasticity and excitotoxicity. The other mGlu receptors couple to G_i/G_o and inhibit neurotransmitter release, most importantly glutamate release.
- Some specific metabotropic glutamate receptor agonists and antagonists are available, as are positive and negative allosteric modulators.

The widespread distribution of GABA – GABA serves as a transmitter at about 30% of all the synapses in the CNS – and the fact that virtually all neurons are sensitive to its inhibitory effect suggests that its function is ubiquitous in the brain. That antagonists such as **bicuculline** induce seizures illustrates the important, ongoing inhibitory role of GABA in the brain.

GABA RECEPTORS: STRUCTURE AND PHARMACOLOGY

GABA acts on two distinct types of receptor: $GABA_A$ receptors are ligand-gated ion channels whereas $GABA_B$ receptors are G protein–coupled.

$GABA_A$ RECEPTORS

$GABA_A$ receptors[9] are members of the *cys-loop* family of receptors that also includes the glycine, nicotinic and $5-HT_3$ receptors (see Ch. 3, Fig. 3.5). The $GABA_A$ receptors are pentamers made up of different subunits.

The reader should not despair when informed that 19 $GABA_A$ receptor subunits have been cloned (α1–6, β1–3, γ1–3, δ, ε, θ, π and ρ1–3) and that splice variants of some subunits also exist. Although the number of possible combinations is large, only a few dozen have been shown to exist. The most common are α1β2γ2 (by far the most abundant), α2β3γ2 and α3β3γ2 subunits. To make up the pentamer, each receptor contains two α, two β and one γ subunit arranged in a circle in the sequence α–β–α–β–γ around the pore when viewed from the extracellular side of the membrane. GABA binds at each of the interfaces between the α and β subunits whereas benzodiazepines (see Ch. 45) bind at the α/γ interface. A novel benzodiazepine binding site at the α/β interface has recently been described but its function is unclear at present. Receptors containing different α and γ subunits exhibit differential sensitivity to benzodiazepines and mediate different behavioural responses to these drugs. This raises the tantalising prospect of developing new agents with greater selectivity and potentially fewer side effects. The $GABA_A$ receptor should therefore be thought of as a group of receptors exhibiting subtle differences in their physiological and pharmacological properties.

$GABA_A$ receptors are primarily located postsynaptically and mediate both fast and tonic postsynaptic inhibition. The $GABA_A$ channel is selectively permeable to Cl^- and because the equilibrium membrane potential for Cl^- is usually negative to the resting potential, increasing Cl^- permeability hyperpolarises the cell as Cl^- ions enter, thereby reducing its excitability.[10] In the postsynaptic cell, $GABA_A$ receptors are located both at areas of synaptic contact and extrasynaptically (Fig. 39.8 and see Farrant & Nusser, 2005).

---

[9]The IUPHAR Nomenclature Committee has recommended (see Olsen & Sieghart, 2008) that the receptors previously referred to as 'GABA$_C$' receptors, because they were insensitive to bicuculline, benzodiazepines and baclofen, should be subtypes of the $GABA_A$ receptor family as they are pentameric Cl^--permeable ligand-gated channels comprising homo- or heteromeric assemblies of ρ subunits. They are referred to as $GABA_A$-rho or $GABA_A$-ρ receptors. Their pharmacology and functional significance is slowly being worked out (see Naffaa et al., 2017).
[10]During early brain development (in which GABA plays an important role), and also in some regions of the adult brain, GABA has an excitatory rather than an inhibitory effect, because the intracellular Cl^- concentration is relatively high, so that the equilibrium potential is positive to the resting membrane potential.

then succinic acid. This reaction is catalysed by GABA transaminase, an enzyme located primarily in astrocytes. It is inhibited by **vigabatrin**, another compound used to treat epilepsy (Ch. 46).

GABA functions as an inhibitory transmitter in many different CNS pathways. About 20% of CNS neurons are GABAergic; most are short interneurons, but there are some long GABAergic tracts, e.g. from the striatum to the substantia nigra and globus pallidus (see Ch. 41 and Fig. 41.4).

Fig. 39.8 **Synaptic and extrasynaptic GABA$_A$ receptors.** (A) Diagram depicting GABA$_A$ receptors at synaptic and extrasynaptic sites in the plasma membrane. The *blue dots* represent GABA molecules. (B) Tonic activation of extrasynaptic GABA$_A$ receptors gives rise to a steady-state inward current *(distance from the baseline indicated by the dashed line)* and increased 'noise' on the trace. The current is blocked on application of the GABA$_A$ receptor antagonist SR95531. (C) Phasic release of GABA from the presynaptic terminal evokes a fast synaptic current *(rapid downward deflection)*. Note the different timescales in (B) and (C). (Figure courtesy M. Usowicz.)

Thus GABA produces inhibition by acting both as a fast 'point-to-point' transmitter and as an 'action-at-a-distance' neuromodulator, as the extrasynaptic GABA$_A$ receptors can be tonically activated by GABA that has diffused away from its site of release. Extrasynaptic GABA$_A$ receptors contain α4 and α6 subunits as well as the δ subunit. They have higher affinity for GABA and show less desensitisation than synaptic receptors, and are also highly sensitive to general anaesthetic agents (see Ch. 42) and ethanol (see Ch. 49),

GABA$_B$ RECEPTORS

GABA$_B$ receptors (see Bettler et al., 2004) are located pre- and postsynaptically. They are class C G protein–coupled receptors that couple through G$_i$/G$_o$ to inhibit voltage-gated Ca^{2+} channels (thus reducing transmitter release), to open potassium channels (thus reducing postsynaptic excitability) and to inhibit adenylyl cyclase.

▼ For GABA$_B$ receptors, the functional receptor is a dimer (see Ch. 3) consisting of two different seven-transmembrane subunits, B1 and B2, held together by a coil/coil interaction between their C-terminal tails. In the absence of B2, the B1 subunit does not traffic to the plasma membrane as it possesses an endoplasmic reticulum retention signal. Interaction of B1 with B2 masks the retention signal and facilitates trafficking to the membrane. Activation of the dimer results from GABA binding to the extracellular, 'Venus fly trap' domain of B1 (even although the B2 subunit possesses a similar domain) whereas it is the B2 subunit that interacts with and activates the G protein (Fig. 39.9).

Fig. 39.9 **Dimeric structure of the GABA$_B$ receptor.** The receptor is made up of two seven-transmembrane domain subunits held together by a coil/coil interaction between their C-terminal tails. Activation of the receptor occurs when GABA binds to the extracellular domain of the B1 subunit (known as the Venus fly trap, because it snaps shut when GABA binds). This produces an allosteric change in the B2 subunit which is coupled to the G protein. (Adapted from Kubo, Y., Tateyama, M., 2005. Towards a view of functioning dimeric metabotropic receptors. Curr. Opin. Neurobiol. 15, 289–295.)

DRUGS ACTING ON GABA RECEPTORS
GABA_A RECEPTORS

GABA$_A$ receptors resemble NMDA receptors in that drugs may act at several different sites (see Fig. 39.5). These include:

- the GABA-binding site
- several modulatory sites
- the ion channel

There is growing evidence that the different receptor subtypes differ in their pharmacological properties.

GABA$_A$ receptors are the target for several important centrally acting drugs, notably benzodiazepines (see Ch. 45), alcohol (see Ch. 49), barbiturates, neurosteroids (see later, Table 39.3) and many general anaesthetics (see Ch. 42). The main agonists, antagonists and modulatory substances that act on GABA receptors are shown in Table 39.3.

Muscimol, derived from a hallucinogenic mushroom, resembles GABA chemically (see Fig. 39.3) and is a powerful GABA$_A$ receptor agonist. A synthetic analogue, **gaboxadol** is a partial agonist that was developed as a hypnotic drug (Ch. 45) but has now been withdrawn. **Bicuculline**, a naturally occurring convulsant compound, is a specific antagonist that blocks the fast inhibitory synaptic potential in most CNS synapses. **Gabazine**, a synthetic GABA analogue, is similar. These compounds are useful experimental tools but have no therapeutic uses.

Benzodiazepines, which have powerful sedative, anxiolytic and anticonvulsant effects (see Ch. 45), selectively potentiate the effects of GABA on some GABA$_A$ receptors depending upon the subunit composition of the receptor. They bind with high affinity to an accessory allosteric site on the GABA$_A$ receptor, in such a way that the binding of GABA is facilitated and its agonist effect is enhanced. Conversely, inverse agonists at the benzodiazepine site (e.g. Ro15-4513) reduce GABA binding and are anxiogenic and proconvulsant – they are unlikely to be therapeutically useful!

Modulators that also enhance the action of GABA, but whose site of action is less well defined than that of benzodiazepines (shown as 'channel modulators' in Fig. 39.5), include other CNS depressants such as barbiturates, anaesthetic agents (Ch. 42) and neurosteroids. Neurosteroids (see Lambert et al., 2009) are compounds that are related to steroid hormones but that act to enhance activation of GABA$_A$ receptors – those containing δ subunits appear most sensitive. Interestingly, they include metabolites of progesterone and androgens that are formed in the nervous system, and are believed to have a physiological role. Synthetic neurosteroids include **alphaxalone**, developed as an anaesthetic agent (Ch. 42).

Table 39.3 Properties of inhibitory amino acid receptors

| | GABA$_A$ | | | | |
	Receptor site	Modulatory site (benzodiazepine)	Modulatory site (others)	GABA$_B$	Glycine
Endogenous agonists	GABA	Unknown, several postulated (see text)	Various neurosteroids (e.g. progesterone metabolites)	GABA	Glycine β-Alanine Taurine
Other agonist(s)	Muscimol Gaboxadol (THIP,[a] a partial agonist)	Anxiolytic benzodiazepines (e.g. diazepam)	Barbiturates Steroid anaesthetics (e.g. alphaxalone)	Baclofen	—
Antagonist(s)	Bicuculline Gabazine	Flumazenil (inverse agonist?)	—	2-Hydroxy-saclofen CGP 35348 and others	Strychnine
Channel blocker	Picrotoxin[b]			Not applicable	—
Effector mechanism(s)	Ligand-gated chloride channel			G protein–coupled receptor; inhibition of Ca^{2+} channels, activation of K$^+$ channels, inhibition of adenylyl cyclase	Ligand-gated chloride channel
Location	Widespread; primarily postsynaptic			Pre- and postsynaptic Widespread	Postsynaptic Mainly in brain stem and spinal cord
Function	Postsynaptic inhibition (fast ipsp and tonic inhibition)			Presynaptic inhibition (decreased Ca^{2+} entry) Postsynaptic inhibition (increased K$^+$ permeability)	Postsynaptic inhibition (fast ipsp)

[a]THIP is an abbreviation of the chemical name of gaboxadol. It is reported to have preference for δ subunit-containing extrasynaptic GABA$_A$ receptors.
[b]Picrotoxin also blocks some glycine receptors.
ipsp, inhibitory postsynaptic potential.

Picrotoxin, a plant product, is a convulsant that acts by blocking the GABA$_A$ receptor chloride channel, thus blocking the postsynaptic inhibitory effect of GABA. It also blocks glycine receptors. It has no therapeutic uses.

GABA$_B$ RECEPTORS

When the importance of GABA as an inhibitory transmitter was recognised, it was thought that a GABA-like substance might prove to be effective in controlling epilepsy and other convulsive states; because GABA itself fails to penetrate the blood–brain barrier, more lipophilic GABA analogues were sought, one of which, **baclofen** (see Fig. 39.3), was introduced in 1972. Unlike GABA, its actions are not blocked by bicuculline. These findings led to the recognition of the GABA$_B$ receptor, for which baclofen is a selective agonist. Baclofen is used to treat spasticity and related motor disorders (Ch. 46); it has been tested for treating alcohol and opioid dependence (see Ch. 50) but results so far are inconclusive.

Competitive antagonists for the GABA$_B$ receptor include a number of experimental compounds (e.g. **2-hydroxy-saclofen** and more potent compounds with improved brain penetration, such as CGP 35348). Tests in animals showed that these compounds produce only slight effects on CNS function (in contrast to the powerful convulsant effects of GABA$_A$ antagonists). The main effect observed, paradoxically, was an anti-epileptic action, specifically in an animal model of absence seizures (see Ch. 46), together with enhanced cognitive performance. However, as in many areas of pharmacology, such preclinical promise has not resulted in the development of a new therapeutic drug.

γ-HYDROXYBUTYRATE

γ-Hydroxybutyrate (**sodium oxybate** or GHB; see Wong et al., 2004) occurs naturally in the brain as a side product of GABA synthesis. As a synthetic drug it can be used to treat narcolepsy and alcoholism. In addition, it has found favour with bodybuilders, based on its ability to evoke the release of growth hormone, and with party-goers, based on its euphoric and disinhibitory effects. It is also used as an intoxicant and 'date rape' drug, but is fatal in higher doses. In common with many abused drugs (see Ch. 50), it activates 'reward pathways' in the brain, and its use is now illegal in most countries. GHB is an agonist at GABA$_A$ receptors containing α4 and δ subunits and a weak partial agonist at GABA$_B$ receptors. A specific GHB receptor has also been postulated but the evidence for its existence is not yet convincing.

GLYCINE

Glycine is an important inhibitory neurotransmitter in the spinal cord and brain stem. It is present in particularly high concentration (5 μmol/g) in the grey matter of the spinal cord. Applied ionophoretically to motor neurons or interneurons, it produces an inhibitory hyperpolarisation that is indistinguishable from the inhibitory synaptic response. **Strychnine,** a convulsant poison that acts mainly on the spinal cord, blocks both the synaptic inhibitory response and the response to glycine. This, together with direct measurements of glycine release in response to nerve stimulation, provides strong evidence for its physiological transmitter role. β-**Alanine** has pharmacological effects and

a pattern of distribution very similar to those of glycine, but its action is not blocked by strychnine.

The inhibitory effect of glycine is quite distinct from its role in facilitating activation of NMDA receptors (see p. 490).

▼ The glycine receptor (see Dutertre et al., 2012) resembles the GABA$_A$ receptor in that it is a cys-loop, pentameric ligand-gated chloride channel. There are no specific metabotropic receptors for glycine. Five glycine receptor subunits have been cloned (α1–4, β) and it appears that in the adult brain the main form of glycine receptor is a heteromeric complex of α and β subunits, probably with a stoichiometry of 2α and 3β. Homomers formed of only α subunits can form and are sensitive to glycine and strychnine, indicating that the binding site for these drugs is on the α subunit. They are also much more sensitive to channel block by **picrotoxin** than are receptors comprised of α and β subunits.

Glycine receptors are involved in the regulation of respiratory rhythms, motor control and muscle tone as well as in the processing of pain signals. Mutations of the receptor have been identified in some inherited neurological disorders associated with muscle spasm and reflex hyperexcitability. There are as yet no therapeutic drugs that act specifically by modifying glycine receptors.

Tetanus toxin, a bacterial toxin resembling **botulinum toxin** (Ch. 14), acts selectively to prevent glycine release from inhibitory interneurons in the spinal cord, causing excessive reflex hyperexcitability and violent muscle spasms (lockjaw).[11]

Glycine is removed from the extracellular space by two transporters, GlyT1 and GlyT2 (Eulenburg et al., 2005). GlyT1 is located primarily on astrocytes and expressed throughout most regions of the CNS. GlyT2, on the other hand is expressed on glycinergic neurons in the spinal cord, brain stem and cerebellum. The GlyT1 inhibitor **bitopertin** failed in phase III clinical trials for the treatment of negative symptoms of schizophrenia (see Ch. 47). GlyT2 inhibitors were thought to have potential as analgesics.

CONCLUDING REMARKS

The study of amino acids and their receptors in the brain has been one of the most active fields of research in the past 30 years, and the amount of information available is prodigious. These signalling systems have been speculatively implicated in almost every kind of neurological and psychiatric disorder, and the pharmaceutical industry has put a great deal of effort into identifying specific ligands – agonists, antagonists, modulators, enzyme inhibitors, transport inhibitors – designed to influence them. While a large number of pharmacologically unimpeachable compounds have emerged, and many clinical trials have been undertaken, due to lack of efficacy and serious adverse effects there have been few therapeutic breakthroughs. The optimistic view is that a better understanding of the particular functions of the many molecular subtypes of these targets, and the design of more subtype-specific ligands, will lead to future breakthroughs. Expectations have, however, undoubtedly dimmed in recent years.

---

[11]Botulinum toxin (also known as botox), then tetanus toxin, hold the prize for the two deadliest substances, with LD$_{50}$s of ~1 and 3 ng/kg. That means 1 g of each is enough to kill over 8 million people, or 935 g could potentially wipe out the entire global population!!

Inhibitory amino acids: GABA and glycine

- GABA is the main inhibitory transmitter in the brain.
- It is present fairly uniformly throughout the brain; there is very little in peripheral tissues.
- GABA is formed from glutamate by the action of glutamic acid decarboxylase. Its action is terminated mainly by reuptake, but also by deamination, catalysed by GABA transaminase.
- There are two main types of GABA receptor: GABA$_A$ and GABA$_B$.
- GABA$_A$ receptors, which occur mainly postsynaptically, are directly coupled to chloride channels, the opening of which reduces membrane excitability.
- **Muscimol** is a specific GABA$_A$ agonist, and the convulsant **bicuculline** is an antagonist.
- Other drugs that interact with GABA$_A$ receptors and channels include:
  - benzodiazepines, which act at an allosteric binding site to facilitate the action of GABA;
  - convulsants such as **picrotoxin**, which block the anion channel;
  - neurosteroids, including endogenous progesterone metabolites;
  - central nervous system depressants, such as barbiturates and many general anaesthetic agents, which facilitate the action of GABA.
- GABA$_B$ receptors are heterodimeric G protein–coupled receptors. They cause pre- and postsynaptic inhibition by inhibiting Ca^{2+} channel opening and increasing K$^+$ conductance. **Baclofen** is a GABA$_B$ receptor agonist used to treat spasticity. GABA$_B$ antagonists are not in clinical use.
- Glycine is an inhibitory transmitter mainly in the spinal cord, acting on its own receptor, structurally and functionally similar to the GABA$_A$ receptor.
- The convulsant drug **strychnine** is a competitive glycine antagonist. Tetanus toxin acts mainly by interfering with glycine release.

REFERENCES AND FURTHER READING

Excitatory amino acids

Bräuner-Osborne, H., Egebjerg, J., Nielsen, E.Ø., Madsen, U., Krogsgaard-Larsen, P., 2000. Ligands for glutamate receptors: design and therapeutic prospects. J. Med. Chem. 43, 2609–2645.

Collingridge, G.L., Olsen, R.W., Peters, J., Spedding, M., 2009. A nomenclature for ligand-gated ion channels. Neuropharmacology 56, 2–5.

Ferraguti, F., Shigemoto, R., 2006. Metabotropic glutamate receptors. Cell Tissue Res. 326, 483–504.

González-Maeso, J., Ang, R.L., Yuen, T., et al., 2008. Identification of a serotonin/glutamate receptor complex implicated in psychosis. Nature 452, 93–99.

Goudet, C., Magnaghi, V., Landry, M., et al., 2009. Metabotropic receptors for glutamate and GABA in pain. Brain Res. Rev. 60, 43–56.

Harvey, R.J., Yee, B.K., 2013. Glycine transporters as novel therapeutic targets in schizophrenia, alcohol dependence and pain. Nat. Rev. Drug Discov. 12, 866–885.

Jensen, A.A., Fahlke, C., Bjørn-Yoshimoto, W.E., Bunch, L., 2015. Excitatory amino acid transporters: recent insights into molecular mechanisms, novel modes of modulation and new therapeutic possibilities. Curr. Opin. Pharmacol. 20, 116–123.

Jane, D.E., Lodge, D., Collingridge, G.L., 2009. Kainate receptors: pharmacology, function and therapeutic potential. Neuropharmacology 56, 90–113.

Lynch, G., 2006. Glutamate-based therapeutic approaches: ampakines. Curr. Opin. Pharmacol. 6, 82–88. (*Report of new allosteric sites on NMDA receptors*)

Nicoletti, F., Bockaert, J., Collingridge, G.L., et al., 2011. Metabotropic glutamate receptors: from the workbench to the bedside. Neuropharmacology 60, 1017–1041. (*Extensive review of the scientific developments in this field and their potential clinical significance in relation to the development of new drugs*)

Traynelis, S.F., Wollmuth, L.P., McBain, C.J., et al., 2010. Glutamate receptor ion channels: structure, regulation and function. Pharmacol. Rev. 62, 405–496.

Watkins, J.C., Jane, D.E., 2006. The glutamate story. Br. J. Pharmacol. 147 (Suppl. 1), S100–S108. (*A brief and engaging history by one of the pioneers in the discovery of glutamate as a CNS transmitter*)

Zhu, S., Paoletti, P., 2015. Allosteric modulators of NMDA receptors: multiple sites and mechanisms. Curr. Opin. Pharmacol. 20, 14–23. (*Review of allosteric sites on NMDA receptors*)

Inhibitory amino acids

Bettler, B., Kaupmann, K., Mosbacher, J., Gassmann, M., 2004. Molecular structure and function of GABA$_B$ receptors. Physiol. Rev. 84, 835–867. (*Comprehensive review article by the team that first cloned the GABA$_B$ receptor and discovered its unusual heterodimeric structure*)

Dutertre, S., Becker, C.M., Betz, H., 2012. Inhibitory glycine receptors: an update. J. Biol. Chem. 287, 40216–40223.

Eulenburg, V., Armsen, W., Betz, H., Gomez, J., 2005. Glycine transporters: essential regulators of neurotransmission. Trends Biochem. Sci. 30, 325–333.

Farrant, M., Nusser, Z., 2005. Variations on an inhibitory theme: phasic and tonic activation of GABA$_A$ receptors. Nat. Rev. Neurosci. 6, 215–229.

Lambert, J.J., Cooper, M.A., Simmons, R.D., Weir, C.J., Belelli, D., 2009. Neurosteroids: endogenous allosteric modulators of GABA(A) receptors. Psychoneuroendocrinology 34 (Suppl. 1), S48–S58.

Naffaa, M.M., Hung, S., Chebib, M., Johnston, G.A.R., Hanrahan, J.R., 2017. GABA-ρ receptors: distinctive functions and molecular pharmacology. Br. J. Pharmacol. 174, 1881–1894.

Olsen, R.W., Sieghart, W., 2008. International Union of Pharmacology. LXX. Subtypes of γ-aminobutyric acid$_A$ receptors: classification on the basis of subunit composition, pharmacology, and function. Update. Pharmacol. Rev. 60, 243–260. (*IUPHAR Nomenclature Subcommittee report containing an extensive discussion of the subtypes of GABA$_A$ receptor depending upon subunit composition. It also contains the recommendation that GABA$_C$ receptors should be considered as subtypes of the GABA$_A$ receptor*)

Wong, C.G.T., Gibson, K.M., Snead, O.C., 2004. From street to brain: neurobiology of the recreational drug gamma-hydroxybutyric acid. Trends Pharmacol. Sci. 25, 29–34. (*Short review article*)

Physiological aspects

Bear, M.F., Connors, B.W., Paradiso, M.A., 2015. Neuroscience: Exploring the Brain, fourth ed. Lippincott, Williams & Wilkins, Baltimore. (*Major neuroscience textbook that discusses in detail long-term potentiation and memory mechanisms*)

Bliss, T.V., Cooke, S.F., 2011. Long-term potentiation and long-term depression: a clinical perspective. Clinics (Sao Paulo) 66 (Suppl. 1), 3–17.

Connor, S.A., Wang, Y.T., 2016. A place at the table: LTD as a mediator of memory genesis. Neuroscientist 22, 359–371. (*An update on the role of LTD in memory*)

Kessels, H.W., Malinow, R., 2009. Synaptic AMPA receptor plasticity and behavior. Neuron 61, 340–350.

Khakh, B.S., Henderson, G., 2000. Modulation of fast synaptic transmission by presynaptic ligand-gated cation channels. J. Auton. Nerv. Syst. 81, 110–121. (*Describes how activation of presynaptic ligand-gated cation channels can either enhance or inhibit neurotransmitter release*)

Massey, P.V., Bashir, Z.I., 2007. Long-term depression: multiple forms and implications for brain function. Trends Neurosci. 30, 176–184.

Nicoll, R.A., 2017. A brief history of long-term potentiation. Neuron 93, 281–290.

Other transmitters and modulators

40

OVERVIEW

The principal 'amine' transmitters in the central nervous system (CNS), namely noradrenaline, dopamine, 5-hydroxytryptamine (5-HT, serotonin) and acetylcholine (ACh), are described in this chapter, with briefer coverage of other mediators, including histamine, melatonin and purines. The monoamines were the first CNS transmitters to be identified, and during the 1960s a combination of neurochemistry and neuropharmacology led to many important discoveries about their role, and about the ability of drugs to influence these systems. Amine mediators differ from the amino acid transmitters discussed in Chapter 39 in being localised to small populations of neurons with cell bodies in the brain stem and basal forebrain, which project diffusely both rostrally to cortical and other areas, and in some cases caudally to the spinal cord. These amine-containing neurons are broadly associated with high-level behaviours (e.g. emotion, cognition and awareness), rather than with localised synaptic excitation or inhibition.[1] More recently, 'gaseotransmitters' - such as nitric oxide (NO), carbon dioxide and hydrogen sulfide (Ch. 21) - and endocannabinoids (Ch. 20) have come on the scene, and they are discussed at the end of the chapter. The other major class of CNS mediators, the neuropeptides (e.g. endorphins, neurokinins and orexins) appear in later chapters in this section.

INTRODUCTION

Although we know much about the many different mediators, their cognate receptors and signalling mechanisms at the cellular level, when describing their effects on brain function and behaviour we fall back on relatively crude terms – psychopharmacologists will be at our throats for so under-rating the sophistication of their measurements – such as 'motor coordination', 'arousal', 'cognitive impairment' and 'exploratory behaviour'. The gap between these two levels of understanding still frustrates the best efforts to link drug action at the molecular level to drug action at the therapeutic level. Modern approaches, such as the use of transgenic animal technology (see Ch. 8) and non-invasive

imaging techniques, are helping to forge links, but there is still a long way to go.

More detail on the content of this chapter can be found in Iversen et al. (2009) and Nestler et al. (2015).

NORADRENALINE

The basic processes responsible for the synthesis, storage and release of noradrenaline are the same in the CNS as in the periphery (Ch. 15). In the CNS, inactivation of released noradrenaline is by neuronal reuptake or by metabolism, largely through the *monamine oxidase, aldehyde reductase* and *catechol-O-methyl transferase* mediated pathway to 3-hydroxy-4-methoxyphenylglycol (MHPG) (see Fig. 15.3).

NORADRENERGIC PATHWAYS IN THE CNS

Although the transmitter role of noradrenaline in the brain was suspected in the 1950s, detailed analysis of its neuronal distribution became possible only when a technique, based on the formation of fluorescent catecholamine derivatives when tissues are exposed to formaldehyde, was devised by Falck and Hillarp. Detailed maps of the pathway of noradrenergic, dopaminergic and serotonergic neurons in laboratory animals were produced and later confirmed in human brains. The cell bodies of noradrenergic neurons occur in small clusters in the *pons* and *medulla*, and they send extensively branching axons to many other parts of the brain and spinal cord (Fig. 40.1). The most prominent cluster is the locus coeruleus (LC), located in the pons. Although it contains only about 10,000 neurons in humans, the axons, running in a discrete *medial forebrain bundle*, give rise to many millions of noradrenergic nerve terminals throughout the cortex, hippocampus, thalamus, hypothalamus and cerebellum. These nerve terminals do not form distinct synaptic contacts but appear to release transmitter somewhat diffusely. The LC also projects to the spinal cord and is involved in the descending control of pain (Ch. 43).

Other noradrenergic neurons lie close to the LC in the pons and project to the amygdala, hypothalamus, hippocampus and other parts of the forebrain, as well as to the spinal cord. A small cluster of adrenergic neurons, which release adrenaline rather than noradrenaline, lies more ventrally in the brain stem. These cells contain phenylethanolamine *N*-methyl transferase, the enzyme that converts noradrenaline to adrenaline (see Ch. 15), and project mainly to the pons, medulla and hypothalamus. Rather little is known about them, but they are believed to be important in cardiovascular control.

[1]They are, if you like, voices from the nether regions, which make you happy or sad, sleepy or alert, cautious or adventurous, energetic or lazy, although you do not quite know why – very much the stuff of mental illness.

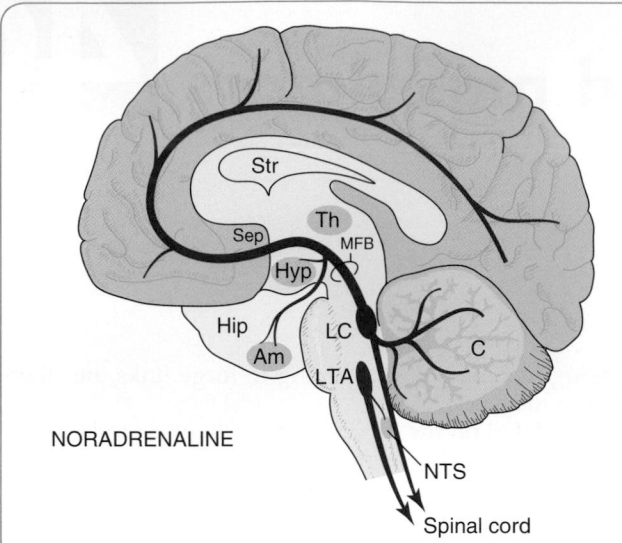

Fig. 40.1 Simplified diagram of the noradrenaline pathways in the brain. The location of the main groups of cell bodies and fibre tracts is in *solid colour*. *Light-shaded areas* show the location of noradrenergic terminals. *Am*, amygdaloid nucleus; *C*, cerebellum; *Hip*, hippocampus; *Hyp*, hypothalamus; *LC*, locus coeruleus; *LTA*, lateral tegmental area, part of the reticular formation; *MFB*, medial forebrain bundle; *NTS*, nucleus of the tractus solitarius (vagal sensory nucleus); *Sep*, septum; *Str*, corpus striatum; *Th*, thalamus.

FUNCTIONAL ASPECTS

With the exception of the β_3 adrenoceptor, all of the adrenoceptors (α_{1A}, α_{1B}, α_{1D}, α_{2A}, α_{2B}, α_{2C}, β_1 and β_2)[2] are expressed in the CNS (see Bylund, 2007). They are G protein–coupled receptors that interact with a variety of effector mechanisms (see Table 15.1). The role of α_1 receptors in the CNS is poorly understood. They are widely distributed, located both on postsynaptic neurons and on glial cells, and may be involved in motor control, cognition and fear. α_2 Adrenoceptors are located on noradrenergic neurons (in both somatodendritic and nerve terminal regions where they function as inhibitory autoreceptors activated by locally released noradrenaline), as well as on postsynaptic non-noradrenergic neurons. They are involved in blood pressure control (see later), sedation (α_2 agonists such as **medetomidine** are used as anaesthetics in veterinary practice) and analgesia. β_1 Receptors are found in the cortex, striatum and hippocampus whereas β_2 receptors are largely found in the cerebellum. They have been implicated in the long-term effects of antidepressant drugs but quite how remains a mystery (see Ch. 48).

Research on the α_2-adrenoceptor antagonist **idazoxan** led to the identification of other putative 'imidazoline receptors' (see Nikolic & Agbaba, 2012). These are the I_1 receptor, which plays a role in the central control of blood pressure (see Ch. 23); the I_2 receptor, which is not a true pharmacological receptor (see Ch. 1) at all but an allosteric binding site on the enzyme monoamine oxidase, and the I_3 receptor, present in the pancreas with a role in regulating insulin secretion.

[2]The α_{1C} receptor was subsequently found to be identical to α_{1A} receptor.

Arousal and mood

Attention has focused mainly on the LC, which is the source of most of the noradrenaline released in the brain, and from which neuronal activity can be measured by implanted electrodes. LC neurons are silent during sleep, and their activity increases with behavioural arousal. 'Wake-up' stimuli of an unfamiliar or threatening kind excite these neurons much more effectively than familiar stimuli. Amphetamine-like drugs, which release catecholamines in the brain, increase wakefulness, alertness and exploratory activity (although, in this case, firing of LC neurons is actually reduced by feedback mechanisms; see Ch. 49).

There is a close relationship between mood and state of arousal; depressed individuals are typically lethargic and unresponsive to external stimuli. The catecholamine hypothesis of depression (see Ch. 48) suggested that it results from a functional deficiency of noradrenaline in certain parts of the brain, while mania results from an excess. This remains controversial, and subsequent findings suggest that 5-HT may be more important than noradrenaline in relation to mood.

Blood pressure regulation

The role of central, as well as peripheral, noradrenergic synapses in blood pressure control is shown by the action of hypotensive drugs such as **clonidine** and **methyldopa** (see Chs 15 and 23), which decrease the discharge of sympathetic nerves emerging from the CNS. They cause hypotension when injected locally into the medulla or fourth ventricle, in much smaller amounts than are required when the drugs are given systemically. Noradrenaline and other α_2-adrenoceptor agonists have the same effect when injected locally. Noradrenergic synapses in the medulla probably form part of the baroreceptor reflex pathway, because stimulation or antagonism of α_2 adrenoceptors in this part of the brain has a powerful effect on the activity of baroreceptor reflexes.

Ascending noradrenergic fibres run to the hypothalamus, and descending fibres run to the lateral horn region of the spinal cord, acting to increase sympathetic discharge in the periphery. It has been suggested that these regulatory neurons may release adrenaline rather than noradrenaline as inhibition of phenylethanolamine *N*-methyl transferase, the enzyme that converts noradrenaline to adrenaline, interferes with the baroreceptor reflex.

Moxonidine and **rilmenidine** are reported to be I_1-receptor agonists with less activity at α_2 adrenoceptors; they act centrally to reduce peripheral sympathetic activity, thus decreasing peripheral vascular resistance (see Ch. 23).

DOPAMINE

Dopamine is particularly important in relation to neuropharmacology, because it is involved in several common disorders of brain function, notably Parkinson's disease, schizophrenia and attention deficit disorder, as well as in drug dependence and certain endocrine disorders. Many of the drugs used clinically to treat these conditions work by influencing dopamine transmission.

The distribution of dopamine in the brain is more restricted than that of noradrenaline. Dopamine is most abundant in the *corpus striatum*, a part of the extrapyramidal motor system concerned with the coordination of movement (see Ch. 41), and high concentrations also occur in certain

Noradrenaline in the central nervous system

- Mechanisms for synthesis, storage, release and reuptake of noradrenaline in the central nervous system (CNS) are essentially the same as in the periphery, as are the receptors (Ch. 15).
- Noradrenergic cell bodies occur in discrete clusters, mainly in the pons and medulla, one important such cell group being the locus coeruleus.
- Noradrenergic pathways, running mainly in the medial forebrain bundle and descending spinal tracts, terminate diffusely in the cortex, hippocampus, hypothalamus, cerebellum and spinal cord.
- The actions of noradrenaline are mediated through α_1, α_2, β_1 and β_2 receptors.
- Noradrenergic transmission is believed to be important in:
  - the 'arousal' system, controlling wakefulness and alertness;
  - blood pressure regulation;
  - control of mood (functional deficiency contributing to depression).
- Psychotropic drugs that act partly or mainly on noradrenergic transmission in the CNS include antidepressants, **cocaine** and **amphetamine**. Some antihypertensive drugs (e.g. **clonidine**, **methyldopa**) act mainly on noradrenergic transmission in the CNS.

Fig. 40.2 The main pathways for dopamine metabolism in the brain. *COMT*, catechol-*O*-methyl transferase; *MAO*, monoamine oxidase.

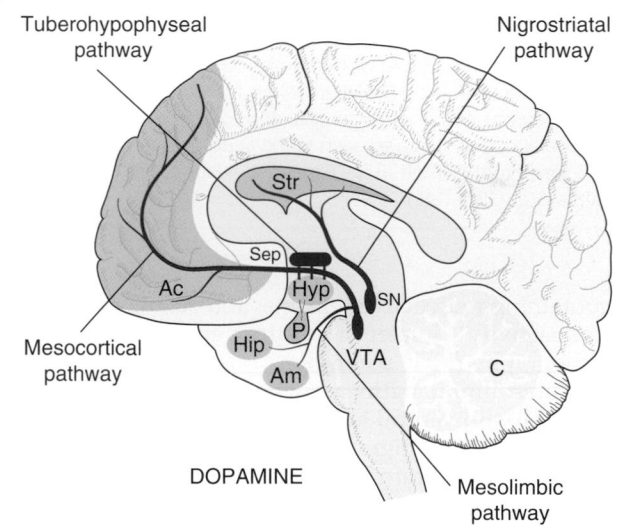

Fig. 40.3 Simplified diagram of the dopamine pathways in the brain, drawn as in Fig. 40.1. The pituitary gland (P) is shown, innervated with dopaminergic fibres from the hypothalamus. *Ac*, nucleus accumbens; *SN*, substantia nigra; *VTA*, ventral tegmental area; other abbreviations as in Fig. 40.1.

parts of the frontal cortex, limbic system and hypothalamus (where its release into the pituitary blood supply inhibits secretion of prolactin; Ch. 34).

The synthesis of dopamine follows the same route as that of noradrenaline (see Fig. 15.1), namely conversion of tyrosine to dopa (the rate-limiting step), followed by decarboxylation to form dopamine. Dopaminergic neurons lack dopamine β-hydroxylase, and thus do not convert dopamine to noradrenaline.

Dopamine is largely recaptured, following its release from nerve terminals, by a specific dopamine transporter, one of the large family of monoamine transporters (see Ch. 15). It is metabolised by monoamine oxidase and catechol-*O*-methyl transferase (Fig. 40.2), the main products being *dihydroxyphenylacetic acid* (DOPAC) and *homovanillic acid* (HVA), the methoxy derivative of DOPAC. The brain content of HVA is often used in animal experiments as an index of dopamine turnover. Drugs that cause the release of dopamine increase HVA, often without changing the content of dopamine. DOPAC and HVA, and their sulfate conjugates, are excreted in the urine, which provides an index of dopamine release in human subjects.

6-Hydroxydopamine, which selectively destroys dopaminergic nerve terminals, is used as a research tool. It is taken up by the dopamine transporter and converted to a reactive metabolite that causes oxidative cytotoxicity.

DOPAMINERGIC PATHWAYS IN THE CNS

There are four main dopaminergic pathways in the brain (Fig. 40.3):

1. The **nigrostriatal pathway**, accounting for about 75% of the dopamine in the brain, consists of cell bodies largely in the substantia nigra whose axons terminate in the corpus striatum. These fibres run in the medial forebrain bundle along with other monoamine-containing fibres. The abundance of dopamine-containing neurons in the human striatum can be appreciated from the image shown in Fig. 40.4, which was obtained by injecting a dopa derivative

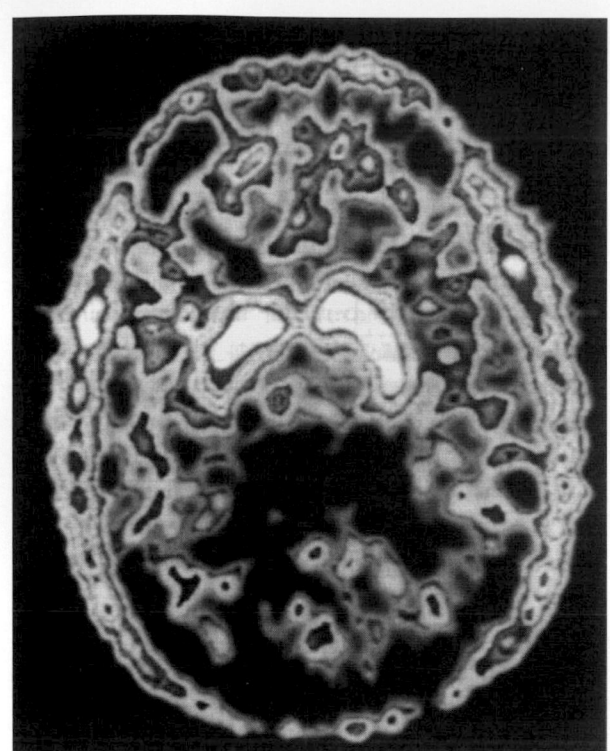

Fig. 40.4 Dopamine in the basal ganglia of a human subject. The subject was injected with 5-fluoro-dopa labelled with the positron-emitting isotope ^{18}F, which was localised 3 h later by the technique of positron emission tomography. The isotope is accumulated *(white areas)* by the dopa uptake system of the neurons of the basal ganglia, and to a smaller extent in the frontal cortex. It is also seen in the scalp and temporalis muscles. (From Garnett, E.S., Firnau, G., Nahmias, C., 1983. Nature 305, 137–138.)

containing radioactive fluorine, and scanning for radioactivity 3 h later by positron emission tomography (PET) scanning.

2. The **mesolimbic pathway**, whose cell bodies occur in the midbrain ventral tegmental area (VTA), adjacent to the substantia nigra, and whose fibres project via the medial forebrain bundle to parts of the limbic system, especially the *nucleus accumbens* and the *amygdaloid nucleus*.

3. The **mesocortical pathway**, whose cell bodies also lie in the VTA and which project via the medial forebrain bundle to the frontal cortex.

4. The **tuberohypophyseal** (or **tuberoinfundibular**) system is a group of short neurons running from the ventral hypothalamus to the median eminence and pituitary gland, the secretions of which they regulate.

There are also dopaminergic neurons in other brain regions and in the retina. For a more complete description, see Björklund and Dunnett (2007). The functions of the main dopaminergic pathways are discussed later.

DOPAMINE RECEPTORS

Two types of receptor, D_1 and D_2, were originally distinguished on pharmacological and biochemical grounds. Gene

cloning revealed further subgroups, D_1 to D_5. The original D_1 family now includes D_1 and D_5, while the D_2 family consists of D_2, D_3 and D_4 (Table 40.1). Splice variants, leading to long and short forms of D_2, and genetic polymorphisms, particularly of D_4, have subsequently been identified.

▼ All belong to the family of G protein–coupled transmembrane receptors described in Chapter 3. D_1 and D_5 receptors link through G_s to stimulate adenylyl cyclase and activate protein kinase A (PKA). PKA mediates many of the effects of D_1 and D_5 receptors by phosphorylating a wide array of proteins, including voltage-activated sodium, potassium and calcium channels, as well as ionotropic glutamate and GABA receptors. D_2, D_3, and D_4 receptors link through G_i/G_o and activate potassium channels as well as inhibiting calcium channels and adenylyl cyclase, and can also affect other cellular second messenger cascades (see Ch. 3). When intracellular cAMP is increased through activation of D_1 receptors, activating PKA, DARPP-32 (a *cAMP-regulated phosphoprotein* also known as *protein phosphatase 1 regulatory subunit 1B*) is phosphorylated. Phosphorylated DARPP-32 inhibits protein phosphatase-1, thus acting in concert with protein kinases as an amplifying mechanism favouring protein phosphorylation. In general, activation of D_2 receptors opposes the effects of D_1 receptor activation.

Dopamine receptors are expressed in the brain in distinct but overlapping areas. D_1 receptors are the most abundant and widespread in areas receiving a dopaminergic innervation (namely the striatum, limbic system, thalamus and hypothalamus; see Fig. 40.3), as are D_2 receptors, which also occur in the pituitary gland. D_2 receptors are found not only on dopaminergic neurons (on the soma, dendrites and nerve terminals), where they function as inhibitory autoreceptors activated by locally released dopamine, but also on glutamatergic, GABAergic and cholinergic nerve terminals (see De Mei et al., 2009). D_3 receptors occur in the limbic system but not in the striatum. The D_4 receptor is much more weakly expressed, mainly in the cortex and limbic systems.

Dopamine receptors also mediate various effects in the periphery (mediated by D_1 receptors), notably renal vasodilatation and increased myocardial contractility (dopamine itself has been used clinically in the treatment of circulatory shock; see Ch. 23).

FUNCTIONAL ASPECTS

The functions of dopaminergic pathways divide broadly into:

- motor control (nigrostriatal system)
- behavioural effects (mesolimbic and mesocortical systems)
- endocrine control (tuberohypophyseal system)

Dopamine and motor systems

Ungerstedt showed, in 1968, that bilateral ablation of the substantia nigra in rats, which destroys the nigrostriatal neurons, causes profound catalepsy, the animals becoming so inactive that they die of starvation unless artificially fed. Parkinson's disease (Ch. 41) is a disorder of motor control, associated with a deficiency of dopamine in the nigrostriatal pathway.

In treating CNS disorders, it is often desired that a certain receptor type be activated or inhibited only in one part of the brain, but the problem is that drugs are rarely brain-region selective and will affect a given receptor type throughout the brain. For example, many antipsychotic drugs (see Ch. 47) are D_2 receptor antagonists, exerting a beneficial effect by blocking D_2 receptors in the mesolimbic

Table 40.1 Dopamine receptors

	Functional role	D$_1$ type		D$_2$ type		
		D$_1$	D$_5$	D$_2$	D$_3$	D$_4$
Distribution						
Cortex	Arousal, mood	+++	—	++	—	+
Limbic system	Emotion, stereotypic behaviour	+++	+	++	+	+
Striatum	Prolactin secretion	+++	+	++	+	+
Ventral hypothalamus and anterior pituitary	Prolactin secretion	—	—	++	+	—
Agonists[a]						
Dopamine		FA	FA	FA	FA	FA
Apomorphine		FA	PA	PA	PA	PA
Bromocriptine		PA	FA	FA	PA	Ant
Quinpirole		Inactive	Inactive	FA	FA	FA
Antagonists						
Chlorpromazine		++	++	++	++	++
Haloperidol		++	+	+++	++	+++
Spiperone		++	+	+++	+++	+++
Sulpiride		—	—	++	++	+
Clozapine		+	+	+	+	++
Aripiprazole		—	—	+++ (PA)	—	++
Raclopride		—	—	+++	++	+
Signal transduction		G$_s$ coupled – activates adenylyl cyclase		G$_i$/G$_o$ coupled – inhibits adenylyl cyclase, activates K$^+$ channels, inhibits Ca^{2+} channels, may also activate phospholipase C		
Effect		Mainly postsynaptic inhibition		Pre- and postsynaptic inhibition Stimulation/inhibition of hormone release		

[a]Agonists generally exhibit lower potency at D$_1$ and D$_5$ receptors compared with D$_2$, D$_3$ and D$_4$ receptors.
Ant, antagonist; *FA*, full agonist; *PA*, partial agonist.
(Data based on that contained in the IUPHAR/BPS Guide to Pharmacology database www.guidetopharmacology.org.)

pathway. However, their D$_2$ antagonist property also gives rise to their major side effect, which is to cause movement disorders, by simultaneously blocking D$_2$ receptors in the nigrostriatal pathway.

Behavioural effects

Administration of **amphetamine** to rats, which releases both dopamine and noradrenaline, causes a cessation of normal 'ratty' behaviour (exploration and grooming), and the appearance of repeated 'stereotyped' behaviour (rearing, gnawing and so on) unrelated to external stimuli. These amphetamine-induced motor disturbances in rats probably reflect hyperactivity in the nigrostriatal dopaminergic system, and are prevented by dopamine antagonists and by destruction of dopamine-containing cell bodies in the midbrain, but not by drugs that inhibit the noradrenergic system.

Amphetamine and **cocaine** (which inhibit the dopamine transporter) and also other drugs of abuse (Chs 49 and 50) activate mesolimbic dopaminergic 'reward' pathways to produce feelings of euphoria in humans. The main receptor involved appears to be D$_1$, and transgenic mice lacking D$_1$ receptors behave as though generally demotivated, with reduced food intake and insensitivity to amphetamine and cocaine.

Neuroendocrine function

The tuberohypophyseal dopaminergic pathway (see Fig. 40.3) inhibits prolactin secretion via dopamine release. This system is of clinical importance. Many antipsychotic drugs (see Ch. 47), by blocking D$_2$ receptors, increase prolactin secretion and can cause breast development and lactation, even in males. **Bromocriptine**, a dopamine-receptor agonist derived from ergot, is used clinically to suppress prolactin secretion by tumours of the pituitary gland.

Growth hormone production is increased in normal subjects by dopamine, but bromocriptine paradoxically inhibits the excessive secretion responsible for acromegaly (probably because it desensitises dopamine receptors, in contrast to the physiological release of dopamine, which is pulsatile) and has a useful therapeutic effect, provided it is given before excessive growth has taken place. It is now rarely used, as other agents are more effective (see Ch. 34). Bromocriptine and other dopamine agonists, such as **cabergoline**, enhance libido and sexual performance.

Vomiting

Pharmacological evidence strongly suggests that dopaminergic neurons have a role in the production of nausea and vomiting. Thus nearly all dopamine-receptor agonists (e.g. bromocriptine) and other drugs that increase dopamine release in the brain (e.g. **levodopa**; Ch. 41) cause nausea and vomiting as side effects, while many dopamine antagonists (e.g. phenothiazines, **metoclopramide**; Ch. 31) have antiemetic activity. D_2 receptors occur in the area of the medulla (the chemoreceptor trigger zone) associated with the initiation of vomiting (Ch. 31), and are assumed to mediate this effect.

Dopamine in the central nervous system

- Dopamine is a neurotransmitter as well as being the precursor for noradrenaline. It is degraded in a similar fashion to noradrenaline, giving rise mainly to dihydroxyphenylacetic acid and homovanillic acid, which are excreted in the urine.
- There are four main dopaminergic pathways:
  - nigrostriatal pathway, important in motor control;
  - mesolimbic pathway, running from groups of cells in the midbrain to parts of the limbic system, especially the nucleus accumbens, involved in emotion and drug-induced reward;
  - mesocortical pathway, running from the midbrain to the cortex, involved in emotion;
  - tuberohypophyseal neurons, running from the hypothalamus to the pituitary gland, whose secretions they regulate.
- There are five dopamine-receptor subtypes. D_1 and D_5 receptors are linked to stimulation of adenylyl cyclase. D_2, D_3 and D_4 receptors are linked to activation of K^+ channels and inhibition of Ca^{2+} channels as well as to inhibition of adenylyl cyclase.
- D_2 receptors may be implicated in the positive symptoms and D_1 receptors in the negative symptoms of schizophrenia.
- Parkinson's disease is associated with a deficiency of nigrostriatal dopaminergic neurons.
- Hormone release from the anterior pituitary gland is regulated by dopamine, especially prolactin release (inhibited) and growth hormone release (stimulated).
- Dopamine acts on the chemoreceptor trigger zone to cause nausea and vomiting.

5-HYDROXYTRYPTAMINE

The occurrence and functions of 5-HT (serotonin) in the periphery are described in Chapter 16. Interest in 5-HT as a possible CNS transmitter dates from 1953, when Gaddum found that **lysergic acid diethylamide** (LSD), a powerful hallucinogen (see Ch. 49), acted as a 5-HT antagonist on peripheral tissues, and suggested that its central effects might also be related to this action. The presence of 5-HT in the brain was demonstrated a few years later. Even though brain 5-HT accounts for only about 1% of the total body content, 5-HT is an important CNS transmitter

(see Iversen et al., 2009; Muller & Jacobs, 2009). 5-HT is involved in various physiological processes, including sleep, appetite, thermoregulation and pain perception as well as in disorders such as migraine, depression, mania, anxiety, obsessive–compulsive disorders, schizophrenia, autism and drug abuse.

In its formation, storage and release, 5-HT resembles noradrenaline. Its precursor is tryptophan, an amino acid derived from dietary protein, the plasma content of which varies considerably according to food intake and time of day. 5-HT does not cross the blood–brain barrier and is synthesised in the CNS. Tryptophan is actively taken up into neurons, converted by tryptophan hydroxylase to 5-hydroxytryptophan (see Fig. 16.1), and then decarboxylated by a non-specific amino acid decarboxylase to form 5-HT. Tryptophan hydroxylase can be selectively and irreversibly inhibited by *p*-**chlorophenylalanine** (PCPA). Availability of tryptophan and the activity of tryptophan hydroxylase are thought to be the main factors that regulate 5-HT synthesis. The decarboxylase is very similar, if not identical, to dopa decarboxylase, and does not play any role in regulating 5-HT synthesis. Following release, 5-HT is largely recovered by neuronal uptake, through a specific transporter (see Ch. 3) similar to, but not identical with, those that take up noradrenaline and dopamine. 5-HT reuptake is specifically inhibited by *selective serotonin reuptake inhibitors* (SSRIs) such as **fluoxetine** and, less specifically, by many of the drugs that inhibit catecholamine uptake (e.g. *tricyclic antidepressants*). SSRIs (see Chs 45 and 48) constitute an important group of antidepressant and antianxiety drugs. 5-HT is degraded almost entirely by monoamine oxidase (Fig. 16.1), which converts it to 5-hydroxyindole acetaldehyde, most of which is then dehydrogenated to form 5-hydroxyindole acetic acid (5-HIAA) and excreted in the urine.

5-HT PATHWAYS IN THE CNS

The distribution of 5-HT-containing neurons (Fig. 40.5) resembles that of noradrenergic neurons. The cell bodies are grouped in the pons and upper medulla, close to the midline (raphe), and are often referred to as raphe nuclei. The rostrally situated nuclei project, via the medial forebrain bundle, to many parts of the cortex, hippocampus, basal ganglia, limbic system and hypothalamus. The caudally situated cells project to the cerebellum, medulla and spinal cord.

5-HT RECEPTORS IN THE CNS

The main 5-HT receptor types are shown in Table 16.1. All are G protein–coupled receptors except for 5-HT_3, which is a ligand-gated cation channel (see later). All are expressed in the CNS, and their functional roles have been extensively analysed. With some 14 identified subtypes plus numerous splice variants, and a large number of pharmacological tools of relatively low specificity, assigning clear-cut functions to 5-HT receptors is not simple. Our present state of knowledge is described by Filip and Bader (2009).

Certain generalisations can be made:

- 5-HT_1 receptors (5-HT_{1A}, 5-HT_{1B}, 5-HT_{1D}, 5-HT_{1E}, 5-HT_{1F})[3] are predominantly inhibitory in their effects.

---

[3]There is no 5-HT_{1C} receptor. The original 5-HT_{1C} receptor has been reclassified as 5-HT_{2C}.

Fig. 40.5 Simplified diagram of the 5-hydroxytryptamine pathways in the brain, drawn as in Fig. 40.1. Abbreviations as in Fig. 40.1.

5-HT$_{1A}$ receptors are expressed on the soma and dendrites of 5-HT neurons in the raphe nuclei and are activated by locally released 5-HT. This inhibitory effect tends to limit the rate of firing of these cells. They are also widely distributed in the limbic system, and are believed to be a major target for drugs used to treat anxiety and depression (see Chs 45 and 48). 5-HT$_{1B}$ and 5-HT$_{1D}$ receptors are found mainly as presynaptic inhibitory receptors on both 5-HT-containing and other nerve terminals in the basal ganglia and cortex. Agonists acting on 5-HT$_{1B}$ and 5-HT$_{1D}$ receptors such as **sumatriptan** are used to treat migraine (see Ch. 16).

- 5-HT$_2$ receptors (5-HT$_{2A}$, 5-HT$_{2B}$ and 5-HT$_{2C}$) are abundant in the cortex and limbic system, where they are located at both pre- and postsynaptic sites. They can exert excitatory or inhibitory effects by enhancing the release of glutamate and GABA. They are believed to be the target of some antidepressants (see Ch. 48) and antipsychotic drugs (see Ch. 47) as well as various hallucinogenic drugs (see Ch. 49). **Lorcaserin**, a 5-HT$_{2C}$ agonist is an anti-obesity drug (see Ch. 33). The use of 5-HT$_2$ receptor antagonists such as **methysergide** in treating migraine is discussed in Chapter 16.
- 5-HT$_3$ receptors are pentameric ligand-gated cation channels that can be either homomeric or heteromeric complexes of different 5-HT$_3$ receptor subunits (see Peters et al., 2005). While 5-HT3A and 5-HT3B subunits are the most extensively studied, the roles of other subunits remain to be fully investigated (see Jensen et al., 2008). In the brain, 5-HT$_3$ receptors are found in the *area postrema* (a region of the medulla involved in vomiting; see Ch. 31) and other parts of the brain stem, extending to the dorsal horn of the spinal cord. They are also present in certain parts of the cortex, as well as in the peripheral nervous system. They are excitatory ionotropic receptors, and specific antagonists (e.g. **granisetron** and **ondansetron**;

see Chs 16 and 31) are used to treat nausea and vomiting.

- 5-HT$_4$ receptors are important in the gastrointestinal (GI) tract (see Chs 16 and 31), and are also expressed in the brain, particularly in the limbic system, basal ganglia, hippocampus and substantia nigra. They are located at both pre- and postsynaptic sites. They exert a presynaptic facilitatory effect, particularly on ACh release, thus enhancing cognitive performance (see Chs 41 and 49). Activation of medullary 5-HT$_4$ receptors opposes the respiratory depressant actions of opioids (see Ch. 43).
- There are two 5-HT$_5$ receptors, 5-HT$_{5A}$ and 5-HT$_{5B}$. In the human, only 5-HT$_{5A}$ is functional. Antagonists may have anxiolytic, antidepressant and antipsychotic activity.
- 5-HT$_6$ receptors occur primarily in the CNS, particularly in the hippocampus, cortex and limbic system. Blockade of 5-HT$_6$ receptors increases glutamate and ACh release and 5HT$_6$-antagonists are considered potential drugs to improve cognition or relieve symptoms of schizophrenia.
- 5-HT$_7$ receptors occur in the hippocampus, cortex, amygdala, thalamus and hypothalamus. They are found on the soma and axon terminals of GABAergic neurons. They are also expressed in blood vessels and the GI tract. Likely CNS functions include thermoregulation and endocrine regulation, as well as suspected involvement in mood, cognitive function and sleep. The antipsychotic drug, **lurasidone** (see Ch. 47), has slightly higher affinity for 5-HT$_7$ receptors than for D$_2$ receptors. Selective antagonists are being developed for clinical use in a variety of potential indications.

FUNCTIONAL ASPECTS

The precise localisation of 5-HT neurons in the brain stem has allowed their electrical activity to be studied in detail and correlated with behavioural and other effects produced by drugs thought to affect 5-HT-mediated transmission. 5-HT cells show an unusual, highly regular, slow discharge pattern, and are strongly inhibited by 5-HT$_1$ receptor agonists, suggesting a local inhibitory feedback mechanism.

In vertebrates, certain physiological and behavioural functions relate particularly to 5-HT pathways, namely:

- hallucinations and behavioural changes
- sleep, wakefulness and mood
- feeding behaviour
- control of sensory transmission (especially pain pathways; see Ch. 43)

Hallucinatory effects

Many hallucinogenic drugs (e.g. LSD; Ch. 49) are agonists at 5-HT$_{2A}$ receptors. It is suggested that a loss of cortical inhibition underlies the hallucinogenic effect. Many antipsychotic drugs (Ch. 47) are antagonists at 5-HT$_{2A}$ receptors in addition to blocking dopamine D$_2$ receptors. The psychostimulant properties of **MDMA** (3,4-methylenedioxymethamphetamine, see Ch. 49) are due partly to its ability to release 5-HT. MDMA is taken up by the serotonin transporter, and displaces 5-HT from storage vesicles – a mechanism analogous to the action of amphetamine on noradrenergic nerve terminals (Ch. 15).

Sleep, wakefulness and mood

Lesions of the raphe nuclei, or depletion of 5-HT by PCPA administration, abolish sleep in experimental animals, whereas microinjection of 5-HT at specific points in the brain stem induces sleep. 5-HT$_7$ receptor antagonists inhibit 'rapid-eye-movement' (REM) sleep and increase the latency to onset of REM sleep. Attempts to cure insomnia in humans by giving 5-HT precursors (tryptophan or 5-hydroxytryptophan) have, however, proved unsuccessful. There is strong evidence that 5-HT, as well as noradrenaline, may be involved in the control of mood (see Ch. 48), and the use of tryptophan to enhance 5-HT synthesis has been tried in depression, with equivocal results.

Feeding and appetite

In experimental animals, 5-HT$_{1A}$ agonists such as 8-hydroxy-2-(di-n-propylamino)-tetralin (8-OH-DPAT) cause hyperphagia, leading to obesity. Antagonists acting on 5-HT$_2$ receptors, including several antipsychotic drugs used clinically, also increase appetite and cause weight gain. However, antidepressant drugs that inhibit 5-HT uptake (see Ch. 48) cause loss of appetite, as does the 5-HT$_{2C}$ receptor agonist **lorcaserin**.

Sensory transmission

After lesions of the raphe nuclei or administration of PCPA, animals show exaggerated responses to many forms of sensory stimulus. They are startled much more easily, and also quickly develop avoidance responses to stimuli that would not normally bother them. It appears that the normal ability to disregard irrelevant forms of sensory input requires intact 5-HT pathways. The 'sensory enhancement' produced by hallucinogenic drugs may be partly due to loss of this gatekeeper function of 5-HT. 5-HT also exerts an inhibitory effect on transmission in the pain pathway, both in the spinal cord and in the brain, and there is a synergistic effect between 5-HT and analgesics such as **morphine** (see Ch. 43). Thus depletion of 5-HT by PCPA, or selective lesions to the descending 5-HT-containing neurons that run to the dorsal horn, antagonise the analgesic effect of morphine, while inhibitors of 5-HT uptake have the opposite effect.

Other roles

Other roles of 5-HT include various autonomic and endocrine functions, such as the regulation of body temperature, blood pressure and sexual function. Further information can be found in Iversen et al. (2009).

CLINICALLY USED DRUGS

Several classes of drugs used clinically influence 5-HT-mediated transmission. They include:

- 5-HT reuptake inhibitors, such as fluoxetine, used as antidepressants (Ch. 48) and anxiolytic agents (Ch. 45)
- 5-HT$_{1D}$ receptor agonists, such as sumatriptan, used to treat migraine (Ch. 16)
- 5-HT$_2$ antagonists, such as pizotifen, used to treat migraine (Ch. 16)
- buspirone, a 5-HT$_{1A}$ receptor agonist used in treating anxiety (Ch. 45)
- 5-HT$_3$ receptor antagonists, such as ondansetron, used as antiemetic agents (see Ch. 31)
- antipsychotic drugs (e.g. clozapine, Ch. 47), which owe their efficacy partly to an action on 5-HT receptors

5-Hydroxytryptamine in the central nervous system

- The processes of synthesis, storage, release, reuptake and degradation of 5-hydroxytryptamine (5-HT) in the brain are very similar to events in the periphery (Ch. 16).
- Availability of tryptophan is the main factor regulating synthesis.
- Urinary excretion of 5-hydroxyindole acetic acid provides a measure of 5-HT turnover.
- 5-HT neurons are concentrated in the midline raphe nuclei in the brain stem projecting diffusely to the cortex, limbic system, hypothalamus and spinal cord, similar to the noradrenergic projections.
- Functions associated with 5-HT pathways include:
  - various behavioural responses (e.g. hallucinatory behaviour, 'wet dog shakes')
  - feeding behaviour
  - control of mood and emotion
  - control of sleep/wakefulness
  - control of sensory pathways, including nociception
  - control of body temperature
  - vomiting
- 5-HT can exert inhibitory or excitatory effects on individual neurons, acting either presynaptically or postsynaptically.
- The main receptor subtypes (see Table 16.1) in the central nervous system (CNS) are 5-HT$_{1A}$, 5-HT$_{1B}$, 5-HT$_{1D}$, 5-HT$_{2A}$, 5-HT$_{2C}$ and 5-HT$_3$. Associations of behavioural and physiological functions with these receptors have been partly worked out. Other receptor types (5-HT$_{4-7}$) also occur in the CNS, but less is known about their function.
- Drugs acting selectively on 5-HT receptors or transporters include:
  - **buspirone**, 5-HT$_{1A}$ receptor agonist used to treat anxiety (see Ch. 45);
  - 'triptans' (e.g. sumatriptan), 5-HT$_{1D}$ agonists used to treat migraine (see Ch. 16);
  - 5-HT$_2$ antagonists (e.g. **pizotifen**) used for migraine prophylaxis (see Ch. 16);
  - selective serotonin uptake inhibitors (e.g. **fluoxetine**) used to treat depression (see Ch. 48);
  - **ondansetron**, a 5-HT$_3$ antagonist, used to treat chemotherapy-induced emesis (see Chs 16 and 31);
  - **MDMA** (ecstasy), a substrate for the 5-HT transporter. It then displaces 5-HT from nerve terminals onto 5-HT receptors to produce its mood-altering effects (see Ch. 49).

ACETYLCHOLINE

There are numerous cholinergic neurons in the CNS, and the basic processes by which ACh is synthesised, stored and released are the same as in the periphery (see Ch. 14). Various biochemical markers have been used to locate cholinergic neurons in the brain, the most useful being

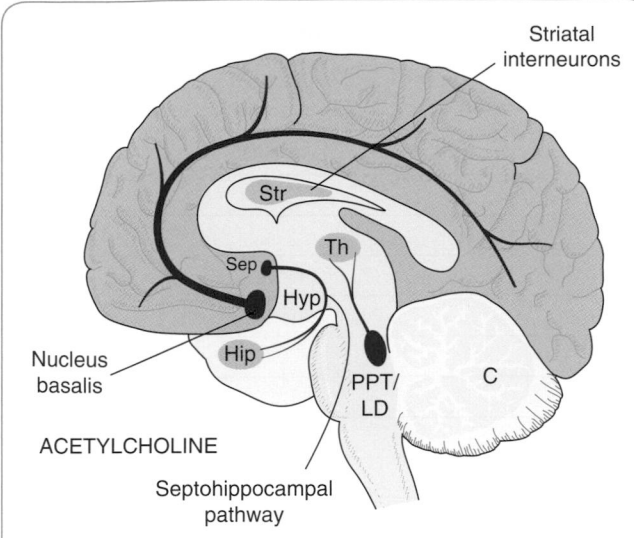

Fig. 40.6 Simplified diagram of the acetylcholine pathways in the brain, drawn as in Fig. 40.1. *PPT/LD*, pedunculopontine and laterodorsal tegmental nuclei; other abbreviations as in Fig. 40.1.

choline acetyltransferase, the enzyme responsible for ACh synthesis, and the transporters that capture choline and package ACh, which can be labelled by immunofluorescence. Biochemical studies on ACh precursors and metabolites are generally more difficult than corresponding studies on other amine transmitters, because the relevant substances, choline and acetate, are involved in many processes other than ACh metabolism.

CHOLINERGIC PATHWAYS IN THE CNS

ACh is very widely distributed in the brain, occurring in all parts of the forebrain (including the cortex), midbrain and brain stem, although there is little in the cerebellum. Cholinergic neurons in the forebrain and brain stem send diffuse projections to many parts of the brain (Fig. 40.6). Cholinergic neurons in the forebrain lie in a discrete area, forming the magnocellular forebrain nuclei (so called because the cell bodies are conspicuously large). Degeneration of one of these, the *nucleus basalis of Meynert*, which projects mainly to the cortex, is associated with Alzheimer's disease (Ch. 41). Another cluster, the *septohippocampal nucleus*, provides the main cholinergic input to the hippocampus, and is also involved in memory. In addition, there are – in contrast to noradrenaline, dopamine and 5-HT-containing pathways – many local cholinergic interneurons, particularly in the corpus striatum, these being important in relation to Parkinson's disease and Huntington's chorea (Ch. 41).

ACETYLCHOLINE RECEPTORS

Acetylcholine acts on both muscarinic (G protein–coupled) and nicotinic (ionotropic) receptors in the CNS (see Ch. 14).

The muscarinic ACh receptors (mAChRs) in the brain are predominantly of the G_q–coupled M_1 class (i.e. M_1, M_3 and M_5 subtypes; see Ch. 14). Activation of these receptors can result in excitation through blockade of M-type (KCNQ/Kv7) K^+ channels (see Delmas & Brown, 2005). G_i/G_o–coupled M_2 and M_4 receptors, however, are inhibitory through activation of inwardly rectifying K^+ channels and

inhibition of voltage-sensitive Ca^{2+} channels. mAChRs on cholinergic terminals function to inhibit ACh release, and muscarinic antagonists, by blocking this inhibition, markedly increase ACh release. Many of the behavioural effects associated with cholinergic pathways seem to be produced by ACh acting on mAChRs. Positive allosteric modulators (see Ch. 2) selective for different muscarinic receptors are under development.

Nicotinic ACh receptors (nAChRs) are ligand-gated cation channels permeable to Na^+, K^+ and Ca^{2+} ions (see Chs 3 and 14). They are pentamers and can be formed as homomeric or heteromeric combinations of α (α2–7) and β (β2–4) subunits (Ch. 3; see Gotti et al., 2008) distributed widely throughout the brain (Table 40.2). Nicotine (see Ch. 49) exerts its central effects by agonist action on nAChRs. The heteromeric α4β2 and the homomeric α7 subtypes are the most extensively characterised. Subtype-specific agonists and positive allosteric modulators have been developed but initial results from clinical trials for cognitive enhancement have so far not lived up to expectation.

nAChRs are located both pre- and postsynaptically. Presynaptic nAChRs act usually to facilitate the release of other transmitters such as glutamate, dopamine and GABA.[4] Postsynaptic nAChRs mediate fast excitatory transmission, as in the periphery (see Ch.14).

Many of the drugs that block nAChRs (e.g. **tubocurarine**; see Ch. 14) do not cross the blood–brain barrier, and even those that do (e.g. **mecamylamine**) produce only modest CNS effects. Various nAChR knock-out mouse strains have been produced and studied. Deletion of the various CNS-specific nAChR subtypes generally has rather little effect, although some cognitive impairment can be detected. Mutations in nAChRs may be the cause of some forms of epilepsy and changes in nAChR expression may occur in disorders such as schizophrenia, attention deficit hyperactivity disorder, depression and anxiety, as well as following neurodegeneration in Alzheimer's and Parkinson's diseases.

FUNCTIONAL ASPECTS

The main functions ascribed to cholinergic pathways are related to arousal, reward, learning and memory, and motor control. The cholinergic projection from the ventral forebrain to the cortex is thought to mediate arousal, whereas the septohippocampal pathway is involved in learning and short-term memory (see Hasselmo, 2006). Cholinergic interneurons in the striatum are involved in motor control (see Ch. 41).

Muscarinic agonists have been shown to partially restore learning and memory deficits induced in experimental animals by lesions of the septohippocampal cholinergic pathway. **Hyoscine**, a muscarinic antagonist, impairs memory in human subjects and causes amnesia when used as preanaesthetic medication. M_1 receptor knock-out mice, however, show only slight impairment of learning and memory (see Wess, 2004).

Nicotine increases alertness and also enhances learning and memory, as do various synthetic agonists at neuronal nAChRs. Conversely, CNS-active nAChR antagonists such as mecamylamine cause detectable, although slight, impairment of learning and memory. Transgenic mice with

---

[4]See Khakh & Henderson (2000) for a description of how presynaptic cation-selective ligand-gated channels can, under different circumstances, facilitate or enhance neurotransmitter release.

Table 40.2 Presence of nicotinic receptors of different subunit composition in selected regions of the central nervous system

Brain region	Nicotinic receptors						
	α7	α3β2	α3β4	α4β2	α4α5β	α6β2β3	α6α4β2β3
Cortex	+			+	+		
Hippocampus	+		+	+	+		
Striatum				+	+	+	+
Amygdala	+			+			
Thalamus				+			
Hypothalamus	+			+			
Substantia nigra	+		+	+	+	+	
Cerebellum	+	+	+	+			
Spinal cord	+	+		+			

α7 may also form heteromeric receptors with β2 subunits. nAChRs comprising α2β2 and α3β3β4 are found in some other areas of the brain.
(Data taken from Gotti et al., 2008.)

disruption of brain nAChRs are only slightly impaired in spatial learning tasks. In the dopaminergic VTA to accumbens 'reward' pathway, nicotine affects neuronal firing at the level of the cell soma in the VTA and modulates dopamine release from terminals in the nucleus accumbens to modify dopamine release in this reward pathway (see Ch. 50).

In conclusion, both nAChRs and mAChRs may play a role in learning and memory, while nAChRs also mediate behavioural arousal. Receptor knock-out mice are surprisingly little affected, suggesting that alternative mechanisms may be able to compensate for the loss of ACh receptor signalling.

The importance of cholinergic neurons in neurodegenerative conditions such as dementia and Parkinson's disease is discussed in Chapter 41. The role of nAChRs in addiction to nicotine is described in Chapter 49 and their role in modulating pain transmission in the CNS is described in Chapter 43.

PURINES

Both adenosine and ATP act as transmitters and/or modulators in the CNS (for review, see Fredholm et al., 2005; Khakh & North, 2012) as they do in the periphery (Ch. 17). Mapping the pathways is difficult, because purinergic neurons are not easily identifiable histochemically. It is likely that adenosine and ATP serve as neuromodulators.

Adenosine is produced intracellularly from ATP. It is not packaged into vesicles but is released mainly by carrier-mediated transport. Because the intracellular concentration of ATP (several mmol/L) greatly exceeds that of adenosine, conversion of a small proportion of ATP results in a large increase in adenosine. ATP is packaged into vesicles and released by exocytosis as a conventional transmitter, but can also leak out of cells in large amounts under conditions of tissue damage. In high concentrations, ATP can act as an excitotoxin (like glutamate; see Ch. 41) and cause further

Acetylcholine in the central nervous system

- Synthesis, storage and release of acetylcholine (ACh) in the central nervous system (CNS) are essentially the same as in the periphery (Ch. 14).
- ACh is widely distributed in the CNS, important pathways being:
  - basal forebrain (magnocellular) nuclei, which send a diffuse projection to most forebrain structures, including the cortex;
  - septohippocampal projection;
  - short interneurons in the striatum and nucleus accumbens.
- Certain neurodegenerative diseases, especially dementia and Parkinson's disease (see Ch. 41), are associated with abnormalities in cholinergic pathways.
- Both nicotinic and muscarinic (predominantly M₁) ACh receptors occur in the CNS. The former mediate the central effects of nicotine. Nicotinic receptors are mainly located presynaptically; there are few examples of transmission mediated by postsynaptic nicotinic receptors.
- Muscarinic receptors appear to mediate the main behavioural effects associated with ACh, namely effects on arousal, and on learning and short-term memory.
- Muscarinic antagonists (e.g. **hyoscine**) cause amnesia.

neuronal damage but it is also quickly converted to adenosine, which exerts a protective effect. These special characteristics of purine metabolism suggest that adenosine serves mainly as a safety mechanism, protecting the neurons from damage when their viability is threatened, for example by ischaemia or seizure activity. It has been suggested that adenosine deficiency may underlie a number of CNS disorders such as some epilepsies as well as Alzheimer's and Parkinson's diseases (Boison & Aronica, 2015).

Adenosine produces its effects through G protein–coupled adenosine A receptors (see Ch. 17). There are four adenosine receptors – A_1, A_{2A}, A_{2B} and A_3 – distributed throughout the CNS. The overall effect of adenosine, or of various adenosine receptor agonists, is inhibitory, leading to effects such as drowsiness and sedation, motor incoordination, analgesia and anticonvulsant activity. Xanthines, such as **caffeine** (Ch. 49), which are antagonists at A_2 receptors, produce arousal and alertness.

For ATP there are two forms of receptor – P2X and P2Y receptors (see Ch. 17 also). P2X receptor subunits (P2X1-7) are trimeric ligand-gated cation channels that can be homomeric or heteromeric in composition. The evidence in favour of ATP acting on postsynaptic P2X receptors mediating fast synaptic transmission in the brain remains weak. P2X receptors are located on the postsynaptic cell membrane away from sites of synaptic contact, on nerve terminals and on astrocytes. Like acetylcholine at nicotinic receptors (see p. 507), ATP acting on nerve terminal P2X receptors appears to play a neuromodulatory role. There are eight P2Y receptors,[5] all are G protein coupled (see Table 17.1).

While there is little doubt that purinergic signalling plays a significant role in CNS function, our understanding is still very limited. There is optimism that purinergic receptor ligands – both agonists and antagonists – will prove useful in a wide range of CNS disorders (see Chen et al., 2013; Jacobson & Müller, 2016).

HISTAMINE

▼ Histamine is present in the brain in much smaller amounts than in other tissues, such as skin and lung, but undoubtedly serves a neurotransmitter role (see Brown et al., 2001). The cell bodies of histaminergic neurons, which also synthesise and release a variety of other transmitters, are restricted to a small part of the hypothalamus, and their axons run to virtually all parts of the brain. Unusually, no uptake mechanism for histamine is present, its action being terminated instead by enzymic methylation. Histamine's prolonged extracellular presence may explain its involvement in homeostatic process such as the sleep/wake cycle, food and water intake and temperature regulation.

Histamine acts on four types of receptor (H_{1-4}; Ch. 18) in the brain. H_1–H_3 occur in most brain regions, H_4 has a more restricted distribution. All are G protein coupled – H_1 receptors to G_q, H_2 to G_s and H_3 and H_4 to G_i/G_o. H_3 receptors are inhibitory receptors on histamine-releasing neurons as well as on terminals releasing other neurotransmitters.

Like other monoamine transmitters, histamine is involved in many different CNS functions. Histamine release follows a distinct circadian pattern, the neurons being active by day and silent by night. H_1 receptors in the cortex and reticular activating system contribute to arousal and wakefulness, and H_1 receptor antagonists that access the CNS produce sedation (see Ch. 45). Antihistamines are widely used to control nausea and vomiting, for example, in motion sickness and middle ear disorders, as well as to induce sleep. Recent pharmaceutical industry activity has centred on the development of selective H_3

---

[5]Unfortunately the nomenclature for P2Y receptors has developed in a rather haphazard manner. There is compelling evidence for the existence of P2Y$_{1,2,4,6,11,12,13}$ and $_{14}$ receptors, but not for others.

receptor antagonists, as they may have potential for the treatment of cognitive impairment associated with Alzheimer's disease (see Ch. 41), schizophrenia (see Ch. 47), attention deficit hyperactivity disorder (see Ch. 49) and Parkinson's disease (see Ch. 41) as well as for the treatment of narcolepsy, obesity and pain states (Ellenbrock & Ghiabi, 2014).

OTHER CNS MEDIATORS

We now move from the familiar neuropharmacological territory of the 'classic' monoamines to some of the odder agents which challenge many of our preconceived ideas of how neurotransmission functions. Useful drugs interacting with some of these mediators are starting to be approved for clinical use.

MELATONIN

▼ Melatonin (N-acetyl-5-methoxytryptamine) (reviewed by Dubocovich et al., 2010) is synthesised exclusively in the pineal, an endocrine gland that plays a role in establishing circadian rhythms. The gland contains two enzymes, not found elsewhere, which convert 5-HT by acetylation and O-methylation to melatonin, its hormonal product.

There are two well-defined melatonin receptors (MT_1 and MT_2) which are G protein–coupled receptors – both coupling to G_i/G_o – found mainly in the brain and retina but also in peripheral tissues (see Jockers et al., 2016). Another type (termed MT_3) has been suggested to be the enzyme quinone reductase 2 (QR2). The function of the interaction between melatonin and QR2 is unclear.

Melatonin secretion (in all animals studied, whether diurnal or nocturnal in their habits) is high at night and low by day. This rhythm is controlled by input from the retina via a noradrenergic retinohypothalamic tract that terminates in the suprachiasmatic nucleus (SCN) in the hypothalamus, a structure often termed the 'biological clock', which generates the circadian rhythm. Activation of MT_1 receptors inhibits neuronal firing in the SCN and prolactin secretion from the pituitary. Activation of MT_2 receptors phase shifts circadian rhythms generated within the SCN. Melatonin has antioxidant properties and may be neuroprotective in Alzheimer's disease and Parkinson's disease (see Ch. 41).

Given orally, melatonin is well absorbed but quickly metabolised, its plasma half-life being a few minutes. Based on its ability to reset the circadian clock, it has been promoted for various uses, such as controlling jet lag, improving the performance of night-shift workers, treating insomnia in the elderly, and controlling sleep disorders in children with autism or attention deficit hyperactivity disorder (ADHD) clinical trials have been unconvincing. **Ramelteon**, an agonist at MT_1 and MT_2 receptors, is used to treat insomnia (see Ch. 45) and **agomelatine**, which also has agonist actions at MT_1 and MT_2 receptors as well as antagonist actions at $5-HT_{2C}$ receptors, is a novel antidepressant drug (see Ch. 48).

NITRIC OXIDE

NO as a peripheral mediator is discussed in Chapter 21. Its significance as an important chemical mediator in the nervous system has demanded a considerable readjustment of our views about neurotransmission and neuromodulation (for review, see Chachlaki et al., 2017). The main defining criteria for transmitter substances – namely that neurons should possess machinery for synthesising and storing the substance, that it should be released from neurons by exocytosis, that it should interact with specific membrane receptors and that there should be mechanisms for its inactivation – do not apply to NO. Moreover, it is an inorganic gas, not at all like the kind of molecule pharmacologists are used to. The mediator function of NO is now well established (Zhou & Zhu, 2009). NO diffuses rapidly through cell membranes, and its action is not highly localised. Its half-life depends greatly on the chemical environment, ranging from seconds in blood to several minutes in normal tissues. The rate of inactivation of NO (see Ch. 21, reaction 21.1) increases disproportionately with NO concentration, so low levels of NO are relatively stable. The presence of superoxide, with which NO reacts (see later), shortens its half-life considerably.

NO in the nervous system is produced mainly by the constitutive neuronal form of *NO synthase* (nNOS; see Ch. 21), which can be detected either histochemically or by immunolabelling. This enzyme is present in roughly 2% of neurons, both short interneurons and long-tract neurons, in virtually all brain areas, with particular concentrations in the cerebellum and hippocampus. It occurs in cell bodies and dendrites, as well as in axon terminals, suggesting that NO may be produced both pre- and postsynaptically. nNOS is calmodulin-dependent and is activated by a rise in intracellular Ca^{2+} concentration, which can occur by many mechanisms (see Ch. 4), including action potential conduction and neurotransmitter action, especially by glutamate activation of NMDA receptors. NO is not stored, but released as it is made. Many studies have shown that NO production is increased by activation of synaptic pathways, or by other events, such as brain ischaemia (see Ch. 41).

NO exerts pre- and postsynaptic actions on neurons as well as acting on glial cells (Garthwaite, 2008). It produces its effects in two main ways:

1. By activation of soluble guanylyl cyclase, leading to the production of cGMP, which itself or through activation of protein kinase G can affect membrane ion channels (Steinert et al., 2010). This 'physiological' control mechanism operates at low NO concentrations of about 0.1 μmol/L.
2. By reacting with the superoxide free radical to generate peroxynitrite, a highly toxic anion that acts by oxidising various intracellular proteins. This requires concentrations of 1–10 μmol/L, which are achieved in brain ischaemia.

There is good evidence that NO plays a role in synaptic plasticity (see Ch. 39), because long-term potentiation and depression are reduced or prevented by NOS inhibitors and are absent in transgenic mice in which the *nNOS* gene has been disrupted.

Based on the same kind of evidence, NO is also believed to play an important part in the mechanisms by which ischaemia causes neuronal death (see Ch. 41). There is also evidence that it may be involved in other processes, including neurodegeneration in Parkinson's disease, senile dementia and amyotrophic lateral sclerosis, and the local control of blood flow linked to neuronal activity.

▼ **Other 'gaseotransmitters'.** These include carbon monoxide, hydrogen sulfide and, more recently, ammonia (see Ch. 21 and Wang, 2014). While evidence is accumulating for their roles in CNS disorders, their pharmacology is still at a very preliminary stage.

Carbon monoxide (CO) is best known as a poisonous gas present in vehicle exhaust, which binds strongly to haemoglobin, causing tissue anoxia. However, it is also formed endogenously and has many features in common with NO. Neurons and other cells contain a CO-generating enzyme, haem oxygenase, and CO, like NO, activates guanylyl cyclase. There is some evidence that CO plays a role in memory mechanisms in the hippocampus (see Cutajar & Edwards, 2007).

Hydrogen sulfide (H_2S) has been postulated to be involved in learning, memory and pain perception but then again so has almost every other neurotransmitter or neuromodulator! It has been suggested that brain H_2S concentrations are lowered in Alzheimer's and Parkinson's diseases but the relevance of such observations still needs to be worked out.

LIPID MEDIATORS

▼ The formation of arachidonic acid, and its conversion to eicosanoids (mainly prostaglandins, leukotrienes and hydroxyeicosatetraenoic acids (HETEs) – see Ch. 18) and to endocannabinoids, anandamide and 2-arachidonoylglycerol (see Ch. 20), also take place in the CNS. Phospholipid cleavage, leading to arachidonic acid production, occurs in neurons in response to receptor activation by many different mediators, including neurotransmitters. The arachidonic acid so formed can act directly as an intracellular messenger, controlling both ion channels and various parts of the protein kinase cascade (see Ch. 3), producing both rapid and delayed effects on neuronal function. Both arachidonic acid itself and its products escape readily from the cell of origin and can affect neighbouring structures, including presynaptic terminals (retrograde signalling) and adjacent cells (paracrine signalling), by acting on receptors or by acting directly as intracellular messengers. Fig. 40.7 shows a schematic view of the variety of different roles these agents can play at the synapse.

Arachidonic acid can be metabolised to eicosanoids, some of which (principally the HETEs) can also act as intracellular messengers acting in the same cell. Eicosanoids can also exert an autocrine effect via membrane receptors expressed by the cell (see Ch. 18). The eicosanoids play important roles in neural function including pain, temperature regulation, sleep induction, synaptic plasticity and spatial learning.

It is now generally accepted that endocannabinoids, such as anandamide and 2-arachidonylglycerol, act as retrograde synaptic messengers in the CNS (see Pertwee, 2015 and Ch. 20). They are synthesised and secreted in response to a rise in intracellular Ca^{2+} and activate presynaptic CB_1 receptors inhibiting the release of neurotransmitters such as glutamate and GABA. CB_1 receptors are widely distributed in the brain and spinal cord, not only on neurons but also on astrocytes and microglia, whereas CB_2 receptor expression is much less but may be up-regulated under pathological conditions. Agonists at CB_1 receptors have therapeutic potential for the treatment of vomiting, pain (CB_2 receptor agonists may also be effective in some pain states), muscle spasms as occur in conditions such as multiple sclerosis and anxiety, as well as in other brain disorders including Alzheimer's disease and tardive dyskinesias. Endocannabinoids released into the extracellular space are removed into cells by facilitated transport, for which inhibitors have been developed, and then metabolised (Cascio & Marini, 2015). Anandamide is metabolised by fatty acid amide hydrolase (FAAH; see Ch. 20). Inhibitors of FAAH potentiate the effects of endocannabinoids and were shown to be effective analgesics in animal models of pain (Roques et al., 2012).[6] The CB_1-receptor antagonist **rimonabant** was introduced as an anti-obesity agent but subsequently had to be withdrawn because of negative effects on mood (see Ch. 20). Endocannabinoids, besides being agonists at cannabinoid receptors, also interact with a variety of ion channels including TRPV1 channels (see Fig. 40.7 and Ch. 43), 5-HT3 receptors (see pp. 504–505), calcium channels and potassium channels (Pertwee, 2015)

Lysophosphatidic acid and sphingosine 1-phosphate are phospholipids with important signalling functions in the brain and elsewhere throughout the body. Their effects are mediated by multiple G protein–coupled receptors (LPA1-6 and S1P1-5). Agonists at S1P1 receptors are in phase III clinical trials for the treatment of multiple sclerosis (see Ch. 41).

---

[6] Readers may recall the tragic phase I clinical trial of one FAAH inhibitor, BIA 10-2474, that caused sudden, severe CNS damage and resulted in one subject being brain dead and four others having permanent brain damage. In this instance the adverse effects were due to actions of the drug on other lipases.

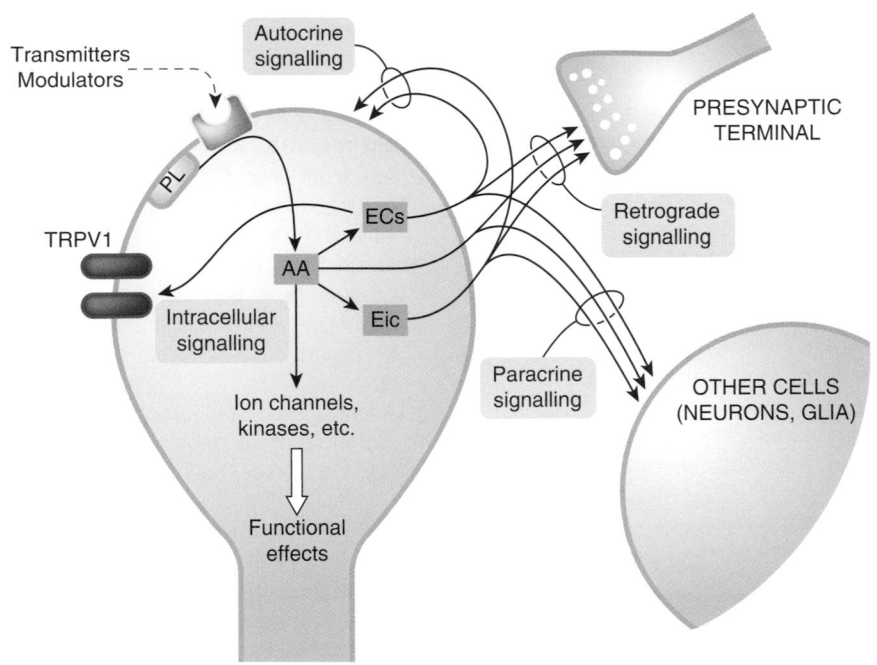

Fig. 40.7 **Postulated modes of signalling by lipid mediators.** Arachidonic acid (AA) is formed by receptor-mediated cleavage of membrane phospholipid. It can act directly as an intracellular messenger on ion channels or components of different kinase cascades, producing various long- and short-term effects. It can also be converted to eicosanoids (prostaglandins, leukotrienes or hydroxyeicosatetraenoic acids [HETEs]) or to the endocannabinoids (ECs), anandamide and 2-arachidonoylglycerol. ECs can also act as intracellular messengers to activate TRPV1 channels. HETEs can also act directly as intracellular messengers. All these mediators also diffuse out of the cell, and exert effects on presynaptic terminals and neighbouring cells, acting either on extracellular receptors or intracellularly. There are examples of most of these modes of signalling, but only limited information about their functional significance in the nervous system. *Eic*, eicosanoids; *PL*, membrane phospholipid.

Other transmitters and modulators

Purines
- ATP functions as a neurotransmitter, being stored in vesicles and released by exocytosis. It acts via ionotropic P2X receptors and metabotropic P2Y receptors.
- Cytosolic ATP is present at relatively high concentration and can be released directly if neuronal viability is compromised (e.g. in stroke). Excessive release may be neurotoxic.
- Released ATP is rapidly converted to ADP, AMP and adenosine.
- Adenosine is not stored in vesicles but is released by carrier mechanisms or generated from released ATP, mainly under pathological conditions.
- Adenosine exerts mainly inhibitory effects, through A_1 and A_2 receptors, resulting in sedative, anticonvulsant and neuroprotective effects, and acting as a safety mechanism.
- Methylxanthines (e.g. **caffeine**) are antagonists at A_2 receptors and increase wakefulness.

Histamine
- Histamine fulfils the criteria for a neurotransmitter. Histaminergic neurons originate in a small area of the hypothalamus and have a widespread distribution.
- H_1, H_2 and H_3 receptors are widespread in the brain.
- The functions of histamine are not well understood, the main clues being that histaminergic neurons are active during waking hours, and H_1 receptor antagonists are strongly sedative.
- H_1 receptor antagonists are antiemetic.

Melatonin
- Melatonin is synthesised from 5-hydroxytryptamine, mainly in the pineal gland, from which it is released as a circulating hormone.
- Secretion is controlled by light intensity, being low by day and high by night. Fibres from the retina run to the suprachiasmatic nucleus ('biological clock'), which controls the pineal gland via its sympathetic innervation.
- Melatonin acts on MT_1 and MT_2 receptors in the brain.
- Agonists at melatonin receptors induce sleep and have antidepressant properties.

Other mediators

Nitric oxide (see Ch. 21)

- Neuronal nitric oxide synthase (nNOS) is present in many central nervous system neurons, and nitric oxide (NO) production is increased by mechanisms (e.g. transmitter action) that raise intracellular Ca^{2+}.
- NO affects neuronal function by increasing cGMP formation, producing both inhibitory and excitatory effects on neurons.
- In larger amounts, NO forms peroxynitrite, which contributes to neurotoxicity.
- Inhibition of nNOS reduces long-term potentiation and long-term depression, probably because NO functions as a retrograde messenger. Inhibition of nNOS also protects against ischaemic brain damage in animal models.

- Carbon monoxide and hydrogen sulfide may also be neural mediators.

Lipid mediators

- Arachidonic acid is produced in neurons by receptor-mediated hydrolysis of phospholipid. It is converted to various eicosanoids and endocannabinoids.
- Arachidonic acid itself, as well as its active products, can produce rapid and slow effects by regulation of ion channels and protein kinase cascades. Such effects can occur in the donor cell or in adjacent cells and nerve terminals.
- Anandamide and 2-arachidonoylglycerol are endogenous activators of cannabinoid CB_1 and CB_2 receptors (Ch. 20) and also of the TRPV1 receptor (Ch. 43).

A FINAL MESSAGE

In the last two chapters we have taken a long and tortuous tour through the brain and its chemistry, with two questions at the back of our minds. What mediators and what receptors play a key role in what brain functions? How does the information relate to existing and future drugs that aim to correct malfunctions? Through the efforts of a huge army of researchers deploying an arsenal of powerful modern techniques, the answers to these questions are slowly being produced. The array of potential CNS targets – comprising multiple receptor subtypes, many with the added complexity of heteromeric assemblies, splice variants, etc., along with regulatory mechanisms that control their expression and localisation – continues to grow in complexity. Speculation about the best target to aim at in order to ameliorate the effect of a particular brain malfunction, such as stroke or schizophrenia, has become less focused, even if better informed, than it was two decades ago. In the ensuing chapters in this section we shall find that most of the therapeutic successes have come from chance discoveries that were followed up empirically; few have followed a logical, mechanism-based route to success. The optimistic view is that this is changing, and that future therapeutic discoveries will depend less on luck and more on molecular logic. But the revolution is slow in coming. One of the key problems, perhaps, is that the brain puts cells, organelles and molecules exactly where they are needed, and uses the same molecules to perform different functions in different locations. Drug discovery scientists are getting quite good at devising molecule-specific ligands (see Ch. 60), but we lack delivery systems able to target them anatomically even to macroscopic brain regions, let alone to specific cells and subcellular structures.

REFERENCES AND FURTHER READING

General references

Iversen, L.L., Iversen, S.D., Bloom, F.E., Roth, R.H., 2009. Introduction to Neuropsychopharmacology. Oxford University Press, New York. (*Clear and well-written textbook giving more detailed information on many topics covered in this chapter*)

Nestler, E.J., Hyman, S.E., Holtzman, M., Malenka, R.C., 2015. Molecular Neuropharmacology: A Foundation for Clinical Neuroscience, third ed. McGraw-Hill, New York. (*Good textbook*)

Noradrenaline

Bylund, D.B., 2007. Receptors for norepinephrine and signal transduction pathways. In: Ordway, G.A., Schwartz, M.A.Frazer, A. (Eds.), Brain Norepinephrine. Cambridge University Press, London.

Nikolic, K., Agbaba, D., 2012. Imidazoline antihypertensive drugs: selective I_1-imidazoline receptor activation. Cardiovasc. Ther. 30, 209–216. (*An update on the potential usefulness of drugs acting at the mysterious imidazoline receptors*)

Dopamine

Björklund, A., Dunnett, S.B., 2007. Dopamine neuron systems in the brain: an update. Trends Neurosci. 30, 194–202. (*Short review of the anatomy of dopaminergic neurons in the central nervous system*)

De Mei, C., Ramos, M., Iitaka, C., Borrelli, E., 2009. Getting specialized: presynaptic and postsynaptic dopamine D_2 receptors. Curr. Opin. Pharmacol. 9, 53–58.

Girault, J.A., Greengard, P., 2004. The neurobiology of dopamine signalling. Arch. Neurol. 61, 641–644. (*Short review article*)

5-Hydroxytryptamine

Filip, M., Bader, M., 2009. Overview of 5-HT receptors and their role in physiology and pathology of the central nervous system. Pharm. Rep. 61, 761–777.

Jensen, A.A., Davies, P.A., Bräuner-Osborne, H., Krzywkowski, K., 2008. 3B but which 3B? And that's just one of the questions: the heterogeneity of human 5-HT$_3$ receptors. Trends Pharmacol. Sci. 29, 437–444. (*Discusses the potential complexity of 5-HT$_3$ receptors now that new subunits have been discovered*)

Muller, C., Jacobs, B., 2009. Handbook of Behavioral Neurobiology of Serotonin, vol. 18, (Handbook of Behavioral Neuroscience). Academic Press, Oxford. (*Extensive coverage of the role of 5-HT in the brain*)

Peters, J.A., Hales, T.G., Lambert, J.J., 2005. Molecular determinants of single-channel conductance and ion selectivity in the Cys-loop family: insights from the 5-HT$_3$ receptor. Trends Pharmacol. Sci. 26, 587–594. (*For those who thought ligand-gated ion channels were just simple pores opened by neurotransmitters, this review will contain a few surprises!*)

Acetylcholine

Delmas, P., Brown, D.A., 2005. Pathways modulating neural KCNQ/M (Kv7) potassium channels. Nat. Rev. Neurosci. 6, 850–862. (*Gives information on the functional significance of the 'M-current' and the therapeutic potential of drugs that modify it*)

Gotti, C., Zoli, M., Clementi, F., 2008. Brain nicotinic acetylcholine receptors: native subtypes and their relevance. Trends Pharmacol. Sci. 27, 482–491.

Hasselmo, M.E., 2006. The role of acetylcholine in learning and memory. Curr. Opin. Neurobiol. 16, 710–715.

Khakh, B.S., Henderson, G., 2000. Modulation of fast synaptic transmission by presynaptic ligand-gated cation channels. J. Auton. Nerv. Syst. 81, 110–121. (*Describes how activation of presynaptic ligand-gated cation channels can either enhance or inhibit neurotransmitter release*)

Wess, J., 2004. Muscarinic acetylcholine receptor knockout mice: novel phenotypes and clinical implications. Annu. Rev. Pharmacol. Toxicol. 44, 423–450. (*Description of functional effects of deleting various peripheral and central mAChR isoforms*)

Other messengers

Boison, D., Aronica, E., 2015. Comorbidities in neurology: is adenosine the common link? Neuropharmacology 97, 18–34.

Brown, R.E., Stevens, D.R., Haas, H.L., 2001. The physiology of brain histamine. Prog. Neurobiol. 63, 637–672. (*Useful review article*)

Buscemi, N., Vandermeer, B., Hooton, N., et al., 2006. Efficacy and safety of exogenous melatonin for secondary sleep disorders and sleep disorders accompanying sleep restriction: meta-analysis. BMJ 332, 385–393.

Cascio, M.G., Marini, P., 2015. Biosynthesis and fate of endocannabinoids. In 'Endocannabinoids', Pertwee R.G. (Ed.), Handb. Exp. Pharmacol. 231, 39–58.

Castillo, P.E., Younts, T.J., Chávez, A.E., Hashimotodani, Y., 2012. Endocannabinoid signaling and synaptic function. Neuron 76, 70–81.

Chachlaki, K., Garthwaite, J., Prevot, V., 2017. The gentle art of saying NO: how nitric oxide gets things done in the hypothalamus. Nat. Rev. Endocrinol. 13, 521–535.

Chen, J.F., Eltzschig, H.K., Fredholm, B.B., 2013. Adenosine receptors as drug targets – what are the challenges? Nat. Rev. Drug Discov. 12, 265–286.

Cutajar, M.C., Edwards, T.M., 2007. Evidence for the role of endogenous carbon monoxide in memory processing. J. Cogn. Neurosci. 19, 557–562.

Dubocovich, M.L., Delagrange, P., Krause, D.N., Sugden, D., Cardinali, D.P., Olcese, J., 2010. International Union of Basic and Clinical Pharmacology. LXXV. Nomenclature, classification, and pharmacology of G protein-coupled melatonin receptors. Pharmacol. Rev. 62, 343–380.

Ellenbroek, B.A., Ghiabi, B., 2014. The other side of the histamine H3 receptor. Trends Neurosci. 37, 191–199.

Fredholm, B.B., Chen, J.F., Masino, S.A., Vaugeois, J.M., 2005. Actions of adenosine at its receptors in the CNS: insights from knockouts and from drugs. Annu. Rev. Pharmacol. Toxicol. 45, 395–412.

Garthwaite, J., 2008. Concepts of neural nitric oxide-mediated transmission. Eur. J. Neurosci. 27, 2783–2802.

Jacobson, K.A., Muller, C.E., 2016. Medicinal chemistry of adenosine, P2Y and P2X receptors. Neuropharmacology 104, 31–49.

Jockers, R., Delagrange, P., Dubocovich, M.L., et al., 2016. Update on melatonin receptors: IUPHAR Review 20. Br. J. Pharmacol. 173, 2702–2725.

Khakh, B.S., North, R.A., 2012. Neuromodulation by extracellular ATP and P2X receptors in the CNS. Neuron 76, 51–69.

Pertwee, R.G., 2015. Endocannabinoids and their pharmacological action. In 'Endocannabinoids', Pertwee R.G. (Ed.), Handb. Exp. Pharmacol. 231, 1–38.

Roques, B.P., Fournié-Zaluski, M.C., Wurm, M., 2012. Inhibiting the breakdown of endogenous opioids and cannabinoids to alleviate pain. Nat. Rev. Drug Discov. 11, 292–310. (*Interesting review of potential for such inhibitors to reduce pain*)

Steinert, J.R., Chernova, T., Forsythe, I.D., 2010. Nitric oxide signaling in brain function, dysfunction, and dementia. Neuroscientist 16, 435–452.

Wang, R., 2014. Gasotransmitters: growing pains and joys. Trends Biochem. Sci. 39, 227–232.

Zhou, L., Zhu, D.Y., 2009. Neuronal nitric oxide synthase: structure, subcellular localization, regulation and clinical implications. Nitric Oxide 20, 223–230.

41 Neurodegenerative diseases

OVERVIEW

As a rule, dead neurons in the adult central nervous system (CNS) are not replaced,[1] nor can their terminals regenerate when their axons are interrupted. Therefore any pathological process causing neuronal death generally has irreversible consequences. At first sight, this appears to be very unpromising territory for pharmacological intervention, and indeed drug therapy is currently very limited, except in the case of Parkinson's disease (PD). Nevertheless, the incidence and social impact of neurodegenerative brain disorders in ageing populations has resulted in a massive research effort in recent years.

In this chapter, a number of neurodegenerative conditions are described: ischaemic brain damage (stroke), Alzheimer's disease (AD), PD, Huntington's disease (HD), amyotrophic lateral sclerosis (ALS), spinal muscular atrophy (SMA) and multiple sclerosis (MS). The main topics discussed in this chapter are:

- **mechanisms responsible for neuronal death, focusing on genetic defects, protein aggregation (e.g. amyloidosis), excitotoxicity, oxidative stress and apoptosis;**
- **pharmacological approaches to neuroprotection, based on the above mechanisms;**
- **pharmacological approaches to compensation for neuronal loss (applicable mainly to AD and PD).**

PROTEIN MISFOLDING AND AGGREGATION IN CHRONIC NEURODEGENERATIVE DISEASES

Protein misfolding and aggregation is the first step in many neurodegenerative diseases (see Peden & Ironside, 2012). Misfolding means the adoption of abnormal conformations, by certain normally expressed proteins, such that they tend to form large insoluble aggregates (Fig. 41.1). The conversion of the linear amino acid chain produced by the ribosome into a functional protein requires it to be folded correctly into a compact conformation with specific amino acids

correctly located on its surface. This complicated stepwise sequence can easily go wrong and lead to misfolded variants that are unable to find a way back to the correct 'native' conformation. The misfolded molecules lack the normal function of the protein, but can nonetheless make mischief within the cell. The misfolding often means that hydrophobic residues that would normally be buried in the core of the protein are exposed on its surface, which gives the molecules a strong tendency to stick to cell membranes and aggregate, initially as oligomers and then as insoluble microscopic aggregates (see Fig. 41.1), leading to the death of neurons. The tendency to adopt such conformations may be favoured by specific mutations of the protein in question, or by infection with prions.[2]

Misfolded conformations can be generated spontaneously at a low rate throughout life, so that aggregates accumulate gradually with age. In the nervous system, the aggregates often form distinct structures, generally known as *amyloid deposits*, that are visible under the microscope and are characteristic of neurodegenerative disease. Although the mechanisms are not clear, such aggregates, or the misfolded protein precursors, lead to neuronal death. Examples of neurodegenerative diseases that are caused by such protein misfolding and aggregation are shown in Table 41.1.

The brain possesses a variety of protective mechanisms that limit the accumulation of such protein aggregates. The main ones involve the production of 'chaperone' proteins, which bind to newly synthesised or misfolded proteins and encourage them to fold correctly, and the 'ubiquitination' reaction, which prepares proteins for destruction within the cell. Accumulation of protein deposits occurs when these protective mechanisms are unable to cope.

MECHANISMS OF NEURONAL DEATH

Acute injury to cells causes them to undergo *necrosis*, recognised pathologically by cell swelling, vacuolisation and lysis, and associated with Ca^{2+} overload of the cells and membrane damage (see p. 516). Necrotic cells typically spill their contents into the surrounding tissue, evoking an inflammatory response. Chronic inflammation is a feature of most neurodegenerative disorders (see Schwab & McGeer, 2008), and a possible target for therapeutic intervention.

Cells can also die by *apoptosis* (programmed cell death, see Ch. 6), a mechanism that is essential for many processes

---

[1]It is recognised that new neurons are formed from progenitor cells (*neurogenesis*) in certain regions of the adult brain and can become functionally integrated, even in primates (see Rakic, 2002; Zhao et al., 2008). Neurogenesis in the hippocampus is thought to play a role in learning and memory, but plays little if any role in brain repair. However, learning how to harness the inherent ability of neuronal progenitors (stem cells) to form new neurons is seen as an obvious approach to treating neurodegenerative disorders.

[2]Such prion diseases include Creutzfeldt–Jakob's disease (CJD) and the new variant CJD that results from eating, or close contact with, beef or human tissue infected with bovine spongiform encephalopathy (BSE). Sadly, no pharmacological treatments that prevent disease progression are yet available and treatment is aimed at ameliorating the symptoms.

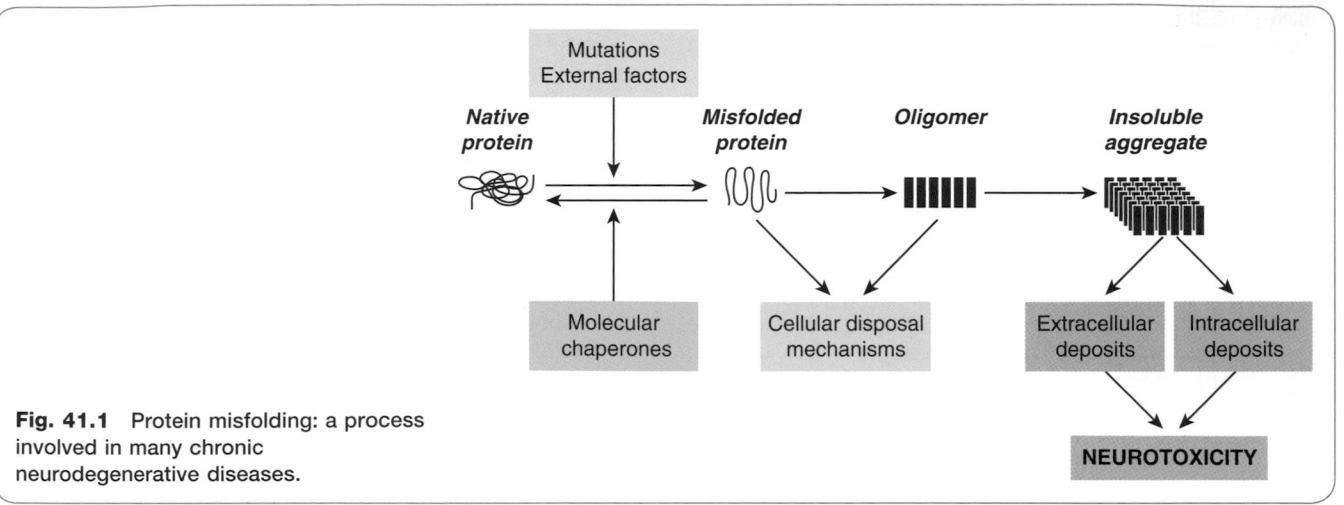

Fig. 41.1 Protein misfolding: a process involved in many chronic neurodegenerative diseases.

Table 41.1 Examples of neurodegenerative diseases associated with protein misfolding and aggregation[a]

Disease	Protein	Characteristic pathology	Notes
Alzheimer's disease	β-Amyloid (Aβ)	Amyloid plaques	Aβ mutations occur in rare familial forms of Alzheimer's disease
	Tau	Neurofibrillary tangles	Implicated in other pathologies ('tauopathies') as well as Alzheimer's disease
Parkinson's disease	α-Synuclein	Lewy bodies	α-Synuclein mutations occur in some types of familial Parkinson's disease
Creutzfeldt–Jakob's disease	Prion protein	Insoluble aggregates of prion protein	Transmitted by infection with prion protein in its misfolded state
Huntington's disease	Huntingtin	No gross lesions	One of several genetic 'polyglutamine repeat' disorders
Amyotrophic lateral sclerosis (a form of motor neuron disease)	Superoxide dismutase	Loss of motor neurons	Mutated superoxide dismutase tends to form aggregates; loss of enzyme function increases susceptibility to oxidative stress

[a]Protein aggregation disorders are often collectively known as amyloidoses and commonly affect organs other than the brain.

Protein misfolding

- Many chronic neurodegenerative diseases involve the misfolding of normal or mutated forms of physiological proteins. Examples include Alzheimer's disease, Parkinson's disease, amyotrophic lateral sclerosis and many less common diseases.
- Misfolded proteins are normally removed by intracellular degradation pathways, which may be altered in neurodegenerative disorders.
- Misfolded proteins tend to aggregate, initially as soluble oligomers, later as large insoluble aggregates that accumulate intracellularly or extracellularly as microscopic deposits, which are stable and resistant to proteolysis.
- Misfolded proteins often present hydrophobic surface residues that promote aggregation and association with membranes.
- The mechanisms responsible for neuronal death are unclear, but there is evidence that both the soluble aggregates and the microscopic deposits may be neurotoxic.

throughout life, including development, immune regulation and tissue remodelling. Apoptosis, as well as necrosis, occurs in both acute neurodegenerative disorders (such as stroke and head injury) and chronic ones (such as Alzheimer's and Parkinson's disease). The distinction between necrosis and apoptosis as processes leading to neurodegeneration is not absolute, for challenges such as excitotoxicity and oxidative stress may be enough to kill cells directly by necrosis or, if less intense, may induce them to undergo apoptosis. Both processes therefore represent possible targets for putative neuroprotective drug therapy. Pharmacological interference with the apoptotic pathway may become possible in the future, but for the present most efforts are directed at the processes involved in cell necrosis, and at compensating pharmacologically for the neuronal loss.

EXCITOTOXICITY

Despite its ubiquitous role as a neurotransmitter, **glutamate** is highly toxic to neurons, a phenomenon dubbed *excitotoxicity* (see Ch. 39). A low concentration of glutamate applied to neurons in culture kills the cells, and the finding in the 1970s that glutamate given orally produces neurodegeneration in vivo caused considerable alarm because of the widespread use of glutamate as a 'taste-enhancing' food additive. The 'Chinese restaurant syndrome' – an acute attack of neck stiffness and chest pain – is well known, but so far, the possibility of more serious neurotoxicity is only hypothetical.

Local injection of the glutamate receptor agonist *kainic acid* is used experimentally to produce neurotoxic lesions. It acts by excitation of local glutamate-releasing neurons, and the release of glutamate, acting on NMDA receptors, and also metabotropic receptors (Ch. 39), leads to neuronal death.

Calcium overload is the essential factor in excitotoxicity. The mechanisms by which this occurs and leads to cell death are as follows (see also Fig. 41.2):

- Glutamate activates NMDA, AMPA and metabotropic receptors (sites 1, 2 and 3 in Fig. 41.2). Activation of AMPA receptors depolarises the cell, which removes the Mg^{2+} block of NMDA channels (see Ch. 39), permitting Ca^{2+} entry. Depolarisation also opens voltage-dependent calcium channels (site 4). Metabotropic receptors cause the release of intracellular Ca^{2+} from the endoplasmic reticulum. Na^+ entry further contributes to Ca^{2+} entry by stimulating Ca^{2+}/Na^+ exchange (site 5). Depolarisation inhibits or reverses glutamate uptake (site 6), thus increasing the extracellular glutamate concentration.
- The mechanisms that normally operate to counteract the rise in cytosolic free Ca^{2+} concentration, $[Ca^{2+}]_i$, include the Ca^{2+} efflux pump (site 7) and, indirectly, the Na^+ pump (site 8).
- The mitochondria and endoplasmic reticulum act as capacious sinks for Ca^{2+} and normally keep $[Ca^{2+}]_i$ under control. Loading of the mitochondrial stores beyond a certain point, however, disrupts mitochondrial function, reducing ATP synthesis, thus reducing the energy available for the membrane pumps and for Ca^{2+} accumulation by the endoplasmic reticulum. Formation of reactive oxygen species (ROS) is also enhanced. This represents the danger point at which positive feedback exaggerates the process.
- Raised $[Ca^{2+}]_i$ affects many processes, the chief ones relevant to neurotoxicity being:
  - increased glutamate release from nerve terminals;
  - activation of proteases (calpains) and lipases, causing membrane damage;
  - activation of nitric oxide synthase; while low concentrations of nitric oxide are neuroprotective, high concentrations in the presence of ROS generate peroxynitrite and hydroxyl free radicals, which damage many important biomolecules, including membrane lipids, proteins and DNA;
  - increased arachidonic acid release, which increases free radical and inflammatory mediator production and also inhibits glutamate uptake (site 6).

Glutamate and Ca^{2+} are arguably the two most ubiquitous chemical signals, extracellular and intracellular, respectively, underlying brain function, so it is disconcerting that such cytotoxic mayhem can be unleashed when they get out of control. Both are stored in dangerous amounts in subcellular organelles, like hand grenades in an ammunition store. Defence against excitotoxicity is clearly essential if our brains are to have any chance of staying alive. Mitochondrial energy metabolism provides one line of defence (see p. 518), and impaired mitochondrial function, by rendering neurons vulnerable to excitotoxic damage, may be a factor in various neurodegenerative conditions, including PD. Furthermore, impaired mitochondrial function can cause release of cytochrome C, which is an important initiator of apoptosis.

The role of excitotoxicity in ischaemic brain damage is well established (see p. 518), and it is also believed to be a factor in other neurodegenerative diseases, such as those discussed below.

▼ There are several examples of neurodegenerative conditions caused by environmental toxins acting as agonists on glutamate receptors. *Domoic acid* is a glutamate analogue produced by mussels, which was identified as the cause of an epidemic of severe mental and neurological deterioration in a group of Newfoundlanders in 1987. On the island of Guam, a syndrome combining the features of dementia, paralysis and PD was traced to an excitotoxic amino acid, β-methylamino-alanine, in the seeds of a local plant. Discouraging the consumption of these seeds has largely eliminated the disease.

Disappointingly, intense effort, based on the mechanisms described earlier, to find effective drugs for a range of neurodegenerative disorders in which excitotoxicity is believed to play a part has had very limited success. **Riluzole** retards to some degree the deterioration of patients with ALS (see p. 528). Its precise mechanism of action is unclear. **Memantine**, a compound first described 40 years ago, is a weak NMDA-receptor antagonist that produces slight improvement in moderate-to-severe cases of AD.

APOPTOSIS

Apoptosis can be initiated by various cell surface signals (see Ch. 6). The cell is systematically dismantled, and the shrunken remnants are removed by macrophages without causing inflammation. Apoptotic cells can be identified by a staining technique that detects the characteristic DNA breaks. Many different signalling pathways can result in apoptosis, but in all cases the final pathway resulting in cell death is the activation of a family of proteases (caspases), which inactivate various intracellular proteins. Neural apoptosis is normally prevented by neuronal growth factors, including *nerve growth factor* and *brain-derived neurotrophic factor*, secreted proteins that are required for the survival of different populations of neurons in the CNS. These growth factors regulate the expression of the two gene products, Bax and Bcl-2, Bax being proapoptotic and Bcl-2 being antiapoptotic (see Ch. 6). Blocking apoptosis by interfering at specific points on these pathways represents an attractive strategy for developing neuroprotective drugs, but one that has yet to bear fruit.

OXIDATIVE STRESS

The brain has high energy needs, which are met almost entirely by mitochondrial oxidative phosphorylation, generating ATP at the same time as reducing molecular O_2 to H_2O. Under certain conditions, highly ROS, for example, oxygen and hydroxyl free radicals and H_2O_2, may be generated as side products of this process (see Barnham et al., 2004). Oxidative stress is the result of excessive

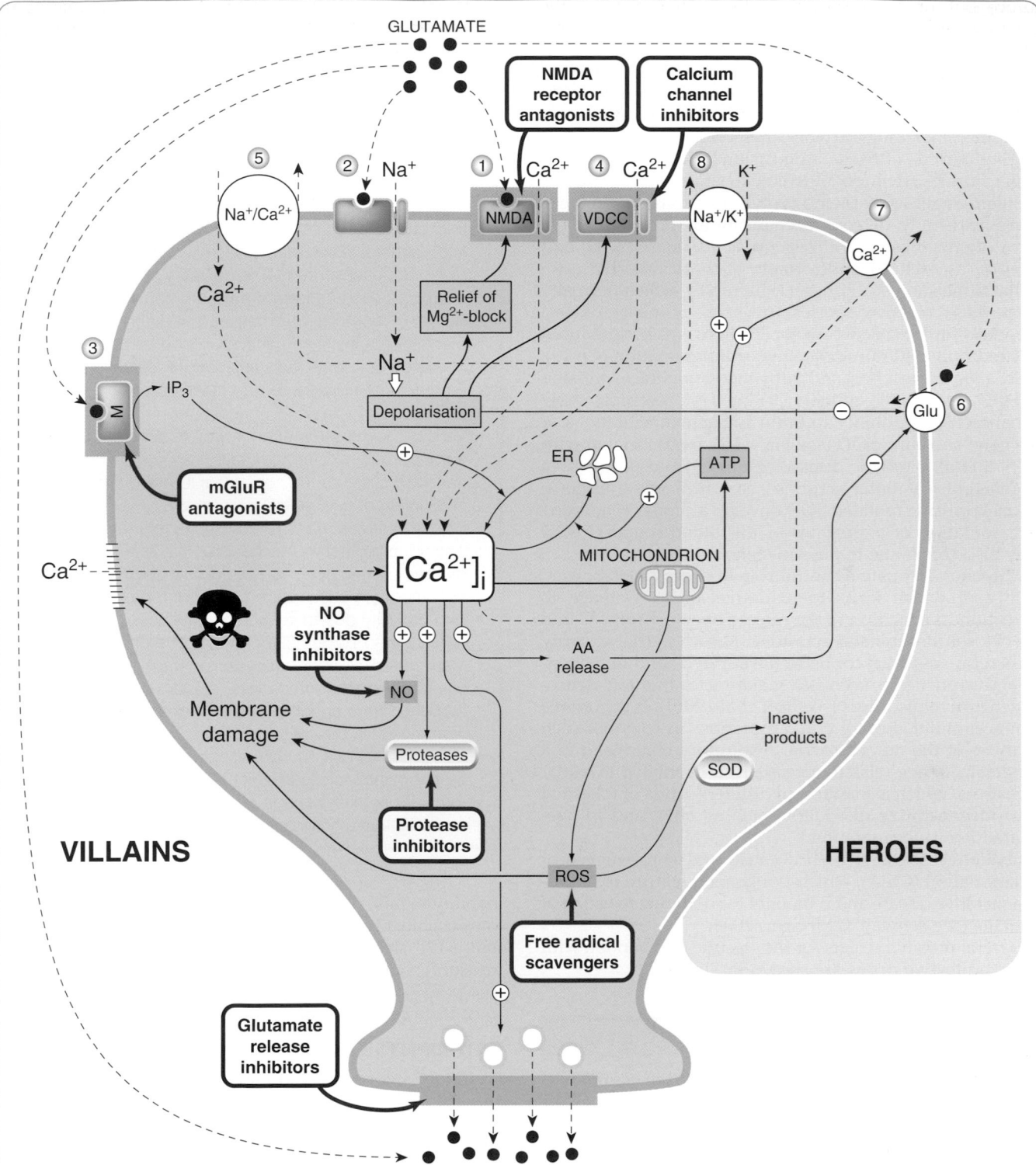

Fig. 41.2 Mechanisms of excitotoxicity. Membrane receptors, ion channels and transporters, identified by numbers 1–8, are discussed in the text. Possible sites of action of neuroprotective drugs (not yet of proven clinical value) are *highlighted*. Mechanisms on the *left* (villains) are those that favour cell death, while those on the *right* (heroes) are protective. See text for details. *AA,* arachidonic acid; *ER,* endoplasmic reticulum; *Glu,* glutamate uptake; *IP$_3$,* inositol trisphosphate; *M, mGluR,* metabotropic glutamate receptor; *NO,* nitric oxide; *ROS,* reactive oxygen species; *SOD,* superoxide dismutase; *VDCC,* voltage-dependent calcium channel.

production of these reactive species. They can also be produced as a byproduct of other biochemical pathways, including nitric oxide synthesis and arachidonic acid metabolism (which are implicated in excitotoxicity; see p. 516), as well as the P450 mono-oxygenase system (see Ch. 10). Unchecked, reactive oxygen radicals attack many key molecules, including enzymes, membrane lipids and DNA. During periods of tissue reperfusion following ischaemia (e.g. in stroke), delinquent leukocytes may exacerbate this problem by releasing their own cytotoxic oxygen products. Not surprisingly, defence mechanisms are provided, in the form of enzymes such as *superoxide dismutase* (SOD) and *catalase*, as well as antioxidants such as ascorbic acid, glutathione and α-tocopherol (vitamin E), which normally keep these reactive species in check. Some cytokines, especially tumour necrosis factor (TNF)-α, which is produced in conditions of brain ischaemia or inflammation (Ch.19), exert a protective effect, partly by increasing the expression of SOD. Transgenic animals lacking TNF receptors show enhanced susceptibility to brain ischaemia. Mutations of the gene encoding SOD (see Fig. 41.2) are associated with ALS, a fatal, paralytic disease resulting from progressive degeneration of motor neurons (see p. 528), and transgenic mice expressing mutated SOD develop a similar condition.[3] Accumulation of aggregates of misfolded mutated SOD may also contribute to neurodegeneration.

Mitochondria play a central role in energy metabolism, failure of which leads to oxidative stress. Damage to mitochondria, leading to the release of cytochrome C into the cytosol, also initiates apoptosis. Mitochondrial integrity is therefore essential for neuronal survival, and mitochondrial dysfunction is seen as a major factor in many neurodegenerative disorders (see Itoh et al., 2013). It is possible that accumulated or inherited mutations in enzymes such as those of the mitochondrial respiratory chain lead to a congenital or age-related increase in susceptibility to oxidative stress, which is manifest in different kinds of inherited neurodegenerative disorders (such as HD), and in age-related neurodegeneration.

Oxidative stress is both a cause and consequence of inflammation (Ch. 7), which is a general feature of neurodegenerative disease and is thought to contribute to neuronal damage (see Schwab & McGeer, 2008).

Several possible targets for therapeutic intervention with neuroprotective drugs are shown in Fig. 41.2.

ISCHAEMIC BRAIN DAMAGE

After heart disease and cancer, strokes are the commonest cause of death in Europe and North America, and the 70% that are non-fatal are the commonest cause of disability. Approximately 85% of strokes are *ischaemic*, usually due to cerebral arterial occlusion caused by local thrombus formation or by a circulating embolus lodging at a narrowing of the vessel. Ischaemic stroke may be preceded by transient ischaemic attacks (TIAs) or 'mini-strokes', resulting from brief episodes of inadequate blood flow. TIAs produce symptoms such as sudden limb or facial muscle weakness,

> ### Excitotoxicity and oxidative stress
>
> - Excitatory amino acids, especially glutamate, can cause neuronal death.
> - Excitotoxicity is associated mainly with activation of NMDA receptors, but other types of excitatory amino acid receptors also contribute.
> - Excitotoxicity results from a sustained rise in intracellular Ca^{2+} concentration (Ca^{2+} overload).
> - Excitotoxicity can occur under pathological conditions (e.g. cerebral ischaemia, epilepsy) in which excessive glutamate release occurs. It can also occur when chemicals such as **kainic acid** are administered.
> - Raised intracellular Ca^{2+} causes cell death by various mechanisms, including activation of proteases, formation of free radicals and lipid peroxidation. Formation of nitric oxide and arachidonic acid are also involved.
> - Various mechanisms act normally to protect neurons against excitotoxicity, the main ones being Ca^{2+} transport systems, mitochondrial function and the production of free radical scavengers.
> - Oxidative stress refers to conditions (e.g. hypoxia) in which the protective mechanisms are compromised, reactive oxygen species accumulate and neurons become more susceptible to excitotoxic damage.
> - Excitotoxicity due to environmental chemicals may contribute to some neurodegenerative disorders.
> - Measures designed to reduce excitotoxicity include the use of glutamate antagonists, calcium channel-blocking drugs and free radical scavengers; none is yet proven for clinical use.
> - Mitochondrial dysfunction, associated with ageing, environmental toxins and genetic abnormalities, leads to oxidative stress and is a common feature of neurodegenerative diseases.

inability to talk, double vision and dizziness. These symptoms usually resolve within 24 hours but serve as a warning that a full stroke may occur in the near future and that measures should be taken to prevent further atherosclerosis (see p. 519). The other type of stroke is *haemorrhagic*, due to rupture of a cerebral artery.

PATHOPHYSIOLOGY

Prolonged interruption of blood supply to the brain initiates the cascade of neuronal events shown in Fig. 41.2, which lead in turn to later consequences, including cerebral oedema and inflammation, which can also contribute to brain damage. Further damage can occur following reperfusion,[4] because of the production of ROS when the oxygenation is restored. Reperfusion injury may be an important component in stroke patients. These secondary processes often take hours to develop, providing a window of opportunity for therapeutic intervention. The lesion produced by occlusion of a major cerebral artery consists of a central core in which the neurons quickly undergo irreversible necrosis,

---

[3]Surprisingly, some SOD mutations associated with ALS are more, rather than less, active than the normal enzyme. The mechanism responsible for neurodegeneration probably involves abnormal accumulation of the enzyme in mitochondria.

[4]Nevertheless, early reperfusion (within 4.5 h of the thrombosis) is clearly beneficial, based on clinical evidence with fibrinolytic drugs.

surrounded by a penumbra of compromised tissue in which inflammation and apoptotic cell death develop over a period of several hours. It is assumed that neuroprotective therapies, given within a few hours, might inhibit this secondary penumbral damage.

Glutamate excitotoxicity plays a critical role in brain ischaemia. Ischaemia causes depolarisation of neurons, and the release of large amounts of glutamate. Ca^{2+} accumulation occurs, partly as a result of glutamate acting on NMDA receptors, as both Ca^{2+} entry and cell death following cerebral ischaemia are inhibited by drugs that block NMDA receptors or channels (see Ch. 39). Nitric oxide is also produced in amounts much greater than result from normal neuronal activity (i.e. to levels that are toxic rather than modulatory).

THERAPEUTIC APPROACHES

The only drug currently approved for treating strokes is a recombinant tissue plasminogen activator, **alteplase**, given intravenously, which helps to restore blood flow by dispersing the thrombus (see Ch. 25). Clinical trials have found that it did not reduce mortality, but gave significant functional benefit to patients who survive. To be effective, it must be given within about 4.5 h of the thrombotic episode. Also, it must not be given in the 15% of cases where the cause is haemorrhage rather than thrombosis, so preliminary computerised tomography (CT) scanning is essential. These stringent requirements seriously limit the use of fibrinolytic agents for treating stroke, except where specialised rapid response facilities are available. The use of intra-arterial clot retrieval devices (mechanical thrombectomy), in combination with alteplase, has yielded greater benefits and this technology is being rolled out in specialised acute stroke treatment centres.

An alternative approach would be to use neuroprotective agents aimed at rescuing cells in the penumbral region of the lesion, which are otherwise likely to die. In animal models involving cerebral artery occlusion, many drugs targeted at the mechanisms shown in Fig. 41.2 (not to mention many others that have been tested on the basis of more far-flung theories) act in this way to reduce the size of the infarct. These include glutamate antagonists, calcium and sodium-channel inhibitors, free radical scavengers, anti-inflammatory drugs, protease inhibitors and others (see Green, 2008). It seems that almost anything works in these animal models. However, of the many drugs that have been tested in over 100 clinical trials, none was effective. The dispiriting list of failures includes calcium- and sodium-channel blockers (e.g. **nimodipine, fosphenytoin**), NMDA-receptor antagonists (**selfotel, eliprodil, dextromethorphan**), drugs that inhibit glutamate release (adenosine analogues, **lubeluzole**), drugs that enhance GABA effects (e.g. **chlormethiazole**), 5-HT antagonists, metal chelators and various free radical scavengers (e.g. **tirilazad**). There was hope that mGlu1-receptor antagonists or negative allosteric modulators might be effective in the treatment of ischaemic brain damage but things have gone quiet on that front recently.

Controlled clinical trials on stroke patients are problematic and very expensive, partly because of the large variability of outcome in terms of functional recovery, which means that large groups of patients (typically thousands) need to be observed for several months. The need to start therapy within hours of the attack is an additional problem.

Stroke treatment is certainly not – so far at least – one of pharmacology's success stories, and medical hopes rest more on prevention (e.g. by controlling blood pressure, taking **aspirin**, **statins** or **ticagrelor** to prevent atherosclerosis [see Ch. 25]) than on treatment.[5]

One area of promise is the use of subanaesthetic doses of **xenon**, which has NMDA-receptor antagonist properties (Ch. 42), in combination with hypothermia to treat hypoxia-induced brain damage in neonates (Esencan et al., 2013).

Stroke

- Associated with intracerebral thrombosis or haemorrhage (less common), resulting in rapid death of neurons by necrosis in the centre of the lesion, followed by more gradual (hours) degeneration of cells in the penumbra due to excitotoxicity and inflammation.
- Spontaneous functional recovery occurs to a highly variable degree.
- Although many types of drug that interfere with excitotoxicity are able to reduce infarct size in experimental animals, none of these has so far proved efficacious in humans.
- Recombinant tissue plasminogen activator (**alteplase**), which disperses blood clots, is beneficial if it is given within 4.5 h; haemorrhagic stroke must be excluded by imaging before its administration.

ALZHEIMER'S DISEASE

Loss of cognitive ability with age is considered to be a normal process whose rate and extent is very variable. AD was originally defined as presenile dementia, but it now appears that the same pathology underlies the dementia irrespective of the age of onset. AD refers to dementia of gradual onset in adulthood, that may follow earlier brain injury, but often has no known antecedent cause. Its prevalence rises sharply with age, from about 2% in those aged 65–69 to 20% in those aged 85–89. Common symptoms of AD are difficulty remembering names and recent events, loss of executive functioning, apathy and depression. Age-related dementia was originally considered to result from the steady loss of neurons that normally goes on throughout life, possibly accelerated by a failing blood supply associated with atherosclerosis. Studies in recent years have, however, revealed specific genetic and molecular mechanisms underlying AD (see Frigero & De Strooper, 2016). These advances raised hopes of more effective treatments, but success has proved elusive, in part because multiple factors rather than a single cause contribute to the disease and because the symptoms of the disease only become obvious after the underlying pathology has progressed.

PATHOGENESIS OF ALZHEIMER'S DISEASE

AD is associated with brain shrinkage and loss of neurons in many brain regions, but especially in the hippocampus

[5]Eating dark chocolate is believed to reduce the risk of stroke. Flavonoids in the chocolate may be protective due to antioxidant, anti-clotting and anti-inflammatory properties. However, this is not a reason to overindulge!

Fig. 41.3 **Pathogenesis of Alzheimer's disease.** (A) Structure of amyloid precursor protein (APP), showing origin of secreted APP (sAPP) and Aβ amyloid protein. The regions involved in amyloidogenic mutations discovered in some cases of familial Alzheimer's disease are shown flanking the Aβ sequence. APP cleavage involves three proteases: secretases α, β and γ. α-Secretase produces soluble APP, whereas β- and γ-secretases generate Aβ amyloid protein. γ-Secretase can cut at different points, generating Aβ peptides of varying lengths, including Aβ40 and Aβ42, the latter having a high tendency to aggregate as amyloid plaques. (B) Processing of APP. The main 'physiological' pathway gives rise to sAPP, which exerts a number of trophic functions. Cleavage of APP at different sites gives rise to Aβ, the predominant form normally being Aβ40, which is weakly amyloidogenic. Mutations in APP or presenilins increase the proportion of APP, which is degraded via the amyloidogenic pathway, and also increase the proportion converted to the much more strongly amyloidogenic form Aβ42. Clearance of Aβ is impaired by mutations in the apoE4 gene. Hyperphosphorylated Tau results in dissociation of Tau from microtubules, misfolding and aggregation to form paired helical filaments, which enhance Aβ toxicity.

and basal forebrain. The loss of cholinergic neurons in the hippocampus and frontal cortex is a feature of the disease, and is thought to underlie the cognitive deficit and loss of short-term memory that occur. Two microscopic features are characteristic of the disease, namely extracellular *amyloid plaques*, consisting of amorphous extracellular deposits of β-amyloid protein (known as Aβ), and intraneuronal *neurofibrillary tangles*, comprising filaments of a phosphorylated form of a microtubule-associated protein (Tau). Both of these deposits are protein aggregates that result from misfolding of native proteins, as discussed previously. They appear also in normal brains, although in smaller numbers. The early appearance of amyloid deposits presages the development of AD, although symptoms may not develop for many years. Altered processing of amyloid protein from its precursor (*amyloid precursor protein*, APP) has been implicated in the pathogenesis of AD. This is based on several lines of evidence, particularly the genetic analysis

of certain, relatively rare, types of familial AD, in which mutations of the APP gene, or of other genes (e.g. for *presenilins* and *sortilin-related receptor 1*) that control amyloid processing, have been discovered.[6]

▼ Amyloid deposits consist of aggregates of Aβ (Fig. 41.3), a 40- or 42-residue segment of APP, generated by the action of specific proteases (*secretases*). Aβ40 is produced normally in small amounts, whereas Aβ42 is overproduced as a result of the genetic mutations mentioned above. Both proteins aggregate to form *amyloid plaques*, but Aβ42 shows a stronger tendency than Aβ40 to do so, and appears to be the main culprit in amyloid formation. APP is a 770-amino acid membrane protein normally expressed by many cells, including CNS neurons. Cleavage by α-secretase releases the large extracellular

---

[6]The APP gene resides on chromosome 21, of which an extra copy is the cause of Down's syndrome, in which early AD-like dementia occurs in association with overexpression of APP.

domain as *soluble APP*, which is believed to serve a physiological trophic function. Formation of Aβ involves cleavage at two different points, including one in the intramembrane domain of APP, by β- and γ-secretases (see Fig. 41.3). γ-Secretase is a clumsy enzyme – actually a large intramembrane complex of several proteins – that lacks precision and cuts APP at different points in the transmembrane domain, generating Aβ fragments of different lengths, including Aβ40 and 42. Mutations in this region of the APP gene affect the preferred cleavage point, tending to favour formation of Aβ42. Mutations of the unrelated presenilin genes result in increased activity of γ-secretase, because the presenilin proteins form part of the γ-secretase complex. These different AD-related mutations increase the ratio of Aβ42:Aβ40, which can be detected in plasma, serving as a marker for familial AD. Mutations in another gene, that for the lipid transport protein ApoE4 which facilitates the clearance of Aβ oligomers, also predispose to AD, probably because the mutant form of ApoE4 proteins are less effective in this function.

It is uncertain exactly how Aβ accumulation would cause neurodegeneration, and whether the damage is done by soluble Aβ monomers or oligomers or by amyloid plaques. There is evidence that the cells die by apoptosis, although an inflammatory response is also evident. Expression of Alzheimer's mutations in transgenic animals (see Götz & Ittner, 2008) causes plaque formation and neurodegeneration, and also increases the susceptibility of CNS neurons to other challenges, such as ischaemia, excitotoxicity and oxidative stress, and this increased vulnerability may be the cause of the progressive neurodegeneration in AD. However, the fact that several novel potential therapies designed to reduce Aβ production (see p. 522) have so far proven to be ineffective in clinical trials on AD patients has led some to question the importance of amyloid plaque formation in AD (see Herrup, 2015 for a critical view).

The other main player on the biochemical stage is *Tau*, the protein of which the neurofibrillary tangles are composed (see Fig. 41.3). Its role in neurodegeneration is unclear, although similar 'tauopathies' occur in many neurodegenerative conditions (see Brunden et al., 2009; Hanger et al., 2009). Tau is a normal constituent of neurons, being associated with the intracellular microtubules that serve as tracks for transporting materials along nerve axons. In AD and other tauopathies, Tau is abnormally phosphorylated by the action of various kinases, including glycogen synthase kinase-3β (GSK-3β) and cyclin-dependent kinase 5 (CDK5), and dissociates from microtubules to be deposited intracellularly as *paired helical filaments* with a characteristic microscopic appearance. When the cells die, these filaments aggregate as extracellular *neurofibrillary tangles*. Tau phosphorylation is enhanced by the presence of Aβ, possibly by activation of kinases. Conversely, hyperphosphorylated Tau favours the formation of amyloid deposits. Whether hyperphosphorylation and intracellular deposition of Tau directly harms the cell is not certain, although it is known that it impairs fast axonal transport, a process that depends on microtubules.

Loss of cholinergic neurons

Although changes in many transmitter systems have been observed, mainly from measurements on postmortem AD brain tissue, a relatively selective loss of cholinergic neurons in the basal forebrain nuclei (Ch. 40) is characteristic. This discovery, made in 1976, implied that pharmacological approaches to restoring cholinergic function might be feasible, leading to the use of cholinesterase inhibitors to treat AD (see later).

Choline acetyl transferase activity, acetylcholine content and acetylcholinesterase and choline transport in the cortex and hippocampus are all reduced considerably in AD but not in other disorders, such as depression or schizophrenia. Muscarinic receptor density, determined by binding studies, is not affected, but nicotinic receptors, particularly in the cortex, are reduced. The reason for the selective loss of cholinergic neurons resulting from Aβ formation is not known.

> ## Alzheimer's disease
>
> - Alzheimer's disease (AD) is a common age-related dementia, distinct from vascular dementia associated with brain infarction.
> - The main pathological features of AD comprise amyloid plaques, neurofibrillary tangles and a loss of neurons (particularly cholinergic neurons of the basal forebrain).
> - Amyloid plaques consist of aggregates of the Aβ fragment of amyloid precursor protein (APP), a normal neuronal membrane protein, produced by the action of β- and γ-secretases. AD is associated with excessive Aβ formation, resulting in neurotoxicity.
> - Familial AD (rare) results from mutations in the APP gene, or in presenilin genes (involved in γ-secretase function), both of which cause increased Aβ formation.
> - Mutations in the lipoprotein ApoE4 increase the risk of developing AD, probably by interfering with Aβ clearance.
> - Neurofibrillary tangles comprise intracellular aggregates of a highly phosphorylated form of a normal neuronal protein (Tau). Hyperphosphorylated Tau and Aβ act synergistically to cause neurodegeneration.
> - Loss of cholinergic neurons is believed to account for much of the learning and memory deficit in AD.

THERAPEUTIC APPROACHES

Currently, cholinesterase inhibitors (see Ch. 14) and **memantine** are the only drugs approved for treating AD. No new treatments have been introduced since 2003 despite intensive research into the underlying causes of the disease and huge investment in drug development. Unravelling the mechanism of neurodegeneration in AD has yet to result in therapies able to retard it and, with some spectacular failures having occurred in expensive clinical trials of new drugs, optimism is waning about an effective new therapy being just around the corner.

CHOLINESTERASE INHIBITORS

Tacrine was the first drug approved for treating AD but because of its hepatotoxicity and the subsequent availability of other anticholinesterase agents use of tacrine has been discontinued. Later compounds include **donepezil, rivastigmine** and **galantamine** (Table 41.2). Clinical trials have demonstrated modest improvements in tests of memory and cognition but no sustained effect on disease progression or improvement in other behavioural and psychological measures that affect quality of life.

Other drugs aimed at improving cholinergic function that are being investigated include other cholinesterase inhibitors and a variety of muscarinic and nicotinic receptor agonists. To date, the lack of selectivity of muscarinic orthosteric agonists has hindered their use to treat CNS disorders due to the incidence of side effects, but the hope is that positive allosteric modulators (see Ch. 3) that are selective (e.g. for the M_1 receptor) will be developed.

MEMANTINE

The other drug currently approved for the treatment of AD is **memantine**, an orally active weak antagonist at

Table 41.2 Cholinesterase inhibitors used in the treatment of Alzheimer's disease[a]

Drug	Type of inhibition	Duration of action and dosage	Main side effects	Notes
Donepezil	CNS, AChE selective	~24 h Once-daily oral dosage	Slight cholinergic side effects	—
Rivastigmine	CNS selective	~8 h Twice-daily oral dosage	Cholinergic side effects that tend to subside with continuing treatment	Gradual dose escalation to minimise side effects Available in a transdermal patch
Galantamine	Affects both AChE and BuChE Also enhances nicotinic ACh receptor activation by allosteric action	~8 h Twice-daily oral dosage	Slight cholinergic side effects	—

[a]Similar level of limited clinical benefit for all drugs. No clinical evidence for retardation of disease process, although animal tests suggest diminution of Aβ and plaque formation by a mechanism not related to cholinesterase inhibition.
AChE, acetylcholinesterase; *BuChE*, butyryl cholinesterase; *CNS*, central nervous system.

NMDA receptors. It was originally introduced as an antiviral drug, and resurrected as a potential inhibitor of excitotoxicity. It produces – surprisingly – a modest cognitive improvement in moderate or severe AD, but does not appear to be neuroprotective. It may work by selectively inhibiting excessive, pathological NMDA-receptor activation while preserving more physiological activation. It has a long plasma half-life, and its adverse effects include headache, dizziness, drowsiness, constipation, shortness of breath and hypertension as well as a raft of less common problems. The potential for other drugs acting as agonists or allosteric modulators at NMDA receptors to enhance cognition is discussed by Collingridge et al. (2013).

Clinical use of drugs in dementia

- Acetylcholinesterase inhibitors and NMDA antagonists detectably improve cognitive impairment in clinical trials but have significant adverse effects and are of limited use clinically. They have not been shown to retard neurodegeneration.
- Efficacy is monitored periodically in individual patients, and administration continued only if the drugs are believed to be working and their effect in slowing functional and cognitive deterioration is judged to outweigh adverse effects.

Acetylcholinesterase inhibitors:
- **Donepezil**, **galantamine**, **rivastigmine**. Unwanted cholinergic effects may be troublesome.
- Used in mild to moderate Alzheimer's disease.

NMDA-receptor antagonists:
- For example, **memantine** (see Ch. 39).
- Used in moderate-to-severe Alzheimer's disease.

Future drug development
▼ For most of the disorders discussed in this chapter, including AD, the Holy Grail, which so far eludes us, would be a drug that retards neurodegeneration. Although several well-characterised targets were identified, such as Aβ formation by β- and γ-secretases, Aβ aggregation and Aβ neurotoxicity, together with a range of transgenic animal models of AD on which compounds can be tested, subsequent clinical trials of drugs targeting these processes have been disappointing. Examples of drugs that proved not to be as effective in stopping or reversing the progress of AD as had been hoped are:

- *verubecestat*, a β-secretase 1 (BACE1) inhibitor;
- *solanezumab*, a monoclonal antibody against Aβ peptide.

There is still some hope that these or similarly acting agents (e.g. **aducanumab)** may prove effective if given at an early stage of disease development.

That treatment strategies targeted at reducing Aβ have failed to reverse the progression of AD suggests that the disease is the result of a more complex pathophysiology and that targeting Aβ alone may not be sufficient to treat AD.

Details of over 100 drugs in various stages of clinical trial for either symptomatic relief or disease-modifying activity in AD are given in Cummings et al. (2017). Cognitive deficits occur in other CNS disorders such as PD, schizophrenia and depression. The development of cognition-enhancing drugs that may be useful across these disorders is described in Chapter 49.

PARKINSON'S DISEASE

FEATURES OF PARKINSON'S DISEASE

PD is a progressive disorder of movement that occurs mainly in the elderly. It was first described in 1817 by James Parkinson. Przedborski (2017) describes in detail how understanding of the disorder and its treatment have evolved over the subsequent 200 years.

The chief symptoms are:

- suppression of voluntary movements (*bradykinesia*), due partly to muscle rigidity and partly to an inherent inertia of the motor system, which means that motor activity is difficult to stop as well as to initiate;
- tremor at rest, usually starting in the hands ('pill-rolling' tremor), which tends to diminish during voluntary activity;
- muscle rigidity, detectable as an increased resistance in passive limb movement;
- a variable degree of cognitive impairment.

Parkinsonian patients walk with a characteristic shuffling gait. They find it hard to start, and once in progress they cannot quickly stop or change direction. PD is commonly associated with dementia, depression, hallucinations and autonomic dysfunction, because the degenerative process is not confined to the basal ganglia but also affects other parts of the brain. Non-motor symptoms may appear before motor symptoms and often predominate in the later stages of the disease.

PD often occurs with no obvious underlying cause, but it may be the result of cerebral ischaemia, viral encephalitis, head injury or other types of pathological damage. The symptoms can also be drug-induced, the main drugs involved being those that block dopamine receptors (e.g. antiemetic and antipsychotic drugs such as **chlorpromazine**; see Chs 31 and 47). There are rare instances of familial early-onset PD, and several gene mutations have been identified, including those encoding *synuclein* and *parkin* (see p. 524). Mutations in the gene encoding leucine-rich repeat kinase 2 (LRRK2) have also been associated with PD. Study of gene mutations has given some clues about the mechanism underlying the neurodegenerative process.

Neurochemical changes

PD affects the basal ganglia, and its neurochemical origin was discovered in 1960 by Hornykiewicz, who showed that the dopamine content of the substantia nigra and corpus striatum (see Ch. 40) in postmortem brains of PD patients was extremely low (usually less than 10% of normal), associated with a loss of dopaminergic neurons in the substantia nigra and degeneration of nerve terminals in the striatum.[7] Neurons containing other monoamines such as noradrenaline and 5-hydroxytryptamine are also affected. Gradual loss of dopamine occurs over several years, with symptoms of PD appearing only when the striatal dopamine content has fallen to 20%–40% of normal. Lesions of the nigrostriatal tract or chemically induced depletion of dopamine in experimental animals also produce symptoms of PD. The symptom most clearly related to dopamine deficiency is *bradykinesia*, which occurs immediately and invariably in lesioned animals. Rigidity and tremor involve more complex neurochemical disturbances of other transmitters (particularly acetylcholine, noradrenaline, 5-hydroxytryptamine and GABA) as well as dopamine. In experimental lesions, two secondary consequences follow damage to the nigrostriatal tract, namely a hyperactivity of the remaining dopaminergic neurons, which show an increased rate of transmitter turnover, and an increase in the number of dopamine receptors, which produces a state of denervation hypersensitivity (see Ch. 13). Neurons in the striatum expresses mainly D_1 (excitatory) and D_2 (inhibitory) receptors (see Ch. 40), but fewer D_3 and D_4 receptors. A simplified diagram of the neuronal circuitry involved, and the pathways primarily affected in PD and HD, is shown in Fig. 41.4.

Cholinergic interneurons of the corpus striatum (not shown in Fig. 41.4) are also involved in PD and HD. Acetylcholine release from the striatum is strongly inhibited by dopamine, and it is suggested that hyperactivity of these cholinergic neurons contributes to the symptoms of PD. The opposite happens in HD, and in both conditions therapies aimed at redressing the balance between the

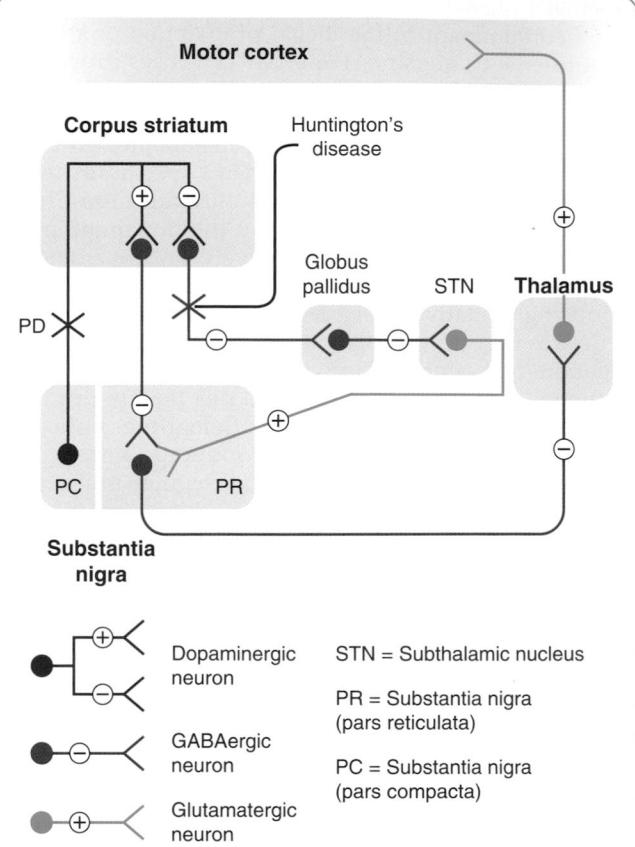

Fig. 41.4 Simplified diagram of the organisation of the extrapyramidal motor system and the defects that occur in Parkinson's disease (PD) and Huntington's disease.
Normally, activity in nigrostriatal dopamine neurons causes excitation of striatonigral neurons and inhibition of striatal neurons that project to the globus pallidus. Because of the different pathways involved, the activity of GABAergic neurons in the substantia nigra is suppressed, releasing the restraint on the thalamus and cortex, causing motor stimulation. In PD, the dopaminergic pathway from the substantia nigra (pars compacta) to the striatum is impaired. In Huntington's disease, the GABAergic striatopallidal pathway is impaired, producing effects opposite to the changes in PD.

dopaminergic and cholinergic neurons are, up to a point, beneficial.

PATHOGENESIS OF PARKINSON'S DISEASE

As with other neurodegenerative disorders, the neuronal damage in PD is caused by protein misfolding and aggregation, aided and abetted by other familiar villains, namely excitotoxicity, mitochondrial dysfunction, oxidative stress, inflammation and apoptosis. Aspects of the pathogenesis and animal models of PD are described by Duty and Jenner (2011).

Neurotoxins

New light was thrown on the possible aetiology of PD by a chance event. In 1982, a group of young drug addicts in California suddenly developed an exceptionally severe form of PD (known as the 'frozen addict' syndrome), and the cause was traced to the compound

---

[7]It is emerging that other types of neuron are also affected. Here we concentrate on the dopaminergic nigrostriatal pathway as it is the most important in relation to current therapies.

1-methyl-4-phenyl-1,2,3,6-tetrahydropyridine (**MPTP**), which was a contaminant in the illegal preparation of a heroin substitute (see Langston, 1985). MPTP causes irreversible destruction of nigrostriatal dopaminergic neurons in various species, and produces a PD-like state in primates. MPTP acts by being converted to a toxic metabolite, MPP^+, by the enzyme monoamine oxidase (MAO, specifically by the MAO-B subtype that is located in glial cells; see Chs 15 and 48). MPP^+ is then taken up by the dopamine transport system, and thus acts selectively on dopaminergic neurons; it inhibits mitochondrial oxidation reactions, producing oxidative stress. MPTP appears to be selective in destroying nigrostriatal neurons and does not affect dopaminergic neurons elsewhere – the reason for this is unknown. It is also less effective in rats than in primates, yet mice show some susceptibility. **Selegiline**, a selective MAO-B inhibitor, prevents MPTP-induced neurotoxicity by blocking its conversion to MPP^+. Selegiline is also used in treating PD (see p. 526); as well as inhibiting dopamine breakdown, it might also work by blocking the metabolic activation of a putative endogenous, or environmental, MPTP-like substance, which is involved in the causation of PD. It is possible that dopamine itself could be the culprit, because oxidation of dopamine gives rise to potentially toxic metabolites. Whether or not the action of MPTP reflects the natural pathogenesis of PD, the MPTP model is a very useful experimental tool for testing possible therapies.

Impaired mitochondrial function is a feature of the disease in humans. Various herbicides, such as **rotenone**, that selectively inhibit mitochondrial function cause a PD-like syndrome in animals. PD in humans is more common in agricultural areas than in cities, suggesting that environmental toxins could be a factor in its causation.

Molecular aspects

▼ PD, as well as several other neurodegenerative disorders, is associated with the development of intracellular protein aggregates known as *Lewy bodies* in various parts of the brain. They consist largely of α-synuclein, a synaptic protein, present in large amounts in normal brains. Recent evidence suggests that α-synuclein may act as a prion-like protein and that PD is in fact a prion-like disease (Olanow & Brundin, 2013). α-Synuclein normally exists in an α-helical conformation. However, under certain circumstances, such as genetic duplication or triplication or genetic mutation, it can undergo a conformational change to a β-sheet-rich structure that polymerises to form toxic aggregates and amyloid plaques. Mutations occur in rare types of hereditary PD (see p. 523). It is believed that misfolding and aggregation renders the protein resistant to degradation within cells, causing it to pile up in Lewy bodies. In parkinsonian patients who received fetal dopaminergic neuron grafts, (see p. 527) the grafted neurons, over time, developed Lewy bodies. Misfolded α-synuclein is thought to have migrated from the native tissue to the grafted tissue.

It is possible (see Lotharius & Brundin, 2002) that the normal function of α-synuclein is related to synaptic vesicle recycling, and that the misfolded form loses this functionality, with the result that vesicular storage of dopamine is impaired. This may lead to an increase in cytosolic dopamine, degradation of which produces ROS and hence neurotoxicity. Consistent with the α-synuclein hypothesis, another mutation associated with PD (*parkin*) also involves a protein that participates in the intracellular degradation of rogue proteins.

▼ Other gene mutations that have been identified as risk factors for early-onset PD code for proteins involved in mitochondrial function,

making cells more susceptible to oxidative stress. Thus, a picture similar to AD pathogenesis is slowly emerging. Misfolded α-synuclein, facilitated by overexpression, genetic mutations or possibly by environmental factors, builds up in the cell as a result of impaired protein degradation (resulting from defective parkin) in the form of Lewy bodies, which, by unknown mechanisms, compromise cell survival. If oxidative stress is increased, as a result of ischaemia, mitochondrial poisons or mutations of certain mitochondrial proteins, the result is cell death.

Parkinson's disease

- Degenerative disease of the basal ganglia causing hypokinesia, tremor at rest and muscle rigidity, often with dementia and autonomic dysfunction.
- Associated with aggregation of α-synuclein (a protein normally involved in vesicle recycling) in the form of characteristic Lewy bodies.
- Often idiopathic but may follow stroke or virus infection; can be drug-induced (antipsychotic drugs). Rare familial forms also occur, associated with various gene mutations, including α-synuclein.
- Associated with degeneration of dopaminergic nigrostriatal neurons that gives rise to the motor symptoms, as well as more general neurodegeneration resulting in dementia and depression.
- Can be induced by 1-methyl-4-phenyl-1,2,3,6-tetrahydropyridine (**MPTP**), a neurotoxin affecting dopamine neurons. Similar environmental neurotoxins, as well as genetic factors, may be involved in human Parkinson's disease.

DRUG TREATMENT OF PARKINSON'S DISEASE

Currently, the main drugs used (Fig. 41.5) are:

- **levodopa** (sometimes in combination with **carbidopa** and **entacapone**);
- dopamine agonists (e.g. **pramipexole, ropinirole, bromocriptine**);
- MAO-B inhibitors (e.g. **selegiline, rasagiline**);
- muscarinic ACh receptor antagonists (e.g. **orphenadrine, procyclidine** and **trihexyphenidyl**) are occasionally used.

None of the drugs used to treat PD affect the progression of the disease.

LEVODOPA

Levodopa is the first-line treatment for PD and is combined with a peripherally acting dopa decarboxylase inhibitor, such as **carbidopa** or **benserazide**, which reduces the dose needed by about 10-fold and diminishes the peripheral side effects. It is well absorbed from the small intestine, a process that relies on active transport, although much of it is inactivated by MAO in the wall of the intestine. The plasma half-life is short (about 2 h). Oral and subcutaneous slow-release preparations have been developed. Conversion to dopamine in the periphery, which would otherwise account for about 95% of the levodopa dose and cause troublesome side effects, is largely prevented by the decarboxylase inhibitor. Decarboxylation occurs rapidly within the brain, because the decarboxylase inhibitors do not penetrate the blood–brain barrier. It is not certain

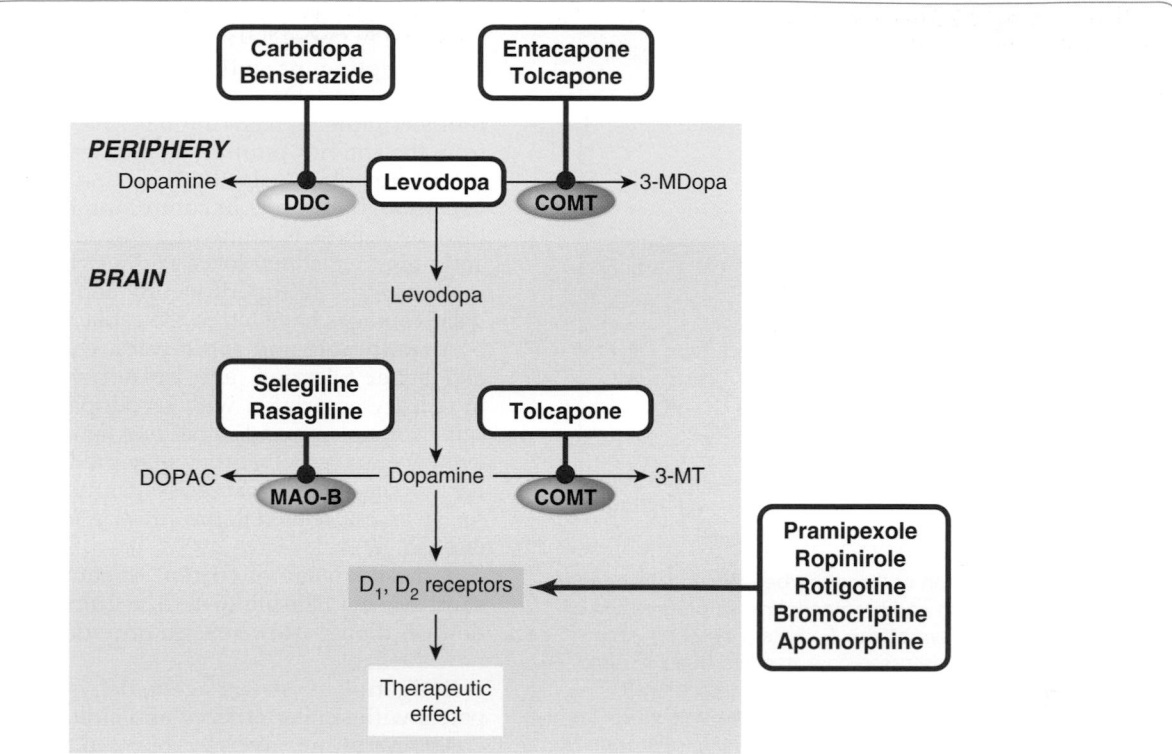

Fig. 41.5 **Sites of action of drugs used to treat Parkinson's disease.** Levodopa enters the brain and is converted to dopamine (the deficient neurotransmitter). Inactivation of levodopa in the periphery is prevented by inhibitors of dopa decarboxylase (DDC) and catechol-*O*-methyl transferase (COMT). Inactivation in the brain is prevented by inhibitors of COMT and monoamine oxidase-B (MAO-B). Dopamine agonists act directly on striatal dopamine receptors. *3-MDopa*, 3-methoxydopa; *3-MT*, 3-methoxytyrosine; *DOPAC*, dihydroxyphenylacetic acid.

whether the effect depends on an increased release of dopamine from the few surviving dopaminergic neurons or on a 'flooding' of the synapse with dopamine formed elsewhere. Because synthetic dopamine agonists (see p. 526) are equally effective, the latter explanation is more likely, and animal studies suggest that levodopa can act even when no dopaminergic nerve terminals are present. On the other hand, the therapeutic effectiveness of levodopa decreases as the disease advances, so part of its action may rely on the presence of functional dopaminergic neurons. Combination of levodopa plus a dopa decarboxylase inhibitor with a catechol-*O*-methyl transferase (COMT) inhibitor (e.g. **entacapone**, **tolcapone** or **opicapone**, see Ch. 15) to inhibit its degradation, is used in patients troubled by 'end of dose' motor fluctuations.

Therapeutic effectiveness

About 80% of patients show initial improvement with levodopa, particularly of rigidity and bradykinesia, and about 20% are restored virtually to normal motor function. As time progresses, the effectiveness of levodopa gradually declines (Fig. 41.6). In a typical study of 100 patients treated with levodopa for 5 years, only 34 were better than they had been at the beginning of the trial, 32 patients having died and 21 having withdrawn from the trial. It is likely that the loss of effectiveness of levodopa mainly reflects the natural progression of the disease, but receptor down-regulation and other compensatory mechanisms may also contribute. There is no evidence that levodopa can actually accelerate the neurodegenerative process through overproduction of dopamine, as was suspected on theoretical grounds. Overall, levodopa increases the life expectancy of PD patients, probably as a result of improved motor function, although some symptoms (e.g. dysphagia, cognitive decline) are not improved.

Unwanted effects

There are two main types of unwanted effect:

1. Involuntary movements (dyskinesia), which do not appear initially but develop in the majority of patients within 2 years of starting levodopa therapy. These movements usually affect the face and limbs, and can become very severe. They occur at the time of the peak therapeutic effect, and the margin between the beneficial and the dyskinetic effect becomes progressively narrower. Levodopa is short acting, and the fluctuating plasma concentration of the drug may favour the development of dyskinesias, as longer-acting dopamine agonists are less problematic in this regard.
2. Rapid fluctuations in clinical state, where bradykinesia and rigidity may suddenly worsen for anything from a few minutes to a few hours, and then improve again. This 'on–off effect' is not seen in untreated PD patients or with other anti-PD drugs. The 'off effect' can be so sudden that the patient stops while walking and feels rooted to the spot, or is unable to rise from a chair,

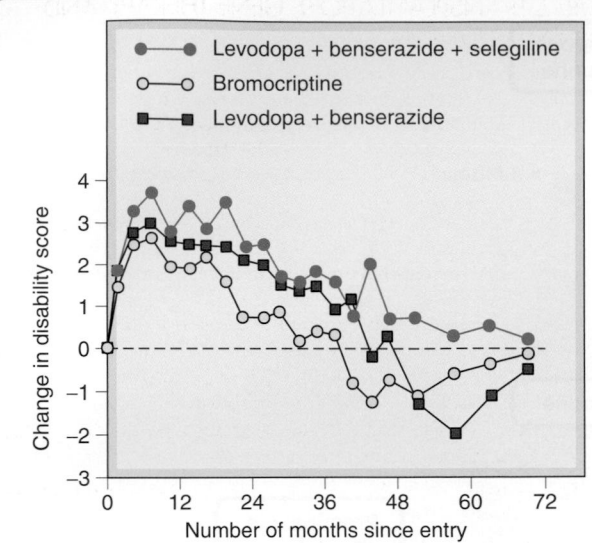

Fig. 41.6 Comparison of levodopa/benserazide, levodopa/benserazide/selegiline and bromocriptine on progression of Parkinson's disease symptoms. Patients (249–271 in each treatment group) were assessed on a standard disability rating score. Before treatment, the average rate of decline was 0.7 units/year. All three treatments produced improvement over the initial rating for 2–3 years, but the effect declined, either because of refractoriness to the drugs or disease progression. Bromocriptine appeared slightly less effective than levodopa regimens, and there was a higher drop-out rate due to side effects in this group. (From Parkinson's Disease Research Group, 1993. Br. Med. J. 307, 469–472.)

having sat down normally a few moments earlier. As with the dyskinesias, the problem seems to reflect the fluctuating plasma concentration of levodopa, and it is suggested that as the disease advances, the ability of neurons to store dopamine is lost, so the therapeutic benefit of levodopa depends increasingly on the continuous formation of extraneuronal dopamine, which requires a continuous supply of levodopa. The use of sustained-release preparations, or co-administration of COMT inhibitors such as **entacapone**, may be used to counteract the fluctuations in plasma concentration of levodopa.

In addition to these slowly developing side effects, levodopa produces several acute effects, which are experienced by most patients at first but tend to disappear after a few weeks. The main ones are as follows:

- Nausea and anorexia. **Domperidone**, a dopamine antagonist that works in the chemoreceptor trigger zone (where the blood–brain barrier is leaky) but does not gain access to the basal ganglia, may be useful in preventing this effect.
- Hypotension. Postural hypotension is a recognised problem, particularly in older patients.
- Psychological effects. Levodopa, by increasing dopamine activity in the brain, can produce a schizophrenia-like syndrome (see Ch. 47) with delusions and hallucinations. More commonly, in about 20% of patients, it causes confusion, disorientation, insomnia or nightmares.

DOPAMINE AGONISTS

Bromocriptine, **pergolide** and **cabergoline** exhibit slight selectivity for $D_{2/3}$ over D_1 receptors (see Ch. 40). Bromocriptine, which inhibits the release of prolactin from the anterior pituitary gland, was first introduced for the treatment of galactorrhoea and gynaecomastia (Ch. 34). Though effective in controlling the symptoms of PD, their usefulness is limited by side effects, such as nausea and vomiting, somnolence and a risk of fibrotic reactions in the lungs, retroperitoneum and pericardium. These disadvantages have led to the replacement of these drugs by **pramipexole** and **ropinirole**, which are $D_{2/3}$ selective and better tolerated, and do not show the fluctuations in efficacy associated with levodopa. They do, however, cause somnolence and sometimes hallucinations, and recent evidence suggests that they may predispose to compulsive behaviours, such as excessive gambling,[8] over-eating and sexual excess, related to the 'reward' functions of dopamine (see Ch. 50).

A disadvantage of current dopamine agonists is their short plasma half-life (6–8 h), requiring three-times daily dosage, though slow-release once-daily formulations are now available.

Rotigotine is a newer agent, delivered as a transdermal patch, with similar efficacy and side effects.

Apomorphine, given by injection, is sometimes used to control the 'off effect' with levodopa. Because of its powerful emetic action, it must be combined with an oral antiemetic drug. It has other serious adverse effects (mood and behavioural changes, cardiac dysrhythmias, hypotension) and is a last resort if other drugs fail.

MAO-B INHIBITORS

Selegiline is a selective MAO-B[9] inhibitor, which lacks the unwanted peripheral effects of non-selective MAO inhibitors used to treat depression (Ch. 48) and, in contrast to them, does not provoke the 'cheese reaction' or interact so frequently with other drugs. Inhibition of MAO-B protects dopamine from extraneuronal degradation and was initially used as an adjunct to levodopa. Long-term trials showed that the combination of selegiline and levodopa was more effective than levodopa alone in relieving symptoms and prolonging life. Recognition of the role of MAO-B in neurotoxicity (see p. 524) suggested that selegiline might be neuroprotective rather than merely enhancing the action of levodopa, but clinical studies do not support this. A large-scale trial (see Fig. 41.6) showed no difference when selegiline was added to levodopa/benserazide treatment. Selegiline is metabolised to amphetamine, and sometimes causes excitement, anxiety and insomnia. **Rasagiline**, a very similar drug, does not have this unwanted effect, and may somewhat retard disease progression, as well as alleviating symptoms (Olanow et al., 2009). **Safinamide** inhibits both MAO-B and dopamine reuptake.

---

[8]In 2008 a plaintiff was awarded $8.2 million damages by a United States court, having become a compulsive gambler (and losing a lot of money) after taking pramipexole for PD – a side effect of which the pharmaceutical company had been aware.
[9]MAO-B in the brain is located mainly in glial cells, and also in 5-HT neurons (though, surprisingly, it does not appear to be expressed in dopamine neurons).

OTHER DRUGS USED IN PARKINSON'S DISEASE

Amantadine

▼ Amantadine was introduced as an antiviral drug and discovered by accident in 1969 to be beneficial in PD. Many possible mechanisms for its action have been suggested based on neurochemical evidence of increased dopamine release, inhibition of amine uptake or a direct action on dopamine receptors. More recently block of NMDA receptors by stabilising closed states of the channel has been described and this may be a novel target for antiparkinsonian drugs.

Amantadine is less effective than levodopa or bromocriptine in treating PD, but it is effective in reducing the dyskinesias induced by prolonged levodopa treatment (see p. 525).

Acetylcholine antagonists

▼ For more than a century, until levodopa was discovered, atropine and related drugs were the main form of treatment for PD. Muscarinic acetylcholine receptors exert an inhibitory effect on dopaminergic nerve terminals, suppression of which compensates for a lack of dopamine. The side effects of muscarinic antagonists (Ch. 14) – dry mouth, constipation, impaired vision, urinary retention – are troublesome, and they are now rarely used, except to treat parkinsonian symptoms in patients receiving antipsychotic drugs (which are dopamine antagonists and thus nullify the effect of levodopa; see Ch. 47). Drugs used are **orphenadrine**, **procyclidine** and **trihexyphenidyl**.

NEW PHARMACOLOGICAL APPROACHES

▼ Potential new treatments for PD at various stages of clinical trial are reviewed by Oertel and Schulz (2016). Active and passive immunisation against α-synuclein and inhibitors or modulators of α-synuclein aggregation may prevent the progression of the disease. Other, pharmacological approaches are aimed at symptomatic relief after the disease has developed. For example, **pimavanserin**, a 5-HT$_{2A}$ receptor inverse agonist, has recently been introduced to treat hallucinations and delusions associated with psychosis in PD. Other potential treatments include adenosine A$_{2A}$ receptor antagonists (e.g. **istradefylline** and **preladenant**), 5-HT$_{1A}$ antagonists (e.g. **sarizotan**) and glutamate receptor antagonists or negative allosteric modulators (acting at mGluR5, AMPA or NMDA receptors) as well as new, improved COMT inhibitors.

Drugs used in Parkinson's disease

- Drugs act by counteracting deficiency of dopamine in basal ganglia or by blocking muscarinic receptors. None of the available drugs affect the underlying neurodegeneration.
- Drugs include:
  - **levodopa** (dopamine precursor; Ch. 15), given with an inhibitor of peripheral dopa decarboxylase (e.g. **carbidopa**) to minimise side effects; sometimes a catechol-*O*-methyl transferase inhibitor (e.g. **entacapone**) is also given, especially to patients with 'end of dose' motor fluctuations;
  - dopamine receptor agonists (**pramipexole**, **ropinirole**, **rotigotine**, **bromocriptine**); **rotigotine** is available as a transdermal patch;
  - monoamine oxidase-B inhibitors (**selegiline**, **rasagiline**);
  - **amantadine** (which may enhance dopamine release);
  - **orphenadrine** (muscarinic receptor antagonist used for parkinsonism caused by antipsychotic drugs).
- Neurotransplantation, still in an experimental phase, may be effective but results are variable, and slowly developing dyskinesias may occur.

NEURAL TRANSPLANTATION, GENE THERAPY AND BRAIN STIMULATION

▼ Parkinson's disease is the first neurodegenerative disease for which neural transplantation was attempted in 1982, amid much publicity. Various transplantation approaches have been tried, based on the injection of dissociated fetal cells (neuroblasts) directly into the striatum. Trials in patients with PD (Barker et al., 2013) have mainly involved injection of midbrain cells from aborted human fetuses. Although such transplants have been shown to survive and establish functional dopaminergic connections, this approach has fallen out of favour recently. Some patients have gone on to develop serious dyskinesias, possibly due to dopamine overproduction. The use of fetal material is, of course, fraught with ethical difficulties (usually cells from five or more fetuses are needed for one transplant) and hopes for the future rest mainly on developing stem cell transplants (Nishimura et al., 2013); small clinical trials are underway.

Gene therapy (see Ch. 5) for PD is aimed at increasing the synthesis of neurotransmitters and neurotrophic factors such as:

- dopamine in the striatum – by expressing tyrosine hydroxylase or dopa decarboxylase;
- GABA in the subthalamic nucleus – by overexpression of glutamic acid decarboxylase (to reduce the excitatory input to the substantia nigra) (see Fig. 41.4);
- neurotrophic factors such as neurturin, a glial-derived neurotrophic factor (GDNF) analogue.

Electrical stimulation of the subthalamic nuclei with implanted electrodes (which inhibits ongoing neural activity, equivalent to reversible ablation) is used in severe cases, and can improve motor dysfunction in PD, but does not improve cognitive and other symptoms and does not stop the neurodegenerative process (see Okun, 2012).

HUNTINGTON'S DISEASE

▼HD is an inherited (autosomal dominant) disorder resulting in progressive brain degeneration, starting in adulthood and causing rapid deterioration and death. As well as dementia, it causes severe motor symptoms in the form of choreiform (i.e. rapid, jerky involuntary) movements, especially of fingers, face or tongue. It is the commonest of a group of so-called *trinucleotide repeat* neurodegenerative diseases, associated with the expansion of the number of repeats of the CAG sequence in specific genes, and hence the number (50 or more) of consecutive glutamine residues at the N-terminal of the expressed protein (see Walker, 2007). The larger the number of repeats, the earlier the appearance of symptoms. The protein coded by the HD gene, *huntingtin*, which normally possesses a chain of fewer than 30 glutamine residues, is a soluble cytosolic protein of unknown function found in all cells. HD develops when the mutant protein contains 40 or more repeats. The long poly-Gln chains reduce the solubility of huntingtin, and favour the formation of aggregates, which are formed by proteolytic cleavage of the mutant protein, releasing N-terminal fragments that include the poly-Gln region. As with AD and PD, aggregation is probably responsible for the neuronal loss, which affects mainly the cortex and the striatum, resulting in progressive dementia and severe involuntary choreiform movements. Studies on postmortem brains showed that the dopamine content of the striatum was normal or slightly increased, while there was a 75% reduction in the activity of glutamic acid decarboxylase, the enzyme responsible for GABA synthesis (Ch. 39). It is believed that the loss of GABA-mediated inhibition in the basal ganglia produces a hyperactivity of dopaminergic synapses, so the syndrome is in some senses a mirror image of PD (see Fig. 41.4).

The effects of drugs that influence dopaminergic transmission are correspondingly the opposite of those that are observed in PD, dopamine antagonists being effective in reducing the involuntary movements, while drugs such as levodopa and bromocriptine make them worse. Drugs used to alleviate the motor symptoms include **tetrabenazine** (an inhibitor of the vesicular monoamine transporter) (see Ch. 15) that reduces dopamine storage, dopamine antagonists such as **chlorpromazine** and **haloperidol** (Ch. 47) and the GABA$_B$

receptor agonist **baclofen** (Ch. 39). Other drug treatments include antidepressants, mood stabilisers (see Ch. 48) and benzodiazepines (see Ch. 45) to reduce the depression, mood swings and anxiety associated with the disorder. None of these drugs affects dementia or retards the course of the disease. It is possible that drugs that inhibit excitotoxicity, antisense to reduce mutant huntingtin expression, or possibly neural transplantation procedures when these become available, may prove useful.

AMYOTROPHIC LATERAL SCLEROSIS

ALS is the most common form of motor neuron disease, in which degeneration of motor neurons leads to paralysis and eventual death. In ALS, degeneration occurs in both upper motor neurons, those projecting from higher centres to the spinal cord and in lower motor neurons, those projecting from the ventral horn of the spinal cord to skeletal muscle. The causes of ALS are not known, but there is evidence that both genetic and environmental factors such as exposure to bacterial toxins, heavy metals, pesticides and trauma are involved.[10] Mutations in several genes – *SOD1*, C9orf72 and NEK1 – have been associated with some cases of familial ALS (see Pochet, 2017).

The drugs currently used in ALS treatment are **riluzole** and **edaravone**. Riluzole may work by reducing glutamate release whereas edaravone may reduce oxidative stress. However, these drugs only provide limited improvement. Antisense oligonucleotide therapies, designed to suppress the expression of mutated genes, and stem cell therapies are undergoing clinical trials.

SPINAL MUSCULAR ATROPHY

SMA is a group of inherited neuromuscular disorders in which there is degeneration of motor neurons and progressive muscle wasting. It is the most common genetic cause of infant death. Motor neurons require expression of a protein, appropriately called *survival motorneuron protein* (SMN), for them to survive and function normally. SMA is caused by a genetic defect in the SMN-1 gene encoding for SMN. **Nusinersen**, introduced in 2016, is a novel gene therapy for the disorder, reported in early trials to halt disease progression in some patients. It is an antisense oligoneucleotide sequence (see Ch. 5) given by intrathecal injection, that facilitates SMN expression, not from the mutated SMN-1 gene but from SMN-2, a 'backup' gene that under normal conditions, due to exon skipping, does not produce much functional SMN. Nusinersen prevents the skipping thus allowing the cell to produce SMN.

MULTIPLE SCLEROSIS

MS is a disease associated with demyelination of nerve axons and neuronal degeneration resulting in lesions that may occur throughout the CNS. Symptoms usually start to develop between 20 and 30 years of age and depend upon the location of the lesions. Common symptoms include problems with vision, dizziness, balance, walking, fatigue, incontinence, muscle stiffness and painful muscle spasms. MS can also affect cognitive processing and mood. It affects almost three times as many women as men. There are two forms of the disease, *relapse–remitting*, in which sufferers have attacks of symptoms which subsequently fade away partially or completely but then relapse at a later date, and *primary progressive*, in which the symptoms persist and increase over time. Relapse–remitting may, however, develop into secondary progressive in later life. The cause of MS is unknown; like other neurodegenerative conditions it may result from a combination of predisposing genetic factors (Hollenbach & Oksenberg, 2015) and exposure to environmental factors such as infection.

MS has long been considered an autoimmune demyelinating disease, although the proteins, lipids and gangliosides in myelin that act as antigens have not been identified. Inflammation (see Ch. 27), enhanced permeability of blood–brain barrier, demyelination and axonal degeneration are common pathological features. It is, however, still unclear whether MS is a primary autoimmune disease that affects the CNS or a neurodegenerative disease with secondary inflammatory demyelination (see Trapp & Nave, 2008). Current therapies are aimed at moderating the acute inflammatory components of MS (Table 41.3), but they are limited in effectiveness. They may reduce the rate of clinical deterioration and incidence of relapses but by and large they do not reverse the neurodegeneration that has occurred. Several (**natalizumab**, **alemtuzumab, daclizumab** and **ocrelizumab**) are monoclonal antibodies that target specific proteins expressed on B and T lymphocytes to limit their spread into the brain and spinal cord where they attack the myelin sheath around motor nerves. Monoclonal antibody therapy does, however, carry the risk of serious autoimmune complications (see Ch. 5) that need to be monitored. The pathological mechanisms underlying the neurodegeneration, which renders the disease irreversible, are still not well understood but may hold the key to finding disease-curing treatments. Symptomatic treatment of MS includes **baclofen** and nabiximols, a botanical extract of cannabis containing tetrahydrocannabinol (THC) and cannabidiol (CBD) (see Ch. 20), for spasticity, **nabiximols** (a botanical extract containing **tetrahydrocannabinol** and **cannabidiol**) for spasticity, and **fampridine** (a potassium-channel blocker that enhances action potential propagation in demyelinated axons) for a modest improvement in walking speed.

---

[10]Intense physical exercise has been suggested to be one potential environmental factor and there are examples of leading sportspersons succumbing to the disease in later life, for example, Joost van der Westhuizen, the great South African scrum half, and Doddie Weir who played for Scotland and the British and Irish Lions.

Drug treatment of multiple sclerosis

Several new and efficacious agents have emerged in the treatment of multiple sclerosis (MS), but these treatments also bring with them a significant risk of serious adverse effects. As the severity and course of MS varies substantially amongst individuals, selection of appropriate therapy must consider not only benefit and harm of the proposed agents, but also the patient's clinical condition and co-morbidities.

Prompt use of disease-modifying therapies is recommended in patients who have clinical and/or radiological evidence of active disease. Examples of therapeutic options for patients with active relapsing–remitting MS are:

- Drugs of moderate efficacy such as **interferon-beta** or **glatiramer acetate** by injection. **Teriflunomide** or **dimethylfumarate** can be used if oral therapy is preferred.
- Drugs of high efficacy such as **natalizumab** or **alemtuzumab** may be considered in those with more active disease.

There is limited evidence for interferon in progressive MS, but **ocrelizumab** is an emerging option for primary progressive disease.

Drugs that are used to manage symptoms or disease complications in multiple sclerosis include **baclofen** (for muscle spasticity) and **amitriptyline** (for emotional lability).

Table 41.3   Disease-modifying treatments for multiple sclerosis

Drug	Mechanism of action	Route(s) and frequency of administration	Notes
Glatiramer acetate	A random polymer (approx. 6 kD) of four amino acids thought to interfere with the immune response to myelin	Subcutaneous (usually administered daily)	Reduces relapses
Dimethyl fumarate	Unknown	Oral (twice a day)	Reduces relapse rate and slows progression
Fingolimod	Inhibits cytotoxic CD8 expressing T cells Phosphorylated derivative is an agonist at S1P receptors.	Oral (daily)	Reduces the rate of relapses Increased risk of progressive multifocal leukoencephalopathy and serious ventricular arrhythmias
Beta interferons (IFN-β) (see Ch. 19)	Modulation of immune function	Subcutaneous (three times a week) Intramuscular (once a week)	Reduce relapses by approximately 30% but not all patients respond
Natalizumab (see Ch. 27)	Humanised monoclonal antibody targeting α4-integrin (see Table 27.3)	Intravenous infusion (every 4 weeks)	Slows the progression of disability in relapsing multiple sclerosis May cause progressive multifocal leukoencephalopathy in some cases
Alemtuzumab (see Chs 27, 57 and Table 27.3)	Humanised monoclonal antibody targeting CD52 on B and T lymphocytes	Intravenous infusion (5-day short courses, 12 months apart)	Also used in the treatment of lymphocytic leukaemia
Daclizumab (see Ch. 27)	Humanised monoclonal antibody targeting CD25, the alpha subunit of the IL-2 receptor on T cells	Subcutaneous (once a month)	Risk of serious liver toxicity; this drug is now restricted to patients who are not suitable for other therapies
Ocrelizumab	Humanised monoclonal antibody targeting CD20 on B lymphocytes	Intravenous infusion (every 6 months after initial treatments)	Superior to beta-interferon in relapsing and progressive multiple sclerosis
Teriflunomide	Immunosuppressant. Active metabolite of leflunomide (see Ch. 27)	Oral (once a day)	Modest efficacy in reducing relapse
Cladribine	Purine nucleoside analogue that has immunosuppressant effects through depletion of lymphocytes	Oral therapy given as two short courses in a 2-year period	Used in rapidly evolving or severe relapsing–remitting MS. Also has a role in hairy cell leukaemia

REFERENCES AND FURTHER READING

General mechanisms of neurodegeneration

Barnham, K.J., Masters, C.L., Bush, A.I., 2004. Neurodegenerative diseases and oxidative stress. Nat. Rev. Drug Discov. 3, 205–214. (*Describes the oxidative stress model of neurodegeneration, including evidence based on various transgenic animal models*)

Brunden, K., Trojanowski, J.O., Lee, V.M.Y., 2009. Advances in Tau-focused drug discovery for Alzheimer's disease and related tauopathies. Nat. Rev. Drug Discov. 8, 783–793. (*Good detailed review of the current status of Tau-directed drug discovery efforts, with a realistic assessment of the problems that have to be overcome*)

Coyle, J.T., Puttfarken, P., 1993. Oxidative stress, glutamate and neurodegenerative disorders. Science 262, 689–695. (*Good review article*)

Hanger, D.P., Anderton, B.H., Noble, W., 2009. Tau phosphorylation: the therapeutic challenge for neurodegenerative disease. Trends Mol. Med. 15, 112–119.

Itoh, K., Nakamura, K., Iijima, M., Sesaki, H., 2013. Mitochondrial dynamics in neurodegeneration. Trends Cell Biol. 23, 64–71. (*Summarises evidence for the involvement of mitochondrial dysfunction in several neurodegenerative diseases*)

Okouchi, M., Ekshyyan, O., Maracine, M., Aw, T.Y., 2007. Neuronal apoptosis in neurodegeneration. Antioxid. Redox Signal. 9, 1059–1096. (*Detailed review describing the role of apoptosis, the factors that induce it and possible therapeutic strategies aimed at preventing it, in various neurodegenerative disorders*)

Peden, A.H., Ironside, J.W., 2012. Molecular pathology in neurodegenerative diseases. Curr. Drug Targets 13, 1548–1559. (*Compares the molecular pathology of neurodegenerative and prion-mediated disorders*)

Zhao, C., Deng, W., Gage, F.H., 2008. Mechanisms and functional implications of adult neurogenesis. Cell 132, 645–660. (*Review by one of the pioneers in this controversial field. Neurogenesis probably contributes to learning, but evidence for involvement in neural repair is weak*)

Alzheimer's disease

Breitner, J.C., Baker, L.D., Montine, T.J., et al., 2011. Extended results of the Alzheimer's disease anti-inflammatory prevention trial. Alzheimers Dement. 7, 402–411. (*Reports on a long-term trial of NSAIDs in AD*)

Brioni, J.D., Esbenshade, T.A., Garrison, T.R., 2011. Discovery of histamine H3 antagonists for the treatment of cognitive disorders and Alzheimer's disease. J. Pharmacol. Exp. Ther. 336, 38–46. (*Reviews preclinical and clinical data on the effectiveness of H3 antagonists to treat a variety of CNS disorders*)

Collingridge, G.L., Volianskis, A., Bannister, N., et al., 2013. The NMDA receptor as a target for cognitive enhancement. Neuropharmacology 64, 13–26. (*Reviews the preclinical evidence that various types of drug acting at the NMDA receptor might improve cognition*)

Corbett, A., Pickett, J., Burns, A., et al., 2012. Drug repositioning for Alzheimer's disease. Nat. Rev. Drug Discov. 11, 833–846. (*Describes recent failures in drug development and discusses how drugs currently used for other conditions might be effective in treating AD*)

Cummings, J., Lee, G., Mortsdorf, T., Ritter, A., Zhong, K., 2017. Alzheimer's disease drug development pipeline. Alzheimers Dement. (N Y) 3, 367–384. (*Describes the drugs in development for AD that are either symptom reducing or disease modifying agents*)

Frigero, C., De Strooper, B., 2016. Alzheimer's disease mechanisms and emerging roads to novel therapeutics. Ann. Rev. Neurosci. 39, 57–79. (*Discusses how genetics, in vitro models and improved animal models will aid the development of new medicines*)

Götz, J., Ittner, L.M., 2008. Animal models of Alzheimer's disease and frontotemporal dementia. Nat. Rev. Neurosci. 9, 532–544. (*Detailed review focusing on transgenic models*)

Herrup, K., 2015. The case for rejecting the amyloid cascade hypothesis. Nat. Nerosci. 18, 794–799. (*Makes a strong case that Alzheimer's disease is not just a disorder resulting from altered amyloid processing*)

Querfurth, H.W., LaFerla, F.M., 2010. Mechanisms of disease: Alzheimer's disease. N. Engl. J. Med. 362, 329–344.

Rakic, P., 2002. Neurogenesis in the primate cortex: an evaluation of the evidence. Nat. Rev. Neurosci. 3, 65–71.

Schenk, D., Barbour, R., Dunn, W., et al., 1999. Immunization with amyloid-beta attenuates Alzheimer-disease-like pathology in the PDAPP mouse. Nature 400, 173–177. (*Report of an ingenious experiment that could have implications for AD treatment in humans*)

Schwab, C., McGeer, P.L., 2008. Inflammatory aspects of Alzheimer's disease and other neurodegenerative disorders. J. Alzheimer Dis. 13, 359–369. (*Discusses the role of inflammation in neurodegeneration and repair*)

Weggen, S., Rogers, M., Eriksen, J., 2007. NSAIDs: small molecules for prevention of Alzheimer's disease or precursors for future drug development. Trends Pharmacol. Sci. 28, 536–543. (*Summarises data relating to effects of NSAIDs on AD and concludes that mechanisms other than cyclo-oxygenase inhibition may be relevant in the search for new anti-AD drugs*)

Parkinson's disease

Barker, R.A., Barrett, J., Mason, S.L., Björklund, A., 2013. Fetal dopaminergic transplantation trials and the future of neural grafting in Parkinson's disease. Lancet Neurol. 12, 84–91. (*Update by pioneers in the field*)

Duty, S., Jenner, P., 2011. Animal models of Parkinson's disease: a source of novel treatments and clues to the cause of the disease. Br. J. Pharmacol. 164, 1357–1391. (*Describes the value of various animal models in the search for new therapies for PD*)

Langston, W.J., 1985. MPTP and Parkinson's disease. Trends Neurosci. 8, 79–83. (*Readable account of the MPTP story by its discoverer*)

Lotharius, J., Brundin, P., 2002. Pathogenesis of Parkinson's disease: dopamine, vesicles and α-synuclein. Nat. Rev. Neurosci. 3, 833–842. (*Review of PD pathogenesis, emphasising the possible role of dopamine itself as a likely source of neurotoxic metabolites*)

Nishimura, K., Takahashi, J., 2013. Therapeutic application of stem cell technology toward the treatment of Parkinson's disease. Biol. Pharm. Bull. 36, 171–175.

Oertel, W., Schulz, J.B., 2016. Current and experimental treatments of Parkinson disease: A guide for neuroscientists. J. Neurochem. 139, S1, 325–337. (*Discusses current therapeutic approaches and drugs recently approved or in clinical trials for treatment of PD*)

Okun, M.S., 2012. Deep-brain stimulation for Parkinson's disease. N. Engl. J. Med. 367, 1529–1538. (*Review of the clinical use of deep brain stimulation to treat Parkinson's disease*)

Olanow, C.W., Brundin, P., 2013. Parkinson's disease and alpha synuclein: is Parkinson's disease a prion-like disorder? Mov. Disord. 28, 31–40.

Olanow, C.W., Rascol, O., Hauser, R., et al., 2009. A double-blind, delayed-start trial of rasagiline in Parkinson's disease. N. Engl. J. Med. 139, 1268–1278. (*Well-conducted trial showing that rasagiline can significantly retard disease progression in patients with early PD*)

Przedborski, S., 2017. The two-century journey of Parkinson disease research. Nat. Rev. Neurosci. 18, 251–259. (*Extensive review of the 200 year timeline of PD research*)

Schapira, A.H.V., 2009. Neurobiology and treatment of Parkinson's disease. Trends Pharmacol. Sci. 30, 41–47. (*Short review of pathophysiology and treatment of PD*)

Stroke

Esencan, E., Yuksel, S., Tosun, Y.B., Robinot, A., Solaroglu, I., Zhang, J.H., 2013. Xenon in medical area: emphasis on neuroprotection in hypoxia and anesthesia. Med. Gas Res. 3, 4. (*Outlines the potential for xenon as a neurprotective agent*)

Green, A.R., 2008. Pharmacological approaches to acute ischaemic stroke: reperfusion certainly, neuroprotection possibly. Br. J. Pharmacol. 153 (Suppl. 1), S325–S338. (*The theories were good but subsequent efforts to develop them into neuroprotective agents for human medicine have proven unsuccessful*)

Huntington's disease

Walker, F.O., 2007. Huntington's disease. Lancet 369, 218–228. (*General review of genetics, pathogenesis and treatment of HD*)

Amyotrophic lateral sclerosis

Pochet, R., 2017. Genetics and ALS: cause for optimism. Cerebrum 2017, 1–13.

Motor neuron disease

Trapp, B.D., Nave, K.A., 2008. Multiple sclerosis: an immune or neurodegenerative disorder. Ann. Rev. Neurosci. 31, 247–269. (*Reviews the evidence for MS being a primary neurodegenerative disorder with secondary inflammation*)

Multiple sclerosis

Hollenbach, J.A., Oksenberg, J.R., 2015. The immunogenetics of multiple sclerosis: A comprehensive review. J. Autoimmun. 64, 13–25.

General anaesthetic agents

42

OVERVIEW

General anaesthesia aims to provide balanced anaesthesia, meeting the requirements of amnesia, analgesia and relaxation tailored for the intended medical procedure. Different general anaesthetic agents provide varying amounts of the components of balanced anaesthesia but they are rarely used nowadays in isolation. Neuromuscular-blocking drugs (Ch. 14), sedative and anxiolytic drugs (Ch. 45), and analgesic drugs (Ch. 43) are frequently co-administered. General anaesthetics are given systemically and exert their main effects on the central nervous system (CNS), in contrast to local anaesthetics (Ch. 44). Although we now take them for granted, general anaesthetics are the drugs that paved the way for modern surgery. Without them, much of modern medicine would be impossible.

In this chapter we first describe the pharmacology of the main agents in current use, which fall into two groups: intravenous agents and inhalation agents (gases and volatile liquids). The use of anaesthetics in combination with other drugs to produce balanced anaesthesia is discussed at the end of the chapter. Detailed information on the clinical pharmacology and use of anaesthetic agents can be found in specialised textbooks (e.g. Aitkenhead et al., 2013).

INTRODUCTION

It was only when inhalation anaesthetics were first discovered, in 1846, that most surgical operations became a practical possibility. Until that time, surgeons relied on being able to operate on struggling patients at lightning speed, and most operations were amputations.

▼ The use of **nitrous oxide** to relieve the pain of surgery was suggested by Humphrey Davy in 1800. He was the first person to make nitrous oxide, and he tested its effects on several people, including himself and the Prime Minister, noting that it caused euphoria, analgesia and loss of consciousness. The use of nitrous oxide, billed as 'laughing gas', became a popular fairground entertainment and came to the notice of an American dentist, Horace Wells, who had a tooth extracted under its influence, while he himself squeezed the inhalation bag. Ether also first gained publicity in a disreputable way, through the spread of 'ether frolics', at which it was used to produce euphoria among the guests. William Morton, also a dentist and a student at Harvard Medical School, used it successfully to extract a tooth in 1846 and then suggested to Warren, the illustrious chief surgeon at Massachusetts General Hospital, that he should administer it for one of Warren's operations. Warren grudgingly agreed, and on 16 October 1846 a large audience was gathered in the main operating theatre[1]; after some preliminary fumbling, Morton's demonstration was a spectacular success. 'Gentlemen, this is no humbug', was the most gracious comment that Warren could bring himself to make to the assembled audience.

In the same year, James Simpson, Professor of Midwifery at Edinburgh University, used chloroform to relieve the pain of childbirth, bringing on himself fierce denunciation from the clergy, one of whom wrote: 'Chloroform is a decoy of Satan, apparently offering itself to bless women; but in the end it will harden society and rob God of the deep, earnest cries which arise in time of trouble, for help.' Opposition was effectively silenced in 1853, when Queen Victoria gave birth to her seventh child under the influence of chloroform, and the procedure became known as *anaesthésie à la reine*.

The second half of the 20th century saw the introduction into clinical practice of a number of new general anaesthetic agents, most notably **isoflurane** and **propofol**, that were markedly superior to earlier agents such as **nitrous oxide** and **thiopental**. Despite the need for further improvement the pipeline has all but dried up in the 21st century, with only **fospropofol** being introduced.

MECHANISM OF ACTION OF ANAESTHETIC DRUGS

Unlike most drugs, anaesthetics, which include substances as diverse as simple gases (e.g. **nitrous oxide** and **xenon**), halogenated hydrocarbons (e.g. **isoflurane**), barbiturates (e.g. **thiopental**) and steroids (e.g. **alphaxalone**), belong to no recognisable chemical class. At one time it appeared that the shape and electronic configuration of the molecule were relatively unimportant, and the pharmacological action required only that the molecule had certain physicochemical properties. We now know much more about how different anaesthetics interact with neuronal membrane proteins and have come to realise that there are multiple mechanisms by which anaesthesia can be produced and that different anaesthetics work by different mechanisms.

As the concentration of an anaesthetic is increased, the switch from being conscious to unconscious occurs over a very narrow concentration range (approximately 0.2 of a log unit). This is a much steeper concentration–response curve than that seen with drugs that interact as agonists or antagonists at classical receptors (see Ch. 2).

LIPID SOLUBILITY

▼ Overton and Meyer, at the turn of the 20th century, showed a close correlation between anaesthetic potency and lipid solubility in a diverse group of simple and unreactive organic compounds that

---

[1]Now preserved as the Ether Dome, a museum piece at Massachusetts General Hospital.

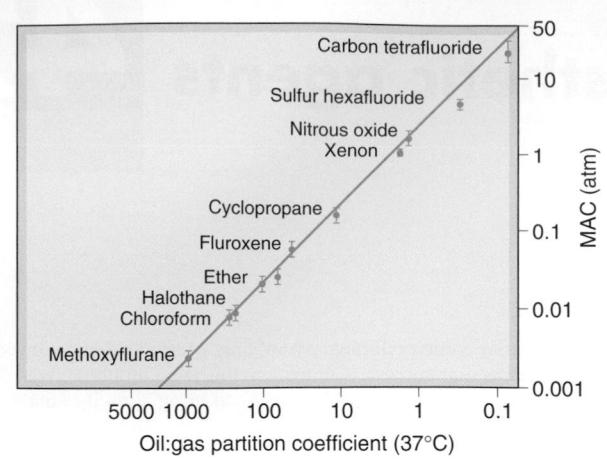

Fig. 42.1 **Correlation of anaesthetic potency with oil:gas partition coefficient.** Anaesthetic potency in humans is expressed as minimum alveolar partial pressure (MAC) required to produce surgical anaesthesia. There is a close correlation with lipid solubility, expressed as the oil:gas partition coefficient. (From Halsey, M.J., 1989. Physicochemical properties of inhalation anaesthetics. In: Nunn, J.F., Utting, J.E., Brown, B.R. (Eds), General Anaesthesia, Butterworth, London.)

Fig. 42.2 **Putative propofol binding site on the β subunit of the GABA_A receptor.** A molecular model showing the approximate binding position of propofol at the interface between the transmembrane domain and the extracellular domain of the β subunit. (Based on the original report by Yip et al., 2013. Nat. Chem. Biol. 9, 715–720.)

were tested for their ability to immobilise tadpoles. This led to a bold theory, formulated by Meyer in 1937: 'Narcosis commences when any chemically indifferent substance has attained a certain molar concentration in the lipids of the cell.'

The relationship between anaesthetic activity and lipid solubility has been repeatedly confirmed for a diverse array of agents. Anaesthetic potency in humans is usually expressed as the minimal alveolar concentration (MAC) required to abolish the response to surgical incision in 50% of subjects. Fig. 42.1 shows the correlation between MAC (inversely proportional to potency) and lipid solubility, expressed as the oil:gas partition coefficient, for a wide range of inhalation anaesthetics. The Overton–Meyer studies did not suggest any particular mechanism, but revealed an impressive correlation, for which any theory of anaesthesia needs to account. Oil:gas partition was assumed to predict partition into membrane lipids, consistent with the suggestion that anaesthesia results from an alteration of membrane function.

How the simple introduction of inert foreign molecules into the lipid bilayer could cause a functional disturbance was not explained. Two possible mechanisms, namely volume expansion and increased membrane fluidity, have been suggested and tested experimentally, but both are now largely discredited and attention has swung from lipids to proteins, the correlation of potency with lipid solubility being explained by molecules of anaesthetic binding to hydrophobic pockets within specific membrane protein targets.

EFFECTS ON ION CHANNELS

Following early studies that showed that anaesthetics can bind to various proteins as well as lipids, it was found that anaesthetics affect several different types of ion channels (see Franks, 2008). For most anaesthetics, there are no known competitive antagonists, so this approach to identify sites of action is denied. Therefore the main criterion for identifying putative mechanisms of action of general anaesthetics is that, for a cellular effect to be relevant to the anaesthetic or analgesic actions of these agents, it must occur at therapeutically relevant concentrations.

Cys-loop ligand-gated ion channels. Almost all anaesthetics (with the exceptions of **cyclopropane**, **ketamine** and

xenon[2]) potentiate the action of GABA at GABA_A receptors (Antkowiak & Rudolph, 2016). As described in detail in Chapter 39, GABA_A receptors are ligand-gated Cl⁻ channels made up of five subunits (generally comprising two α, two β and one γ or δ subunit). Anaesthetics can bind to hydrophobic pockets within different GABA_A receptor subunits to act as positive allosteric modulators.

▼ Specific mutations of the amino acid sequence of the α subunit inhibit the actions of volatile anaesthetics but not those of intravenous anaesthetics, whereas mutations of the β subunit inhibit both volatile and intravenous anaesthetics (see Franks, 2008). This suggest that volatile anaesthetics may bind at the interface between α and β subunits (analogous to benzodiazepines that bind at the interface between α and γ/δ subunits, see Ch. 39), whereas the intravenous anaesthetics such as propofol may bind only on the β subunit (Fig. 42.2). However, photoaffinity labelling experiments suggest that **etomidate** may bind to amino acid residues on both the α and β subunits. A further level of complexity arises because there are different subtypes of each subunit (see Ch. 39). Different subunit compositions give rise to subtly different subtypes of GABA_A receptor and these may be involved in different aspects of anaesthetic action. GABA_A receptors clustered at

---

[2]There is some controversy about whether or not xenon potentiates GABA_A responses but at present the weight of evidence suggests it does not.

the synapse have different pharmacological and kinetic properties from those that are distributed elsewhere across the cell (extrasynaptic receptors; see Ch. 39). Extrasynaptic GABA$_A$ receptors contain α4 and α6 subunits as well as the δ subunit, and anaesthetics appear to have a greater potentiating effect on these extrasynaptic GABA$_A$ receptors.

General anaesthetics also affect other neuronal cys-loop ligand-gated channels such as those activated by glycine (Ch. 39), acetylcholine and 5-hydroxytryptamine (Ch. 40). Their actions on these channels are similar to those on GABA$_A$ receptors but the relative importance of such actions to general anaesthesia is still to be determined.

Two-pore domain K$^+$ channels. These belong to a family of 'background' K$^+$ channels that modulate neuronal excitability. They are homomeric or heteromeric assemblies of a family of structurally related subunits (Bayliss & Barrett, 2008). Channels made up of TREK1, TREK2, TASK1, TASK3 or TRESK (see Ch. 4, Table 4.2) subunits can be directly activated by low concentrations of volatile and gaseous anaesthetics, thus reducing membrane excitability (see Franks, 2008). This may contribute to the analgesic, hypnotic and immobilising effects of these agents. Two-pore domain K$^+$ channels do not appear to be affected by intravenous anaesthetics.

NMDA receptors. **Glutamate**, the major excitatory neurotransmitter in the CNS, activates three main classes of ionotropic receptor – AMPA, kainate and NMDA receptors (see Ch. 39). NMDA receptors are an important site of action for anaesthetics such as **nitrous oxide**, **xenon** and **ketamine** which act, in different ways, to reduce NMDA receptor-mediated responses. Xenon appears to inhibit NMDA receptors by competing with glycine for its regulatory site on this receptor whereas ketamine blocks the pore of the channel (see Ch. 39). Other inhalation anaesthetics may also exert effects on the NMDA receptor in addition to their effects on other proteins such as the GABA$_A$ receptor.

Other ion channels. Anaesthetics may also exert actions at cyclic nucleotide-gated K$^+$ channels and K$_{ATP}$ channels. Some general anaesthetics inhibit certain subtypes of voltage-gated Na$^+$ channels. Inhibition of presynaptic Na$^+$ channels may give rise to the inhibition of transmitter release at excitatory synapses.

It may be overly simplistic to think of each anaesthetic as having only one mechanism of action: individual anaesthetics differ in their actions and affect cellular function in several different ways, so a single mechanism is unlikely to be sufficient.

Comprehensive reviews of the molecular and cellular actions of general anaesthetics can be found in Schüttler and Schwilden (2008).

EFFECTS ON THE NERVOUS SYSTEM

At the cellular level, the effects of anaesthetics are to enhance tonic inhibition (through enhancing the actions of GABA), reduce excitation (opening K$^+$ channels) and to inhibit excitatory synaptic transmission (by depressing transmitter release and inhibiting ligand-gated ion channels). Effects on axonal conduction are relatively unimportant.

The anaesthetised state comprises several components, including *unconsciousness*, loss of reflexes (*muscle relaxation*) and *analgesia*. Much effort has gone into identifying the brain regions on which anaesthetics act to produce these effects. The most sensitive regions appear to be the midbrain reticular formation, thalamic sensory relay nuclei and, to

> ## Theories of anaesthesia
>
> - Many simple, unreactive compounds produce general anaesthesia, the extreme example being the inert gas **xenon**.
> - Anaesthetic potency is closely correlated with lipid solubility (Overton–Meyer correlation), not with chemical structure.
> - Earlier theories of anaesthesia postulated interaction with the lipid membrane bilayer. Recent work favours interaction with membrane ion channels.
> - Most anaesthetics enhance the activity of inhibitory GABA$_A$ receptors and other cys-loop ligand-gated ion channels. Other important effects are the activation of a subfamily of potassium channels (the two-pore domain K$^+$ channels) and inhibition of excitatory NMDA receptors.

a lesser extent, parts of the cortex. Inhibition of these regions results in unconsciousness and analgesia. Some anaesthetics – particularly volatile anaesthetics – cause inhibition at the spinal level, producing a loss of reflex responses to painful stimuli, although, in practice, neuromuscular-blocking drugs (Ch. 14) are used as an adjunct to produce muscle relaxation rather than relying on the anaesthetic alone. Anaesthetics, even in low concentrations, cause short-term amnesia. It is likely that interference with hippocampal function produces this effect, because the hippocampus is involved in short-term memory, and certain hippocampal synapses are highly susceptible to inhibition by anaesthetics.

As the anaesthetic concentration is increased, all brain functions are progressively affected, including motor control and reflex activity, respiration and autonomic regulation. Therefore it is not possible to identify a critical 'target site' in the brain responsible for all the phenomena of anaesthesia.

High concentrations of any general anaesthetic affect all parts of the CNS, causing profound inhibition which, in the absence of artificial respiration, leads to death from respiratory failure. The margin between surgical anaesthesia and potentially fatal respiratory and circulatory depression is quite narrow, requiring careful monitoring by the anaesthetist and adjustment of the level of anaesthesia.

EFFECTS ON THE CARDIOVASCULAR AND RESPIRATORY SYSTEMS

Most anaesthetics decrease cardiac contractility, but their effects on cardiac output and blood pressure vary because of concomitant actions on the sympathetic nervous system and vascular smooth muscle. **Isoflurane** and other halogenated anaesthetics inhibit sympathetic outflow, reduce arterial and venous tone and thus decrease arterial pressure and venous pressure. By contrast, **nitrous oxide** and **ketamine** increase sympathetic discharge and plasma noradrenaline concentration and, if used alone, increase heart rate and maintain blood pressure.

Halogenated anaesthetics cause ventricular extrasystoles. The mechanism involves sensitisation to adrenaline. Electrocardiogram monitoring shows that extrasystolic beats occur commonly in patients under anaesthesia, with no harm coming to the patient. If catecholamine secretion is excessive, however (*par excellence* in phaeochromocytoma, a neuroendocrine tumour that secretes catecholamines into the circulation; see Ch. 15), there is a risk of precipitating ventricular fibrillation.

With the exception of **nitrous oxide, ketamine** and **xenon**, all anaesthetics depress respiration markedly and increase arterial P_{CO_2}. Nitrous oxide has much less effect, in part because its low potency prevents very deep anaesthesia from being produced with this drug. Some inhalation anaesthetics are pungent, particularly **desflurane**, which is liable to cause coughing, laryngospasm and bronchospasm, so desflurane is not used for induction of anaesthesia but only for maintenance.

Pharmacological effects of anaesthetic agents

- Anaesthesia involves three main neurophysiological changes: unconsciousness, loss of response to painful stimulation and loss of reflexes (motor and autonomic).
- At supra-anaesthetic doses, all anaesthetic agents can cause death by loss of cardiovascular reflexes and respiratory paralysis.
- At the cellular level, anaesthetic agents affect synaptic transmission and neuronal excitability rather than axonal conduction. GABA-mediated inhibitory transmission is enhanced by most anaesthetics. The release of excitatory transmitters and the response of the postsynaptic receptors are also inhibited.
- Although all parts of the nervous system are affected by anaesthetic agents, the main targets appear to be the cortex, thalamus, hippocampus, midbrain reticular formation and spinal cord.
- Most anaesthetic agents (with the exception of **ketamine**, **nitrous oxide** and **xenon**) produce similar neurophysiological effects and differ mainly in respect of their pharmacokinetic properties and toxicity.
- Most anaesthetic agents cause cardiovascular depression by effects on the myocardium and blood vessels, as well as on the nervous system. Halogenated anaesthetic agents are likely to cause cardiac dysrhythmias, accentuated by circulating catecholamines.

INTRAVENOUS ANAESTHETIC AGENTS

Even the fastest-acting inhalation anaesthetics take a few minutes to act and cause a period of excitement before anaesthesia is induced. Intravenous anaesthetics act more rapidly, producing unconsciousness in about 20 s, as soon as the drug reaches the brain from its site of injection. These drugs (e.g. **propofol**, **thiopental** and **etomidate**) are normally used for induction of anaesthesia. They are preferred by many patients because injection generally lacks the menacing quality associated with a face mask in an apprehensive individual. With propofol, recovery is also fast due to rapid metabolism.

Although many intravenous anaesthetics are not suitable for maintaining anaesthesia because their elimination from the body is relatively slow compared with that of inhalation agents, propofol can be used as a continuous infusion, and

the duration of action of ketamine is sufficient that it can be administered as a single bolus for short operations without the need for an inhalation agent. Under these circumstances a short-acting opioid such as **alfentanil** or **remifentanil** (Ch. 43) may be co-administered to provide analgesia.

The properties of the main intravenous anaesthetics are summarised in Table 42.1.[3]

PROPOFOL

Propofol, introduced in 1983, has now largely replaced thiopental as an induction agent. It has a rapid onset of action (approximately 30 s) and a rapid rate of redistribution ($t_{1/2}$ 2–4 min), which makes it short acting. Because of its low water solubility, it is administered as an oil-in-water emulsion, which can cause pain on injection, and supports microbial growth. **Fospropofol** is a recently developed water-soluble derivative that is less painful on injection and rapidly converted by alkaline phosphatases to propofol in the body. Propofol metabolism to inactive conjugates and quinols follows first-order kinetics, in contrast to thiopental (see later), resulting in more rapid recovery and less hangover effect than occurs with thiopental. It has a cardiovascular depressant effect that may lead to hypotension and bradycardia. Respiratory depression may also occur. It is particularly useful for day-case surgery, especially as it causes less nausea and vomiting than do inhalation anaesthetics.

There have been reports of a propofol infusion syndrome occurring in approximately 1 in 300 patients when it has been given for a prolonged period to maintain sedation, particularly to sick patients – especially children in whom it is contraindicated in this setting – in intensive care units. This is characterised by severe metabolic acidosis, skeletal muscle necrosis (rhabdomyolysis), hyperkalaemia, lipaemia, hepatomegaly, renal failure, arrhythmia and cardiovascular collapse.

Propofol can be taken as a drug of abuse, especially by those, such as anaesthetists, who have ready access to the drug. Using propofol to obtain a sedative high is a risky business given its steep concentration–response curve.[4]

THIOPENTAL

Thiopental is the only remaining barbiturate in common use. It has very high lipid solubility, and this accounts for the speed of onset and transience of its effect when it is injected intravenously. The free acid is insoluble in water, so thiopental is given as the sodium salt. On intravenous injection, thiopental causes unconsciousness within about 20 s, lasting for 5–10 min. The anaesthetic effect closely parallels the concentration of thiopental in the blood reaching the brain, because its high lipid solubility allows it to cross the blood–brain barrier without noticeable delay.

The blood concentration of thiopental declines rapidly, by about 80% within 1–2 min, following the initial peak after intravenous injection, because the drug is redistributed, first to tissues with a large blood flow (liver, kidneys, brain,

---

[3]**Propanidid** and **alphaxalone** were withdrawn because of allergic reactions including hypotension and bronchoconstriction – probably attributable to the solvent Cremophor – but a new formulation of alphaxalone has been reintroduced to veterinary medicine and is thought to be less allergenic.
[4]Propofol is referred to as the 'milk of amnesia'. The singer Michael Jackson died of a propofol overdose.

Table 42.1 Properties of intravenous anaesthetic agents

Drug	Speed of induction and recovery	Main unwanted effect(s)	Notes
Propofol	Fast onset, very fast recovery	Cardiovascular and respiratory depression	Rapidly metabolised Possible to use as continuous infusion Causes pain at injection site Fospropofol is a prodrug, less painful on injection
Thiopental	Fast (accumulation occurs, giving slow recovery) 'Hangover'	Cardiovascular and respiratory depression	Largely replaced by propofol Causes pain at injection site Risk of precipitating porphyria in susceptible patients
Etomidate	Fast onset, fairly fast recovery	Excitatory effects during induction and recovery Adrenocortical suppression	Less cardiovascular and respiratory depression than with thiopental Causes pain at injection site
Ketamine	Slow onset, after effects common during recovery	Psychotomimetic effects following recovery Postoperative nausea, vomiting and salivation Raised intracranial pressure	Produces good analgesia and amnesia with little respiratory depression
Midazolam	Slower than other agents	—	Amnesia, but little analgesia Little respiratory or cardiovascular depression

etc.) and more slowly to muscle. Uptake into body fat, although favoured by the high lipid solubility of thiopental, occurs only slowly, because of the low blood flow to this tissue. After several hours, however, most of the thiopental present in the body will have accumulated in body fat, the rest having been metabolised. Recovery from the anaesthetic effect of a bolus dose occurs within about 5 min, governed entirely by redistribution of the drug to well-perfused tissues; very little is metabolised in this time. After the initial rapid decline, the blood concentration drops more slowly, over several hours, as the drug is taken up by body fat and metabolised in the liver. Consequently, thiopental produces a long-lasting hangover. Thiopental metabolism shows saturation kinetics (see Ch. 11). Because of this, large doses or repeated intravenous doses cause progressively longer periods of anaesthesia, as the plateau in blood concentration becomes progressively more elevated as more drug accumulates in the body and metabolism saturates. For this reason, thiopental is not used to maintain surgical anaesthesia but only as an induction agent. It is also still used to terminate status epilepticus (see Ch. 46) or (in patients with a secured airway) to lower intracranial pressure.

Thiopental binds to plasma albumin (roughly 85% of the blood content normally being bound). The fraction bound is less in states of malnutrition, liver disease or renal disease, which affect the concentration and drug-binding properties of plasma albumin, and this can appreciably reduce the dose needed for induction of anaesthesia.

If thiopental – a strongly alkaline solution – is accidentally injected around rather than into a vein, or into an artery, this can cause pain, local tissue necrosis and ulceration or severe arterial spasm that can result in gangrene.

The actions of thiopental on the nervous system are very similar to those of inhalation anaesthetics, although it has little analgesic effect and can cause profound respiratory depression, even in amounts that fail to abolish reflex responses to painful stimuli. Its long after-effect, associated with a slowly declining plasma concentration, means that drowsiness and some degree of respiratory depression persist for some hours.

Thiopental, like other barbiturates, induces production of various liver enzymes, including those involved in haem synthesis, and can precipitate attacks of porphyria in patients suffering from this genetic disorder.

ETOMIDATE

Etomidate has gained favour over thiopental on account of the larger margin between the anaesthetic dose and the dose needed to produce cardiovascular depression. It is more rapidly metabolised than thiopental, and thus less likely to cause a prolonged hangover. It causes less hypotension than propofol or thiopental. In other respects, etomidate is very similar to thiopental, although involuntary movements during induction, postoperative nausea and vomiting, and pain at the injection site are problems with its use. Etomidate suppresses the production of adrenal steroids, an effect that has been associated with an increase in mortality in severely ill patients. It should be avoided in patients at risk of having adrenal insufficiency, e.g. in sepsis. It is preferable to thiopental in patients at risk of circulatory failure.

OTHER INTRAVENOUS AGENTS
KETAMINE

▼ **Ketamine** closely resembles **phencyclidine**, both chemically and pharmacologically. Both are used recreationally for their pronounced effects on sensory perception (see Ch. 49). Both drugs are believed to act by blocking activation of the NMDA receptor (see Ch. 39). They produce a similar anaesthesia-like state and profound analgesia, but ketamine produces less euphoria and sensory distortion than phencyclidine and is thus more useful in anaesthesia. Ketamine can be used in lower doses as an analgesic (Ch. 43) and as an acute treatment for depression (Ch. 48).

Given intravenously, ketamine takes effect more slowly (1–2 min) than thiopental, and produces a different effect, known as 'dissociative anaesthesia', in which there is a marked sensory loss and analgesia, as well as amnesia, without complete loss of consciousness. During induction and recovery, involuntary movements and peculiar sensory experiences often occur. Ketamine does not act simply as a CNS depressant, and it produces cardiovascular and respiratory effects quite different from those of most anaesthetics. Blood pressure and heart rate are usually increased, and respiration is unaffected by effective anaesthetic doses. This makes it relatively safe to use in low-technology healthcare situations or in accident and emergency situations where it can be administered intramuscularly if intravenous administration is not possible.[5] However, ketamine, unlike other intravenous anaesthetic drugs, can increase intracranial pressure, so it should not be given to patients with raised intracranial pressure or at risk of cerebral ischaemia. The other main drawback of ketamine is that hallucinations, and sometimes delirium and irrational behaviour, are common during recovery. These after effects limit the usefulness of ketamine but are said to be less marked in children,[6] and ketamine, often in conjunction with a benzodiazepine, is sometimes still used for minor procedures in paediatrics.

MIDAZOLAM

Midazolam, a benzodiazepine (see Ch. 45), is slower in onset and offset than the drugs discussed above but, like ketamine, causes less respiratory or cardiovascular depression. Midazolam (or **diazepam**) is often used as a preoperative sedative and during procedures such as endoscopy, where full anaesthesia is not required. It can be administered in combination with an analgesic such as **alfentanil**. In the event of overdose it can be reversed by **flumazenil** (see Ch. 45).

INHALATION ANAESTHETICS

Many inhalation anaesthetics that were once widely used, such as ether, chloroform, trichloroethylene, cyclopropane, methoxyflurane and enflurane, have now been replaced in clinical practice, particularly by **isoflurane**, **sevoflurane** and **desflurane**, which have improved pharmacokinetic properties, fewer side effects and are non-flammable. Of the older agents, nitrous oxide is still used widely (especially in obstetric practice), and **halothane** now only occasionally.

PHARMACOKINETIC ASPECTS

An important characteristic of an inhalation anaesthetic is the speed at which the arterial blood concentration, which governs the pharmacological effect in the brain, follows changes in the partial pressure of the drug in the inspired gas mixture. Ideally, the blood concentration should follow as quickly as possible, so that the depth of anaesthesia can be controlled rapidly. In particular, the blood concentration should fall to a subanaesthetic level rapidly when administration is stopped, so that the patient recovers consciousness with minimal delay. A prolonged semi-comatose state, in which vomiting is likely and respiratory reflexes are weak or absent, is particularly hazardous.

The lungs are the only quantitatively important route by which inhalation anaesthetics enter and leave the body.

Intravenous anaesthetic agents

- Most commonly used for induction of anaesthesia, followed by inhalation agent. **Propofol** can also be used to maintain anaesthesia during surgery.
- **Propofol**, **thiopental** and **etomidate** are most commonly used; all act within 20–30 s if given intravenously.
- **Propofol:**
  - potent;
  - rapid onset and distribution;
  - rapidly metabolised;
  - very rapid recovery, limited cumulative effect;
  - useful for day-case surgery;
  - low incidence of nausea and vomiting;
  - risk of bradycardia;
  - may induce an adverse 'propofol infusion syndrome' when administered at high doses for prolonged periods of time.
- **Thiopental:**
  - barbiturate with very high lipid solubility;
  - rapid action due to rapid transfer across blood–brain barrier; short duration (about 5 min) due to redistribution, mainly to muscle;
  - reduces intracranial pressure;
  - slowly metabolised and liable to accumulate in body fat, therefore may cause prolonged effect if given repeatedly;
  - narrow margin between anaesthetic dose and dose causing cardiovascular depression;
  - risk of tissue damage if accidentally injected extravascularly or into an artery;
  - can precipitate an attack of porphyria in susceptible individuals (see Ch. 12).
- **Etomidate:**
  - similar to thiopental but more quickly metabolised;
  - less risk of cardiovascular depression;
  - may cause involuntary movements during induction and high incidence of nausea;
  - possible risk of adrenocortical suppression.
- **Ketamine:**
  - analogue of **phencyclidine**, with similar properties;
  - action differs from other agents, probably related to inhibition of NMDA receptors;
  - onset of effect is relatively slow (1–2 min);
  - powerful analgesic;
  - produces 'dissociative' anaesthesia, in which the patient may remain conscious although amnesic and insensitive to pain;
  - high incidence of dysphoria, hallucinations, etc. during recovery; used mainly for minor procedures in children;
  - can raise intracranial pressure.

---

[5]An anaesthetist colleague tells of coming across a motorway accident where most of a victim was hidden under a mass of distorted metal but enough of a limb was available for an injection of ketamine to be given.
[6]A cautionary note: many adverse effects are claimed to be less marked in children, perhaps because they cannot verbalise their experiences. At one time, muscle relaxants alone were used without anaesthesia during cardiac surgery in neonates. The babies did not complain of pain, but their circulating catecholamines reached extreme levels.

For modern inhalation anaesthetics, metabolic degradation is generally insignificant in determining their duration of action. Inhalation anaesthetics are all small, lipid-soluble molecules that readily cross alveolar membranes. It is therefore the rates of delivery of drug to and from the lungs, via (respectively) the inspired air and bloodstream, which determine the overall kinetic behaviour of an anaesthetic. The reason that anaesthetics vary in their kinetic behaviour is that their relative solubilities in blood, and in body fat, vary between one drug and another.

The main factors that determine the speed of induction and recovery can be summarised as follows:

- Properties of the anaesthetic:
  - blood:gas partition coefficient (i.e. solubility in blood)
  - oil:gas partition coefficient (i.e. solubility in fat)
- Physiological factors:
  - alveolar ventilation rate
  - cardiac output

SOLUBILITY OF INHALATION ANAESTHETICS

Inhalation anaesthetics can be regarded physicochemically as ideal gases: their solubility in different media is expressed as *partition coefficients*, defined as the ratio of the concentration of the agent in two phases at equilibrium.

The *blood:gas partition coefficient* is the main factor that determines the rate of induction and recovery of an inhalation anaesthetic, and the lower the blood:gas partition coefficient, the faster is induction and recovery (Table 42.2).

This is because it is the partial pressure of the gas in the alveolar space that governs the concentration in the blood. The lower the blood:gas partition coefficient, the more rapidly the partial pressure of the gas in the alveolar space will equal that being administered in the inspired air (see later).

The *oil:gas partition coefficient*, a measure of fat solubility, determines the potency of an anaesthetic (as already discussed) and also influences the kinetics of its distribution in the body, the main effect being that high lipid solubility, by causing accumulation in body fat, delays recovery from anaesthesia. Values of blood:gas and oil:gas partition coefficients for some anaesthetics are given in Table 42.2.

INDUCTION AND RECOVERY

Cerebral blood flow is a substantial fraction of cardiac output (~15%), and the blood–brain barrier is freely permeable to anaesthetics, so the concentration of anaesthetic in the brain closely tracks that in the arterial blood. The kinetics of transfer of anaesthetic between the inspired air and the arterial blood therefore determine the kinetics of the pharmacological effect.

When a volatile anaesthetic is first administered, the initial breaths are diluted into the residual gas volume in

Table 42.2 Characteristics of inhalation anaesthetics

Drug	Partition coefficient Blood:gas	Oil:gas	Minimum alveolar concentration (% v/v)	Induction/ recovery	Main adverse effect(s) and disadvantage(s)	Notes
Nitrous oxide	0.5	1.4	100[a]	Fast	Few adverse effects Risk of anaemia (with prolonged or repeated use) Accumulation in gaseous cavities	Good analgesic effect Low potency precludes use as sole anaesthetic agent – normally combined with other inhalation agents
Isoflurane	1.4	91	1.2	Medium	Few adverse effects Possible risk of coronary ischaemia in susceptible patients	Widely used Has replaced halothane
Desflurane	0.4	23	6.1	Fast	Respiratory tract irritation, cough, bronchospasm	Used for day-case surgery because of fast onset and recovery (comparable with nitrous oxide)
Sevoflurane	0.6	53	2.1	Fast	Few reported Theoretical risk of renal toxicity owing to fluoride	Similar to desflurane
Halothane	2.4	220	0.8	Medium	Hypotension Cardiac arrhythmias Hepatotoxicity (with repeated use) Malignant hyperthermia (rare)	Little used nowadays Significant metabolism to trifluoracetate
Enflurane	1.9	98	1.7	Medium	Risk of convulsions (slight) Malignant hyperthermia (rare)	Has declined in use May induce seizures
Ether	12.0	65	1.9	Slow	Respiratory irritation Nausea and vomiting Explosion risk	Now obsolete, except where modern facilities are lacking

[a]Theoretical value based on experiments under hyperbaric conditions.

the lungs resulting in a reduction in the alveolar partial pressure of the anaesthetic as compared with the inspired gas mixture. With subsequent breaths, the alveolar partial pressure rises towards equilibrium. For an anaesthetic with a low blood:gas partition coefficient, the absorption into the blood will be slower, so with repeated breaths the partial pressure in the alveolar space will rise faster than with an agent of high blood:gas partition coefficient. Thus a smaller number of breaths (i.e. a shorter time) will be needed to reach equilibrium. Therefore, contrary to what one might intuitively suppose, the *lower* the solubility in blood, the *faster* is the process of equilibration. Fig. 42.3 shows the much faster equilibration for **nitrous oxide**, a low-solubility agent, than for **ether**, a high-solubility agent.

▼ The rate of absorption into the blood can be enhanced by administering a volatile anaesthetic along with nitrous oxide. The rapid movement of nitrous oxide from the alveoli into the blood concentrates the volatile anaesthetic in the alveoli which will increase its movement into the blood – referred to as the *concentration effect*. Furthermore, the volume of nitrous oxide taken up from the alveoli into the blood is replaced by inspired gas, thus augmenting the delivery to the alveoli of the volatile anaesthetic, and speeding its absorption – referred to as the *second gas effect*.

The transfer of anaesthetic between blood and tissues also affects the kinetics of equilibration. Fig. 42.4 shows a very simple model of the circulation, in which two tissue compartments are included. Body fat has a low blood flow but has a high capacity to take up anaesthetics, and constitutes about 20% of the volume of a non-obese human. Therefore for a drug such as **halothane**, which is about 100 times more soluble in fat than in water, the amount present in fat after complete equilibration would be roughly 95% of the total amount in the body. Because of the low blood flow to adipose tissue, it takes many hours for the drug to enter and leave the fat, which results in a pronounced slow phase of equilibration following the rapid phase associated with the blood–gas exchanges (see Fig. 42.3). The more fat-soluble the anaesthetic and the fatter

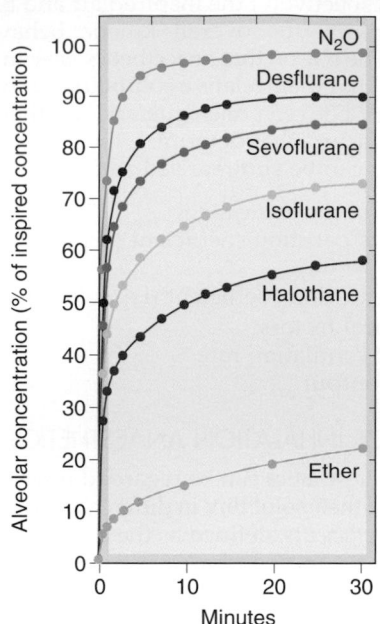

Fig. 42.3 Rate of equilibration of inhalation anaesthetics in humans. The curves show alveolar concentration (which closely reflects arterial blood concentration) as a function of time during induction. The initial rate of equilibration reflects solubility in blood. There is also a slow phase of equilibration, most marked with highly lipid-soluble drugs (ether and halothane), owing to the slow transfer between blood and fat (see Fig. 42.4). (Adapted from Yasuda, N., Lockhart, S.H., Eger, E.I. II et al., 1991. Comparison of kinetics of sevoflurane and isoflurane in humans. Anesth. Analg. 72, 316–324.)

Fig. 42.4 Factors affecting the rate of equilibration of inhalation anaesthetics in the body. The body is represented as two compartments. Lean tissues, including the brain, have a large blood flow and low partition coefficient for anaesthetics, and therefore equilibrate rapidly with the blood. Fat tissues have a small blood flow and large partition coefficient, and therefore equilibrate slowly, acting as a reservoir of drug during the recovery phase.

the patient, the more pronounced this slow phase becomes and recovery will also be delayed.

Of the physiological factors affecting the rate of equilibration of inhalation anaesthetics, alveolar ventilation is the most important. The greater the minute volume (respiration rate × tidal volume), the faster is equilibration, particularly for drugs that have high blood:gas partition coefficients. Respiratory depressant drugs such as **morphine** (see Ch. 43) can thus retard recovery from anaesthesia. The effect of changes in cardiac output on the rate of equilibration is more complex. By reducing alveolar perfusion, a reduction of cardiac output reduces alveolar absorption of the anaesthetic, and thus speeds up induction, but this is partially offset by a reduction of cerebral blood flow slowing down delivery to the brain.

Recovery from anaesthesia involves the same processes as induction but in reverse, the rapid phase of recovery being followed by a slow 'hangover'. Because of these kinetic factors, the search for improved inhalation anaesthetics has focused on agents with low blood and tissue solubility. Newer drugs, which show kinetic properties similar to those of nitrous oxide but have higher potency, include **sevoflurane** and **desflurane** (see Table 42.2 and Fig. 42.3).

METABOLISM AND TOXICITY

Metabolism, although not quantitatively important as a route of elimination of inhalation anaesthetics, can generate toxic metabolites (Ch. 58).[7] This is the main reason that agents that are now obsolete or obsolescent, such as chloroform, methoxyflurane and halothane, have been replaced by the less toxic alternatives described below.

Malignant hyperthermia is an important but rare *idiosyncratic reaction* (see Ch. 58), caused by heat production in skeletal muscle, due to excessive release of Ca^{2+} from the sarcoplasmic reticulum. The result is muscle contracture, acidosis, increased metabolism and an associated dramatic rise in body temperature that can be fatal unless treated promptly. Triggers include halogenated anaesthetics and depolarising neuromuscular-blocking drugs (see Ch. 14). Susceptibility has a genetic basis, being associated with mutations in the gene encoding the ryanodine receptor, which controls Ca^{2+} release from the sarcoplasmic reticulum (Ch. 4). Malignant hyperthermia is treated with **dantrolene**, a muscle relaxant drug that blocks these calcium-release channels.

INDIVIDUAL INHALATION ANAESTHETICS

The main inhalation anaesthetics currently used in developed countries are **isoflurane**, **desflurane** and **sevoflurane**, sometimes used in combination with **nitrous oxide**. Due to its relatively rapid onset of action and pleasant smell, sevoflurane is used, under some circumstances, on its own to induce anaesthesia, e.g. in paediatrics or in adults frightened by the prospect of venous cannulation. **Xenon**, an inert gas shown many years ago to have anaesthetic properties, is making something of a comeback in the clinic because – not surprisingly for an inert gas – it lacks toxicity,

---

> ## Pharmacokinetic properties of inhalation anaesthetics
>
> - Rapid induction and recovery are important properties of an anaesthetic agent, allowing flexible control over the depth of anaesthesia.
> - Speed of induction and recovery are determined by two properties of the anaesthetic: solubility in blood (blood:gas partition coefficient) and solubility in fat (lipid solubility).
> - Agents with low blood:gas partition coefficients produce rapid induction and recovery (e.g. **nitrous oxide**, **desflurane**); agents with high blood:gas partition coefficients show slow induction and recovery.
> - Agents with high lipid solubility accumulate gradually in body fat and may produce a prolonged 'hangover' if used for a long operation.
> - Some halogenated anaesthetics (especially **halothane** and **methoxyflurane**) are metabolised. This is not very important in determining their duration of action, but contributes to toxicity (e.g. renal toxicity associated with fluoride production with **methoxyflurane** – no longer used).

but its relatively low potency and high cost are disadvantages. It may also be neuroprotective in neonatal hypoxia (see Ch. 41).

ISOFLURANE, DESFLURANE, SEVOFLURANE, ENFLURANE AND HALOTHANE

Isoflurane is now the most widely used volatile anaesthetic. It is not appreciably metabolised and lacks the proconvulsive property of enflurane. It can cause hypotension and is a powerful coronary vasodilator. Paradoxically, this can exacerbate cardiac ischaemia in patients with coronary disease, because of the 'steal' phenomenon (see Ch. 22).

Desflurane is chemically similar to isoflurane, but its lower solubility in blood and fat means that adjustment of anaesthetic depth and recovery are faster, so it is increasingly used as an anaesthetic in obese patients undergoing bariatric surgery and for day-case surgery. It is not appreciably metabolised. It is less potent than the drugs described above. At the concentrations used for induction of anaesthesia (about 10%), desflurane causes some respiratory tract irritation, which can lead to coughing and bronchospasm. Rapid increases in the depth of desflurane anaesthesia can be associated with a striking increase in sympathetic activity, which is undesirable in patients with ischaemic heart disease.

Sevoflurane resembles desflurane but is more potent and does not cause the same degree of respiratory irritation. It is partially (about 3%) metabolised, and detectable levels of fluoride are produced, although this does not appear to be sufficient to cause toxicity.

Enflurane has a moderate speed of induction but is little used nowadays. It was originally introduced as an alternative to methoxyflurane. It can cause seizures, either during induction or following recovery from anaesthesia, especially in patients suffering from epilepsy. In this connection, it is interesting that a related substance, the fluorine-substituted

---

[7]The problem of toxicity of low concentrations of anaesthetics inhaled over long periods by operating theatre staff was at one time a cause for concern. Strict measures are now used to minimise the escape of anaesthetics into the air of operating theatres.

diethyl-ether hexafluoroether, is a powerful convulsant agent, although the mechanism is not understood.

Halothane was an important drug in the development of volatile inhalation anaesthetics, but its use has declined in favour of isoflurane due to the potential for accumulation of toxic metabolites. Halothane has a marked relaxant effect on the uterus which can cause postpartum bleeding and limits its usefulness for obstetric purposes.

NITROUS OXIDE

Nitrous oxide (N_2O, not to be confused with nitric oxide, NO) is an odourless gas with many advantageous features for anaesthesia. It is rapid in onset of action because of its low blood:gas partition coefficient (see Table 42.2), and is an effective analgesic in concentrations too low to cause unconsciousness. Its potency is low. It is used as a 50:50 mixture with O_2 to reduce pain during childbirth. It must never be given as 100% of the inspired gas as patients do need to breathe oxygen! Even at 80% in the inspired gas mixture, nitrous oxide does not produce surgical anaesthesia. It is not therefore used on its own as an anaesthetic, but is used (as 70% nitrous oxide in oxygen) as an adjunct to volatile anaesthetics to speed up induction – see description of the second gas effect (p. 538). During recovery from nitrous oxide anaesthesia, the transfer of the gas from the blood into the alveoli can be sufficient to reduce, by dilution, the alveolar partial pressure of oxygen, producing transient hypoxia (known as *diffusional hypoxia*). This is important for patients with respiratory disease.

Nitrous oxide tends to enter gaseous cavities in the body causing them to expand. This can be dangerous if a pneumothorax or vascular air embolus is present, or if the intestine is obstructed.

Given for brief periods, nitrous oxide is devoid of any serious toxic effects, but prolonged exposure (>6 h) causes inactivation of methionine synthase, an enzyme required for DNA and protein synthesis, resulting in bone marrow depression that may cause anaemia and leukopenia, so its use should be avoided in patients with anaemia related to vitamin B_{12} deficiency. Bone marrow depression does not occur with brief exposure to nitrous oxide, but prolonged or repeated use (for example, in intermittently painful conditions such as sickle cell anaemia) should be avoided. Nitrous oxide 'sniffers' are subject to this danger.

BALANCED ANAESTHESIA

Only in simple, short surgical procedures would a single anaesthetic be used on its own. In complex surgery, an array of drugs will be given at various times throughout the procedure. These may include a sedative or anxiolytic premedication (e.g. a benzodiazepine, see Ch. 45), an intravenous anaesthetic for rapid induction (e.g. **propofol**), a perioperative opioid analgesic (e.g. **alfentanil** or **remifentanil**, see Ch. 43), an inhalation anaesthetic to maintain anaesthesia during surgery (e.g. **nitrous oxide** and **isoflurane**), a neuromuscular-blocking agent to produce adequate muscle relaxation (e.g. **vecuronium**, see Ch. 14) for access to the abdominal cavity for example, an antiemetic agent (e.g. **ondansetron**, see Ch. 31) and a muscarinic antagonist to prevent or treat bradycardia or to reduce bronchial and salivary secretions (e.g. **atropine** or **glycopyrrolate**, see Ch. 14). Towards the end of the procedure, an anticholinesterase agent (e.g. **neostigmine**, see Ch. 14) to reverse the

Individual inhalation anaesthetics

- The main agents in current use in developed countries are **isoflurane**, **desflurane** and **sevoflurane**, sometimes supplemented with **nitrous oxide**.
- As a rare but serious hazard, inhalation anaesthetics can cause malignant hyperthermia.
- **Nitrous oxide:**
  - low potency, therefore must be combined with other agents
  - rapid induction and recovery
  - good analgesic properties
  - risk of bone marrow depression with prolonged administration
  - accumulates in gaseous cavities
- **Isoflurane:**
  - similar to **enflurane** but lacks epileptogenic property
  - may precipitate myocardial ischaemia in patients with coronary disease
  - irritant to respiratory tract
- **Desflurane**:
  - similar to **isoflurane** but with faster onset and recovery
  - respiratory irritant, so liable to cause coughing and laryngospasm
  - useful for day-case surgery
- **Sevoflurane**:
  - similar to **desflurane**, with lack of respiratory irritation

Clinical uses of general anaesthetics

- *Intravenous anaesthetics* are used for:
  - induction of anaesthesia (e.g. **propofol** or **thiopental**);
  - maintenance of anaesthesia throughout surgery ('total intravenous anaesthesia', e.g. **propofol** sometimes in combination with muscle relaxants and analgesics).
- *Inhalational anaesthetics* (gases or volatile liquids) are used for maintenance of anaesthesia. Points to note are that:
  - volatile anaesthetics (e.g. **isoflurane**, **sevoflurane**) are delivered in air, oxygen or oxygen–nitrous oxide mixtures as the carrier gas;
  - **nitrous oxide** must always be given with oxygen;
  - because of its potential for inducing hepatotoxicity, **halothane** has largely been replaced by newer volatile anaesthetics such as **isoflurane**;
  - all inhalational anaesthetics can trigger *malignant hyperthermia* in susceptible individuals.

neuromuscular blockade (**sugammadex**, which binds and inactivates steroidal neuromuscular-blocking drugs, can also be used for this purpose) and an analgesic for postoperative pain relief (e.g. an opioid such as **morphine** and/or a non-steroidal anti-inflammatory drug, see Ch. 43). Such combinations of drugs result in much faster induction and recovery, avoiding long (and potentially hazardous) periods of semiconsciousness, good analgesia and muscle relaxation and it enables surgery to be carried out with less undesirable cardiorespiratory depression.

Low doses of general anaesthetics may be used to provide sedation where a local anaesthetic (Ch. 44), administered intrathecally, is used to provide analgesia and relaxation needed to perform surgery to the lower parts of the body.

REFERENCES AND FURTHER READING

Aitkenhead, A.R., Moppett, I., Thompson, J., 2013. Smith & Aitkenhead's Textbook of Anaesthesia, sixth ed. Churchill Livingstone/Elsevier, Edinburgh. (*Major textbook of anaesthesia*)

Antkowiak, B., Rudolph, U., 2016. New insights in the systemic and molecular underpinnings of general anesthetic actions mediated by γ-aminobutyric acid A receptors. Cur. Opin. In: Anaesth, vol. 29. pp. 447–453. (*Useful update on the interaction of general anaesthetics with the GABA$_A$ receptor*)

Bayliss, D.A., Barrett, P.Q., 2008. Emerging roles for two-pore-domain potassium channels and their potential therapeutic impact. Trends Pharmacol. Sci. 29, 566–575.

Franks, N.P., 2008. General anaesthesia: from molecular targets to neuronal pathways of sleep and arousal. Nat. Rev. Neurosci. 9, 370–386. (*Detailed discussion of the sites of action of general anaesthetics on specific ion channels*)

Schüttler, J., Schwilden, H., 2008. Modern anesthetics. Handb. Exp. Pharmacol. 182. (*Entire volume given over to multiauthor reviews of the mechanisms of action of general anaesthetics*)

43 Analgesic drugs

OVERVIEW

Pain is a disabling accompaniment of many acute and chronic medical conditions, and pain control is one of the most important therapeutic priorities.

In this chapter, we discuss the neural mechanisms responsible for different types of pain, and the various drugs that are used to reduce it. The 'classic' analgesic drugs, notably opioids and non-steroidal anti-inflammatory drugs (NSAIDs; described in Ch. 27), have their origins in natural products that have been used for centuries. The original compounds, typified by morphine and aspirin, are still in widespread use, but many synthetic compounds that act by the same mechanisms have been developed. Opioid analgesics are described in detail in this chapter. We also consider various other drug classes, such as antidepressants and antiepileptic drugs, which clinical experience has shown to be effective in certain types of pain.

NEURAL MECHANISMS OF PAIN

Pain is a subjective experience, hard to define exactly, even though we all know what we mean by it. Typically, it is a direct response to an untoward event associated with tissue damage, such as injury, inflammation or cancer, but severe pain can arise independently of any obvious predisposing cause (e.g. trigeminal neuralgia), or persist long after the precipitating injury has healed (e.g. phantom limb pain). It can also occur as a consequence of brain or nerve injury (e.g. following a stroke or herpes infection, and as a consequence of diabetes or multiple sclerosis). Painful conditions of the latter kind, not directly linked to tissue injury, are often described as 'neuropathic pains'. They are very common and a major cause of disability and distress. Their cause is often uncertain and in general they respond less well to conventional analgesic drugs. In these cases, we need to think of pain in terms of disordered neural function rather than simply as a 'normal' response to tissue injury. The perception of noxious stimuli (termed *nociception* by Sherrington) is not the same thing as pain, which is a subjective experience and includes a strong emotional (affective) component, especially in people suffering from chronic pain.

Though clinical pain is broadly categorised as 'acute' and 'chronic', these terms are a bit misleading (e.g. the pain occurring with cancer, while described as acute, can be experienced for some considerable time). The following mechanistic classification is more relevant when considering analgesic drugs.

- Pain associated with tissue pathology (e.g. trauma, inflammation, tumours).
- Neuropathic pain associated with nervous system pathology (e.g. herpes, diabetes, stroke).
- Musculo-skeletal pain (e.g. back pain) and pain of unknown cause assumed by default to be psychogenic (e.g. fibromyalgia).

Good accounts of the neural basis of pain can be found in McMahon et al. (2013).

NOCICEPTIVE AFFERENT NEURONS

Under normal conditions, pain is associated with impulse activity in small-diameter (C and Aδ) primary afferent fibres of peripheral nerves. These nerves have sensory endings in peripheral tissues and are activated by stimuli of various kinds (mechanical, thermal, chemical). The majority of non-myelinated (C) fibres are associated with *polymodal nociceptive* endings and convey a dull, diffuse burning pain, whereas myelinated (Aδ) fibres convey a sensation of sharp, well-localised pain. C and Aδ fibres convey nociceptive information from muscle and viscera as well as from the skin.

With many pathological conditions, tissue injury is the immediate cause of the pain and results in the local release of a variety of chemicals that act on the nerve terminals, either activating them directly or enhancing their sensitivity to other forms of stimulation (Fig. 43.1). The pharmacological properties of nociceptive nerve terminals are discussed in more detail later.

The cell bodies of spinal nociceptive afferent fibres lie in dorsal root ganglia; fibres enter the spinal cord via the dorsal roots, ending in the grey matter of the dorsal horn (see Fig. 43.4). Most of the nociceptive afferents terminate in the superficial region of the dorsal horn, the C fibres and some Aδ fibres innervating cell bodies in laminae I and II (also known as the *substantia gelatinosa* [SG]), while other A fibres penetrate deeper into the dorsal horn (lamina V). The SG is rich in both endogenous opioid peptides and opioid receptors, and may be an important site of action for morphine-like drugs. Cells in laminae I and V give rise to the main projection pathways from the dorsal horn to the thalamus. For a more detailed account of dorsal horn circuitry, see Todd and Koerber (2013).

The nociceptive afferent neurons release glutamate and possibly ATP as the fast neurotransmitters at their central synapses in the dorsal horn. Glutamate acting on AMPA receptors is responsible for fast synaptic transmission at the first synapse in the dorsal horn. There is also a slower NMDA receptor-mediated response, which is important in relation to the phenomenon of 'wind-up' (Fig. 43.2). The nociceptive afferent neurons also contain several

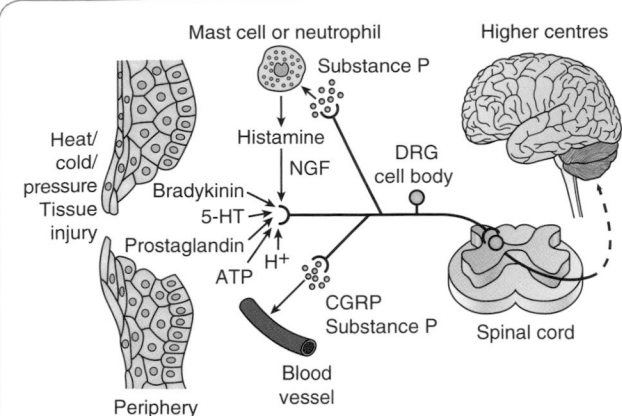

Fig. 43.1 Activation of nociceptive neurons. Various stimuli (physical and chemical), some shown here, can initiate or enhance the rate of action potential firing in nociceptive primary afferent neurons (i.e. induce pain). These afferent fibres project to the dorsal horn of the spinal cord where they synapse on neurons projecting to higher centres. *5-HT*, 5-hydroxytryptamine; *CGRP*, calcitonin gene-related peptide; *DRG*, dorsal root ganglion; *NGF*, nerve growth factor. (Adapted from Julius, D., Basbaum, A.I., 2001. Nature 413, 203–210.)

Fig. 43.2 Effect of glutamate and substance P antagonists on nociceptive transmission in the rat spinal cord. The rat paw was inflamed by ultraviolet irradiation 2 days before the experiment, a procedure that induces hyperalgesia and spinal cord facilitation. The synaptic response was recorded from the ventral root, in response to stimulation of C fibres in the dorsal root with (A) single stimuli or (B) repetitive stimuli. The effects of the NMDA receptor antagonist D-AP-5 (see Ch. 39) and the substance P antagonist RP 67580 (selective for neurokinin type 2, (NK_2) receptors) are shown. The slow component of the synaptic response is reduced by both antagonists (A), as is the 'wind-up' in response to repetitive stimulation (B). These effects are much less pronounced in the normal animal. Thus both glutamate, acting on NMDA receptors, and substance P, acting on NK_2 receptors, are involved in nociceptive transmission, and their contribution increases as a result of inflammatory hyperalgesia. (Records kindly provided by L. Urban and S.W. Thompson.)

neuropeptides (see Ch. 19), particularly substance P and calcitonin gene-related peptide (CGRP). These are released as mediators at both the central and the peripheral terminals, and play an important role in the pathology of pain. In the periphery, substance P and CGRP produce some of the features of neurogenic inflammation. CGRP antagonists have potential for the treatment of migraine (see Ch. 16) but have not proved effective for other pain states. In animal models, substance P acting on NK_1 receptors was shown to be involved in wind-up and central sensitisation in the dorsal horn (see Fig. 43.2). Surprisingly, however, antagonists of substance P at NK_1 receptors turned out to be ineffective as analgesics in humans, although they do have antiemetic activity (Ch. 31).

MODULATION IN THE NOCICEPTIVE PATHWAY

Pain resulting from trauma, inflammation or cancer is generally well accounted for in terms of nociception – an excessive noxious stimulus giving rise to an intense and unpleasant sensation. In contrast, neuropathic pain states are associated with aberrations of the normal physiological pathway, giving rise to *hyperalgesia* (an increased amount of pain associated with a mild noxious stimulus) and *allodynia* (pain evoked by a non-noxious stimulus). Some of the main mechanisms are summarised in Fig. 43.3.

HYPERALGESIA AND ALLODYNIA

▼ Anyone who has suffered a burn or sprained ankle has experienced hyperalgesia and allodynia. Hyperalgesia involves both sensitisation of peripheral nociceptive nerve terminals and central facilitation of transmission at the level of the dorsal horn and thalamus. The peripheral component is due to the action of mediators such as bradykinin and prostaglandins acting on the nerve terminals. The central component reflects facilitation of synaptic transmission in the dorsal horn of the spinal cord (see Yaksh, 1999). The synaptic responses of dorsal horn neurons to nociceptive inputs display the phenomenon of 'wind-up' – i.e. the synaptic potentials steadily increase in amplitude

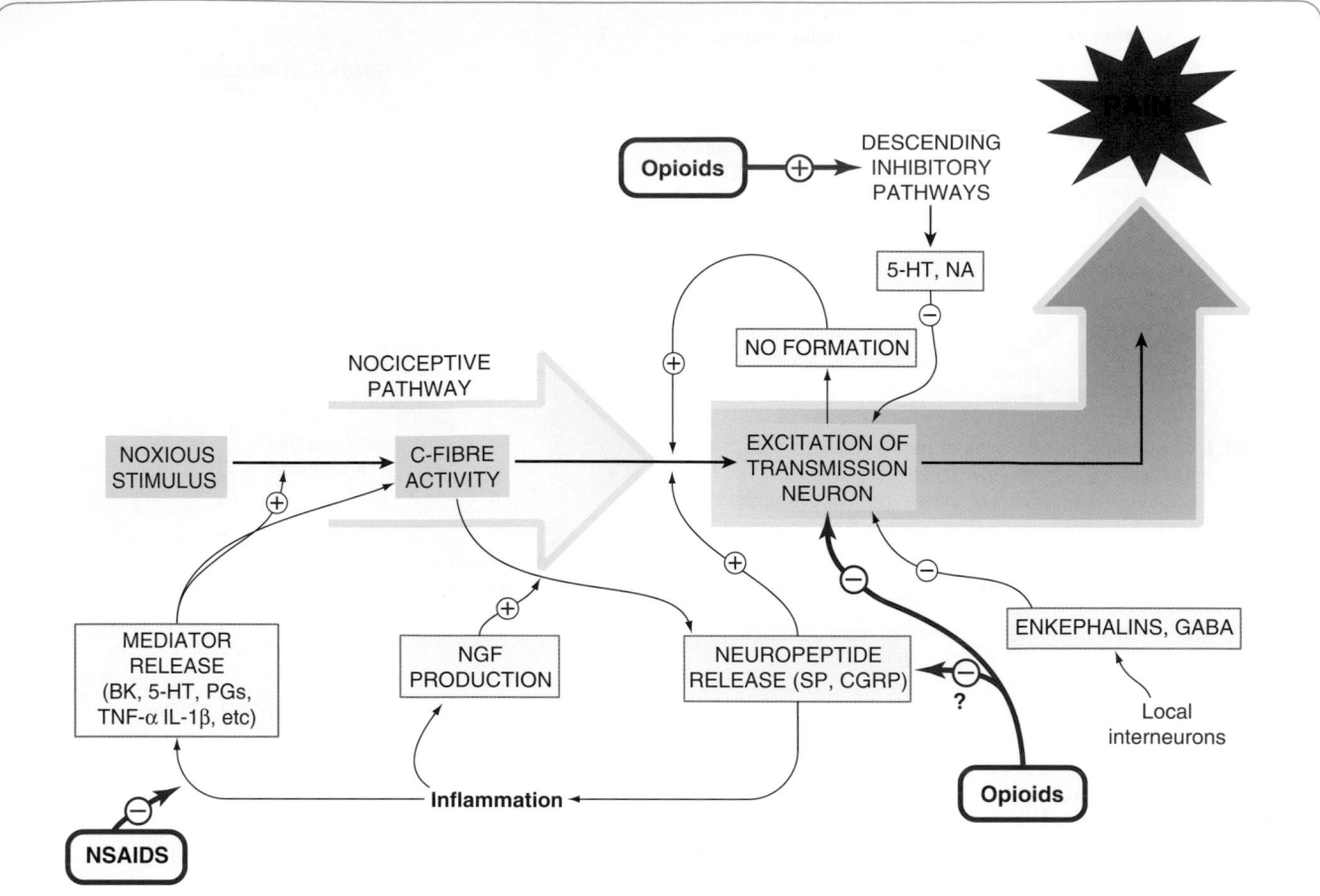

Fig. 43.3 Summary of modulatory mechanisms in the nociceptive pathway. *5-HT*, 5-hydroxytryptamine; *BK*, bradykinin; *CGRP*, calcitonin gene-related peptide; *IL-1β*, interleukin; *NA*, noradrenaline; *NGF*, nerve growth factor; *NO*, nitric oxide; *NSAID*, non-steroidal anti-inflammatory drug; *PG*, prostaglandin; *SP*, substance P; *TNF-α*, tumour necrosis factor-α.

with each stimulus – when repeated stimuli are delivered at physiological frequencies. This activity-dependent facilitation of transmission has features in common with the phenomenon of long-term potentiation, described in Chapter 39, and the chemical mechanisms underlying it may also be similar. In the dorsal horn, the facilitation is blocked by antagonists and also in part by antagonists of substance P and by inhibitors of nitric oxide (NO) synthesis (see Figs 43.2 and 43.3).

Substance P and CGRP released from primary afferent neurons (see Fig. 43.1) also act in the periphery, promoting inflammation by their effects on blood vessels and cells of the immune system (Ch. 19). This mechanism, known as *neurogenic inflammation*, amplifies and sustains the inflammatory reaction and the accompanying activation of nociceptive afferent fibres.

Central facilitation is an important component of pathological hyperalgesia (e.g. that associated with inflammatory responses). The mediators responsible for central facilitation include substance P, CGRP, brain-derived neurotrophic factor (BDNF) and NO, as well as many others. For example, nerve growth factor (NGF), a cytokine-like mediator produced by peripheral tissues, particularly in inflammation, acts on a kinase-linked receptor (known as TrkA) on nociceptive afferent neurons, increasing their electrical excitability, chemosensitivity and peptide content, and also promoting the formation of synaptic contacts. Increased NGF production may be an important mechanism by which nociceptive transmission becomes facilitated by tissue damage, leading to hyperalgesia (see Mantyh et al., 2011). Increased gene expression in sensory neurons is induced by NGF and other inflammatory mediators; the up-regulated genes include those for neuropeptides and neuromodulators (e.g. CGRP, substance P and

BDNF) as well as for receptors (e.g. transient receptor potential TRPV1 and the ATP receptor P2X) and sodium channels, and have the overall effect of facilitating transmission at the first synaptic relay in the dorsal horn. BDNF released from primary afferent nerve terminals activates the kinase-linked TrkB receptor on postsynaptic dorsal horn neurons leading to phosphorylation of the NMDA subunit GluN1 and thus sensitisation of these glutamate receptors, resulting in synaptic facilitation, in the dorsal horn.

Excitation of nociceptive sensory neurons depends, as in other neurons (see Ch. 4), on voltage-gated sodium channels. Individuals who express non-functional mutations of $Na_v1.7$ are unable to experience pain. The expression and/or activity of certain sodium-channel subtypes (e.g. $Na_v1.3$, $Na_v1.7$, $Na_v 1.8$ and $Na_v1.9$ channels) is increased in sensory neurons in various pathological pain states and their enhanced activity underlies the sensitisation to external stimuli that occurs in inflammatory pain and hyperalgesia (see Ch. 4 for more detail on voltage-activated sodium channels). Consistent with this hypothesis is the fact that many antiepileptic and antidysrhythmic drugs, which act by blocking sodium channels (see Chs 22 and 46), also find clinical application as analgesics.

TRANSMISSION OF PAIN TO HIGHER CENTRES

From the dorsal horn, ascending nerve axons travel in the contralateral spinothalamic tracts, and synapse on neurons in the ventral and medial parts of the thalamus, from which there are further projections to the somatosensory cortex. In the medial thalamus in particular, many cells respond specifically to noxious stimuli in the periphery, and lesions in this area cause analgesia. Functional brain imaging studies in conscious subjects have been performed to localise regions involved in pain processing. These include sensory, discriminatory areas such as primary and secondary somatosensory cortex, thalamus and posterior parts of insula as well as affective, cognitive areas such as the anterior parts of insula, anterior cingulate cortex and prefrontal cortex (see Apkarian et al., 2013).

DESCENDING INHIBITORY CONTROLS

Descending pathways (Fig. 43.4) control impulse transmission in the dorsal horn. A key part of this descending system is the *periaqueductal grey* (PAG) area of the midbrain, a small area of grey matter surrounding the central canal. In 1969, Reynolds found that electrical stimulation of this brain area in the rat caused analgesia sufficiently intense that abdominal surgery could be performed without anaesthesia and without eliciting any marked response. The responses to non-painful stimuli were unaffected. The PAG receives inputs from many other brain regions, including the hypothalamus, amygdala and cortex, and is the main pathway through which cortical and other inputs act to control the nociceptive 'gate' in the dorsal horn.

The PAG projects first to the rostroventral medulla (RVM) and thence via the dorsolateral funiculus of the spinal cord to the dorsal horn. Two important transmitters in this pathway are 5-hydroxytryptamine (5-HT; serotonin) and the enkephalins, which act directly or via interneurons to inhibit the discharge of spinothalamic neurons (see Fig. 43.4).

The descending inhibitory pathway is probably an important site of action for opioid analgesics. Both PAG and SG are particularly rich in enkephalin-containing neurons, and opioid antagonists such as naloxone (see p. 549) can prevent analgesia induced by PAG stimulation, which would suggest that endogenous opioid peptides may function as transmitters in this system. The physiological role of opioid peptides in regulating pain transmission has been controversial, mainly because under normal conditions naloxone has relatively little effect on pain threshold. Under pathological conditions, however, when stress is present, naloxone causes hyperalgesia, implying that the opioid system is active.

Interneurons in the dorsal horn release GABA (see Ch. 39), which inhibits transmitter release from primary afferent terminals.

There is also a noradrenergic pathway from the *locus coeruleus* (LC; see Ch. 40), which has a similar inhibitory effect on transmission in the dorsal horn. Surprisingly, opioids inhibit rather than activate this pathway. The use of tricyclic antidepressants to control pain (see p. 559) probably depends on potentiating this pathway.

It is thought that descending inhibitory purinergic pathways may release adenosine on to A_1 receptors on dorsal horn neurons to produce analgesia.

PLACEBO ANALGESIA

Placebo analgesia is the phenomenon of reduced sensation of pain when the subject believes that they have been given a drug that will suppress pain, when in fact no drug has been administered at all. It is often a substantial effect that poses problems in clinical trials of analgesic drugs. Placebo analgesia is reduced by administration of an opioid antagonist such as **naloxone**, indicating that it involves the release of endogenous opioid peptides. Brain imaging

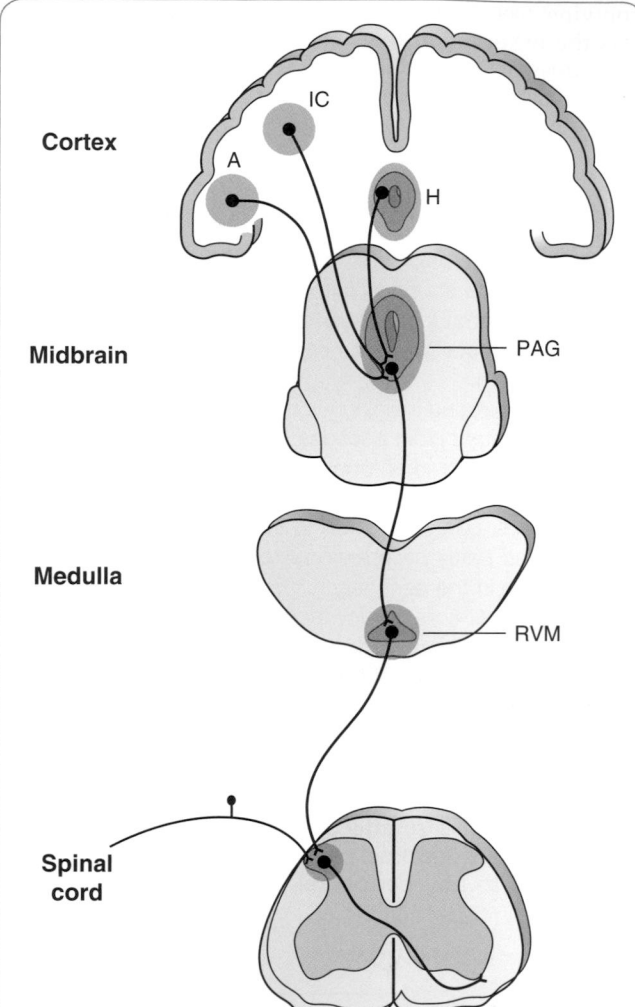

Fig. 43.4 **The descending pain control system and sites of action of opioids to relieve pain.** Opioids induce analgesia when microinjected into the insular cortex (IC), amygdala (A), hypothalamus (H), periaqueductal grey (PAG) region and rostroventral medulla (RVM), as well as into the dorsal horn of the spinal cord. The PAG receives input from higher centres and is the main output centre of the limbic system. It projects to the RVM. From the RVM, descending inhibitory fibres, some of which contain 5-hydroxytryptamine, project to the dorsal horn of the spinal cord. *Pink shaded areas* indicate regions expressing μ opioid receptors. The pathways shown in this diagram represent a considerable oversimplification. (Adapted from Fields, H., 2001. Prog. Brain Res. 122, 245–253. For a fuller account of the descending pain modulating pathways, see Todd & Koerber, 2013.)

studies have revealed that the placebo response results from changes in neuronal activity in the prefrontal cortex and PAG, resulting in activation of descending inhibitory pathways to the spinal cord to suppress the processing of pain information.

Expectation can also modify the response when an analgesic drug is given. Subjects receiving an intravenous infusion of remifentanil, an opioid analgesic, showed more pain relief when they were told they were receiving the drug than when the drug was administered without them knowing (see Bingel et al., 2012). Even more surprising was the observation that when the subjects received the same dose of remifentanyl, but were told the infusion was of a substance that would exacerbate pain, they did not show any analgesic response to the opioid.

Modulation of pain transmission

- Descending pathways from the midbrain and brain stem exert a strong inhibitory effect on dorsal horn transmission. Electrical stimulation of the midbrain periaqueductal grey area causes analgesia through this mechanism.
- The descending inhibition is mediated mainly by endogenous opioid peptides, 5-hydroxytryptamine (serotonin), noradrenaline and adenosine. Opioids cause analgesia partly by activating these descending pathways, partly by inhibiting transmission in the dorsal horn and partly by inhibiting excitation of sensory nerve terminals in the periphery.
- Repetitive C-fibre activity facilitates transmission through the dorsal horn ('wind-up') by mechanisms involving activation of NMDA and substance P receptors.

NEUROPATHIC PAIN

Neurological disease affecting the sensory pathway can produce severe chronic pain – termed *neuropathic pain* – unrelated to any peripheral tissue injury. This occurs with central nervous system (CNS) disorders such as stroke and multiple sclerosis, or with conditions associated with peripheral nerve damage, such as mechanical injury, diabetic neuropathy or herpes zoster infection (shingles). The pathophysiological mechanisms underlying this kind of pain are poorly understood, although spontaneous activity in damaged sensory neurons, due to overexpression or redistribution of voltage-gated sodium channels, is thought to be a factor. In addition, central sensitisation occurs. The sympathetic nervous system also plays a part, because damaged sensory neurons can express α_1 adrenoceptors and develop a sensitivity to noradrenaline that they do not possess under normal conditions. Thus, physiological stimuli that evoke sympathetic responses can produce severe pain, a phenomenon described clinically as sympathetically mediated pain. Neuropathic pain responds poorly to conventional analgesic drugs but can be relieved by some antidepressant and antiepileptic agents (see p. 559).

CHEMICAL SIGNALLING IN THE NOCICEPTIVE PATHWAY
CHEMOSENSITIVITY OF NOCICEPTIVE NERVE ENDINGS

In most cases, stimulation of nociceptive endings in the periphery is chemical in origin. Excessive mechanical or thermal stimuli can obviously cause acute pain, but the persistence of such pain after the stimulus has been removed, or the pain resulting from inflammatory or ischaemic changes in tissues, generally reflects an altered chemical environment of the pain afferents. The current state of knowledge is summarised in Fig. 43.5.

Fig. 43.5 **Channels, receptors and transduction mechanisms of nociceptive afferent terminals.** Only the main channels and receptors are shown. Ligand-gated channels include acid-sensitive ion channels (ASICs), ATP-sensitive channels (P2X receptors) and the capsaicin-sensitive channel (TRPV1), which is also sensitive to protons and to temperature. Various facilitatory and inhibitory G protein–coupled receptors (GPCRs) are shown, which regulate channel function through various second messenger systems. Growth factors such as nerve growth factor (NGF) act via kinase-linked receptors (TrkA) to control ion channel function and gene expression. *B₂ receptor,* bradykinin type 2 receptor; *PKA,* protein kinase A; *PKC,* protein kinase C.

Table 43.1 Thermosensitive TRP channels expressed on sensory neurons

Channel type	TRPA1	TRPM8	TRPV4	TRPV3	TRPV1	TRPV2
Activation temperature (°C)	<17	8–28	>27	>33	>43	>52
Chemical activators	Icilin Wintergreen oil Mustard oil	Menthol Icilin Eucalyptol Geraniol	4αPDD	Camphor Menthol Eugenol	Capsaicin Protons Anandamide Camphor Resiniferatoxin Eugenol	Δ⁹-THC

4αPDD, 4 alpha-phorbol 12,13-didecanoate; *Δ⁹-THC*, Δ⁹-tetrahydrocannabinol; *TRP*, transient receptor protein.

TRP channels – thermal sensation and pain

The *transient receptor potential* (TRP) channel family comprises some 27 or more structurally related ion channels that serve a wide variety of physiological functions (see Nilius & Szallasi, 2014). Within this family are a group of channels present on sensory neurons that are activated both by thermal stimuli across a wide range of temperatures and by chemical agents (Table 43.1). With respect to pain, the most important channels are TRPV1, TRPM8 and TRPA1.

▼ **Capsaicin**, the substance in chilli peppers that gives them their pungency, selectively excites nociceptive nerve terminals, causing intense pain if injected into the skin or applied to sensitive structures such as the cornea.[1] It produces this effect by activating TRPV1.[2] Agonists such as capsaicin open the channel, which is permeable to Na^+, Ca^{2+} and other cations, causing depolarisation and initiation of action potentials. The large influx of Ca^{2+} into peripheral nerve terminals also results in peptide release (mainly substance P and CGRP), causing intense vascular and other physiological responses. The Ca^{2+} influx may be enough to cause nerve degeneration (see Ch. 41). Applied topically, capsaicin reduces neuropathic and osteoarthritic pain by this mechanism, but the initial strong irritant effect is a major disadvantage.

TRPV1 responds not only to capsaicin-like agonists but also to other stimuli (see Table 43.1), including temperatures in excess of about 42°C (the threshold for pain) and proton concentrations in the micromolar range (pH 5.5 and below), which also cause pain. The receptor thus has unusual 'polymodal' characteristics and is believed to play a central role in nociception. TRPV1 is, like many other ionotropic receptors, modulated by phosphorylation, and several of the pain-producing substances that act through G protein–coupled receptors (e.g. bradykinin) work by sensitising TRPV1. A search for endogenous ligands for TRPV1 revealed, surprisingly, that **anandamide** (a lipid mediator previously identified as an agonist at cannabinoid receptors; see Ch. 20) is also a TRPV1 agonist, although less potent than capsaicin. TRPV1 knock-out mice show reduced responsiveness to noxious heat and also fail to show thermal hyperalgesia in response to inflammation. The latter observation is interesting, because TRPV1 expression is known to be increased by inflammation and this may be a key mechanism by which hyperalgesia is produced. A number of pharmaceutical companies developed TRPV1 agonists – to act as desensitising agents – and antagonists as analgesic agents. However, TRPV1 agonists were found to induce hypothermia, associated with activation of hypothalamic thermosensitive neurons, and TRPV1 antagonists were found to induce hyperthermia, consistent with a role of TRPV1 in body temperature control as well as nociception.

TRPM8 and TRPA1 respond to cold rather than heat (see Table 43.1).

Fig. 43.6 Response of a nociceptive afferent neuron to bradykinin and prostaglandin. Recordings were made from a nociceptive afferent fibre supplying a muscle, and drugs were injected into the arterial supply. Upper records: single-fibre recordings showing discharge caused by bradykinin (Brad) alone *(left)*, and by bradykinin following injection of prostaglandin *(right)*. Lower trace: ratemeter recording of single-fibre discharge, showing long-lasting enhancement of response to bradykinin after an injection of prostaglandin E_2 (PGE_2). Prostaglandin itself did not evoke a discharge. (From Mense, S., 1981. Brain Res. 225, 95.)

TRPM8 is important in cold hypersensitivity, which is often a feature of neuropathic pain. TRPA1 is activated in some experimental settings by noxious cold temperatures, calcium, pain-producing substances and inflammatory mediators; it can therefore also be considered to be a polymodal sensor. It may be important for the analgesic and antipyretic actions of paracetamol (see p. 559).

Kinins

When applied to sensory nerve endings, *bradykinin* and *kallidin* (see Ch. 19) induce intense pain. These two closely related peptides are produced under conditions of tissue injury by the proteolytic cleavage of the active kinins from a precursor protein contained in the plasma. Bradykinin acts partly by release of prostaglandins, which strongly enhance the direct action of bradykinin on the nerve terminals (Fig. 43.6). Bradykinin acts on B_2 receptors on nociceptive neurons. B_2 receptors are coupled to activation of a specific isoform of protein kinase C (PKCε), which phosphorylates TRPV1 and facilitates opening of the TRPV1 channel.

▼ Bradykinin is converted in tissues by removal of a terminal arginine residue to *des-Arg9 bradykinin*, which acts selectively on B_1 receptors. B_1 receptors are normally expressed at very low levels, but their expression is strongly up-regulated in inflamed tissues. Transgenic knock-out animals lacking either type of receptor show reduced inflammatory hyperalgesia. Specific competitive antagonists for both

---

[1]Anyone who has rubbed their eyes after cutting up chilli peppers will know this.
[2]The receptor was originally known as the vanilloid receptor because many capsaicin-like compounds are based on the structure of vanillic acid.

B_1 and B_2 receptors have been developed, such as the B_2 antagonist **icatibant**, used in the treatment of angioedema (Ch. 19), but none have yet been developed as analgesic agents.

Prostaglandins

Prostaglandins do not themselves cause pain, but they strongly enhance the pain-producing effect of other agents such as 5-HT or bradykinin (see Fig. 43.6). Prostaglandins of the E and F series are released in inflammation (Ch. 18) and also during tissue ischaemia. Antagonists at EP_1 receptors decrease inflammatory hyperalgesia in animal models. Prostaglandins sensitise nerve terminals to other agents, partly by inhibiting potassium channels and partly by facilitating – through second messenger-mediated phosphorylation reactions (see Ch. 3) – the cation channels opened by noxious agents. It is of interest that bradykinin itself causes prostaglandin release, and thus has a powerful 'self-sensitising' effect on nociceptive afferents. Other eicosanoids, including prostacyclin, leukotrienes and the unstable hydroxyeicosatetraenoic acid (HETE) derivatives (Ch. 18), may also be important. The analgesic effects of NSAIDs (Ch. 27) result from inhibition of prostaglandin synthesis.

Other peripheral mediators

Pro-inflammatory cytokines such as tumour necrosis factor-α (TNF-α) and interleukin-1β (IL-1β) (described in detail in Ch. 27) are released from macrophages to activate and sensitise nociceptive neurons (see Fig. 43.3) and contribute to persistent pain states.

Various metabolites and substances are released from damaged or ischaemic cells, or inflamed tissues, including ATP, protons (produced by lactic acid), 5-HT, histamine and K^+, many of which affect nociceptive nerve terminals.

ATP excites nociceptive nerve terminals (see Fig. 43.5) by acting on homomeric $P2X_3$ receptors or heteromeric $P2X_2/P2X_3$ receptors (see Ch. 17), ligand-gated ion channels that are selectively expressed by these neurons. Down-regulation of $P2X_3$ receptors, by antisense DNA, reduces inflammatory pain.[3] Antagonists at this receptor were developed as potential analgesic drugs. In a surprising development one such $P2X_3$ antagonist, **gefapixant** (formerly known as AF-219), has been shown to be effective in treating refractory cough (see Ch. 29). Other P2X receptors ($P2X_4$ and $P2X_7$) are expressed on microglia in the spinal cord; activation results in the release of cytokines and chemokines that then act on neighbouring neurons to promote hypersensitivity. ATP and other purine mediators, such as adenosine, also play a role in the dorsal horn, and other types of purinoceptor may also be targeted by analgesic drugs in the future. In the periphery adenosine exerts dual effects – acting on A_1 receptors it causes analgesia but on A_2 receptors it does the opposite.

Low pH excites nociceptive afferent neurons partly by opening proton-activated cation channels (acid-sensitive ion channels, ASICs) and partly by activation of TRPV1 (see p. 547).

5-HT causes excitation, but studies with antagonists suggest that it plays at most a minor role. Histamine is also active but causes itching rather than pain. Both these substances are released locally in inflammation (see Chs 16 and 18).

In summary, nociceptive nerve endings can be activated or sensitised by a wide variety of endogenous mediators, the receptors for which are often up- or down-regulated under pathophysiological conditions.

Mechanisms of pain and nociception

- Nociception is the mechanism whereby noxious peripheral stimuli are transmitted to the central nervous system. Pain is a subjective experience not always associated with nociception.
- Polymodal nociceptors (PMNs) are the main type of peripheral sensory neuron that responds to noxious stimuli. The majority are non-myelinated C fibres whose endings respond to thermal, mechanical and chemical stimuli.
- Chemical stimuli acting on PMNs to cause pain include bradykinin, protons, ATP and vanilloids (e.g. **capsaicin**). PMNs are sensitised by prostaglandins, which explains the analgesic effect of **aspirin**-like drugs, particularly in the presence of inflammation.
- The TRPV1 receptor responds to noxious heat as well as to **capsaicin**-like agonists.
- Nociceptive fibres terminate in the superficial layers of the dorsal horn, forming synaptic connections with transmission neurons running to the thalamus.
- PMN neurons release glutamate (fast transmitter) and various peptides that act as slow transmitters. Peptides are also released peripherally and contribute to neurogenic inflammation.
- Neuropathic pain, associated with damage to neurons of the nociceptive pathway rather than an excessive peripheral stimulus, is frequently a component of chronic pain states and may respond poorly to opioid analgesics.

ANALGESIC DRUGS

OPIOID DRUGS

Opium is an extract of the juice of the poppy *Papaver somniferum* that contains **morphine**, the prototypic opioid agonist, and other related alkaloids. It has been used for social and medicinal purposes for thousands of years as an agent to produce euphoria, analgesia and sleep, and to prevent diarrhoea. It was introduced in Britain at the end of the 17th century, usually taken orally as 'tincture of laudanum', addiction to which acquired a certain social cachet during the next 200 years. The situation changed when the hypodermic syringe and needle were invented in the mid-19th century, and opioid dependence began to take on a more sinister significance (see Ch. 50).

The history of opioid research is reviewed by Corbett et al. (2006).

CHEMICAL ASPECTS

The structure of morphine (Fig. 43.7) was determined in 1902, and since then many semisynthetic compounds (some

---

[3]P2X₃ knock-out mice are, in contrast, fairly normal in this respect, presumably because other mechanisms take over.

Fig. 43.7 **Chemical structures of morphine and related drugs.** The *shaded area* indicates the part of the morphine molecule that is structurally similar to tyrosine, the N-terminal amino acid in the endorphins. Carbon atoms 3 and 6 in the morphine structure are indicated. Diamorphine (heroin) is 3,6-diacetylmorphine, and morphine is metabolised by addition of a glucuronide moiety at either position 3 or position 6.

produced by chemical modification of morphine) and fully synthetic opioids have been developed in attempts to develop better analgesic drugs devoid of the unwanted side effects of morphine.

Morphine is a phenanthrene derivative with two planar rings and two aliphatic ring structures, which occupy a plane roughly at right-angles to the rest of the molecule (see Fig. 43.7). The most important parts of the molecule for opioid activity are the free hydroxyl on the benzene ring that is linked by two carbon atoms to a nitrogen atom. Variants of the morphine molecule have been produced by substitution at one or both of the hydroxyls (e.g. **diamorphine**[4] 3,6-diacetylmorphine, **codeine** 3-methoxymorphine and **oxycodone**). **Pethidine** and **fentanyl** represent more dramatic changes to the basic morphine structure whereas **methadone** and the novel opioid analgesics, **oliceridine** and **PZM21**, bear little obvious chemical relationship to morphine. Substitution of a bulky substituent on the nitrogen atom of morphine introduces antagonist activity to the molecule (e.g. **naloxone**).

OPIOID RECEPTORS

The proposal that opioids produce analgesia and their other effects by interacting with specific receptors first arose in the 1950s, based on the strict structural and stereochemical requirements essential for activity. It was, however, only with the development of molecules with antagonist activity (e.g. naloxone) that the notion of a specific receptor became accepted. Martin and co-workers then provided pharmacological evidence for multiple types of opioid receptors. They proposed three different types of receptor, called μ, κ and σ.[5] Subsequently, in the early 1970s, radioligand

Opioid analgesics

- Terminology:
  - *opioid*: any substance, whether endogenous or synthetic, that produces **morphine**-like effects that are blocked by antagonists such as **naloxone**;
  - *opiate*: compounds such as **morphine** and **codeine** that are found in the opium poppy;
  - *narcotic analgesic*: old term for opioids; *narcotic* refers to their ability to induce sleep. Unfortunately, the term narcotic has subsequently been hijacked and used inappropriately by some to refer generically to drugs of abuse (see Ch. 50).
- Important structurally related agonists include **diamorphine**, **oxycodone** and **codeine**.
- Synthetic analogues include **pethidine**, **fentanyl**, **methadone**, **buprenorphine**.
- Opioid analgesics may be given orally, by injection or intrathecally to produce analgesia.

binding (see Ch. 2) was used to demonstrate the presence of μ receptors in the brain.

Why are there specific receptors in the brain for morphine, a drug that is present in the opium poppy? Hughes and Kosterlitz argued that there must be an endogenous substance or substances in the brain that activated these receptors.[6] In 1975 they reported the isolation and characterisation of the first endogenous ligands, the *enkephalins*. We now know that the enkephalins are only two members of a larger family of endogenous opioid peptides known collectively as the *endorphins*, all of which possess a tyrosine residue at their N-terminus. The chemical structure of tyrosine includes an amine group separated from a phenol ring by two carbon atoms. This same structure (phenol-2 carbon atom chain-amine) is also contained within the

---

[4]While 'diamorphine' is the recommended International Nonproprietary Name (rINN), this drug is widely known as heroin.
[5]The σ 'receptor' is no longer considered to be an opioid receptor. It was originally postulated in order to account for the dysphoric effects (anxiety, hallucinations, bad dreams, etc.) produced by some opioids. It is now accepted that these effects result from drug-induced block of the NMDA receptor channel pore, an effect that is also produced by agents such as ketamine (see Ch. 42). Novel σ receptors – σ₁ and σ₂ subtypes – have now been cloned and characterized. They are not structurally related to other receptor types and little is known about their physiological role, but they have been suggested as novel drug targets for psychiatric disorders.

[6]It may seem obvious today that if there is a receptor then there is likely also to be an endogenous ligand for that receptor but it was the search for, and subsequent discovery of, the enkephalins that gave credence to this idea.

morphine structure (see Fig. 43.7). It is probably just chance (good or bad luck depending on one's viewpoint) that the opium poppy synthesises a semi-rigid alkaloid molecule, morphine, part of which structurally resembles the tyrosine residue in the endogenous opioid peptides.

Following on from the discovery of the enkephalins, pharmacological and ligand-binding studies revealed another receptor, δ, and the three recognised receptor types (μ, δ and κ) were cloned. Later, another opioid receptor (ORL$_1$) that had a high a degree of amino acid sequence homology (>60%) towards the μ, δ and κ opioid receptors was identified by cloning techniques, although the antagonist, naloxone, did not bind to this new receptor. The terminology used for opioid receptors has over the years been through several revisions; in this chapter we shall use the classical terminology. The four opioid receptors, μ, δ, κ and NOP (originally referred to as opioid receptor like receptor 1 or ORL$_1$) are all G protein–coupled receptors (see Ch. 3).[7] The main behavioural effects resulting from their activation are summarised in Table 43.2. The interaction of various endogenous opioid peptides with the various receptor types is summarised in Table 43.3. Some agents that are used as experimental tools for distinguishing the different receptor types are also shown.

The development of transgenic mouse strains lacking each of the three main opioid receptor types has revealed that the major pharmacological effects of morphine, including analgesia, are mediated by the μ receptor.

All four opioid receptors appear to form homomeric as well as heteromeric receptor complexes (see Ch. 3). Opioid receptors are, in fact, quite promiscuous and can form heteromers with non-opioid receptors. Heteromerisation between opioid receptors has been shown to result in pharmacological characteristics distinct from those observed with the monomeric receptors and may explain some of the subtypes of each receptor that have been proposed (see Fujita et al., 2014). Another level of complexity may reflect 'bias' (see Ch. 3), whereby different ligands acting on the same opioid receptor can elicit different cellular responses and differential receptor trafficking (see Kelly, 2013).[8]

MECHANISM OF ACTION OF OPIOIDS

The opioids have probably been studied more intensively than any other group of drugs in the effort to understand their powerful effects in molecular, cellular and physiological terms, and to use this understanding to develop new drugs as analgesics with significant advantages over morphine. Even so, morphine – described by Osler as 'God's own medicine' – remains the standard against which any new analgesic is assessed.

---

[7]The opioid receptors are unusual among G protein–coupled receptors. First, in that there are many (20 or more) opioid peptides but only four receptors. In contrast, 5-hydroxytryptamine (5-HT), for example, is a single mediator interacting with many (about 14) receptors, which is the more common pattern. Second, all four receptors couple to the same types of G protein (G$_i$/G$_o$) and therefore activate the same spectrum of cellular effector mechanisms. In contrast, other receptor families (e.g. muscarinic receptors) couple to different types of G proteins and therefore give rise to different cellular responses (see Ch. 14).

[8]Claims have been made recently that 'G protein biased' μ opioid receptor ligands will show a reduced side-effect profile in comparison to morphine which is 'unbiased', but time will tell if this is indeed true.

Table 43.2 Functional effects associated with the main types of opioid receptor

Receptor	μ	δ	κ	NOP
Analgesia				
Supraspinal	+++	—?	—	Anti-opioid[a]
Spinal	++	++	+	++
Peripheral	++	—	++	—
Respiratory depression	+++	++	—	—
Pupil constriction	++	—	+	—
Reduced gastrointestinal motility	++	++	+	—
Euphoria	+++	—	—	—
Dysphoria and hallucinations	—	—	+++	—
Sedation	++	—	++	—
Catatonia	—	—	—	++
Physical dependence	+++	—	—	—

[a]NOP receptor agonists were originally thought to produce nociception or hyperalgesia but it was later shown that they reverse the supraspinal analgesic effects of endogenous and exogenous μ receptor agonists.

Cellular actions

All four types of opioid receptor belong to the family of G$_i$/G$_o$ protein–coupled receptors. Opioids thus exert powerful effects on ion channels on neuronal membranes through a direct G protein coupling to the channel. Opioids promote the opening of potassium channels (see Ch. 4) and inhibit the opening of voltage-gated calcium channels. These membrane effects decrease neuronal excitability (because the increased K$^+$ conductance causes hyperpolarisation of the membrane making the cell less likely to fire action potentials) and reduce transmitter release (due to inhibition of Ca^{2+} entry). The overall effect is therefore inhibitory at the cellular level. Nonetheless, opioids do increase activity in some neuronal pathways (see p. 545, Fig. 43.4). They cause excitation of projection neurons by suppressing the activity of inhibitory interneurons that tonically inhibit the projection neurons (see Ch. 38, Fig. 38.2).

At the biochemical level, all four receptor types inhibit adenylyl cyclase and cause MAP kinase (ERK) activation (see Ch. 3). These cellular responses are likely to be important in mediating the long-term adaptive changes that occur in response to prolonged receptor activation and which, for μ receptor agonists, may underlie the phenomenon of physical dependence (see Ch. 50).

At the cellular level, therefore, all four types of opioid receptor mediate very similar effects. It is their heterogeneous anatomical distributions across the CNS that give rise to the different behavioural responses seen with selective agonists for each type of receptor.

Table 43.3 Endogenous opioid peptides and receptor-selective drugs

	μ	δ	κ	NOP
Endogenous peptides				
β-Endorphin	+++	+++	+	–
Leu-enkephalin	(++)	+++	+	–
Met-enkephalin	++	+++	+	–
Dynorphin	+	+	+++	–
Orphanin FQ/nociceptin[a]	–	–	–	+++
Research tools				
AGONISTS				
DAMGO[b]	+++	–	–	–
DPDPE[b]	–	++	–	–
Enadoline	–	–	+++	–
Ro64-6198	–	–	–	+++
Antagonists				
CTOP[b]	+++	–	–	–
Naltrindole	–	+++	+	–
Nor-binaltorphimine	+	+	+++	–
SB 612111	–	–	–	+++

Note: + symbols represent agonist or antagonist activity; partial agonists in parentheses; – symbols represent weak or no activity.

[a]The endogenous ligand for the NOP receptor is referred to in the literature both as orphanin FQ and as nociceptin.
[b]DAMGO, DPDPE and CTOP are synthetic peptides.

Opioid receptors

- μ Receptors are responsible for most of the analgesic effects of opioids, and for some major unwanted effects (e.g. respiratory depression, constipation, euphoria, sedation and dependence).
- δ Receptor activation results in analgesia but also can be proconvulsant.
- κ Receptors contribute to analgesia at the spinal level and may elicit sedation, dysphoria and hallucinations. Some analgesics are mixed κ agonists/μ antagonists.
- NOP receptors are also members of the opioid-receptor family. Activation results in an antiopioid effect (supraspinal), analgesia (spinal), immobility and impairment of learning.
- σ Receptors are not true opioid receptors but are the site of action of certain psychotomimetic drugs, with which some opioids also interact.
- All opioid receptors are linked through G_i/G_o proteins and thus open potassium channels (causing hyperpolarisation) and inhibit the opening of calcium channels (inhibiting transmitter release). In addition, they inhibit adenylyl cyclase and activate the MAP kinase (ERK) pathway.
- Functional heteromers, formed by combination of different types of opioid receptor or with other types of G protein–coupled receptor, may occur and give rise to further pharmacological diversity.

Sites of action of opioids to produce analgesia

Opioid receptors are widely distributed in the brain and spinal cord. Opioids are effective as analgesics when injected in minute doses into a number of specific brain nuclei (such as the insular cortex, amygdala, hypothalamus, PAG region and RVM) as well as into the dorsal horn of the spinal cord (see Fig. 43.4). There is evidence to suggest that supraspinal opioid analgesia involves endogenous opioid peptide release both at supraspinal and spinal sites and that at the spinal level there is also a component of the analgesia that results from the release of serotonin (5-HT) from descending inhibitory fibres. Surgical interruption of the descending pathway from the RVM to the spinal cord reduces analgesia induced by morphine that has been given systemically or microinjected into supraspinal sites, implying that a combination of effects at supraspinal and spinal sites contribute to the analgesic response.

At the spinal level, morphine inhibits transmission of nociceptive impulses through the dorsal horn and suppresses nociceptive spinal reflexes, even in patients with spinal cord transection. It can act presynaptically to inhibit release of various neurotransmitters from primary afferent terminals in the dorsal horn as well as acting postsynaptically to reduce the excitability of dorsal horn neurons.

There is also evidence (see Sawynok, 2003) that opioids inhibit the discharge of nociceptive afferent terminals in the periphery, particularly under conditions of inflammation, in which the expression of opioid receptors by sensory neurons is increased. Injection of morphine into the knee joint following surgery to the joint provides effective analgesia, undermining the age-old belief that opioid analgesia is exclusively a central phenomenon.

PHARMACOLOGICAL ACTIONS

Morphine is typical of many opioid analgesics and will be taken as the reference compound. Its effects are mediated predominately through μ receptors.

The most important effects of morphine are on the CNS and the gastrointestinal tract, although numerous effects of lesser significance on many other systems have been described.

Effects on the CNS

Analgesia

Morphine and other opioids are highly effective in most kinds of acute pain as well as in 'end of life' pain resulting from cancer. They are less effective in treating neuropathic and other chronic pain states.

Hyperalgesia

In both animal studies and in patients receiving opioids for pain relief, prolonged exposure to opioids may paradoxically induce a state of hyperalgesia in which pain sensitisation or allodynia occurs (see Lee et al., 2011). This can appear as a reduced analgesic response to a given dose of opioid but should not be confused with tolerance, which is a reduced responsiveness due in large part to µ receptor desensitisation (see p. 553) and occurs with other opioid-induced effects such as euphoria and to a lesser extent respiratory depression. Hyperalgesia appears to have peripheral, spinal and supraspinal components. At the neuronal level, an array of mediators and mechanisms have been proposed to contribute to this phenomenon (Roeckel et al., 2016). These include NO, PKC and NMDA receptor activation. In addition, $P2X_4$ receptor expression in microglia is up-regulated resulting in BDNF release, TrkB signalling and down-regulation of the K^+/Cl^- co-transporter KCC2. In mice in which BDNF has been deleted from microglia, hyperalgesia to morphine does not occur, whereas antinociception and tolerance are unaffected. Opioid-induced hyperalgesia can be reduced by ketamine (an NMDA antagonist), propofol (an intravenous anaesthetic), α_2-adrenoceptor agonists and COX-2 inhibitors. Switching to another opioid can also reduce hyperalgesia; in this regard, methadone may be a good choice as it is a weak NMDA-receptor antagonist.

Euphoria

Morphine causes a powerful sense of contentment and well-being (see also Ch. 50). This may contribute to its analgesic effect. If morphine or diamorphine (heroin) is given intravenously, the result is a sudden 'rush' likened to an 'abdominal orgasm'. The euphoria produced by morphine depends considerably on the circumstances. In patients who are distressed, it is pronounced, but in patients who become accustomed to chronic pain, morphine causes analgesia with little or no euphoria. Some patients report restlessness rather than euphoria under these circumstances.

Euphoria is mediated through µ receptors, whereas κ receptor activation produces dysphoria and hallucinations (see Table 43.2). Thus, different opioid drugs vary greatly in the amount of euphoria that they produce. It does not occur with codeine to any marked extent. There is evidence that antagonists at the κ receptor have antidepressant properties which may indicate that release of endogenous κ agonists may occur in depression.

Respiratory depression

Respiratory depression, resulting in increased arterial $P\text{CO}_2$, occurs with a normal analgesic dose of morphine or related compounds, although in patients in severe pain the degree of respiratory depression produced may be less than anticipated. Respiratory depression is mediated by µ receptors. The depressant effect is associated with a decrease in the sensitivity of the respiratory centres to arterial $P\text{CO}_2$ and an inhibition of respiratory rhythm generation. Changes in $P\text{CO}_2$ are detected by chemosensitive neurons in a number of brain stem and medullary nuclei. Increased arterial CO_2 (hypercapnia) thus normally results in a compensatory increase in minute ventilation rate (V_E). In some of the chemosensitive regions, opioids exert a depressant effect on the hypercapnic response, making the increase in V_E insufficient to counteract the increased CO_2. Respiratory movements originate from activity of a rhythm generator (the *pre-Bötzinger complex*) within the ventral respiratory column of the medulla. µ opioid receptors are located in this region, and local injection of opioid agonists decreases respiratory frequency.

Respiratory depression by opioids is not accompanied by depression of the medullary centres controlling cardiovascular function (in contrast to the action of general anaesthetics and other CNS depressants). This means that respiratory depression produced by opioids is much better tolerated than a similar degree of depression caused by, say, a barbiturate. Nonetheless, respiratory depression is a dangerous unwanted effect of these drugs and, unlike that due to general CNS depressant drugs, it occurs at therapeutic doses. It is the commonest cause of death in acute opioid poisoning.

Depression of cough reflex

Cough suppression (antitussive effect; see also Ch. 29), surprisingly, does not correlate closely with the analgesic and respiratory depressant actions of opioids, and its mechanism at the receptor level is unclear. In general, increasing substitution on the phenolic hydroxyl group of morphine increases antitussive relative to analgesic activity. **Codeine** and **pholcodine** suppress cough in subanalgesic doses but they cause constipation as an unwanted effect.

▼ **Dextromethorphan**, the dextro-isomer of the opioid analgesic **levorphanol**, suppresses cough but has very low affinity for opioid receptors and its cough suppressing action, unlike that of opioids, is not antagonised by naloxone. It is an uncompetitive NMDA receptor antagonist – this might explain why at high doses it evokes CNS effects similar to ketamine and may be abused – and has putative actions at σ receptors. It is believed to work at various sites in the brain stem and medulla to suppress cough. In addition to its antitussive action, dextromethorphan is neuroprotective (see Ch. 41) and has an analgesic action in neuropathic pain.

Nausea and vomiting

Nausea and vomiting occur in up to 40% of patients to whom morphine is given, and do not seem to be separable from the analgesic effect among a range of opioid analgesics. The site of action is the *area postrema* (chemoreceptor trigger zone), a region of the medulla where chemical stimuli of many kinds may initiate vomiting (see Ch. 31).[9] Nausea and vomiting following morphine injection are usually transient and disappear with repeated administration, although in some individuals they persist and can limit patient compliance.

Pupillary constriction

Pupillary constriction is caused by µ and κ receptor-mediated stimulation of the oculomotor nucleus. Pinpoint pupils are an important diagnostic feature in opioid poisoning,[10] because most other causes of coma and respiratory depression produce pupillary dilatation. Tolerance does not develop to the pupillary constriction induced by opioids and therefore can be observed in opioid-dependent drug users who may have been taking opioids for a considerable time.

Effects on the gastrointestinal tract

Opioids increase tone and reduce motility in many parts of the gastrointestinal system, resulting in constipation, which may be severe and very troublesome to the patient.[11]

---

[9]The chemically related compound apomorphine is more strongly emetic than morphine, through its action as a dopamine agonist; despite its name, it is inactive on opioid receptors.

[10]The exception is pethidine, which causes pupillary dilatation because it blocks muscarinic receptors.

[11]In treating pain, constipation is regarded as an undesirable side effect. However, opiates such as codeine and morphine can be used to treat diarrhoea.

The resulting delay in gastric emptying can considerably retard the absorption of other drugs. Pressure in the biliary tract increases because of contraction of the gall bladder and constriction of the biliary sphincter. Opioids should be avoided in patients suffering from biliary colic due to gallstones, in whom pain may be increased rather than relieved. The rise in intrabiliary pressure can cause a transient increase in the concentration of amylase and lipase in the plasma.

The action of morphine on visceral smooth muscle is probably mediated mainly through the intramural nerve plexuses, because the increase in tone is reduced or abolished by atropine. It is also partly mediated by a central action, because intracerebroventricular injection of morphine inhibits propulsive gastrointestinal movements. **Methylnal-trexone bromide** (see also Ch. 9) **alvimopan** and **naloxegol** are opioid antagonists that do not cross the blood–brain barrier. They have been developed to reduce unwanted peripheral side effects of opioids, such as constipation, without significantly reducing analgesia or precipitating withdrawal in dependent individuals.

Other actions of opioids

Morphine releases histamine from mast cells by an action unrelated to opioid receptors. Pethidine and fentanyl do not produce this effect. The release of histamine can cause local effects, such as urticaria and itching at the site of the injection, or systemic effects, namely bronchoconstriction and hypotension.

Hypotension and bradycardia occur with large doses of most opioids, due to an action on the medulla. With morphine and similar drugs, histamine release may contribute to the hypotension.

Effects on smooth muscle other than that of the gastrointestinal tract and bronchi are slight, although spasms of the ureters, bladder and uterus sometimes occur. Opioids also exert complex immunosuppressant effects, which may be important as a link between the nervous system and immune function. The pharmacological significance of this is not yet clear, but there is evidence in humans that the immune system is depressed by long-term opioid use, and that in addicts suffering from AIDS the use of opioids may exacerbate the immune deficiency.

TOLERANCE AND DEPENDENCE

Tolerance to many of the actions of opioids (i.e. an increase in the dose needed to produce a given pharmacological effect) develops within a few days during repeated administration. There is some controversy over whether significant tolerance develops to the analgesic effects of morphine, especially in palliative care patients with severe cancer pain (see McQuay, 1999; Ballantyne & Mao, 2003). Drug rotation (changing from one opioid to another) is frequently used clinically to overcome loss of effectiveness. As tolerance is likely to depend upon the level of receptor occupancy, the degree of tolerance observed may reflect the response being assessed (e.g. analgesia versus respiratory depression), the intrinsic efficacy of the drug and the dose being administered (see Hayhurst & Durieaux, 2016).

Physical dependence refers to a state in which withdrawal of the drug causes adverse physiological effects, i.e. the abstinence syndrome.

Different adaptive cellular mechanisms underlie tolerance and dependence (see Williams et al., 2013; see also Chs 2 and 50). These phenomena occur to some degree whenever

Actions of morphine

- The main pharmacological effects are:
  - analgesia
  - euphoria and sedation
  - respiratory depression
  - suppression of cough
  - nausea and vomiting
  - pupillary constriction
  - reduced gastrointestinal motility, causing constipation
  - histamine release, causing itch, bronchoconstriction and hypotension
- The most troublesome unwanted effects are nausea and vomiting, constipation and respiratory depression.
- Acute overdosage with **morphine** produces coma and respiratory depression.
- **Diamorphine** (heroin) is inactive at opioid receptors but is rapidly cleaved in the brain to 6-acetylmorphine and **morphine**.
- **Codeine** is also converted to **morphine** but more slowly by liver metabolism.

opioids are administered for more than a few days. They must not be confused with addiction (see Ch. 50), in which physical dependence is much more pronounced and psychological dependence (or 'craving') is the main driving force.

Tolerance

In animal experiments, tolerance can be detected even with a single dose of morphine. Tolerance extends to most of the pharmacological effects of morphine, including analgesia, emesis, euphoria and respiratory depression, but affects the constipating and pupil-constricting actions much less. Therefore, addicts may take 50 times the normal analgesic dose of morphine with relatively little respiratory depression but marked constipation and pupillary constriction.

The cellular mechanisms responsible for tolerance are discussed in Chapter 2. Tolerance results in part from desensitisation of the μ receptors (i.e. at the level of the drug target) as well as from long-term adaptive changes at the cellular, synaptic and network levels (see Williams et al., 2013). Tolerance is a general phenomenon of opioid receptor ligands, irrespective of which type of receptor they act on. Cross-tolerance occurs between drugs acting at the same receptor, but not between opioids that act on different receptors. In clinical settings, the opioid dose required for effective pain relief may increase as a result of developing tolerance, but it does not constitute a major problem.

Physical dependence

Physical dependence is characterised by a clear-cut abstinence syndrome. In experimental animals (e.g. rats), abrupt withdrawal of morphine after repeated administration for a few days, or the administration of an antagonist such as naloxone, causes an increased irritability, diarrhoea, loss of weight and a variety of abnormal behaviour patterns, such as body shakes, writhing, jumping and signs of aggression. These reactions decrease after a few days, but abnormal irritability and aggression persist for many weeks. The signs of physical dependence are much less intense if the opioid is withdrawn gradually. Humans often experience an abstinence syndrome when opioids are withdrawn after being used for pain relief over days or weeks, with symptoms of restlessness, runny nose, diarrhoea, shivering and piloerection.[12]

Many physiological changes have been described in relation to the abstinence syndrome. For example, spinal reflex hyperexcitability occurs in morphine-dependent animals and can be produced by chronic intrathecal as well as systemic administration of morphine. The noradrenergic pathways emanating from the LC (see Ch. 40) may also play an important role in causing the abstinence syndrome. The rate of firing of LC neurons is reduced by opioids and increased during the abstinence syndrome. The α_2-adrenoceptor agonist **lofexidine** (Ch. 15) can be used to alleviate withdrawal symptoms. In animal models, and also in humans, the abstinence syndrome can also be reduced by giving NMDA receptor antagonists (e.g. ketamine).

Tolerance and dependence

- Tolerance develops rapidly.
- The mechanism of tolerance involves receptor desensitisation. It is not pharmacokinetic in origin.
- Dependence comprises two components:
  - physical dependence, associated with the withdrawal syndrome and lasting for a few days;
  - psychological dependence, associated with craving and lasting for months or years; it rarely occurs in patients being given opioids as analgesics.
- Physical dependence, characterised by a withdrawal syndrome on cessation of drug administration, occurs with μ receptor agonists.
- The withdrawal syndrome is precipitated by μ receptor antagonists.
- Long-acting μ receptor agonists such as **methadone** and **buprenorphine** may be used to relieve withdrawal symptoms.
- Certain opioid analgesics, such as **codeine**, **buprenorphine** and **tramadol**, are much less likely to cause physical or psychological dependence.

PHARMACOKINETIC ASPECTS

Table 43.4 summarises the pharmacokinetic properties of the main opioid analgesics. The absorption of morphine congeners by mouth is variable. Morphine itself is slowly and erratically absorbed, and is commonly given by intravenous injection to treat acute severe pain; oral morphine is, however, often used in treating chronic pain, and slow-release preparations are available to increase its duration of action. Oxycodone is also available as a slow-release oral preparation. Codeine is well absorbed and normally given by mouth. Most morphine-like drugs undergo considerable first-pass metabolism, and are therefore markedly less potent when taken orally than when injected.

The plasma half-life of most morphine analogues is 3–6 h. Hepatic metabolism is the main mode of inactivation, usually by conjugation with glucuronide. This occurs at the 3- and 6-OH groups (see Fig. 43.7), and these glucuronides constitute a considerable fraction of the drug in the bloodstream. Morphine-6-glucuronide is more active as an analgesic than morphine itself, and contributes to the pharmacological effect. Morphine-3-glucuronide has been claimed to antagonise the analgesic effect of morphine, but the significance of this experimental finding is uncertain, as this metabolite has little or no affinity for opioid receptors. Morphine glucuronides are excreted in the urine, so the dose needs to be reduced in cases of renal failure. Glucuronides also reach the gut via biliary excretion, where they are hydrolysed, most of the morphine being reabsorbed (enterohepatic circulation). Because of low conjugating capacity in neonates, morphine-like drugs have a much longer duration of action; because even a small degree of respiratory depression can be hazardous, morphine congeners should not be used in the neonatal period, nor used as analgesics during childbirth. Pethidine (see p. 557) is a safer alternative for this purpose.

Analogues that have no free hydroxyl group in the 3 position (i.e. diamorphine, codeine) are converted to morphine, which accounts for all or part of their pharmacological activity. With heroin the conversion occurs rapidly in the brain but with codeine the effect is slower and occurs by metabolism in the liver. Morphine produces very effective analgesia when administered intrathecally, and is used in this way by anaesthetists, the advantage being that the sedative and respiratory depressant effects are reduced, although not completely avoided. **Remifentanil** is rapidly hydrolysed and eliminated with a half-life of 3–4 min. The advantage of this is that when given by intravenous infusion during general anaesthesia, the level of the drug can be manipulated rapidly when required (see Ch. 11 for a description of how, for intravenous infusion, both the rate of rise and the rate of decay of the plasma concentration are determined by the half-time of elimination).

In postoperative and cancer pain, opioids are often given 'on demand' (patient-controlled analgesia). The patients are provided with an infusion pump that they control, the maximum possible rate of administration being limited to avoid acute toxicity. Patients show little tendency to use excessively large doses and become dependent; instead, the dose is adjusted to achieve analgesia without excessive sedation, and is reduced as the pain subsides. Being in control of their own analgesia, the patients' anxiety and distress are reduced, and analgesic consumption actually tends to decrease. In chronic pain, patients often experience sudden, sharp increases in the level of pain they are experiencing. This is referred to as breakthrough pain. To combat this, there is a therapeutic need to be able to increase rapidly the amount of opioid being administered. This has led to the development of touch-sensitive transdermal patches containing potent opioids such as fentanyl that rapidly release drug into the bloodstream. Fentanyl lozenges and lollipops, producing rapid absorption through the buccal mucosa, are also used.

The opioid antagonist, naloxone, has a shorter biological half-life than most opioid agonists. In the treatment of opioid overdose, it must be given repeatedly to avoid the respiratory depressant effect of the agonist reoccurring once the naloxone has been eliminated. Naltrexone has a longer biological half-life.

---

[12]Causing goose pimples. This is the origin of the phrase 'cold turkey' used to describe the effect of morphine withdrawal.

Table 43.4 Characteristics of the main opioid analgesic drugs

Drug	Use(s)	Route(s) of administration	Pharmacokinetic aspects	Main adverse effects	Notes
Morphine	Widely used for acute and chronic pain	Oral, including sustained-release form Injection[a] Intrathecal	Half-life 3–4 h Converted to active metabolite (morphine-6-glucuronide)	Sedation Respiratory depression Constipation Nausea and vomiting Itching (histamine release) Tolerance and dependence Euphoria	Tolerance and withdrawal effects not common when used for analgesia
Diamorphine (heroin)	Acute and chronic pain	Oral Injection	Acts more rapidly than morphine because of rapid brain penetration.	As morphine	Not available in all countries Metabolised to morphine and other active metabolites
Hydromorphone	Acute and chronic pain	Oral Injection	Half-life 2–4 h No active metabolites	As morphine but allegedly less sedative	Levorphanol is similar, with longer duration of action
Oxycodone	Acute and chronic pain	Oral, including sustained-release form Injection	Half-life 3–4.5 h	As morphine	Has become a major drug of abuse Hydrocodone, used primarily in the United States, is similar
Methadone	Chronic pain Maintenance of addicts	Oral Injection	Long half-life (>24 h) Slow onset	As morphine but less euphoric effect Accumulation may occur	Slow recovery results in attenuated withdrawal syndrome because of long half-life
Pethidine	Acute pain	Oral Intramuscular injection	Half-life 2–4 h Active metabolite (norpethidine) may account for stimulant effects	As morphine Anticholinergic effects Risk of excitement and convulsions	Known as meperidine in United States Interacts with monoamine oxidase inhibitors (Ch. 48)
Buprenorphine	Acute and chronic pain Maintenance of addicts	Sublingual Injection Transdermal patch Intrathecal	Half-life about 12 h Slow onset Inactive orally because of first-pass metabolism	As morphine but less pronounced Respiratory depression not reversed by naloxone (therefore not suitable for obstetric use) May precipitate opioid withdrawal (partial agonist)	Useful in chronic pain with patient-controlled injection systems

Continued

Table 43.4 Characteristics of the main opioid analgesic drugs—cont'd

Drug	Use(s)	Route(s) of administration	Pharmacokinetic aspects	Main adverse effects	Notes
Dipipanone	Moderate to severe pain	Oral	Half-life 3.5 h (although there are longer values quoted)	In addition to effects similar to morphine it produces psychosis	Marketed in combination with cyclazine (Diconal) and became a popular intravenous drug of abuse
Fentanyl	Acute pain Anaesthesia	Intravenous Sublingual Transdermal patch	Half-life 1–2 h	As morphine	High potency allows transdermal administration Sufentanil is similar
Remifentanil	Anaesthesia	Intravenous infusion	Half-life 5 min	Respiratory depression	Very rapid onset and recovery
Codeine	Mild pain	Oral	Acts as prodrug Metabolised to morphine and other active metabolites	Mainly constipation Low dependence liability	Effective only in mild pain Also used to suppress cough Dihydrocodeine is similar
Dextropropoxyphene	Mild pain	Mainly oral	Half-life ~4 h Active metabolite (norpropoxyphene) with half-life ~24 h	Respiratory depression May cause convulsions (possibly by action of norpropoxyphene)	Similar to codeine No longer recommended
Tramadol	Acute (mainly postoperative) and chronic pain	Oral Intravenous	Well absorbed Half-life 4–6 h	Dizziness May cause convulsions No respiratory depression	Mechanism of action uncertain Weak agonist at opioid receptors Also inhibits monoamine uptake. Tapentadol is similar

[a]Injections may be given intravenously, intramuscularly or subcutaneously for most drugs.

UNWANTED EFFECTS

The main unwanted effects of morphine and related drugs are listed in Table 43.4.

Acute overdosage with morphine results in coma and respiratory depression, with characteristically constricted pupils. It is treated by giving naloxone intramuscularly or intravenously. This also serves as a diagnostic test, for failure to respond to naloxone suggests a cause other than opioid poisoning for the comatose state.[13] There is a danger of precipitating a severe withdrawal syndrome with naloxone, because opioid poisoning occurs mainly in addicts.

Individual variability

▼ Individuals vary by as much as 10-fold in their sensitivity to opioid analgesics. This can be due to altered metabolism or altered sensitivity of the receptors (for extensive review, see Rollason et al., 2008). For morphine, reduced responsiveness may result from mutations in a number of genes including that for the drug transporter, P-glycoprotein (see Chs 10 and 12), for glucuronyltransferase that metabolises morphine and for the μ receptor itself. Mutations of various cytochrome P450 (CYP) enzymes influence the metabolism of codeine, oxycodone, methadone, tramadol and dextromethorphan. Genotyping could in principle be used to identify opioid-resistant individuals, but first the contribution of genotype to clinical outcome must be confirmed in the population at large.

OTHER OPIOID ANALGESICS

Diamorphine (heroin) is 3,6-diacetylmorphine; it can be considered as a prodrug because its high analgesic potency is attributable to rapid conversion to 6-monoacetylmorphine and morphine. Its effects are indistinguishable from those of morphine following oral administration. However, because of its greater lipid solubility, it crosses the blood–brain barrier more rapidly than morphine and gives a greater 'buzz' when injected intravenously. It is said to be less emetic than morphine, but the evidence for this is slight. It is still available in Britain for use as an analgesic, although it is banned in many countries. Its only advantage over morphine is its greater solubility, which allows smaller volumes to be given orally, subcutaneously or intrathecally. It exerts the same respiratory depressant effect as morphine and, if given intravenously, is more likely to cause dependence.

Codeine (3-methoxymorphine) is also a prodrug but, unlike heroin, undergoes demethylation by CYP2D6 in the liver to produce morphine. It has 20% or less of the analgesic potency of morphine, as a large proportion of the absorbed drug is not converted to morphine but instead undergoes hepatic glucuronidation and is then excreted. Its analgesic effect does not increase appreciably at higher dose levels, presumably because of limited conversion to morphine, and so it is sometimes referred to as a weak agonist. It is more reliably absorbed by mouth than morphine and is therefore used mainly as an oral analgesic for mild types of pain (headache, backache, etc.). About 10% of the population is resistant to the analgesic effect of codeine, because they lack the demethylating enzyme that converts it to morphine. Unlike morphine, it causes little or no euphoria and is rarely addictive. It is often combined with **paracetamol** in proprietary analgesic preparations (see later section on combined use of opioids and NSAIDs). In relation to its analgesic effect, codeine produces the same degree of respiratory depression as morphine, but the limited response, even at high doses, means that it is seldom a problem in practice. It does, however, cause constipation. Codeine has marked antitussive activity and is often used in cough mixtures (see Ch. 29). **Dihydrocodeine** is pharmacologically very similar, having no substantial advantages or disadvantages over codeine.

Oxycodone is used in the treatment of acute and chronic pain. The suggestion that it acts on a subtype of κ opioid receptor is not generally accepted. Claims that it has less euphoric effect and less abuse potential are unfounded. It is available as a slow-release oral preparation, as is **hydrocodone** which is similar in action. Misprescribing of these drugs has led to them becoming major drugs of abuse, especially in North America (see Ch. 50).

Fentanyl, **alfentanil**, **sufentanil** and **remifentanil** are highly potent phenylpiperidine derivatives, with actions similar to those of morphine but with a more rapid onset and shorter duration of action, particularly remifentanil. They are used extensively in anaesthesia, and they may be given intrathecally. **Carfentanil** is a more potent analogue used to sedate large animals. Fentanyl, alfentanil and sufentanil are also used in patient-controlled infusion systems and in severe chronic pain, when they are administered via patches applied to the skin. The rapid onset is advantageous in breakthrough pain. Fentanyl has minimal cardiovascular effects and does not release histamine. In recent years, illegally produced fentanyl, carfentanil and a range of other analogues have become major drugs of abuse, especially in the United States (See Ch. 50). Unlike other opioids, they are easily synthesised, without the need to harvest poppies.

Methadone is orally active and pharmacologically similar to morphine, the main difference being that its duration of action is considerably longer (plasma half-life >24 h). The increased duration seems to occur because the drug is bound in the extravascular compartment and slowly released. On withdrawal, the physical abstinence syndrome is less acute than with morphine, although the psychological dependence is no less pronounced. Methadone is widely used as a means of treating heroin addiction (see Ch. 50). It is possible to wean addicts from heroin by giving regular oral doses of methadone – an improvement, if not a cure.[14] Methadone has actions at other sites in the CNS, including block of potassium channels, NMDA receptors and 5-HT receptors, that may explain its CNS side-effect profile. There is also interindividual variation in the response to methadone, probably due to genetic variability between individuals in its metabolism.

Pethidine (meperidine) is very similar to morphine in its pharmacological effects, except that it tends to cause restlessness rather than sedation. It was originally investigated as a new antimuscarinic agent but was found to have opioid analgesic activity; its residual antimuscarinic action being responsible for its side effects of dry mouth and blurring of vision. It produces a very similar euphoric effect and is equally liable to cause dependence. Its duration of action is the same or slightly shorter than that of

---

[13]Naloxone is less effective in reversing the effects of buprenorphine as this agonist dissociates very slowly from the receptors.

[14]The benefits come mainly from removing the risks of self-injection and the need to finance the drug habit through crime.

morphine, but the route of metabolic degradation is different. Pethidine is partly *N*-demethylated in the liver to norpethidine, which has hallucinogenic and convulsant effects. These become significant with large oral doses of pethidine, producing an overdose syndrome rather different from that of morphine. Pethidine is preferred to morphine for analgesia during labour, because it does not reduce the force of uterine contraction. Pethidine is only slowly eliminated in the neonate, and naloxone may be needed to reverse respiratory depression in the newborn (morphine is even more problematic in this regard, because the conjugation reactions on which the excretion of morphine, but not of pethidine, depends are deficient in the newborn). Severe reactions, consisting of excitement, hyperthermia and convulsions, have been reported when pethidine is given to patients receiving monoamine oxidase inhibitors. This seems to be due to inhibition of an alternative metabolic pathway, leading to increased norpethidine formation, but the details are unclear.

Etorphine is a morphine analogue with a potency more than 1000 times that of morphine, but otherwise very similar in its actions. Its high potency confers no particular human clinical advantage, but it is used in veterinary practice, especially in large animals. It can be used in conjunction with sedative agents (neuroleptanalgesia) to immobilise wild animals for trapping.[15]

Buprenorphine is a partial agonist on μ receptors that produces strong analgesia but there is a ceiling to its respiratory depressant effect. Because of its antagonist actions, it can produce mild withdrawal symptoms in patients dependent on other opioids. It dissociates slowly from the receptors and so has a long duration of action and can be difficult to reverse with naloxone. It has abuse liability but, like methadone, it is also used in the treatment of heroin addiction. When heroin is injected 'on top' of buprenorphine, less euphoria is obtained because buprenorphine is a partial agonist. It is marketed as a sublingual preparation combined with naloxone for the management of opioid dependence; when administered as intended the naloxone is not absorbed and does not influence the effect of the buprenorphine, but if it is administered parenterally the effects of the buprenorphine are hopefully reduced by the naloxone, discouraging such abuse. How effective this is in practice has been questioned.

Meptazinol is an opioid of unusual chemical structure. It can be given orally or by injection and has a duration of action shorter than that of morphine. It seems to be relatively free of morphine-like side effects, causing neither euphoria nor dysphoria, nor severe respiratory depression. It does, however, produce nausea, sedation and dizziness, and has atropine-like actions. Because of its short duration of action and lack of respiratory depression, it may have advantages for obstetric analgesia.

Tramadol and **tapentadol** are widely used as analgesics for postoperative pain. Tramadol comprises two structural enantiomers – (+)-tramadol inhibits 5-HT reuptake and (−)-tramadol inhibits NA reuptake – and the major metabolite of (+)-tramadol, O-desmethyltramadol activates the μ receptor. Tapentadol inhibits NA reuptake and activates the μ receptor. They are effective analgesics and appear to have a better side-effect profile than most opioids, although

psychiatric reactions have been reported. They are given by mouth or by intramuscular or intravenous injection for acute and chronic pain, including musculoskeletal pain and the pain associated with diabetic neuropathy.

Nalbuphine is an analgesic that has activity at κ, μ, and to a lesser extent, δ receptors. It acts as an agonist at κ receptors and as a partial agonist at μ receptors. **Pentazocine**, rarely used clinically nowadays, also combines a degree of κ agonist and μ antagonist (or weak partial agonist) activity. These agents are thought to produce less euphoria than μ receptor agonists. **Cebranopadol**, currently in late stages of clinical trials, is an agonist at all four opioid receptors.

Loperamide is a μ receptor agonist that is effectively extruded from the brain by P-glycoprotein and therefore lacks analgesic activity. It inhibits peristalsis, and is used to control diarrhoea (see Ch. 31).

OPIOID ANTAGONISTS

Naloxone was the first pure opioid antagonist, with affinity for all three classic opioid receptors (μ > κ ≥ δ). It blocks the actions of endogenous opioid peptides as well as those of morphine-like drugs and has been extensively used as an experimental tool to determine the physiological role of these peptides, particularly in pain transmission.

Given on its own, naloxone produces very little effect in normal subjects but produces a rapid reversal of the effects of morphine and other opioids. It has little effect on pain threshold under normal conditions but causes hyperalgesia under conditions of stress or inflammation, when endogenous opioids are produced. This occurs, for example, in patients undergoing dental surgery, or in animals subjected to physical stress. Naloxone also inhibits acupuncture analgesia, which is known to be associated with the release of endogenous opioid peptides, but does not reduce meditation-induced analgesia. Analgesia produced by PAG stimulation is also prevented by naloxone.

The main clinical uses of naloxone are to treat respiratory depression caused by opioid overdosage (see Ch. 50), and occasionally to reverse the effect of opioid analgesics, used during labour, on the respiration of the newborn baby. It can be administered nasally, intramuscularly or intravenously, and its effects are rapid in onset. It is rapidly metabolised by the liver, and its effect lasts only 2–4 h, which is considerably shorter than that of most morphine-like drugs and therefore it may have to be given repeatedly.

Naloxone has no important unwanted effects of its own but precipitates withdrawal symptoms in addicts. It can be used to detect opioid addiction.

Naltrexone is very similar to naloxone but with the advantage of a much longer duration of action (half-life about 10 h). It may be of value in addicts who have been 'detoxified', because it nullifies the effect of a dose of opioid should the patient's resolve fail. For this purpose, it is available in a slow-release subcutaneous implant formulation. It is also effective in reducing alcohol consumption in heavy drinkers (see Ch. 50), the rationale being that part of the high from alcohol comes from the release of endogenous opioid peptides. **Nalmefene**, another non-selective opioid antagonist, is also used to treat alcoholics. Naltrexone may also have beneficial effects in septic shock. It is effective in treating chronic itching (pruritus), as occurs in chronic liver disease. Again, this may indicate the involvement of endogenous opioid peptides in the pathophysiology of such itch conditions.

---

[15]The required dose of etorphine, even for an elephant, is small enough to be incorporated into a dart or pellet.

Methylnaltrexone bromide, **alvimopan** and **naloxegol** are μ receptor antagonists that do not cross the blood–brain barrier. They can be used in combination with opioid agonists to block unwanted effects, most notably reduced gastrointestinal motility, nausea and vomiting.

Specific antagonists at μ, δ and κ receptors are available for experimental use (see Table 43.3) but they are not used clinically.

Opioid antagonists

- Pure antagonists include **naloxone** (short acting) and **naltrexone** (longer acting). They block μ, δ and κ receptors. Selective antagonists are available as experimental tools.
- **Alvimopan** and naloxegol are μ receptor antagonists that do not cross the blood–brain barrier. They block opioid-induced constipation, nausea and vomiting.
- **Naloxone** does not affect pain threshold normally but blocks stress-induced analgesia and can exacerbate clinical pain.
- **Naloxone** rapidly reverses opioid-induced analgesia and respiratory depression, and is used mainly to treat opioid overdose or to improve breathing in newborn babies affected by opioids given to the mother.
- **Naloxone** precipitates withdrawal symptoms in **morphine**-dependent patients or animals. **Buprenorphine** (a partial agonist) can also precipitate withdrawal due to its antagonist action against higher efficacy opioid agonists.

PARACETAMOL

Non-steroidal antiinflammatory drugs (NSAIDs, covered in detail in Ch. 27) are widely used to treat painful inflammatory conditions and to reduce fever. **Paracetamol** (known as **acetaminophen** in the United States) deserves special mention here. It was first synthesised more than a century ago, and since the 1950s has (alongside aspirin and ibuprofen) been the most widely used over-the-counter remedy for minor aches and pains. Paracetamol differs from other NSAIDs in producing analgesic and antipyretic effects while lacking anti-inflammatory effects. It also lacks the tendency of other NSAIDs to cause gastric ulceration and bleeding. The reason for the difference between paracetamol and other NSAIDs is unclear. Biochemical tests showed it to be only a weak cyclo-oxygenase (COX) inhibitor, with some selectivity for brain COX, possibly because of the unique reducing environment in neurones (see Ch. 27). Interestingly, the antinociceptive and antipyretic effects of paracetamol are absent in mice lacking the TRPA1 receptor (see p. 547). These effects appear to be mediated by a metabolite (*N*-acetyl-*p*-benzoquinoneimine), not by paracetamol itself. This activates TRPA1 and thus reduces voltage-gated calcium and sodium currents in primary sensory neurons.

Paracetamol is well absorbed by mouth, and its plasma half-life is about 3 h. It is metabolised by hydroxylation, conjugated mainly as glucuronide, and excreted in the urine. In therapeutic doses, it has few adverse effects. However, in overdose, paracetamol causes severe liver damage, which is commonly fatal (see Chs 27 and 58), and the drug is often used in attempted suicide.

USE OF OPIOIDS AND NSAIDS IN COMBINATION

The rationale behind co-administration of two drugs that produce analgesia by different mechanisms is that, if the effects are additive, less of each drug can therefore be given but the same degree of analgesia produced. This has the effect of reducing the intensity of the unwanted side effects produced by each drug. In the case of opioids (e.g. codeine) in combination with paracetamol or aspirin, the combination appears to produce synergy rather than simple additivity. The combination of dextropropoxyphene and paracetamol has been withdrawn in the United Kingdom due to concerns about overdosing.

TREATMENT OF CHRONIC PAIN

Chronic pain, that which persists beyond normal healing time and which includes pain of musculoskeletal or neuropathic origin, involves not only the processing of nociceptive information but also comprises emotional and psychosocial components (e.g. mood, circumstance, stress, duration, meaning, acceptance, expectation and fear), more so than acute or cancer-related pain (see Stannard, 2016). These other components may render opioid drugs less effective in the long-term treatment of chronic pain (i.e. treatment lasting more than 12 weeks)[16]. The British Medical Association have concluded that 'There is a lack of good-quality evidence to support a strong clinical recommendation for the long-term use of opioids for patients with chronic pain' (see BMA, 2017).

Several non-opioid drugs that are also used clinically for effects other than analgesia have been found to be effective in neuropathic pain (see Dworkin et al., 2010; BMA, 2017), largely as a result of serendipitous observations rather than a rational programme of drug discovery.

Tricyclic antidepressants, particularly **amitriptyline**, **nortriptyline** and **desipramine** (Ch. 48) are widely used. These drugs act centrally by inhibiting noradrenaline reuptake and are effective in relieving neuropathic pain in some, but not all, cases. Their action is independent of their antidepressant effects. Drugs such as **duloxetine** and **venlafaxine**, which inhibit serotonin and noradrenaline uptake, are also effective and have a different side-effect profile, but selective serotonin reuptake inhibitors show little or no benefit.

Gabapentin and its congener, **pregabalin**, are antiepileptic drugs (Ch. 46) that are also effective in the treatment of neuropathic pain. They reduce the expression of α2δ subunits of voltage-activated calcium channels on the nerve membrane (see Ch. 4) and reduce neurotransmitter release. The α2δ subunits are up-regulated in damaged sensory neurons, which may explain why these agents are more effective across a range of pain states associated with nerve damage than in other forms of pain.

Carbamazepine, another type of anti-epileptic drug, is effective in trigeminal neuralgia but evidence for effectiveness against other neuropathic pains is lacking. Carbamazepine blocks voltage-gated sodium channels

---

[16]Over the past 30 years there has been widespread long-term prescribing of opioids for chronic pain in the developed world leading to an alarming increase in addiction to prescription opioids and to overdose deaths (see Ch 50).

(see Ch. 4) being slightly more potent in blocking $Na_v1.8$ than $Na_v1.7$ and $Na_v1.3$ channels; all of these channel subtypes are thought to be up-regulated by nerve damage and contribute to the sensation of pain. At higher concentrations, it inhibits voltage-activated calcium channels. **Phenytoin** administered intravenously is sometimes used in a crisis.

Other antiepileptic agents such as **valproic acid**, **lamotrigine**, **oxcarbazepine**, **topiramate** and **levetiracetam** may have efficacy in some neuropathic pain states.

Lidocaine (lignocaine), a local anaesthetic drug (Ch. 44), can be used topically to relieve neuropathic pain. It probably acts by blocking spontaneous discharges from damaged sensory nerve terminals. Some antidysrhythmic drugs (e.g. **mexiletine**, **tocainide**, **flecainide**; see Ch. 22) are effective orally.

The abundance of drugs and mechanisms deployed to alleviate chronic pain reflects the current lack of drugs that work effectively and reliably in this common and serious condition, the cause of which is often unclear. Psychological treatments are often used in addition to drugs.

Drugs used to treat neuropathic pain

- Various antidepressants (e.g. **amitriptyline**, **duloxetine**) provide therapeutic benefit.
- **Gabapentin** and **pregabalin** are now used more to relieve neuropathic pain than as antiepileptic agents.
- **Carbamazepine**, as well as some other antiepileptic agents that block sodium channels, can be effective in treating trigeminal neuralgia.
- **Lidocaine** may provide relief when applied topically.

TREATMENT OF FIBROMYALGIA

Fibromyalgia is a chronic disorder characterised by widespread musculoskeletal pain, fatigue and insomnia. Its cause is unknown, with no obvious characteristic pathology being apparent. It is associated with allodynia. Classical analgesics (i.e. NSAIDs and opioids), while bringing some relief, are not very effective in treating this disorder. Various antidepressant drugs (e.g. amitriptyline, **citalopram**, **milnacipran**, duloxetine, venlafaxine; see Ch. 48), antiepileptic agents (e.g. gabapentin, pregabalin; see Ch. 46), benzodiazepines (e.g. **clonazepam**, **zopiclone**; see Ch. 45) are currently used for this disorder – this long list reflecting their uncertain efficacy.

OTHER PAIN-RELIEVING DRUGS

Nefopam, an inhibitor of amine uptake with some sodium channel-blocking properties is used in the treatment of persistent pain unresponsive to opioid drugs. It does not depress respiration but does produce sympathomimetic and antimuscarinic side effects.

Ketamine, a dissociative anaesthetic (Ch. 42), **memantine** and **dextromethorphan** work by blocking NMDA receptor channels, and probably reduce the wind-up phenomenon in the dorsal horn (see Fig. 43.2). Given intrathecally, ketamine's effects on memory and cognitive function are largely

avoided. It is used for acute pain relief rather than long-term treatment.

Ziconotide, a synthetic analogue of the N-type calcium-channel blocking peptide ω-conotoxin MVIIA, is effective when administered by the intrathecal route. It is used in patients whose pain does not respond to other analgesic agents. Blockers of low voltage-activated T-type calcium channels may also be effective analgesics in some pain states.

Cannabinoids (see Ch. 20) acting at CB_1 receptors are effective pain-relieving agents in animal pain models, including models of acute, antinociceptive, inflammatory and neuropathic pain. There is also mounting evidence that these agents are effective in reducing pain in humans (see Barnes & Barnes, 2016). The strongest evidence of therapeutic benefit is for central neuropathic pain in multiple sclerosis. Effective cannabinoids include synthetic agents such as **nabilone** and **dronabinol** as well as natural cannabinoids such as **nabiximols** (formerly known by its trade name **Sativex**). **Nabiximols** is an extract of the cannabis plant containing Δ^9-tetrahydrocannabinol (THC) and cannabidiol that has been suggested to have improved therapeutic efficacy. CB_2 receptor agonists may also be potential analgesic agents.

In addition, cannabinoids and related drugs that lack agonist action at CB_1 receptors have been observed to induce analgesia by potentiating the actions of the inhibitory amino acid glycine at the ionotropic glycine receptor (see Ch. 39) in the spinal cord. This may lead to the development of new therapeutic agents lacking the unwanted effects of CB_1 agonism.

Botulinum toxin injections are effective in relieving back pain and the pain associated with spasticity. This effect is due mainly to a relief of muscle spasm (Ch. 14).

Ropinirole, **pramipexole** and **rotigotine**, dopamine-receptor agonists (see Ch. 40), are used to treat restless leg syndrome, which can be painful in some individuals.

Other analgesic drugs

- **Paracetamol** resembles non-steroidal anti-inflammatory drugs and is effective as an analgesic, but it lacks anti-inflammatory activity. It may act by inhibiting cyclo-oxygenase (COX)-3, a splice variant of COX-1, but probably has other effects as well. In overdose, it causes hepatotoxicity.
- **Nefopam** is an amine uptake inhibitor that can be used to treat opioid-resistant pain.
- The NMDA receptor antagonist **ketamine** is occasionally used as a short-term treatment.

NEW APPROACHES

▼ As in other fields of neuropharmacology, increasing knowledge of the various chemical mediators and signalling pathways responsible for pain sensation suggests many new approaches to the control of pain. Pain treatment is currently far from perfect, and a vast array of novel approaches, too numerous be covered in detail here, are currently being explored (see Gilron & Dickenson, 2014; McEntire et al., 2016).

Clinical uses of analgesic drugs (1)

- Analgesics are used to treat and prevent pain, for example:
  - pre- and postoperatively
  - common painful conditions including headache, dysmenorrhoea, labour, trauma and burns
  - many medical and surgical emergencies (e.g. myocardial infarction and renal colic)
  - terminal disease (especially metastatic cancer)
- Opioid analgesics are used in some non-painful conditions, for example acute heart failure (because of their haemodynamic effects) and terminal chronic heart failure (to relieve distress).
- The choice and route of administration of analgesic drugs depends on the nature and duration of the pain.
- A progressive approach is often used, starting with non-steroidal anti-inflammatory drugs (NSAIDs), supplemented first by weak opioid analgesics and then by strong opioids.
- In general, severe acute pain is treated with strong opioids (e.g. **morphine**, **fentanyl**) given by injection. Mild inflammatory pain (e.g. sprains, mild arthralgia) is treated with NSAIDs (e.g. **ibuprofen**) or by **paracetamol** supplemented by weak opioids (e.g. **codeine**). Severe pain (e.g. cancer pain) is treated with strong opioids given orally, intrathecally, epidurally or by subcutaneous injection. Patient-controlled infusion systems are useful postoperatively.
- Chronic neuropathic pain is less responsive to opioids and can be treated with tricyclic antidepressants (e.g. **amitriptyline**) or anticonvulsants (e.g. **carbamazepine**, **gabapentin**).

Clinical uses of analgesic drugs (2)

- Non-steroidal anti-inflammatory drugs (see first clinical box), including **paracetamol**, are useful for musculoskeletal and dental pain and for dysmenorrhoea. They reduce opioid requirements in acute (e.g. postoperative) and chronic (e.g. bone metastasis) pain.
- Weak opioids (e.g. **codeine**) combined with **paracetamol** are useful in moderately severe pain if non-opioids are not sufficient. **Tramadol** and **tapentadol** (a weak opioid with additional action on 5-hydroxytryptamine and noradrenaline uptake) are alternatives.
- Strong opioids (e.g. **morphine**) are used for severe pain, particularly of visceral origin.
- Note that:
  - the intravenous route provides rapid relief from pain and distress;
  - the intravenous dose is much lower than the oral dose because of presystemic metabolism;
  - **morphine** is given orally as a solution or as 'immediate-release' tablets every 4 h;
  - dose is titrated; when the daily requirement is apparent, the preparation is changed to a modified-release formulation to allow once- or twice-daily dosing;
  - **morphine** and **oxycodone** can be given orally in slow-release tablet form;
  - transdermal administration (e.g. patches of **fentanyl**) is an alternative, rapid means of pain relief;
  - adverse effects (nausea, constipation) are anticipated and treated pre-emptively;
  - addiction is not an issue in the setting of terminal care.
- Subanaesthetic doses of **nitrous oxide** (Ch. 42) are analgesic, and self-administration of a mixture of **nitrous oxide** with oxygen is widely used during labour or for painful dressing changes.

REFERENCES AND FURTHER READING

General

Apkarian, A.V., Bushnell, M.C., Schweinhardt, P., 2013. Representation of pain in the brain. In: McMahon, S.B., Koltzenburg, M., Tracey, I., Turk, D.C. (Eds.), Wall & Melzack's Textbook of Pain, sixth ed. Elsevier, Philadelphia, pp. 111–128. (*Detailed account of central pathways that inhibit or enhance transmission in the dorsal horn*)

Todd, A.J., Koerber, H.R., 2013. Neuroanatomical substrates of spinal nociception. In: McMahon, S.B., Koltzenburg, M., Tracey, I., Turk, D.C. (Eds.), Wall & Melzack's Textbook of Pain, sixth ed. Elsevier, Philadelphia, pp. 77–93. (*Detailed account of central pathways that inhibit or enhance transmission in the dorsal horn*)

McMahon, S.B., Koltzenburg, M., Tracey, I., Turk, D.C. (Eds.), 2013. Wall & Melzack's Textbook of Pain, sixth ed. Elsevier, Philadelphia. (*Large multiauthor reference book*)

Yaksh, T.L., 1999. Spinal systems and pain processing: development of novel analgesic drugs with mechanistically defined models. Trends Pharmacol. Sci. 20, 329–337. (*Good general review article on spinal cord mechanisms – more general than its title suggests*)

TRP channels

Nilius, B., Szallasi, A., 2014. Transient receptor potential channels as drug targets: from the science of basic research to the art of medicine. Pharmacol. Rev. 66, 676–814. (*Extensive review of the potential of TRP channels for drug development*)

BDNF and TrkA

Mantyh, P.W., Koltzenburg, M., Mendell, L.M., Tive, L., Shelton, D.L., 2011. Antagonism of nerve growth factor-TrkA signaling and the relief of pain. Anesthesiology 115, 189–204.

Opioids

Ballantyne, J.C., Mao, J., 2003. Opioid therapy for chronic pain. N. Engl. J. Med. 349, 1943–1953. (*Considers whether or not tolerance is a problem when opioids are used to treat chronic pain*)

Bingel, U., Tracey, I., Wiech, K., 2012. Neuroimaging as a tool to investigate how cognitive factors influence analgesic drug outcomes. Neurosci. Lett. 520, 149–155.

BMA, 2017. Chronic pain: supporting safer prescribing of analgesics. Available at https://www.bma.org.uk/collective-voice/policy-and-research/public-and-population-health/analgesics-use.

Corbett, A.D., Henderson, G., McKnight, A.T., et al., 2006. 75 years of opioid research: the exciting but vain search for the holy grail. Br. J. Pharmacol. 147, S153–S162. (*Comprehensive historical review of opioid research*)

Fujita, W., Gomes, I., Devi, L.A., 2014. Revolution in GPCR signalling: opioid receptor heteromers as novel therapeutic targets: IUPHAR review 10. Br. J. Pharmacol. 171, 4155–4176.

Hayhurst, C.J., Durieux, M.E., 2016. Differential opioid tolerance and opioid-induced hyperalgesia: a clinical reality. Anesthesiology 124, 483–488. (*Discusses the potential adverse consequences of tolerance developing more to the analgesic that respiratory depressant effects of opioids*)

Kelly, E., 2013. Efficacy and ligand bias at the μ-opioid receptor. Br. J. Pharmacol. 169, 1430–1446. (*Gentle introduction to the topic of ligand bias*)

Lee, M., Silverman, S.M., Hansen, H., Patel, V.B., Manchikanti, L., 2011. A comprehensive review of opioid-induced hyperalgesia. Pain Physician 14, 145–161.

McQuay, H., 1999. Opioids in pain management. Lancet 353, 2229–2232. (*Discusses whether or not tolerance occurs to opioids in clinical situations*)

Roeckel, L.A., Le Coz, G.M., Gavériaux-Ruff, C., Simonin, F., 2016. Opioid-induced hyperalgesia: cellular and molecular mechanisms. Neuroscience 338, 160–182.

Rollason, V., Samer, C., Piquet, V., et al., 2008. Pharmacogenetics of analgesics: towards the personalization of prescription. Pharmacogenomics 9, 905–933.

Sawynok, J., 2003. Topical and peripherally acting analgesics. Pharmacol. Rev. 55, 1–20. (*Review of the numerous mechanisms by which drugs interfere with nociceptive mechanisms in the periphery*)

Stannard, C., 2016. Opioids and chronic pain: using what we know to change what we do. Curr. Opin. Support. Palliat. Care 10, 129–136. (*An interesting article that tries to explain why opioids are not very effective in the treatment of chronic pain*)

Williams, J.T., Ingram, S.L., Henderson, G., et al., 2013. Regulation of μ-opioid receptors: desensitization, phosphorylation, internalization, and tolerance. Pharmacol. Rev. 65, 223–254. (*Very comprehensive review of the molecular and cellular mechanisms underlying opioid tolerance*)

Neuropathic pain and new drug targets

Barnes, M.P., Barnes, J.C., 2016. Cannabis: the evidence for medical use. All Party Parliamentary Group on Drug Policy Reform report. Available at https://drive.google.com/file/d/0B0c_8hkDJu0DUDZMUzhoY1RqMG8/view. (*A very comprehensive review of clinical trials of natural and synthetic cannabinoids for a range of disorders including pain*)

Dworkin, R.H., O'Connor, A.B., Audette, J., et al., 2010. Recommendations for the pharmacological management of neuropathic pain: an overview and literature update. Mayo Clin. Proc. 85 (3 Suppl.), S3–S14. (*An evaluation of the clinical effectiveness of current drugs used to treat neuropathic pain*)

Gilron, I., Dickenson, A.H., 2014. Emerging drugs for neuropathic pain. Expert Opin. Emerg. Drugs 19, 329–341. (*Contains details on a range of new drugs in development for the treatment of neuropathic pain*)

McEntire, D.M., Kirkpatrick, D.R., Dueck, N.P., et al., 2016. Pain transduction: a pharmacologic perspective. Expert Rev. Clin. Pharmacol. 9, 1069–1080. (*Reviews the development of analgesic drugs interacting with TRP, ASIC and Na^+ channels*)

Local anaesthetics and other drugs affecting sodium channels

OVERVIEW

As described in Chapter 4, the property of electrical excitability is what enables the membranes of nerve and muscle cells to generate propagated action potentials, which are essential for communication in the nervous system and for the initiation of mechanical activity in striated muscle. Initiation of the action potential depends on voltage-gated sodium channels, which open transiently when the membrane is depolarised. Here we discuss local anaesthetics, which act mainly by blocking sodium channels, and mention briefly other drugs that affect sodium-channel function.

There are, broadly speaking, two ways in which channel function may be modified, namely block of the channels and modification of gating behaviour. Blocking sodium channels reduces excitability. On the other hand, different types of drugs can either facilitate channel opening and thus increase excitability, or inhibit channel opening and reduce excitability.

LOCAL ANAESTHETICS

Although many drugs can, at high concentrations, block voltage-sensitive sodium channels and inhibit the generation of the action potential, the only drugs used clinically for this effect are the local anaesthetics, various antiepileptic and analgesic drugs (see Chs 43 and 46) and class I antidysrhythmic drugs (see Ch. 22).

HISTORY

Coca leaves have been chewed for their psychotropic effects for thousands of years (see Ch. 49) by South American Indians, who knew about the numbing effect they produced on the mouth and tongue. **Cocaine** was isolated in 1860 and proposed as a local anaesthetic for surgical procedures. Sigmund Freud, who tried unsuccessfully to make use of its 'psychic energising' power, gave some cocaine to his ophthalmologist friend in Vienna, Carl Köller, who reported in 1884 that reversible corneal anaesthesia could be produced by dropping cocaine on to the eye. The idea was rapidly taken up, and within a few years cocaine anaesthesia was introduced into dentistry and general surgery. A synthetic substitute, **procaine**, was discovered in 1905, and many other useful compounds were later developed.

CHEMICAL ASPECTS

Local anaesthetic molecules consist of an aromatic part linked by an ester or amide bond to a basic side chain (Fig. 44.1). They are weak bases, with pK_a values mainly in the range 8–9, so that they are mainly, but not completely, ionised at physiological pH (see Ch. 9 for an explanation of how pH influences the ionisation of weak bases). This is important in relation to their ability to penetrate the nerve sheath and axon membrane; quaternary derivatives such as QX-314, which are fully ionised irrespective of pH, are ineffective as local anaesthetics but have important experimental uses. **Benzocaine**, an atypical local anaesthetic, has no basic group.

The presence of the ester or amide bond in local anaesthetic molecules is important because of its susceptibility to metabolic hydrolysis. The ester-containing compounds are fairly rapidly inactivated in the plasma and tissues (mainly liver) by non-specific esterases. Amides are more stable, and these anaesthetics generally have longer plasma half-lives.

MECHANISM OF ACTION

Local anaesthetics block the initiation and propagation of action potentials by preventing the voltage-dependent increase in Na^+ conductance (see Ch. 4 and Strichartz & Ritchie, 1987; Hille, 2001). At low concentrations they decrease the rate of rise of the action potential, increasing its duration, and increase the refractory period thus reducing the firing rate. At higher concentrations they prevent action potential firing. Currently available local anaesthetic agents do not, by and large, distinguish between different sodium-channel subtypes, although their potencies vary (see Ch. 4). They block sodium channels by physically plugging the transmembrane pore, interacting with various amino acid residues of the S6 transmembrane helical domain of the channel protein (see Catterall & Swanson, 2015).

▼ Local anaesthetic activity is strongly pH-dependent, being increased at alkaline extracellular pH (i.e. when the proportion of ionised molecules is low) and reduced at acid pH. This is because the compound needs to penetrate the nerve sheath and the axon membrane to reach the inner end of the sodium channel (where the local anaesthetic-binding site resides). Because the ionised form is not membrane-permeant, penetration is very poor at acid pH. Once inside the axon, it is primarily the ionised form of the local anaesthetic molecule that binds to the channel and blocks it (Fig. 44.2), the unionised form having only weak channel-blocking activity. This pH dependence can be clinically important, because the extracellular fluid of inflamed tissues is often relatively acidic and such tissues are thus somewhat resistant to local anaesthetic agents.

Further analysis of local anaesthetic action (see Strichartz & Ritchie, 1987) has shown that many drugs exhibit the property of 'use-dependent' block of sodium channels, as well as affecting, to some extent, the gating of the channels. Use-dependence means that the more the channels are opened, the greater the block becomes. It is a prominent feature of the action of many class I antidysrhythmic drugs (Ch. 22) and antiepileptic drugs (Ch. 46), and occurs because the blocking

563

Fig. 44.1   Structures of local anaesthetics. The general structure of local anaesthetic molecules consists of an aromatic group *(left)*, ester or amide group *(shaded blue)* and amine group *(right)*.

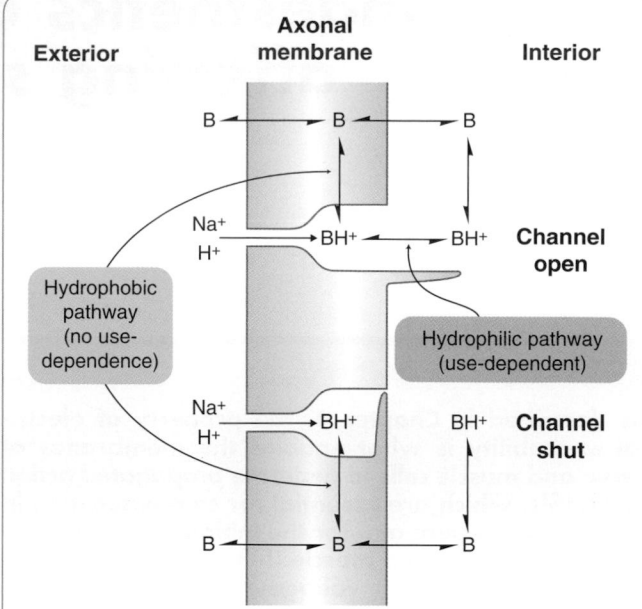

Fig. 44.2   Interaction of local anaesthetics with sodium channels. The blocking site within the channel can be reached via the open channel gate on the inner surface of the membrane by the charged species BH$^+$ (hydrophilic pathway), or directly from the membrane through fenestrations in the channel wall by the uncharged species B (hydrophilic pathway).

effect by reducing the number of channels available for opening, and by prolonging the refractory period following an action potential. The passage of a train of action potentials, for example, in response to a painful stimulus, causes the channels to cycle through the open and inactivated states, both of which are more likely to bind local anaesthetic molecules than the resting state; thus both mechanisms contribute to use dependence, which explains in part why pain transmission may be blocked more effectively than other sensory modalities.

Quaternary amine local anaesthetics only work when applied to the inside of the membrane and the channels must be cycled through their open state a few times before the blocking effect appears. With tertiary amine local anaesthetics, block can develop even if the channels are not open, and it is likely that the blocking molecule (uncharged) can reach the channel either directly from the membrane phase through fenestrations in the channel protein that allow uncharged molecules to access the pore of the channel in the resting (closed) state or from the intracellular side via the open gate (see Fig. 44.2). The relative importance of these two blocking pathways – the hydrophobic pathway via the membrane and the hydrophilic pathway via the inner mouth of the channel – varies according to the lipid solubility of the drug.

In general, local anaesthetics block conduction in small-diameter nerve fibres more readily than in large fibres. Because nociceptive impulses are carried by Aδ and C fibres (Ch. 43), pain sensation is blocked more readily than other sensory modalities (touch, proprioception, etc.). Motor axons, being large in diameter, are also relatively resistant. The differences in sensitivity among different nerve fibres, although easily measured experimentally, are not of much practical importance, and it is not possible to block pain sensation without affecting other sensory modalities.

Local anaesthetics, as their name implies, are mainly used to produce local nerve block. At low concentrations, they are also able to suppress the spontaneous action potential discharge in sensory neurons that occurs in neuropathic pain. The properties of individual local anaesthetic drugs are summarised in Table 44.1.

molecule enters the channel much more readily when the channel is open than when it is closed. Furthermore, for local anaesthetics that rapidly dissociate from the channel, block only occurs at high frequencies of action potential firing when the time between action potentials is too short for drug dissociation from the channel to occur. The channel can exist in three functional states: resting, open and inactivated (see Ch. 4). Many local anaesthetics bind most strongly to the inactivated state of the channel. Therefore, at any given membrane potential, the equilibrium between resting and inactivated channels will, in the presence of a local anaesthetic, be shifted in favour of the inactivated state, and this factor contributes to the overall blocking

Table 44.1 Properties of local anaesthetics

Drug	Onset	Duration	Tissue penetration	Plasma half-life (h)	Main unwanted effects	Notes
Cocaine	Medium	Medium	Good	~1	Cardiovascular and CNS effects owing to block of amine uptake	Rarely used, only as spray for upper respiratory tract
Procaine	Medium	Short	Poor	<1	CNS: restlessness, shivering, anxiety, occasionally convulsions followed by respiratory depression Cardiovascular system: bradycardia and decreased cardiac output; vasodilatation, which can cause cardiovascular collapse	The first synthetic agent No longer used **Chloroprocaine** is also short acting and is used to produce intrathecal anaesthesia
Lidocaine (lignocaine)	Rapid	Medium	Good	~2	As procaine but less tendency to cause CNS effects	Widely used for local anaesthesia Also used intravenously for treating ventricular dysrhythmias though no longer as first choice (Ch. 22)
Mepivacaine	Rapid	Medium	Good	~2	As procaine	Less vasodilatation (may be administered without a vasoconstrictor)
Tetracaine (amethocaine)	Very slow	Long	Moderate	~1	As lidocaine	Used mainly for anaesthesia before venipuncture or venous cannulation
Bupivacaine	Slow	Long	Moderate	~2	As lidocaine but greater cardiotoxicity	Widely used because of long duration of action Ropivacaine is similar, with less cardiotoxicity Levobupivacaine causes less cardiotoxicity and CNS depression than the racemate, bupivacaine
Prilocaine	Medium	Medium	Moderate	~2	No vasodilator activity Can cause methaemoglobinaemia	Widely used; not for obstetric analgesia because of risk of neonatal methaemoglobinaemia
Articaine	Rapid	Short	Good	~0.5	As lidocaine	Used in dentistry While its chemical structure contains an amide linkage it also has an ester group on a side chain (see Fig. 44.1). Hydrolysis of the side chain inactivates the drug

CNS, central nervous system.

UNWANTED EFFECTS

When used clinically as local anaesthetics, the main unwanted effects involve the central nervous system (CNS) and the cardiovascular system (see Table 44.1). Their action on the heart can also be of use in treating cardiac arrhythmias (see Ch. 22). Although local anaesthetics are usually administered in such a way as to minimise their spread to other parts of the body, they are ultimately absorbed into the systemic circulation. They may also be injected into veins or arterioles in error.

Most local anaesthetics produce a mixture of depressant and stimulant effects on the CNS. Depressant effects predominate at low plasma concentrations, giving way to stimulation at higher concentrations, resulting in restlessness, tremor and sometimes convulsions, accompanied by subjective effects ranging from confusion to extreme agitation. Further increasing the dose produces profound CNS

---

depression and death due to respiratory depression. The only local anaesthetic with markedly different CNS effects is **cocaine** (see Ch. 49), which produces euphoria at doses well below those that cause other CNS effects. This relates to its specific effect to inhibit monoamine uptake, an effect not shared by other local anaesthetics. **Procaine** is particularly liable to produce unwanted central effects, and has been superseded in clinical use by agents such as **lidocaine** and **prilocaine**. Studies with **bupivacaine**, a widely used long-acting local anaesthetic prepared as a racemic mixture of two optical isomers, suggested that its CNS and cardiac effects were mainly due to the $S(+)$ isomer. The $R(-)$ isomer (**levobupivacaine**) has a better margin of safety.

Actions of local anaesthetics

- Local anaesthetics block action potential generation by blocking sodium channels.
- Local anaesthetics are amphiphilic molecules with a hydrophobic aromatic group and a basic amine group.
- Local anaesthetics are weak bases that act in their cationic form but must reach their site of action by penetrating the nerve sheath and axonal membrane as un-ionised species.
- Many local anaesthetics show use-dependence (depth of block increases with action potential frequency). This arises:
  - because anaesthetic molecules gain access to the channel more readily when the channel is open;
  - because anaesthetic molecules have higher affinity for inactivated than for resting channels.
- Use-dependence is mainly of importance in relation to antidysrhythmic and antiepileptic effects of sodium-channel blockers.
- Local anaesthetics block conduction in peripheral nerves in the following order: small myelinated axons, non-myelinated axons, large myelinated axons. Nociceptive and sympathetic transmission is thus blocked first.
- Sodium-channel block in cardiac muscle and in central nervous system neurons is exploited in the therapy of cardiac dysrhythmias (Ch. 22) and epilepsy (Ch. 46).

The adverse cardiovascular effects of local anaesthetics are due mainly to myocardial depression, conduction block and vasodilatation. Reduction of myocardial contractility probably results indirectly from an inhibition of the Na^+ current in cardiac muscle (see Ch. 22). The resulting decrease of $[Na^+]_i$ in turn reduces intracellular Ca^{2+} stores (see Ch. 4), and this reduces the force of contraction. Interference with atrioventricular conduction can result in partial or complete heart block, as well as other types of dysrhythmia. **Ropivacaine** has less cardiotoxicity than bupivacaine.

Vasodilatation, mainly affecting arterioles, is due partly to a direct effect on vascular smooth muscle, and partly to inhibition of the sympathetic nervous system. This leads to a fall in blood pressure, which may be sudden and life-threatening. Cocaine is an exception in respect of its cardiovascular effects, because of its ability to inhibit noradrenaline reuptake (see Ch. 15). This enhances sympathetic activity, leading to tachycardia, increased cardiac output, vasoconstriction and increased arterial pressure.

Hypersensitivity reactions sometimes occur with local anaesthetics, usually in the form of allergic dermatitis but rarely as an acute anaphylactic reaction. Other unwanted effects that are specific to particular drugs include mucosal irritation (cocaine) and methaemoglobinaemia (which occurs after large doses of prilocaine, because of the production of a toxic metabolite).

PHARMACOKINETIC ASPECTS

Local anaesthetics vary a good deal in the rapidity with which they penetrate tissues, and this affects the rate at which they cause nerve block when injected into tissues, and the rate of onset of, and recovery from, anaesthesia (see Table 44.1; see Becker & Reed, 2012). It also affects their usefulness as surface anaesthetics for application to mucous membranes.

Most of the ester-linked local anaesthetics (e.g. **tetracaine**) are rapidly hydrolysed by plasma cholinesterase, so their plasma half-life is short. Procaine – now rarely used – is hydrolysed to *p*-aminobenzoic acid, a folate precursor that interferes with the antibacterial effect of sulfonamides (see Ch. 52). The amide-linked drugs (e.g. lidocaine and prilocaine) are metabolised mainly in the liver, usually by *N*-dealkylation rather than cleavage of the amide bond, and the metabolites are often pharmacologically active.

Benzocaine is an unusual local anaesthetic of very low solubility, which is used as a dry powder to dress painful skin ulcers, or as throat lozenges. The drug is slowly released and produces long-lasting surface anaesthesia.[1]

The routes of administration, uses and main adverse effects of local anaesthetics are summarised in Table 44.2.

Most local anaesthetics have a direct vasodilator action, which increases the rate at which they are absorbed into the systemic circulation, thus increasing their potential toxicity and reducing their local anaesthetic action. **Adrenaline** (**epinephrine**), **phenylephrine** or **felypressin**, a short-acting vasopressin analogue (see Ch. 34), may be added to local anaesthetic solutions injected locally to cause vasoconstriction. Adrenaline and phenylephrine absorbed into the circulation may induce unwanted cardiovascular effects such as tachycardia and vasoconstriction, and felypressin may cause coronary artery constriction. Their use in patients with cardiovascular disease is contraindicated.

NEW APPROACHES

Blocking specific sodium-channel subtypes is seen as a promising therapeutic strategy for a variety of clinical conditions, including epilepsy (see Ch. 46), neurodegenerative diseases and stroke (see Ch. 41), neuropathic pain (see Ch. 43) and myopathies (see Ch. 22). As our understanding of the role of specific sodium-channel subtypes in different pathophysiological situations increases, so too will be the likelihood that selective blocking agents can be developed for use in different clinical situations.

▼ Charged local anaesthetics do not cross the plasma membrane and thus when applied to the outside of nerves do not inhibit action potential firing. They can, however, enter cells via the pore of TRP channels such as TRPV1 (see Ch. 43). As TRPV1 channels are primarily localised on sensory neurons carrying pain information, this raises

---

[1]Benzocaine is also used in 'endurance' condoms to delay ejaculation.

Table 44.2 Methods of administration, uses and adverse effects of local anaesthetics

Method	Uses	Drug(s)	Notes and adverse effects
Surface anaesthesia	Nose, mouth, bronchial tree (usually in spray form), cornea, urinary tract, uterus (for hysteroscopy) Not very effective for skin[a]	Lidocaine, tetracaine, (amethocaine), dibucaine, benzocaine	Risk of systemic toxicity when high concentrations and large areas are involved **Chloroethane** (ethyl chloride) applied to the skin produces a mild chilling and local numbing. It can be used for minor surgical procedures
Infiltration anaesthesia	Direct injection into tissues to reach nerve branches and terminals Used in minor surgery	Most	Adrenaline (epinephrine) or felypressin often added as vasoconstrictors (not with fingers or toes, for fear of causing ischaemic tissue damage) Suitable for only small areas, otherwise serious risk of systemic toxicity
Intravenous regional anaesthesia	LA injected intravenously distal to a pressure cuff to arrest blood flow; remains effective until the circulation is restored Used for limb surgery	Mainly lidocaine, prilocaine	Risk of systemic toxicity when cuff is released prematurely; risk is small if cuff remains inflated for at least 20 min
Nerve block anaesthesia	LA is injected close to nerve trunks (e.g. brachial plexus, intercostal or dental nerves) to produce a loss of sensation peripherally Used for surgery, dentistry, analgesia	Most	Less LA needed than for infiltration anaesthesia Accurate placement of the needle is important Onset of anaesthesia may be slow Duration of anaesthesia may be increased by addition of vasoconstrictor
Spinal anaesthesia[b]	LA injected into the subarachnoid or intrathecal space (containing cerebrospinal fluid) to act on spinal roots and spinal cord Sometimes formulated with glucose ('hyperbaricity') so that spread of LA can be controlled by tilting patient Used for surgery to abdomen, pelvis or leg LA can be used alone or in conjunction with a general anaesthetic to reduce stress Provides good postoperative pain relief	Mainly lidocaine	Main risks are bradycardia and hypotension (owing to sympathetic block), respiratory depression (owing to effects on phrenic nerve or respiratory centre); avoided by minimising cranial spread Postoperative urinary retention (block of pelvic autonomic outflow) is common
Epidural anaesthesia[c]	LA injected into epidural space, blocking spinal roots Uses as for spinal anaesthesia; also for painless childbirth	Mainly lidocaine, bupivacaine	Unwanted effects similar to those of spinal anaesthesia but less probable, because longitudinal spread of LA is reduced Postoperative urinary retention common

LA, local anaesthetic.
[a]Surface anaesthesia does not work well on the skin, although a non-crystalline mixture of lidocaine and prilocaine (eutectic mixture of local anaesthetics or EMLA) has been developed for application to the skin, producing complete anaesthesia in about 1 h. Lidocaine is available in a patch preparation that can be applied to the skin to reduce pain in conditions such as post-herpetic neuralgia (shingles).
[b]Use of spinal anaesthesia is declining in favour of epidural administration.
[c]Intrathecal or epidural administration of LA in combination with an opioid (see Ch. 43) produces more effective analgesia than can be achieved with the opioid alone. Only a small concentration of LA is needed, insufficient to produce appreciable loss of sensation or other side effects. The mechanism of this synergism is unknown, but the procedure has proved useful in pain treatment.

the possibility of applying a charged local anaesthetic such as QX-314 along with a TRPV1 activator, thus allowing the local anaesthetic to enter and block sodium channels only on nociceptive neurons, resulting in the block of pain sensation without affecting motor, autonomic or other sensory nerves.

OTHER DRUGS THAT AFFECT SODIUM CHANNELS

TETRODOTOXIN AND SAXITOXIN

▼ Tetrodotoxin (TTX) is produced by a marine bacterium and accumulates in the tissues of a poisonous Pacific fish, the puffer fish. The puffer fish is regarded in Japan as a special delicacy, partly because of the mild tingling sensation that follows eating its flesh. To serve it in public restaurants, however, the chef must be registered as sufficiently skilled in removing the toxic organs (especially liver and ovaries) to make the flesh safe to eat. Accidental TTX poisoning is quite common, nonetheless. Historical records of long sea voyages often contained reference to attacks of severe weakness, progressing to complete paralysis and death, caused by eating puffer fish. It was suggested that the powders used by voodoo practitioners to induce zombification may contain TTX but this is disputed.

Saxitoxin (STX) is produced by a marine microorganism that sometimes proliferates in very large numbers and even colours the sea, giving the *red tide* phenomenon. At such times, marine shellfish can accumulate the toxin and become poisonous to humans.

These toxins, unlike conventional local anaesthetics, act exclusively from the outside of the membrane. Both are complex molecules, bearing a positively charged guanidinium moiety. The guanidinium ion is able to permeate voltage-sensitive sodium channels, and this

Unwanted effects and pharmacokinetics of local anaesthetics

- Local anaesthetics are either esters or amides. Esters are rapidly hydrolysed by plasma and tissue esterases, and amides are metabolised in the liver. Plasma half-lives are generally short, about 1–2 h.
- Unwanted effects are due mainly to escape of local anaesthetics into the systemic circulation.
- Main unwanted effects are:
  - central nervous system effects, namely agitation, confusion, tremors progressing to convulsions and respiratory depression;
  - cardiovascular effects, namely myocardial depression and vasodilatation, leading to fall in blood pressure;
  - occasional hypersensitivity reactions.
- Local anaesthetics vary in the rapidity with which they penetrate tissues, and in their duration of action. **Lidocaine** (lignocaine) penetrates tissues readily and is suitable for surface application; **bupivacaine** has a particularly long duration of action.

part of the TTX or STX molecule lodges in the channel, while the rest of the molecule blocks its outer mouth. In the manner of its blockade of sodium channels, TTX can be likened to a champagne cork. In contrast to the local anaesthetics, there is no interaction between the gating and blocking reactions with TTX or STX – their association and dissociation are independent of whether the channel is open or closed. Some voltage-sensitive sodium channels expressed in cardiac muscle or up-regulated in sensory neurons in neuropathic pain (i.e. $Na_V1.5$, $Na_V1.8$ and $Na_V1.9$) are relatively insensitive to TTX (see Ch. 43).

Both TTX and STX are unsuitable for clinical use as local anaesthetics, being expensive to obtain from their exotic sources and poor at penetrating tissues because of their very low lipid solubility. They have, however, been important as experimental tools for the isolation and cloning of sodium channels (see Ch. 4).

AGENTS THAT AFFECT SODIUM-CHANNEL GATING

▼ Various substances modify sodium-channel gating in such a way as to *increase* the probability of opening of the channels (see Hille, 2001). They include various toxins, mainly from frog skin (e.g. batrachotoxin), scorpion or sea anemone venoms; plant alkaloids such as **veratridine**; and insecticides such as DDT and the pyrethrins. They facilitate sodium-channel activation so that sodium channels open at more negative potentials close to the normal resting potential; they also inhibit inactivation, so that the channels fail to close if the membrane remains depolarised. The membrane thus becomes hyper-excitable, and the action potential is prolonged. Spontaneous discharges occur at first, but the cells eventually become permanently depolarised and inexcitable. All these substances affect the heart, producing extrasystoles and other dysrhythmias, culminating in fibrillation; they also cause spontaneous discharges in nerve and muscle, leading to twitching and convulsions. The very high lipid solubility of substances like DDT makes them effective as insecticides, for they are readily absorbed through the integument. Drugs in this class are useful as experimental tools for studying sodium channels but have no clinical uses.

Clinical uses of local anaesthetics

- Local anaesthetics may be injected into soft tissue (e.g. of gums) or to block a nerve or nerve plexus.
- Co-administration of a vasoconstrictor (e.g. **adrenaline**) prolongs the local effect.
- Lipid-soluble drugs (e.g. **lidocaine**) are absorbed from mucous membranes and are used as surface anaesthetics.
- **Bupivacaine** has a slow onset but long duration. It is often used for epidural blockade (e.g. to provide continuous epidural blockade during labour) and spinal anaesthesia. Its isomer **levobupivacaine** is less cardiotoxic if it is inadvertently administered into a blood vessel.

REFERENCES AND FURTHER READING

Becker, D.E., Reed, K.L., 2012. Local anesthetics: review of pharmacological considerations. Anesth. Progr. 59, 90–102. (*Brief review of local anaesthetic pharmacology from a dental perspective*)

Catterall, W.A., Swanson, T.M., 2015. Structural basis for pharmacology of voltage-gated sodium and calcium channels. Mol. Pharmacol. 88, 141–150. (*Reviews recent advances in our knowledge of the structure of sodium channels that explains how local anaesthetics enter and bind to the pore region of the channel*)

Hille, B., 2001. Ionic Channels of Excitable Membranes. Sinauer, Sunderland. (*Excellent, clearly written textbook. The information it contains is still very relevant today*)

Strichartz, G.R., Ritchie, J.M., 1987. The action of local anaesthetics on ion channels of excitable tissues. Handb. Exp. Pharmacol. 81, 21–52. (*Excellent review of actions of local anaesthetics – other articles in the same volume cover more clinical aspects*)

Anxiolytic and hypnotic drugs

OVERVIEW

In this chapter we discuss the nature of anxiety and the drugs used to treat it (anxiolytic drugs), as well as drugs used to treat insomnia (hypnotic drugs). Historically there was overlap between these two groups, reflecting the fact that older anxiolytic drugs commonly caused a degree of sedation and drowsiness. Newer anxiolytic drugs show much less sedative effect and other hypnotic drugs have been introduced that lack specific anxiolytic effects. Many of the drugs now used to treat anxiety were first developed, and are still used, to treat other disorders such as depression (Ch. 48), epilepsy (Ch. 46) and schizophrenia (Ch. 47). Here we will focus on their use as anxiolytics.

THE NATURE OF ANXIETY AND ITS TREATMENT

The normal fear response to threatening stimuli comprises several components, including defensive behaviours, autonomic reflexes, arousal and alertness, corticosteroid secretion and negative emotions. In anxiety states, these reactions occur in an anticipatory manner, often independently of external events. The distinction between a 'pathological' and a 'normal' state of anxiety is not clear-cut but represents the point at which the symptoms interfere with normal productive activities. The term 'anxiety' is applied to several distinct disorders. A useful division of anxiety disorders that may help to explain why different types of anxiety respond differently to different drugs is into (i) disorders that involve *fear* (panic attacks and phobias) and (ii) those that involve a more general feeling of *anxiety* (often categorised as general anxiety disorder).

Anxiety disorders recognised clinically include the following:

- *generalised anxiety disorder* (an ongoing state of excessive anxiety lacking any clear reason or focus)
- *social anxiety disorder* (fear of being with and interacting with other people)
- *phobias* (strong fears of specific objects or situations, e.g. snakes, open spaces, flying)
- *panic disorder* (sudden attacks of overwhelming fear that occur in association with marked somatic symptoms, such as sweating, tachycardia, chest pains, trembling and choking). Such attacks can be induced even in normal individuals by infusion of sodium lactate, and the condition appears to have a genetic component.

Related disorders include:

- *post-traumatic stress disorder* (PTSD; distress triggered by recall of past stressful experiences)
- *obsessive–compulsive disorder* (compulsive ritualistic behaviour driven by irrational anxiety, e.g. fear of contamination).

Extensive descriptions of anxiety disorders can be found in DSM-5.[1]

It should be stressed that the treatment of such disorders generally involves psychological approaches as well as drug treatment. Over the last decade, the drug treatment of anxiety has changed from using traditional anxiolytic/hypnotic agents (i.e. benzodiazepines and barbiturates) to using a range of drugs that are also used to treat other central nervous system (CNS) disorders (e.g. antidepressant, antiepileptic and antipsychotic drugs) or 5-hydroxytryptamine (5-HT)$_{1A}$-receptor agonists (e.g. **buspirone**) that have no hypnotic effect. Furthermore, benzodiazepines, while being effective anxiolytic drugs, have the disadvantages of producing unwanted side effects such as amnesia, and of inducing tolerance and physical dependence, as well as being drugs of abuse. They are also ineffective in treating any depression that may occur along with anxiety. Unlike antidepressants and buspirone, which require treatment for three or more weeks to show any therapeutic effect, benzodiazepines act within 30 minutes, so they can be useful for patients who need acute treatment, and can be taken on an 'as needed' basis.

In recent years a number of over-the-counter 'relaxation' drinks containing CNS neurotransmitters, their precursors or other hormones and amino acids have been marketed, without any evidence of efficacy.[2]

MEASUREMENT OF ANXIOLYTIC ACTIVITY

ANIMAL MODELS OF ANXIETY

In addition to the subjective (emotional) component of human anxiety, there are measurable behavioural and physiological effects that also occur in experimental animals. In biological terms, anxiety induces a particular form of behavioural inhibition that occurs in response to novel environmental events that are threatening or painful. In animals, this behavioural inhibition may take the form of

[1]DSM-5: Diagnostic and Statistical Manual of Mental Disorders, 2013. fifth ed. American Psychiatric Association, Washington, DC.
[2]Because 'relaxation' drinks are classified as dietary supplements they are not subject to the same efficacy and safety tests as drugs (see Editorial in Nature Neuroscience, 2012, vol. 15, p. 497).

Fig. 45.1 Anxiety testing. (A) Illustration of the elevated plus maze with open and closed arms. (B) Effect of diazepam on time spent by rats in the open arms of the elevated plus maze. Each bar represents time spent with movement in the open arms during a 5-min test period. (C) and (D) Effect of a 7.5% CO_2 challenge for 20 minutes on anxiety, measured on a visual analogue scale (VAS), and salivary cortisol levels in human subjects. (Panel [B], data taken from Kapus et al., 2008. Psychopharmacology 198, 2231–2241; panels [C] and [D], data taken from K. Seddon et al., 2011. J. Psychopharmacol. 25, 43–51.)

immobility or suppression of a behavioural response, such as bar pressing to obtain food. A rat placed in an unfamiliar environment normally responds by remaining immobile although alert (behavioural suppression) for a time, which may represent 'anxiety' produced by the strange environment. This immobility is reduced if anxiolytic drugs are administered. The 'elevated cross maze' is a widely used test model (Fig. 45.1). Two arms of the raised horizontal cross are closed in, and the others are open. Normally, rats spend most of their time in the closed arms and avoid the open arms (afraid, possibly, of falling off or being attacked). Administration of anxiolytic drugs increases the time spent in the open arms and also increases the number of entries made into the open arm but without an increase in motor activity.

Conflict tests can also be used. For example, a rat trained to press a bar repeatedly to obtain a food pellet normally achieves a high and consistent response rate. A conflict element is then introduced: at intervals, indicated by an auditory signal, bar pressing results in an occasional 'punishment' in the form of an electric shock in addition to the reward of a food pellet. Normally, the rat ceases

pressing the bar (behavioural inhibition), and thus avoids the shock, while the signal is sounding. The effect of an anxiolytic drug is to relieve this suppressive effect, so that the rats continue bar pressing for reward despite the 'punishment'. Other types of psychotropic drug are not effective, nor are analgesic drugs. Other evidence confirms that anxiolytic drugs affect the level of behavioural inhibition produced by the 'conflict situation', rather than simply raising the pain threshold.

Some of these anxiety models may measure fear rather than general anxiety, which occurs in humans in the absence of specific stimuli. To develop new anxiolytic drugs, it is important to have animal tests that give a good guide to efficacy in humans, and much ingenuity has gone into developing and validating such tests (see Ramos, 2008; Ennaceur & Chazot, 2016).

TESTS ON HUMANS

Various subjective *anxiety scale* tests have been devised based on standard patient questionnaires. Galvanic skin reactions – a measure of sweat secretion – are also used to monitor anxiety. Neuropsychological tests have been

Table 45.1 Characteristics of benzodiazepines in humans

Drug(s)	Half-life of parent compound (h)	Active metabolite	Half-life of metabolite (h)	Overall duration of action	Main use(s)
Midazolam[a]	2–4	Hydroxylated derivative	2	Ultrashort (<6 h)	Hypnotic Midazolam used as intravenous anaesthetic and anticonvulsant
Zolpidem[b]	2	No	—	Ultrashort (~4 h)	Hypnotic
Lorazepam, oxazepam, temazepam, lormetazepam	8–12	No	—	Short (12–18 h)	Anxiolytic, hypnotic. Lorazepam used as anticonvulsant
Alprazolam	6–12	Hydroxylated derivative	6	Medium (24 h)	Anxiolytic, antidepressant
Nitrazepam	16–40	No	—	Medium	Anxiolytic, hypnotic[c]
Diazepam, chlordiazepoxide	20–40	Nordazepam	60	Long (24–48 h)	Anxiolytic, muscle relaxant Diazepam used as anticonvulsant
Flurazepam	1	Desmethyl-flurazepam	60	Long	Anxiolytic, hypnotic[c]
Clonazepam	50	No	—	Long	Anticonvulsant, anxiolytic (especially mania)

[a]Another short-acting benzodiazepine, triazolam, has been withdrawn from use in the United Kingdom on account of side effects.
[b]Zolpidem is not a benzodiazepine but acts in a similar manner. Zopiclone and zaleplon are similar.
[c]Due to their long half-life, drowsiness is common on waking.

developed to investigate emotional and attentional biases associated with responses to emotive faces and words. An experience akin to a panic attack can be induced in many subjects by breathing an increased level of CO_2, usually prolonged breathing of 7.5% CO_2 or a single inhalation of 35% CO_2 (see Fig. 45.1). Such tests have confirmed the efficacy of many anxiolytic drugs, but placebo treatment often also produces highly significant responses.

A human version of the conflict test described above involves the substitution of money for food pellets, and the use of graded electric shocks as punishment. As with rats, administration of diazepam increases the rate of button pressing for money during the periods when the punishment was in operation, although the subjects reported no change in the painfulness of the electric shock.

DRUGS USED TO TREAT ANXIETY

The main groups of drugs are as follows:

- Antidepressants (see Ch. 48 for details). Selective serotonin (5-HT) reuptake inhibitors (SSRIs; e.g. **escitalopram, sertraline** and **paroxetine**) and serotonin/noradrenaline reuptake inhibitors (SNRIs; e.g. **venlafaxine and duloxetine**) are effective in the treatment of generalised anxiety disorder, phobias, social anxiety disorder, post-traumatic stress disorder and obsessive–compulsive disorder. Older antidepressants (tricyclic antidepressants and monoamine oxidase inhibitors [MAOIs]) are also

effective, but a lower side-effect profile favours the use of SSRIs. These agents have the additional advantage of reducing depression, which is not uncommonly associated with anxiety.

- **Benzodiazepines.** Used to treat acute anxiety. Those used to treat anxiety have a long biological half-life (Table 45.1). They may be co-administered during stabilisation of a patient on an SSRI.
- **Gabapentin** and **pregabalin** are used to treat general anxiety disorder, although trial data on gabapentin are limited. Other antiepileptic drugs such as **tiagabine, valproate** and **levetiracetam** (see Ch. 46), may also be effective in treating generalised anxiety disorder.
- **Buspirone.** This 5-HT_{1A} receptor agonist is effective in generalised anxiety disorder but ineffective in the treatment of phobias or severe anxiety states.
- Some atypical antipsychotic agents (see Ch. 47) such as **olanzapine, risperidone, quetiapine** and **ziprasidone** may be effective in generalised anxiety disorder and post-traumatic stress disorder.
- β-Adrenoceptor antagonists (e.g. **propranolol**; Ch. 15). These are used to treat some forms of anxiety, particularly where physical symptoms such as sweating, tremor and tachycardia are troublesome.[3] Their effectiveness depends on block of peripheral sympathetic responses rather than on any central effects.

---

[3]β-Blockers are sometimes used by actors and musicians to reduce the symptoms of stage fright, but their use by snooker players to minimise tremor is banned as unsportsmanlike.

Antidepressants (Ch. 48), antiepileptics (Ch. 46), anti-psychotics Ch. 47) and β-adrenoceptor antagonists (Ch. 15) are described in detail elsewhere in this book. Here we will first focus on how SSRIs and buspirone exert their anxiolytic activity and then discuss in detail the benzo-diazepines, the primary use of which is to treat anxiety.

Classes of anxiolytic drugs

- Antidepressant drugs (selective serotonin reuptake inhibitors [SSRIs], serotonin/noradrenaline reuptake inhibitors [SNRIs], tricyclic antidepressants and monoamine oxidase inhibitors [MAOIs] – see Ch. 48) are effective anxiolytic agents.
- Benzodiazepines are used for treating acute anxiety and insomnia.
- **Gabapentin** and **pregabalin** drugs have anxiolytic properties.
- **Buspirone** is a 5-hydroxytryptamine (5-HT)$_{1A}$-receptor agonist with anxiolytic activity but little sedative effect.
- Some atypical antipsychotic agents (e.g. **quetiapine**) can be useful to treat some forms of anxiety, but have significant unwanted effects.
- β-Adrenoceptor antagonists (e.g. **propranolol**) are used mainly to reduce physical symptoms of anxiety (tremor, palpitations, etc.); no effect on affective component.

DELAYED ANXIOLYTIC EFFECT OF SSRIs AND BUSPIRONE

The anxiolytic effects of SSRIs (e.g. **escitalopram** and **sertraline**) and **buspirone** are not immediate but take days or weeks to develop after commencing drug therapy, suggesting that adaptive responses to the initial effects of these drugs that develop over time are important.

Buspirone is a partial agonist at 5-HT$_{1A}$ receptors (Ch. 16) and also binds to dopamine receptors, but it is likely that its 5-HT-related actions are important in relation to anxiety suppression, because related experimental compounds (e.g. ipsapirone and gepirone), which are highly specific for 5-HT$_{1A}$ receptors, show similar anxiolytic activity in experimental animals.

5-HT$_{1A}$ receptors are expressed on the soma and dendrites of 5-HT-containing neurons, where they function as inhibitory autoreceptors, as well as being expressed on other types of neuron (e.g. noradrenergic locus coeruleus neurons) where, along with other types of 5-HT receptor (see Ch. 40), they mediate the postsynaptic actions of 5-HT. Postsynaptic 5-HT$_{1A}$ receptors are highly expressed within the cortico-limbic circuits implicated in emotional behaviour. One theory of how SSRIs and buspirone produce their delayed anxiolytic effect is that over time they induce desensitisation of somatodendritic 5-HT$_{1A}$ autoreceptors, resulting in heightened excitation of serotonergic neurons and enhanced 5-HT release (Ch. 48, Fig. 48.3). This might also explain why early in treatment, anxiety can be worsened by these drugs due to the initial activation of 5-HT$_{1A}$ autoreceptors and inhibition of 5-HT release. This receptor desensitisation theory would predict that a 5-HT$_{1A}$ antagonist that would rapidly block the action of 5-HT at 5-HT$_{1A}$

autoreceptors – and thus swiftly enhance 5-HT release – might be anxiolytic without delayed onset. Drugs with combined 5-HT$_{1A}$ antagonism and SSRI properties have been developed but have not been found to be effective in man, perhaps because they block both 5HT$_{1A}$ autoreceptors and postsynaptic receptors, the latter effect occluding the beneficial effect of the former. Elevated 5-HT levels may also induce other postsynaptic adaptations. 5-HT$_2$ receptors have also been implicated, down-regulation of which may be important for anxiolytic action. Drugs with 5-HT$_2$ and 5-HT$_3$ receptor antagonist activity are in clinical trials for treating anxiety.

Buspirone inhibits the activity of noradrenergic locus coeruleus neurons (Ch. 40) and thus interferes with arousal reactions. It has side effects quite different from those of benzodiazepines. It does not cause sedation or motor incoordination, nor have tolerance or withdrawal effects been reported. Its main side effects are nausea, dizziness, headache and restlessness, which generally seem to be less troublesome than the side effects of benzodiazepines. Buspirone does not suppress the benzodiazepine withdrawal syndrome (see p. 576), presumably because it acts by a different mechanism. Hence, when switching from benzo-diazepine treatment to buspirone treatment, the benzo-diazepine dose still needs to be reduced gradually.

Antidepressants and 5-HT$_{1A}$ agonists as anxiolytic drugs

- Anxiolytic effects take days or weeks to develop.
- Antidepressants (selective serotonin reuptake inhibitors [SSRIs], serotonin/noradrenaline reuptake inhibitors [SNRIs], tricyclic antidepressants and monoamine oxidase inhibitors [MAOIs] – see Ch. 48):
  - effective treatments for generalised anxiety disorder, phobias, social anxiety disorder and post-traumatic stress disorder;
  - may also reduce depression associated with anxiety.
- **Buspirone** is a potent agonist at 5-hydroxytryptamine (5-HT)$_{1A}$ receptors:
  - it is an effective treatment for generalised anxiety disorder but not phobias
  - side effects appear less troublesome than with benzodiazepines; they include dizziness, nausea, headache, but not sedation or loss of coordination.

BENZODIAZEPINES AND RELATED DRUGS

▼ The first benzodiazepine, **chlordiazepoxide**, was synthesised by accident in 1961, the unusual seven-membered ring having been produced as a result of a reaction that went wrong in the laboratories of Hoffman–La Roche. Its unexpected pharmacological activity was recognised in a routine screening procedure, and benzodiazepines quite soon became the most widely prescribed drugs in the pharmacopoeia.

The basic chemical structure of benzodiazepines consists of a seven-membered ring fused to an aromatic ring, with four main substituent groups that can be modified without loss of activity. Thousands of compounds have been made and tested, and about 20 are available for clinical use, the most important ones being listed in Table 45.1. They are basically similar in their pharmacological actions, although some degree of selectivity has been reported. For example, some, such as **clonazepam**, show anticonvulsant activity with less marked

Fig. 45.2 Potentiating effect of benzodiazepines and chlordiazepoxide on the action of GABA. Drugs were applied by iontophoresis to mouse spinal cord neurons grown in tissue culture, from micropipettes placed close to the cells. The membrane was hyperpolarised to −90 mV, and the cells were loaded with Cl⁻ from the recording microelectrode, so inhibitory amino acids (GABA and glycine [Gly]), as well as excitatory ones (glutamate [Glu]), caused depolarising responses. The potentiating effect of diazepam is restricted to GABA responses, glutamate and glycine responses being unaffected. *Con*, Control.

▼ The GABA$_A$ receptor is a ligand-gated ion channel (see Ch. 3) consisting of a pentameric assembly of different subunits, the main ones being α, β and γ (see Ch. 39). The GABA$_A$ receptor should actually be thought of as a family of receptors as there are six different subtypes of α subunit, three subtypes of β and three subtypes of γ. Although the potential number of combinations is therefore large, certain combinations predominate in the adult brain (see Ch. 39). The various combinations occur in different parts of the brain, have different physiological functions and have subtle differences in their pharmacological properties.

Benzodiazepines bind across the interface between the α and γ subunits but only to receptors that contain γ2 and α1, α2, α3 or α5 subunits. Genetic approaches have been used to study the roles of different subunits in the different behavioural effects of benzodiazepines. Behavioural analysis of mice with various mutations of the GABA$_A$ receptor subunit indicates that α1-containing receptors mediate the anticonvulsant, sedative/hypnotic and addictive effects but not the anxiolytic effect of benzodiazepines, whereas α2-containing receptors mediate the anxiolytic effect, α2-, α3- and α5-containing receptors mediate muscle relaxation and α1- and α5-containing receptors mediate the amnesic effects (Tan et al., 2011).

The obvious next step was to try to develop subunit-selective drugs. Unfortunately, this has proved difficult, due to the structural similarity between the benzodiazepine binding site on different α subunits. The α-subunit selectivity of some benzodiazepines is given in Table 45.2. It was hoped that selective efficacy at α2-containing receptors would produce anxiolytic drugs lacking the unwanted effects of sedation and amnesia. However, such compounds have not yet translated into human therapeutic agents (Skolnick, 2012). **Pagoclone**, reported to be a full agonist at α3 with less efficacy at α1, α2 and α5, has little or no sedative/hypnotic or amnesic actions. Clinical trials of this drug as a treatment for stammering proved unsuccessful.

Peripheral benzodiazepine-binding sites, not associated with GABA receptors, are present in many tissues. The target is a protein known as *translocator protein* located primarily on mitochondrial membranes.

ANTAGONISM AND NEGATIVE ALLOSTERIC MODULATION

Flumazenil is a benzodiazepine-like compound that competes with benzodiazepines at their binding site on GABA$_A$ receptors and thus antagonises their effects. This compound was originally reported to lack effects on behaviour or on drug-induced convulsions when given on its own, although it was later found to possess some 'anxiogenic' and proconvulsant activity which may indicate that it possesses weak negative allosteric modulatory activity. Flumazenil can be used to reverse the effect of benzodiazepine overdosage

sedative effects. From a clinical point of view, differences in pharmacokinetic behaviour among different benzodiazepines (see Table 45.1) are more important than differences in profile of activity. Drugs with a similar structure have been discovered that reverse the effects of the benzodiazepines, for example, **flumazenil** (see later).

The term 'benzodiazepine' refers to a distinct chemical structure. Also discussed here are 'Z-drugs' such as **zaleplon**, **zolpidem** and **zopiclone**[4] as well as **abecarnil** – a β-carboline (not licensed for clinical use) – which have different chemical structures, but bind to the same sites as the benzodiazepines.

MECHANISM OF ACTION

Benzodiazepines act selectively on GABA$_A$ receptors (Ch. 39), which mediate inhibitory synaptic transmission throughout the CNS. They act as positive allosteric modulators (see Ch. 2) to facilitate the opening of GABA-activated chloride channels thus enhancing the response to GABA (Ch. 39, Fig. 39.5). They bind specifically to a modulatory site on the receptor, distinct from the GABA-binding sites (see Fig. 45.3), and act allosterically to increase the affinity of GABA for the receptor. Single-channel recordings show an increase in the frequency of channel opening by a given concentration of GABA, but no change in the conductance or mean open time, consistent with an effect on GABA binding rather than the channel-gating mechanism. Benzodiazepines do not affect receptors for other amino acids, such as glycine or glutamate (Fig. 45.2).

Table 45.2 GABA$_A$-receptor α-subunit selectivity of some therapeutically used benzodiazepines

Drug	Subunit selectivity
Diazepam	α1, α2, α3, α4, α5, α6
Flunitrazepam	α1, α2, α5
Midazolam	α1, α2, α3, α4, α5, α6
Zolpidem	α1
Flumazenil	Antagonist at α1, α2, α3, α4, α5, α6

(Adapted from Tan, K.R., Rudolph, U., Lüscher, C., 2011. Hooked on benzodiazepines: GABA$_A$-receptor subtypes and addiction. Trends Neurosci. 34, 188–197.)

---

[4]Z-drugs are used primarily to induce sleep and so should perhaps be called 'Zzzzzz drugs'.

(normally used only if respiration is severely depressed), or to reverse the effect of benzodiazepines such as midazolam used for minor surgical procedures. Flumazenil acts quickly and effectively when given by injection, but its action lasts for only about 2 h, so drowsiness tends to return. Convulsions may occur in patients treated with flumazenil, and this is more common in patients receiving tricyclic antidepressants (Ch. 48). Reports that flumazenil improves the mental state of patients with severe liver disease (hepatic encephalopathy) and alcohol intoxication have not been confirmed in controlled trials.

▼ Drugs that bind to the benzodiazepine site and exert the opposite effect to that of conventional benzodiazepines (negative allosteric modulators, see Ch. 2), produce signs of increased anxiety and convulsions. These include ethyl-β-carboline-3-carboxylate (βCCE) and diazepam-binding inhibitor (see later), as well as some benzodiazepine analogues. It is possible (Fig. 45.3) to explain these complexities in terms of the two-state model discussed in Chapter 2, by postulating that the receptor exists in two distinct conformations, only one of which (A) can bind GABA molecules and open the chloride channel. The other conformation (B) cannot bind GABA. Normally, with no benzodiazepine ligand present, there is an equilibrium between these two conformations; sensitivity to GABA is present but submaximal. Positive allosteric modulators (e.g. diazepam) are postulated to bind preferentially to conformation (A), thus shifting the equilibrium in favour of (A) and enhancing GABA sensitivity. Negative allosteric modulators bind selectively to (B) and have the opposite effect.

Fig. 45.3 Model of benzodiazepine/GABA$_A$-receptor interaction. Benzodiazepines and related drugs bind to a modulatory site on the GABA$_A$ receptor distinct from the GABA-binding site. This model envisages a conformational equilibrium between states in which the benzodiazepine site binds positive allosteric modulators (PAMs) (A) and negative allosteric modulators (NAMs) (B). In the latter state, the GABA$_A$ receptor has a much reduced affinity for GABA; consequently, the chloride channel remains closed.

IS THERE AN ENDOGENOUS BENZODIAZEPINE-LIKE MEDIATOR?

▼ Despite considerable scientific effort, the question of whether or not there are endogenous ligands for the benzodiazepine site, whose function is to regulate the action of GABA, remains unanswered.

That **flumazenil** produces responses both in vivo and in vitro in the absence of any exogenous benzodiazepines has been cited to support the view that there must be ongoing benzodiazepine-like action produced by endogenous ligand(s). However, it is possible that it has positive or negative modulatory activity at subtypes of GABA$_A$ receptor (depending on the α subunit present), or in some pathological conditions in which the GABA$_A$ receptors have become modified.

Several endogenous compounds that act at the benzodiazepine site have been isolated, including β-carbolines (e.g. βCCE), structurally related to tryptophan, and diazepam-binding inhibitor, a 10-kDa peptide. Whether these molecules exist in the brain (i.e. are endogenous) or are generated during the processes involved in extracting them from the tissue is an open issue. Interestingly, both βCCE and diazepam-binding inhibitor have the opposite effect to benzodiazepines, i.e. they are negative allosteric modulators and inhibit chloride channel opening by GABA and, in the whole animal, exert anxiogenic and proconvulsant effects. There was also a suggestion that benzodiazepines themselves may occur naturally in the brain, but the origin of these compounds and how biosynthesis occurs is unclear. At present there is no general agreement on the identity and function of endogenous ligands for the benzodiazepine site. Other possible endogenous modulators of GABA$_A$ receptors include steroid metabolites, but they bind to a different site from benzodiazepines (see Ch. 39).

PHARMACOLOGICAL EFFECTS AND USES

The main effects of benzodiazepines are:

- reduction of anxiety and aggression;
- induction of sleep (see section on hypnotic drugs, p. 577);
- reduction of muscle tone;
- anticonvulsant effect;
- anterograde amnesia.

Reduction of anxiety and aggression

Benzodiazepines show anxiolytic effects in animal tests, as described previously, and also exert a marked 'taming' effect, allowing animals to be handled more easily.[5] With the possible exception of alprazolam (see Table 45.1), benzodiazepines do not have antidepressant effects. Benzodiazepines may paradoxically produce an increase in irritability and aggression in some individuals. This appears to be particularly pronounced with the ultrashort-acting drug triazolam (and led to its withdrawal in the United Kingdom and some other countries), and is generally more common with short-acting compounds. It is probably a manifestation of the benzodiazepine withdrawal syndrome, which occurs with all these drugs (see p. 576) but is more acute with drugs whose action wears off rapidly.

Benzodiazepines are now used mainly for treating acute anxiety states, behavioural emergencies and during procedures such as endoscopy. They are also used as premedication before surgery (both medical and dental). Under these circumstances their anxiolytic, sedative and amnesic

---

[5]This depends on the species. Cats actually become more excitable (and hungry), as a colleague of one of the authors discovered to his cost when attempting to sedate a tiger in the Baltimore zoo.

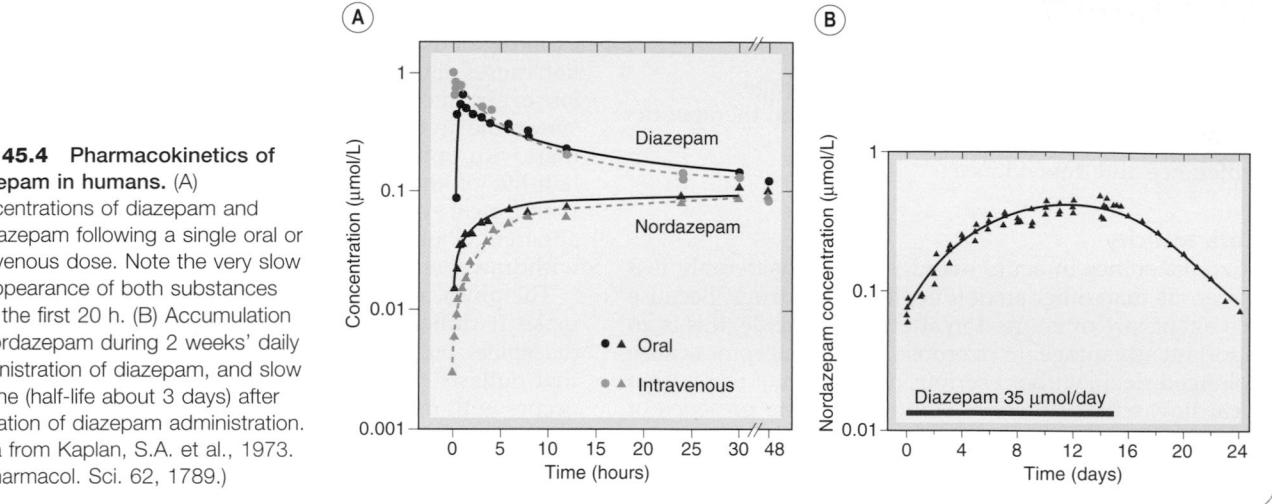

Fig. 45.4 Pharmacokinetics of diazepam in humans. (A) Concentrations of diazepam and nordazepam following a single oral or intravenous dose. Note the very slow disappearance of both substances after the first 20 h. (B) Accumulation of nordazepam during 2 weeks' daily administration of diazepam, and slow decline (half-life about 3 days) after cessation of diazepam administration. (Data from Kaplan, S.A. et al., 1973. J. Pharmacol. Sci. 62, 1789.)

properties may be beneficial. Intravenous midazolam can be used to induce anaesthesia (see Ch. 42).

Reduction of muscle tone
Benzodiazepines reduce muscle tone by a central action on GABA_A receptors, primarily in the spinal cord.

Increased muscle tone is a common feature of anxiety states in humans and may contribute to the aches and pains, including headache, that often trouble anxious patients. The relaxant effect of benzodiazepines may therefore be clinically useful. A reduction of muscle tone appears to be possible without appreciable loss of coordination. However, with intravenous administration in anaesthesia and in overdose when these drugs are being abused, airway obstruction may occur. Other clinical uses of muscle relaxants are discussed in Chapter 14.

Anticonvulsant effects
All the benzodiazepines have anticonvulsant activity in experimental animal tests. They are highly effective against chemically induced convulsions caused by **pentylenetetrazol**, **bicuculline** and similar drugs that act by blocking GABA_A receptors (see Chs 39 and 46) but less so against electrically induced convulsions.

Clonazepam (see Table 45.1), **diazepam, midazolam** and **lorazepam** are used to treat epilepsy (Ch. 46). They can be given intravenously to control life-threatening seizures in status epilepticus. Diazepam can be administered rectally to children to control acute seizures. Tolerance develops to the anticonvulsant actions of benzodiazepines (see p. 576).

Anterograde amnesia
Benzodiazepines prevent memory of events experienced while under their influence, an effect not seen with other CNS depressants. Minor surgical or invasive procedures can thus be performed without leaving unpleasant memories. **Flunitrazepam** (better known to the general public by one of its trade names, Rohypnol) is infamous as a date rape drug and victims frequently have difficulty in recalling exactly what took place during the attack.

Amnesia is thought to be due to benzodiazepines binding to GABA_A receptors containing the α5 subunit. α5-Knock-out mice show an enhanced learning and memory

phenotype. This raises the possibility that an α5 subunit-selective negative allosteric modulator could be memory enhancing.

PHARMACOKINETIC ASPECTS
Benzodiazepines are well absorbed when given orally, usually giving a peak plasma concentration in about 1 h. Some (e.g. oxazepam, lorazepam) are absorbed more slowly. They bind strongly to plasma protein, and their high lipid solubility causes many of them to accumulate gradually in body fat. They are normally given by mouth but can be given intravenously (e.g. diazepam in status epilepticus, midazolam in anaesthesia), buccally, or rectally. Intramuscular injection often results in slow absorption.

Benzodiazepines are all metabolised and eventually excreted as glucuronide conjugates in the urine. They vary greatly in duration of action and can be roughly divided into short-, medium- and long-acting compounds (see Table 45.1). Duration of action influences their use, short-acting compounds being useful hypnotics with reduced hangover effect on wakening, long-acting compounds being more useful for use as anxiolytic and anticonvulsant drugs. Several are converted to active metabolites such as N-desmethyldiazepam (**nordazepam**), which has a half-life of about 60 h, and which accounts for the tendency of many benzodiazepines to produce cumulative effects and long hangovers when they are given repeatedly. The short-acting compounds are those that are metabolised directly by conjugation with glucuronide. Fig. 45.4 shows the gradual build up and slow disappearance of nordazepam from the plasma of a human subject given diazepam daily for 15 days.

▼ Advancing age affects the rate of oxidative reactions more than that of conjugation reactions. Thus the effect of the long-acting benzodiazepines tends to increase with age, and it is common for drowsiness and confusion to develop insidiously for this reason.[6]

---

[6]At the age of 91 years, the grandmother of one of the authors was growing increasingly forgetful and mildly dotty, having been taking nitrazepam for insomnia regularly for years. To the author's lasting shame, it took a canny general practitioner to diagnose the problem. Cancellation of the nitrazepam prescription produced a dramatic improvement.

UNWANTED EFFECTS

These may be divided into:

- toxic effects resulting from acute overdosage;
- unwanted effects occurring during normal therapeutic use;
- tolerance and dependence.

Acute toxicity

Benzodiazepines in acute overdose are considerably less dangerous than other anxiolytic/hypnotic drugs. Because such agents are often used in attempted suicide, this is an important advantage. In overdose, benzodiazepines cause prolonged sleep, without serious depression of respiration or cardiovascular function. However, in the presence of other CNS depressants, particularly alcohol, benzodiazepines can cause severe, even life-threatening, respiratory depression. This is a frequent problem when benzodiazepines are abused (see Chs 50 and 59). The availability of an effective antagonist, flumazenil, means that the effects of an acute overdose can be counteracted,[7] which is not possible for most CNS depressants.

Side effects during therapeutic use

The main side effects of benzodiazepines are drowsiness, confusion, amnesia and impaired coordination, which considerably impairs manual skills such as driving performance. Benzodiazepines enhance the depressant effect of other drugs, including alcohol, in a more than additive way. The long and unpredictable duration of action of many benzodiazepines is important in relation to side effects. Long-acting drugs such as nitrazepam are rarely used as hypnotics, and even shorter-acting compounds such as lorazepam can produce a substantial day-after impairment of job performance and driving skill.

Tolerance and dependence

Tolerance (i.e. a gradual escalation of dose needed to produce the required effect) occurs with all benzodiazepines, as does dependence, which is their main drawback. They share these properties with other sedatives. Tolerance appears to represent a change at the receptor level, but the mechanism is not well understood. There may be selective loss of membrane $GABA_A$ receptors containing the α2 subunit (Jacob et al., 2012).

At the receptor level, the degree of tolerance will be governed both by the number of sites occupied (i.e. the dose) and the duration of site occupancy (which may vary according to the therapeutic use). Therefore marked tolerance develops when benzodiazepines are used continuously to treat epilepsy, whereas less tolerance occurs to the sleep-inducing effect of short-acting agents when the subject is relatively drug free during the day. It is not clear to what degree tolerance develops to the anxiolytic effect.

Benzodiazepines produce dependence, and this is a major problem. In human subjects and patients, abrupt cessation of benzodiazepine treatment after weeks or months causes a rebound heightened anxiety, together with tremor, dizziness, tinnitus, weight loss and disturbed sleep due to enhanced REM sleep (see p. 578). It is recommended that benzodiazepines be withdrawn gradually by stepwise lowering of the dose. Withdrawal after chronic administration causes physical symptoms, namely nervousness, tremor, loss of appetite and sometimes convulsions.[8] The withdrawal syndrome, in both animals and humans, is slower in onset than with opioids, probably because of the long plasma half-life of most benzodiazepines. With diazepam, the withdrawal symptoms may take up to 3 weeks to become apparent. Short-acting benzodiazepines cause more abrupt withdrawal effects.

The physical and psychological withdrawal symptoms make it difficult for patients to give up taking benzodiazepines, but craving (i.e. severe psychological dependence that outlasts the physical withdrawal syndrome), which occurs with many drugs of abuse (Ch. 50), is not a major problem.

Abuse potential

Benzodiazepines are widely abused drugs, often taken in combination with other drugs such as opioids or alcohol (see Ch. 50). Most illicit use comes from diversion of prescribed benzodiazepines. They induce a feeling of calm and reduced anxiety, with users describing a dream state where they are cushioned from reality. The risk of overdose is greatly increased when used in combination with alcohol. Tolerance and physical dependence occur as described above.

OTHER POTENTIAL ANXIOLYTIC DRUGS

Post-traumatic stress disorder (PTSD) is caused by experiencing stressful, frightening or distressing events. Sufferers often relive the traumatic events through nightmares and flashbacks, and may experience feelings of isolation, irritability and guilt. Symptoms include anxiety, depression and insomnia. If treatment with psychological therapies is unsuccessful then drug therapy with anxiolytic/antidepressant drugs (see Ch. 48) such as SSRIs (e.g. **paroxetine**, **sertraline** and **mirtazapine)**, a tricyclic antidepressant (**amitriptyline**) or a monoamine oxidase inhibitor (**phenelzine**) may be tried. In addition hypnotic agents (see later) may aid sleeping.

A recent development has been the realisation that the unpleasant, negative memories that underlie fear are not necessarily permanent. When such memories are reactivated (recalled) they return transiently to a labile state that can be disrupted. In humans, propranolol administered before memory reactivation may erase negative memories (see Lonergan et al., 2013). Ketamine, psilocybin, lysergic acid diethylamide (LSD) and 3,4-methylenedioxymethamphetamine (MDMA or ecstasy) may have a similar effect. Disrupting unpleasant memories in this way may provide a new treatment for PSTD.

Besides the GABA and 5-HT mechanisms discussed before, many other transmitters and hormones have been implicated in anxiety and panic disorders, particularly noradrenaline, glutamate, melatonin, corticotrophin-releasing factor, cholecystokinin (CCK), substance P, neuropeptide Y, galanin, orexins and neurosteroids. Anxiolytic drugs

---

[7]In practice, patients are usually left to sleep it off, because there is a risk of seizures with flumazenil; however, flumazenil may be useful diagnostically to rule out coma of other causes.

[8]Withdrawal symptoms can be more severe. A relative of one of the authors, advised to stop taking benzodiazepines after 20 years, suffered hallucinations and one day tore down all the curtains, convinced that they were on fire.

Benzodiazepines

- Act by binding to a specific allosteric modulatory site on the GABA$_A$ receptor, thus enhancing the inhibitory effect of GABA. Subtypes of the GABA$_A$ receptor exist in different regions of the brain and differ in their functional effects.
- Anxiolytic benzodiazepines are agonists at this modulatory site. Other benzodiazepines (e.g. **flumazenil**) are antagonists or weak negative allosteric modulators and prevent the actions of the anxiolytic benzodiazepines. Strong negative allosteric modulators (not used clinically) are anxiogenic and proconvulsant.
- Anxiolytic effects are mediated by GABA$_A$ receptors containing the α2 subunit, while sedation occurs through those with the α1 subunit.
- Benzodiazepines cause:
  - reduction of anxiety and aggression
  - sedation, leading to improvement of insomnia
  - muscle relaxation and loss of motor coordination
  - suppression of convulsions (antiepileptic effect)
  - anterograde amnesia
- Differences in the pharmacological profile of different benzodiazepines are minor; **clonazepam** appears to have more anticonvulsant action in relation to its other effects.
- Benzodiazepines are active orally and differ mainly in respect of their duration of action. Short-acting agents (e.g. **lorazepam** and **temazepam**, half-lives 8–12 h) are metabolised to inactive compounds and are used mainly as sleeping pills. Some long-acting agents (e.g. **diazepam** and **chlordiazepoxide**) are converted to a long-lasting active metabolite (**nordazepam**).
- Some are used intravenously, for example, **diazepam and lorazepam** in status epilepticus, **midazolam** in anaesthesia.
- Benzodiazepines are relatively safe in overdose. Their main disadvantages are interaction with alcohol, long-lasting 'hangover' effects and the development of tolerance and physical dependence – characteristic withdrawal syndrome on cessation of use.

Clinical use of drugs as anxiolytics

- Antidepressants (selective serotonin reuptake inhibitors [SSRIs] or serotonin/noradrenaline reuptake inhibitors [SNRIs]) are now the main drugs used to treat anxiety, especially when this is associated with depression. Their effects are slow in onset (>2 weeks).
- Benzodiazepines are now considered only as a short-term measure, usually limited to acute relief of severe and disabling anxiety.
- **Buspirone** (5-hydroxytryptamine [5-HT]$_{1A}$ agonist) has a different pattern of adverse effects from benzodiazepines and much lower abuse potential. Its effect is slow in onset (>2 weeks). It is licensed for short-term use, but specialists may use it for several months.

aimed at these targets are in development (see Murrough et al., 2015). Some cannabinoids (see Ch. 20) may have anxiolytic properties.

DRUGS USED TO TREAT INSOMNIA (HYPNOTIC DRUGS)

Insomnia can be *transient*, in people who normally sleep well but have to do shift work or have jet lag, *short-term*, usually due to illness or emotional upset, or *chronic*, where there is an underlying cause such as anxiety, depression, drug abuse, pain, pruritus or dyspnoea. While in anxiety and depression the underlying psychiatric condition should be treated, improvement of sleep patterns can improve the underlying condition. The drugs used to treat insomnia are:

- Benzodiazepines. Short-acting benzodiazepines (e.g. lorazepam and temazepam) are used for treating insomnia as they have little hangover effect. Diazepam, which is longer-acting, can be used to treat insomnia associated with daytime anxiety.
- Z-drugs (e.g. **zaleplon**, **zolpidem** and **zopiclone**). Although chemically distinct, these short-acting hypnotics act at the benzodiazepine site on GABA$_A$ receptors containing the α1 subunit. They lack appreciable anxiolytic activity. **Eszopiclone** is the active stereoisomer of zopiclone.
- **Clomethiazole**. It acts as a positive allosteric modulator of GABA$_A$ receptors acting at a site distinct from the benzodiazepines.
- Melatonin receptor agonists. **Melatonin**, **ramelteon** and **tasimelteon** are agonists at MT$_1$ and MT$_2$ receptors (see Ch. 40). They are effective in treating insomnia in the elderly and autistic children as well as in totally blind individuals.
- Orexin receptor antagonist. **Suvorexant** is an antagonist of OX$_1$ and OX$_2$ receptors which mediate the actions of the orexins, peptide transmitters in the CNS that are important in setting diurnal rhythm. Orexin levels are normally high in daylight and low at night, so the drug reduces wakefulness.
- Antihistamines[9] (see Ch. 27; e.g. **diphenhydramine** and **promethazine**) can be used to induce sleep. They are included in various over-the-counter preparations. **Doxepin** is an SNRI antidepressant (see Ch. 48) with histamine H$_1$- and H$_2$-receptor antagonist properties and **quetiapine** is an antipsychotic drug with a wide spectrum of activity (see Table 47.1) including H$_1$ antagonism; both are used to treat insomnia.
- Miscellaneous other drugs (e.g. **chloral hydrate** and **meprobamate**). They are no longer recommended, but therapeutic habits die hard and they are occasionally used. **Methaqualone**, used as a hypnotic and once popular as a drug of abuse, has been discontinued.

[9]This is an interesting example of an initial unwanted side effect – sedation is undesired when treating hay fever – subsequently becoming a therapeutic use.

Fig. 45.5 Effects of long-term benzodiazepine treatment on sleep quality. A group of 100 poor sleepers were given, under double-blind conditions, lormetazepam 5 mg, nitrazepam 2 mg or placebo nightly for 24 weeks, the test period being preceded and followed by 4 weeks of placebo treatment. They were asked to assess, on a subjective rating scale, the quality of sleep during each night, and the results are expressed as a 5-day rolling average of these scores. The improvement in sleep quality was maintained during the 24-week test period, and was followed by a 'rebound' worsening of sleep when the test period ended. (From Oswald, I. et al., 1982. Br. Med. J. 284, 860–864.)

INDUCTION OF SLEEP BY BENZODIAZEPINES

Benzodiazepines decrease the time taken to get to sleep, and increase the total duration of sleep, although the latter effect occurs only in subjects who normally sleep for less than about 6 h each night. With agents that have a short duration of action (e.g. zolpidem or temazepam), a pronounced hangover effect on wakening can be avoided.

▼ On the basis of electroencephalography measurements, several levels of sleep can be recognised. Of particular psychological importance are REM sleep, which is associated with dreaming, and slow-wave sleep, which corresponds to the deepest level of sleep when the metabolic rate and adrenal steroid are at their lowest and the secretion of growth hormone is at its highest (see Ch. 34). Most hypnotic drugs reduce the proportion of REM sleep, although benzodiazepines affect it less than other hypnotics, and zolpidem least of all. Artificial interruption of REM sleep causes irritability and anxiety, even if the total amount of sleep is not reduced, and the lost REM sleep is made up for at the end of such an experiment by a rebound increase. The same rebound in REM sleep is seen at the end of a period of administration of benzodiazepines or other hypnotics. The proportion of slow-wave sleep is significantly reduced by benzodiazepines, although growth hormone secretion is unaffected.

Fig. 45.5 shows the improvement of subjective ratings of sleep quality produced by a benzodiazepine, and the rebound decrease at the end of a 32-week period of drug treatment. It is notable that, although tolerance to objective effects such as reduced sleep latency occurs

within a few days, this is not obvious in the subjective ratings.

Benzodiazepines are now, however, only recommended for short courses of treatment of insomnia. Tolerance develops over 1–2 weeks with continuous use, and on cessation rebound insomnia and withdrawal occurs.

Hypnotic drugs

- Drugs that potentiate the action of GABA at GABA$_A$ receptors (e.g. benzodiazepines, **zolpidem**, **zopiclone**, **zaleplon** and **clomethiazole**) are used to induce sleep.
- Drugs with shorter half-lives in the body reduce the incidence of hangover the next morning.
- Drugs with H$_1$-receptor antagonist properties induce sedation and sleep.
- Drugs with novel mechanisms of action have been developed, e.g. melatonin receptor agonists and orexin receptor antagonists.

Clinical use of hypnotics ('sleeping tablets')

- The cause of insomnia should be established before administering hypnotic drugs. Common causes include alcohol or other drug misuse (see Ch. 50) and physical or psychiatric disorders (especially depression).
- Tricyclic antidepressants (Ch. 48) cause drowsiness, so can kill two birds with one stone if taken at night by depressed patients with sleep disturbance.
- Optimal treatment of chronic insomnia is often by changing behaviour (e.g. increasing exercise, staying awake during the day) rather than with drugs.
- Benzodiazepines should be used only for short periods (<4 weeks) and for severe insomnia. They can be useful for a few nights when transient factors such as admission to hospital, jet lag or an impending procedure cause insomnia.
- Drugs used to treat insomnia include:
  - benzodiazepines (e.g. **temazepam**) and related drugs (e.g. **zolpidem**, **zopiclone**, which also act at the benzodiazepine binding site);
  - **chloral hydrate** and **triclofos**, which were used formerly in children, but this is seldom justified;
  - sedating antihistamines (e.g. **promethazine**), which cause drowsiness (see Ch. 27) are less suitable for treating insomnia. They can impair performance the next day.

REFERENCES AND FURTHER READING

Ennaceur, A., Chazot, P.L., 2016. Preclinical animal anxiety research – flaws and prejudices. Pharmacol. Res. Perspect. 4, e00223. (*An interesting critique of animal models of anxiety*)

Jacob, T.C., Michels, G., Silayeva, L., Haydonm, J., Succol, F., Moss, S.J., 2012. Benzodiazepine treatment induces subtype-specific changes in GABA$_A$ receptor trafficking and decreases synaptic inhibition. Proc.

Natl. Acad. Sci. U. S. A. 109, 18595–18600. (*At last the mechanism of benzodiazepine tolerance is beginning to be explained*)

Lonergan, M.H., Olivera-Figueroa, L.A., Pitman, R.K., Brunet, A., 2013. Propranolol's effects on the consolidation and reconsolidation of long-term emotional memory in healthy participants: a meta-analysis. J. Psychiatry Neurosci. 38, 222–231. (*A meta analysis of a number of trials examining the ability of propranolol to disrupt negative memories*)

Murrough, J.W., Yaqubi, S., Sayed, S., Charney, D.S., 2015. Emerging drugs for the treatment of anxiety. Expert Opin. Emerg. Drugs 20, 393–406. (*This review focuses on the potential for development of novel treatments for anxiety*)

Ramos, A., 2008. Animal models of anxiety: do I need multiple tests? Trends Pharmacol. Sci. 29, 493–498. (*Describes the need for animal models in the testing of anxiolytic drugs*)

Skolnick, P., 2012. Anxioselective anxiolytics: on a quest for the Holy Grail. Trends Pharmacol. Sci. 33, 611–620.

Tan, K.R., Rudolph, U., Lüscher, C., 2011. Hooked on benzodiazepines: $GABA_A$ receptor subtypes and addiction. Trends Neurosci. 34, 188–197. (*Don't be fooled by the title, this review also contains information on how different $GABA_A$-receptor subunits mediate the different effects of benzodiazepines*)

46 Antiepileptic drugs

OVERVIEW

In this chapter we describe the nature of epilepsy, the neurobiological mechanisms underlying it and the animal models that can be used to study it. We then proceed to describe the various classes of drugs that are used to treat it, the mechanisms by which they work and their pharmacological characteristics.
 Centrally acting muscle relaxants are discussed briefly at the end of the chapter.

INTRODUCTION

Epilepsy is a very common disorder, characterised by *seizures*, which take various forms and result from episodic neuronal discharges, the form of the seizure depending on the part of the brain affected. Epilepsy affects 0.5%–1% of the population, i.e. ~50 million people worldwide. It may be genetic in origin (often referred to as idiopathic) or develop after brain damage, such as trauma, stroke, infection or tumour growth, or other kinds of neurological disease. In some instances the cause is unknown. Epilepsy is treated mainly with drugs, although brain surgery may be used for suitable severe cases. Current antiepileptic drugs are effective in controlling seizures in about 70% of cases, but their use is often limited by side effects. In addition to their use in patients with epilepsy, antiepileptic drugs are used to treat or prevent convulsions caused by other brain disorders, for example trauma (including following neurosurgery), infection (as an adjunct to antibiotics), brain tumours and stroke. For this reason, they are sometimes termed anticonvulsants rather than antiepileptics. Increasingly, some antiepileptic drugs have been found to have beneficial effects in non-convulsive disorders such as neuropathic pain (Ch. 43), bipolar depression (Ch. 48) and anxiety (Ch. 45). Many new antiepileptic drugs have been developed over the past 25 or so years in attempts to improve their efficacy and side-effect profile, for example by modifying their pharmacokinetics. Improvements have been steady rather than spectacular, and epilepsy remains a difficult problem, despite the fact that controlling reverberative neuronal discharges would seem, on the face of it, to be a much simpler problem than controlling those aspects of brain function that determine emotions, mood and cognitive function.

THE NATURE OF EPILEPSY

The term 'epilepsy' is used to define a group of neurological disorders, all of which exhibit periodic seizures. For information on the underlying causes of epilepsy and factors that precipitate periodic seizures see Browne and Holmes (2008). As explained later, not all seizures involve convulsions. Seizures are associated with episodic high-frequency discharge of impulses by a group of neurons (sometimes referred to as the *focus*) in the brain. What starts as a local abnormal discharge may then spread to other areas of the brain. The site of the primary discharge and the extent of its spread determine the symptoms that are produced, which range from a brief lapse of attention to a full convulsive fit lasting for several minutes, as well as odd sensations or behaviours. The particular symptoms produced depend on the function of the region of the brain that is affected. Thus, involvement of the motor cortex causes convulsions, involvement of the hypothalamus causes peripheral autonomic discharge, and involvement of the reticular formation in the upper brain stem leads to loss of consciousness.

Abnormal electrical activity during and following a seizure can be detected by electroencephalography (EEG) recording from electrodes distributed over the surface of the scalp. Various types of seizure can be recognised on the basis of the nature and distribution of the abnormal discharge (Fig. 46.1). Modern brain imaging techniques, such as magnetic resonance imaging and positron emission tomography, are now routinely used in the evaluation of patients with epilepsy (Fig. 46.2) to identify structural abnormalities (e.g. ischaemic lesions, tumours; see Deblaere & Achten, 2008).

TYPES OF EPILEPSY

The clinical classification of epilepsy is done on the basis of the characteristics of the seizure rather than on the cause or underlying pathology. There are two major seizure categories, namely *partial* (localised to part of the brain) and *generalised* (involving the whole brain).

PARTIAL SEIZURES

Partial (focal) seizures are those in which the discharge begins locally and often remains localised. The symptoms depend on the brain region or regions involved, and include involuntary muscle contractions, abnormal sensory experiences or autonomic discharge, or effects on mood and behaviour – often termed *psychomotor epilepsy* – which may arise from a focus within a temporal lobe. The EEG discharge in this type of epilepsy is normally confined to one hemisphere (see Fig. 46.1D). Partial seizures can often be attributed to local cerebral lesions, and their incidence increases with age. In complex partial seizures, loss of consciousness may occur at the outset of the attack, or somewhat later, when the discharge has spread from its site of origin to regions of the brain stem reticular formation. In some individuals, a partial seizure can, during the seizure,

(A) Normal

(B) Generalised seizure (grand mal) — tonic–clonic type

(C) Generalised seizure (petit mal) — absence seizure type

(D) Partial seizure

Fig. 46.1 **Electroencephalography (EEG) records in epilepsy.** (A) Normal EEG recorded from frontal *(F)*, temporal *(T)* and occipital *(O)* sites on both sides, as shown in the inset diagram. The α rhythm (10/s) can be seen in the occipital region. (B) Sections of EEG recorded during a generalised tonic–clonic (grand mal) seizure: *1*, normal record; *2*, onset of tonic phase; *3*, clonic phase; *4*, postconvulsive coma. (C) Generalised absence seizure (petit mal) showing sudden brief episode of 3/s 'spike-and-wave' discharge. (D) Partial seizure with synchronous abnormal discharges in left frontal and temporal regions. (From Eliasson, S.G. et al., 1978. Neurological Pathophysiology, second ed. Oxford University Press, New York.)

Fig. 46.2 **Positron emission tomography (PET) image using [^{18}F]-fluoro-2-deoxyglucose (FDG) of the brain of a female patient suffering from temporal lobe epilepsy.** The interictal area of hypometabolism in the left temporal lobe *(indicated by the arrow)* is suggestive of the site of the epileptic focus. (Image kindly provided by Prof. John Duncan and Prof. Peter Ell, UCL Institute of Neurology, London.)

become generalised when the abnormal neuronal activity spreads across the whole brain.

An epileptic focus in the motor cortex results in attacks, sometimes called *Jacksonian epilepsy,*[1] consisting of repetitive jerking of a particular muscle group, beginning on one side of the body, often in the thumb, big toe or angle of the mouth, which spreads and may involve much of the body within about 2 min before dying out. The patient loses voluntary control of the affected parts of the body but does not necessarily lose consciousness. In *psychomotor epilepsy* the attack may consist of stereotyped purposive movements such as rubbing or patting movements, or much more complex behaviour such as dressing, walking or hair combing. The seizure usually lasts for a few minutes, after which the patient recovers with no recollection of the event. The behaviour during the seizure can be bizarre and accompanied by a strong emotional response.

GENERALISED SEIZURES

Generalised seizures involve the whole brain, including the reticular system, thus producing abnormal electrical activity throughout both hemispheres. Immediate loss of consciousness is characteristic of generalised seizures. There are a number of types of generalised seizure – two important categories are *tonic–clonic* seizures (formerly referred to as grand mal, see Fig. 46.1B) and *absence seizures* (petit mal, see Fig. 46.1C); others include myoclonic, tonic, atonic and clonic seizures.

A *tonic–clonic seizure* consists of an initial strong contraction of the whole musculature, causing a rigid extensor spasm and an involuntary cry. Respiration stops, and

[1]After Hughlings Jackson, a distinguished 19th-century Yorkshire neurologist who published his outstanding work in the *Annals of the West Riding Lunatic Asylum.*

defecation, micturition and salivation often occur. This tonic phase lasts for about 1 min, during which the face is suffused and becomes blue (an important clinical distinction from syncope, the main disorder from which fits must be distinguished, where the face is ashen pale), and is followed by a series of violent, synchronous jerks that gradually die out in 2–4 min. The patient stays unconscious for a few more minutes and then gradually recovers, feeling ill and confused. Injury may occur during the convulsive episode. The EEG shows generalised continuous high-frequency activity in the tonic phase and an intermittent discharge in the clonic phase (see Fig. 46.1B).

Absence seizures occur in children; they are much less dramatic but may occur more frequently (many seizures each day) than tonic–clonic seizures. The patient abruptly ceases whatever he or she was doing, sometimes stopping speaking in mid-sentence, and stares vacantly for a few seconds, with little or no motor disturbance. Patients are unaware of their surroundings and recover abruptly with no after effects. The EEG pattern shows a characteristic rhythmic discharge during the period of the seizure (see Fig. 46.1C). The rhythmicity appears to be due to oscillatory feedback between the cortex and the thalamus, the special properties of the thalamic neurons being dependent on the T-type calcium channels that they express (see Shin, 2006). The pattern differs from that of partial seizures, where a high-frequency asynchronous discharge spreads out from a local focus. Accordingly, the drugs used specifically to treat absence seizures act mainly by blocking T-type calcium channels, whereas drugs effective against other types of epilepsy act mainly by blocking sodium channels or enhancing GABA-mediated inhibition.

A particularly severe kind of epilepsy, *Lennox–Gastaut syndrome*, occurs in children and is associated with progressive mental retardation, possibly a reflection of excitotoxic neurodegeneration (see Ch. 41).

About one-third of cases of epilepsy are familial and involve genetic mutations. While some are due to a single mutation, most result from polygenetic mutations (see Pandolfo, 2011). Most genes associated with familial epilepsies encode neuronal ion channels closely involved in controlling action potential generation (see Ch. 4), such as voltage-gated sodium and potassium channels, GABA receptors and nicotinic acetylcholine receptors. Some other genes encode proteins that interact with ion channels.

Status epilepticus refers to continuous uninterrupted seizures, requiring emergency medical treatment.

NEURAL MECHANISMS AND ANIMAL MODELS OF EPILEPSY

▼ The underlying neuronal abnormality in epilepsy is poorly understood. In general, excitation will naturally tend to spread throughout a network of interconnected neurons but is normally prevented from doing so by inhibitory mechanisms. Thus *epileptogenesis* can arise if excitatory transmission is facilitated or inhibitory transmission is reduced (exemplified by GABA$_A$ receptor antagonists causing convulsions; see Ch. 39). In certain respects, epileptogenesis resembles long-term potentiation (Ch. 39), and similar types of use-dependent synaptic plasticity may be involved. Neurons from which the epileptic discharge originates display an unusual type of electrical behaviour, termed the paroxysmal depolarising shift (PDS), during which the membrane potential suddenly decreases by about 30 mV and remains depolarised for up to a few seconds before returning to normal. A burst of action potentials often accompanies this depolarisation (Fig. 46.3). This event probably results from the abnormally exaggerated and prolonged action of an excitatory transmitter. Activation of NMDA

Fig. 46.3 'Paroxysmal depolarising shift' (PDS) compared with experimental activation of glutamate receptors of the NMDA type. (A) PDS recorded with an intracellular microelectrode from cortical neurons of anaesthetised cats. Seizure activity was induced by topical application of penicillin. (B) Intracellular recording from the caudate nucleus of an anaesthetised cat. The glutamate analogue NMDA was applied by ionophoresis from a nearby micropipette. (Panel [A] from Matsumoto, H., Marsan, C.A., 1964. Exp. Neurol. 9, 286; panel [B] from Herrling, P.L. et al., 1983. J. Physiol. 339, 207.)

receptors (see Ch. 39) produces 'plateau-shaped' depolarising responses very similar to the PDS.

Because detailed studies are difficult to carry out on epileptic patients, many different animal models of epilepsy have been investigated (see Bialer & White, 2010; Grone & Baraban, 2015). Transgenic mouse strains have been reported that show spontaneous seizures. They include knock-out mutations of various ion channels, receptors and other synaptic proteins. Local application of penicillin crystals to the cerebral cortex results in focal seizures, probably by interfering with inhibitory synaptic transmission. Convulsant drugs (e.g. **pentylenetetrazol** [PTZ]) are often used, as are seizures caused by electrical stimulation of the whole brain. In the *kainate model* a single injection of the glutamate receptor agonist kainic acid into the amygdaloid nucleus of a rat can produce spontaneous seizures 2–4 weeks later that continue indefinitely. This is believed to result from excitotoxic damage to inhibitory neurons.

In the *kindling model*, brief low-intensity electrical stimulation of certain regions of the limbic system, such as the amygdala, normally produces no seizure response but if repeated daily for several days the response gradually increases until very low levels of stimulation will evoke a full seizure, and eventually seizures occur spontaneously. This kindled state can persist indefinitely but is prevented by NMDA receptor antagonists or deletion of the neurotrophin receptor, TrkB.

In human focal epilepsies, surgical removal of a damaged region of cortex may fail to cure the condition, as though the abnormal discharge from the region of primary damage had somehow produced a secondary hyperexcitability elsewhere in the brain. Furthermore, following severe head injury, prophylactic treatment with antiepileptic drugs reduces the incidence of post-traumatic epilepsy, which suggests that a phenomenon similar to kindling may underlie this form of epilepsy.

Most recently, zebrafish have been used to study epileptic phenotypes resulting from genetic manipulation, both gene knock-out and knock-in of specific mutations. There is promise for this approach in the screening of drugs with activity against specific forms of genetic epilepsies (Grone & Baraban, 2015)

ANTIEPILEPTIC DRUGS

Antiepileptic (sometimes known as *anticonvulsant*) drugs are used to treat epilepsy as well as non-epileptic convulsive disorders.

Nature of epilepsy

- Epilepsy affects about 0.5% of the population.
- The characteristic event is the seizure, which may be associated with convulsions but may take other forms.
- The seizure is caused by an asynchronous high-frequency discharge of a group of neurons, starting locally and spreading to a varying extent to affect other parts of the brain. In absence seizures, the discharge is regular and oscillatory.
- Partial seizures affect localised brain regions, and the attack may involve mainly motor, sensory or behavioural phenomena. Unconsciousness occurs when the reticular formation is involved.
- Generalised seizures affect the whole brain. Two common forms of generalised seizure are the tonic–clonic fit and the absence seizure. Status epilepticus is a life-threatening condition in which seizure activity is uninterrupted.
- Partial seizures can become secondarily generalised if the localised abnormal neuronal activity subsequently spreads across the whole brain.
- Many animal models have been devised, including electrically and chemically induced generalised seizures, production of local chemical damage and kindling. These provide good prediction of antiepileptic drug effects in humans.
- The neurochemical basis of the abnormal discharge is not well understood. It may be associated with enhanced excitatory amino acid transmission, impaired inhibitory transmission or abnormal electrical properties of the affected cells. Several susceptibility genes, mainly encoding neuronal ion channels, have been identified.
- Repeated epileptic discharge can cause neuronal death (excitotoxicity).
- Current drug therapy is effective in 70%–80% of patients.

With optimal drug therapy, epilepsy is controlled completely in about 75% of patients, but about 10% (50,000 in Britain) continue to have seizures at intervals of 1 month or less, which severely disrupts their life and work. There is therefore a need to improve the efficacy of therapy.

Patients with epilepsy usually need to take drugs continuously for many years, so avoidance of side effects is particularly important. Nevertheless, some drugs that have considerable adverse effects are still quite widely used even though they are not drugs of choice for newly diagnosed patients.[2] There is a need for more specific and effective drugs, and a number of new drugs have recently been introduced for clinical use or are in late stages of clinical trials. Long-established antiepileptic drugs are listed in

Table 46.1. Newer drugs (see Table 46.2) with similar mechanisms of action to older drugs or novel mechanisms of action may offer advantages in terms of efficacy in drug-resistant epilepsies, better pharmacokinetic profile, improved tolerability, lower potential for interaction with other drugs (see Ch. 58) and fewer adverse effects. The appropriate use of drugs from this large available menu depends on many clinical factors (see Shih et al., 2017).

MECHANISM OF ACTION

Antiepileptic drugs aim to inhibit the abnormal neuronal discharge rather than to correct the underlying cause. Three main mechanisms of action appear to be important:

1. Enhancement of GABA action.
2. Inhibition of sodium channel function.
3. Inhibition of calcium channel function.

More recently, newer drugs with other, novel mechanisms of action have been developed.

Antiepileptic drugs may exert more than one beneficial action, prime examples being **valproate** and **topiramate** (see Tables 46.1 and 46.2). The relative importance and contribution of each of these actions to the therapeutic effect is somewhat uncertain.

As with drugs used to treat cardiac dysrhythmias (Ch. 22), the aim is to prevent the paroxysmal discharge without affecting normal transmission. It is clear that properties such as use-dependence and voltage-dependence of channel-blocking drugs (see Ch. 4) are important in achieving this selectivity, but our understanding remains fragmentary.

Enhancement of GABA action

Several antiepileptic drugs (e.g. **phenobarbital** and **benzodiazepines**) enhance the activation of $GABA_A$ receptors, thus facilitating the GABA-mediated opening of chloride channels (see Chs 3 and 45).[3] **Vigabatrin** acts by irreversibly inhibiting the enzyme GABA transaminase that is responsible for inactivating GABA (see Ch. 39) in astrocytes and GABAergic nerve terminals. **Tiagabine** is an inhibitor of the 'neuronal' GABA transporter GAT1 that is expressed on GABAergic nerve terminals, and, to a lesser extent, on neighbouring astrocytes, thus inhibiting the removal of GABA from the synapse. It elevates the extracellular GABA concentration, as measured in microdialysis experiments, and also potentiates and prolongs GABA-mediated synaptic responses in the brain.

Inhibition of sodium channel function

Many antiepileptic drugs (e.g. **carbamazepine, phenytoin** and **lamotrigine**; see Tables 46.1 and 46.2) affect membrane excitability by an action on voltage-dependent sodium channels (see Chs 4 and 44), which carry the inward membrane current necessary for the generation of an action potential. Their blocking action shows the property of use-dependence; in other words, they block preferentially the excitation of cells that are firing repetitively, and the higher the frequency of firing, the greater the block produced. This characteristic, which is relevant to the ability of drugs to block the high-frequency discharge that occurs in an epileptic fit without unduly interfering with the

---

[2]Bromide was the first antiepileptic agent. Its propensity to induce sedation and other unwanted side effects has resulted in it being largely withdrawn from human medicine, although it is still approved for human use in some countries and may have uses in drug-resistant childhood epilepsies. It is still widely used in veterinary practice to treat epilepsy in dogs and cats.

[3]Absence seizures, paradoxically, are often exacerbated by drugs that enhance GABA activity and better treated by drugs acting by different mechanisms such as T-type calcium-channel inhibition.

Table 46.1 Properties of long-established antiepileptic drugs

Drug	Site of action				Main uses	Main unwanted effect(s)	Pharmacokinetics
	Sodium channel	GABA_A receptor	Calcium channel	Other			
Carbamazepine[a]	+	—	—	—	All types except absence seizures Especially focal seizures such as temporal lobe epilepsy Also trigeminal neuralgia	Sedation, ataxia, blurred vision, water retention, hypersensitivity reactions, leukopenia, liver failure (rare)	Half-life 12–18 h (longer initially) Strong induction of liver enzymes, so risk of drug interactions
Phenytoin[b]	+	—	—	—	All types except absence seizures	Ataxia, vertigo, gum hypertrophy, hirsutism, megaloblastic anaemia, fetal malformation, hypersensitivity reactions	Half-life ~24 h Saturation kinetics, therefore unpredictable plasma levels Plasma monitoring often required
Valproate	+	?+	+	GABA transaminase inhibition	Most types, including absence seizures	Generally less than with other drugs Nausea, hair loss, weight gain, fetal malformations	Half-life 12–15 h
Ethosuximide[c]	—	—	+	—	Absence seizures May exacerbate tonic–clonic seizures	Nausea, anorexia, mood changes, headache	Long plasma half-life (~60 h)
Phenobarbital[d]	?+	+	—	—	All types except absence seizures	Sedation, depression	Long plasma half-life (>60 h) Strong induction of liver enzymes, so risk of drug interactions (e.g. with phenytoin)
Benzodiazepines (e.g. clonazepam, clobazam, lorazepam, diazepam)	—	+	—	—	Lorazepam used intravenously to control status epilepticus	Sedation Withdrawal syndrome (see Ch. 45)	See Ch. 45

[a]Oxcarbazepine and eslicarbazepine, recently introduced, are similar; claimed to have fewer side effects.
[b]Fosphenytoin is a water-soluble phenytoin prodrug that is safer than phenytoin when given by injection.
[c]Trimethadione is similar to ethosuximide in that it acts selectively against absence seizures but has greater toxicity (especially the risk of severe hypersensitivity reactions and teratogenicity).
[d]Primidone is pharmacologically similar to phenobarbital and is converted to phenobarbital in the body. It has no clear advantages and is more liable to produce hypersensitivity reactions, so is now rarely used.

low-frequency firing of neurons in the normal state, arises from the ability of blocking drugs to discriminate between sodium channels in their resting, open and inactivated states (see Chs 4 and 44). Depolarisation of a neuron (such as occurs in the PDS described previously) increases the proportion of the sodium channels in the inactivated state. Antiepileptic drugs bind preferentially to channels in this state, preventing them from returning to the resting state, and thus reducing the number of functional channels

available to generate subsequent action potentials. **Lacosamide** enhances sodium channel inactivation, but unlike other antiepileptic drugs it appears to affect slow rather than rapid inactivation processes.

Inhibition of calcium channels

Drugs that are used to treat absence seizures (e.g. **ethosuximide** and **valproate**) share the ability to block T-type low-voltage-activated calcium channels. T-type channel

Table 46.2 Properties of newer antiepileptic drugs[a]

Drug	Site of action				Main uses	Main unwanted effect(s)	Pharmacokinetics
	Sodium channel	GABA$_A$ receptor	Calcium channel	Other			
Vigabatrin	—	—	—	GABA transaminase inhibition	All types Appears to be effective in patients resistant to other drugs	Sedation, behavioural and mood changes (occasionally psychosis) Visual field defects	Short plasma half-life, but enzyme inhibition is long-lasting
Lamotrigine	+	—	?+	Inhibits glutamate release	All types	Dizziness, sedation, rashes	Plasma half-life 24–36 h
Gabapentin Pregabalin	—	—	+	—	Partial seizures	Few side effects, mainly sedation	Plasma half-life 6–9 h
Felbamate	+	+	?+	? NMDA receptor block	Used mainly for severe epilepsy (Lennox–Gastaut syndrome) because of risk of adverse reaction	Few acute side effects but can cause aplastic anaemia and liver damage (rare but serious)	Plasma half-life ~20 h Excreted unchanged
Tiagabine	—	—	—	Inhibits GABA uptake	Partial seizures	Sedation Dizziness, lightheadedness	Plasma half-life ~7 h Liver metabolism
Topiramate	+	?+	?+	AMPA-receptor block	Partial and generalised tonic–clonic seizures. Lennox–Gastaut syndrome	Sedation Fewer pharmacokinetic interactions than phenytoin Fetal malformation	Plasma half-life ~20 h Excreted unchanged
Levetiracetam[a]	—	—	—	Binds to SV2A protein	Partial and generalised tonic–clonic seizures	Sedation (slight)	Plasma half-life ~7 h Excreted unchanged
Zonisamide	+	?+	+	—	Partial seizures	Sedation (slight) Appetite suppression, weight loss	Plasma half-life ~70 h
Rufinamide	+	—	—	?+ Inhibits GABA reuptake	Partial seizures	Headache, dizziness, fatigue	Plasma half-life 6–10 h
Lacosamide	+	—	—	—	Partial seizures	Nausea and vomiting dizziness, visual disturbances impaired coordination mood changes	Plasma half-life 13 h
Perampanel	—	—	—	Non-competitive AMPA antagonist	Partial seizures	Dizziness, weight gain, sedation impaired coordination changes in mood and behaviour	Plasma half-life 70–100 h

[a]Brivaracetam is a structural analogue.
SV2A, synaptic vesicle protein 2A.

activity is important in determining the rhythmic discharge of thalamic neurons associated with absence seizures (Khosravani et al., 2004).

Gabapentin, though designed as a simple analogue of GABA that would be sufficiently lipid soluble to penetrate the blood–brain barrier, owes its antiepileptic effect mainly to an action on P/Q-type calcium channels. By binding to a particular channel subunit ($\alpha2\delta1$), both gabapentin and **pregabalin** (a related analogue) reduce the trafficking to the plasma membrane of calcium channels containing this subunit, thereby reducing calcium entry into the nerve terminals and reducing the release of various neurotransmitters and modulators.

Other mechanisms

Many of the newer antiepileptic drugs were developed empirically on the basis of activity in animal models. Their mechanism of action at the cellular level is not fully understood.

Levetiracetam is believed to interfere with neurotransmitter release by binding to synaptic vesicle protein 2A (SV2A), which is involved in synaptic vesicle docking and fusion. **Brivaracetam**, a related antiepileptic agent, also binds to SV2A with 10-fold higher affinity.

While a drug may appear to work by one of the major mechanisms described, close scrutiny often reveals other actions that may also be therapeutically relevant. For example, **phenytoin** not only causes use-dependent block of sodium channels (see p. 583) but also affects other aspects of membrane function, including calcium channels and post-tetanic potentiation, as well as intracellular protein phosphorylation by calmodulin-activated kinases, which could also interfere with membrane excitability and synaptic function.

Antagonism at ionotropic excitatory amino acid receptors has been a major focus in the search for new antiepileptic drugs. Despite showing efficacy in animal models, by and large they did not prove useful in the clinic, because the margin between the desired anticonvulsant effect and unacceptable side effects, such as loss of motor coordination, was too narrow. However, **perampanel**, a non-competitive AMPA-receptor antagonist, has been approved as an add on treatment for partial seizures.

Mechanism of action of antiepileptic drugs

- The major antiepileptic drugs are thought to act by three main mechanisms:
  - reducing electrical excitability of cell membranes, mainly through use-dependent block of sodium channels;
  - enhancing GABA-mediated synaptic inhibition; this may be achieved by an enhanced postsynaptic action of GABA, by inhibiting GABA transaminase or by inhibiting GABA uptake into neurons and glial cells;
  - inhibiting T-type calcium channels (important in controlling absence seizures).
- Newer drugs act by other mechanisms, some yet to be elucidated.

CARBAMAZEPINE

Carbamazepine is chemically related to the tricyclic antidepressant drugs (see Ch. 48) and was found in a routine screening test to inhibit electrically evoked seizures in mice. Pharmacologically and clinically, its actions resemble those of phenytoin, although it appears to be particularly effective in treating certain partial seizures (e.g. psychomotor epilepsy). It is also used to treat other conditions, such as neuropathic pain (Ch. 43) and manic-depressive illness (Ch. 48).

Pharmacokinetic aspects

Carbamazepine is slowly but well absorbed after oral administration. Its plasma half-life is about 30 h when it is given as a single dose, but it is a strong inducer of hepatic enzymes, and the plasma half-life shortens to about 15 h when it is given repeatedly. Some of its metabolites have antiepileptic properties. A slow-release preparation is used for patients who experience transient side effects coinciding with plasma concentration peaks following oral dosing.

Unwanted effects

Carbamazepine produces a variety of unwanted effects ranging from drowsiness, dizziness and ataxia to more severe mental and motor disturbances.[4] It can also cause water retention (and hence hyponatraemia; Ch. 30) and a variety of gastrointestinal and cardiovascular side effects. The incidence and severity of these effects is relatively low, however, compared with other drugs. Treatment is usually started with a low dose, which is built up gradually to avoid dose-related toxicity. Severe bone marrow depression, causing neutropenia, and other severe forms of hypersensitivity reaction can occur, especially in people of Asian origin (see Ch. 12).

Carbamazepine is a powerful inducer of hepatic microsomal enzymes, and thus accelerates the metabolism of many other drugs, such as phenytoin, oral contraceptives, warfarin and corticosteroids, as well as of itself. When starting treatment, the opposite of a 'loading dose' strategy is employed: small initial doses are gradually increased, as when dosing is initiated, metabolising enzymes are not induced and so even low doses may give rise to adverse effects (notably ataxia); as enzyme induction occurs, increasing doses are needed to maintain therapeutic plasma concentrations. In general, it is inadvisable to combine it with other antiepileptic drugs, and interactions with other drugs (e.g. warfarin) metabolised by cytochrome P450 (CYP) enzymes are common and clinically important. **Oxcarbazepine** is a prodrug that is metabolised to a compound closely resembling carbamazepine, with similar actions but less tendency to induce drug-metabolising enzymes. Another structurally related drug, **eslicarbazepine** may have less effect on metabolising enzymes.

PHENYTOIN

Phenytoin is the most important member of the hydantoin group of compounds, which are structurally related to the barbiturates. It is highly effective in reducing the intensity

---

[4]One of the authors who was a keen hockey player played in a team with a goalkeeper who sometimes made silly errors early in the match. It turned out that he suffered from epilepsy and had taken his dose of carbamazepine too close to the start of the match.

and duration of electrically induced convulsions in mice, although ineffective against PTZ-induced convulsions. Owing to its many side effects and unpredictable pharmacokinetic behaviour, phenytoin usage is declining. Phenytoin is effective against various forms of partial and generalised seizures, although not against absence seizures, which it may even worsen.

Pharmacokinetic aspects

Phenytoin has certain pharmacokinetic peculiarities that need to be taken into account when it is used clinically. It is well absorbed when given orally, and about 80%–90% of the plasma content is bound to albumin. Other drugs, such as salicylates, phenylbutazone and valproate, inhibit this binding competitively (see Ch. 58). This increases the free phenytoin concentration but also increases hepatic clearance of phenytoin, so may enhance or reduce the effect of the phenytoin in an unpredictable way. Phenytoin is metabolised by the hepatic mixed function oxidase system and excreted mainly as glucuronide. It causes enzyme induction, and thus increases the rate of metabolism of other drugs (e.g. oral anticoagulants). The metabolism of phenytoin itself can be either enhanced or competitively inhibited by various other drugs that share the same hepatic enzymes. **Phenobarbital** produces both effects, and because competitive inhibition is immediate whereas induction takes time, it initially enhances and later reduces the pharmacological activity of phenytoin. **Ethanol** has a similar dual effect.

The metabolism of phenytoin shows the characteristic of saturation (see Ch. 11), which means that over the therapeutic plasma concentration range the rate of inactivation does not increase in proportion to the plasma concentration. The consequences of this are that:

- the plasma half-life (approximately 20 h) increases as the dose is increased
- the steady-state mean plasma concentration, achieved when a patient is given a constant daily dose, varies disproportionately with the dose. Fig. 46.4 shows that, in one patient, increasing the dose by 50% caused the steady-state plasma concentration to increase more than four-fold.

The range of plasma concentration over which phenytoin is effective without causing excessive unwanted effects is quite narrow (approximately 40–100 μmol/L). The very steep relationship between dose and plasma concentration, and the many interacting factors, mean that there is considerable individual variation in the plasma concentration achieved with a given dose. Regular monitoring of plasma concentration has helped considerably in achieving an optimal therapeutic effect. The past tendency was to add further drugs in cases where a single drug failed to give adequate control. It is now recognised that much of the unpredictability can be ascribed to pharmacokinetic variability, and regular monitoring of plasma concentration has reduced the use of polypharmacy.

Unwanted effects

Side effects of phenytoin begin to appear at plasma concentrations exceeding 100 μmol/L and may be severe above about 150 μmol/L. The milder side effects include vertigo, ataxia, headache and nystagmus, but not sedation. At higher plasma concentrations, marked confusion with intellectual deterioration occurs; a paradoxical increase in seizure frequency is a particular trap for the unwary prescriber. These effects occur acutely and are quickly reversible. Hyperplasia of the gums often develops gradually, as does hirsutism and coarsening of the features, which probably result from increased androgen secretion. Megaloblastic anaemia, associated with a disorder of folate metabolism, sometimes occurs, and can be corrected by giving folic acid (Ch. 26). Hypersensitivity reactions, mainly rashes, are quite common. Phenytoin has also been implicated as a cause of the increased incidence of fetal malformations in children born to epileptic mothers, particularly the occurrence of cleft palate, associated with the formation of an epoxide metabolite. Severe idiosyncratic reactions, including hepatitis, skin reactions and neoplastic lymphocyte disorders, occur in a small proportion of patients.

VALPROATE

Valproate is a simple monocarboxylic acid usually administered as the sodium salt. It is chemically unrelated to any other class of antiepileptic drug, and in 1963 it was discovered quite accidentally to have anticonvulsant properties

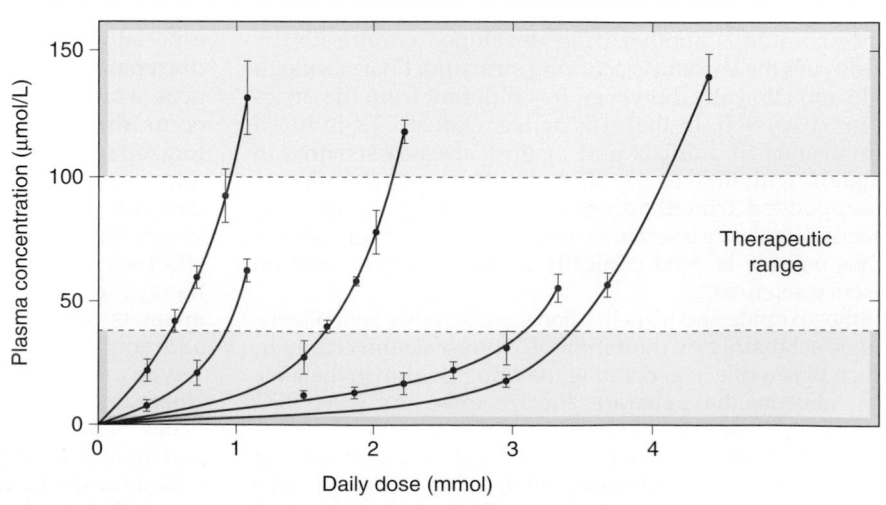

Fig. 46.4 **Non-linear relationship between daily dose of phenytoin and steady-state plasma concentration in five individual human subjects.** The daily dose required to achieve the therapeutic range of plasma concentrations (40–100 μmol/L) varies greatly between individuals, and for any one individual the dose has to be adjusted rather precisely to keep within the acceptable plasma concentration range. (Redrawn from Richens, A., Dunlop, A., 1975. Lancet 2, 247.)

in mice. It inhibits most kinds of experimentally induced convulsions and is effective in many kinds of epilepsy, being particularly useful in certain types of infantile epilepsy, where its low toxicity and lack of sedative action are important, and in adolescents who exhibit both tonic–clonic or myoclonic seizures as well as absence seizures, because valproate (unlike most antiepileptic drugs) is effective against each. Like carbamazepine, valproate is also used in psychiatric conditions such as bipolar depressive illness (Ch. 48).

Valproate works by several mechanisms (see Table 46.1), the relative importance of which remains to be clarified. It causes a significant increase in the GABA content of the brain and is a weak inhibitor of the enzyme system that inactivates GABA, namely GABA transaminase and succinic semialdehyde dehydrogenase (Ch. 39), but in vitro studies suggest that these effects would be very slight at clinical dosage. Other more potent inhibitors of these enzymes (e.g. **vigabatrin**; see p. 589) also increase GABA content and have an anticonvulsant effect in experimental animals. There is some evidence that it enhances the action of GABA by a postsynaptic action, but no clear evidence that it affects inhibitory synaptic responses. It inhibits sodium channels, but less so than phenytoin, and inhibits T-type calcium channels, which might explain why it is effective against absence seizures.

Valproate is well absorbed orally and excreted, mainly as the glucuronide, in the urine, the plasma half-life being about 15 h.

Unwanted effects

Valproate is contra-indicated in women of childbearing age because it is a potent teratogen (even more so than other anticonvulsants that tend to share this secondary pharmacology) (see p. 590), causing spina bifida and other neural tube defects.

Another serious but rare side effect is hepatotoxicity. An increase in plasma glutamic oxaloacetic transaminase, which signals liver damage of some degree, commonly occurs, but proven cases of valproate-induced hepatitis are rare. The few cases of fatal hepatitis in valproate-treated patients may well have been caused by other factors. More commonly, valproate causes thinning and curling of the hair, in about 10% of patients. Analogues of valproate with potentially reduced side effects are in development.

ETHOSUXIMIDE

Ethosuximide is another drug developed empirically by modifying the barbituric acid ring structure. Pharmacologically and clinically, however, it is different from the drugs so far discussed, in that it is active against PTZ-induced convulsions in animals and against absence seizures in humans, with little or no effect on other types of epilepsy. It supplanted **trimethadione**, the first drug found to be effective in absence seizures, which had major side effects. Ethosuximide is used clinically for its selective effect on absence seizures.

Ethosuximide and trimethadione, unlike other antiepileptic drugs, act mainly by inhibition of T-type calcium channels, which play a role in generating the firing rhythm in thalamic relay neurons that generates the 3/s spike-and-wave EEG pattern characteristic of absence seizures.

Ethosuximide is well absorbed, and metabolised and excreted much like phenobarbital, with a plasma half-life of about 60 h. Its main side effects are nausea and anorexia, sometimes lethargy and dizziness, and it is said to precipitate tonic–clonic seizures in susceptible patients. Very rarely, it can cause severe hypersensitivity reactions.

PHENOBARBITAL

▼ Phenobarbital was one of the first barbiturates to be developed but is rarely used nowadays. Its clinical effectiveness closely resembles that of phenytoin; it affects the duration and intensity of artificially induced seizures, rather than the seizure threshold, and is (like phenytoin) ineffective in treating absence seizures. **Primidone**, also now rarely used, acts by being metabolised to phenobarbital. It often causes hypersensitivity reactions. The clinical uses of phenobarbital are virtually the same as those of phenytoin, but it is seldom used now because it causes sedation. For some years, phenobarbital was widely used in children, including as prophylaxis following febrile convulsions in infancy, but it can cause behavioural disturbances and hyperkinesias. It is, however, widely used in veterinary practice.

Pharmacokinetic aspects

▼ Phenobarbital is well absorbed, and about 50% of the drug in the blood is bound to plasma albumin. It is eliminated slowly from the plasma (half-life 50–140 h). About 25% is excreted unchanged in the urine. Because phenobarbital is a weak acid, its ionisation and hence renal elimination are increased if the urine is made alkaline (see Ch. 10). The remaining 75% is metabolised, mainly by oxidation and conjugation, by hepatic microsomal enzymes. Phenobarbital is a powerful inducer of liver CYP enzymes, and it lowers the plasma concentration of several other drugs (e.g. steroids, oral contraceptives, warfarin, tricyclic antidepressants) to an extent that is clinically important.

Unwanted effects

▼ The main unwanted effect of phenobarbital is sedation, which often occurs at plasma concentrations within the therapeutic range for seizure control. This is a serious drawback, because the drug may have to be used for years on end. Some degree of tolerance to the sedative effect seems to occur, but objective tests of cognition and motor performance show impairment even during long-term treatment. Other unwanted effects that may occur with clinical dosage include megaloblastic anaemia (similar to that caused by phenytoin), mild hypersensitivity reactions and osteomalacia. Like other barbiturates, it must not be given to patients with porphyria (see Ch. 12). In overdose, phenobarbital depresses brain stem function, producing coma and respiratory and circulatory failure, as do all barbiturates.

BENZODIAZEPINES

Benzodiazepines can be used to treat both acute seizures, especially in children – midazolam given buccally or **diazepam** being administered rectally – and status epilepticus (a life-threatening condition in which epileptic seizures occur almost without a break) for which agents such as **lorazepam**, diazepam, or **clonazepam** are administered intravenously. The advantage in status epilepticus is that they act very rapidly compared with other antiepileptic drugs. With most benzodiazepines (see Ch. 45), the sedative effect is too pronounced for them to be used for maintenance therapy and tolerance develops over 1–6 months. **Clonazepam** is unique among the benzodiazepines in that in addition to acting at the GABA$_A$ receptor, it also inhibits T-type calcium channels. Both it and the related compound **clobazam** are claimed to be relatively selective as antiepileptic drugs. Sedation is the main side effect of these compounds, and an added problem may be the withdrawal syndrome, which results in an exacerbation of seizures if the drug is stopped abruptly.

NEWER ANTIEPILEPTIC DRUGS
VIGABATRIN

Vigabatrin, the first 'designer drug' in the epilepsy field, is a vinyl-substituted analogue of GABA that was designed as an irreversible inhibitor of the GABA-metabolising enzyme GABA transaminase. In animal studies, vigabatrin increases the GABA content of the brain and also increases the stimulation-evoked release of GABA, implying that GABA transaminase inhibition can increase the releasable pool of GABA and effectively enhance inhibitory transmission. In humans, vigabatrin increases the content of GABA in the cerebrospinal fluid. Although its plasma half-life is short, it produces a long-lasting effect because the enzyme is blocked irreversibly, and the drug can be given by mouth once daily.

Vigabatrin's licence is restricted to patients with resistant epilepsy who have not responded or tolerated other appropriate drug combinations. A major drawback of vigabatrin is the development of irreversible peripheral visual field defects in a proportion of patients on long-term therapy, thus necessitating systematic screening examinations of the visual fields at regular intervals. Vigabatrin may cause depression, and occasionally psychotic disturbances and hallucinations, in a minority of patients.

LAMOTRIGINE

Lamotrigine, although chemically unrelated, resembles phenytoin and carbamazepine in its pharmacological effects but it appears that, despite its similar mechanism of action, lamotrigine has a broader therapeutic profile than the earlier drugs, with significant efficacy against absence seizures (it is also used to treat unrelated psychiatric disorders). Its main side effects are nausea, dizziness and ataxia, and hypersensitivity reactions (mainly mild rashes, but occasionally more severe). Its plasma half-life is about 24 h, with no particular pharmacokinetic anomalies, and it is taken orally.

FELBAMATE

Felbamate is an analogue of an obsolete anxiolytic drug, **meprobamate**. It is active in many animal seizure models and has a broader clinical spectrum than earlier antiepileptic drugs, but its mechanism of action at the cellular level is uncertain. Its acute side effects are mild, mainly nausea, irritability and insomnia, but it occasionally causes severe reactions resulting in aplastic anaemia or hepatitis. For this reason, its recommended use is limited to intractable epilepsy (e.g. in children with Lennox–Gastaut syndrome) that is unresponsive to other drugs. Its plasma half-life is about 24 h, and it can enhance the plasma concentration of other antiepileptic drugs given concomitantly.

GABAPENTIN AND PREGABALIN

Gabapentin and pregabalin are effective against partial seizures. Side effects (sleepiness, headache, fatigue, dizziness and weight gain) are less severe than with many antiepileptic drugs. The absorption of gabapentin from the intestine depends on the L-amino acid carrier system and shows the property of saturability, which means that increasing the dose does not proportionately increase the amount absorbed. Its plasma half-life is about 6 h, requiring dosing two to three times daily. Pregabalin is more readily absorbed from the gut and has a longer half-life (6–12 h).

As these drugs are excreted unchanged in the urine they must be used with care in patients whose renal function is impaired. Both drugs are also used as analgesics to treat neuropathic pain (Ch. 43) and as anxiolytics in the treatment of general anxiety disorders (see Ch. 45). Recently they have become drugs of abuse especially popular amongst heroin users and may contribute to opioid overdose deaths (see Ch. 50).

TIAGABINE

Tiagabine is an analogue of GABA that is able to penetrate the blood–brain barrier. It has a short plasma half-life and is mainly used as an add-on therapy for partial seizures. Its main side effects are drowsiness and confusion, dizziness, fatigue, agitation and tremor.

TOPIRAMATE

Topiramate is a drug that appears to do a little of everything, blocking sodium and calcium channels, enhancing the action of GABA, blocking AMPA receptors and, for good measure, weakly inhibiting carbonic anhydrase. Its clinical effectiveness resembles that of phenytoin, and it is claimed to produce less severe side effects, as well as being devoid of the pharmacokinetic properties that cause trouble with phenytoin. Currently, it is mainly used as add-on therapy in refractory cases of partial and generalised seizures.

LEVETIRACETAM

Levetiracetam was developed as an analogue of **piracetam**, a drug developed to improve cognitive function, and discovered by accident to have antiepileptic activity in animal models. Unusually, it lacks activity in conventional models such as electroshock and PTZ tests, but is effective in the audiogenic and kindling models (see p. 582). Levetiracetam is excreted unchanged in the urine. Common side effects include headaches, inflammation of the nose and throat, sleepiness, vomiting and irritability. **Brivaracetam** is similar to levetiracetam.

ZONISAMIDE

Zonisamide is a sulfonamide compound originally intended as an antibacterial drug and found accidentally to have antiepileptic properties. It is mainly free of major unwanted effects, although it causes drowsiness, and of serious interaction with other drugs. It tends to suppress appetite and cause weight loss, and is sometimes used for this purpose. Zonisamide has a long plasma half-life of 60–80 h, and is partly excreted unchanged and partly converted to a glucuronide metabolite. It is licensed for use as an adjunct treatment of partial and generalised seizures but may be effective as a monotherapy.

RUFINAMIDE

Rufinamide is a triazole derivative structurally unrelated to other antiepileptic drugs. It is licensed for treating Lennox–Gastaut syndrome and may also be effective in partial seizures. It has low plasma protein binding and is not metabolised by CYP enzymes.

PERAMPANEL

Perampanel is effective in refractory partial seizures. Side effects include dizziness, sedation, fatigue, irritability, weight gain, and loss of motor coordination. There is a risk of serious psychiatric problems (violent, even homicidal, thoughts and threatening behaviour) in some individuals.

LACOSAMIDE

Lacosamide is used to treat partial seizures. Side effects include nausea, dizziness, sedation and fatigue. It produces relief of pain due to diabetic neuropathy.

STIRIPENTOL

Stiripentol has some efficacy as an adjunctive therapy in children. It enhances GABA release and prolongs GABA-mediated synaptic events in a manner similar to pheno-barbital. It also inhibits lactate dehydrogenase (LDH) which may reduce the metabolic energy production required to maintain seizures.

NEW DRUGS

There are a number of new antiepileptic agents with novel mechanism of action approved or in late stages of clinical trials.[5] Ganaxolone, structurally resembling endogenous neurosteroids (see Ch. 39), is a positive allosteric modulator of GABA$_A$ receptors containing δ subunits that has recently been approved for the treatment of CDLK5 disorder, a rare form of genetic epilepsy predominantly affecting young girls. Cannabidiol, the major non-psychoactive component of cannabis (see Ch. 20), has recently been approved in the USA for the treatment of Dravet syndrome and Lennox–Gastaut syndrome. The mechanisms underlying its anti-epileptic efficacy are unclear as it has low affinity for CB$_1$ and CB$_2$ cannabinoid receptors. Other phytocannabinoids are reported to have anticonvulsant properties – an area to watch. Everolimus, an inhibitor of mammalian target of rapamycin (mTOR, see Ch. 27) is in phase III clinical trial for partial seizures. Tonabersat is a novel neuronal gap junction inhibitor that shows early promise.

The identification of epileptogenic mutations of genes encoding specific ion channels and other functional proteins (see Weber & Lerche, 2008) has for some time been expected to lead to new drugs aimed at these potential targets, but we are still waiting.

OTHER USES OF ANTIEPILEPTIC DRUGS

Antiepileptic drugs have proved to have much wider clinical applications than was originally envisaged, and clinical trials have shown many of them to be effective in the following conditions:

- bipolar disorder (**valproate**, carbamazepine, oxcarbazepine, lamotrigine, topiramate; Ch. 48)
- migraine prophylaxis (**valproate, gabapentin, topiramate**; Ch. 16)
- anxiety disorders (**gabapentin, pregabalin**; Ch. 45)
- neuropathic pain (**gabapentin, pregabalin, carbamazepine, lamotrigine**; Ch. 43)

This surprising multiplicity of clinical indications may reflect the fact that similar neurobiological mechanisms, involving synaptic plasticity and increased excitability of interconnected populations of neurons, underlie each of these disorders.

[5]The Epilepsy Foundation website (http://www.epilepsy.com/accelerating-new-therapies/new-therapies-pipeline#drugs) gives details of the large number of drugs currently in development for the treatment of epilepsies.

ANTIEPILEPTIC DRUGS AND PREGNANCY

There are several important implications for women taking antiepileptic drugs. By inducing hepatic CYP3A4 enzymes, some antiepileptic drugs may increase oral contraceptive metabolism, thus reducing their effectiveness (see Ch. 36). Taken during pregnancy, drugs such as phenytoin, carba-mazepine, lamotrogine, topiramate and valproate are thought to have some risk of teratogenic effects, although the magnitude of risk appears greatest with valproate. It remains to be clarified if newer agents also have this problem. Induction of CYP enzymes may result in vitamin K deficiency in the newborn (Ch. 26).

Clinical uses of antiepileptic drugs

- Generalised tonic–clonic seizures:
  - **valproate, lamotrigine** or **carbamazepine**;
  - use of a single drug is preferred, when possible, to avoid pharmacokinetic interactions;
  - newer agents include **topiramate, levetiracetam**.
- Partial (focal) seizures: **carbamazepine**, or **lamotrigine**; alternatives include **valproate, levetiracetam, clobazam, gabapentin, topiramate, levetiracetam**.
- Absence seizures: **ethosuximide, valproate**
  - **valproate** is the first-choice drug when absence seizures coexist with tonic–clonic seizures, because most other drugs used for tonic–clonic seizures can worsen absence seizures.
- Myoclonic seizures: **valproate, topiramate, levetiracetam**
- Status epilepticus: **lorazepam** intravenously or (in absence of accessible veins, intramuscular or oromucosal **midazolam**, or **diazepam** rectally).
- Neuropathic pain: for example **carbamazepine, gabapentin** (see Ch. 43).
- To stabilise mood in mono- or bipolar affective disorder (as an alternative to **lithium**): for example, **carbamazepine, valproate** (see Ch. 48).

MUSCLE SPASM AND MUSCLE RELAXANTS

Many diseases of the brain and spinal cord produce an increase in muscle tone, which can be painful and disabling. Spasticity resulting from birth injury or cerebral vascular disease, and the paralysis produced by spinal cord lesions, are examples. Multiple sclerosis is a neurodegenerative disease that is triggered by inflammatory attack on the central nervous system (see Ch. 41). When the disease has progressed for some years it can cause muscle stiffness and spasms, as well as other symptoms such as pain, fatigue, difficulty passing urine and tremors. Local injury or inflam-mation, as in arthritis, can also cause muscle spasm, and chronic back pain is also often associated with local muscle spasm.

Certain centrally acting drugs are available that have the effect of reducing the background tone of the muscle without seriously affecting its ability to contract transiently under voluntary control. The distinction between voluntary movements and 'background tone' is not clear-cut, and the selectivity of those drugs is not complete. Postural control, for example, is usually jeopardised by centrally acting muscle relaxants. Furthermore, drugs that affect motor control generally produce rather widespread effects on the central nervous system, and drowsiness and confusion turn out to be very common side effects of these agents.

Baclofen (see Ch. 39) is a chlorophenyl derivative of GABA originally prepared as a lipophilic GABA-like agent in order to assist penetration of the blood–brain barrier, which is impermeable to GABA itself. Baclofen is a selective agonist at $GABA_B$ receptors (see Ch. 39). The antispastic action of baclofen is exerted mainly on the spinal cord, where it inhibits both monosynaptic and polysynaptic activation of motor neurons. It is effective when given by mouth, and is used in the treatment of spasticity associated with multiple sclerosis or spinal injury. However, it is ineffective in cerebral spasticity caused by birth injury.

Baclofen produces various unwanted effects, particularly drowsiness, motor incoordination and nausea, and it may also have behavioural effects. It is not useful in epilepsy.

Benzodiazepines are discussed in detail in Chapter 45. They produce muscle relaxation by an effect in the spinal cord. They are also anxiolytic.

Tizanidine is an α_2-adrenoceptor agonist that relieves spasticity associated with multiple sclerosis and spinal cord injury.

For many years anecdotal evidence suggested that smoking **cannabis** (Ch. 20) relieves the painful muscle spasms associated with multiple sclerosis. **Sativex**, a cannabis extract containing Δ^9-tetrahydrocannabinol (also known as THC or **dronabinol**; see Ch. 20) and cannabidiol, is licensed in some countries as a treatment for spasticity in multiple sclerosis. It also has pain-relieving properties (see Chs 20 and 43).

Methocarbamol is used to treat muscle pain and stiffness. Its mechanism of action is unclear.

Dantrolene acts peripherally rather than centrally to produce muscle relaxation (see Ch. 4).

Botulinum toxin (see Ch. 14) injected into a muscle, inhibits acetylcholine release, causing long-lasting paralysis confined to the site of injection; its use to treat local muscle spasm is increasing. Its non-medicinal use as a 'beauty' treatment has become widespread.

REFERENCES AND FURTHER READING

General
Browne, T.R., Holmes, G.L., 2008. Handbook of Epilepsy. Lippincott, Williams & Wilkins, Philadelphia. (*A compact textbook covering most areas of epilepsy and its treatment*)

Pathogenesis and types of epilepsy
Deblaere, K., Achten, E., 2008. Structural magnetic resonance imaging in epilepsy. Eur. Radiol. 18, 119–129. (*Describes the use of brain imaging in the diagnosis of epilepsy*)
Grone, B.P., Baraban, S.C., 2015. Animal models in epilepsy research: legacies and new directions. Nat. Neurosci. 18, 339–343. (*Good description of older animal models of epilepsy and of the use of newer invertebrate models to study genetic idiopathic epilepsies*)
Khosravani, H., Altier, C., Simms, B., et al., 2004. Gating effects of mutations in the Ca$_v$3.2 T-type calcium channel associated with childhood absence epilepsy. J. Biol. Chem. 279, 9681–9684. (*Study showing that calcium channel mutations seen in childhood absence seizures cause abnormal neuronal discharges in transgenic mice*)

Pandolfo, M., 2011. Genetics of epilepsy. Semin. Neurol. 31, 506–518.
Shin, H.S., 2006. T-type Ca^{2+} channels and absence epilepsy. Cell Calcium 40, 191–196.
Weber, Y.G., Lerche, H., 2008. Genetic mechanisms in idiopathic epilepsies. Dev. Med. Child Neurol. 50, 648–654. (*Reviews how mutations in voltage- and ligand-gated ion channels are associated with idiopathic epilepsy syndromes*)

Antiepileptic drugs
Bialer, M., White, H.S., 2010. Key factors in the discovery and development of new antiepileptic drugs. Nat. Rev. Drug Discov. 9, 68–82. (*Interesting account of avenues for antiepileptic drug discovery*)
Shih, J.J., Whitlock, J.B., Chimato, N., Vargas, E., Karceski, S.C., Frank, R.D., 2017. Epilepsy treatment in adults and adolescents. Epilepsy Behav. 69, 186–222. (*Brings together the views of a number of acknowledged experts in epilepsy treatment on current drug therapies for different forms of epilepsy*)

47 Antipsychotic drugs

OVERVIEW

In this chapter we focus on schizophrenia and the drugs used to treat it. We start by describing the illness and what is known of its pathogenesis, including the various neurochemical hypotheses and their relation to the actions of the main types of antipsychotic drugs that are in use or in development. Further information can be found in Gross and Geyer (2012).

INTRODUCTION

Psychotic illnesses include various disorders, but the term antipsychotic drugs – previously known as *neuroleptic drugs*, *antischizophrenic drugs* or *major tranquillisers* – conventionally refers to those used to treat schizophrenia, one of the most common and debilitating forms of mental illness. These same drugs are also used to treat mania (Ch. 48) and other acute behavioural disturbances. Pharmacologically, most are dopamine receptor antagonists, although many of them also act on other targets, particularly 5-hydroxytryptamine (5-HT) receptors, which may contribute to their clinical efficacy. Existing drugs have many drawbacks in terms of their efficacy and side effects. Gradual improvements have been achieved with newer drugs, but radical new approaches will require a better understanding of the causes and underlying pathology of the disease, which are still poorly understood.[1]

THE NATURE OF SCHIZOPHRENIA

Schizophrenia[2] (see Stahl, 2008) affects about 1% of the population. It is one of the most important forms of psychiatric illness, because it affects young people, is often chronic and is usually highly disabling.[3] There is a strong hereditary factor in its aetiology, and evidence suggestive of a fundamental biological disorder. The main clinical features of the disease are as follows.

Positive symptoms
- Delusions (often paranoid in nature).
- Hallucinations (often in the form of voices, which may be exhortatory in their message).
- Thought disorder (comprising wild trains of thought, delusions of grandeur, garbled sentences and irrational conclusions).
- Abnormal, disorganised behaviour (such as stereotyped movements, disorientation and occasionally aggressive behaviours).
- Catatonia (can be apparent as immobility or purposeless motor activity).

Negative symptoms
- Withdrawal from social contacts.
- Flattening of emotional responses.
- Anhedonia (an inability to experience pleasure).
- Reluctance to perform everyday tasks.

Cognition
- Deficits in cognitive function (e.g. attention, memory).

In addition, anxiety, guilt, depression and self-punishment are often present, leading to suicide attempts in up to 50% of cases, about 10% of which are successful. The clinical phenotype varies greatly, particularly with respect to the balance between positive and negative symptoms, and this may have a bearing on the efficacy of antipsychotic drugs in individual cases. Schizophrenia can present dramatically, usually in young people, with predominantly positive features such as hallucinations, delusions and uncontrollable behaviour, or more insidiously in older patients with negative features such as flat mood and social withdrawal. The latter may be more debilitated than those with a florid presentation, and the prognosis is generally worse. Cognitive impairment may be evident even before the onset of other symptoms. Schizophrenia can follow a relapsing and remitting course, or be chronic and progressive, particularly in cases with a later onset. Chronic schizophrenia used to account for most of the patients in long-stay psychiatric hospitals; following the closure of many of these in the United Kingdom, it now accounts for many of society's outcasts.

A characteristic feature of schizophrenia is a defect in 'selective attention'. Whereas a normal individual quickly accommodates to stimuli of a familiar or inconsequential nature, and responds only to stimuli that are unexpected or significant, the ability of schizophrenic patients to

---

[1]In this respect, the study of schizophrenia lags some years behind that of Alzheimer's disease (Ch. 41), where understanding of the pathogenesis has progressed rapidly to the point where promising drug targets have been identified. On the other hand, pragmatists can argue that drugs against Alzheimer's disease are so far only marginally effective, whereas current antipsychotic drugs deliver great benefits even though we do not quite know how they work.

[2]Schizophrenia is a condition where the patient exhibits symptoms of psychosis (e.g. delusions, hallucinations and disorganized behaviour). Psychotic episodes may also occur as a result of taking certain recreational drugs (see Ch. 49); as an adverse effect of drug treatment, for example steroid-induced psychoses; or in disorders such as mania, depression (see Ch. 48) and Alzheimer's disease (see Ch. 41).

[3]A compelling account of what it is like to suffer from schizophrenia is contained in Kean (2009) Schizophrenia Bulletin 35, 1034–1036. The author is a pharmacology graduate.

discriminate between significant and insignificant stimuli seems to be impaired. Thus the ticking of a clock may command as much attention as the words of a companion; a chance thought, which a normal person would dismiss as inconsequential, may become an irresistible imperative.

AETIOLOGY AND PATHOGENESIS OF SCHIZOPHRENIA
GENETIC AND ENVIRONMENTAL FACTORS

The causes of schizophrenia remain unclear but involve a combination of genetic and environmental factors. Thus a person may have a genetic makeup that predisposes them to schizophrenia, but exposure to environmental factors may be required for schizophrenia to develop. The different forms that gene–environment interaction can take are discussed in detail in Ayhan et al. (2016).

The disease shows a strong, but incomplete, hereditary tendency. In first-degree relatives, the risk is about 10%, but even in monozygotic (identical) twins, one of whom has schizophrenia, the probability of the other being affected is only about 50%, pointing towards the importance of environmental factors. Genetic linkage studies have identified more than 100 genetic regions (loci) associated with a risk of schizophrenia (see Ripke et al., 2014; Sekar et al., 2016). There are significant associations between polymorphisms in individual genes and the likelihood of an individual developing schizophrenia but there appears to be no single gene that has an overriding influence. Some of the genes implicated in schizophrenia are also associated with bipolar disorder (see Ch. 48).

▼ The most robust associations are with genes that control neuronal development, synaptic connectivity and glutamatergic neurotransmission. These include *complement component 4A (C4A), neuregulin, dysbindin, DISC-1, TCF4* and *NOTCH4*. Increases in C4A expression result in increased synaptic pruning (the process of synapse elimination that occurs between early childhood and the onset of puberty) and may help explain the reduced numbers of synapses in the brains of schizophrenics. Transgenic mice that underexpress neuregulin-1, a protein involved in synaptic development and plasticity and which controls NMDA receptor expression, show a phenotype resembling human schizophrenia in certain respects. Malfunction of NMDA receptors is further implicated by genetic association with the genes for D-amino acid oxidase (DAAO), the enzyme responsible for metabolising D-serine, an allosteric modulator of NMDA receptors (see Ch. 39), and for DAAO activator (G72). Dysbindin is located in postsynaptic density domains and may be involved in tethering receptors including NMDA receptors. DISC-1 – which stands for disrupted in schizophrenia-1 – is a protein that associates with cytoskeletal proteins and is involved with cell migration, neurite outgrowth and receptor trafficking. Population genetic studies have suggested that *NOTCH4*, a developmentally expressed gene, and TCF-4, a gene also associated with mental retardation, are strongly associated with susceptibility for schizophrenia but their precise roles in its aetiology remain to be elucidated. Among other suggested susceptibility genes, some (such as the genes for monoamine oxidase A [MAO-A], tyrosine hydroxylase and the D_2 dopamine receptor) are involved in monoamine transmission in the central nervous system. However, the weight of current evidence seems to suggest that schizophrenia may result from abnormal glutamatergic transmission, involving a decrease in NMDA receptor function (see p. 594).

Some environmental influences early in development have been identified as possible predisposing factors, particularly maternal virus infections. This and other evidence suggests that schizophrenia is associated with a neurodevelopmental disorder affecting mainly the cerebral cortex and occurring in the first few months of prenatal development. This view is supported by brain imaging studies showing

cortical atrophy apparent in the early course of the disease which may increase with time and correlate with the progression of the disorder (van Haren et al., 2007). Studies of postmortem schizophrenic brains show evidence of misplaced cortical neurons with abnormal morphology. Other environmental factors such as cannabis consumption in adolescence and early adulthood (see Chs 20 and 49) may also reveal schizophrenia.

THE NEUROANATOMICAL AND NEUROCHEMICAL BASIS OF SCHIZOPHRENIA

Different symptoms of schizophrenia appear to result from malfunctions in different neuronal circuits. Changes in the mesolimbic pathway (the neuronal projection from the ventral tegmental area (VTA) to the nucleus accumbens, amygdala and hippocampus) being associated with positive symptoms, whereas negative symptoms are associated with changes in the prefrontal cortex which receives input from the VTA via the mesocortical pathway and which projects to the nucleus accumbens and dorsal striatum.

The main neurotransmitters thought to be involved in the pathogenesis of schizophrenia are dopamine and glutamate.

Dopamine

The original dopamine theory of schizophrenia was proposed by Carlson – awarded a Nobel Prize in 2000 – on the basis of indirect pharmacological evidence in humans and experimental animals. **Amphetamine** releases dopamine in the brain and can produce in humans a behavioural syndrome reminiscent of an acute schizophrenic episode. Also, hallucinations are a side effect of levodopa and dopamine agonists used for Parkinson's disease (see Ch. 41). In animals, dopamine release causes a specific pattern of stereotyped behaviour that resembles the repetitive behaviours sometimes seen in schizophrenic patients. Potent D_2 receptor agonists, such as **bromocriptine**, produce similar effects in animals, and these drugs, like amphetamine, exacerbate the symptoms of schizophrenic patients. Furthermore, dopamine antagonists and drugs that block neuronal dopamine storage (e.g. **reserpine**) are effective in controlling the positive symptoms of schizophrenia, and in preventing amphetamine-induced behavioural changes.

▼ It is now believed that positive symptoms result from *overactivity* in the mesolimbic dopaminergic pathway activating D_2 receptors (for a more detailed description of the dopamine pathways in the brain, see Ch. 40) whereas negative symptoms may result from a *decreased activity* in the mesocortical dopaminergic pathway where D_1 receptors predominate. Other dopaminergic pathways in the brain (i.e. nigrostriatal and tuberoinfundibular; see Ch. 40) appear to function normally in schizophrenia.

There is a strong correlation between antipsychotic potency in reducing positive symptoms and activity in blocking D_2 receptors (Fig. 47.1) and receptor imaging studies have shown that clinical efficacy of antipsychotic drugs is consistently achieved when D_2 receptor occupancy reaches about 80%.[4] Furthermore, brain imaging studies have revealed an increased dopamine synthesis and release in the striatum of schizophrenic patients (Laruelle et al., 1999). Similar changes have also been reported in non-schizophrenic close relatives, indicating that such changes may indicate predisposition to schizophrenia rather than the exhibition of symptoms. Injection of amphetamine caused dopamine release that was greater by a factor of two or more in

---

[4]There are, however, exceptions to this simple rule. Up to one-third of schizophrenic patients fail to respond even when D_2 receptor blockade exceeds 90%, and clozapine (see Table 47.1) can be effective at much lower levels of block.

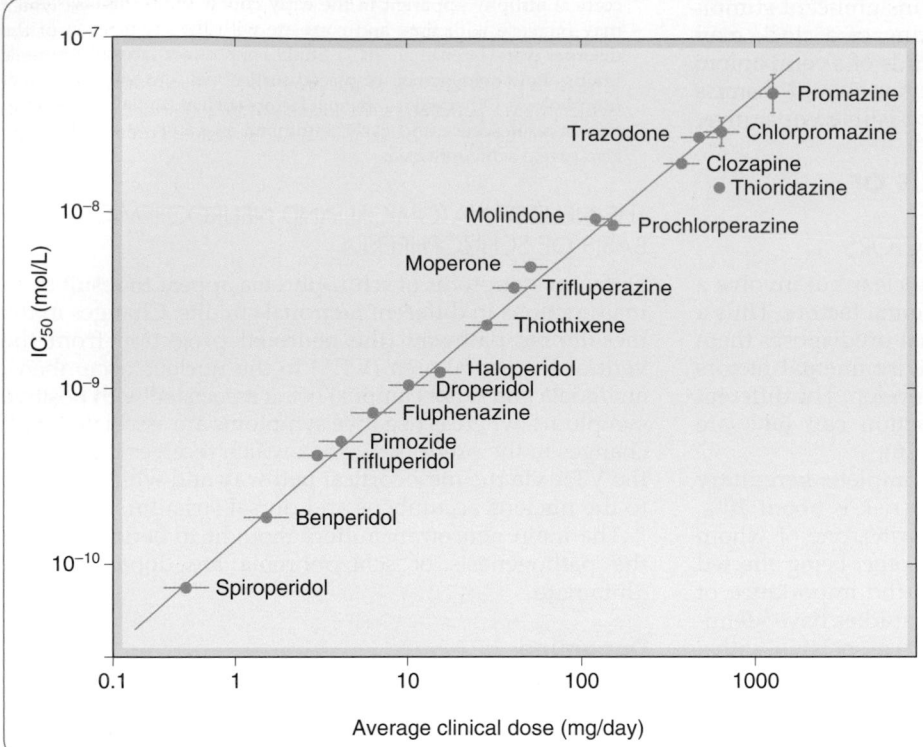

Fig. 47.1 Correlation between the clinical potency and affinity for dopamine D_2 receptors among antipsychotic drugs. Clinical potency is expressed as the daily dose used in treating schizophrenia, and binding activity is expressed as the concentration needed to produce 50% inhibition of haloperidol binding. (From Seeman, P. et al., 1976. Nature 361, 717.)

schizophrenic subjects compared with control subjects. The effect was greatest in schizophrenic individuals during acute attacks, and absent during spontaneous remissions – clear evidence linking dopamine release to the symptomatology.

An increase in dopamine receptor density in schizophrenia has been reported in some studies, but not consistently, and the interpretation is complicated by the fact that chronic antipsychotic drug treatment is known to increase dopamine receptor expression.

Thus, therapeutically it might be desirable to *inhibit* dopaminergic transmission in the limbic system yet *enhance* dopaminergic transmission in the prefrontal cortex (how this might be achieved is discussed later).

Glutamate

In humans, NMDA receptor antagonists such as **phencyclidine**, **ketamine** and **dizocilpine** (Ch. 39) can produce positive, negative and cognitive deficit symptoms – in contrast to amphetamine, which produces only positive symptoms. In the brains from schizophrenic patients, expression of the glutamate uptake transporter VGLUT1 is reduced, which may indicate a disruption of glutamatergic nerve terminals. It has therefore been postulated that schizophrenia may result from disruption of glutamatergic neurotransmission, evident as a reduction in the function of NMDA receptors (the NMDA hypofunction hypothesis; see Coyle 2017). Consistent with this hypothesis, transgenic mice in which NMDA receptor expression is reduced (not abolished, because this is fatal) show stereotypic behaviours and reduced social interaction that are features of human schizophrenia and that respond to antipsychotic drugs.

▼ Glutamatergic neurons and GABAergic neurons play complex roles in controlling the level of activity in neuronal pathways involved in schizophrenia. NMDA receptor hypofunction is thought to *reduce* the level of activity in mesocortical dopaminergic neurons. This would result in a decrease in dopamine release in the prefrontal cortex and could thus give rise to negative symptoms of schizophrenia.

NMDA receptor hypofunction in the cortex may affect GABAergic interneurons and alter cortical processing, giving rise to cognitive impairment. In addition, NMDA receptor hypofunction on GABAergic neurons would reduce inhibition of the excitatory cortical input to the VTA and thus *enhance* activity in the mesolimbic dopaminergic pathway. Thus NMDA receptor hypofunction could give rise to enhanced dopamine release in limbic areas such as the nucleus accumbens, resulting in the production of positive symptoms.

Given the evidence that schizophrenic symptoms may be due to a reduction in NMDA receptor function, efforts have been made to develop new drugs to enhance NMDA receptor function but not to a level where it becomes neurotoxic (see Ch. 41), e.g. by activating the facilitatory glycine site on the NMDA receptor (see Ch. 39) with an agonist or by raising extracellular glycine levels by inhibiting the GlyT1 transporter. However, **bitopertin**, a GlyT1 inhibitor, failed as an antipsychotic drug in clinical trials.

Other glutamate pathways thought to be involved in schizophrenia are the corticostriatal, thalamocortical, corticothalamic and cortico-brain stem pathways. The thalamus normally functions as a sensory filter to limit unnecessary sensory input to the cortex. Disruption of the normal inputs to the thalamus, for example from a reduction in glutamatergic or GABAergic transmission, disables this 'sensory gate' function, allowing uninhibited input to reach the cortex. The role of the thalamus in schizophrenia is reviewed by Pergola et al. (2015).

The hope is that a fuller understanding of the altered function of glutamate transmission in schizophrenia will lead to the development of new, improved antipsychotic drugs.

Animal models

There is a need for the development of animal models of schizophrenia that simulate the positive, negative and cognitive deficit components of this disorder. Schizophrenia presents as a heterogeneous disorder with sufferers exhibiting different combinations of symptoms that may result from different neuronal abnormalities. Traditional models by and large reflect behaviours resulting from heightened dopaminergic transmission in the brain. Thus they were likely to show positive results with drugs that have dopamine receptor-antagonist activity. Models based on inhibition of NMDA function by **phencyclidine** (PCP) and related drugs have become popular in recent years. Also, various genetic models are being examined. These have focused on proteins such as DISC-1 that are implicated in schizophrenia and on receptors and transporters for neurotransmitters such as glutamate and dopamine. However, as described earlier, the genetic basis of schizophrenia is multifactorial and environmental factors are also important. Thus mutation of a single gene may provide only limited information. Models of cognitive deficits and negative symptoms are lacking. The development of such models is a major challenge that requires a better understanding of the pathophysiological processes that underlie different symptoms. For further details on the development of new animal models of schizophrenia see Pratt et al. (2012) and Sigardsson (2015).

The nature of schizophrenia

- Psychotic illness characterised by delusions, hallucinations and thought disorder (positive symptoms), together with social withdrawal and flattening of emotional responses (negative symptoms), and cognitive impairment.
- Acute episodes (mainly positive symptoms) frequently recur and may develop into chronic schizophrenia, with predominantly negative symptoms.
- Incidence is about 1% of the population, with a significant hereditary component. Genetic linkage studies suggest involvement of multiple genes, but no single 'schizophrenia gene'.
- Pharmacological evidence is generally consistent with dopamine dysregulation and glutamate underactivity hypotheses, supported by biochemical findings, clinical efficacy and imaging studies.

ANTIPSYCHOTIC DRUGS

CLASSIFICATION OF ANTIPSYCHOTIC DRUGS

More than 80 different antipsychotic drugs are available for clinical use. These have been divided into two groups – those drugs that were originally developed (e.g. **chlorpromazine**, **haloperidol** and many similar compounds), often referred to as *first-generation*, *typical* or *conventional antipsychotic drugs*, and more recently developed agents (e.g. **clozapine**, **risperidone**), which are termed *second-generation* or *atypical antipsychotic drugs*. Table 47.1 summarises the main drugs that are in clinical use.[5]

▼ The term 'atypical' has been widely used but not clearly defined. In effect, it refers to the diminished tendency of later compounds to cause unwanted motor side effects, but it is also used to describe compounds with a different pharmacological profile from first-generation compounds. In practice, however, it often serves – not

very usefully – to distinguish the large group of similar first-generation dopamine antagonists from the more diverse group of later compounds.

The therapeutic activity of the prototype drug, **chlorpromazine**, in schizophrenic patients was discovered through the acute observations of a French surgeon, Laborit, in 1947. He tested various substances, including **promethazine**, for their ability to alleviate signs of stress in patients undergoing surgery, and concluded that promethazine had a calming effect that was different from mere sedation. Elaboration of the phenothiazine structure led to chlorpromazine, the antipsychotic effect of which was demonstrated in man, at Laborit's instigation, by Delay and Deniker in 1953. This drug was unique in controlling the symptoms of psychotic patients. The clinical efficacy of phenothiazines was discovered long before their mechanism was guessed at, let alone understood.

Pharmacological investigation showed that phenothiazines, the first-generation antipsychotic agents, block many different mediators, including histamine, catecholamines, acetylcholine and 5-HT, and this multiplicity of actions led to the trade name Largactil for chlorpromazine. It is now clear (see Fig. 47.1) that antagonism of dopamine is the main determinant of antipsychotic action.

Classification of antipsychotic drugs

- Main categories are:
  - first-generation ('typical', 'classical' or 'conventional') antipsychotics (e.g. **chlorpromazine**, **haloperidol**, **fluphenazine**, **flupentixol**, **zuclopenthixol**);
  - second-generation ('atypical') antipsychotics (e.g. **clozapine**, **risperidone**, **quetiapine**, **amisulpride**, **aripiprazole**, **ziprasidone**).
- Distinction between first- and second-generation drugs is not clearly defined but rests on:
  - receptor profile;
  - incidence of extrapyramidal side effects (less in second-generation group);
  - efficacy (specifically of **clozapine**) in 'treatment-resistant' group of patients;
  - efficacy against negative symptoms.

CLINICAL EFFICACY IN TREATMENT OF SCHIZOPHRENIA

The clinical efficacy of antipsychotic drugs in enabling schizophrenic patients to lead more normal lives has been demonstrated in many controlled trials (see Leucht et al., 2013). The inpatient population (mainly chronic schizophrenics) of mental hospitals declined sharply in the 1950s and 1960s. The introduction of antipsychotic drugs was a significant enabling factor, as well as the changing public and professional attitudes towards hospitalisation of the mentally ill.

Antipsychotic drugs have severe drawbacks that include:

- Not all schizophrenic patients respond to drug therapy. It is recommended to try **clozapine** in patients who are resistant to other antipsychotic drugs. The 30% of patients who do not respond are classed as 'treatment resistant' and present a major therapeutic problem. The reason for the difference between responsive and unresponsive patients is unknown at present, although there is some evidence

[5]Wikipedia (https://en.wikipedia.org/wiki/List_of_antipsychotics) lists no fewer than 49 first-generation and 32 second-generation agents approved for clinical use. Despite this huge investment by the pharmaceutical industry and plethora of me-too compounds, clinical benefits have been modest.

Table 47.1 Characteristics of some major antipsychotic drugs

Drug	Receptor affinity						Main side effects				Notes
	D_1	D_2	α_1	H_1	mACh	5-HT$_{2A}$	EPS	Sed	Hypo	Other	
Chlorpromazine	++	++	+++	+++	++	+++	++	+++	++	Increased prolactin (gynaecomastia)	Phenothiazine class
										Hypothermia	Perphenazine and prochlorperazine are similar. Fluphenazine, trifluoperazine are similar but:
										Anticholinergic effects	• do not cause jaundice
										Hypersensitivity reactions	• cause less hypotension • cause more EPS
										Obstructive jaundice	
											Fluphenazine available as depot preparation
											Pericyazine causes less EPS probably due to its greater muscarinic antagonist actions. Pipotiazine has been withdrawn
Haloperidol	++	+++	++	+	—	++	+++	—	+	As chlorpromazine but does not cause jaundice	Butyrophenone class
										Fewer anticholinergic side effects	Widely used antipsychotic drug
											Strong EPS tendency
											Available as depot preparation
Flupentixol	+++	+++		+++	—	+	++	+	+	Increased prolactin (gynaecomastia)	Thioxanthine class
										Restlessness	Zuclopenthixol is similar
											Available as depot preparation
Amisulpride	—	++	—	—	—	—	+	+	—	Increased prolactin (gynaecomastia)	Benzamide class (includes sulpiride)
											Selective D_2/D_3 antagonist
											Less EPS than haloperidol (reason for this unclear, but could result from action at D_3 or very weak partial agonism at D_2)
											Increases alertness in apathetic patients
											Poorly absorbed
											Amisulpride and pimozide (long-acting) are similar
Clozapine	+	+	+++	++++	++	+++	—	++	++	Risk of agranulocytosis (~1%): regular blood counts required	Dibenzodiazepine class
										Seizures	No EPS (first second-generation antipsychotic)

Table 47.1 Characteristics of some major antipsychotic drugs—cont'd

Drug	Receptor affinity						Main side effects				Notes
	D_1	D_2	α_1	H_1	mACh	$5\text{-}HT_{2A}$	EPS	Sed	Hypo	Other	
Clozapine, cont'd										Salivation	Shows efficacy in 'treatment-resistant' patients and reduces incidence of suicide
										Anticholinergic side effects	Effective against negative and positive symptoms
										Weight gain	Olanzapine is somewhat less sedative, without risk of agranulocytosis, but questionable efficacy in treatment-resistant patients
Risperidone	+	+++	+++	++	—	++++ (IA?)	+	++	++	Weight gain	Significant risk of EPS
										EPS at high doses	? Effective against negative symptoms
										Hypotension	Potent on D_4 receptors
											Available as depot preparation
											Paliperidone is a metabolite of risperidone
											Iloperidone reported to have low incidence of EPS and weight gain
Quetiapine	+	+	+++	+++	+	+	—	++	++	Tachycardia	Low incidence of EPS
										Drowsiness	No increase in prolactin secretion
										Dry mouth	$5\text{-}HT_{1A}$ partial agonist
										Constipation	Short-acting (plasma half-life ~6 h)
										Weight gain	
Aripiprazole	+	++++ (PA)	++	++	—	+++	—	+	—	—	Long-acting (plasma half-life ~3 days)
											Unusual D_2 partial agonist profile may account for paucity of side effects
											Also a $5HT_{1A}$ partial agonist
											No effect on prolactin secretion
											No weight gain
											Available as a depot preparation
											Brexpiprazole may also be useful in the treatment of depression
Ziprasidone	++	+++	+++	++	—	++++	+	—	+	Tiredness	Low incidence of EPS
										Nausea	No weight gain
											Lurasidone is similar
											? Effective against negative symptoms
											Short-acting (plasma half-life ~8 h) but a depot preparation is available

+, pKi 5–7; ++, pKi 7–8; +++, pKi 8–9; +++, pKi >9; *5-HT₁A, 5-HT₂A*, 5-hydroxytryptamine types 1A and 2A receptors; *α₁, α₁* adrenoceptor; *D₁, D₂, D₃, D₄*, dopamine types 1, 2, 3 and 4 receptor, respectively; *ECG*, electrocardiograph; *EPS*, extrapyramidal side effects; *H₁*, histamine type 1 receptor; *Hypo*, hypotension; *IA*, inverse agonist; *mACh*, muscarinic acetylcholine receptor; *PA*, partial agonist; *Sed*, sedation.

(Table based on data contained in Guide to Pharmacology (http://www.guidetopharmacology.org/) and NIMH Psychoactive Drug Screening Program database (http://pdsp.med.unc.edu/). Where available, data obtained on human receptors are given.)

(not conclusive) that polymorphisms within the family of dopamine and 5-HT receptors may be involved.
- While they control the positive symptoms (thought disorder, hallucinations, delusions, etc.) effectively, most are ineffective in relieving the negative symptoms (emotional flattening, social isolation) and cognitive impairment.
- They induce a range of side effects that include extrapyramidal motor, endocrine and sedative effects (see Table 47.1) that can be severe and limit patient compliance.
- They may produce unwanted cardiac (pro-arrhythmic) effects (see Ch. 22).

Second-generation antipsychotic drugs were believed to overcome these shortcomings to some degree. However, a meta-analysis (Leucht et al., 2013) concluded that only some of the second-generation antipsychotic drugs examined showed better overall efficacy. There is a definite need for the development of new treatments.

Abrupt cessation of antipsychotic drug administration may lead to a rapid onset psychotic episode distinct from the underlying illness.

OTHER USES OF ANTIPSYCHOTIC DRUGS

A common emerging theme with centrally acting drugs is that while they were initially developed to treat one brain disorder they have been subsequently found to be effective in treating other disorders. This is also the case with antipsychotic drugs, which are now used to treat a range of disorders, including:

- bipolar disorder, mania and depression (see Ch. 48)
- psychomotor agitation and severe anxiety (**chlorpromazine** and **haloperidol**)
- agitation and restlessness in the elderly (**risperidone**), although this is highly questionable
- psychosis associated with Parkinson's disease (**primavanserin**) (see Ch. 41)
- restlessness and pain in palliative care (**levomepromazine**)
- nausea and vomiting (e.g. **chlorpromazine** and **haloperidol**) reflecting antagonism at dopamine, muscarinic, histamine and possibly 5-HT receptors
- motor tics and intractable hiccup (**chlorpromazine** and **haloperidol**)
- antisocial sexual behaviour (**benperidol**)
- involuntary movements caused by Huntington's disease (mainly **haloperidol**; see Ch. 41)

PHARMACOLOGICAL PROPERTIES
DOPAMINE RECEPTORS

The classification of dopamine receptors in the central nervous system is discussed in Chapter 40 (see Table 40.1). There are five subtypes, which fall into two functional classes: the D_1 type, comprising D_1 and D_5, and the D_2 type, comprising D_2, D_3 and D_4. Antipsychotic drugs owe their therapeutic effects mainly to blockade of D_2 receptors.[6] As stated previously, antipsychotic effects require about 80%

---

[6]The D_4 receptor attracted attention on account of the high degree of genetic polymorphism that it shows in human subjects, and because some of the newer antipsychotic drugs (e.g. clozapine) have a high affinity for this receptor subtype. However, a specific D_4 receptor antagonist proved ineffective in clinical trials.

block of D_2 receptors. The first-generation compounds show some preference for D_2 over D_1 receptors, whereas some of the later agents (e.g. **sulpiride**, **amisulpride**,) are highly selective for D_2 receptors. D_2 antagonists that dissociate rapidly from the receptor (e.g. **quetiapine**) and D_2 partial agonists (e.g. **aripiprazole**) were introduced in an attempt to reduce extrapyramidal motor side effects (see p. 599). **Cariprazine**, a new antipsychotic drug, is a D_2 and D_3 partial agonist with higher affinity for D_3 than D_2 receptors.

It is the antagonism of D_2 receptors in the mesolimbic pathway that is believed to relieve the positive symptoms of schizophrenia. Unfortunately, systemically administered antipsychotic drugs do not discriminate between D_2 receptors in distinct brain regions and D_2 receptors in other brain pathways will also be blocked. Thus antipsychotic drugs produce unwanted motor effects (block of D_2 receptors in the nigrostriatal pathway), enhance prolactin secretion (block of D_2 receptors in the tuberoinfundibular pathway), reduce pleasure (block of D_2 receptors in the reward component of the mesolimbic pathway) and perhaps even worsen the negative symptoms of schizophrenia (block of D_2 receptors in the prefrontal cortex, although these are only expressed at a low density – D_1 receptors being in greater abundance). While all antipsychotic drugs block D_2 receptors and should therefore in theory induce all of these unwanted effects, some have additional pharmacological activity (e.g. mACh receptor antagonism and 5-HT_{2A} receptor antagonism) that, to varying degrees, ameliorate unwanted effects. 5-HT_{2A} antagonism may also help to alleviate the negative and cognitive impairments of schizophrenia.

Antipsychotic drugs have classically been thought to have a delayed onset to their therapeutic actions, even though their dopamine receptor-blocking action is immediate. This view has, however, been called into question (Kapur et al., 2005; Leucht et al., 2005). In animal studies, chronic antipsychotic drug administration does produce compensatory changes in the brain, for example, a reduction in the activity of dopaminergic neurons and proliferation of dopamine receptors, detectable as an increase in haloperidol binding, with a pharmacological supersensitivity to dopamine reminiscent of the phenomenon of denervation supersensitivity (Ch. 13). The mechanism(s) of these delayed effects are poorly understood. They are likely to contribute to the development of unwanted *tardive dyskinesias*. The sedating effect of antipsychotic drugs is immediate, allowing them to be used in acute behavioural emergencies.

> ### Mechanism of action of antipsychotic drugs
>
> - Most antipsychotic drugs are antagonists or partial agonists at D_2 dopamine receptors, but they also block a variety of other receptors.
> - Antipsychotic potency generally runs parallel to activity on D_2 receptors, but activities at other receptors (e.g. 5-HT_{2A} and muscarinic) may reduce extrapyramidal side effects.
> - Activity at muscarinic, H_1 and α receptors may determine unwanted side effect profile.
> - Imaging studies suggest that therapeutic effect requires about 80% occupancy of D_2 receptors.

5-HYDROXYTRYPTAMINE RECEPTORS

The idea that 5-HT dysfunction could be involved in schizophrenia has drifted in and out of favour many times. It was originally based on the fact that LSD, a partial agonist at 5-HT$_{2A}$ receptors (see Chs 16 and 49), produces hallucinations. Conventional wisdom was that 5-HT is not directly involved in the pathogenesis of schizophrenia. Nevertheless, pharmacological manipulation of 5-HT receptor activity, combined with D$_2$ receptor antagonism, has resulted in new drugs with improved therapeutic profiles (see Table 47.1).[7] There is a plethora of 5-HT receptors (see Chs 16 and 40), with disparate functions in the body. It is the 5-HT$_{2A}$ receptor and, to a lesser extent, the 5-HT$_{1A}$ receptor that are important in the treatment of schizophrenia.

5-HT$_{2A}$ receptors are G$_i$/G$_o$-coupled receptors and their activation produces neuronal inhibition (through decreased neuronal excitability at the soma and decreased transmitter release at the nerve terminals; see Ch. 40). In this way, in the nigrostriatal pathway, 5-HT$_{2A}$ receptors control the release of dopamine. Drugs with 5-HT$_{2A}$ antagonist properties (e.g. **olanzapine** and risperidone) enhance dopamine release in the striatum by reducing the inhibitory effect of 5-HT. This will reduce extrapyramidal side effects (see later). In contrast, in the mesolimbic pathway, the combined effects of D$_2$ and 5-HT$_{2A}$ antagonism are thought to counteract the increased dopamine function that gives rise to positive symptoms of schizophrenia. Further, enhancing both dopamine and glutamate release in the mesocortical circuit, 5-HT$_{2A}$ receptor antagonism may improve the negative symptoms of schizophrenia (Stahl, 2008). **Primavanserin**, a drug recently introduced for the treatment of psychosis associated with Parkinson's disease (see Ch. 41) and which may be beneficial as an adjunct to other antipsychotic drugs in the treatment of schizophrenia, is an inverse agonist at the 5-HT$_{2A}$ receptor and has no activity at dopaminergic receptors.

5-HT$_{1A}$ receptors are somatodendritic autoreceptors that inhibit 5-HT release (see Ch. 40). Antipsychotic drugs that are agonists or partial agonists at 5-HT$_{1A}$ receptors (e.g. **quetiapine**; see Table 47.1) may work by decreasing 5-HT release, thus enhancing dopamine release in the striatum and prefrontal cortex.

The concept of 5-HT receptors as targets for novel antipsychotic drug development is discussed further at the end of this chapter.

MUSCARINIC ACETYLCHOLINE RECEPTORS

Some phenothiazine antipsychotic drugs (e.g. **pericyazine**) have been reported to produce fewer extrapyramidal side effects than others, and this was thought to correlate with their muscarinic antagonist actions. Also, some second-generation drugs possess muscarinic antagonist properties (e.g. olanzapine). In the striatum, dopaminergic nerve terminals are thought to innervate cholinergic interneurons that express inhibitory D$_2$ receptors (Pisani et al., 2007). It is suggested that there is normally a balance between D$_2$ receptor activation and muscarinic receptor activation. Blocking D$_2$ receptors in the striatum with an antipsychotic agent will result in enhanced acetylcholine release on to muscarinic receptors, thus producing extrapyramidal side effects, which are counteracted if the D$_2$ antagonist also has muscarinic antagonist activity. Maintaining the dopamine/acetylcholine balance was also the rationale for the use of the muscarinic antagonist **benztropine** to reduce extrapyramidal effects of antipsychotic drugs. Muscarinic antagonist activity does, however, induce side effects such as constipation, dry mouth and blurred vision.

UNWANTED EFFECTS
EXTRAPYRAMIDAL MOTOR DISTURBANCES

Antipsychotic drugs produce two main kinds of motor disturbance in humans: *acute dystonias* and *tardive dyskinesias*, collectively termed *extrapyramidal side effects*. These all result directly or indirectly from D$_2$ receptor blockade in the nigrostriatal pathway. Extrapyramidal side effects constitute one of the main disadvantages of first-generation antipsychotic drugs. Second-generation drugs were thought to have less tendency to produce extrapyramidal side effects. However, a long-term study of olanzapine, risperidone, quetiapine and **ziprasidone** concluded that they too can induce extrapyramidal side effects (see Lieberman & Stroup, 2011). Even aripiprazole, which is a D$_2$ partial agonist, has been reported to produce this unwanted effect.

Acute dystonias are involuntary movements (restlessness, muscle spasms, protruding tongue, fixed upward gaze, neck muscle spasm), often accompanied by symptoms of Parkinson's disease (Ch. 41). They occur commonly in the first few weeks, often declining with time, and are reversible on stopping drug treatment. The timing is consistent with block of the dopaminergic nigrostriatal pathway. Concomitant block of muscarinic receptors and 5-HT$_{2A}$ receptors mitigates the motor effects of dopamine receptor antagonists (see earlier).

Tardive dyskinesia (see Klawans et al., 1988) develops after months or years (hence 'tardive') in 20%–40% of patients treated with first-generation antipsychotic drugs, and is one of the main problems of antipsychotic therapy. Its seriousness lies in the fact that it is a disabling and often irreversible condition, which often gets worse when antipsychotic therapy is stopped and is resistant to treatment. The syndrome consists of involuntary movements, often of the face and tongue, but also of the trunk and limbs, which can be severely disabling. It resembles that seen after prolonged treatment of Parkinson's disease with **levodopa** (see Ch. 41). The incidence depends greatly on drug, dose and age (being commonest in patients who are over 50 years of age).

▼ There are several theories about the mechanism of tardive dyskinesia (see Casey, 1995). One is that it is associated with a gradual increase in the number of D$_2$ receptors in the striatum, which is less marked during treatment with second-generation than with first-generation antipsychotic drugs. Another possibility is that chronic block of inhibitory dopamine receptors enhances catecholamine and/or glutamate release in the striatum, leading to excitotoxic neurodegeneration (Ch. 41).

Drugs that rapidly dissociate from D$_2$ receptors (e.g. clozapine, olanzapine) induce less severe extrapyramidal side effects. A possible explanation for this (see Kapur & Seeman, 2001) is that with a rapidly

---

[7]Early antipsychotic drugs (e.g. chlorpromazine) had actions at various receptors but also had unwanted side effects that resulted from activity at other receptors. Towards the end of the 20th century, drug development, not just of antipsychotic drugs, was focused largely on developing agents with a single action with the intention of reducing unwanted side effects. This philosophy drove the search for selective D$_4$ receptor antagonists, which proved ineffective. What is now apparent is that drugs with selected multiple actions (e.g. a combination of D$_2$ antagonism and 5-HT$_{2A}$ antagonism) may have a better therapeutic profile.

dissociating compound, a brief surge of dopamine can effectively overcome the block by competition (see Ch. 2), whereas with a slowly dissociating compound, the level of block takes a long time to respond to the presence of endogenous dopamine, and is in practice non-competitive. Adverse motor effects may be avoided if fractional receptor occupation by the antagonist falls during physiological surges of dopamine. An extension of this idea is that perhaps a little D_2 receptor activation may be beneficial. This could be produced, for example, by drugs that are D_2 partial agonists (e.g. aripiprazole) in contrast to simple antagonists. It is thought that partial agonists reduce D_2 hyperactivation in the mesolimbic pathway, thus alleviating positive symptoms of schizophrenia, but provide enough D_2 receptor stimulation in the mesocortical pathway to prevent negative symptoms, and in the nigrostriatal pathway to lower the incidence of extrapyramidal side effects.

Antipsychotic-induced motor disturbances

- Major problem of antipsychotic drug treatment.
- Two main types of disturbance occur:
  - acute, reversible dystonias and Parkinson-like symptoms (indeed, antipsychotic drugs generally worsen Parkinson's disease and block the actions of drugs used to treat the disorder);
  - slowly developing tardive dyskinesia, often irreversible.
- Acute symptoms comprise involuntary movements, tremor and rigidity, and are probably the direct consequence of block of nigrostriatal dopamine receptors.
- Tardive dyskinesia comprises mainly involuntary movements of the face and limbs, appearing after months or years of antipsychotic treatment. It may be associated with proliferation of dopamine receptors in the corpus striatum. Treatment is generally unsuccessful.
- Incidence of acute dystonias and tardive dyskinesia is less with newer, second-generation antipsychotics, and particularly low with **clozapine**, **aripiprazole** and **zotepine**.

ENDOCRINE EFFECTS

Dopamine, released in the median eminence by neurons of the tuberohypophyseal pathway (see Chs 34 and 40), acts physiologically via D_2 receptors to inhibit prolactin secretion. Blocking D_2 receptors by antipsychotic drugs can therefore increase the plasma prolactin concentration (Fig. 47.2), resulting in breast swelling, pain and lactation (known as 'galactorrhoea'), which can occur in men as well as in women. As can be seen from Fig. 47.2, the effect is maintained during chronic antipsychotic administration, without any habituation. Other less pronounced endocrine changes have also been reported, including a decrease of growth hormone secretion, but these, unlike the prolactin response, are believed to be relatively unimportant clinically. Because of its D_2 receptor partial agonist action aripiprazole, unlike other antipsychotic drugs, reduces prolactin secretion.

OTHER UNWANTED EFFECTS

Most antipsychotic drugs block a variety of receptors, particularly acetylcholine (muscarinic), histamine (H_1),

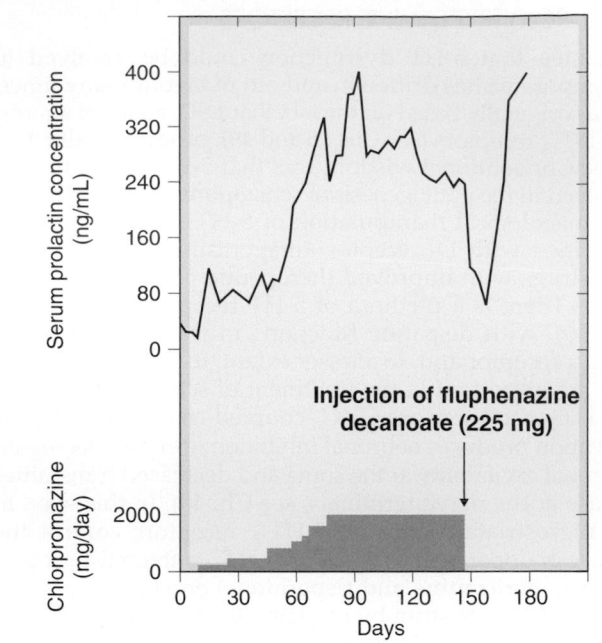

Fig. 47.2 **Effects of antipsychotic drugs on prolactin secretion in a schizophrenic patient.** When daily dosage with chlorpromazine was replaced with a depot injection of fluphenazine, the plasma prolactin initally dropped, because of the delay in absorption, and then returned to a high level. (From Meltzer, H.Y. et al., 1978. In: Lipton et al. (Eds). Psychopharmacology: A Generation in Progress. Raven Press, New York.)

noradrenaline (α) and 5-HT receptors (see Table 47.1). This gives rise to a wide range of side effects.

They can produce sexual dysfunction – decreased libido and decreased arousal as well as erection and ejaculation difficulties in men – through block of dopamine, muscarinic and α_1 receptors.

Drowsiness and sedation, which tend to decrease with continued use, occur with many antipsychotic drugs. Antihistamine (H_1) activity is a property of some phenothiazine antipsychotics (e.g. chlorpromazine and **methotrimeprazine**) and contributes to their sedative and antiemetic properties (see Ch. 31), but not to their antipsychotic action.

While block of muscarinic receptors produces a variety of peripheral effects, including blurring of vision and increased intraocular pressure, dry mouth and eyes, constipation and urinary retention (see Ch. 14), it may, however, also be beneficial in relation to extrapyramidal side effects (see p. 599).

Blocking α adrenoceptors causes *orthostatic hypotension* (see Ch. 15) but does not seem to be important for their antipsychotic action.

Weight gain is a common and troublesome side effect. Increased risk of diabetes and cardiovascular disease occurs with several second-generation antipsychotic drugs. These effects are probably related to their antagonist actions at H_1, 5-HT and muscarinic receptors.

Antipsychotic drugs can prolong the QT interval in the heart (see Ch. 22) giving rise to arrhythmia and risk of sudden death (Jolly et al., 2009). As such, a range of baseline measurements are usually recommended prior to starting antipsychotic drugs; these include weight, blood pressure, blood glucose, and electrocardiogram.

Various idiosyncratic and hypersensitivity reactions can occur, the most important being the following:

- *Jaundice*, which occurs with older phenothiazines such as chlorpromazine. The jaundice is usually mild, associated with elevated serum alkaline phosphatase activity (an 'obstructive' pattern), and disappears quickly when the drug is stopped or substituted by a chemically unrelated antipsychotic.
- *Leukopenia* and *agranulocytosis* are rare but potentially fatal, and occur in the first few weeks of treatment. The incidence of leukopenia (usually reversible) is less than 1 in 10,000 for most antipsychotic drugs, but much higher (1%–2%) with clozapine, whose use therefore requires regular monitoring of blood cell counts. Provided the drug is stopped at the first sign of leukopenia or anaemia, the effect is reversible. Olanzapine appears to be free of this disadvantage.
- *Urticarial skin reactions* are common but usually mild. Excessive sensitivity to ultraviolet light may also occur.
- *Antipsychotic malignant syndrome* is a rare but serious complication similar to the malignant hyperthermia syndrome seen with certain anaesthetics (see Ch. 42). Muscle rigidity is accompanied by a rapid rise in body temperature and mental confusion. It is usually reversible, but death from renal or cardiovascular failure occurs in 10%–20% of cases.

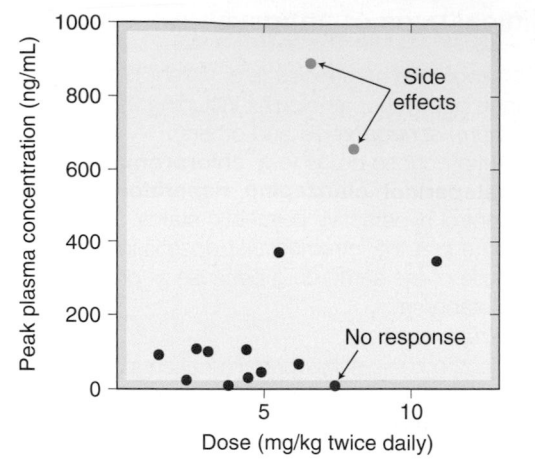

Fig. 47.3 Individual variation in the relation between dose and plasma concentration of chlorpromazine in a group of schizophrenic patients. (Data from Curry, S.H. et al., 1970. Arch. Gen. Psychiatry 22, 289.)

This is made even more difficult by the fact that at least 40% of schizophrenic patients fail to take drugs as prescribed. It is remarkably fortunate that the acute toxicity of antipsychotic drugs is slight, given the unpredictability of the clinical response.

The plasma half-life of most antipsychotic drugs is 15–30 h, clearance depending entirely on hepatic transformation by a combination of oxidative and conjugative reactions.

Most antipsychotic drugs can be given orally or in urgent situations by intramuscular injection. Slow-release (depot) preparations of many are available, in which the active drug is esterified with heptanoic or decanoic acid and dissolved in oil. Given as an intramuscular injection, the drug acts for 2–4 weeks, but initially may produce acute side effects. These preparations are widely used to minimise compliance problems.

Unwanted effects of antipsychotic drugs

- Important side effects common to many drugs are:
  - motor disturbances (see *Antipsychotic-induced motor disturbances* box);
  - endocrine disturbances (increased prolactin release);
  - these are secondary to dopamine receptor block.
- Sedation, hypotension and weight gain are common.
- Obstructive jaundice sometimes occurs with phenothiazines.
- Other side effects (dry mouth, blurred vision, hypotension, etc.) are due to block of other receptors, particularly muscarinic receptors and α adrenoceptors.
- Some antipsychotic drugs cause agranulocytosis as a rare and serious idiosyncratic reaction. With **clozapine**, leukopenia is common and requires routine monitoring.
- Antipsychotic malignant syndrome is a rare but potentially dangerous idiosyncratic reaction.

PHARMACOKINETIC ASPECTS

Chlorpromazine, in common with other phenothiazines, is erratically absorbed after oral administration. Fig. 47.3 shows the wide range of variation of the peak plasma concentration as a function of dosage in 14 patients. Among four patients treated at the high dosage level of 6–8 mg/kg, the variation in peak plasma concentration was nearly 90-fold; two showed marked side effects, one was well controlled and one showed no clinical response.

The relationship between the plasma concentration and the clinical effect of antipsychotic drugs is highly variable, and the dosage has to be adjusted on a trial-and-error basis.

FUTURE DEVELOPMENTS

The cognition enhancer **modafinil** (see Ch. 49) may be useful in treating the cognitive deficit in schizophrenia.

Preclinical and clinical studies have provided encouraging evidence that orthosteric and allosteric agonists of mGluR$_2$ and mGluR$_3$ metabotropic glutamate receptors (see Ch. 39) are effective in the treatment of the positive symptoms of schizophrenia. Paradoxically, activating presynaptic mGluR$_2$ and mGluR$_3$ autoreceptors reduces glutamate release but this may result in a compensatory up-regulation of NMDA receptors which might be beneficial. mGluR$_2$ receptors form heteromers with 5-HT$_{2A}$ receptors (see Ch. 3) with altered intracellular signalling properties and targeting the dimer may offer hope for future drug development. Agonists at postsynaptic mGluR$_5$ receptors may improve positive and negative symptoms as well as cognitive function. mGluR$_5$ receptors are closely associated with NMDA receptors and activation of mGluR$_5$ may enhance NMDA receptor function by increasing NMDA receptor phosphorylation.

A number of current antipsychotic drugs have, among their myriad of actions, 5-HT$_6$ and 5-HT$_7$ receptor antagonist properties; more specific antagonists at these receptors are

Clinical uses of antipsychotic drugs

- *Behavioural emergencies* (e.g. violent patients with a range of psychopathologies including *mania*, *toxic delirium*, *schizophrenia* and others):
  - Antipsychotic drugs (e.g. **chlorpromazine, haloperidol, olanzapine, risperidone**) can rapidly control hyperactive psychotic states.
  - Note that the intramuscular dose is lower than the oral dose of the same drug because of presystemic metabolism.
- *Schizophrenia*:
  - Many chronic schizophrenic patients are treated with first-generation antipsychotic drugs. Depot injections (e.g. **flupentixol decanoate**) may be useful for maintenance treatment when compliance with oral treatment is a problem

- **Flupentixol** has antidepressant properties distinct from its antipsychotic action.
- Newer antipsychotic drugs (e.g. **amisulpride, olanzapine, risperidone**) are used if extrapyramidal symptoms are troublesome or if symptom control is inadequate.
- **Clozapine** can cause *agranulocytosis* but is distinctively effective against 'negative' features of schizophrenia. It is reserved for patients whose condition remains inadequately controlled despite previous use of two or more antipsychotic drugs, of which at least one is a second-generation drug. Blood count is monitored weekly for the first 18 weeks, and less frequently thereafter.

being investigated; their ability to produce cognitive improvement is controversial.

Also in various stages of development are inhibitors of phosphodiesterase (PDE10), α_7 nicotinic receptor agonists, histamine H_3 antagonists and 5-HT$_6$ antagonists. Selective agonist action at M_1 muscarinic receptors (either orthosteric

or allosteric) has significant potential for cognition enhancement in both schizophrenia and Alzheimer's disease, but to date drug development has been hampered by a lack of selectivity across muscarinic receptor subtypes (e.g. **xanomeline** is an M_1 and M_4 agonist and M_5 antagonist) that gives rise to significant unwanted effects.

REFERENCES AND FURTHER READING

General reading

Gross, G., Geyer, M.A., 2012. Current antipsychotics. Handb. Exp. Pharmacology 212, Springer Verlag. (*Multi-authored volume containing individual chapters on current drugs*)

Stahl, S.M., 2008. Antipsychotics and Mood Stabilizers, third ed. Cambridge University Press, New York. (*Highly readable, yet detailed, description of the biology of schizophrenia and of the mechanisms of action of the drugs used to treat the disorder*)

Pathogenesis of schizophrenia

Ayhan, Y., McFarland, R., Pletnikov, M.V., 2016. Animal models of gene-environment interaction in schizophrenia: a dimensional perspective. Prog. Neurobiol. 136, 1–27. (*Don't be deceived by the title, this paper contains a wealth of information from human studies of gene-environment interactions in the development of schizophrenia*)

Ripke, S., Neale, B.M., Corvin, A., et al., 2014. Biological insights from 108 schizophrenia-associated genetic loci. Nature 511, 421–427. (*Extensive study on the human genetic basis of schizophrenia*)

Sekar, A., Bialas, A.R., de Rivera, H., et al., 2016. Schizophrenia risk from complex variation of complement component 4. Nature 530, 177–183. (*Major gene-wide association study (GWAS) demonstrating the importance of compliment component 4 in schizophrenia*)

Pergola, G., Selvaggi, P., Trizio, S., et al., 2015. The role of the thalamus in schizophrenia from a neuroimaging perspective. Neurosci. Biobehav. Rev. 54, 57–75.

van Haren, N.E., Hulshoff Pol, H.E., Schnack, H.G., et al., 2007. Focal gray matter changes in schizophrenia across the course of the illness: a 5-year follow-up study. Neuropsychopharmacology 32, 2057–2066.

Dopamine, glutamate and 5-hydroxytryptamine

Coyle, J.T., 2017. Schizophrenia: basic and clinical. Adv. Neurobiol. 15, 255–280. (*Discusses the importance of NMDA receptor hypofunction in schizophrenia*)

Laruelle, M., Abi-Dargham, A., Gil, R., et al., 1999. Increased dopamine transmission in schizophrenia: relationship to illness phases. Biol. Psychiatry 46, 56–72. (*The first direct evidence for increased dopamine function as a cause of symptoms in schizophrenia*)

Animal models

Pratt, J., Winchester, C., Dawson, N., Morris, B., 2012. Advancing schizophrenia drug discovery: optimizing rodent

models to bridge the translational gap. Nat. Rev. Drug Discov. 11, 560–579.

Sigurdsson, T., 2015. Neural circuit dysfunction in schizophrenia: insights from animal models. Neuroscience 321, 42–65.

Antipsychotic drugs

Jolly, K., Gammage, M.D., Cheng, K.K., Bradburn, P., Banting, M.V., Langman, M.J., 2009. Sudden death in patients receiving drugs tending to prolong the QT interval. Br. J. Clin. Pharmacol. 68, 743–751. (*Compares the risk of sudden death in patients receiving various antipsychotic and antidepressant therapies*)

Kapur, S., Seeman, P., 2001. Does fast dissociation from the dopamine D_2 receptor explain the action of atypical antipsychotics? A new hypothesis. Am. J. Psychiatry 158, 360–369. (*Suggests that differences in dissociation rates, rather than receptor selectivity profiles, may account for differing tendency of drugs to cause motor side effects*)

Kapur, S., Arenovich, T., Agid, O., et al., 2005. Evidence for onset of antipsychotic effects within the first 24 hours of treatment. Am. J. Psychiatry 162, 939–946.

Leucht, S., Busch, R., Hamann, J., Kissling, W., Kane, J.M., 2005. Early-onset hypothesis of antipsychotic drug action: a hypothesis tested, confirmed and extended. Biol. Psychiatry 57, 1543–1549.

Leucht, S., Cipriani, A., Spineli, L., et al., 2013. Comparative efficacy and tolerability of 15 antipsychotic drugs in schizophrenia: a multiple-treatments meta-analysis. Lancet 382, 951–962. (*Meta-analysis of major antipsychotic drugs examining their efficacy and side effects*)

Extrapyramidal side effects

Casey, D.E., 1995. Tardive dyskinesia: pathophysiology. In: Bloom, F.E., Kupfer, D.J. (Eds.), Psychopharmacology: A Fourth Generation of Progress. Raven Press, New York.

Klawans, H.L., Tanner, C.M., Goetz, C.G., 1988. Epidemiology and pathophysiology of tardive dyskinesias. Adv. Neurol. 49, 185–197.

Lieberman, J.A., Stroup, T.S., 2011. The NIMH-CATIE Schizophrenia Study: what did we learn? Am. J. Psychiatry 68, 770–775. (*A comprehensive review of the effectiveness and side effect profiles of antipsychotic drugs*)

Pisani, A., Bernardi, G., Ding, J., Surmeier, D.J., 2007. Re-emergence of striatal cholinergic interneurons in movement disorders. Trends Neurosci. 30, 545–553.

Antidepressant drugs

48

OVERVIEW

Depression is an extremely common psychiatric condition, about which a variety of neurochemical theories exist, and for which a corresponding variety of different types of drug are used in treatment. It is a field in which therapeutic empiricism has led the way, with mechanistic understanding tending to lag behind, part of the problem being that it has been difficult to develop animal models that replicate the characteristics that define the human condition. In this chapter, we discuss the current understanding of the nature of the disorder, and describe the major drugs that are used to treat it.

THE NATURE OF DEPRESSION

Depression is the most common of the *affective disorders* (defined as disorders of mood); it may range from a very mild condition, bordering on normality, to severe (psychotic) depression accompanied by hallucinations and delusions. Worldwide, depression is a major cause of disability and premature death. In addition to the significant suicide risk, depressed individuals are more likely to die from other causes, such as heart disease or cancer. Depression is a heterogeneous disorder, with patients presenting with one or more core symptoms, and depression is often associated with other psychiatric conditions, including anxiety, eating disorders, schizophrenia, Parkinson's disease and drug addiction.

The symptoms of depression include emotional and biological components. Emotional symptoms include:

- low mood, excessive rumination of negative thought, misery, apathy and pessimism
- low self-esteem: feelings of guilt, inadequacy and ugliness
- indecisiveness, loss of motivation
- anhedonia, loss of reward

Biological symptoms include:

- retardation of thought and action
- loss of libido
- sleep disturbance and loss of appetite

There are two distinct types of depressive syndrome, namely *unipolar depression*, in which the mood changes are always in the same direction, and *bipolar disorder*, in which depression alternates with mania. Mania is in most respects exactly the opposite, with excessive exuberance, enthusiasm and self-confidence, accompanied by impulsive actions, these signs often being combined with irritability, impatience and aggression, and sometimes with grandiose delusions of the Napoleonic kind. As with depression, the mood and actions are inappropriate to the circumstances.

Unipolar depression is commonly (about 75% of cases) non-familial, clearly associated with stressful life events, and usually accompanied by symptoms of anxiety and agitation; this type is sometimes termed *reactive depression*. Other cases (about 25%, sometimes termed *endogenous depression*) show a familial pattern, unrelated to obvious external stresses and with a somewhat different symptomatology. This distinction is made clinically, but there is little evidence that antidepressant drugs show significant selectivity between these conditions. After an inauspicious start, population genetic studies have begun to identify novel genetic variations associated with depression (see Mullins & Lewis, 2017), but depression is probably a polygenic disorder where a number of individual genetic variations as well as environmental factors contribute to the disorder.

Depression cannot be attributed to altered neuronal activity within a single brain region; rather, the circuitry linking different parts of the brain may be affected. Brain-imaging studies have indicated that the prefrontal cortex, amygdala and hippocampus may all be involved in different components of these disorders.

Bipolar disorder, which usually appears in early adult life, is less common and results in oscillating depression and mania over a period of a few weeks. It can be difficult to differentiate between mild bipolar disorder and unipolar depression. Also, bipolar manic episodes can be confused with episodes of schizophrenic psychosis (see Ch. 47). There is a strong hereditary tendency, and gene-wide association studies (GWAS) have identified a number of new susceptibility genes that may have an effect on the brain functions affected in bipolar disorder (Soronen et al., 2010) but to date these have not impacted on drug therapy of the disorder.

THEORIES OF DEPRESSION

Several theories have been proposed to explain the causes of depression. None fully explain all of the observations and evidence of pathological changes that occur with depression. Here we summarise the main theories as they relate to the mechanisms of action of current drug therapies. A more comprehensive review and analysis is provided by Harmer et al. (2017).

THE MONOAMINE THEORY

The monoamine theory of depression, first proposed by Schildkraut in 1965, states that depression is caused by a functional deficit of the monoamine transmitters, noradrenaline and 5-hydroxytryptamine (5-HT) at certain sites in the brain, while mania results from a functional excess.

The monoamine hypothesis grew originally out of associations between the clinical effects of various drugs that cause or alleviate symptoms of depression and their known neurochemical effects on monoaminergic transmission in the

Table 48.1 Pharmacological evidence supporting the monoamine hypothesis of depression

Drug(s)	Principal action	Effect in depressed patients
Tricyclic antidepressants	Block noradrenaline and 5-HT reuptake	Mood ↑
MAO inhibitors	Increase stores of noradrenaline and 5-HT	Mood ↑
Reserpine	Inhibits noradrenaline and 5-HT storage	Mood ↓
α-Methyltyrosine	Inhibits noradrenaline synthesis	Mood ↓ (calming of manic patients)
Methyldopa	Inhibits noradrenaline synthesis	Mood ↓
Electroconvulsive therapy	? Increases central nervous system responses to noradrenaline and 5-HT	Mood ↑
Tryptophan (5-hydroxytryptophan)	Increases 5-HT synthesis	Mood ? ↑ in some studies
Tryptophan depletion	Decreases brain 5-HT synthesis	Induces relapse in SSRI-treated patients

5-HT, 5-hydroxytryptamine; *MAO*, monoamine oxidase; *SSRI*, selective serotonin reuptake inhibitor.

brain. This pharmacological evidence, which is summarised in Table 48.1, gives general support to the monoamine hypothesis, although there are several anomalies. Attempts to obtain more direct evidence, by studying monoamine metabolism in depressed patients or by measuring changes in the number of monoamine receptors in postmortem brain tissue, have tended to give inconsistent and equivocal results, and the interpretation of these studies is often problematic, because the changes described are not specific to depression. Similarly, investigation by functional tests of the activity of known monoaminergic pathways (e.g. those controlling pituitary hormone release) in depressed patients have also given equivocal results.

The pharmacological evidence does not enable a clear distinction to be drawn between the noradrenaline and 5-HT theories of depression. Clinically, it seems that inhibitors of noradrenaline reuptake and of 5-HT reuptake are equally effective as antidepressants, although individual patients may respond better to one or the other.

Other evidence in support of the monoamine theory is that agents known to block noradrenaline or 5-HT synthesis consistently lower mood and reverse the therapeutic effects of antidepressant drugs that act selectively on these two transmitter systems (see Table 48.1).

Any theory of depression has to take account of the fact that the direct neurochemical effects of most antidepressant drugs appear very rapidly (minutes to hours), whereas their antidepressant effects take weeks to develop. A similar situation exists in relation to antipsychotic drugs (Ch. 47) and some anxiolytic drugs (Ch. 45). To explain this phenomenon, proponents of the monoamine theory have suggested that secondary, adaptive changes in the brain (see p. 611), rather than the primary drug effect, are responsible for the clinical improvement and that the drug-induced effects on brain monoamine systems result in longer-term trophic effects, the time course of which is paralleled by mood changes.

NEGATIVE AFFECTIVE BIAS

People suffering from depression tend to perceive events in a negative way, focus on negative information and recall information in a negative rather than positive manner – a behaviour pattern that psychologists term *negative affective bias*. Studies comparing healthy volunteers and depressed patients suggest that antidepressant drugs may indeed exert acute effects on the way information is processed (cognitive processing), leading to a positive effect on emotional behaviour. For example, when presented with a series of pictures showing facial expression of different levels of happiness or sadness, depressed patients consider fewer of the faces to be happy than do healthy volunteers presented with the same faces (Fig. 48.1). But after a single dose of an antidepressant the depressed patients now consider more of the same faces to be happy (i.e. their perception of what is happy [positive] has changed). It is suggested that depressed patients may not initially be consciously aware of the effect the antidepressant drug has produced, but over time, and with prolonged drug administration, they subconsciously recalibrate what they perceive to be happy and thus their mood improves.

NEUROENDOCRINE MECHANISMS

Various attempts have been made to test for a functional deficit of monoamine pathways in depression. Hypothalamic neurons controlling pituitary function receive noradrenergic and 5-HT inputs, which control the discharge of these cells. Hypothalamic cells release corticotrophin-releasing factor (CRF; also known as *corticotrophin-releasing hormone*), which stimulates pituitary cells to secrete adrenocorticotrophic hormone (ACTH), leading in turn to cortisol secretion (Ch. 34). The plasma cortisol concentration is usually high in depressed patients. Other hormones in plasma are also affected, for example, growth hormone concentration is reduced and prolactin is increased. While these changes are consistent with deficiencies in monoamine transmission, they are not specific to depressive syndromes.

CRF is widely distributed in the brain and has behavioural effects that are distinct from its endocrine functions. Injected into the brain of experimental animals, CRF mimics some aspects of depression in humans, such as diminished activity, loss of appetite and increased signs of anxiety. Furthermore, CRF concentrations in the brain and cerebrospinal fluid of depressed patients are increased. Therefore CRF hyperfunction, as well as monoamine hypofunction, may be associated with depression. Raised CRF levels are associated with

Fig. 48.1 **Recognition of happy facial expressions by depressed patients.** (A) An illustrative sample of sad and happy facial expressions. (B) When presented with an array of faces, such as those in (A), depressed patients considered fewer faces to be happy than did control subjects. After an acute dose of reboxetine, depressed patients considered more of the facial expressions to be happy. (Faces in panel [A] are reprinted from the P1vital Oxford Emotional Test Battery, P1vital Products Ltd. Data in panel [B] are adapted from Harmer et al., 2009. Am. J. Psychiatry. 166:1178–1184.)

stress and, in many cases, depression is preceded by periods of chronic stress. However, CRF$_1$ receptor antagonists have so far not proven to be effective antidepressant drugs.

TROPHIC EFFECTS AND NEUROPLASTICITY

It has been suggested that lowered levels of brain-derived neurotrophic factor (BDNF) or malfunction of its receptor, TrkB, plays a significant role in the pathology of depression. Depressive behaviour is often associated with a reduction in BDNF expression and treatment with antidepressants elevates BDNF levels. Glycogen synthase kinase 3 (GSK3β) has been implicated in the pathogenesis of depression following its identification as a target of the mood stabiliser **lithium** (see p. 620).

Changes in glutamatergic neurotransmission may also be involved in depression. Sufferers from depression have been shown to have elevated cortical levels of glutamate. Antidepressant treatment may reduce glutamate release and depress NMDA receptor function. Indeed ketamine, an NMDA antagonist, has antidepressant activity (see p. 618). The effects of antidepressants on activity-induced long-term potentiation (LTP; see Ch. 39) at hippocampal glutamatergic synapses is complex – both depression and facilitation have been observed and may occur rapidly after antidepressant administration.

Another view (see Racagni & Popoli, 2008) is that major depression is associated with neuronal loss in the hippocampus and prefrontal cortex, and that antidepressant therapies of different kinds act by inhibiting or actually reversing this loss by stimulating neurogenesis.[1] This surprising idea is supported by various lines of evidence:

- Brain imaging and postmortem studies show ventricular enlargement as well as shrinkage of the hippocampus and prefrontal cortex of depressed patients, with loss of neurons and glia. Functional imaging reveals reduced neuronal activity in these regions.
- In animals, the same effect is produced by chronic stress of various kinds, or by administration of glucocorticoids, mimicking the increased cortisol secretion in human depression. Excessive glucocorticoid secretion in humans (Cushing's syndrome; see Ch. 34) often causes depression.
- In experimental animals, antidepressant drugs, or other treatments such as electroconvulsions (see later section on Brain Stimulation Therapies), promote neurogenesis in these regions, and (as in humans) restore functional activity. Preventing hippocampal neurogenesis prevents the behavioural effects of antidepressants in rats.

---

[1]Neurogenesis (see Ch. 41) – the formation of new neurons from stem cell precursors – occurs to a significant degree in the adult hippocampus, and possibly elsewhere in the brain, contradicting the old dogma that it occurs only during brain development.

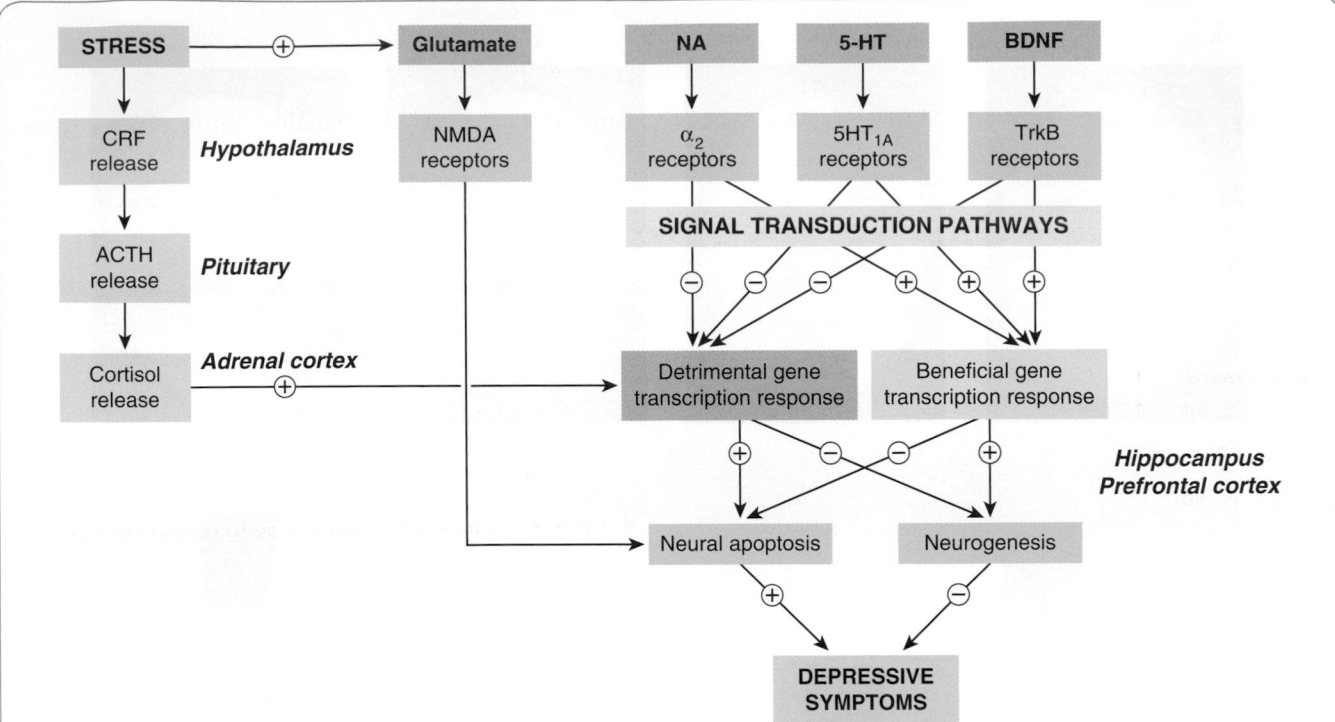

Fig. 48.2 Simplified diagram showing mechanisms believed to be involved in the pathophysiology of depression. The main prodepressive pathways involve the hypothalamic–pituitary–adrenal axis, which is activated by stress and in turn enhances the excitotoxic action of glutamate, mediated by NMDA receptors (see Ch. 39), and switches on the expression of genes that promote neural apoptosis in the hippocampus and prefrontal cortex. The antidepressive pathways involve the monoamines noradrenaline (NA) and 5-hydroxytryptamine (5-HT), which act on G protein–coupled receptors, and the brain-derived neurotrophic factor (BDNF), which acts on a kinase-linked receptor (TrkB), switching on genes that protect neurons against apoptosis and also promote neurogenesis. *ACTH*, adrenocorticotrophic hormone; *CRF*, corticotrophin-releasing factor. (For further detail, see Charney & Manji (2004) Science STKE 2004, re5.)

- 5-HT and noradrenaline, whose actions are enhanced by many antidepressants, promote neurogenesis, probably through activation of 5-HT$_{1A}$ receptors and α$_2$ adrenoceptors, respectively. This effect may be mediated by BDNF.
- Exercise has been shown to promote neurogenesis in animals and to be effective in some patients with mild to moderate depression.

Fig. 48.2 summarises the possible mechanisms involved. It should be stressed that these hypotheses are far from proven, but the diagram emphasises the way in which the field has moved on since the formulation of the monoamine hypothesis, suggesting a range of possible targets for the next generation of antidepressant drugs.[2]

---

[2]Cynics may feel that these mechanisms, in which glutamate, neurotrophic factors, monoamines and steroids all interact to control neuronal death, survival and plasticity, are being invoked just as enthusiastically to account for almost every neurological and psychiatric disorder that you can think of, from stroke and Parkinson's disease to schizophrenia. 'Are we missing something,' they may feel, 'or are all these diseases basically the same? If so, why are their effects so different? Is this just a scientific bandwagon, or does this mechanistic convergence point to some fundamental principles of neural organisation?' We do not have the answers, of course, but it is a field worth watching.

ANTIDEPRESSANT DRUGS

TYPES OF ANTIDEPRESSANT DRUG

Antidepressant drugs fall into the following categories.

Inhibitors of monoamine uptake
- Selective serotonin (5-HT) reuptake inhibitors (SSRIs) (e.g. **fluoxetine, fluvoxamine, paroxetine, sertraline, citalopram, escitalopram, vilazodone**).
- Classic tricyclic antidepressants (TCAs) (e.g. **imipramine, desipramine, amitriptyline, nortriptyline, clomipramine**). These vary in their activity and selectivity with respect to inhibition of noradrenaline and 5-HT reuptake.
- Newer, mixed 5-HT and noradrenaline reuptake inhibitors (e.g. **venlafaxine** [somewhat selective for 5-HT, although less so than SSRIs], **desvenlafaxine, duloxetine**).
- Noradrenaline reuptake inhibitors (e.g. **reboxetine, atomoxetine, bupropion**).
- The herbal preparation St John's wort, the main active ingredient of which is hyperforin: it has similar clinical efficacy to most of the prescribed

Theories of depression

- The monoamine theory, first proposed in 1965, suggests that depression results from functionally deficient monoaminergic (noradrenaline and/or 5-hydroxytryptamine) transmission in the central nervous system.
- The theory is based on the ability of most antidepressant drugs (tricyclic antidepressants and monoamine oxidase inhibitors) to facilitate monoaminergic transmission, and of drugs such as **reserpine** to cause depression.
- Biochemical studies on depressed patients do not clearly support the monoamine hypothesis in its simple form.
- Although the monoamine hypothesis in its simple form is insufficient as an explanation of depression, pharmacological manipulation of monoamine transmission remains the most successful therapeutic approach.
- The *negative affective bias theory* of depression suggests that drugs may produce immediate behavioural changes but patients receiving the drugs need time to become aware of the improvements in their mood.
- Recent evidence suggests that depression may be associated with neurodegeneration and reduced neurogenesis in the hippocampus.
- Current approaches focus on other mediators, signal transduction pathways, growth factors, etc., but theories remain imprecise.

antidepressants. It is a weak monoamine uptake inhibitor but also has other actions.[3]

Monoamine receptor antagonists
- Drugs such as **mirtazapine**, **trazodone**, **mianserin** are non-selective and inhibit a range of amine receptors including α_2 adrenoceptors and 5-HT$_2$ receptors. They may also have weak effects on monoamine uptake.

Monoamine oxidase inhibitors (MAOIs)
- Irreversible, non-competitive inhibitors (e.g. **phenelzine**, **tranylcypromine**), which are non-selective with respect to the MAO-A and -B subtypes.
- Reversible, MAO-A-selective inhibitors (e.g. **moclobemide**).

Melatonin receptor agonist
- **Agomelatine** is an agonist at MT$_1$ and MT$_2$ melatonin receptors, and a weak 5-HT$_{2C}$ antagonist.

---

[3]Although relatively free of acute side effects, hyperforin activates cytochrome P450, resulting in loss of efficacy (Ch. 10), with serious consequences, of several important drugs, including ciclosporine, oral contraceptives, some anti-HIV and anticancer drugs, and oral anticoagulants – underlining the principle that herbal remedies are not inherently safe, and must be used with the same degree of informed caution as any other drug.

Miscellaneous agents
- **Ketamine** is a non-competitive NMDA channel blocker.

Table 48.2 summarises the main features of these types of drug. Mention should also be made of electroconvulsive therapy (ECT), electromagnetic therapy, deep brain stimulation and vagus stimulation, which are effective and usually act more rapidly than antidepressant drugs (see p. 619).

To some extent, the term 'antidepressant drug' is misleading, as many of these drugs are now also used to treat disorders other than depression. These include:

- neuropathic pain (e.g. amitriptyline, nortriptyline, duloxetine; Ch. 43)
- anxiety disorders (e.g. SSRIs, venlafaxine, duloxetine; Ch. 45)
- fibromyalgia (e.g. duloxetine, venlafaxine, SSRIs, TCAs; Ch. 43)
- bipolar disorder (e.g. fluoxetine in conjunction with **olanzapine**; see later)
- smoking cessation (e.g. bupropion; Ch. 50)
- attention deficit/hyperactivity disorder (e.g. atomoxetine; Ch. 49)

Types of antidepressant drugs

- Main types are:
  - monoamine uptake inhibitors (tricyclic antidepressants, selective serotonin reuptake inhibitors, newer inhibitors of noradrenaline and 5-HT reuptake);
  - monoamine receptor antagonists;
  - monoamine oxidase (MAO) inhibitors.
- Monoamine uptake inhibitors act by inhibiting uptake of noradrenaline and/or 5-HT by monoaminergic nerve terminals.
- α_2-Adrenoceptor antagonists can indirectly elevate 5-HT release.
- MAO inhibitors inhibit one or both forms of brain MAO, thus increasing the cytosolic stores of noradrenaline and 5-HT in nerve terminals. Inhibition of type A MAO correlates with antidepressant activity. Most are non-selective; **moclobemide** is specific for MAO-A.
- Most antidepressant drugs appear to take at least 2 weeks to produce any perceived beneficial effects.
- Ketamine (not yet approved as an antidepressant), given as a single intravenous dose, is reported to produce a rapid response lasting for several days

TESTING OF ANTIDEPRESSANT DRUGS
ANIMAL MODELS

Progress in unravelling the neurochemical mechanisms is, as in so many areas of psychopharmacology, limited by the lack of good animal models of the clinical condition. There is no known animal condition corresponding to the inherited form of depression in humans. Procedures involving mild stress (e.g. the forced swim test, inescapable foot shock) produce behavioural states in animals (withdrawal from social interaction, loss of appetite, reduced motor activity, etc.) that mimic aspects of human depression (see O'Leary & Cryan, 2013). In such tests, current antidepressant

Table 48.2 Types of antidepressant drugs and their characteristics

Type and examples	Action(s)	Unwanted effects	Risk of overdose	Pharmacokinetics	Notes
Monoamine uptake inhibitors					
(1) SSRIs	All highly selective for 5-HT	Nausea, diarrhoea, agitation, insomnia, anorgasmia Inhibit metabolism of other drugs, so risk of interactions	Low risk in overdose but must not be used in combination with MAO inhibitors	—	—
Fluoxetine	As above	As above	As above	Long $t_{1/2}$ (24–96 h)	—
Fluvoxamine	As above	As above	As above	$t_{1/2}$ 18–24 h	Less nausea than with other SSRIs
Paroxetine	As above	As above	As above	$t_{1/2}$ 18–24 h	Withdrawal reaction
Citalopram	As above	As above	As above	$t_{1/2}$ 24–36 h	—
Escitalopram	As above	As above	As above	$t_{1/2}$ 24–36 h	Active S isomer of citalopram Fewer side effects
Sertraline	As above	As above	As above	$t_{1/2}$ 24–36 h	—
Vilazodone	As above. Also has 5-HT$_{1A}$ receptor partial agonist activity	As above	As above	$t_{1/2}$ 25 h	—
Vortioxetine	As above. Also has partial agonist activity at 5-HT$_{1A}$ and 5-HT$_{1B}$ receptors and antagonist activity at 5-HT$_{3A}$ receptors.	As above	As above	$t_{1/2}$ >60 h	—
(2) Classical TCA group[a]	Inhibition of NA and 5-HT reuptake	Sedation Anticholinergic effects (dry mouth, constipation, blurred vision, urinary retention, etc.) Postural hypotension Seizures Impotence Interaction with CNS depressants (especially alcohol, MAO inhibitors)	Ventricular dysrhythmias High risk in combination with CNS depressants	—	'First-generation' antidepressants, still very widely used, although newer compounds generally have fewer side effects and lower risk with overdose
Imipramine	Non-selective Converted to desipramine	As above	As above	$t_{1/2}$ 4–18 h	—
Desipramine	NA selective	As above	As above	$t_{1/2}$ 12–24 h	—
Amitriptyline	Non-selective	As above	As above	$t_{1/2}$ 12–24 h; converted to nortriptyline	Widely used, also for neuropathic pain (Ch. 43)
Nortriptyline	NA selective (slight)	As above	As above	Long $t_{1/2}$ (24–96 h)	Long duration, less sedative
Clomipramine	Non-selective	As above	As above	$t_{1/2}$ 18–24 h	Also used for anxiety disorders

[a]Other TCAs include dosulepin, doxepin, lofepramine, trimipramine.

Table 48.2 Types of antidepressant drugs and their characteristics—cont'd

Type and examples	Action(s)	Unwanted effects	Risk of overdose	Pharmacokinetics	Notes
(3) Other 5-HT/NA uptake inhibitors[b]					
Venlafaxine	Weak non-selective NA/5-HT uptake inhibitor Also, non-selective receptor-blocking effects	As SSRIs Withdrawal effects common and troublesome if doses are missed	Safe in overdose	Short $t_{1/2}$ (~5 h) Converted to desvenlafaxine which inhibits NA uptake	Claimed to act more rapidly than other antidepressants, and to work better in 'treatment-resistant' patients Usually classed as non-selective NA/5-HT uptake blocker, although in vitro data show selectivity for 5-HT
Duloxetine	Potent non-selective NA/5-HT uptake inhibitor No action on monoamine receptors	Fewer side effects than venlafaxine Sedation, dizziness, nausea Sexual dysfunction	See SSRIs above	$t_{1/2}$ ~14 h	Also used to treat urinary incontinence (see Ch. 30) and for anxiety disorders
St John's wort (active principle: hyperforin)	Weak non-selective NA/5-HT uptake inhibitor Also, non-selective receptor-blocking effects	Few side effects reported Risk of drug interactions due to enhanced drug metabolism (e.g. loss of efficacy of ciclosporin, antidiabetic drugs, etc.)	—	$t_{1/2}$ ~12 h	Freely available as crude herbal preparation Similar efficacy to other antidepressants, with fewer acute side effects but risk of serious drug interactions
(4) NA-selective inhibitors					
Bupropion	Selective inhibitor of NA over 5-HT uptake but also inhibits dopamine uptake Converted to active metabolites (e.g. radafaxine)	Headache, dry mouth, agitation, insomnia	Seizures at high doses	$t_{1/2}$ ~12 h Plasma half-life ~20 h	Used in depression associated with anxiety Slow-release formulation used to treat nicotine dependence (Ch. 50)
Reboxetine	Selective NA uptake inhibitor	Dizziness Insomnia Anticholinergic effects	Safe in overdose (low risk of cardiac dysrhythmia)	$t_{1/2}$ ~12 h	Less effective than TCAs The related drug atomoxetine now used mainly to treat ADHD (Ch. 49)
Maprotiline	Selective NA uptake inhibitor	As TCAs; no significant advantages	As TCAs	Long $t_{1/2}$ ~40 h	No significant advantages over TCAs
Monoamine receptor antagonists					
Mirtazapine	Blocks α_2, 5-HT_{2C} and 5-HT_3 receptors	Dry mouth Sedation Weight gain	No serious drug interactions	$t_{1/2}$ 20–40 h	Claimed to have faster onset of action than other antidepressants
Trazodone	Blocks 5-HT_{2A} and 5-HT_{2C} receptors as well as H_1 receptors Weak 5-HT uptake inhibitor (enhances NA/5-HT release)	Sedation Hypotension Cardiac dysrhythmias	Safe in overdose	$t_{1/2}$ 6–12 h	Nefazodone is similar

[b]Other 5-HT/NA uptake inhibitors include milnacipran and levomilnacipran.

Continued

Table 48.2   Types of antidepressant drugs and their characteristics—cont'd

Type and examples	Action(s)	Unwanted effects	Risk of overdose	Pharmacokinetics	Notes
Mianserin	Blocks α_1, α_2, 5-HT$_{2A}$ and H$_1$ receptors	Milder antimuscarinic and cardiovascular effects than TCAs Agranulocytosis, aplastic anaemia	—	t$_{1/2}$ 10–35 h	Blood count advised in early stages of use
MAO inhibitors	Inhibit MAO-A and/or MAO-B Earlier compounds have long duration of action due to covalent binding to enzyme				
Phenelzine	Non-selective	'Cheese reaction' to tyramine-containing foods (see text) Anticholinergic side effects Hypotension Insomnia Weight gain Liver damage (rare)	Many interactions (TCAs, opioids, sympathomimetic drugs) – risk of severe hypertension due to 'cheese reaction'	t$_{1/2}$ 1–2 h Long duration of action due to irreversible binding	—
Tranylcypromine	Non-selective	As phenelzine	As phenelzine	t$_{1/2}$ 1–2 h Long duration of action due to irreversible binding	—
Isocarboxazid	Non-selective	As phenelzine	As phenelzine	Long t$_{1/2}$ ~36 h	—
Moclobemide	MAO-A selective Short acting	Nausea, insomnia, agitation	Interactions less severe than with other MAO inhibitors; no 'cheese reactions' reported	t$_{1/2}$ 1–2 h	Safer alternative to earlier MAO inhibitors
Melatonin agonist					
Agomelatine	MT$_1$ and MT$_2$ receptor agonist. Weak 5-HT$_{2C}$ antagonist	Headache, dizziness, drowsiness, fatigue, sleep disturbance, anxiety, nausea, GI disturbances, sweating	Limited data available at present	t$_{1/2}$ 1–2 h	Should not be combined with ethanol Usually taken once daily before bed
NMDA antagonist					
Ketamine	NMDA-channel blocker	Psychotomimetic at higher doses (see Ch. 49) Prolonged use of high doses can cause cystitis	Deaths from overdose are rare	t$_{1/2}$ 2–4 h Given intravenously.	Rapid onset antidepressant action lasting for a few days after single i.v. dose Effective in patients resistant to other antidepressants Potentially metabolites of ketamine are responsible for the antidepressant effects

5-HT, 5-hydroxytryptamine; *ADHD*, attention deficit/hyperactivity disorder; *CNS*, central nervous system; *GI*, gastrointestinal; *i.v.*, intravenous; *MAO*, monoamine oxidase; *NA*, noradrenaline; *SSRI*, selective serotonin reuptake inhibitor; *TCA*, tricyclic antidepressant.

drugs reverse the symptoms of depression. However, we need new drugs to treat forms of depression that are resistant to current drugs and thus new animal models are required. Genetically modified mice (e.g. knock-down of 5-HT, noradrenaline and glutamate transporters, mutations or knock-down of 5-HT receptors, etc.) have been extensively studied to mimic various aspects of the disorder. However, a good animal model of drug-resistant depression has still to be developed (Willner & Belzung, 2015).

TESTS ON HUMANS

Clinically, the effect of antidepressant drugs is usually measured by a subjective rating scale such as the Hamilton Rating Scale or the Beck Depression Inventory. Clinical depression takes many forms, and the symptoms vary between patients and over time. Quantitation is therefore difficult, and the many clinical trials of antidepressants have generally shown rather weak effects, after allowance for quite large placebo responses. There is also a high degree of individual variation, with 30%–40% of patients failing to show any improvement, possibly due to genetic factors (see later section on Clinical Effectiveness).

MECHANISM OF ACTION OF ANTIDEPRESSANT DRUGS
CHRONIC ADAPTIVE CHANGES

Given the discrepancy between the fast onset of the neurochemical effects of most antidepressant drugs and the slow onset of their antidepressant effects, efforts have been made to determine whether the therapeutic benefits arise from slow adaptive changes induced by chronic exposure to these drugs (Racagni & Popoli, 2008).

This approach led to the discovery that certain monoamine receptors, in particular β_1 and α_2 adrenoceptors, are consistently down-regulated following chronic antidepressant treatment and, in some cases, by ECT too. This can be demonstrated in experimental animals as a reduction in the number of binding sites, as well as by a reduction in the functional response to agonists (e.g. stimulation of cAMP formation by β-adrenoceptor agonists). Receptor down-regulation probably also occurs in humans, because endocrine responses to **clonidine**, an α_2-adrenoceptor agonist, are reduced by long-term antidepressant treatment. However, the relevance of these findings to the antidepressant response is unclear. Loss of β adrenoceptors as a factor in alleviating depression does not fit comfortably with theory, because β-adrenoceptor antagonists are not antidepressant.

On acute administration, one would expect inhibition of 5-HT uptake (e.g. by SSRIs) to increase the level of 5-HT at the synapse by inhibiting reuptake into the nerve terminals. However, the increase in synaptic 5-HT levels has been observed to be less than expected. This is because increased activation of $5-HT_{1A}$ receptors on the soma and dendrites of 5-HT-containing raphe neurons (Fig. 48.3A) inhibits these neurons and thus reduces 5-HT release, thus cancelling out to some extent the effect of inhibiting reuptake into the terminals. On prolonged drug treatment, the elevated level of 5-HT in the somatodendritic region desensitises the $5-HT_{1A}$ receptors, reducing their inhibitory effect on 5-HT release from the nerve terminals.

NORADRENERGIC CONTROL OF 5-HT RELEASE

Block of presynaptic α_2 autoreceptors on noradrenergic nerve terminals throughout the central nervous system (CNS) will reduce the negative feedback from released noradrenaline and thus enhance further noradrenaline release (see Chs 15 and 38). In addition, α_2-adrenoceptor antagonists can indirectly enhance 5-HT release.

The effect of α_2-adrenoceptor antagonists on synaptic noradrenaline and 5-HT levels would be rapid in onset and so these changes must somehow induce other, slower adaptive responses that give rise to the slowly developing antidepressant effects.

GENE EXPRESSION AND NEUROGENESIS

More recently, interest has centred on intracellular signalling pathways, changes in gene expression and neurogenesis. Much attention has been focused on how antidepressants may activate the transcription factor, CREB, a cAMP response element-binding protein. The role of other transcription factors, such as those of the Fos family and NF-κB, have been less extensively studied. As described earlier, several antidepressant drugs appear to promote neurogenesis in the hippocampus, a mechanism that could account for the slow development of the therapeutic effect. The role of raised synaptic noradrenaline and 5-HT levels in inducing changes in gene expression and neurogenesis, and the mechanisms involved, await further elucidation.

MONOAMINE UPTAKE INHIBITORS
SELECTIVE 5-HYDROXYTRYPTAMINE UPTAKE INHIBITORS

These are the most commonly prescribed group of antidepressants. Examples include **fluoxetine**, **fluvoxamine**, **paroxetine**, **citalopram**, **escitalopram** and **sertraline** (see Table 48.2). As well as showing selectivity with respect to 5-HT over noradrenaline uptake (Fig. 48.4), they are less likely than TCAs to cause anticholinergic side effects and are less dangerous in overdose. In contrast to MAOIs, they do not cause 'cheese reactions'. They are also used to treat anxiety disorders (see Ch. 45) and premature ejaculation. **Vortioxetine** is a novel SSRI that also has partial agonist activity at $5-HT_{1A}$ and $5-HT_{1B}$ receptors and is an antagonist at other 5-HT receptors including $5-HT_{3A}$ receptors.

Individual patients may respond more favourably to one SSRI than another. This may reflect other pharmacological properties of each individual drug as none is devoid of other actions. Fluoxetine has $5-HT_{2C}$ antagonist activity, a property it shares with other non-SSRI antidepressants such as **mirtazapine**. Sertraline is a weak inhibitor of dopamine uptake. Escitalopram is the *S* isomer of racemic citalopram. It lacks the antihistamine and CYP2D6 inhibitory properties of the *R* isomer.

Pharmacokinetic aspects
The SSRIs are well absorbed when given orally, and most have plasma half-lives of 18–24 h (fluoxetine is longer acting: 24–96 h). Paroxetine and fluoxetine are not used in combination with TCAs, whose hepatic metabolism they inhibit through an interaction with CYP2D6, for fear of increasing TCA toxicity.

Unwanted effects
Common side effects include nausea, anorexia, insomnia, loss of libido and failure of orgasm.[4] Some of these unwanted

---

[4] Thus, conversely, SSRIs can be used to treat premature ejaculation. Dapoxetine has a short half-life and is taken 1–3 hours before sex.

effects result from the enhanced stimulation of postsynaptic 5-HT receptors as a result of the drugs increasing the levels of extracellular 5-HT. This can be either stimulation of the wrong type of 5-HT receptor (e.g. $5\text{-}HT_2$, $5\text{-}HT_3$ and $5\text{-}HT_4$ receptors) or stimulation of the same receptor that gives therapeutic benefit (e.g. postsynaptic $5\text{-}HT_{1A}$ receptors) but in the wrong brain region (i.e. enhanced stimulation of 5-HT receptors can result in both therapeutic and adverse responses).

In combination with MAOIs, SSRIs can cause a 'serotonin syndrome' characterised by tremor, agitation, increased reflexes, hyperthermia and cardiovascular collapse, from which deaths have occurred.

There have been reports of increased aggression, and occasionally violence, in patients treated with fluoxetine, but these have not been confirmed by controlled studies. The use of SSRIs is not recommended for treating depression in children under 18, in whom efficacy is doubtful and adverse effects, including excitement, insomnia and aggression in the first few weeks of treatment, may occur. The possibility of increased suicidal ideation is a concern in this age group (see p. 619).

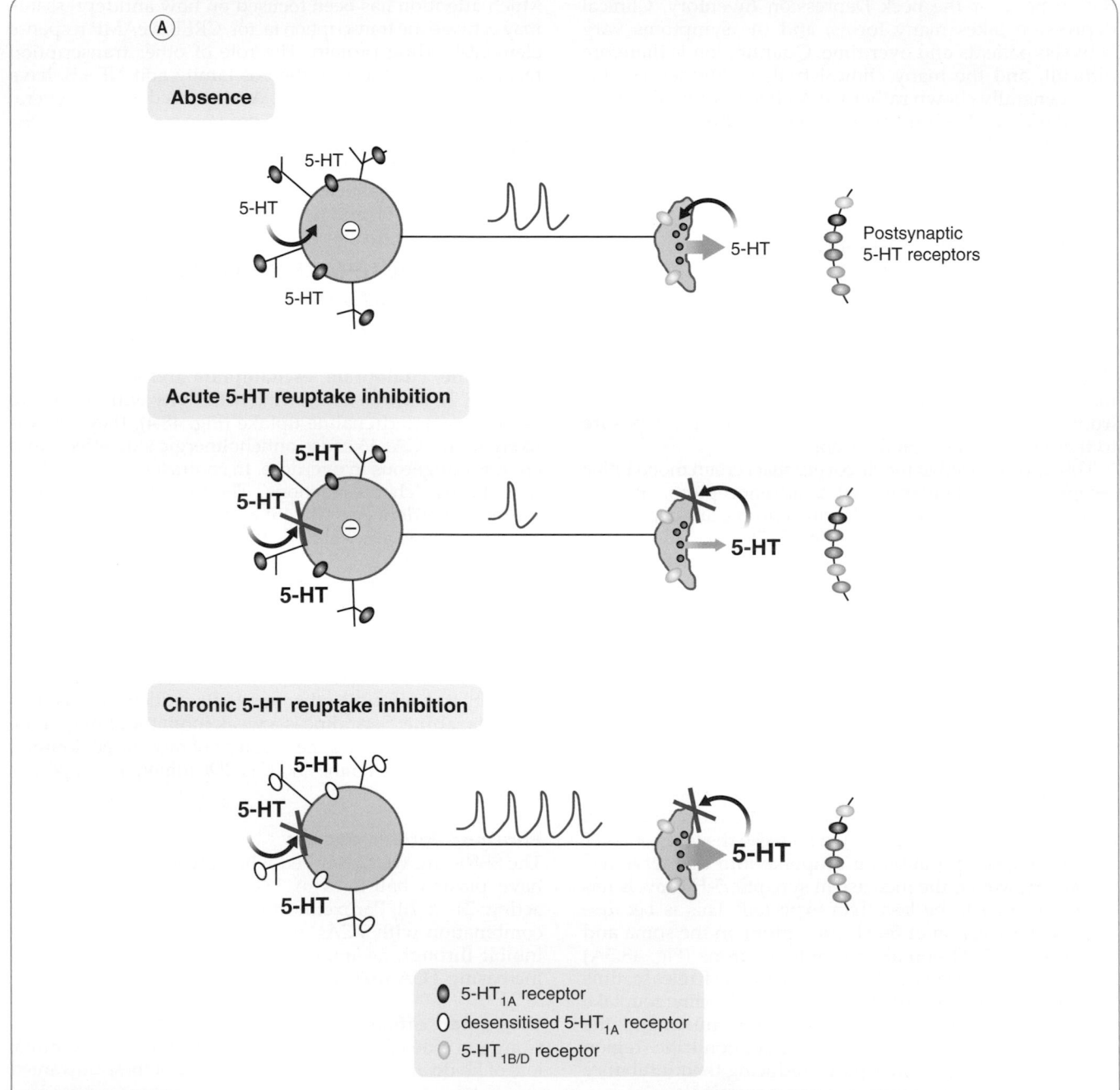

Fig. 48.3 Control of 5-hydroxytryptamine (5-HT) release. (A) 5-HT release is controlled by the inhibitory action of 5-HT on somatodendritic $5\text{-}HT_{1A}$ receptors. Acute inhibition of 5-HT reuptake results in increased extracellular levels of 5-HT but this increases somatodendritic $5\text{-}HT_{1A}$ receptor-mediated inhibition, hence synaptic 5-HT levels do not rise as much as expected. $5\text{-}HT_{1A}$ receptors eventually desensitise, resulting in reduced inhibition and thus greater 5-HT release.

Fig. 48.3, cont'd (B) 5-HT release is controlled by both an excitatory action of noradrenaline (NA) on somatodendritic α_1 adrenoceptors and an inhibitory action on α_2 adrenoceptors on serotonergic nerve terminals. Block of α_2 adrenoceptors located on noradrenergic neurons (not shown) enhances noradrenaline release resulting in further excitation of serotonergic neurons, while block of α_2 adrenoceptors on serotonergic neurons removes presynaptic inhibition and thus 5-HT release is enhanced.

Despite the apparent advantages of 5-HT uptake inhibitors over TCAs in terms of side effects, the combined results of many trials show little overall difference in terms of patient acceptability (Cipriani et al., 2009).

They are relatively safe in overdose, compared with TCAs (see p. 619) but can prolong the cardiac QT interval, giving rise to ventricular arrhythmias (see Ch. 22) and risk of sudden death (Jolly et al., 2009).

5-HT uptake inhibitors are used in a variety of other psychiatric disorders, as well as in depression, including anxiety disorders and obsessive–compulsive disorder (see Ch. 45).

TRICYCLIC ANTIDEPRESSANT DRUGS

TCAs (**imipramine, desipramine, amitriptyline, nortriptyline, clomipramine**) are still widely used. They are, however, far from ideal in practice, and it was the need for drugs that act more quickly and reliably, produce fewer side effects and are less hazardous in overdose that led to the introduction of newer 5-HT reuptake inhibitors and other antidepressants.

TCAs are closely related in structure to the phenothiazines (Ch. 47) and were initially synthesised (in 1949) as potential

Selective serotonin reuptake inhibitors (SSRIs)

- Examples include **fluoxetine, fluvoxamine, paroxetine, sertraline, citalopram, escitalopram**.
- Antidepressant actions are similar in efficacy and time course to tricyclic antidepressants (TCAs).
- Acute toxicity (especially cardiotoxicity) is less than that of monoamine oxidase inhibitors (MAOIs) or TCAs, so overdose risk is reduced.
- Side effects include nausea, insomnia and sexual dysfunction. SSRIs are less sedating and have fewer antimuscarinic side effects than the older TCAs.
- No food reactions, but dangerous 'serotonin reaction' (hyperthermia, muscle rigidity, cardiovascular collapse) can occur if given with MAOIs.
- There is concern about the use of SSRIs in children and adolescents, due to reports of an increase in suicidal thoughts on starting treatment.
- Also used for some other psychiatric indications (e.g. anxiety and obsessive–compulsive disorder).

Fig. 48.4 Selectivity of inhibition of noradrenaline (NA) and 5-hydroxytryptamine (5-HT) uptake by various antidepressants.

Table 48.3 Inhibition of neuronal noradrenaline (NA) and 5-hydroxytryptamine (5-HT) uptake by tricyclic antidepressants and their metabolites

Drug/metabolite	NA uptake	5-HT uptake
Imipramine	+++	++
Desmethylimipramine (DMI) (also known as desipramine)	++++	+
Hydroxy-DMI	+++	—
Clomipramine (CMI)	++	+++
Desmethyl-CMI	+++	+
Amitriptyline (AMI)	++	++
Nortriptyline (desmethyl-AMI)	+++	++
Hydroxynortriptyline	++	++

antipsychotic drugs. Several are tertiary amines and are quite rapidly demethylated in vivo (Fig. 48.5) to the corresponding secondary amines (e.g. imipramine to desipramine, amitriptyline to nortriptyline), which are themselves active and may be administered as drugs in their own right. Other tricyclic derivatives with slightly modified bridge structures include **doxepin**. The pharmacological differences between these drugs are not very great and relate mainly to their side effects, which are discussed later.

Some TCAs are also used to treat neuropathic pain (see Ch. 43).

Mechanism of action

As discussed previously, the main immediate effect of TCAs is to block the uptake of amines by nerve terminals, by competition for the binding site of the amine transporter (Ch. 15). Most TCAs inhibit noradrenaline and 5-HT uptake (see Fig. 48.4) but have much less effect on dopamine uptake. It has been suggested that improvement of emotional symptoms reflects mainly an enhancement of 5-HT-mediated transmission, whereas relief of biological symptoms results from facilitation of noradrenergic transmission. Interpretation is made difficult by the fact that the major metabolites of TCAs have considerable pharmacological activity (in some cases greater than that of the parent drug) and often differ from the parent drug in respect of their noradrenaline/5-HT selectivity (Table 48.3).

In addition to their effects on amine uptake, most TCAs affect other receptors, including muscarinic acetylcholine receptors, histamine receptors and 5-HT receptors. The antimuscarinic effects of TCAs are responsible for various side effects (see next section).

Unwanted effects

In non-depressed human subjects, TCAs cause sedation, confusion and motor incoordination. These effects occur also in depressed patients in the first few days of treatment, but tend to wear off in 1–2 weeks as the antidepressant effect develops.

TCAs produce a number of troublesome side effects, mainly due to interference with autonomic control.

Anti-muscarinic effects include dry mouth, blurred vision, constipation and urinary retention. These effects are strong with amitriptyline and much weaker with desipramine. Postural hypotension occurs with TCAs. This may seem anomalous for drugs that enhance noradrenergic transmission, and possibly results from an effect on adrenergic transmission in the medullary vasomotor centre. The other common side effect is sedation, and the long duration of action means that daytime performance is often affected by drowsiness and difficulty in concentrating.

TCAs, particularly in overdose, may cause ventricular dysrhythmias associated with prolongation of the QT interval (see Ch. 22). Usual therapeutic doses of TCAs increase, slightly but significantly, the risk of sudden cardiac death.

Interactions with other drugs

TCAs are particularly likely to cause adverse effects when given in conjunction with other drugs (see Ch. 58). They rely on hepatic metabolism by microsomal cytochrome P450 (CYP) enzymes for elimination, and this may be inhibited by competing drugs (e.g. antipsychotic drugs and some steroids).

TCAs potentiate the effects of alcohol and anaesthetic agents, for reasons that are not well understood, and deaths have occurred as a result of this, when severe respiratory depression has followed a bout of drinking. TCAs also interfere with the action of various antihypertensive drugs (see Ch. 23), with potentially dangerous consequences, so their use in hypertensive patients requires close monitoring.

Acute toxicity

TCAs are dangerous in overdose, and were at one time commonly used for suicide attempts, which was an important factor prompting the introduction of safer antidepressants. The main effects are on the CNS and the heart. The initial effect of TCA overdosage is to cause excitement and delirium, which may be accompanied by convulsions. This is followed by coma and respiratory depression lasting for

Fig. 48.5 Metabolism of imipramine, which is typical of that of other tricyclic antidepressants. *The hydroxylating enzyme CYP2D6 is subject to genetic polymorphism, which may account for individual variation in response to tricyclic antidepressants (see Ch. 12).

some days. Atropine-like effects are pronounced, including dry mouth and skin, mydriasis and inhibition of gut and bladder. Anticholinesterase drugs have been used to counter atropine-like effects but are no longer recommended. Cardiac dysrhythmias are common, and sudden death (rare) may occur from ventricular fibrillation.

Pharmacokinetic aspects

TCAs are all rapidly absorbed when given orally and bind strongly to plasma albumin, most being 90%–95% bound at therapeutic plasma concentrations. They also bind to extravascular tissues, which accounts for their generally very large distribution volumes (usually 10–50 L/kg; see Ch. 9) and low rates of elimination. Extravascular sequestration, together with strong binding to plasma albumin, means that haemodialysis is ineffective as a means of increasing drug elimination.

TCAs are metabolised in the liver by two main routes, N-demethylation and ring hydroxylation (see Fig. 48.5). Both the desmethyl and the hydroxylated metabolites commonly retain biological activity (Table 48.4). During prolonged treatment with TCAs, the plasma concentration of these metabolites is usually comparable to that of the parent drug, although there is wide variation between individuals. Inactivation of the drugs occurs by glucuronide conjugation of the hydroxylated metabolites, the glucuronides being excreted in the urine.

The overall half-times for elimination of TCAs are generally long, ranging from 10 to 20 h for imipramine and desipramine to about 80 h for **protriptyline**. They are even

Table 48.4 Substrates and inhibitors for type A and type B monoamine oxidase

	Type A	Type B
Preferred substrates	Noradrenaline 5-Hydroxytryptamine	Phenylethylamine Benzylamine
Non-specific substrates	Dopamine Tyramine	Dopamine Tyramine
Specific inhibitors	Clorgyline Moclobemide	Selegiline
Non-specific inhibitors	Pargyline Tranylcypromine Isocarboxazid	Pargyline Tranylcypromine Isocarboxazid

longer in elderly patients. Therefore gradual accumulation is possible, leading to slowly developing side effects.

SEROTONIN AND NORADRENALINE UPTAKE INHIBITORS (SNRIS)

These drugs are relatively non-selective for 5-HT and noradrenaline uptake. They include **venlafaxine**, **desvenlafaxine** and **duloxetine** (see Table 48.2).

As the dose of venlafaxine is increased, its efficacy also increases, which has been interpreted as demonstrating that its weak action to inhibit noradrenaline reuptake may add

Tricyclic antidepressants

- Tricyclic antidepressants are chemically related to phenothiazine antipsychotic drugs (Ch. 47), and some have similar non-selective receptor-blocking actions.
- Important examples are **imipramine**, **amitriptyline** and **clomipramine**.
- Most are long acting, and they are often converted to active metabolites.
- Important side effects: sedation (H_1 block); postural hypotension (α-adrenoceptor block); dry mouth, blurred vision, constipation (muscarinic block); occasionally mania and convulsions. Risk of ventricular dysrhythmias.
- Dangerous in acute overdose: confusion and mania, cardiac dysrhythmias.
- Liable to interact with other drugs (e.g. alcohol, anaesthetics, hypotensive drugs and non-steroidal anti-inflammatory drugs; should not be given with monoamine oxidase inhibitors).
- Also used to treat neuropathic pain.

Other monoamine uptake inhibitors

- **Venlafaxine** is a 5-HT uptake inhibitor, but less selective for 5-HT versus noradrenaline than SSRIs. It is metabolised to **desvenlafaxine**, which is also antidepressant.
- **Duloxetine** inhibits noradrenaline and 5-HT uptake.
- **Bupropion** is a noradrenaline and dopamine uptake inhibitor.
- Generally similar to tricyclic antidepressants but lack major receptor-blocking actions, so fewer side effects.
- Less risk of cardiac effects, so safer in overdose than tricyclic antidepressants.
- Can be used to treat other disorders:
  - **venlafaxine**, **desvenlafaxine** and **duloxetine** – anxiety disorders
  - **duloxetine** – neuropathic pain and fibromyalgia
  - **duloxetine** – urinary incontinence
  - **bupropion** – nicotine dependence

to its 5-HT uptake inhibition that occurs at lower doses, the combination providing additional therapeutic benefit. They are all active orally; slow-release formulations are available that reduce the incidence of nausea. Venlafaxine, desvenlafaxine and duloxetine are effective in some anxiety disorders (see Ch. 45). Desvenlafaxine may be useful in treating some perimenopausal symptoms such as hot flushes and insomnia. Duloxetine is also used in the treatment of neuropathic pain and fibromyalgia (see Ch. 43) and urinary incontinence.

Venlafaxine and duloxetine are metabolised by CYP2D6. Venlafaxine is converted to desvenlafaxine, which shows greater inhibition of noradrenaline reuptake. Unwanted effects of these drugs – largely due to enhanced activation of adrenoceptors – include headache, insomnia, sexual dysfunction, dry mouth, dizziness, sweating and decreased appetite. The most common symptoms in overdose are CNS depression, serotonin toxicity, seizure and cardiac conduction abnormalities. Duloxetine has been reported to cause hepatotoxicity and is contraindicated for patients with hepatic impairment.

OTHER NORADRENALINE UPTAKE INHIBITORS

Bupropion inhibits both noradrenaline and dopamine (but not 5-HT) uptake but, unlike cocaine and amphetamine (see Ch. 49), does not induce euphoria and has so far not been observed to have abuse potential. It is metabolised to active metabolites. It is also used to treat nicotine dependence (see Ch. 50). At high doses it may induce seizures. **Reboxetine** and **atomoxetine** are highly selective inhibitors of noradrenaline uptake but their efficacy in depression is less than that of TCAs. Atomoxetine is approved for the treatment of attention deficit/hyperactivity disorder (see Ch. 49).

MONOAMINE RECEPTOR ANTAGONISTS

Mirtazapine blocks not only α_2 adrenoreceptors but also other receptors, including 5-HT$_{2C}$ receptors, which may contribute to its antidepressant actions. Block of α_2 adrenoceptors will not only increase noradrenaline release but will also enhance 5-HT release (see Fig. 48.3B); however, by simultaneously blocking 5-HT$_{2A}$ and 5-HT$_3$ receptors,

Monoamine receptor antagonist antidepressant drugs

- **Mirtazapine** blocks α_2 adrenoceptors and 5-HT$_{2C}$ receptors, enhancing noradrenaline and 5-HT release.
- **Mirtazapine** may act more rapidly than other antidepressants, and causes less nausea and sexual dysfunction than SSRIs.
- **Trazodone** blocks 5-HT$_{2A}$ and 5-HT$_{2C}$ receptors and blocks 5-HT reuptake.
- **Mianserin** is an antagonist at multiple 5-HT receptors (including 5-HT$_{2A}$) as well as at α_1 and α_2 receptors. It is also an inverse agonist at H_1 receptors. Use is declining because of risk of bone marrow depression. Regular blood counts are advisable.
- Cardiovascular side effects of these drugs are fewer than those of tricyclic antidepressants.
- **Vortioxetine** has both 5-HT uptake inhibition and multiple 5-HT receptor partial agonist or antagonist actions.

it will reduce unwanted effects mediated through these receptors (e.g. sexual dysfunction and nausea) but leave intact stimulation of postsynaptic 5-HT$_{1A}$ receptors. It also blocks histamine H_1 receptors, which may cause sedation. **Trazodone** combines 5-HT$_{2A}$ and 5-HT$_{2C}$ receptor antagonism with 5-HT reuptake inhibition.

Mianserin, another α_2-adrenoceptor antagonist that also blocks H_1, 5-HT$_{2A}$ and α_1 adrenoreceptors, can cause bone marrow depression, requiring regular blood counts, so its use has declined in recent years.

MONOAMINE OXIDASE INHIBITORS

MAOIs were among the first drugs to be introduced clinically as antidepressants but were largely superseded by other types of antidepressants, whose clinical efficacies were considered better and whose side effects are generally less than those of MAOIs. The main examples are **phenelzine**, **tranylcypromine** and **iproniazid**. These drugs cause irreversible inhibition of the enzyme and do not distinguish between the two main isozymes (see later). The discovery of reversible inhibitors that show isozyme selectivity has rekindled interest in this class of drug. Although several studies have shown a reduction in platelet MAO activity in certain groups of depressed patients, there is no clear evidence that abnormal MAO activity is involved in the pathogenesis of depression.

Monoamine oxidase (see Ch. 15) is found in nearly all tissues, and exists in two similar molecular forms coded by separate genes (see Table 48.4). MAO-A has a substrate preference for 5-HT and noradrenaline, and is the main target for the antidepressant MAOIs. MAO-B has a substrate preference for phenylethylamine and dopamine. Type B is selectively inhibited by **selegiline**, which is used in the treatment of Parkinson's disease (see Ch. 41). Disruption of the MAO-A gene in mice causes increased brain accumulation of 5-HT and, to a lesser extent, noradrenaline, along with aggressive behaviour. A family has been reported with an inherited mutation leading to loss of MAO-A activity, whose members showed mental retardation and violent behaviour patterns. Most antidepressant MAOIs act on both forms of MAO, but clinical studies with subtype-specific inhibitors have shown clearly that antidepressant activity, as well as the main side effects of MAOIs, is associated with MAO-A inhibition. MAO is located intracellularly, mostly associated with mitochondria, and has two main functions:

1. Within nerve terminals, MAO regulates the free intraneuronal concentration of noradrenaline or 5-HT. It is not involved in the inactivation of released transmitter.
2. MAO in the gut wall is important in the inactivation of endogenous and ingested amines such as tyramine that would otherwise produce unwanted effects.

Chemical aspects

MAOIs are substrate analogues with a phenylethylamine-like structure, and most contain a reactive group (e.g. hydrazine, propargylamine, cyclopropylamine) that enables the inhibitor to bind covalently to the enzyme, resulting in a non-competitive and long-lasting inhibition. Recovery of MAO activity after inhibition takes several weeks with most drugs, but is quicker after **tranylcypromine**, which forms a less stable bond with the enzyme. **Moclobemide** acts as a reversible competitive inhibitor.

MAOIs are not specific in their actions, and inhibit a variety of other enzymes as well as MAO, including many enzymes involved in the metabolism of other drugs. This is responsible for some of the many clinically important drug interactions associated with MAOIs.

Pharmacological effects

Monoamine oxidase inhibitors cause a rapid and sustained increase in the 5-HT, noradrenaline and dopamine content of the brain, 5-HT being affected most and dopamine least. Similar changes occur in peripheral tissues such as heart, liver and intestine, and increases in the plasma concentrations of these amines are also detectable. Although these increases in tissue amine content are largely due to accumulation within neurons, transmitter release in response to nerve activity is not increased. In contrast to the effect of TCAs,

MAOIs do not increase the response of peripheral organs, such as the heart and blood vessels, to sympathetic nerve stimulation. The main effect of MAOIs is to increase the cytoplasmic concentration of monoamines in nerve terminals, without greatly affecting the vesicular stores that are releasable by nerve stimulation. The increased cytoplasmic pool results in an increased rate of spontaneous leakage of monoamines, and also an increased release by indirectly acting sympathomimetic amines such as amphetamine and tyramine (see Ch. 15 and Fig. 15.7). Tyramine thus causes a much greater rise in blood pressure in MAOI-treated animals than in controls. This mechanism is important in relation to the 'cheese reaction' produced by MAOIs in humans (see later).

In normal human subjects, MAOIs cause an immediate increase in motor activity; euphoria and excitement develop over the course of a few days. This is in contrast to TCAs, which cause only sedation and confusion when given to non-depressed subjects. The effects of MAOIs on amine metabolism develop rapidly, and the effect of a single dose lasts for several days. There is a clear discrepancy, as with SSRIs and TCAs, between the rapid biochemical response and the delayed antidepressant effect.

Unwanted effects and toxicity

Many of the unwanted effects of MAOIs result directly from MAO inhibition, but some are produced by other mechanisms.

Hypotension is a common side effect; indeed, **pargyline** was at one time used as an antihypertensive drug. One possible explanation for this effect – the opposite of what might have been expected – is that amines such as dopamine or octopamine accumulate within peripheral sympathetic nerve terminals and displace noradrenaline from the storage vesicles, thus reducing noradrenaline release associated with sympathetic activity.

Excessive central stimulation may cause tremors, excitement, insomnia and, in overdose, convulsions.

Increased appetite, leading to weight gain, can be so extreme as to require the drug to be discontinued.

Atropine-like side effects (dry mouth, blurred vision, urinary retention, etc.) are common with MAOIs, although they are less of a problem than with TCAs.

MAOIs of the hydrazine type (e.g. phenelzine and iproniazid) produce, very rarely (less than 1 in 10,000), severe hepatotoxicity, which seems to be due to the hydrazine moiety of the molecule. Their use in patients with liver disease is therefore unwise.

Interaction with other drugs and foods

Interaction with other drugs and foods is the most serious problem with MAOIs and is the main factor that caused their clinical use to decline. The special advantage claimed for the new reversible MAOIs, such as moclobemide, is that these interactions are reduced.

The 'cheese reaction' is a direct consequence of MAO inhibition and occurs when normally innocuous amines (mainly tyramine) produced during fermentation are ingested. Tyramine is normally metabolised by MAO in the gut wall and liver, and little dietary tyramine reaches the systemic circulation. MAO inhibition allows tyramine to be absorbed, and also enhances its sympathomimetic effect, as discussed earlier. The result is acute hypertension, giving rise to a severe throbbing headache and occasionally even to intracranial haemorrhage. Although many foods contain some tyramine, it appears that at least 10 mg of tyramine needs to be ingested to produce such a response, and the main danger is from ripe cheeses and from concentrated yeast products such as Marmite. Administration of indirectly acting sympathomimetic amines (e.g. **ephedrine** – a nasal decongestant – or amphetamine – a drug of abuse) also causes severe hypertension in patients receiving MAOIs; directly acting agents such as noradrenaline (used, for example, in conjunction with local anaesthetics; see Ch. 44) are not hazardous. Moclobemide, a specific MAO-A inhibitor, does not cause the 'cheese reaction', probably because tyramine can still be metabolised by MAO-B.

Hypertensive episodes have been reported in patients given TCAs and MAOIs simultaneously. The probable explanation is that inhibition of noradrenaline reuptake further enhances the cardiovascular response to dietary tyramine, thus accentuating the 'cheese reaction'. This combination of drugs can also produce excitement and hyperactivity.

Monoamine oxidase inhibitors can interact with **pethidine** (see Ch. 43) to cause severe hyperpyrexia, with restlessness, coma and hypotension. The mechanism is uncertain, but it is likely that an abnormal pethidine metabolite is produced because of inhibition of demethylation.

MELATONIN AGONIST

Agomelatine is a potent agonist at MT_1 and MT_2 receptors (see Ch. 40) with weak antagonist activity at 5-$HT_{2A,2B,2C}$ receptors (almost 1000-fold lower potency). It has a short biological half-life and does not give rise to the side effects associated with other antidepressant drugs. Used to treat severe depression, it is usually taken once daily before bed and may work by correcting disturbances in circadian rhythms often associated with depression. There are reports of hepatotoxicity in a few patients, and it should not be used in patients with liver disease.

KETAMINE

Small clinical trials suggest that a single, intravenous, sub-anaesthetic dose of **ketamine** may produce a rapid but short-lasting decrease in depressive symptoms lasting from a few hours up to 14 days, without the 3- to 4-week delay in onset of action seen with other antidepressant drugs (see Malhi et al., 2016). Though not approved for use in this indication, ketamine is claimed to improve mood in patients suffering from depression resistant to other forms of antidepressant therapy. Clinical trials of intranasal **esketamine**, the S isomer of ketamine, are underway, as are larger, longer-term studies of ketamine itself. The muscarinic antagonist, **scopolamine** (see Ch. 14), may also have rapid onset antidepressant effects but further, large clinical trials are required to substantiate this claim.

Ketamine is a non-competitive NMDA channel blocker (see Ch. 42), however, memantine, which also blocks NMDA receptors has not been shown to be antidepressant. There is controversy surrounding whether the putative antidepressant effect is produced by ketamine itself or by its metabolite, R,R-hydroxynorketamine. Hydroxynorketamine would have the added advantage that, unlike ketamine, it may not produce psychotomimetic effects as it has low affinity for the NMDA receptor, and thus would be unlikely to be abused (see Ch. 50).

OTHER ANTIDEPRESSANT APPROACHES

Methylfolate, given as a dietary supplement, may be effective in depressed individuals who have lowered folate levels.

Monoamine oxidase inhibitors (MAOIs)

- Main examples are **phenelzine**, **tranylcypromine**, **isocarboxazid** (irreversible, long-acting, non-selective between MAO-A and -B) and **moclobemide** (reversible, short-acting, MAO-A selective).
- Long-acting MAOIs:
  - main side effects: postural hypotension (sympathetic block); atropine-like effects (as with tricyclic antidepressants [TCAs]); weight gain; central nervous system (CNS) stimulation, causing restlessness, insomnia; hepatotoxicity and neurotoxicity (rare);
  - acute overdose causes CNS stimulation, sometimes convulsions;
  - 'cheese reaction', i.e. severe hypertensive response to tyramine-containing foods (e.g. cheese, beer, wine, well-hung game, yeast or soy extracts); such reactions can occur up to 2 weeks after treatment is discontinued.
- Interaction with other amines (e.g. **ephedrine** in over-the-counter decongestants, **clomipramine** and other TCAs) and some other drugs (e.g. **pethidine**) are also potentially lethal.
- **Moclobemide** is used for major depression and social phobia. 'Cheese reaction' and other drug interactions are less severe and shorter lasting than with irreversible MAOIs.
- MAOIs are used much less than other antidepressants because of their adverse effects and serious interactions. They are indicated for major depression in patients who have not responded to other drugs.

Oestrogen, which is known to elevate mood in perimenopausal women, may also be of value for the treatment of postnatal depression. Its effectiveness in treating other forms of depression is unclear. In addition to its well-documented hormonal actions in the body (see Ch. 36), it also has actions on monoaminergic, GABAergic and glutamatergic systems in the brain (see Chs 39 and 40).

Novel-acting antidepressants

- **Agomelatine** is an agonist at MT_1 and MT_2 melatonin receptors that improves mood, probably by improving sleep patterns.
- **Ketamine**, an NMDA receptor channel blocker, produces rapid onset antidepressant effects in patients resistant to other therapies.

CLINICAL EFFECTIVENESS OF ANTIDEPRESSANT TREATMENTS

The overall clinical efficacy of antidepressants is generally accepted for severe depression, though there is concern that the published clinical trials evidence may be misleading, because many negative trials have gone unreported. However, 30%–40% of depressed patients fail to show improvement, and those that do may only show partial improvement, re-inforcing the need for new drugs with novel mechanisms of action. Clear evidence of benefit from current antidepressant drugs in mild to moderate depression is lacking. Interpretation of trials data is complicated by a high placebo response, and spontaneous recovery independent of any treatment. Clinical trial data do not suggest that drugs currently in use differ in terms of efficacy. Nevertheless, clinical experience suggests that individual patients may, for unknown reasons, respond better to one drug than another. Current treatment guidelines recommend evidence-based psychological procedures as first-line treatments in most cases, before antidepressant drugs.

Pharmacogenetic factors

▼ The individual variation in response to antidepressants and the incidence of adverse effects may be partly due to genetic factors (Crisafulli et al., 2014). Two genetic factors have received particular attention, namely:

- polymorphism of cytochrome P450 genes, especially *CYP2D6* and *CYP2C19*, which are responsible for hydroxylation and demethylation of TCAs and SSRIs;
- polymorphism of serotonin and noradrenaline transporter genes.

Up to 10% of Caucasians possess a dysfunctional *CYP2D6* gene, and consequently may be susceptible to side effects of antidepressants and various other drugs (see Ch. 12) that are metabolised by this route. The opposite effect, caused by duplication of the gene, is common in Eastern European and East African populations, and may account for a lack of clinical efficacy in some individuals. There is some evidence to suggest that responsiveness to SSRIs and SNRIs is related to polymorphism of the serotonin and noradrenaline transporter genes.

Although genotyping may prove to be a useful approach in the future to individualising antidepressant therapy, its practical realisation is still some way off.

Suicide and antidepressants

▼ SSRI and SNRI antidepressants can increase the risk of 'suicidality' and increase aggression in children, adolescents and young adults (see Sharma et al., 2016). The term *suicidality* encompasses suicidal thoughts and planning as well as unsuccessful attempts; actual suicide, although one of the major causes of death in young people, is much rarer than suicidality. The risk is less in older age groups. However, the risk has to be balanced against the beneficial effects of these drugs, not only on depression but also on anxiety, panic and obsessive–compulsive disorders (see Ch. 45).

FUTURE ANTIDEPRESSANT DRUGS

Considerable effort is being made to develop drugs that combine a number of pharmacological effects thought to contribute towards antidepressant actions in one chemical entity (e.g. drugs inhibiting 5-HT, noradrenaline and dopamine uptake as well as having one or more of the following properties: β_3 adrenoceptor agonism, D_2 dopamine receptor agonism or antagonism, 5-HT_{1A} receptor agonism or partial agonism and 5-HT_{2A} receptor antagonism).

Interest in developing drugs acting as antagonists at different subtypes of NMDA receptor (Ch. 39) has been stimulated by reports that ketamine rapidly alleviates depression. The drive is to find a drug devoid of ketamine's unwanted psychotomimetic effects.

Drugs acting at these and other novel targets are discussed in detail by Ionescu and Papakostas (2017).

Clinical uses of drugs in depression

- Mild depression is often best treated initially with non-drug measures (such as cognitive behavioural therapy), with antidepressant drugs being used in addition if the response is poor.
- The use of antidepressant drugs is advisable in the treatment of moderate to severe depression.
- The clinical efficacy of antidepressant drugs is limited, and varies between individuals. Clinical trials have produced inconsistent results, because of placebo responses and spontaneous fluctuations in the level of depression.
- Different classes of antidepressant drugs have similar efficacy but different side effects.
- Choice of drug is based on individual aspects including concomitant disease treatment, suicide risk and previous response to treatment. Other things being equal, a SSRI is preferred as these are usually better tolerated and are less dangerous in overdose.
- Antidepressant drugs take several weeks before taking effect, so decisions on dose increment or switching to another class should not be made precipitately. Use of MAOIs is managed by specialists.
- An effective regimen should be continued for at least 2 years.
- In urgent situations, specialist consideration should be given to possible use of electroconvulsive therapy.
- Anxiolytic (e.g. benzodiazepine, Ch. 45), or antipsychotic drugs (Ch. 47) are useful adjuncts in some patients.

BRAIN STIMULATION THERAPIES

A number of brain stimulation techniques are now being used or developed to treat depression. Bright light stimulation has been proposed as a treatment for seasonal affective disorder. The most established brain stimulation techniques are electroconvulsive therapy (ECT) and repetitive transcranial magnetic stimulation (TMS). Brain stimulation treatments are often used as the therapeutic approach of last resort for patients who have not responded to antidepressant drugs.

ECT involves stimulation through electrodes placed on either side of the head, with the patient lightly anaesthetised, paralysed with a short-acting neuromuscular-blocking drug (e.g. **suxamethonium**; Ch. 14) to avoid physical injury, and artificially ventilated. Controlled trials have shown ECT to be at least as effective as antidepressant drugs, with response rates ranging between 60% and 80%; it appears to be an effective treatment for severe suicidal depression and has the advantage of producing a fast-onset response. The main disadvantage of ECT is that it often causes confusion and memory loss lasting for days or weeks. TMS gives electrical stimulation without anaesthesia or convulsion and does not produce cognitive impairment, but comparative studies suggest that its antidepressant efficacy is less than that of conventional ECT.

The effect of ECT on experimental animals has been carefully analysed to see if it provides clues as to the mode of action of antidepressant drugs, but the clues it gives are enigmatic. 5-HT synthesis and uptake are unaltered, and noradrenaline uptake is somewhat increased (in contrast to the effect of TCAs). Decreased β adrenoceptor responsiveness, both biochemical and behavioural, occurs with both ECT and long-term administration of antidepressant drugs, but changes in 5-HT-mediated responses tend to go in opposite directions.

There have been reports that deep brain stimulation, which has also been used in the treatment of Parkinson's disease (see Ch. 41), in which stimulation is delivered in a specific brain region through surgically implanted electrodes, is effective in patients not responding to other treatments (see Mayberg et al., 2005). The effectiveness of another technique, vagal stimulation, in producing long-term benefit in depression is still unclear.

DRUG TREATMENT OF BIPOLAR DISORDER

A range of drugs are now used to control the mood swings characteristic of manic–depressive (bipolar) illness. The major drugs are:

- **lithium**;
- several antiepileptic drugs, e.g. **carbamazepine**, **valproate**, **lamotrigine**;
- some antipsychotic drugs, e.g. **olanzapine**, **risperidone**, **quetiapine**, **aripiprazole**, **brexpiprazole**, **cariprazine**.

When used to treat bipolar disorder, lithium and antiepileptic agents are often referred to as *mood-stabilising* drugs.

Other agents that may have some beneficial effects in the treatment of bipolar disorder are benzodiazepines (to calm, induce sleep and reduce anxiety), **memantine**, **amantadine** and **ketamine**. The use of antidepressant drugs in bipolar disorder is somewhat controversial. It is recommended that they are given in combination with an antimanic agent because, in some patients, they may induce or enhance mania.

Used prophylactically in bipolar disorder, drugs prevent the swings of mood and thus can reduce both the depressive and the manic phases of the illness. They are given over long periods, and their beneficial effects take 3–4 weeks to develop. Given in an acute attack, they are effective only in reducing mania, but not the depressive phase (although lithium is sometimes used as an adjunct to antidepressants in severe cases of unipolar depression).

LITHIUM

The psychotropic effect of lithium was discovered in 1949 by Cade, who had predicted that urate salts should prevent the induction by uraemia of a hyperexcitability state in guinea pigs. He found lithium urate to produce an effect, quickly discovered that it was due to lithium rather than urate, and went on to show that lithium produced a rapid improvement in a group of manic patients.

Anti-epileptic and atypical antipsychotic drugs (see later) are equally effective in treating acute mania; they act more quickly and are considerably safer, so the clinical use of lithium is mainly confined to prophylactic control of

manic–depressive illness. The use of lithium is declining.[5] It is relatively difficult to use, as plasma concentration monitoring is required, and there is the potential for problems in patients with renal impairment and for drug interactions, for example with diuretics (see Ch. 58). Lithium may have beneficial effects in neurodegenerative diseases such as Alzheimer's disease (see Ch. 41).

Pharmacological effects and mechanism of action
Lithium is clinically effective at a plasma concentration of 0.5–1 mmol/L, and above 1.5 mmol/L it produces a variety of toxic effects, so the therapeutic window is narrow. In normal subjects, 1 mmol/L lithium in plasma has no appreciable psychotropic effects. It does, however, produce many detectable biochemical changes, and it is still unclear how these may be related to its therapeutic effect.

Lithium is a monovalent cation that can mimic the role of Na^+ in excitable tissues, being able to permeate the voltage-gated Na^+ channels that are responsible for action potential generation (see Ch. 4). It is, however, not pumped out by the Na^+-K^+-ATPase, and therefore tends to accumulate inside excitable cells, leading to a partial loss of intracellular K^+, and depolarisation of the cell.

The biochemical effects of lithium are complex, and it inhibits many enzymes that participate in signal transduction pathways. Those that are thought to be relevant to its therapeutic actions are as follows:

- Inhibition of inositol monophosphatase, which blocks the phosphatidylinositol (PI) pathway (see Ch. 3) at the point where inositol phosphate is hydrolysed to free inositol, resulting in depletion of PI. This prevents agonist-stimulated inositol trisphosphate formation through various PI-linked receptors, and therefore blocks many receptor-mediated effects.
- Inhibition of glycogen synthase kinase 3 (GSK3) isoforms, possibly by competing with magnesium for its association with these kinases. GSK3 isoforms phosphorylate a number of key enzymes involved in pathways leading to apoptosis and amyloid formation (see Phiel & Klein, 2001). Lithium can also affect GSK3 isoforms indirectly by interfering with their regulation by Akt, a closely related serine/threonine kinase regulated through PI-mediated signalling and by arrestins (see Ch. 3; Beaulieu et al., 2009).

Lithium inhibits G protein function, thus reducing K^+ channel activation and hormone-induced cAMP production. It also blocks other cellular responses (e.g. the response of renal tubular cells to antidiuretic hormone, and of the thyroid to thyroid-stimulating hormone; see Chs 30 and 35, respectively). This is not, however, a pronounced effect in the brain.

The cellular selectivity of lithium appears to depend on its selective uptake, reflecting the activity of sodium channels in different cells. This could explain its relatively selective action in the brain and kidney, even though many other tissues use the same second messengers. Notwithstanding such insights, our ignorance of the nature of the disturbance underlying the mood swings in bipolar disorder leaves us groping for links between the biochemical and prophylactic effects of lithium.

---

[5]The decline in lithium use may have been influenced by the imbalance in the marketing of this simple inorganic ion versus more profitable pharmacological agents.

Pharmacokinetic aspects and toxicity

Lithium is given by mouth as the carbonate salt and is excreted by the kidney. About half of an oral dose is excreted within about 12 h – the remainder, which presumably represents lithium taken up by cells, is excreted over the next 1–2 weeks. This very slow phase means that, with regular dosage, lithium accumulates slowly over 2 weeks or more before a steady state is reached. The narrow therapeutic window means that monitoring of the plasma concentration is essential. Na⁺ depletion reduces the rate of excretion by increasing the reabsorption of lithium by the proximal tubule, and thus increases the likelihood of toxicity. Diuretics that act distal to the proximal tubule (Ch. 30) also have this effect, and renal disease also predisposes to lithium toxicity.

The main toxic effects that may occur during treatment are as follows:

- nausea, vomiting and diarrhoea;
- tremor;
- renal effects: polyuria (with resulting thirst) resulting from inhibition of the action of antidiuretic hormone. At the same time, there is some Na⁺ retention associated with increased aldosterone secretion. With prolonged treatment, serious renal tubular damage may occur, making it essential to monitor renal function regularly in lithium-treated patients;
- thyroid enlargement, sometimes associated with hypothyroidism;
- weight gain;
- hair loss.

Acute lithium toxicity results in various neurological effects, progressing from confusion and motor impairment to coma, convulsions and death if the plasma concentration reaches 3–5 mmol/L.

ANTIEPILEPTIC DRUGS

Carbamazepine, **valproate** and **lamotrigine** (see Ch. 46) have fewer side effects than lithium and have proved efficacious in the treatment of bipolar disorder.

It is assumed that the mechanisms of action of anticonvulsant drugs in reducing bipolar disorder are related to their anticonvulsant activity. While each drug has multiple actions (see Table 46.1), the antiepileptic drugs effective in bipolar disorder share the property of sodium-channel blockade, although there are subtle differences in their effectiveness against the different phases of bipolar disorder. Valproate and carbamazepine are effective in treating acute attacks of mania and in the long-term treatment of the disorder, although carbamazepine may not be as effective in treating the depression phase. Valproate is sometimes given along with other drugs such as lithium. Lamotrigine is effective in preventing the recurrence of both mania and depression.

SECOND-GENERATION ANTIPSYCHOTIC DRUGS

An ever-increasing number of second-generation antipsychotic drugs (e.g. **olanzapine**, **risperidone**, **quetiapine**, **aripiprazole**, **cariprazine**, **brexpiprazole**, **asenapine**), (see Ch. 47), are proving effective in the treatment of bipolar depression. These agents have D₂-dopamine and 5-HT$_{2A}$ receptor antagonist properties as well as actions on other receptors and amine transporters that may contribute to their effectiveness. All appear to be effective against mania while some may also be effective against bipolar depression.

In bipolar depression, they are often used in combination with lithium or valproate. Olanzapine is given in combination with the antidepressant fluoxetine. Haloperidol, a first-generation antipsychotic drug is also sometimes used to treat bipolar depression.

Treatment of bipolar disorder

- **Lithium**, an inorganic ion, taken orally as lithium carbonate.
- Mechanism of action is not understood. The main biochemical possibilities are:
  - interference with inositol trisphosphate formation
  - inhibition of kinases
- Antiepileptic drugs (e.g. **carbamazepine**, **valproate**, **lamotrigine**):
  - better side effect and safety profile.
- Atypical antipsychotic drugs (e.g. **olanzapine**, **risperidone**, **quetiapine**, **aripiprazole**) and also **haloperidol**.

Clinical uses of mood-stabilising drugs

- **Lithium** (as the carbonate) is the classical drug. It is used:
  - in prophylaxis and treatment of *mania*, and in the prophylaxis of *bipolar* or *unipolar disorder* (manic depression or recurrent depression).
- Points to note include the following:
  - there is a narrow therapeutic window and long duration of action;
  - acute toxic effects include cerebellar effects, nephrogenic *diabetes insipidus* (see Ch. 30) and renal failure;
  - dose must be adjusted according to the plasma concentration;
  - elimination is via the kidney and is reduced by proximal tubular reabsorption. Diuretics increase the activity of the reabsorptive mechanism and hence can precipitate lithium toxicity;
  - *thyroid disorders* and mild *cognitive impairment* occur during chronic use.
- **Carbamazepine valproate** and **lamotrigine** (sodium-channel blockers with antiepileptic actions; Ch. 46) are used for:
  - the prophylaxis and treatment of manic episodes in patients with *bipolar disorder*;
  - the treatment of *bipolar disorder* (**valproate**, **lamotrigine**).
- **Olanzapine**, **risperidone**, **quetiapine**, **aripiprazole** (atypical antipsychotic drugs) are primarily used to treat *mania*.

REFERENCES AND FURTHER READING

Pathogenesis of depressive illness

Harmer, C.J., Duman, R.S., Cowen, P.J., 2017. How do antidepressants work? New perspectives for refining future treatment approaches. Lancet Psychiatry 4, 409–418. (*Reviews the various theories of how antidepressant drugs produce their effects*)

Ionescu, D.F., Papakostas, G.I., 2017. Experimental medication treatment approaches for depression. Transl. Psychiatry. 7, e1068. (*Describes new targets for antidepressant drugs*)

Mullins, N., Lewis, C.M., 2017. Genetics of depression: progress at last. Curr. Psychiatry Rep. 19, 43. (*Describes recent developments in determining the genetic causes of depression*)

O'Leary, O.F., Cryan, J.F., 2013. Towards translational rodent models of depression. Cell Tissue Res. 354, 141–153. (*Describes current animal models for depression*)

Soronen, P., Ollila, H.M., Antila, M., et al., 2010. Replication of GWAS of bipolar disorder: association of SNPs near *CDH7* with bipolar disorder and visual processing. Mol. Psychiatry 15, 4–6. (*A major study of potential genetic influences on depression*)

Willner, P., Belzung, C., 2015. Treatment-resistant depression: are animal models of depression fit for purpose? Psychopharmacology (Berl) 232, 3473–3495. (*Detailed discussion of animal models of depression*)

Antidepressant treatments

Cipriani, A., Santilli, C., Furukawa, T.A., et al., 2009. Escitalopram versus other antidepressive agents for depression. Cochrane Database Syst. Rev. (2), Art. No.: CD006532, doi:10.1002/14651858.CD006532. pub2.

Crisafulli, C., Drago, A., Calabro, M., et al., 2014. Pharmacogenetics of antidepressant drugs: an update. Hospital Pharmacology 1, 33–51.

Jolly, K., Gammage, M.D., Cheng, K.K., Bradburn, P., Banting, M.V., Langman, M.J., 2009. Sudden death in patients receiving drugs tending to prolong the QT interval. Br. J. Clin. Pharmacol. 68, 743–751. (*Compares the risk of sudden death in patients receiving various antipsychotic and antidepressant therapies*)

Malhi, G.S., Byrow, Y., Cassidy, F., et al., 2016. Ketamine: stimulating antidepressant treatment? Brit J. Psychiatry Open 2, e5–e9. (*Brings together the views of a wide range of experts on the effectiveness of ketamine as an antidepressant*)

Mayberg, H.S., Lozano, A.M., Voon, V., et al., 2005. Deep brain stimulation for treatment-resistant depression. Neuron 45, 651–660.

Racagni, G., Popoli, M., 2008. Cellular and molecular mechanisms in the long-term action of antidepressants. Dialogues Clin. Neurosci. 10, 385–400. (*An extensive review of long-term changes induced in the brain by antidepressant drugs that may be responsible for producing the therapeutic benefit*)

Sharma, T., Guski, L.S., Freund, N., Gøtzsche, P.C., 2016. Suicidality and aggression during antidepressant treatment: systematic review and meta-analyses based on clinical study reports. Brit. Med. J. 352, i65. (*Detailed analysis of published papers that concludes SSRI and NRI can induce suicidality and aggression in younger people*)

Lithium

Beaulieu, J.M., Gainetdinov, R.R., Caron, M.G., 2009. Akt/GSK3 signaling in the action of psychotropic drugs. Annu. Rev. Pharmacol. Toxicol. 49, 327–347.

Phiel, C.J., Klein, P.S., 2001. Molecular targets of lithium action. Annu. Rev. Pharmacol. Toxicol. 41, 789–813. (*Review of a topic that is still little understood*)

Psychoactive drugs **49**

OVERVIEW

In its broadest sense, the term 'psychoactive drug' would cover all drugs that act on the brain to produce changes in perception, mood, consciousness and behaviour, and would thus include anaesthetic, anxiolytic, antipsychotic and antidepressant drugs, which are described elsewhere in this book. Here we describe psychoactive drugs that are not covered in detail elsewhere. Some of these drugs have proven therapeutic usefulness in the treatment of behavioural disorders such as attention deficit/hyperactive disorder and narcolepsy. Others may prove to have clinical potential as cognition enhancers.

Many psychoactive drugs described in this chapter are used to alter mood and perception, or to satisfy addiction, and are drugs of abuse. This aspect is also discussed in Chapters 50 and 59.

Further information on psychoactive drugs is contained in Miller (2015).

INTRODUCTION

Attempting to classify psychoactive drugs according to their pharmacological mechanisms of action and their behavioural effects is a challenging task. Several of the drugs exert more than one important pharmacological action, drugs with apparently similar pharmacological activity can induce different subjective experiences (e.g. amphetamine and MDMA) and for a single drug the behavioural response may change with dose (e.g. ethanol induces excitement at low doses but is depressant at higher doses). Here, for convenience, we have grouped psychoactive drugs as

- Psychomotor stimulants
- Psychedelics
- Ketamine and related drugs
- Depressants
- Synthetic cannabinoids

The 21st century has seen an explosion in the availability of novel psychoactive substances (NPS). By and large, these have been developed to circumvent legal restrictions on more established drugs (e.g. amphetamines, cocaine, MDMA and cannabinoids) and were for a time referred to as 'legal highs'. This has led to changes in the law in the United Kingdom to make any NPS illegal. NPS are appearing so rapidly – over 600 were recorded between 2008 and 2015 – that any catalogue of them would likely be out of date by the time it had been compiled. In this chapter we concentrate on psychoactive drugs for which good evidence

PSYCHOMOTOR STIMULANTS

Table 49.1 lists the major psychomotor stimulants, their mechanisms of action and clinical uses.

AMPHETAMINES[1]

DL-amphetamine (*speed* or *billy whizz*), its active dextroisomer **dextroamphetamine** (*dexies*), and **methamphetamine** (*crystal meth* or *ice*) have very similar chemical and pharmacological properties (Fig. 49.1).

Pharmacological effects

The amphetamines act by releasing monoamines, primarily dopamine and noradrenaline, from nerve terminals in the brain. They do this in a number of ways. They are substrates for the neuronal plasma membrane monoamine uptake transporters DAT and NET but not SERT (see Chs 15, 16 and 40), and thus act as competitive inhibitors, reducing the reuptake of dopamine and noradrenaline. In addition, they enter nerve terminals via the uptake processes or by diffusion and interact with the vesicular monoamine pump VMAT-2 to inhibit the uptake into synaptic vesicles of cytoplasmic dopamine and noradrenaline. The amphetamines are taken up into the storage vesicles by VMAT-2 and displace the endogenous monoamines from the vesicles into the cytoplasm. At high concentrations, amphetamines can inhibit monoamine oxidase, which otherwise would break down cytoplasmic monoamines, and monoamine oxidase inhibitors (see Ch. 48) potentiate the effects of amphetamine. The cytoplasmic monoamines can then be transported out of the nerve endings via the plasma membrane DAT and NET transporters working in reverse, a process that is thought to be facilitated by amphetamine binding to these transporters. All of the above will combine to increase the concentration of extracellular dopamine and noradrenaline in the vicinity of the synapse (see Chs 15 and 40).

In animals, prolonged administration results in degeneration of monoamine-containing nerve terminals and eventually cell death. This effect is observed with toxic doses and is probably due to the accumulation of reactive metabolites of the parent compounds within the nerve terminals. In human brain-imaging studies a reduction in the levels of

---

[1]As discussed in the Preface to this book, in Chapters 49 and 50, where mainly illicit drug use is being described, we use common drug names and spellings (e.g. amphetamine and heroin) rather than their recommended international non-proprietary names (amfetamine and 3,6-diacetyl morphine).

Table 49.1 Major central nervous system psychomotor stimulants

Drugs	Mode(s) of action	Clinical significance	Notes
Amphetamine and related compounds (e.g. dexamphetamine, methamphetamine)	Release of DA and NA Inhibition of DA and NA uptake	Dexamphetamine used to treat ADHD in children; otherwise very limited clinical use Some use to treat narcolepsy	Risk of dependence, sympathomimetic side effects and pulmonary hypertension Mainly important as drugs of abuse **Fenethylline** is a prodrug that is broken down to release both amphetamine and theophylline. It is a popular drug of abuse in Arab countries
Methylphenidate	Inhibition of DA and NA uptake	Used to treat ADHD in children.	Structurally related to amphetamines (see Fig. 49.1) **Ethylphenidate** has similar actions
Modafinil	Inhibition of DA reuptake	May have use to reduce fatigue and enhance cognition	—
Cocaine	Inhibition of DA, 5-HT and NA uptake Local anaesthetic	Risk of fetal damage Occasionally used for nasopharyngeal and ophthalmic anaesthesia (see Ch. 44)	Major drug of abuse
MDMA (ecstasy)	Releases 5-HT and inhibits uptake	May have potential in the treatment of post-traumatic stress disorder	Other related drugs are **3,4-methylenedioxyamphetamine** (MDA), **4-bromo-2,5-dimethoxyphenethylamine** (2CB) and **4-methylthioamphetamine** (4-MTA)
Paramethoxyamphetamine (PMA)	Releases 5-HT and blocks uptake	—	Often added to, or sold as, MDMA, **paramethoxymethamphetamine** (PMMA) is similar but less potent
Methylone	Inhibits NA, DA and 5-HT uptake	—	Cathinone derivative containing the dioxy ring of MDMA **Ethylone** and **butylone** are similar
Benzofuran derivatives	Releases 5-HT and NA and inhibit uptake	—	Have both MDMA and amphetamine-like properties Examples include **1-(benzofuran-5-yl)-propan-2-amine** (5APB) and **1-(benzofuran-6-yl)-propan-2-amine** (6APB)
Mephedrone	Inhibition of DA and 5-HT uptake	—	Drug of abuse Derived from cathinone **Methedrone** and **mexedrone** are similar
Benzylpiperazine (BZP)	Inhibition of DA, NA and 5-HT uptake α_2-adrenoceptor agonist, 5-HT$_{2A}$ agonist	—	Drug of abuse
Methylxanthines (e.g. caffeine, theophylline)	Inhibition of phosphodiesterase Antagonism of adenosine A$_2$ receptors	Theophylline used for action on cardiac and bronchial muscle (see Chs 22 and 29)	Caffeine is a constituent of beverages and tonics. It is also available in tablet form
Nicotine	Stimulates and desensitises nicotinic receptors (see Chs 14 and 40)	—	—
Arecoline	Muscarinic agonist	—	Mild stimulant contained in betel nut. Use is widespread in India, Thailand, Indonesia and other Asian countries

ADHD, attention deficit/hyperactivity disorder; *DA,* dopamine; *5-HT,* 5-hydroxytryptamine; *NA,* noradrenaline.

Fig. 49.1 Structures of amphetamine, MDMA and related drugs.

DAT and D_2 receptors has been observed in the brains of amphetamine users. It is unclear, however, whether this is due to long-term exposure to the drug inducing nerve damage or is an underlying pathology that was responsible for drug-seeking in the first instance.

The main central effects of amphetamine-like drugs are:

- locomotor stimulation
- euphoria and excitement
- insomnia
- increased stamina
- anorexia
- long-term psychological effects: psychotic symptoms, anxiety, depression and cognitive impairment

In addition, amphetamines have peripheral sympathomimetic actions (Ch. 15), producing a rise in blood pressure and inhibition of gastrointestinal motility.

In humans, amphetamines cause euphoria; with intravenous injection, this can be so intense as to be described as 'orgasmic'. Rats quickly learn to press a lever in order to obtain a dose of amphetamine – an indication that the drug is rewarding. Humans become confident, hyperactive and talkative, and sex drive is said to be enhanced. Fatigue, both physical and mental, is reduced. Amphetamines (and similar drugs such as **dexfenfluramine** and **sibutramine**) cause marked anorexia, but with continued administration this effect wears off and food intake returns to normal. They are no longer used clinically for weight reduction (Ch. 33). They are ineffective in producing maintained weight loss, and their central nervous system (CNS) and cardiovascular effects are harmful.

Adverse effects of amphetamines include feelings of anxiety, irritability and restlessness. High doses may induce panic and paranoia.

The locomotor and rewarding effects of amphetamine are due mainly to release of dopamine rather than noradrenaline, since destruction of the dopamine-containing nucleus accumbens (see Ch. 40) or administration of D_2-receptor antagonists (see Ch. 47) inhibit these responses, which are absent in mice genetically engineered to lack DAT.

Chronic use, tolerance and dependence

If amphetamines are taken repeatedly over a few days, a state of 'amphetamine psychosis' can develop, resembling an acute schizophrenic attack (see Ch. 47), with hallucinations, paranoia and aggressive behaviour. At the same time, repetitive stereotyped behaviour may develop. The close similarity of this condition to schizophrenia, and the effectiveness of antipsychotic drugs in controlling it, is consistent with the dopamine theory of schizophrenia (see Ch. 47).

Tolerance develops rapidly to euphoric and anorexic effects of amphetamines, but more slowly to the other effects. Presumably tolerance is due to depletion of dopamine in nerve terminals.

Psychological dependence on amphetamines, a consequence of the insistent memory of euphoria, is very strong (see Ch. 50). When drug taking is stopped there is usually a period of deep sleep, and on awakening the subject feels lethargic, depressed, anxious, irritable (sometimes even suicidal) and hungry. These after effects may be the result of depletion of the normal stores of dopamine and noradrenaline. It is estimated that about 10%–15% of users progress to full dependence, the usual pattern being that the dose is increased as tolerance develops, and then uncontrolled 'binges' occur in which the user takes the drug repeatedly over a period of a day or more, remaining continuously intoxicated. Large doses may be consumed in such binges, with a high risk of acute toxicity, and the demand for the drug displaces all other considerations.

Experimental animals, given unlimited access to amphetamine, take it in such large amounts that they die from the cardiovascular effects within a few days. Given limited amounts, they too develop a binge pattern of dependence.

Pharmacokinetic aspects

Amphetamines are readily absorbed from the gastrointestinal tract, but to increase the intensity of the hit the drugs can be snorted or injected. In crystal form, the free base of methamphetamine can be ignited and smoked in a manner similar to crack cocaine (see p. 627). Amphetamines freely penetrate the blood–brain barrier. They do this more readily than other indirectly acting sympathomimetic amines such as **ephedrine** or **tyramine** (Ch. 15), which probably explains why they produce more marked central effects than those drugs. Amphetamines are mainly excreted unchanged in the urine, and the rate of excretion is increased when the urine is made more acidic (see Fig. 10.6).

METHYLPHENIDATE

Methylphenidate (*Ritalin*) inhibits the NET and DAT transporters on the neuronal plasma membrane. Unlike the amphetamines, methylphenidate is not a substrate for these transporters and thus does not enter the nerve terminals to facilitate noradrenaline (NA) and dopamine (DA) release (Heal et al., 2009). It nevertheless produces a profound and sustained elevation of extracellular NA and DA.

Methylphenidate is orally active, being absorbed from the intestine, but it undergoes presystemic metabolism such that only ~20% enters the systemic circulation. Absorption is slow following oral administration – T_{max} ~2 hours – which may limit the intensity of any euphoric response to the drug. It is metabolised by carboxylesterase and has a half-life of ~2–4 h. It is used therapeutically to treat attention deficit/hyperactivity disorder (ADHD; see p. 626) and may also have cognition-enhancing effects (see p. 633).

Amphetamines

- The main effects are:
  - increased motor activity
  - euphoria and excitement
  - insomnia
  - anorexia
  - with prolonged administration, stereotyped and psychotic behaviour
- Effects are due mainly to release of catecholamines, especially dopamine and noradrenaline.
- Stimulant effect lasts for a few hours and is followed by depression and anxiety.
- Tolerance to the stimulant effects develops rapidly, although peripheral sympathomimetic effects may persist.
- Amphetamines induce strong psychological dependence.
- Amphetamine psychosis, which closely resembles schizophrenia, can develop after prolonged use.
- Amphetamines may be useful in treating narcolepsy, and also (paradoxically) to control hyperkinetic children. They are no longer prescribed as appetite suppressants.
- Their main importance is in drug abuse.

MODAFINIL

Modafinil is the primary metabolite of **adrafinil**, a drug that was introduced as a treatment for narcolepsy in the 1980s. Since 1994, modafinil has been available as a drug in its own right. It inhibits dopamine reuptake by binding to DAT but with low potency. In the human brain, modafinil blocks DAT and increases extracellular dopamine levels in the caudate, putamen and nucleus accumbens. It also produces a number of other effects including α_1-drenoceptor activation, enhanced release of 5-hydroxytryptamine (5-HT), glutamate and histamine, and inhibition of GABA release, as well as enhanced electrotonic coupling between neurons. The contribution of each action to the behavioural effects of modafinil remains to be clarified. Modafinil enhances some aspects of cognitive performance (see p. 633), and has gained popularity as a 'lifestyle drug' (see Ch. 59) for this reason.

Modafinil is well absorbed from the gut, metabolised in the liver and has a half-life of 10–14 h. While reported to 'brighten mood' there is little evidence that modafinil produces significant levels of euphoria when administered by mouth, but tablets can be crushed and snorted to obtain a quicker onset of effect. Modafinil is too insoluble for intravenous injection to be practical.

CLINICAL USE OF STIMULANTS

Attention deficit/hyperactivity disorder (ADHD)

The main use of amphetamines and methylphenidate is in the treatment of ADHD, a common and increasingly diagnosed condition, estimated as occurring in up to 9% of children whose overactivity and limited attention span disrupt their education and social development. The efficacy of drug treatment (e.g. with methylphenidate) has been confirmed in controlled trials, but there is concern as to possible long-term adverse effects since treatment is

sometimes continued into adolescence and beyond. Drug treatment should be part of a programme that includes psychological intervention if available, and is started after the diagnosis has been confirmed by an expert. Disorders of noradrenaline and dopamine pathways in the frontal cortex and basal ganglia are thought to underlie ADHD symptomatology, but there is still controversy over the relative importance of each monoamine and the specific brain regions involved in the actions of drugs used to alleviate the symptoms of ADHD.

Slow-release formulations of amphetamine and methylphenidate have been developed to deliver more stable concentrations of drug, lower than that required to produce euphoria. D-amphetamine conjugated to lysine (**lisdexamphetamine**) is an inactive prodrug that, following oral administration, is cleaved enzymatically to release D-amphetamine, resulting in a slower onset of action and potentially a reduced abuse potential.

▼ Other drug treatments for ADHD include the noradrenaline reuptake inhibitor **atomoxetine** (Ch. 48), and α_2-adrenoceptor agonists such as **clonidine** and **guanfacine**. The monoamine uptake inhibitor modafinil is not approved for paediatric use but may be effective in adult ADHD, as is **bupropion**. **Melatonin** (Ch. 40) improves sleep patterns in ADHD sufferers. The pharmacology of drugs used to treat ADHD is reviewed by Heal et al. (2009).

Narcolepsy

This is a rare, disabling sleep disturbance in which the patient suddenly and unpredictably falls asleep at frequent intervals during the day, while suffering nocturnal insomnia. Amphetamine is helpful but not completely effective. Modafinil is also effective in reducing attacks. Narcolepsy is often accompanied by *cataplexy* (abrupt onset of paralysis of variable extent often triggered by emotion, sometimes with 'frozen' posture). Treatment is usually with **fluoxetine**, a selective 5-HT reuptake inhibitor or **venlafaxine**, a 5-HT and norepinephrine reuptake inhibitor (see Ch. 48). **Sodium oxybate**, the sodium salt of γ-hydroxybutyrate (also known as GHB and frequently abused, see Ch. 39), is a CNS depressant that paradoxically is used to prevent cataplexy.

Clinical uses of CNS stimulants

- Central nervous system (CNS) stimulants have few legitimate therapeutic indications. Where appropriate they are usually initiated by experts.
- Attention deficit/hyperactivity disorder (ADHD): **methylphenidate**, **atomoxetine** (see Ch. 48). **Dexamphetamine** is an alternative in children who do not respond.
- Narcolepsy: **modafinil** for the excessive sleepiness; **oxybate** to reduce cataplexy (which can be associated with narcolepsy).
- Apnoea of prematurity: *xanthine alkaloids* (under expert supervision in hospital) are effective; **caffeine** is preferred to **theophylline**.

COCAINE

Cocaine is found in the leaves of the South American shrub coca. These leaves are used for their stimulant properties by natives of South America, particularly those in mountainous areas, who use it to reduce fatigue during work at high altitude.

Considerable mystical significance was attached to the powers of cocaine to boost the flagging human spirit, and Freud tested it extensively on his patients and his family, publishing an influential monograph in 1884 advocating its use as a psychostimulant.[2] Freud's ophthalmologist colleague, Köller, obtained supplies of the drug and discovered its local anaesthetic action (Ch. 44), but the psychostimulant effects of cocaine have not proved to be clinically useful. On the other hand, they led to it becoming a widespread drug of abuse in Western countries. The mechanisms and treatment of cocaine abuse are discussed in Chapter 50.

Pharmacological effects

Cocaine binds to and inhibits the transporters NET, DAT and SERT (see Chs 15, 16 and 40), thereby producing a marked psychomotor stimulant effect, and enhancing the peripheral effects of sympathetic nerve activity.

In humans, cocaine produces euphoria, garrulousness, increased motor activity and a magnification of pleasure. Users feel alert, energetic and physically strong and believe they have enhanced mental capabilities. Its effects resemble those of amphetamines, although it has less tendency to produce stereotyped behaviour, delusions, hallucinations and paranoia. Evidence from transgenic knock-out mice indicates that the euphoric effects of cocaine involve inhibition of both dopamine and 5-HT reuptake. The peripheral sympathomimetic actions lead to tachycardia, vasoconstriction and an increase in blood pressure. Body temperature may increase, owing to the increased motor activity coupled with reduced heat loss. With excessive dosage, tremors and convulsions, followed by respiratory and vasomotor depression, may occur.

Experimental animals rapidly learn to press a lever to self-administer cocaine and will consume toxic amounts of the drug if access is not limited. In transgenic mice lacking the D_2 receptor, the enhanced locomotor effects of cocaine are reduced, but surprisingly self-administration of cocaine is increased, in contrast to what is found with other self-administered drugs such as ethanol and morphine.

Chronic use, dependence and tolerance

Cocaine undoubtedly causes strong psychological dependence (see Ch. 50), but there is some debate about whether or not its continued use induces tolerance and physical dependence. Users may increase their intake of the drug but this may reflect a desire for an increased effect rather than the development of tolerance. In experimental animals, sensitisation (the opposite of tolerance) can be observed but the relevance of this to the situation in humans is unclear. Cocaine does not produce a clear-cut withdrawal syndrome but depression, dysphoria and fatigue may be experienced following the initial stimulant effect. Cocaine induces

psychological dependence where users crave the drug's euphoric and stimulatory effects. The cellular mechanisms underlying craving, and pharmacological approaches to reduce craving, are discussed in Chapter 50. The pattern of dependence, evolving from occasional use through escalating dosage to compulsive binges, is similar to that seen with amphetamines.

Pharmacokinetic aspects

Cocaine is readily absorbed by many routes. For many years illicit supplies have consisted of the hydrochloride salt, which could be taken by nasal inhalation or intravenously. The latter route produces an intense and immediate euphoria, whereas nasal inhalation produces a less dramatic sensation and also tends to cause atrophy and necrosis of the nasal mucosa and septum.

Cocaine use increased dramatically when the free-base form ('crack') became available as a street drug. When an aqueous solution of cocaine hydrochloride is heated with sodium bicarbonate, free-base cocaine, water, CO_2 and NaCl are produced. The free-base cocaine is insoluble in water, precipitates out and can then be rolled into 'rocks' of crack. Free-base cocaine vaporises at around 90°C, much lower than the melting point of cocaine hydrochloride (190°C), which burns rather than vaporises. Thus crack can be smoked, with the uncharged free base being rapidly absorbed across the large surface area of the alveolae, giving rise to a greater CNS effect than that obtained by snorting cocaine. Indeed, the effect is nearly as rapid as that of intravenous administration. The social, economic and even political consequences of this small change in formulation have been far-reaching.

The duration of its stimulant effect, about 30 min, is much shorter than that of amphetamine. It is rapidly metabolised in the liver. Heroin users may inject cocaine and heroin together intravenously (known as *speedballing*) to obtain the rapid effect of cocaine before the prolonged effect of heroin kicks in.

A cocaine metabolite is deposited in hair, and analysis of its content along the hair shaft allows the pattern of cocaine consumption to be monitored, a technique that has revealed a much higher incidence of cocaine use than was voluntarily reported. Cocaine exposure in utero can be estimated from analysis of the hair of neonates.

Cocaine is still occasionally used topically as a local anaesthetic, mainly in ophthalmology and minor nose and throat surgery, where its local vasoconstrictor action is an advantage, but has no other clinical uses.

Adverse effects

Toxic effects occur commonly in cocaine abusers. The main acute dangers are serious cardiovascular events (cardiac dysrhythmias, aortic dissection, and myocardial or cerebral infarction or haemorrhage). Progressive myocardial damage can lead to heart failure, even in the absence of a history of acute cardiac effects.

Cocaine can severely impair brain development in utero. The brain size is significantly reduced in babies exposed to cocaine in pregnancy, and neurological and limb malformations are increased. The incidence of ischaemic and haemorrhagic brain lesions, and of sudden infant death, is also higher in cocaine-exposed babies. Interpretation of the data is difficult because many cocaine abusers also take other illicit drugs that may affect fetal development, but the probability is that cocaine is highly detrimental.

---

[2]In the 1860s a Corsican pharmacist, Mariani, devised cocaine-containing beverages, Vin Mariani and Thé Mariani, which were sold very successfully as tonics. Imitators soon moved in, and Thé Mariani became the forerunner of Coca-Cola. In 1903, cocaine was removed from Coca-Cola because of its growing association with addiction and criminality.

Dependence, the main psychological adverse effect of amphetamines and cocaine, has potentially severe effects on quality of life (Ch. 50).

Cocaine

- **Cocaine** acts by inhibiting catecholamine uptake (especially dopamine) by nerve terminals.
- Behavioural effects of cocaine are very similar to those of amphetamines, although psychotomimetic effects are rarer. Duration of action is shorter.
- **Cocaine** used in pregnancy impairs fetal development and may produce fetal malformations.
- **Cocaine** produces strong psychological dependence.

MDMA

MDMA (3,4-methylenedioxymethamphetamine, 'ecstasy' or 'molly') and related drugs are widely used as 'party drugs' because of the feelings of empathy and euphoria, and the loss of inhibitions, heightened sensations and energy surge, that they produce. They are sometimes referred to as 'empathogens' or 'enactogens'. They also have mild hallucinogenic effects. Common examples are listed in Table 49.1. In conjunction with psychotherapy, MDMA is in phase III clinical trials for the treatment of post-traumatic stress disorder.

Pharmacological effects

Although an amphetamine derivative (see Fig. 49.1), MDMA affects monoamine function in a different manner from the amphetamines. It inhibits monoamine transporters, principally the 5-HT transporter, and also releases 5-HT, the net effect being a large increase in free 5-HT in certain brain regions, followed by depletion. Similar but smaller changes occur in relation to dopamine and noradrenaline release. Simplistically, the effects on 5-HT function determine the psychotomimetic effects, while dopamine and noradrenaline changes account for the initial euphoria and later rebound dysphoria. MDMA does not induce psychological or physical dependence but its use carries serious risks. Unintentional consumption of high doses may occur if pills have a higher than expected MDMA content or when MDMA is taken in powdered form. Also, illicit MDMA tablets or powders may be contaminated with or entirely substituted with **para-methoxyamphetamine** (PMA) a more dangerous psychoactive agent.

Common adverse effects of MDMA ingestion are:

- Acute hyperthermia (Fig. 49.2), resulting in damage to skeletal muscle and consequent renal failure. It is still unclear how hyperthermia is produced in humans. It may be mediated centrally through release of 5-HT, dopamine and noradrenaline acting on various receptors for these monoamines (Docherty & Green, 2010). It could also reflect an action of MDMA on mitochondrial function. It is exacerbated by energetic dancing and high ambient temperature and certain individuals may be particularly susceptible to this danger.
- Excess water intake and water retention. Users may consume large amounts of water as a result of increased physical activity and feeling hot. In

Fig. 49.2 A single injection of MDMA causes a dose-related increase in body temperature in rats. Drug administered at time zero. (Reproduced with permission from Green et al., 2004. Eur. J. Pharmacol. 500, 3–13.)

addition, MDMA causes inappropriate secretion of antidiuretic hormone (see Ch. 34). This can lead to overhydration and hyponatraemia ('water intoxication'). Symptoms include dizziness and disorientation, leading to collapse into coma.
- Heart failure in individuals with an undiagnosed heart condition.

The after effects of MDMA persist for a few days and comprise depression, anxiety, irritability and increased aggression – the 'mid-week blues'. There is also evidence of long-term deleterious effects on memory and cognitive function in heavy MDMA users. In animal studies, MDMA can cause degeneration of 5-HT and dopamine neurons, but whether this occurs in humans is uncertain (see Green et al., 2012).

MDMA (ecstasy)

- **MDMA** is an amphetamine analogue that has powerful psychostimulant as well as mild psychotomimetic effects.
- **MDMA** inhibits monoamine transporters, principally the 5-hydroxytryptamine (5-HT) transporter, and releases 5-HT.
- **MDMA** can cause an acute hyperthermic reaction as well as overhydration and hyponatraemia, sometimes fatal.
- **MDMA** does not cause physical dependence.

CATHINONES

Cathinone and **cathine** are the active ingredients in the khat shrub. Chewing the leaves is popular in parts of Africa, such as Ethiopia and Somalia, and its use is spreading through immigrant populations in Western countries.

Synthetic cathinone derivatives have become popular street drugs as they produce feelings of elevated mood and improved mental function. **Mephedrone** elevates extracellular levels of both dopamine and 5-HT, possibly by inhibiting reuptake and enhancing release.

METHYLXANTHINES

Various beverages, particularly tea, coffee and cocoa, contain methylxanthines, to which they owe their mild central stimulant effects. The main compounds responsible are **caffeine** and **theophylline**. The nuts of the cola plant also contain caffeine, which is present in cola-flavoured soft drinks. However, the most important sources, by far, are coffee and tea, which account for more than 90% of caffeine consumption. Further information on the pharmacology and toxicology of caffeine is presented by Fredholm et al. (1999).

Pharmacological effects

Methylxanthines have the following major pharmacological actions:

- CNS stimulation
- mild diuresis, not clinically significant
- stimulation of cardiac muscle (see Ch. 22)
- relaxation of smooth muscle, especially bronchial muscle (see Ch. 29)

The latter two effects resemble those of β-adrenoceptor stimulation (see Chs 15, 22 and 29). This is thought to be because methylxanthines (especially **theophylline**) inhibit phosphodiesterase, which is responsible for the intracellular metabolism of cAMP (Ch. 3). They thus increase intracellular cAMP and produce effects that mimic those of mediators that stimulate adenylyl cyclase. Methylxanthines also antagonise many of the effects of adenosine, acting on both A_1 and A_2 receptors (see Ch. 17). Transgenic mice lacking functional A_2 receptors are abnormally active and aggressive, and fail to show increased motor activity in response to caffeine, suggesting that antagonism at A_2 receptors accounts for part, at least, of its CNS stimulant action. Caffeine also sensitises ryanodine receptors (see Ch. 4) but this effect occurs at higher concentrations (>10 mmol/L) than those achieved by recreational intake of caffeine. The concentration of caffeine reached in plasma and brain after two or three cups of strong coffee – about 100 µmol/L – is sufficient to produce appreciable adenosine receptor block and a small degree of phosphodiesterase inhibition. Adenosine receptor block probably causes the diuretic effect by reducing proximal tubular reabsorption of sodium.

Caffeine and theophylline have very similar stimulant effects on the CNS. Human subjects experience a reduction of fatigue, with improved concentration and a clearer flow of thought. This is confirmed by objective studies, which have shown that caffeine reduces reaction time and produces an increase in the speed at which simple calculations can be performed (although without much improvement in accuracy). Performance at motor tasks, such as typing and simulated driving, is also improved, particularly in fatigued subjects. Mental tasks, such as syllable learning, association tests and so on, are also facilitated by moderate doses (up to about 200 mg of caffeine, or about two cups of coffee) but impaired by larger doses. Insomnia is common. By comparison with amphetamines, methylxanthines produce less locomotor stimulation and do not induce euphoria, stereotyped behaviour patterns or a psychotic state, but their effects on fatigue and mental function are similar.

Tolerance and habituation develop to a small extent, but much less than with amphetamines; withdrawal effects are modest but can be troublesome.[3] Caffeine is not self-administered by animals, and it cannot be classified as a dependence-producing drug.

Clinical use and unwanted effects

There are few clinical uses for caffeine. It is included with aspirin in some preparations for treating headaches and other aches and pains, and with ergotamine in some antimigraine preparations, the objective being to produce a mildly agreeable sense of alertness. Methylxanthines are effective respiratory stimulants in the treatment of apnoea of prematurity (a developmental disorder caused by immaturity of central respiratory control), for which indication caffeine is preferred to theophylline because of its long half-life and safety. Theophylline (formulated as **aminophylline**) is used mainly as a bronchodilator in treating severe asthmatic attacks (see Ch. 29). In vitro tests show that it has mutagenic activity, and large doses are teratogenic in animals. However, epidemiological studies have shown no evidence of carcinogenic or teratogenic effects of tea or coffee drinking in humans.

Methylxanthines

- **Caffeine** and **theophylline** produce psychomotor stimulant effects.
- Average **caffeine** consumption from beverages is about 200 mg/day.
- Main psychological effects are reduced fatigue and improved mental performance, without euphoria. Even large doses do not cause stereotyped behaviour or psychotomimetic effects.
- Methylxanthines act mainly by antagonism at A_2 purine receptors, and partly by inhibiting phosphodiesterase.
- Peripheral actions are exerted mainly on heart, smooth muscle and kidney.
- **Theophylline** is used clinically as a bronchodilator; **caffeine** is used as a respiratory stimulant for apnoea of prematurity and as an additive in many beverages and over-the-counter analgesics.

NICOTINE

Nicotine[4] is the psychoactive ingredient in tobacco.

Tobacco growing, chewing and smoking was indigenous throughout the American subcontinent and Australia at the time that European explorers first visited these places. Smoking spread through Europe during the 16th century,

---

[3]Caffeine withdrawal symptoms are a well-recognised cause of adverse events (headache, irritability) in residential phase I clinical trial units where caffeine-containing beverages are routinely prohibited.
[4]From the plant *Nicotiana*, named after Jean Nicot, French ambassador to Portugal, who presented seeds to the French king in 1560, having been persuaded by natives of South America of the medical value of smoking tobacco leaves. Smoking was believed to protect against illness, particularly the plague.

coming to England mainly as a result of its enthusiastic espousal by Walter Raleigh at the court of Elizabeth I. James I strongly disapproved of both Raleigh and tobacco, and in the early 17th century initiated the first antismoking campaign, with the support of the Royal College of Physicians. Parliament responded by imposing a substantial duty on tobacco, thereby giving the state an economic interest in the continuation of smoking at the same time that its official expert advisers were issuing emphatic warnings about its dangers.

Until the latter half of the 19th century, tobacco was smoked in pipes, and primarily by men. Cigarette manufacture began at the end of the 19th century. Filter cigarettes (which give a lower delivery of carcinogenic tars and nicotine than standard cigarettes) and 'low-tar' cigarettes (which are also low in nicotine) became available in the 1950s and were thought to be less harmful.[5] More recently, the use of electronic cigarettes (e-cigarettes) to deliver nicotine, without the carcinogenic tars of cigarette smoke, has become popular. Laws banning smoking in public places and the increased use of e-cigarettes has led to a reduction in cigarette consumption in the United Kingdom.

PHARMACOLOGICAL EFFECTS OF NICOTINE
EFFECTS ON THE CNS

At the neuronal level, nicotine acts on nicotinic acetylcholine receptors (nAChRs) (see Ch. 40), which are widely expressed in the brain, particularly in the cortex and hippocampus, and are believed to play a role in cognitive function, as well as in the ventral tegmental area (VTA), from which dopaminergic neurons project to the nucleus accumbens (the reward pathway, Fig. 40.3). nAChRs are ligand-gated cation channels located both pre- and postsynaptically, causing, respectively, enhanced transmitter release and neuronal excitation (see Wonnacott et al., 2005). Nicotine increases the firing rate and phasic activity of VTA dopaminergic neurons (see Fig. 49.3). Of the various subtypes of nAChR (see Table 40.2), the α4β2, α6β2 and α7 subtypes have received most attention, but other subtypes may also be involved in the rewarding effects of nicotine. As well as activating the receptors, nicotine also causes desensitisation, so the effects of a dose of nicotine are diminished in animals after sustained exposure to the drug. Chronic nicotine administration leads to a substantial increase in the number of nAChRs (an effect opposite to that produced by sustained administration of most receptor agonists), which may represent an adaptive response to prolonged receptor desensitisation. It is likely that the overall effect of nicotine reflects a balance between activation of nAChRs, causing neuronal excitation, and desensitisation, causing synaptic block.

The higher level functioning of the brain, as reflected in the subjective sense of alertness or by the electroencephalography (EEG) pattern, can be affected in either direction by nicotine, according to dose and circumstances. Nicotine wakes people up when they are drowsy and calms them down when they are tense, and EEG recordings broadly bear this out. It also seems that small doses of nicotine tend to cause arousal, whereas large doses do the reverse. Tests of motor and sensory performance (e.g. reaction time measurements or vigilance tests) in humans generally show improvement with nicotine, and nicotine enhances learning

Fig. 49.3 Nicotine alters action potential firing characteristics of VTA dopaminergic neurons in freely moving rats. (A) Neuronal firing rate increases after nicotine injection i.p. (B) Action potential firing is phasic after nicotine injection. (Adapted from De Biasi et al., 2011.)

in rats. Nicotine and other nicotinic agonists such as **epibatidine** (Ch. 43) have significant analgesic activity in animal models, but, taken in the form of tobacco smoke or administered by other delivery systems such as patch or nasal spray, has only a weak analgesic effect in man.

Peripheral effects

The peripheral effects of small doses of nicotine result from stimulation of autonomic ganglia (see Ch. 14) and of peripheral sensory receptors, mainly in the heart and lungs. Stimulation of these receptors produces tachycardia, increased cardiac output and arterial pressure, sweating, and a reduction of gastrointestinal motility. When people take nicotine for the first time, they usually experience nausea and sometimes vomit, probably because of stimulation of sensory receptors in the stomach. All these effects decline with repeated dosage, although the central effects remain. Secretion of adrenaline and noradrenaline from the adrenal medulla contributes to the cardiovascular effects,

---

[5]Smokers, however, adapt by smoking more low-tar cigarettes and inhaling more deeply to maintain their nicotine consumption.

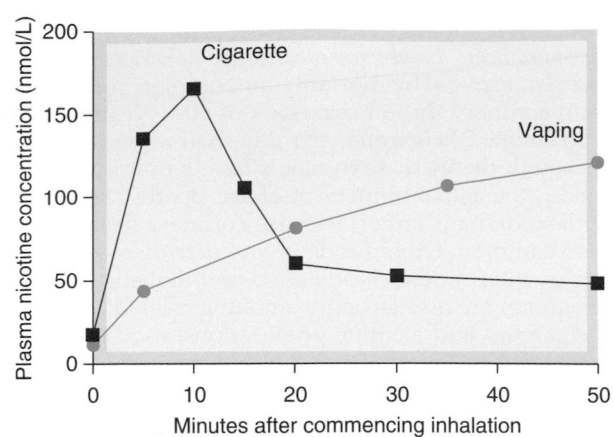

Fig. 49.4 **Nicotine concentration in plasma during smoking or vaping.** The subjects were habitual users who inhaled from a traditional cigarette or an e-cigarette according to their usual habit. (Data from Bowman, W.C., Rand, M., 1980. Chapter 4. In: Textbook of Pharmacology. Blackwell, Oxford and Farsalinos et al., 2015. Sci. Rep. 5, 11269.)

and release of antidiuretic hormone from the posterior pituitary causes a decrease in urine flow.[6] The plasma concentration of free fatty acids is increased, probably owing to sympathetic stimulation and adrenaline secretion. Smokers weigh, on average, about 4 kg less than non-smokers, mainly because of reduced food intake; giving up smoking usually causes weight gain associated with increased food intake.

PHARMACOKINETIC ASPECTS

Nicotine is rapidly absorbed from the lungs but less readily from the mouth and nasopharynx.[7] Therefore inhalation is required to give appreciable absorption of nicotine, each puff delivering a distinct bolus of drug to the CNS. The amount of nicotine absorbed varies greatly with the habits of the user and the way in which nicotine is self-administered.

An average cigarette, smoked over 10 min, causes the plasma nicotine concentration to rise to 15–30 ng/mL (100–200 nmol/L), falling to about half within 10 min and then more slowly over the next 1–2 h (Fig. 49.4). The rapid decline results mainly from redistribution between the blood and other tissues; the slower decline is due to hepatic metabolism, mainly by oxidation to an inactive ketone metabolite, *cotinine*. This has a long plasma half-life, and measurement of urinary cotinine provides a useful indication of nicotine consumption.

E-cigarettes work by heating a liquid (usually propylene glycol and glycerin) to generate a vapour containing nicotine which is then inhaled (a process commonly referred to as vaping). Vaping avoids inhalation of the toxic chemicals present in tobacco smoke. Early e-cigarette devices were found to deliver only minimal amounts of nicotine to the user. However, the technology has advanced rapidly and

new-generation devices have been developed that deliver more nicotine more rapidly, but as yet, not quite as fast as a traditional cigarette (see Fig. 49.4).

Other routes of nicotine administration that provide a more sustained delivery are used by smokers trying to quit. A transdermal nicotine patch applied for 24 h causes the plasma concentration of nicotine to rise to 75–150 nmol/L over 6 h and to remain fairly constant for about 20 h. Administration by nasal spray or chewing gum results in a time course intermediate between that of smoking and the nicotine patch.

TOLERANCE AND DEPENDENCE

As with other dependence-producing drugs, three separate processes – psychological dependence, physical dependence and tolerance – contribute to the overall state of dependence, in which taking the drug becomes compulsive. For reviews on nicotine and addiction see De Biasi et al. (2011) and Leslie et al. (2013).

The effects of nicotine associated with peripheral ganglionic stimulation show rapid tolerance, perhaps as a result of desensitisation of nAChRs. With large doses of nicotine, this desensitisation produces a block of ganglionic transmission (see Ch. 14). Tolerance to the central effects of nicotine (e.g. in the arousal response) is much less than in the periphery. The increase in the number of nAChRs in the brain produced by chronic nicotine administration in animals also occurs in heavy smokers. Because the cellular effects of nicotine are diminished, it is possible that the additional binding sites represent desensitised rather than functional receptors.

The addictiveness of nicotine is due to the effects of the drug combined with the ritual of taking it (see Le Foll & Goldberg, 2005). Rats choose to drink dilute nicotine solution in preference to water if given a choice, and in a situation in which lever pressing causes an injection of nicotine to be delivered – admittedly at high doses – they quickly learn to self-administer it. Similarly, monkeys who have been trained to smoke, by providing a reward in response to smoking behaviour, will continue to do so spontaneously (i.e. unrewarded) if the smoking medium contains nicotine, but not if nicotine-free tobacco is offered instead. Humans, however, are unlikely to become addicted to nicotine delivered from patches, suggesting that other factors are also involved, such as the controlled pulsatile delivery associated with smoking and vaping.

Like other addictive drugs, nicotine causes excitation of the mesolimbic reward pathway and increased dopamine release in the nucleus accumbens. Transgenic mice lacking the β2 subunit of the nAChR lose the rewarding effect of nicotine and its dopamine-releasing effect, confirming the importance of the β2-containing nAChR subtypes and mesolimbic dopamine release in the response to nicotine. In contrast to normal mice, the mutant mice could not be induced to self-administer nicotine, even though they did so with cocaine.

In contrast to euphoria, induction of physical dependence involves nicotinic receptors containing α5 and β4 subunits in the medial habenula–interpeduncular nucleus pathway. A physical withdrawal syndrome occurs in humans on cessation of smoking. Its main features are increased irritability, impaired performance of psychomotor tasks, aggressiveness and sleep disturbance. The withdrawal syndrome is much less severe than that produced by opioids, and can be alleviated by replacement nicotine. It lasts for 2–3

---

[6]This may explain why, in years gone by, men smoked cigars while chatting over drinks after dinner.

[7]Nicotine absorbed from cigar smoke is via the buccal mucosa but cigars deliver a much higher dose per puff than cigarettes, so a substantial amount gets in despite a low fraction absorbed.

weeks, although the craving for cigarettes persists for much longer than this; relapses during attempts to quit occur most commonly at a time when the physical withdrawal syndrome has long since subsided.

Pharmacology of nicotine

- At the cellular level, **nicotine** acts on nicotinic acetylcholine receptors (nAChRs) to enhance neurotransmitter release and increase neuronal excitation. Its central effects are blocked by receptor antagonists such as **mecamylamine**.
- At the behavioural level, nicotine produces a mixture of inhibitory and excitatory effects.
- **Nicotine** shows reinforcing properties, associated with increased activity in the mesolimbic dopaminergic pathway, and self-administration can be elicited in animal studies.
- Electroencephalography changes show an arousal response, and subjects report increased alertness accompanied by a reduction of anxiety and tension.
- Learning, particularly under stress, is facilitated by **nicotine**.
- Peripheral effects of **nicotine** are due mainly to ganglionic stimulation: tachycardia, increased blood pressure and reduced gastrointestinal motility. Tolerance develops rapidly to these effects.
- **Nicotine** is metabolised to cotinine, mainly in the liver, within 1–2 h.
- **Nicotine** gives rise to tolerance, physical dependence and psychological dependence (craving). Attempts at long-term cessation succeed in only about 20% of cases.
- **Nicotine** replacement therapy (e-cigarettes, chewing gum or skin patch preparations) improves the chances of giving up smoking when combined with active counselling.

HARMFUL EFFECTS OF TOBACCO SMOKING

The life expectancy of smokers is shorter than that of non-smokers. Smoking causes almost 90% of deaths from lung cancer, about 80% of deaths from bronchitis and emphysema, and 17% of deaths from heart disease. The increased use of e-cigarettes should reduce the number of such deaths. About one-third of all cancer deaths can be attributed to smoking. Smoking is, by a large margin, the biggest preventable cause of death, responsible for about 1 in 10 adult deaths worldwide. Despite the introduction of e-cigarettes, deaths from smoking worldwide are continuing to rise. In 2015, it was estimated that smoking was responsible for some 6.4 million deaths (and approximately 800,000 additional deaths of non-smokers from involuntary secondary inhalation).

The main health risks are as follows:

- *Cancer, particularly of the lung and upper respiratory tract but also of the oesophagus, pancreas and bladder.* Smoking 20 cigarettes per day is estimated to increase the risk of lung cancer about 10-fold. Tar, rather than nicotine, is responsible for the cancer risk. Genetic variants of nicotinic-receptor subunits have been associated with lung cancer although the mechanisms behind this association are unclear (see Hung et al., 2008).
- *Coronary heart disease and other forms of peripheral vascular disease.* The mortality among men aged 55–64 from coronary thrombosis is about 60% greater in men who smoke 20 cigarettes per day than in non-smokers. Although the increase in risk is less than it is for lung cancer, the actual number of excess deaths associated with smoking is larger, because coronary heart disease is so common. Other kinds of vascular disease (e.g. stroke, intermittent claudication and diabetic gangrene) are also strongly smoking related. E-cigarettes and nicotine preparations, used to help smokers give up cigarettes, are not thought to carry a serious risk. Carbon monoxide (see later) could be a factor. However, there is no clear increase in ischaemic heart disease in pipe and cigar smokers, even though similar blood nicotine and carboxyhaemoglobin concentrations are reached, suggesting that other factors may be responsible for the risk associated with cigarettes.
- *Chronic obstructive pulmonary disease* (COPD; see Ch. 29) is a major global health problem. Cigarette smoking is the main cause. Stopping smoking slows the progression of the disease. Bronchitis, inflammation of the mucous membranes of the bronchi, is much more common in smokers than in non-smokers. These effects are probably due to tar and other irritants rather than nicotine.
- *Harmful effects in pregnancy.* Smoking, particularly during the latter half of pregnancy, significantly reduces birth weight (by about 8% in women who smoke 25 or more cigarettes per day during pregnancy) and increases perinatal mortality (by an estimated 28% in babies born to mothers who smoke in the last half of pregnancy). There is evidence that children born to smoking mothers remain behind, in both physical and mental development, for at least 7 years. By 11 years of age, the difference is no longer significant. These effects of smoking, although measurable, are much smaller than the effects of other factors, such as social class and birth order. Various other complications of pregnancy are also more common in women who smoke, including spontaneous abortion (increased 30%–70% by smoking), premature delivery (increased about 40%) and placenta praevia (where the placenta obstructs normal vaginal delivery, increased 25%–90%). Nicotine is excreted in breast milk in sufficient amounts to cause tachycardia in the infant.

The agents probably responsible for the harmful effects are as follows:

- Tar and irritants, such as nitrogen dioxide and formaldehyde. Cigarette smoke tar contains many known carcinogenic hydrocarbons, as well as tumour promoters, which together account for the high cancer risk. It is likely that the various irritant substances are also responsible for the increase in bronchitis and emphysema.
- Nicotine probably accounts for retarded fetal development because of its vasoconstrictor properties.
- Carbon monoxide. Cigarette smoke contains about 3% carbon monoxide. Carbon monoxide has a high

affinity for haemoglobin, and the average carboxyhaemoglobin content in the blood of cigarette smokers is about 2.5% (compared with 0.4% for non-smoking urban dwellers). In very heavy smokers, up to 15% of haemoglobin may be carboxylated, a level that affects fetal development in rats. Fetal haemoglobin has a higher affinity for carbon monoxide than adult haemoglobin, and the proportion of carboxyhaemoglobin is higher in fetal than in maternal blood.

- Increased oxidative stress may contribute to atherogenesis (Ch. 24) and COPD (Ch. 29).

OTHER EFFECTS OF TOBACCO SMOKING

Parkinson's disease is approximately twice as common in non-smokers as in smokers. It is possible that this reflects a protective effect of nicotine. Ulcerative colitis appears to be a disease of non-smokers. Former smokers are at high risk for developing ulcerative colitis, while current smokers have the least risk. This tendency indicates that smoking cigarettes may prevent the onset of ulcerative colitis. In contrast, smoking tends to worsen the effects of Crohn's disease (another type of inflammatory bowel disease). Earlier reports that Alzheimer's disease is less common in smokers have not been confirmed; indeed there is evidence that smoking may increase the occurrence of Alzheimer's disease in some genetic groups.

Effects of tobacco smoking

- Smoking accounts for more than 10% of deaths worldwide, mainly due to:
  - cancer, especially lung cancer, of which about 90% of cases are smoking related; carcinogenic tars are responsible;
  - chronic bronchitis; tars are mainly responsible.
- Smoking in pregnancy reduces birth weight and retards childhood development. It also increases abortion rate and perinatal mortality. **Nicotine** and possibly carbon monoxide are responsible.
- Use of e-cigarettes (vaping) avoids the inhalation of tar and carbon monoxide that occurs with smoking.
- The incidence of Parkinson's disease is lower in smokers than in non-smokers.

COGNITION-ENHANCING DRUGS

'Cognition' embraces many aspects of mental function, including memory, reasoning and problem-solving skills, situational judgements, decision-making and executive function. A variety of different test batteries have been designed to measure these functions in humans (e.g. Cambridge Neuropsychological Test Automated Battery, CANTAB) and test the effects of drugs. Many clinical disorders, such as Alzheimer's disease (Ch. 41), schizophrenia (Ch. 47), depression (Ch. 48) and drug addiction (Ch. 50) impair these functions, and the hope is to develop cognition-enhancing drugs to restore them. Progress has been limited, though much hyped, as much with the questionable aim of 'improving' mental function in healthy humans, as in alleviating deficits in the sick.

Drugs currently available have been shown to:

- alter memory processing (i.e. enhance memory);
- reduce fatigue (stimulants), thus permitting the user to function for longer (i.e. perform complex tasks, study for examinations, overcome jet lag);
- increase motivation, energy, confidence and concentration.

They are also referred to as 'smart drugs' or 'nootropics'

Drugs reported to enhance cognitive performance are caffeine, amphetamines, methylphenidate, modafinil, arecoline, **donepezil**, **vortioxetine** and **piracetam** but the clinical efficacy of these drugs is limited, and development of more effective cognition enhancers could have significant benefits for many patient groups.

Cognition-enhancing drugs are also used by healthy individuals aiming to enhance their performance e.g. in revising for and taking examinations (d'Angelo et al., 2017) or in demanding professional roles. The use of drugs by healthy individuals to enhance academic performance does raise ethical issues in relation to fairness, academic pressure and fears of coercion by 'pushy' parents. There are also safety issues. Although many of the drugs taken are available as medicines (i.e. have gone through standard drug safety testing) there is still a lack of information on their acute and long-term effects in children and adolescents whose brains are still in development. In healthy individuals, cognitive performance can be enhanced by improved sleep and mood as well as reduced anxiety. It would seem more appropriate to achieve this by lifestyle changes and behavioural therapy rather than resorting to the use of drugs.[8]

EFFECTIVENESS

While the effectiveness of cognition enhancers on healthy individuals is often trumpeted by individuals who use them and in the media, their actual effectiveness as assessed in scientific studies is somewhat inconclusive and ambiguous. Also, drugs may affect different forms of memory differently (d'Angelo et al., 2017). It is important to distinguish between drugs that only improve a subject's abilities when they are fatigued and those that might improve cognitive ability in non-fatigued individuals.

Many studies have shown that amphetamines improve mental performance in fatigued subjects. Mental performance is improved for simple tedious tasks much more than for difficult tasks. Amphetamines are thought to increase ability to focus and maintain self-control. In addition to reducing fatigue, methylphenidate has a positive effect on long-term memory consolidation. Amphetamines and modafinil have been used to improve the performance of soldiers, military pilots and others who need to remain alert under extremely fatiguing conditions. Modafinil appears to enhance cognition in non-fatigued individuals (Battleday & Brem, 2015) while also improving wakefulness, memory and executive functions in sleep-deprived individuals. Evidence for efficacy in patients with chronic cognitive impairment is controversial.

[8]A new phenomenon is 'microdosing' with very small quantities of psychedelic drugs such as LSD, psilocybin or mescaline (see p. 634) every few days with the aim of improving concentration, creativity and problem solving. At such low doses users do not experience psychedelic effects. Properly controlled scientific studies are required to determine whether this form of drug taking really is effective.

NON-STIMULANT DRUGS

The novel antidepressant, vortioxetine (see Ch. 48), improves cognitive dysfunction in patients suffering from major depression.

Piracetam, which is a positive allosteric modulator at AMPA receptors (see Ch. 39), enhances memory in non-fatigued adults, and there is limited clinical evidence of reading improvement in dyslexic children. **Phenylpiracetam** is said to be more potent and may also have nicotinic antagonist properties. As with many CNS disorders, the possible importance of glutamate and its receptors is widely speculated on, but new, effective drugs acting on the glutamatergic system are still awaited (see, for example, Collingridge et al., 2013; Harms et al., 2013).

PSYCHEDELIC DRUGS

Psychedelic drugs (also sometimes referred to as *halluci-nogenic* or *psychotomimetic* drugs) affect thought, perception and mood, without causing marked psychomotor stimula-tion or depression (see Nichols, 2004). Thoughts and percep-tions tend to become distorted and dream-like, rather than being merely sharpened or dulled, and the change in mood is likewise more complex than a simple shift in the direction of euphoria or depression. Importantly, psychedelic drugs do not cause dependence. Common psychedelic drugs are listed in Table 49.2.

LSD, PSILOCYBIN AND MESCALINE

Lysergic acid diethylamide (LSD) is an exceptionally potent psychotomimetic drug capable of producing strong effects in humans in doses less than 1 µg/kg. It is a chemical derivative of lysergic acid, which occurs in the cereal fungus ergot (see Ch. 16).

▼ LSD was first synthesised by Hoffman in 1943. Hoffman deliberately swallowed about 250 µg of LSD (the threshold dose is now known to be around 20 µg) and wrote 30 years later of the experience: 'the faces of those around me appeared as grotesque coloured masks … marked motoric unrest, alternating with paralysis … heavy feeling in the head, limbs and entire body, as if they were filled with lead … clear recognition of my condition, in which state I sometimes observed, in the manner of an independent observer, that I shouted half insanely.' These effects lasted for a few hours, after which Hoffman fell asleep, 'and awoke next morning feeling perfectly well.' Apart from these dramatic psychological effects, LSD has few physiological effects in humans at doses that cause hallucinations.

Mescaline, which is derived from the Mexican peyote cactus and has been known as a hallucinogenic agent for many centuries, was made famous by Aldous Huxley in *The Doors of Perception*.

Psilocybin is obtained from fungi ('magic mushrooms'). It is rapidly dephosphorylated to psilocin, the active moiety. Its effects are similar to those experienced with LSD. The potential of psilocybin as a treatment for depression and some forms of anxiety is debated in Carhart-Harris and Gregory (2017).

Pharmacological effects

The main effects of these drugs are on mental function, most notably an alteration of perception in such a way that sights and sounds appear distorted and fantastic. Hallucina-tions – visual, auditory, tactile or olfactory – also occur, and sensory modalities may become confused, so that sounds are perceived as visions. Thought processes tend to become illogical and disconnected, but subjects retain insight into the fact that their disturbance is drug-induced, and generally find the experience exhilarating. Occasionally, especially if the user is already anxious, LSD produces a syndrome that is extremely disturbing (the 'bad trip'), in which the hallucinatory experience takes on a menacing quality and may be accompanied by paranoid delusions. 'Flashbacks' of the hallucinatory experience have been reported weeks or months later.

LSD acts on various 5-HT-receptor subtypes (see Chs 16 and 40); its psychotomimetic effects are thought to be mediated mainly by its 5-HT$_{2A}$-receptor agonist actions (see Nichols, 2004). It inhibits the firing of 5-HT-containing neurons in the raphe nuclei (see Ch. 40), apparently by acting as an agonist on the inhibitory somatodendritic 5-HT$_{1A}$ receptors on these cells. The significance of this response to its psychotomimetic effects is unclear. Psilocybin is dephosphorylated to psilocin, which is a weak agonist at several 5-HT receptors including the 5-HT$_{2A}$ receptor. The mechanism of action of mescaline is less well defined. There are contradictory reports about its activity at 5-HT$_{2A}$ recep-tors. It has also been reported to act as an inhibitor of monoamine transport.

Dependence and adverse effects

LSD, psilocybin and mescaline are seldom self-administered by experimental animals. Indeed, in contrast to most of the drugs that are widely abused by humans, they have aversive rather than reinforcing properties in behavioural tests. Tolerance to their effects develops quite quickly, but there is no physical withdrawal syndrome in animals or humans.

Table 49.2 Major psychedelic drugs

Drugs	Mode(s) of action	Notes
LSD	Interacts with 5-HT and DA receptors. Psychedelic effects are thought to be mainly through 5-HT$_{2A}$ receptor activation	No current clinical use
Mescaline	Agonist at 5-HT$_{2A}$ and other 5-HT receptors. Chemically related to amphetamine	No current clinical use. Found in Peyote cactus plant
Psilocybin	Rapidly metabolised to psilocin, a partial agonist at 5-HT$_{2A}$ receptors. Chemically related to 5-HT	No current clinical use. May have potential for the treatment of depression and some forms of anxiety
Salvinorin A	κ Opioid receptor agonist (see Ch. 43)	No clinical use. Found in *Salvia divinorum* (plant)

5-HT, 5-hydroxytryptamine; *DA*, dopamine; *LSD*, lysergic acid diethylamide.

The main effects of these psychedelic drugs are subjective, so it is not surprising that animal tests that reliably predict psychedelic activity in humans have not been devised.[9].

OTHER PSYCHEDELIC DRUGS

Salvinorin A is a hallucinogenic agent contained in the American sage plant *Salvia divinorum*, a member of the mint family. It was originally used by the Mazatecs in Mexico; in recent years its use has spread and it has become known as *herbal ecstasy*. It is a κ opioid receptor agonist (see Ch. 43).[10] It also produces dissociative effects (see later) and at high doses, delirium.

Other hallucinogens include **α–MT** (methyltryptamine) and **DMT** (dimethyltryptamine), which are naturally occurring, and **DPT** (dipropyltryptamine) and **DOM** (2,5-dimethoxy-4-methylamphetamine).

Muscarinic receptor antagonists (see Chs 14 and 40), **hyoscine, hyoscyamine** and **atropine** are contained in various plants, including henbane and mandrake. Consumption can cause hallucinations, drowsiness and disorientation.

Ibogaine is contained in the root bark of iboga shrubs in Africa, South America and Australia. At high doses, it is hallucinogenic. Users have reported experiencing a reduced desire to take other drugs such as cocaine and heroin, leading to ibogaine being investigated as a potential treatment for drug craving (see Ch. 50).

Psychedelic drugs

- The main types are lysergic acid diethylamide (LSD), psilocybin and mescaline.
- They act as 5-hydroxytryptamine (5-HT)$_{2A}$ receptor agonists.
- They cause sensory distortion and hallucinatory experiences.
- **LSD** is exceptionally potent, producing a long-lasting sense of dissociation and disordered thought. Hallucinatory episodes can recur after a long interval.
- In animal behavioural tests, they exhibit aversive rather than rewarding properties.
- **Salvinorin A** is a κ opioid receptor agonist that causes hallucinatory and dissociative effects.

KETAMINE AND RELATED DRUGS

Ketamine ('Special K'), a dissociative anaesthetic (Ch. 42), is also used for its psychoactive properties (see Morgan & Curran, 2012). Its fore-runner **phencyclidine** (PCP, 'angel dust'), was a popular hallucinogen in the 1970s but its use has declined. These drugs produce a feeling of euphoria. At higher doses they cause hallucinations and feelings of detachment, disorientation and numbness. PCP was reported

to cause psychotic episodes and is used in experimental animals to produce a model of schizophrenia (see Ch. 47 and Morris et al., 2005).

Pharmacological effects

Their main pharmacological effect is non-competitive block of the NMDA-receptor channel (see Ch. 39). **Methoxetamine**, a chemical derivative of ketamine, is an NMDA antagonist as well as an inhibitor of 5-HT reuptake, which may contribute to its CNS effects.

Adverse effects

Tolerance develops with repeated use of ketamine, resulting in higher doses being taken to achieve the same effect. Repeated use is associated with serious and persistent toxic effects, including abdominal pain, ulcerative cystitis (with associated severe bladder pain), liver damage and cognitive impairment (Morgan & Curran, 2012). Combination of ketamine with depressant drugs such as **alcohol**, **barbiturates** and **heroin** can result in dangerous overdose.

Nitrous oxide is a weak general anaesthetic that acts as an antagonist at NMDA receptors (see Ch. 42). At low doses it produces feelings of euphoria – it is often referred to as 'laughing gas' – relaxation and dissociation.

DEPRESSANTS

Many CNS depressant drugs (Table 49.3) that are used for their psychoactive effects also have important therapeutic uses that are described in detail elsewhere in this book. Here we will concentrate on ethanol, which has little or

Table 49.3 Depressant drugs

Drugs	Described in detail in Chapter	Notes
Benzodiazepines (diazepam, temazepam, diclazepam)	45	Etizolam and pyrazolam are derived from benzodiazepines and act similarly
Zopiclone and other Z drugs	45	Short acting but similar effects to benzodiazepines
Gabapentin and pregabalin	46	Often taken in high doses to induce a feeling of drunkenness and stupor May enhance likelihood of overdose in opioid users
γ-Hydroxybutyric acid (GHB)	39	γ-Butyrolactone (GBL) and 1,4-butanediol (BD) are broken down to GHB in the body
Ethanol	This chapter	
Propofol	42	Sub-anaesthetic doses induce a general feeling of well-being, euphoria, and sexual disinhibition

[9]One of the more bizarre attempts involves spiders, whose normal elegantly symmetrical webs become jumbled and erratic if the animals are treated with LSD. Search the web (worldwide rather than arachnid) for 'spiders LSD' to see images.
[10]In phase I clinical trials of synthetic κ-opioid-receptor agonists as potential analgesic agents, the drugs were reported to induce a feeling of dysphoria. Perhaps the 'normal' volunteers in those trials were disturbed by the hallucinations they probably experienced. Interesting then that a naturally occurring κ agonist has now become a drug of abuse.

no therapeutic value but is widely used in many countries for its psychoactive properties.

ETHANOL

It may at first seem strange to categorise ethanol as a depressant drug[11] given that its consumption in alcoholic beverages can make people excited, garrulous and violent. However, as with general anaesthetics (see Ch. 42), at low concentrations ethanol depresses inhibitions resulting in apparent behavioural stimulation whereas at higher concentrations all brain functions are depressed.

Judged on a molar basis, the consumption of ethanol far exceeds that of any other drug. The ethanol content of various drinks ranges from about 2.5% (weak beer) to about 55% (strong spirits), and the size of the normal measure is such that a single drink usually contains about 8–12 g (0.17–0.26 mol) of ethanol. Its low pharmacological potency is reflected in the range of plasma concentrations needed to produce pharmacological effects: minimal effects occur at about 10 mmol/L (46 mg/100 mL), and 10 times this concentration may be lethal. The average per capita consumption of ethanol in the United Kingdom doubled between 1970 and 2007, but has fallen slightly since then. There has been an increase in non-drinkers, mainly amongst young people. Amongst those who do drink, the main changes have been a growing consumption of wine in preference to beer among adults, greater consumption in the home and an increasing tendency for binge drinking, especially among young people.

For practical purposes, ethanol intake is often expressed in terms of units. One unit is equal to 8 g (10 mL) of ethanol, and is the amount contained in half a pint of normal strength beer, one measure of spirits or one small glass of wine. The current UK government's guidelines state that for both men and women it is safest not to drink regularly more than 14 units per week, and that if as much as 14 units per week are drunk, it is best to spread this evenly over 3 days or more. It is estimated that in the United Kingdom, about 31% of men and 16% of women exceed these levels. Governments in most developed countries are attempting to curb alcohol consumption.

An excellent detailed review of all aspects of alcohol and alcoholism is provided by Spanagel (2009).

PHARMACOLOGICAL EFFECTS OF ETHANOL

Effects on CNS neurons

The main effects of ethanol are on the CNS, where its depressant actions resemble those of volatile anaesthetics (Ch. 42). At a neuronal level, the effect of ethanol is depressant, although it increases neuronal activity – presumably by disinhibition – in some parts of the CNS, notably in the mesolimbic dopaminergic pathway that is involved in reward. The main acute cellular effects of ethanol that occur at concentrations (5–100 mmol/L) relevant to alcohol consumption by humans are:

- enhancement of both GABA- and glycine-mediated inhibition
- inhibition of Ca^{2+} entry through voltage-gated calcium channels
- activation of certain types of K^+ channel

- inhibition of ionotropic glutamate receptor function
- inhibition of adenosine transport

For review, see Harris et al. (2008).

Ethanol enhances the action of GABA on $GABA_A$ receptors in a similar way to benzodiazepines (see Ch. 45). Its effect is, however, smaller and less consistent than that of benzodiazepines, and no clear effect on inhibitory synaptic transmission in the CNS has been demonstrated for ethanol. This may be because the effect of ethanol is seen only on some subtypes of $GABA_A$ receptor (see Ch. 39) e.g. the extrasynaptic $\alpha6\beta3\delta$ $GABA_A$ receptor subtype has been reported to be sensitive to ethanol. Ethanol may also act presynaptically to enhance GABA release.

Ethanol enhances glycine receptor function, due both to a direct interaction with the $\alpha1$ subunit of the glycine receptor and to indirect effects mediated through protein kinase C (PKC) activation. Ethanol can also enhance glycine release from nerve terminals.

Ethanol reduces transmitter release in response to nerve terminal depolarisation by inhibiting the opening of voltage-gated calcium channels in neurons. It also reduces neuronal excitability by activating G protein-activated inwardly rectifying K^+ (GIRK) channels as well as potentiating calcium-activated potassium (BK) channel activity.

The excitatory effects of glutamate are inhibited by ethanol at concentrations that produce CNS depressant effects in vivo. NMDA receptor activation is inhibited at lower ethanol concentrations than are required to affect AMPA receptors (see Ch. 39). Other effects produced by ethanol include an enhancement of the excitatory effects produced by activation of nAChRs and $5-HT_3$ receptors. The relative importance of these various effects in the overall effects of ethanol on CNS function is not clear.

The depressant effects of ethanol on neuronal function resemble those of adenosine acting on A_1 receptors (see Ch. 17). Ethanol in cell culture systems increases extracellular adenosine by inhibiting adenosine uptake, and there is some evidence that inhibition of the adenosine transporter may account for some of its CNS effects.

Endogenous opioids also play a role in the CNS effects of ethanol, because both human and animal studies show that the opioid receptor antagonist **naltrexone** reduces the reward associated with ethanol.

Behavioural effects

The effects of acute ethanol intoxication in humans are well known and include slurred speech, motor incoordination, increased self-confidence and euphoria. The effect on mood varies among individuals, most becoming louder and more outgoing, but some becoming morose and withdrawn. At higher levels of intoxication, the mood tends to become highly labile, with euphoria and melancholy, aggression and submission, often occurring successively. The association between alcohol consumption and violence is well documented.

Intellectual and motor performance and sensory discrimination are impaired by ethanol, but subjects are generally unable to judge this for themselves.[12] Much effort has gone

---

[11]In some countries ethanol is classed as a food, not a drug! This reflects the lobbying power of the alcohol industry. Ethanol meets the criteria for 'What is a drug?' given in Chapter 1.

[12]Bus drivers were asked to drive through a gap that they selected as the minimum for their bus to pass through; ethanol caused them not only to hit the barriers more often at any given gap setting, but also to set the gap to a narrower dimension, often narrower than the bus.

into measuring the effect of ethanol on driving performance in real life, as opposed to artificial tests under experimental conditions. In a US study of city drivers, it was found that the probability of being involved in an accident was unaffected at blood ethanol concentrations up to 50 mg/100 mL (10.9 mmol/L); by 80 mg/100 mL (17.4 mmol/L) the probability was increased about four-fold, and by 150 mg/100 mL (32.6 mmol/L) about 25-fold. In Scotland, driving with a blood ethanol concentration greater than 50 mg/100 mL is illegal whereas in the rest of the United Kingdom the legal limit is 80 mg/100 mL.

The relationship between plasma ethanol concentration and effect is highly variable. A given concentration produces a larger effect when the concentration is rising than when it is steady or falling. A substantial degree of cellular tolerance develops in habitual drinkers, with the result that a higher plasma ethanol concentration is needed to produce a given effect. In one study, 'gross intoxication' (assessed by a battery of tests that measured speech, gait and so on) occurred in 30% of subjects between 50 and 100 mg/100 mL and in 90% of subjects with more than 150 mg/100 mL. Coma generally occurs at about 400 mg/100 mL, and death from respiratory failure is likely at levels exceeding 500 mg/100 mL.

Ethanol significantly enhances – sometimes to a dangerous extent – the CNS depressant effects of many other drugs, including benzodiazepines, antidepressants, antipsychotic drugs and opioids.

Neurotoxicity

In addition to the acute effects of ethanol on the nervous system, chronic administration also causes irreversible neurological damage (see Harper & Matsumoto, 2005). This may be due to ethanol itself, or to metabolites such as acetaldehyde or fatty acid esters, or to dietary deficiencies (e.g. of thiamine) that are common in alcoholics. Binge drinking is thought to produce greater damage; probably due to the high brain concentrations of ethanol achieved and to repeated phases of withdrawal between binges. Heavy drinkers often exhibit convulsions and may develop irreversible dementia and motor impairment associated with thinning of the cerebral cortex (apparent as ventricular enlargement) detectable by brain-imaging techniques. Degeneration of the cerebellar vermis, the mammillary bodies and other specific brain regions can also occur, as well as peripheral neuropathy.

Effects on other systems

The main acute cardiovascular effect of ethanol is to produce cutaneous vasodilatation, central in origin, which causes a warm feeling but actually increases heat loss.[13] It has been proposed that mild consumption of ethanol reduces the incidence of coronary heart disease, by increasing circulating levels of high-density lipoproteins (HDL) thus reducing the incidence of atherosclerosis (see Ch. 24). The much hyped notion that a glass of red wine each day (red wine contains the antioxidant, resveratrol) reduces coronary

artery disease has come in for criticism in recent years. Moderate ethanol consumption may protect against ischaemic heart disease, especially in older people, perhaps partly by inhibiting platelet aggregation. This effect occurs at ethanol concentrations in the range achieved by moderate drinking (10–20 mmol/L) and probably results from inhibition of arachidonic acid formation from phospholipid. However, chronic or intermittent drinking of excessive amounts of ethanol causes raised blood pressure, which is one of the most important risk factors for having a heart attack or a stroke.

Diuresis is a familiar effect of ethanol. It is caused by inhibition of antidiuretic hormone secretion, and tolerance develops rapidly, so that the diuresis is not sustained. There is a similar inhibition of oxytocin secretion, which can delay parturition.

Ethanol increases salivary and gastric secretion, perhaps a reason in some cultures for the popularity of a glass of sherry before dinner. However, heavy consumption of spirits causes damage directly to the gastric mucosa, causing chronic gastritis. Both this and the increased acid secretion are factors in the high incidence of gastric bleeding in alcoholics. CNS depression predisposes to aspiration pneumonia and lung abscess formation. Acute pancreatitis may become chronic with pseudocyst formation (collections of fluid in the peritoneal sac), fat malabsorption and ultimately loss of B-cell function, and insulin-dependent diabetes mellitus.

Ethanol produces a variety of endocrine effects. In particular, it increases the output of adrenal steroid hormones by stimulating the anterior pituitary gland to secrete adrenocorticotrophic hormone. However, the increase in plasma hydrocortisone usually seen in alcoholics (producing a 'pseudo-Cushing's syndrome' [Ch. 34]) is due partly to inhibition by ethanol of hydrocortisone metabolism in the liver.

Acute toxic effects on muscle are exacerbated by seizures and prolonged immobility; severe myositis ('rhabdomyolysis') with myoglobinuria can cause acute renal failure. Chronic toxicity affects particularly cardiac muscle, giving rise to alcoholic cardiomyopathy and chronic heart failure.

Chronic ethanol consumption may also result in immunosuppression, leading to increased incidence of infections such as pneumonia (immunisation with pneumococcal vaccine is important in chronic alcoholics); and increased cancer risk, particularly of the mouth, larynx and oesophagus.

Male alcoholics are often impotent and show signs of feminisation. This is associated with impaired testicular steroid synthesis, but induction of hepatic microsomal enzymes by ethanol, and hence an increased rate of testosterone inactivation, also contributes.

Effects of ethanol on the liver

Together with brain damage, liver damage is the most common serious long-term consequence of excessive ethanol consumption (see Lieber, 1995). Ethanol increases fat accumulation in the liver even after a single dose. Increased fat accumulation (fatty liver) progresses to hepatitis (i.e. inflammation of the liver) and eventually to irreversible hepatic necrosis and fibrosis. Cirrhosis is an end stage, with extensive fibrosis and foci of regenerating hepatocytes that are not correctly 'plumbed in' to the blood and biliary systems. Diversion of portal blood flow around the cirrhotic liver often causes portal hypertension and the development of oesophageal varices, which can bleed suddenly and catastrophically.

---

[13]The image of a large St Bernard dog carrying a small keg of brandy around its neck to revive avalanche victims is an apocryphal one created by the English painter Edwin Landseer, who in 1820 produced a painting called 'Alpine Mastiffs Reanimating a Distressed Traveller'. With their keen sense of smell, such dogs were useful in searching for people buried in the snow, but taking a tot of brandy would only have enhanced the victim's heat loss.

With chronic ethanol consumption, many other factors contribute to the liver damage. One is malnutrition, for alcoholic individuals may satisfy much of their calorie requirement from ethanol itself. Three hundred grams of ethanol (equivalent to one bottle of whisky) provides about 2000 kcal but, unlike a normal diet, it provides no vitamins, amino acids or fatty acids. Thiamine deficiency is an important factor in causing chronic neurological damage. Folate deficiency (Ch. 26) is also common in alcoholics, often associated with macrocytosis of red blood cells.

The overall incidence of chronic liver disease is a function of cumulative ethanol consumption over many years. An increase in the plasma concentration of the liver enzyme γ-glutamyl transpeptidase (a marker of cytochrome P450 induction, Ch. 10) often raises the suspicion of ethanol-related liver damage, although not specific to ethanol.

The effect of ethanol on fetal development

Drinking alcohol, especially in the first 3 months of pregnancy, increases the risk of miscarriage, premature birth and low birth weight. The adverse effect of heavier ethanol consumption during pregnancy on fetal development was demonstrated in the early 1970s, when the term *fetal alcohol syndrome* (FAS) was coined.

The features of full FAS include:

- abnormal facial development, with wide-set eyes, short palpebral fissures and small cheekbones;
- reduced cranial circumference;
- retarded growth;
- mental retardation and behavioural abnormalities, often taking the form of hyperactivity and difficulty with social integration;
- other anatomical abnormalities, which may be major or minor (e.g. congenital cardiac abnormalities, malformation of the eyes and ears).

A lesser degree of impairment, termed *alcohol-related neurodevelopmental disorder* (ARND), results in behavioural problems, and cognitive and motor deficits, often associated with reduced brain size. Full FAS occurs in about 3 per 1000 live births and affects about 30% of children born to alcoholic mothers. It is rare with mothers who drink less than about 5 units/day, and most common in binge drinkers who sporadically consume much larger amounts, resulting in high peak levels of ethanol. ARND is about three times as common. Although there is no clearly defined safe threshold, there is no evidence that amounts less than about 2 units/day are harmful. There is no critical period during pregnancy when ethanol consumption is likely to lead to FAS, although one study suggests that FAS incidence correlates most strongly with ethanol consumption very early in pregnancy, even before pregnancy is recognised, implying that not only pregnant women, but also women who are likely to become pregnant, should be advised not to drink heavily. Experiments on rats and mice suggest that the effect on facial development may be produced very early in pregnancy (up to 4 weeks in humans), while the effect on brain development is produced rather later (up to 10 weeks).

PHARMACOKINETIC ASPECTS

Metabolism of ethanol

Ethanol is rapidly absorbed, an appreciable amount being absorbed from the stomach. A substantial fraction is cleared by first-pass hepatic metabolism. Hepatic metabolism of

Effects of ethanol

- **Ethanol** acts as a general central nervous system depressant, similar to volatile anaesthetic agents, producing the familiar effects of acute intoxication.
- Several cellular mechanisms are postulated: enhancement of GABA and glycine action, inhibition of calcium channel opening, activation of potassium channels and inhibition at NMDA receptors.
- Effective plasma concentrations:
  - threshold effects: about 20 mg/100 mL (5 mmol/L)
  - severe intoxication: about 150 mg/100 mL
  - death from respiratory failure: about 500 mg/100 mL
- Main peripheral effects are self-limiting diuresis (reduced antidiuretic hormone secretion), and cutaneous vasodilatation.
- Neurological degeneration occurs with heavy and binge drinking, causing dementia and peripheral neuropathies.
- Long-term ethanol consumption causes liver disease, progressing to cirrhosis and liver failure.
- Excessive consumption in pregnancy causes impaired fetal development, associated with small size, abnormal facial development and other physical abnormalities, and mental retardation.
- Psychological dependence, physical dependence and tolerance all occur with **ethanol**.

ethanol shows saturation kinetics (see Chs 10 and 11) at quite low ethanol concentrations, so the fraction of ethanol removed decreases as the concentration reaching the liver increases. Thus, if ethanol absorption is rapid and portal vein concentration is high, most of the ethanol escapes into the systemic circulation, whereas with slow absorption more is removed by first-pass metabolism. This is one reason why drinking ethanol on an empty stomach produces a much greater pharmacological effect. Ethanol is quickly distributed throughout the body water, the rate of its redistribution depending mainly on the blood flow to individual tissues, as with volatile anaesthetics (see Ch. 42).

Ethanol is about 90% metabolised, 5%–10% being excreted unchanged in expired air and in urine. This fraction is not pharmacokinetically significant but provides the basis for estimating blood ethanol concentration from measurements on breath or urine. The ratio of ethanol concentrations in blood and alveolar air, measured at the end of deep expiration, is relatively constant, 80 mg/100 mL of ethanol in blood producing 35 μg/100 mL in expired air; this being the basis of the breathalyser test. The concentration in urine is more variable and provides a less accurate measure of blood concentration.

Ethanol metabolism occurs almost entirely in the liver, and mainly by a pathway involving successive oxidations, first to acetaldehyde and then to acetic acid (Fig. 49.5). Since ethanol is often consumed in large quantities (compared with most drugs), 1–2 mol daily being by no means unusual, it constitutes a substantial load on the hepatic oxidative systems. The oxidation of 2 mol of ethanol consumes about 1.5 kg of the co-factor nicotinamide adenine dinucleotide (NAD^+). Availability of NAD^+ limits the rate of ethanol oxidation to about 8 g/h in a normal adult,

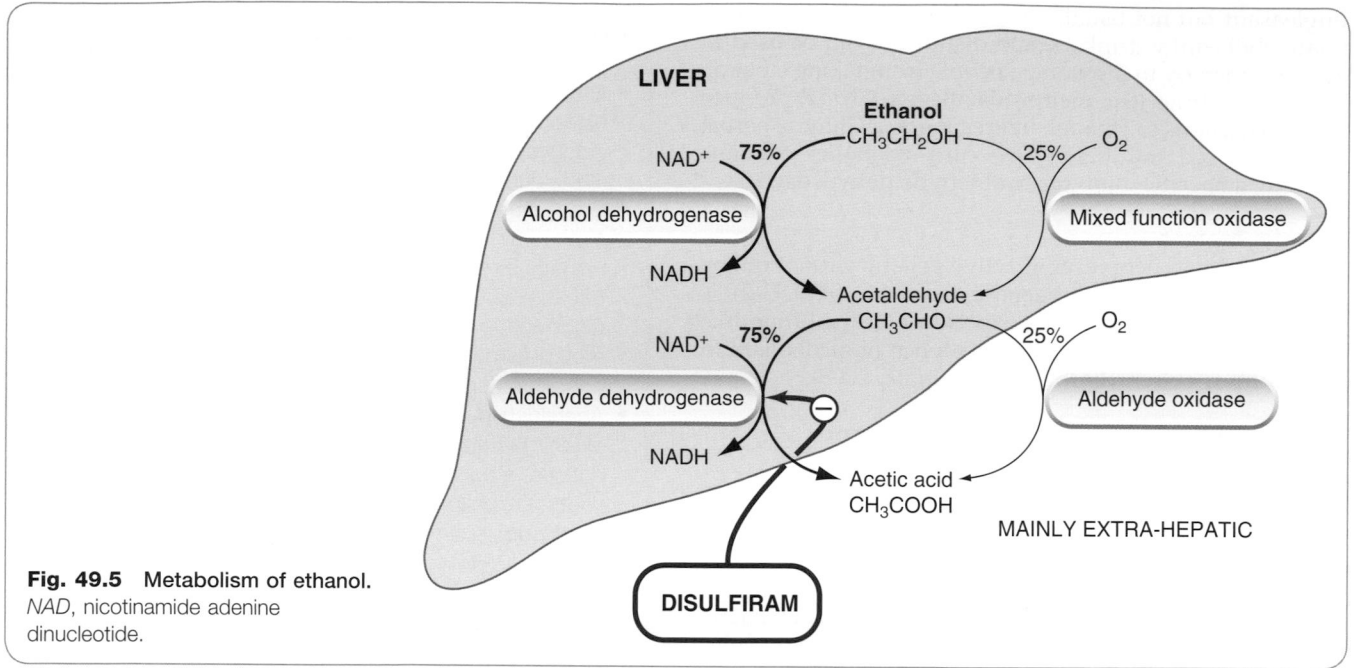

Fig. 49.5 Metabolism of ethanol.
NAD, nicotinamide adenine dinucleotide.

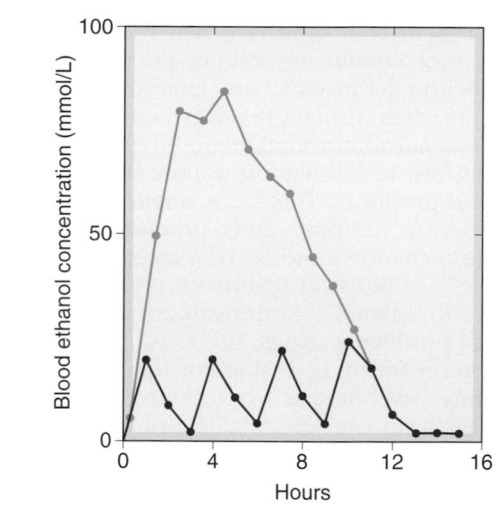

Fig. 49.6 Zero-order kinetics of ethanol elimination in rats. Rats were given ethanol orally (104 mmol/kg) either as a single dose or as four divided doses. The single dose results in a much higher and more sustained blood ethanol concentration than the same quantity given as divided doses. Note that, after the single dose, ethanol concentration declines linearly, the rate of decline being similar after a small or large dose, because of the saturation phenomenon. (From Kalant, H. et al., 1975. Biochem. Pharmacol. 24, 431.)

with various fatty acids also occurs in the tissues, and these esters may also contribute to long-term toxicity.

Alcohol dehydrogenase is a soluble cytoplasmic enzyme, confined mainly to liver cells, which oxidises ethanol at the same time as reducing NAD$^+$ to NADH (see Fig. 49.5). Ethanol metabolism causes the ratio of NAD$^+$ to NADH to fall, and this has other metabolic consequences (e.g. increased lactate and slowing down of the Krebs cycle). The limitation on ethanol metabolism imposed by the limited rate of NAD$^+$ regeneration has led to attempts to find a 'sobering up' agent that works by regenerating NAD$^+$ from NADH. One such agent is fructose, which is reduced by an NADH-requiring enzyme. In large doses, it causes a measurable increase in the rate of ethanol metabolism, but not enough to have a useful effect on the rate of return to sobriety.

Normally, only a small amount of ethanol is metabolised by the microsomal mixed function oxidase system (see Ch. 10), but induction of this system occurs in alcoholics. Ethanol can affect the metabolism of other drugs that are metabolised by the mixed function oxidase system (e.g. **phenobarbital**, **warfarin** and **steroids**), with an initial inhibitory effect produced by competition, followed by enhancement due to enzyme induction.

Nearly all the acetaldehyde produced is converted to acetate in the liver by *aldehyde dehydrogenase* (see Fig. 49.5). Normally, only a little acetaldehyde escapes from the liver, giving a blood acetaldehyde concentration of 20–50 µmol/L after an intoxicating dose of ethanol in humans. The circulating acetaldehyde usually has little or no effect, but the concentration may become much larger under certain circumstances and produce toxic effects. This occurs if aldehyde dehydrogenase is inhibited by drugs such as **disulfiram**. In the presence of disulfiram, which produces no marked effect when given alone, ethanol consumption is followed by a severe reaction comprising flushing, tachycardia, hyperventilation and considerable panic and distress, which is due to excessive acetaldehyde accumulation in the bloodstream. This reaction is extremely

independently of ethanol concentration (Fig. 49.6), causing the process to show saturating kinetics (Ch. 11). It also leads to competition between the ethanol and other metabolic substrates for the available NAD$^+$ supplies, which may be a factor in ethanol-induced liver damage (see Ch. 58). The intermediate metabolite, acetaldehyde, is a reactive and toxic compound, and this may also contribute to the hepatotoxicity. A small degree of esterification of ethanol unpleasant but not usually harmful, at least in otherwise relatively healthy drinkers, and disulfiram can be used as aversion therapy to discourage people from taking ethanol. Some other drugs (e.g. **metronidazole**; see Ch. 52) produce similar reactions to ethanol. Interestingly, a Chinese herbal medicine used traditionally to cure alcoholics contains **daidzin**, a specific inhibitor of aldehyde dehydrogenase.[14]

Genetic factors

In 50% of Asian people, an inactive genetic variant of one of the aldehyde dehydrogenase isoforms (ALDH-2) is expressed; these individuals experience a disulfiram-like reaction after alcohol, and the incidence of alcoholism in this group is extremely low (see Tyndale, 2003).

Metabolism and toxicity of methanol and ethylene glycol

▼ Methanol is metabolised in the same way as ethanol but produces formaldehyde instead of acetaldehyde from the first oxidation step. Formaldehyde is more reactive than acetaldehyde and reacts rapidly with proteins, causing the inactivation of enzymes involved in the tricarboxylic acid cycle. It is converted to another toxic metabolite, formic acid. This, unlike acetic acid, cannot be utilised in the tricarboxylic acid cycle and is liable to cause tissue damage. Conversion of alcohols to aldehydes occurs not only in the liver but also in the retina, catalysed by the dehydrogenase responsible for retinol–retinal conversion. Formation of formaldehyde in the retina accounts for one of the main toxic effects of methanol, namely blindness, which can occur after ingestion of as little as 10 g. Formic acid production and derangement of the tricarboxylic acid cycle also produce severe acidosis.

Methanol is used as an industrial solvent and also to adulterate industrial ethanol in order to make it unfit to drink. Methanol poisoning is quite common, and used to be treated by administration of large doses of ethanol, which acts to retard methanol metabolism by competition for alcohol dehydrogenase. **Fomepizole** inhibits alcohol dehydrogenase and is now preferred, if available. Such treatment may be in conjunction with haemodialysis to remove unchanged methanol, which has a small volume of distribution.

Poisoning with ethylene glycol, used in automobile antifreeze and brake fluid, is a medical emergency. It is rapidly absorbed from the gut and metabolised to glycolate and then more slowly to oxalate. Glycolate interferes with metabolic processes and produces metabolic acidosis. It affects the brain, heart and kidneys. Treatment is with fomepizole or, with caution, ethanol,[15] and haemodialysis.

TOLERANCE AND DEPENDENCE

Tolerance to the effects of ethanol can be demonstrated in both humans and experimental animals, to the extent of a two- to three-fold reduction in potency occurring over 1–3 weeks of continuing ethanol administration. A small component of this is due to the more rapid elimination of ethanol. The major component is cellular tolerance, which accounts for a roughly two-fold decrease in potency and which can be observed in vitro (e.g. by measuring the inhibitory effect of ethanol on transmitter release from

Metabolism of ethanol

- **Ethanol** is metabolised mainly by the liver, first by alcohol dehydrogenase to acetaldehyde, then by aldehyde dehydrogenase to acetate. About 25% of the acetaldehyde is metabolised extrahepatically.
- Small amounts of **ethanol** are excreted in urine and expired air.
- Hepatic metabolism shows saturation kinetics, mainly because of limited availability of nicotinamide adenine dinucleotide (NAD⁺). Maximal rate of **ethanol** metabolism is about 10 mL/h. Thus plasma concentration falls linearly rather than exponentially.
- Acetaldehyde may produce toxic effects. Inhibition of aldehyde dehydrogenase by **disulfiram** accentuates nausea, etc., caused by acetaldehyde, and can be used in aversion therapy.
- **Methanol** is similarly metabolised to formic acid, which is toxic, especially to the retina.
- Asian people show a high rate of genetic polymorphism of alcohol and aldehyde dehydrogenase, associated with alcoholism and alcohol intolerance, respectively.

synaptosomes) as well as in vivo. The mechanism of this tolerance is not known for certain. Ethanol tolerance is associated with tolerance to many anaesthetic agents, and alcoholics are often difficult to anaesthetise.

Chronic ethanol administration produces various changes in CNS neurons, which tend to oppose the acute cellular effects that it produces. There is a small reduction in the density of GABA$_A$ receptors, and a proliferation of voltage-gated calcium channels and NMDA receptors.

A well-defined physical abstinence syndrome develops in response to ethanol withdrawal. As with most other dependence-producing drugs, this is probably important as a short-term factor in sustaining the drug habit, but other (mainly psychological) factors are more important in the longer term (see Ch. 50). The physical abstinence syndrome usually subsides in a few days, but the craving for ethanol and the tendency to relapse last for very much longer. Treatment of alcohol dependence is described in Chapter 50.

The physical abstinence syndrome in humans, in severe form, develops after about 8 h. In the first stage, the main symptoms are tremor, nausea, sweating, fever and sometimes hallucinations. These last for about 24 h. This phase may be followed by seizures ('rum fits'). Over the next few days, the condition of 'delirium tremens' develops, in which the patient becomes confused, agitated and often aggressive, and may suffer much more severe hallucinations. Treatment of this medical emergency is by sedation with large doses of a benzodiazepine such as **chlordiazepoxide** (Ch. 45) together with large doses of thiamine.

SYNTHETIC CANNABINOIDS

The endogenous cannabinoid system and cannabinoids contained in the *Cannabis sativa* plant (phytocannabinoids) are described in detail in Chapter 20. Here we will focus on synthetic cannabinoids, which have names such as *Spice,*

---

[14]In hamsters (which spontaneously consume alcohol in amounts that would defeat even the hardest two-legged drinker, while remaining, as far as one can tell in a hamster, completely sober), daidzin markedly inhibits alcohol consumption.

[15]When presented with a late evening emergency poisoning of a dog with ethylene glycol, a veterinarian colleague of one of the authors ran to the local supermarket and purchased a bottle of vodka – the dog survived!

K2 or *Black Mamba.* The chemical structures of synthetic cannabinoids are diverse, with over 10 chemical families having been described (see Davidson et al., 2017). Some originated from legitimate attempts by pharmaceutical companies to develop new analgesic compounds but more recently others have been developed purely for non-medicinal purposes. Synthetic cannabinoids are commonly sprayed on herbal material and smoked but are also available in crystal and powder form. They are agonists at the CB_1 cannabinoid receptor, the target through which Δ^9-tetrahydrocannabinol (THC), the major psychoactive ingredient in cannabis, has its effects. Synthetic cannabinoids are said to exert a 'more forceful' activation of the CB_1 receptor, in that users often become 'zombie-like' or cataleptic. This may explain their popularity amongst the homeless and prisoners in jail, allowing them a period of escape from their daily lives.

Unlike cannabis itself, synthetic cannabinoids are quite harmful and can induce hallucinations, psychotic episodes, seizures and death. The precise reasons for these toxic effects are not known. They may have 'off-target' effects unrelated to their actions on CB_1 receptors. Furthermore, when smoked, the parent compounds are subject to pyrolysis giving rise to unexpected derivatives, which may be responsible for some of the damaging effects. Quality control is not a priority for the producers of these agents and so there may be toxic contaminants in occasional batches of chemicals.

REFERENCES AND FURTHER READING

General reference
Miller, R.J., 2015. Drugged: The Science and Culture Behind Psychotropic Drugs. Oxford University Press. (*A lively account of psychoactive drug use*)

Stimulants
Docherty, J.R., Green, A.R., 2010. The role of monoamines in the changes in body temperature induced by 3,4-methylene-dioxymethamphetamine (MDMA, ecstasy) and its derivatives. Br. J. Pharmacol. 160, 1029–1044.
Fredholm, B.B., Battig, K., Holmes, J., et al., 1999. Actions of caffeine in the brain with special reference to factors that contribute to its widespread use. Pharmacol. Rev. 51, 83–133. (*Comprehensive review article covering pharmacological, behavioural and social aspects*)
Green, A.R., King, M.V., Shortall, S.E., Fone, K.C., 2012. Lost in translation: preclinical studies on 3,4-methylenedioxy-methamphetamine provide information on mechanisms of action, but do not allow accurate prediction of adverse events in humans. Br. J. Pharmacol. 166, 1523–1536.
Heal, D.J., Cheetham, S.C., Smith, S.L., 2009. The neuropharmacology of ADHD drugs in vivo: insights on efficacy and safety. Neuropharmacology 57, 608–618. (*Reviews various aspects of the pharmacology of drugs used to treat ADHD*)

Nicotine
De Biasi, M., Dani, J.A., 2011. Reward, addiction, withdrawal to nicotine. Annu. Rev. Neurosci. 34, 105–130.
Hung, R.J., McKay, J.D., Gaborieau, V., et al., 2008. A susceptibility locus for lung cancer maps to nicotinic acetylcholine receptor subunit genes on 15q25. Nature 452, 633–637. (*Original paper showing a genetic link between cancer and single nucleotide polymorphisms in the nicotinic receptor*)
Le Foll, B., Goldberg, S.R., 2005. Control of the reinforcing effects of nicotine by associated environmental stimuli in animals and humans. Trends Pharmacol. Sci. 26, 287–293.
Leslie, F.M., Mojica, C.Y., Reynaga, D.D., 2013. Nicotinic receptors in addiction pathways. Mol. Pharmacol. 83, 753–758.
Wonnacott, S., Sidhpura, N., Balfour, D.J.K., 2005. Nicotine: from molecular mechanisms to behaviour. Curr. Opin. Pharmacol. 5, 53–59. (*Useful review on the acute and long-term CNS effects of nicotine*)

Cognition enhancers
Battleday, R.M., Brem, A.K., 2015. Modafinil for cognitive neuroenhancement in healthy non-sleep-deprived subjects: a systematic review. Eur. Neuropsychopharmacol. 25, 1865–1881. (*A systematic review of published research papers evaluating the effect of modafinil in non-fatigued individuals*)
Collingridge, G.L., Volianskis, A., Bannister, N., et al., 2013. The NMDA receptor as a target for cognitive enhancement. Neuropharmacology 64, 13–26.
De Mei, C., Ramos, M., Litaka, C., Borrelli, E., 2009. Getting specialized: presynaptic and postsynaptic dopamine D_2 receptors. Curr. Opin. Pharmacol. 9, 53–58.
D'Angelo, L.S.C., Savulich, D., Sahakian, B.J., 2017. Lifestyle use of drugs by healthy people for enhancing cognition, creativity, motivation and pleasure. Br. J. Pharmacol. 174, 3257–3267.

Harms, J.E., Benveniste, M., Maclean, J.K., Partin, K.M., Jamieson, C., 2013. Functional analysis of a novel positive allosteric modulator of AMPA receptors derived from a structure-based drug design strategy. Neuropharmacology 64, 45–52.

Psychedelics
Carhart-Harris, R.L., Goodwin, G.M., 2017. The therapeutic potential of psychedelic drugs: past, present, and future. Neuropsychopharmacol. 42, 2105–2113. (*An interesting discussion between two leading scientists with differing views on the topic*)
Nichols, D.E., 2004. Hallucinogens. Pharmacol. Ther. 101, 131–181. (*Comprehensive review article focusing on 5-HT$_{2A}$ receptors as the target of psychotomimetic drugs*)

Ethanol
Garbutt, J.C., 2009. The state of pharmacotherapy for the treatment of alcohol dependence. J. Subst. Abuse Treat. 36, S15–S21. (*Reviews current treatments and potential new approaches*)
Harper, C., Matsumoto, I., 2005. Ethanol and brain damage. Curr. Opin. Pharmacol. 5, 73–78. (*Describes deleterious effects of long-term alcohol abuse on brain function*)
Harris, R.A., Trudell, J.R., Mihic, S.J., 2008. Ethanol's molecular targets. Sci. Signal. 1, re7. (*Short review of potential molecular actions of alcohol relevant to its effects on the brain*)
Lieber, C.S., 1995. Medical disorders of alcoholism. N. Engl. J. Med. 333, 1058–1065. (*Review focusing on ethanol-induced liver damage in relation to ethanol metabolism*)
Spanagel, R., 2009. Alcoholism: a systems approach from molecular physiology to addictive behaviour. Physiol. Rev. 89, 649–705. (*Comprehensive review article, very useful for reference*)
Tyndale, R.F., 2003. Genetics of alcohol and tobacco use in humans. Ann. Med. 35, 94–121. (*Detailed review of the many genetic factors implicated in alcohol and nicotine consumption habits*)

Dissociative drugs
Morgan, C.J., Curran, H.V., 2012. Ketamine use: a review. Addiction 107, 27–38. (*Extensive review of current use of ketamine and the harms associated with its use*)
Morris, B.J., Cochran, S.M., Pratt, J.A., 2005. PCP: from pharmacology to modelling schizophrenia. Curr. Opin. Pharmacol. 5, 101–106. (*Review arguing that NMDA channel block by phencyclidine closely models human schizophrenia*)

Synthetic cannabinoids
Davidson, C., Opacka-Juffry, J., Arevalo-Martin, A., Garcia-Ovejero, D., Molina-Holgado, E., Molina-Holgado, F., 2017. Spicing up pharmacology: a review of synthetic cannabinoids from structure to adverse events. Adv. Pharmacol. 80, 135–168. (*Gives details of the chemical structures of synthetic cannabinoids and describes their adverse effects*)

50 Drug abuse and dependence

OVERVIEW

In other chapters, we have considered how drugs that are taken (abused) because they are pleasurable (hedonic) exert their profound effects. In this chapter, we now focus on factors that relate specifically to drug abuse (e.g. routes of administration, harms involved in drug taking) and on why some drugs of abuse produce dependence (addiction). Finally, pharmacological treatments for drug dependence are described. The use of drugs in sport and bodybuilding is discussed in Chapter 59.

The reasons why the use of a particular drug is viewed as a problem to society – and hence may be considered 'drug abuse' – are complex and largely outside the scope of this book. The drug and its pharmacological activity are only the starting point. For many, but not all, drugs of abuse, continued use leads to dependence (addiction).

DRUG USE AND ABUSE

A number of terms are used, sometimes interchangeably and sometimes incorrectly, to describe drug use and the consequences of self-administration of drugs. Terms that are best avoided are listed in Table 50.1. Other, more useful, terms are defined in the text.

A vast and ever-increasing array of drugs is used to alter mood and perception.[1] These include drugs that are also used as medicines, e.g. anxiolytics (Ch. 45), opioids (Ch. 43) and general anaesthetics (Ch. 42), as well as cannabinoids (Ch. 20) and the range of non-medicinal drugs described in Chapter 49. Volatile organic solvents (present in glues and aerosols), taken by inhalation, also feature as abused drugs. The popularity of each varies between different societies across the world, and within societies popularity differs among different groups of individuals.[2] Frequently, users will take more than one drug concomitantly (e.g. heroin users will inject cocaine and heroin together, an activity known as *speedballing*) or sequentially. Sequential use is often intended to reduce adverse effects when coming down off the first drug (e.g. use of benzodiazepines when coming down from stimulants). Polydrug use is a very under-researched area in regard to why it is done, how

---

[1]Most are illegal in many countries, though there are strong lobbies to legalise some that are considered less harmful.
[2]A survey in one UK city showed that among Friday-night clubbers, the choice of drug was associated with the type of music the clubs played (Measham & Moore, 2009).

different drugs may interact and the potential harm that may arise from such practices. For example, ethanol alters cocaine metabolism, resulting in the production of *cocaethylene*, which is more potent than cocaine and has potentially greater cardiovascular toxicity.

Drugs of abuse are an extremely heterogeneous pharmacological group; we can find little in common at the molecular and cellular level between say, **morphine**, **cocaine** and **LSD** (lysergic acid diethylamide). What links them is that people find their effects pleasurable (hedonic) and tend to want to repeat the experience. The drug experience may take the form of intense euphoria, mood elevation, hallucinations, stimulation, sedation or calming, depending upon the specific drug taken. In this regard, drug use can be described as *thrill seeking*. Many drug users, however, have existing mental health problems and for them drug taking is a means of escaping reality and this can be described as *self-medicating*.

The popularity and availability of drugs change with time. For example, over the last 20 years the opioid epidemic in the United States has been fuelled first by the ease of obtaining prescription opioids such as **oxycodone**, and more recently by the availability of illicitly produced **fentanyls**, such that in 2016 in the United States, of over 50,000 deaths due to opioid overdose, some 38% were due to fentanyl and related drugs, 27% to prescription opioids and only 29% to **heroin** (official name diamorphine). The situation is different in other countries such as the United Kingdom, where oxycodone and fentanyl abuse is still fairly uncommon.

Drug use involves effects on the brain that can be both acute and chronic (Fig. 50.1). The immediate, acute effect on mood is the reason the drug is taken. For some drugs (e.g. **amphetamines**, Ch. 49), this may be followed by a rebound negative or depressed phase. Persistent use of a drug may lead to compulsive drug use (addiction – a complex state that involves both psychological and physiological dependence) and to the development of tolerance. Psychological dependence can give rise to intense craving for the drug even when the user has been drug-free for months or years.

DRUG ADMINISTRATION

For drugs that induce strong feelings of euphoria, there are two components to the experience: an initial rapid effect (the *rush* or *buzz*) and a more prolonged pleasurable effect (the *high*) that may for some drugs (e.g. **gabapentin/pregabalin** or opioids) be accompanied by a period of sedation (*gouching*). The intensity of the initial effect is determined by how fast the drug enters the brain and activates its effector mechanism. For many casual drug users, ease of administration defines how the drug is taken (e.g. smoking, swallowing or snorting a drug is relatively easy). However, for other

Table 50.1 Glossary of frequently used and 'abused' terms

Addict	Person for whom the desire to experience a drug's effects overrides any consideration for the serious physical, social or psychological problems that the drug may cause to the individual or others. Often used in non-scientific circles to convey criminal intent and so has fallen out of favour with those involved in treating people with drug problems
Drug misuse	Non-medicinal drug use (although some would not consider taking drugs to alter mood/induce hallucinations as 'misuse' or 'abuse')
Junkie	Pejorative term for someone who is dependent upon a drug
Narcotics	Originally used as a term to describe opioids as they induce sleep (narcosis). Subsequently this term has been used by non-scientists to describe a wide range of drugs of abuse (including cocaine, which is a stimulant!)
Recreational drug use	Originally used to describe all drug abuse, it is now sometimes used to describe drug use in the bar/club/dance scene
Substance use	Some governments do not consider ethanol or chemical solvents to be drugs, hence 'substance use' (or 'substance abuse') is used to include these agents

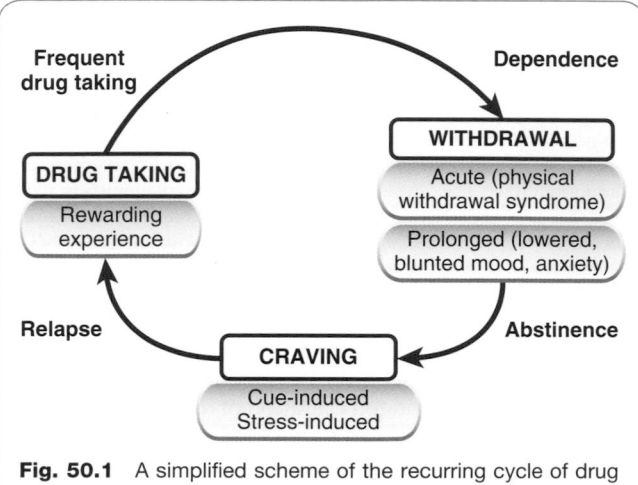

Fig. 50.1 A simplified scheme of the recurring cycle of drug dependence.

drug users chasing a more intense experience, the route of administration and the choice of individual drug become important. Intravenous injection or smoking results in faster absorption of a drug than when it is taken orally. Heroin, cocaine, amphetamines, tobacco and cannabis are all taken by one or other of these routes. Heroin is more popular as a drug of abuse than morphine. This is because it enters the brain more rapidly than morphine. However, heroin itself does not interact with opioid receptors but is rapidly deacetylated to 6-acetylmorphine and morphine, μ opioid–receptor agonists (see Ch. 43).

DRUG HARM

All drugs of abuse are harmful to a varying extent. Adverse effects can be the result of drug overdose (e.g. respiratory depression produced by opioids), of effects on tissues other than the brain (e.g. necrosis of the nasal septum resulting from chronic cocaine use), of the route of administration (e.g. HIV and other infections in drug users who share needles), of effects unrelated to the specific actions of the drug (e.g. carcinogenicity of tobacco smoke, severe bladder pain in regular **ketamine** users) or of use for illegal purposes (e.g. **flunitrazepam** or **γ-hydroxybutyrate [GHB]** as

date-rape drugs). Many major harms relate to the ability of some drugs to induce dependence (e.g. psychostimulants, opioids, ethanol and tobacco) or to reveal a susceptibility to psychotic illness in some individuals (e.g. amphetamines and cannabis).

An attempt to produce a rational scale of harm, based on assessment by an expert panel of physical risk, dependence liability and social cost, was reported by Nutt et al. (2010), who have argued that such ratings should influence how governments police and punish people for supplying and using particular drugs. As might be expected, ethanol, heroin and cocaine were judged to be the most harmful, with cannabis, LSD and ecstasy (**MDMA**, see Ch. 49) much less so – an order that is not reflected in the classification of these drugs under UK law.[3]

DRUG DEPENDENCE

Drug dependence (addiction) describes the human condition in which:

- drug taking becomes compulsive, taking precedence over other needs;
- there is a loss of control of the amount of drug taken;
- physical and psychological changes occur when access to drug is denied.

Dependence thus involves both psychological and physiological components and can be considered as a three-stage process around which dependent individuals recycle (see Fig. 50.1). The neurobiology of drug dependence is described in detail by Koob and Volkow (2016).

Dependence becomes a problem when the want becomes so insistent that it dominates the lifestyle of the individual and damages his or her quality of life, and the habit itself causes actual harm to the individual or the community. Examples of the latter are the mental incapacity and liver damage caused by ethanol, the many diseases associated

---

[3]In determining society's attitude towards drugs, the media play an influential role. In the United Kingdom, deaths following consumption of ecstasy (63 in 2016) are often widely reported in the press and on television, but deaths due to heroin overdose, which are much more prevalent (1209 in 2016), are largely ignored unless the victim is famous.

with smoking tobacco, the high risk of infection when injecting intravenously (especially HIV and hepatitis C), the serious risk of overdose with most opioids and the criminal behaviour resorted to when drug users need to finance their drug taking.

Not all psychoactive drugs induce severe dependence. Major dependence-inducing drugs are nicotine, ethanol, opioids, cocaine, amphetamine and benzodiazepines. Cannabis, MDMA and psychedelic drugs are less dependence inducing.

Not everyone who takes a drug progresses to become dependent upon it. Family studies show clearly that susceptibility to dependence is an inherited characteristic. Around 50% of the risk of becoming dependent is genetic, with the remainder being developmental (adolescents are more at risk than adults) and environmental, e.g. stress, social pressures and drug availability. Variants of many different genes may each make a small contribution to the overall susceptibility of an individual to addiction – a familiar scenario that provides few pointers for therapeutic intervention. Polymorphisms in ethanol-metabolising genes (see Ch. 49) are the best example of genes that directly affect the tendency to abuse a drug.

DRUG-INDUCED REWARD

The common feature of the various types of psychoactive drugs that are addictive is that all produce a *rewarding* experience (e.g. an elevation of mood or a feeling of euphoria or calmness).

In animal studies, where the state of mood cannot be inferred directly, reward is manifest as *positive reinforcement*, i.e. an increase in the probability of occurrence of any behaviour that is associated with the drug experience. In *conditioned place preference* studies, animals receive a drug or placebo and are then placed in different environments. Subsequently, when tested in a drug-free state, they will spend more time in the environment associated with a previous rewarding drug experience. Another way of determining if a drug is rewarding is to test whether or not animals will self-administer the drug by pressing a lever to obtain it. All dependence-producing drugs are self-administered by experimental animals. Psychedelic drugs are not, however, normally self-administered by experimental animals, which may indicate that, unlike humans, they find the experience non-rewarding.

Humans have a choice as to whether or not they wish to experiment with and continue taking drugs – there may therefore be an element of risk-taking when experimenting with drugs. In behavioural tests, some rats are observed to be much more impulsive than others (Jupp et al., 2013). These impulsive rats show a higher rate of cocaine, nicotine, alcohol and methylphenidate self-administration and have a lower level of expression of D_2 and D_3 dopamine receptors in the nucleus accumbens (see later for the importance of this brain region in drug use). Impulsive rats are not, however, more prone to self-administering opioids.

REWARD PATHWAYS

▼ Virtually all of the major dependence-producing drugs so far tested, including opioids, nicotine, amphetamines, ethanol and cocaine, activate the *reward pathway* – the mesolimbic dopaminergic pathway (see Ch. 40), that runs, via the medial forebrain bundle, from the ventral tegmental area (VTA) of the midbrain to the nucleus accumbens and limbic region. Even though for some of these drugs their primary sites of action may be elsewhere in the brain, they all increase the

extracellular level of dopamine in the nucleus accumbens, as shown by microdialysis in animals and in vivo brain-imaging techniques in humans. Opioids enhance the firing of VTA dopaminergic neurons by reducing the level of GABAergic inhibition (disinhibition) within the VTA, whereas amphetamine and cocaine act on dopaminergic nerve terminals in the nucleus accumbens to release dopamine or prevent its reuptake (see Ch. 15). Given that dopamine release in the nucleus accumbens is also enhanced by naturally rewarding stimuli, such as food, water, sex and nurturing, it would appear that drugs are simply activating, or overactivating, the body's own pleasure system. In experienced drug users the anticipation of the effect may become sufficient to elicit the release of dopamine. Paradoxically, brain-imaging studies have revealed that in chronic users the increase in dopamine may be less than expected when compared with what is seen in naïve individuals, even though the subjective high is still intense. This may reflect some degree of sensitisation, but the mechanism is not well understood.

Chemical or surgical interruption of the VTA–accumbens dopaminergic pathway impairs drug-seeking behaviours in many experimental situations. Deletion of D_2 receptors in a transgenic mouse strain was shown to eliminate the rewarding properties of morphine administration without reducing other opioid effects, and it did not prevent the occurrence of physical withdrawal symptoms in morphine-dependent animals (Maldonado et al., 1997), suggesting that the dopaminergic pathway is responsible for the positive reward but not for the negative withdrawal effects. However, D_2-receptor antagonists (antipsychotic drugs; see Ch. 47) have not been successful in treating addiction, and more recent evidence suggests that D_1 receptors activated by steep increases in dopamine release and possibly also D_3 receptors play important roles. The development of D_3-receptor antagonists or partial agonists as potential treatments for drug abuse is ongoing (see Maramai et al., 2016).

PHYSICAL DEPENDENCE

This is characterised by a *withdrawal* or *abstinence syndrome* whereby on cessation of drug administration or on administering an antagonist, adverse physiological effects are experienced. On prolonged cessation of drug administration the withdrawal effects can persist for a period of days or weeks, the precise withdrawal responses being characteristic of the type of drug taken. The intensity of the withdrawal syndrome also varies between drugs of the same type according to their pharmacokinetic characteristics. The desire to avoid or suppress the withdrawal syndrome increases the drive to retake the drug. In individuals undergoing treatment for drug dependence (detox) pharmacological intervention can be used to reduce the intensity of drug withdrawal (Table 50.2).

▼ The mechanisms responsible for the withdrawal syndrome have been most fully characterised for opioid dependence but similar mechanisms may apply to cocaine and ethanol withdrawal. At the cellular level, opioids inhibit cAMP formation, and withdrawal results in a rebound increase as a result of 'superactivation' of adenylyl cyclase, as well as up-regulation of the amount of this enzyme. This results in activation of protein kinase A (PKA), in an increase in adenosine as a consequence of the conversion of cAMP to adenosine, and in activation of a transcription factor – cAMP response element binding protein (CREB). The rise in PKA activity increases the excitability of nerve terminals by phosphorylating neurotransmitter transporters to increase their ionic conductance (see Bagley et al., 2005), as well as increasing neurotransmitter release by a direct action on the secretory process (Williams et al., 2001). Withdrawal results in enhanced GABA release in various parts of the brain, probably through the mechanisms described above (see Bagley et al., 2011). The release of other neurotransmitters is also likely to be enhanced. On the other hand, the enhanced extracellular levels of adenosine, acting on presynaptic A_1 receptors (see Ch. 17), inhibits glutamate release at excitatory synapses, and thus counteracts the neuronal hyperexcitability that occurs during drug withdrawal, suggesting

Table 50.2 Pharmacological approaches to treating drug dependence

Mechanism	Example(s)
Substitution therapies	• Methadone (orally active opioid agonist with long biological half-life) and buprenorphine (sublingually absorbed opioid partial agonist) or legal heroin to maintain opioid-dependent patients • Nicotine patches or chewing gum to alleviate nicotine withdrawal symptoms
Blocking pleasurable response	• Naltrexone (non-selective opioid antagonist) to block opioid effects in drug-withdrawn patients • Naltrexone and nalmefene (non-selective opioid agonist/weak partial agonist) to reduce ethanol use (presumably by blocking the effects of endogenous opioids released by ethanol in the brain) • Mecamylamine (nicotinic antagonist) to block nicotine effects • Immunisation against nicotine, cocaine and heroin to produce circulating antibodies (still being developed)
Aversive therapies	• Disulfiram (aldehyde dehydrogenase inhibitor) to induce unpleasant response to ethanol
To alleviate withdrawal symptoms	• Methadone or buprenorphine used short term to blunt opioid withdrawal • Ibogaine (a naturally occurring psychoactive agent) used by some to reduce opioid withdrawal symptoms • α_2-Adrenoceptor agonists (e.g. clonidine, lofexidine) to diminish opioid, alcohol and nicotine withdrawal symptoms • β-Adrenoceptor antagonists (e.g. propranolol) to diminish excessive peripheral sympathetic activity • Varenicline ($\alpha4\beta2$ nicotinic receptor partial agonist) to alleviate nicotine withdrawal symptoms. Treatment can be continued in abstinent individuals to reduce risk of relapse • Benzodiazepines (e.g. chlordiazepoxide), clomethiazole, topiramate and GHB to blunt alcohol withdrawal symptoms
Reducing continued drug use (may act by reducing craving)	• Bupropion (antidepressant with some nicotinic receptor antagonist activity) and nortriptyline (noradrenaline reuptake inhibiting antidepressant) to reduce tobacco use • Clonidine (α_2-adrenoceptor agonist) to reduce craving for nicotine[a] • Acamprosate (NMDA receptor antagonist) to treat alcoholism[a] • Topiramate and lamotrigine (antiepileptic agents) to treat alcoholism and cocaine use[a] • GHB reported to reduce craving for alcohol and cocaine[a] • Baclofen (GABA$_B$ receptor agonist) reported to reduce opioid, alcohol and stimulant use[a] • Modafinil (dopamine reuptake inhibitor) to reduce cocaine use[a] • Ibogaine (natural product hallucinogen) reported to reduce craving for stimulants and opioids[a]

[a]The effectiveness of these agents at reducing the continued use of other drugs of abuse over and above the ones listed remains to be determined.

Notes: Antidepressant, mood stabilising, anxiolytic and antipsychotic medications are useful when treating patients who, in addition to their drug use, also suffer from other mental disorders. The cannabinoid CB$_1$-receptor antagonist rimonabant, in addition to its antiobesity effects, also reduces nicotine, ethanol, stimulant and opioid consumption. However, it also induces depression and its use has been discontinued.

GHB, γ-hydroxybutyric acid.

the possibility – not yet clinically proven – that adenosine agonists might prove useful in treating drug dependence. CREB, which is up-regulated in the nucleus accumbens by prolonged administration of opioids or cocaine, plays a key role in regulating various components of cAMP signalling pathways, and transgenic animals lacking CREB show reduced withdrawal symptoms (see Chao & Nestler, 2004).

Several types of therapeutic drug, including antidepressant and antipsychotic agents, also produce withdrawal symptoms on cessation of administration, but it is important to distinguish this type of commonly observed 'rebound' phenomenon from the physical dependence associated with drugs of abuse. A degree of physical dependence is common when patients receive opioid analgesics in hospital for several days, but this rarely leads to addiction.

PSYCHOLOGICAL DEPENDENCE

During periods of drug withdrawal, individuals experience irritability, stress, anxiety, low mood and blunted responses to experiences that would normally be pleasurable. These aversive behavioural changes can be long lasting and contribute to the drive to retake the drug to escape from what is a negative emotional state (*negative affect*).

The memory of previous drug-induced experiences can be very intense and long lasting, giving rise to *craving*; it may drive an individual to take the drug again – referred to as *relapse* – even after a prolonged period of abstinence (see Weiss, 2005). Craving may be triggered by stress or by cues, such as experiencing the environment that a person associates with previously taking the drug or the sight of drug administration paraphernalia e.g. a crack pipe or syringe. This suggests that associative learning may be an important factor in psychological dependence (Robbins et al., 2008). It has been suggested that drugs alter memory formation to enhance the recollection of previous drug experience. In this regard, it is of interest that several drugs produce changes in synaptic plasticity, a cellular correlate of memory formation (see Ch. 39). While cocaine, morphine, nicotine and ethanol enhance long-term potentiation (LTP) in the VTA by increasing the expression of AMPA receptors on the plasma membrane, cocaine also increases long-term depression (LTD) in the nucleus accumbens (Hyman et al., 2006).

The psychological factors in drug dependence are discussed in detail by Koob and Volkow (2016) and summarised in Fig. 50.2.

Drug dependence

- Dependence occurs when, as a result of repeated administration of the drug, the desire to experience the effects of a drug again becomes compulsive.
- Dependence occurs with a wide range of psychotropic drugs, acting by many different mechanisms.
- The common feature of the major dependence-inducing drugs is that they have a positive reinforcing action ('reward') associated with activation of the mesolimbic dopaminergic pathway.
- Dependence can be subdivided into physical and psychological components.
- Physical dependence is characterised by a withdrawal syndrome, which varies in type and intensity for different classes of drug.
- Psychological dependence comprises both mood changes – irritability, stress, anxiety, and blunted responses to normally rewarding experiences – and craving.
- Craving can be triggered by stress or cues relating to previous drug experience and may occur in individuals who have been drug free for some considerable time.
- On repeated administration, tolerance may occur to the effects of the drug.
- Although genetic factors contribute to drug-seeking behaviour, no specific genes have yet been identified.

TOLERANCE

Tolerance (see Ch. 2) describes the decrease in pharmacological effect on repeated administration of a drug – it develops over time, as does the state of dependence. It does not occur with all drugs of abuse. Contrary to earlier thinking, physical dependence and tolerance are now thought to involve different mechanisms (see Bailey & Connor, 2005).

▼ For drugs such as opioids that are agonists at specific receptors (see Ch. 43), cellular tolerance results in part from desensitisation of the receptors. On prolonged activation by an agonist, the μ receptor is phosphorylated by various intracellular kinases (Williams et al., 2013) – which either directly desensitises the receptor or causes the binding to the receptor of other proteins, such as arrestins, that uncouple the receptor from its G protein (see Ch. 3). In the intact animal, inhibition or knock-out of these kinases reduces the level of tolerance.).

PHARMACOLOGICAL APPROACHES TO TREATING DRUG DEPENDENCE

There are a number of different approaches taken to treat drug dependence. Specific examples of the drugs used in each are given in Table 50.2.

- Substitution therapy, in which a replacement medicinal grade drug (e.g. methadone or buprenorphine for opioid users) is provided long term to '*maintain*' the individual, preventing them from going into withdrawal and reducing the need/drive to take illicit drug(s). This form of treatment has been shown to reduce illegal activities to fund illicit drug purchase and to reduce associated health hazards such as HIV and hepatitis C infection.
- Facilitating drug withdrawal (detox) by either substituting a drug in the same class from which subsequent withdrawal is less intense or by

Fig. 50.2 A simplified scheme of some of the psychological factors involved in drug dependence.

administration of other drugs during the withdrawal process that reduce the intensity of the withdrawal symptoms.

- Blocking the effects of an abused drug by prior administration of an antagonist so that if the individual has detoxed but relapses and retakes the drug again they will not experience the pleasurable effects of the drug. For this to be successful, the antagonist has to be long lasting or administered in the form of an implant that releases the antagonist over a prolonged period.
- Blocking the effects of an abused drug by immunisation to produce circulating antibodies. Vaccines against nicotine, heroin or cocaine, to induce antibody formation that would mop up these drugs when they enter the blood stream are in early clinical development, although progress has been slow.
- Making the drug experience unpleasant. The best example of this approach is for ethanol which is rapidly metabolised to acetic acid by a two-step process (see Ch. 49, Fig. 49.5). Disulfiram, an aldehyde dehydrogenase inhibitor, inhibits the second step, resulting in the build-up of acetaldehyde which elicits an unpleasant response when ethanol is consumed.
- Reducing craving for a drug. A range of drugs have been suggested to reduce craving for various drugs. Their effectiveness is an ongoing area of debate and research.

For intravenous drug users, the provision of sterile needles reduces needle sharing and the spread of blood-borne diseases such as HIV and hepatitis C. Opioid overdose results in severe respiratory depression that can lead to death. Opioid-induced respiratory depression is rapidly reversed by intramuscular injection of the opioid antagonist, **naloxone**. Supervised injection rooms and the distribution of naloxone injection kits within the drug using community are ways to reduce opioid overdose deaths.

Drug abuse involves many psychosocial and some genetic factors, as well as neuropharmacological mechanisms, and so while pharmacological approaches to drug treatment are important, they are only one component of the therapeutic approaches that are used. For information on other approaches to the treatment of drug addiction, readers are advised to consult the National Institute on Drug Abuse (NIDA) website at http://www.nida.nih.gov/.

Clinical use of drugs in substance dependence

Tobacco dependence

- Short-term **nicotine** is an adjunct to behavioural therapy in smokers committed to giving up; **varenicline** is also used as an adjunct but has been linked to suicidal ideation.
- **Bupropion** is also effective but lowers seizure threshold, so is contraindicated in people with risk factors for seizures (and also if there is a history of eating disorder).

Alcohol dependence

- Long-acting benzodiazepines (e.g. **chlordiazepoxide**) can be used to reduce withdrawal symptoms and the risk of seizures; they should be tapered over 1–2 weeks and then discontinued because of their abuse potential.
- **Disulfiram** is used as an adjunct to behavioural therapy in suitably motivated alcoholics after detoxification; it is contraindicated for patients in whom hypotension would be dangerous (e.g. those with coronary or cerebral vascular disease).
- **Acamprosate** can help to maintain abstinence; it is started as soon as abstinence has been achieved and maintained if relapse occurs, and it is continued for 1 year.

Opioid dependence

- **Naloxone**, a competitive opioid antagonist, has become available for use in community settings to reverse respiratory depression from opioid overdose. It can be administered as a nasal spray or by intramuscular injection.
- Opioid agonists or partial agonists (e.g., respectively, **methadone** or **buprenorphine**) administered orally or sublingually may be substituted for injectable narcotics, many of whose harmful effects are attributable to the route of administration.
- **Naltrexone**, a long-acting opioid antagonist, is used as an adjunct to help prevent relapse in detoxified addicts (opioid free for at least 1 week).
- **Lofexidine**, an α_2 agonist (cf. **clonidine**; Ch. 15), is used short term (usually up to 10 days) to ameliorate symptoms of opioid withdrawal, and is then tapered over a further 2–4 days.

REFERENCES AND FURTHER READING

General

Chao, J., Nestler, E.J., 2004. Molecular neurobiology of addiction. Annu. Rev. Med. 55, 113–132. (*Useful review article by leading scientists in addiction research*)

Koob, G.F., Volkow, N.D., 2016. Neurobiology of addiction: a neurocircuitry analysis. Lancet Psychiatry 3, 760–773. (*Describes in detail the components of drug dependence as well as the neuronal pathways and neurotransmitters involved*)

Measham, F., Moore, K., 2009. Repertoires of distinction. Exploring patterns of weekend polydrug use within local leisure scenes across the English night time economy. Criminol. Crim. Justice. 9, 437–464.

Nutt, D., King, L.A., Phillips, L.D., 2010. Drug harms in the UK: a multicriteria decision analysis. Lancet 376, 558–565.

Reward

Hyman, S.E., Malenka, R.C., Nestler, E.J., 2006. Neural mechanisms of addiction: the role of reward-related learning and memory. Annu. Rev. Neurosci. 29, 565–598. (*Extensive review on how drugs of abuse can alter memory and learning processes*)

Jupp, B., Caprioli, D., Dalley, J.W., 2013. Highly impulsive rats: modelling an endophenotype to determine the neurobiological, genetic and environmental mechanisms of addiction. Dis. Model. Mech. 6, 302–311 (*An extensive review of impulsivity and how it relates to drug seeking*)

Maldonado, R., Saiardi, A., Valverde, O., et al., 1997. Absence of opiate rewarding effects in mice lacking dopamine D2 receptors. Nature 388, 586–589. (*Use of transgenic animals to demonstrate role of dopamine receptors in reward properties of opiates*)

Maramai, S., Gemma, S., Brogi, S., et al., 2016. Dopamine D3 receptor antagonists as potential therapeutics for the treatment of neurological diseases. Front. Neurosci. 10, 451. (*Discusses the development and potential uses of selective D_3 antagonists in the treatment of drug abuse*)

Dependence and tolerance

Bagley, E.E., Gerke, M.B., Vaughan, C.W., et al., 2005. GABA transporter currents activated by protein kinase A excite midbrain neurons during opioid withdrawal. Neuron 45, 433–445.

Bagley, E.E., Hacker, J., Chefer, V.I., et al., 2011. Drug-induced GABA transporter currents enhance GABA release to induce opioid withdrawal behaviors. Nat. Neurosci. 14, 1548–1554. (*Describes the cellular mechanism underlying the opioid withdrawal response*)

Bailey, C.P., Connor, M., 2005. Opioids: cellular mechanisms of tolerance and physical dependence. Curr. Opin. Pharmacol. 5, 60–68.

Robbins, T.W., Ersche, K.D., Everitt, B.J., 2008. Drug addiction and the memory systems of the brain. Ann. N. Y. Acad. Sci. 1141, 1–21. (*Review of how different forms of memory play important roles in drug dependence*)

Weiss, F., 2005. Neurobiology of craving, conditioned reward and relapse. Curr. Opin. Pharmacol. 5, 9–19. (*Review of recent studies on the neurobiology of addiction, focusing mainly on animal models*)

Williams, J.T., Christie, M.J., Manzoni, O., 2001. Cellular and synaptic adaptations mediating opioid dependence. Physiol. Rev. 81, 299–343.

Williams, J.T., Ingram, S.L., Henderson, G., et al., 2013. Regulation of μ-opioid receptors: desensitization, phosphorylation, internalization, and tolerance. Pharmacol. Rev. 65, 223–254.

Basic principles of antimicrobial chemotherapy

51

OVERVIEW

The term *chemotherapy* was originally used to describe the use of drugs that were 'selectively toxic' to pathogens (including bacteria, viruses, protozoa, fungi and helminths) while having minimal effects on the host. It also refers to the use of drugs to treat tumours and, in the public mind at least, is usually associated with those cytotoxic anticancer drugs that cause distressing and unwanted effects such as loss of hair, nausea and vomiting. In this chapter, we focus on antimicrobial chemotherapy: anticancer drugs are covered in Chapter 57. The feasibility of the selective toxicity strategy depends on the ability to exploit such biochemical differences as may exist between the infecting organism and the host. While the bulk of this section of the book describes the drugs used to combat such infections, in this introductory chapter we consider the nature of these biochemical differences, outline the molecular targets of drug action and discuss the grave problem of antibiotic resistance.

BACKGROUND

All living organisms are vulnerable to infection. Humans, being no exception, are susceptible to diseases caused by certain viruses, bacteria, protozoa, fungi and helminths (collectively referred to as *pathogens*). The use of chemotherapeutic agents dates back to the work of Ehrlich and others and to the development of selectively toxic arsenical drugs such as salvarsan for the treatment of syphilis.[1] Indeed, it was Ehrlich himself who coined the term *chemotherapy* to describe the use of synthetic chemicals to destroy such pathogens. In recent years the definition of the term has been broadened to include *antibiotics* – strictly speaking, substances produced by microorganisms (although latterly by pharmaceutical chemists as well) that kill or inhibit the growth of other microorganisms. The successful development of such agents during the past 80 years, particularly during the 'golden age' of antibiotic research (1940s–1970s), constitutes one of the most important therapeutic advances in the history of medicine.

Unhappily, our success in developing drugs to neutralise these invaders has been paralleled by their own success in counteracting their effects, resulting in the emergence of *drug resistance*. And at present, the invaders – particularly some bacteria – seem close to getting the upper hand. This is a very important problem, and so we will devote some space to the mechanisms of resistance and the means by which it is spread.

THE MOLECULAR BASIS OF CHEMOTHERAPY

Chemotherapeutic agents, then, are chemicals intended to be toxic to the pathogenic organism but innocuous to the host. It is important to remember that many microorganisms share our body spaces (e.g. the gut[2]) without causing disease (these are called *commensals*), although they may become pathogenic under adverse circumstances (i.e. if the host is immunocompromised or if barrier breakdown results in them setting up shop in an inappropriate location elsewhere in our bodies).

All living organisms can be classified as either *prokaryotes*, cells without nuclei (e.g. bacteria), or *eukaryotes*, cells with nuclei (e.g. protozoa, fungi, helminths). In a separate category are the viruses, which need to utilise the metabolic machinery of the host cell to replicate, and they thus present a particular kind of problem for chemotherapeutic attack. Lurking in the taxonomic shadows, there remain those mysterious proteinaceous agents, *prions* (see Ch. 40), which cause disease but resist all attempts at classification and treatment.

Virtually all creatures, host and parasite alike, have the same basic DNA blueprint (an exception being the RNA viruses), so many biochemical processes are common to most, if not all, organisms. Finding agents that affect pathogens but not other human cells necessitates finding either qualitative or quantitative biochemical differences between them.

BACTERIA

Bacteria are a common cause both of mild and severe infectious disease, and Fig. 51.1 shows, in simplified diagrammatic form, the main components of a notional bacterial cell and their functions. Surrounding the bacterium is the *cell wall*, which characteristically contains *peptidoglycan* (except in *Mycoplasma*). Peptidoglycan is unique to prokaryotic cells and has no counterpart in eukaryotes. Within the cell wall is the *plasma membrane*, which, like that of eukaryotic cells, consists of a phospholipid bilayer and proteins. It

---

[1]Mercury-containing compounds were also once commonly used for treating syphilis. 'One night with Venus, a lifetime with Mercury' was a saying prior to the advent of the antibiotic era.

[2]Humans harbour about 2 kg of bacteria in the gut, comprising a large 'forgotten organ' in the body which has important metabolic functions and which, together with the commensals living on our skin and other organs, are collectively known as the *microbiome*.

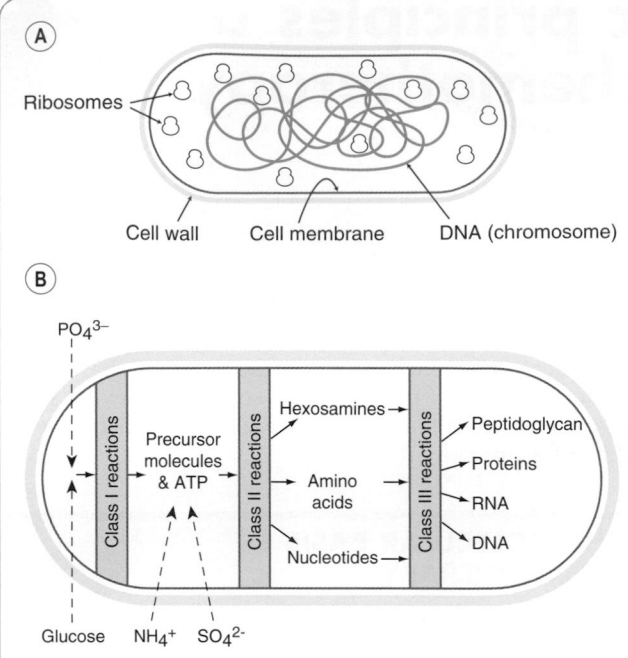

Fig. 51.1 Diagram of the structure and metabolism of a 'typical' bacterial cell. (A) Schematic representation of a bacterial cell. (B) Flow diagram showing the synthesis of the main types of macromolecule of a bacterial cell. Class I reactions result in the synthesis of the precursor molecules necessary for class II reactions, which result in the synthesis of the constituent molecules; these are then assembled into macromolecules by class III reactions. (Modified from Mandelstam, J., McQuillen, K., Dawes, I. (Eds) 1982. Biochemistry of Bacterial growth. Blackwell Scientific, Oxford.)

functions as a selectively permeable membrane with specific transport mechanisms for various nutrients. However, in bacteria the plasma membrane does not contain any *sterols* (e.g. cholesterol), and this may alter the penetration of some chemicals.

The cell wall supports the underlying plasma membrane, which is subject to an internal osmotic pressure of about 5 atmospheres in *gram-negative* organisms, and about 20 atmospheres in *gram-positive* organisms (see Ch. 52 for a full explanation of Gram staining). The plasma membrane and cell wall together comprise the *bacterial envelope*.

As in eukaryotic cells, the plasma membrane surrounds the *cytoplasm* and cellular organelles. Bacterial cells have no nucleus or mitochondria. Instead, the genetic material, in the form of a single *chromosome* containing all the genetic information, lies in the cytoplasm with no surrounding nuclear membrane and cellular energy is generated by enzyme systems located in the plasma membrane rather than dedicated organelles.

Biochemical reactions that are potential targets for antibacterial drugs are shown in Fig. 51.1. These can be classified into three groups:

- *Class I*: those catabolic reactions involved in the utilisation of glucose, or some alternative carbon source, for the generation of energy (ATP) and synthesis of simple carbon compounds used as precursors in the next class of reactions.

- *Class II*: synthetic pathways which utilise these precursors in an energy-dependent synthesis of all the amino acids, nucleotides, phospholipids, amino sugars, carbohydrates and growth factors required by the cell for survival and growth.
- *Class III*: anabolic reactions which assemble these small molecules into macromolecules – proteins, RNA, DNA, polysaccharides and peptidoglycan.

Other potential drug targets include *formed structures*, for example, the cell membrane, the *microtubules* in fungi or muscle tissue in helminths. In considering these targets, emphasis will be placed on bacteria, but reference will also be made to protozoa, helminths, fungi and viruses. The classification that follows is not rigid; a drug may affect more than one class of reactions or more than one subgroup of reactions within a class.

The molecular basis of antibacterial chemotherapy

- Chemotherapeutic drugs should be toxic to invading organisms and innocuous to the host. Such selective toxicity depends on the identification of biochemical differences between the pathogen and the host that can be appropriately exploited.
- Three general classes of biochemical reaction are potential targets for chemotherapy of bacteria:
  - *class I*: biochemical reactions that utilise glucose and other carbon sources to produce ATP and simple carbon compounds
  - *class II*: metabolic pathways utilising energy and class I compounds to make small molecules (e.g. amino acids and nucleotides)
  - *class III*: anabolic pathways that convert small molecules into macromolecules such as proteins, nucleic acids and peptidoglycan

BIOCHEMICAL REACTIONS AS POTENTIAL TARGETS

CLASS I REACTIONS

Class I reactions are not promising targets for two reasons. First, bacterial and human cells use similar mechanisms to obtain energy from glucose (the *Embden–Meyerhof pathway* and the *tricarboxylic acid cycle*). Second, even if glucose oxidation is blocked, many other compounds (amino acids, lactate, etc.) can be utilised by bacteria as an alternative energy source.

CLASS II REACTIONS

Class II reactions are better targets because some pathways exist in pathogens, but not in human cells. There are several examples, with one of the most significant being the folate biosynthesis pathway.

Folate biosynthesis and utilisation

Folate is required for DNA synthesis in both bacteria and in humans (see Chs 26 and 52) but in humans, which have no biosynthetic pathway, it must be obtained from the diet and concentrated in cells by specific uptake

Table 51.1 Specificity of inhibitors of dihydrofolate reductase

Inhibitor	IC$_{50}$ (µmol/L) for dihydrofolate reductase		
	Human	Protozoal	Bacterial
Trimethoprim	260	0.07	0.005
Pyrimethamine	0.7	0.0005	2.5
Methotrexate	0.001	~0.1[a]	Inactive

[a]Tested on *Plasmodium berghei*, a rodent malaria.

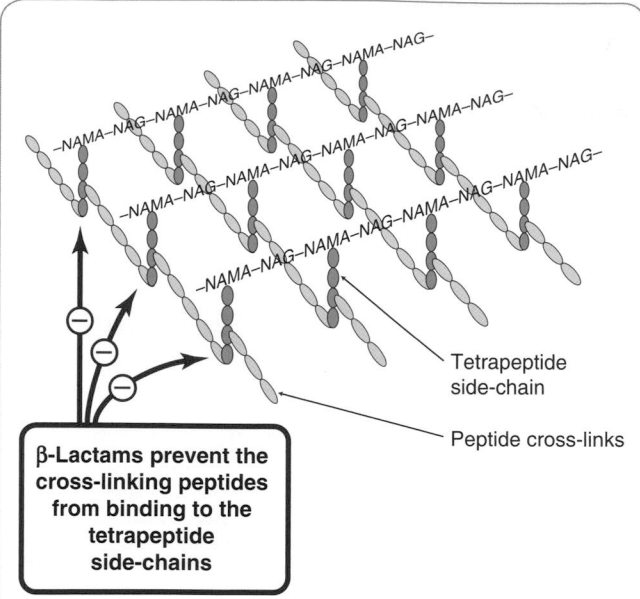

β-Lactams prevent the cross-linking peptides from binding to the tetrapeptide side-chains

Fig. 51.2 Schematic diagram of a single layer of peptidoglycan from a bacterial cell (e.g. *Staphylococcus aureus*), showing the site of action of the β-lactam antibiotics. In *S. aureus* the peptide cross-links consist of five glycine residues. Gram-positive bacteria have several layers of peptidoglycan. More detail in Fig. 51.3. *NAG*, N-acetylglucosamine; *NAMA*, N-acetylmuramic acid.

mechanisms. By contrast, most species of bacteria, as well as the asexual forms of malarial protozoa, lack these transport mechanisms. Therefore they cannot make use of preformed folate but must synthesise this de novo. **Sulfonamides** contain the sulfanilamide moiety – a structural analogue of *p*-aminobenzoic acid (PABA), which is essential in bacterial synthesis of folate (see Ch. 52, Fig. 52.1). Sulfonamides therefore compete with PABA, and thus inhibit bacterial growth without impairing mammalian cell function.

The intracellular utilisation of folate, in the form of *tetrahydrofolate*, as a co-factor in thymidylate synthesis is a good example of a pathway where human and bacterial enzymes exhibit a differential sensitivity to chemicals (Table 51.1; see Volpato & Pelletier, 2009). Although the pathway is virtually identical in microorganisms and humans, one of the key enzymes, *dihydrofolate reductase*, which reduces dihydrofolate to tetrahydrofolate (Ch. 52, Fig. 52.2), is many times more sensitive to the inhibitor **trimethoprim** in bacteria than in humans. In some malarial protozoa, this enzyme is somewhat less sensitive than the bacterial enzyme to trimethoprim but more sensitive to **pyrimethamine** and **proguanil**, which are used as antimalarial agents (Ch. 55). The relative IC$_{50}$ values (the concentration causing 50% inhibition) for bacterial, malarial, protozoal and mammalian enzymes are given in Table 51.1. The human enzyme, by comparison, is very sensitive to the effect of the folate analogue **methotrexate**, which is used to treat inflammatory arthritis (Ch. 27), severe psoriasis (Ch. 28) and cancer (Ch. 57).

▼ The use of sequential blockade with a combination of two drugs that affect the same pathway at different points, for example sulfonamides and the folate antagonists, may be more successful than the use of either alone. Thus, pyrimethamine and a sulfonamide (**sulfadoxine**) are used to treat *falciparum* malaria (Ch. 55). **Co-trimoxazole** is an antibacterial formulation that contains both a sulfonamide and trimethoprim. Once widely used, this combination has become less popular for treating bacterial infections because trimethoprim alone is similarly effective and does not cause sulfonamide-specific adverse effects; its use is now mainly restricted to treatment of *Pneumocystis jirovecii*, for which high doses are required (Ch. 55).

CLASS III REACTIONS

As pathogen cells cannot take up their own unique macromolecules, class III reactions are particularly good targets for selective toxicity, and there are distinct differences between mammalian cells and parasitic cells in this respect. Once again, there are several examples.

The synthesis of peptidoglycan

The cell wall of bacteria contains *peptidoglycan*, a substance that does not occur in eukaryotes and which contains D-amino acids and unusual sugars. It is the equivalent of a non-stretchable string bag enclosing the whole bacterium. In gram-negative bacteria, this bag consists of a single thickness, but in gram-positive bacteria there may be as many as 40 layers of peptidoglycan. Each layer consists of multiple backbones of amino sugars – alternating N-acetylglucosamine and N-acetylmuramic acid residues (Fig. 51.2) – the latter having short peptide side-chains that are cross-linked to form a polymeric lattice, which may constitute up to 10%–15% of the dry weight of the cell and is strong enough to resist the high internal osmotic pressure. The cross-links differ in different species. In staphylococci, for example, they consist of five glycine residues.

▼ To build up this very large insoluble peptidoglycan layer on the outside of the cell membrane, the bacterial cell has the problem of how to transport the hydrophilic cytoplasmic 'building blocks' through the hydrophobic cell membrane structure. This is accomplished by linking them to a very large lipid carrier, containing 55 carbon atoms, which 'tows' them across the membrane. The process of peptidoglycan synthesis is outlined in Fig. 51.3. First, N-acetylmuramic acid, attached to uridine diphosphate (UDP) and a pentapeptide, is transferred to the C$_{55}$ lipid carrier in the membrane, with the release of uridine monophosphate. This is followed by a reaction with UDP–N-acetylglucosamine, resulting in the formation of a disaccharide–pentapeptide complex attached to the carrier. This complex is the basic building block of the peptidoglycan. In *Staphylococcus aureus*, the five glycine residues are attached to the peptide chain at this stage. The building block is now transported out of the cell and added to the growing end of the peptidoglycan, the 'acceptor', with the release of the C$_{55}$ lipid, which still has two phosphates attached. The lipid carrier then loses one phosphate group and thus becomes available for another

Fig. 51.3 Schematic diagram of the biosynthesis of peptidoglycan in a bacterial cell (e.g. *Staphylococcus aureus*), with the sites of action of various antibiotics. The hydrophilic disaccharide–pentapeptide is transferred across the lipid cell membrane attached to a large lipid (C_{55} lipid) by a pyrophosphate bridge (–P–P–). On the outside, it is enzymically attached to the 'acceptor' (the growing peptidoglycan layer). The final reaction is a transpeptidation, in which the loose end of the (Gly) 5 chain is attached to a peptide side-chain of an M in the acceptor and during which the terminal amino acid (alanine) is lost. The lipid is regenerated by loss of a phosphate group (Pi) before functioning again as a carrier. *G*, N-acetylglucosamine; *M*, N-acetylmuramic acid; *UDP*, uridine diphosphate; *UMP*, uridine monophosphate.

cycle. Cross-linking between the peptide side-chains of the sugar residues in the peptidoglycan layer then occurs, the hydrolytic removal of the terminal alanine supplying the requisite energy.

This synthesis of peptidoglycan is a vulnerable step and can be blocked at several points by antibiotics (see Fig. 51.3 and Ch. 52). **Cycloserine**, which is a structural analogue of D-alanine, prevents the addition of the two terminal alanine residues to the initial tripeptide side-chain on N-acetylmuramic acid by competitive inhibition. **Vancomycin** inhibits the release of the building block unit from the carrier, thus preventing its addition to the growing end of the peptidoglycan. **Bacitracin** interferes with the regeneration of the lipid carrier by blocking its dephosphorylation. **Penicillins**, **cephalosporins** and other β-lactams inhibit the final transpeptidation by forming covalent bonds with *penicillin-binding proteins* that have transpeptidase and carboxypeptidase activities, thus preventing formation of the cross-links.

Protein synthesis

Another class III target is protein synthesis. This takes place on the ribosomes but eukaryotic and prokaryotic ribosomes are different, and this provides the basis for the selective antimicrobial action of some antibiotics. The bacterial ribosome consists of a 50S subunit and a 30S subunit (Fig.

51.4), whereas in the mammalian ribosome the subunits are 60S and 40S. The other elements involved in peptide synthesis are messenger RNA (mRNA), which forms the template for protein synthesis, and transfer RNA (tRNA), which specifically transfers the individual amino acids to the ribosome. The ribosome has three binding sites for tRNA, termed the A, P and E sites.

A simplified version of protein synthesis in bacteria is shown in Fig. 51.4. To initiate translation, mRNA, transcribed from the DNA template, is attached to the 30S subunit of the ribosome. The 50S subunit then binds to the 30S subunit to form a 70S subunit,[3] which moves along the mRNA such that successive codons of the messenger pass along the ribosome from the A position to the P position. Antibiotics may affect protein synthesis at any one of these stages (see Fig. 51.4 and Ch. 52).

---

[3]You query whether 30S + 50S = 70S? Yes it does, because we are talking about *Svedberg units*, which measure sedimentation *rate*, which is only partly dependent on *mass*.

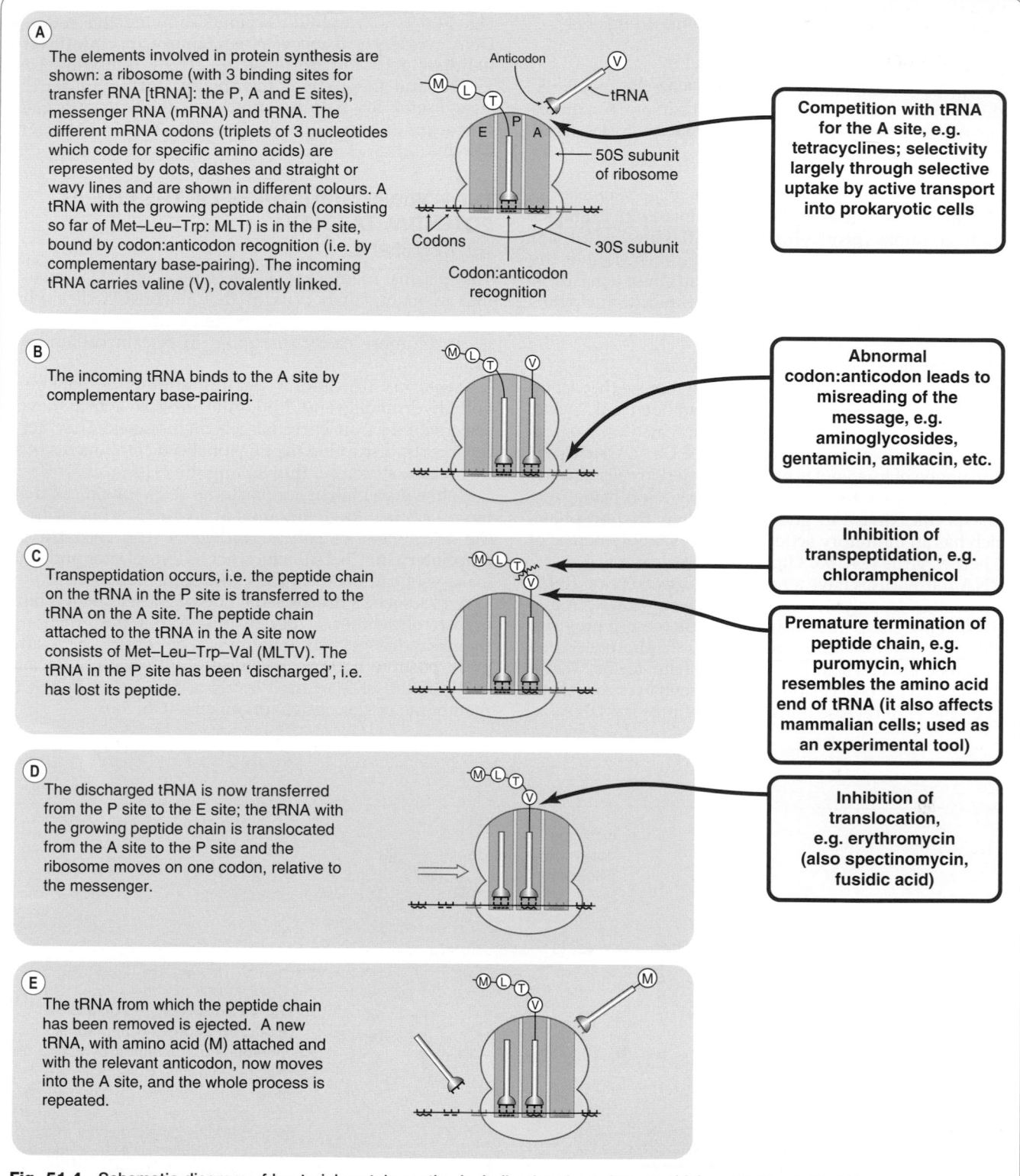

Fig. 51.4 Schematic diagram of bacterial protein synthesis, indicating the points at which antibiotics inhibit the process.

Nucleic acid synthesis

Gene expression and cell division also require nucleic acid synthesis, and this class III reaction is an important site of action of many chemotherapeutic drugs. It is possible to interfere with nucleic acid synthesis in five different ways:

- by inhibiting the synthesis of the nucleotides;
- by altering the base-pairing properties of the DNA template;
- by inhibiting either DNA or RNA polymerase;
- by inhibiting DNA gyrase, which uncoils supercoiled DNA to allow transcription;

- by a direct effect on DNA itself. Some anticancer drugs, but no antimicrobial drugs, work in this way.

Inhibition of the synthesis of nucleotides
This can be accomplished by an effect on the metabolic pathways that generate nucleotide precursors. Examples of agents that have such an effect have been described under class II reactions.

Alteration of the base-pairing properties of the template
Agents that intercalate in the DNA have this effect. Examples include acridines (**proflavine** and **acriflavine**), which are used topically as antiseptics. The acridines double the distance between adjacent base pairs and cause a *frameshift mutation*, whereas some purine and pyrimidine analogues cause base *mispairing*.

Inhibition of either DNA or RNA polymerase
Specific inhibitors of bacterial RNA polymerase that act by binding to this enzyme in prokaryotic, but not in eukaryotic, cells include **rifamycin** and **rifampicin**, which are particularly useful for treating tuberculosis (see Ch. 52). **Aciclovir** (an analogue of guanine) is phosphorylated in cells infected with herpes virus, the initial phosphorylation being by a virus-specific kinase to give the aciclovir trisphosphate, which has an inhibitory action on the DNA polymerase of the herpes virus (Ch. 53; Fig. 51.5).

RNA retroviruses have a *reverse transcriptase* (viral RNA-dependent DNA polymerase) that copies the viral RNA into DNA that integrates into the host cell genome as a provirus. Various agents (**zidovudine**, **didanosine**) are phosphorylated by cellular enzymes to the trisphosphate forms, which compete with the host cell precursors essential for the formation by the viral reverse transcriptase of proviral DNA.

Inhibition of DNA gyrase
Fig. 51.6 is a simplified scheme showing the action of DNA gyrase. The *fluoroquinolones* (**cinoxacin**, **ciprofloxacin**, **nalidixic acid** and **norfloxacin**) act by inhibiting DNA gyrase, and these chemotherapeutic agents are particularly useful for treating infections with gram-negative organisms (Ch. 52). They are selective for the bacterial enzyme.

THE FORMED STRUCTURES OF THE CELL AS POTENTIAL TARGETS
THE MEMBRANE
The plasma membrane of bacterial cells is similar to that in mammalian cells in that it consists of a phospholipid bilayer in which proteins are embedded, but it can be more easily disrupted in certain bacteria and fungi.

Polymixins are cationic peptide antibiotics, containing both hydrophilic and lipophilic groups, which have a selective effect on bacterial cell membranes. They act as detergents, disrupting the phospholipid components of the membrane structure, thus killing the cell.

Unlike mammalian and bacterial cells, fungal cell membranes contain large amounts of *ergosterol*. This facilitates the attachment of *polyene antibiotics* (e.g. **nystatin** and **amphotericin**; Ch. 54), which act as ionophores and cause leakage of cations from the cytoplasm.

Azoles such as **itraconazole** kill fungal cells by inhibiting ergosterol synthesis, thereby disrupting the function of membrane-associated enzymes. The azoles also affect gram-positive bacteria, their selectivity being associated with the presence of high levels of free fatty acids in the membrane of susceptible organisms (Ch. 54).

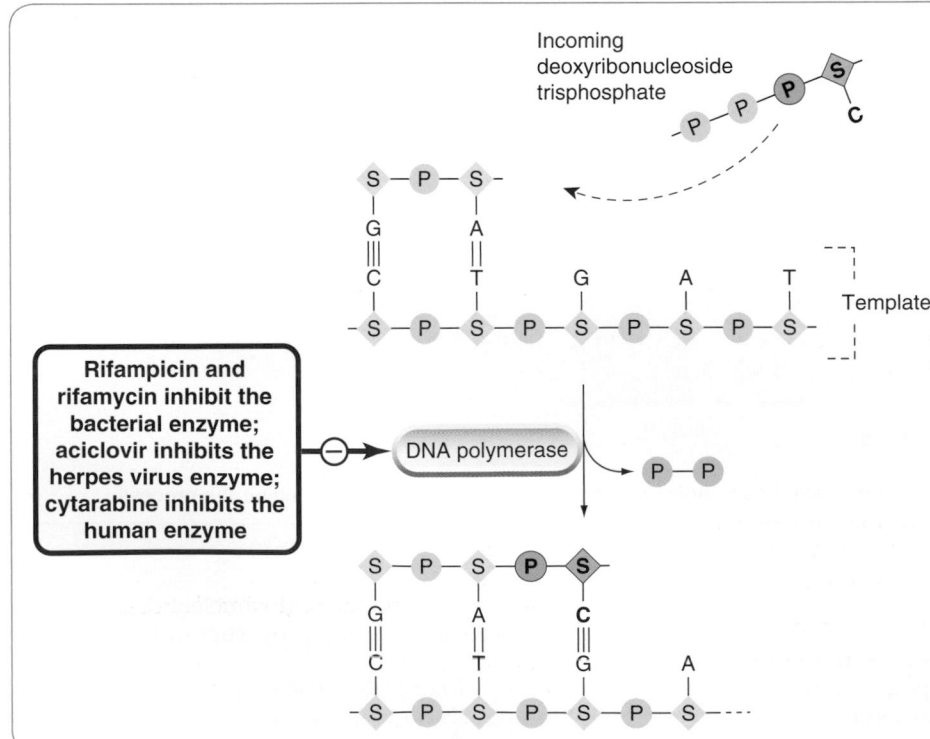

Fig. 51.5 Schematic diagram of DNA replication, showing some antibiotics that inhibit it by acting on DNA polymerase. Nucleotides are added, one at a time, by base pairing to an exposed template strand, and are then covalently joined together in a reaction catalysed by DNA polymerase. The units that pair with the complementary residues in the template consist of a base linked to a sugar and three phosphate groups. Condensation occurs with the elimination of two phosphates. The elements added to the template are shown in *darker colours* and *bold type*. A, adenine; C, cytosine; G, guanine; P, phosphate; S, sugar; T, thymine.

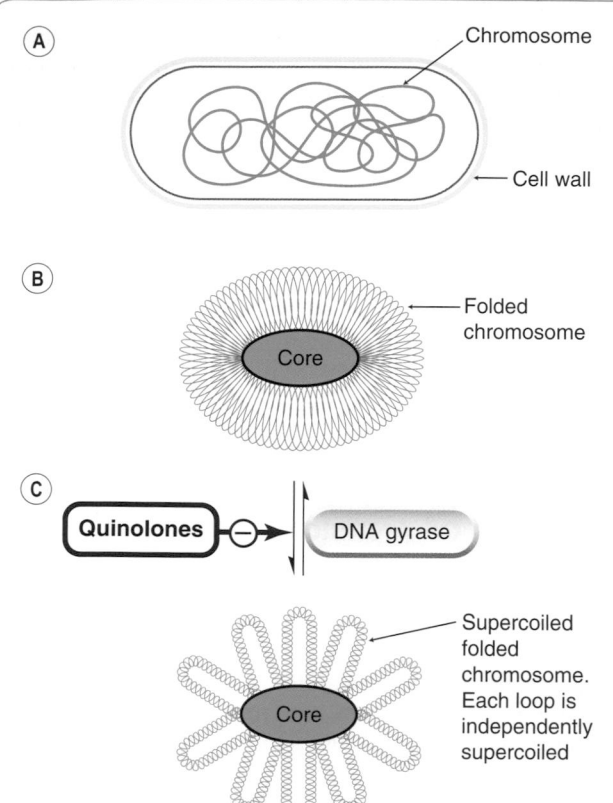

Fig. 51.6 Schematic diagram of the action of DNA gyrase: the site of action for quinolone antibacterials. (A) Conventional diagram used to depict a bacterial cell and chromosome (e.g. *Escherichia coli*). Note that the *E. coli* chromosome is 1300 mm long and is contained in a cell envelope of 2 μm × 1 μm; this is approximately equivalent to a 50 m length of cotton folded into a matchbox. (B) Chromosome folded around RNA core, and then (C), supercoiled by DNA gyrase (topoisomerase II). Quinolone antibacterials interfere with the action of this enzyme. (Modified from Smith, J.T., 1985. In: Greenwood, D., O'Grady., F. (Eds). Scientific Basis of Antimicrobial Therapy. Cambridge University Press, Cambridge, p. 69.)

INTRACELLULAR ORGANELLES[4]

Microtubules and/or microfilaments

The benzimidazoles (e.g. **albendazole**) exert their antihelminthic action by binding selectively to parasite tubulin and preventing microtubule formation (Ch. 56).

Food vacuoles

The erythrocytic form of the malaria plasmodium feeds on host haemoglobin, which is digested by proteases in the parasite food vacuole, the final product, haem, being detoxified by polymerisation. **Chloroquine** and several other antimalarials exert their antimalarial actions by inhibiting plasmodial haem polymerase (Ch. 55).

---

[4]Bacteria do not contain mitochondria so drugs such as atovaquine (see Ch. 55) that target these organelles in parasites are ineffective in bacteria. However, they can damage the host mitochondria (which originated from bacteria during eukaryote evolution) and contribute to the toxicity encountered during their use.

> **Biochemical reactions as potential targets for chemotherapy**
>
> - Class I reactions are poor targets.
> - Class II reactions are better targets:
>   - *folate synthesis* in bacteria is inhibited by sulphonamides;
>   - *folate utilisation* is inhibited by folate antagonists, for example **trimethoprim** (bacteria), **pyrimethamine** (malarial parasite).
> - Class III reactions are important targets:
>   - *peptidoglycan synthesis* in bacteria can be selectively inhibited by β-lactam antibiotics (e.g. **penicillin**);
>   - *bacterial protein synthesis* can be selectively inhibited by antibiotics that prevent binding of tRNA (e.g. tetracyclines), promote misreading of mRNA (e.g. aminoglycosides), inhibit transpeptidation (e.g. **chloramphenicol**) or inhibit translocation of tRNA (e.g. **erythromycin**);
>   - *nucleic acid synthesis* can be inhibited by altering base pairing of DNA template (e.g. the antiviral **vidarabine**), by inhibiting DNA polymerase (e.g. the antivirals **aciclovir** and **foscarnet**) or by inhibiting DNA gyrase (e.g. the antibacterial **ciprofloxacin**).

Muscle fibres

Some antihelminthic drugs have a selective action on helminth muscle cells (Ch. 56). **Piperazine** acts as an agonist on parasite-specific chloride channels gated by GABA in nematode muscle, hyperpolarising the muscle fibre membrane and paralysing the worm; **avermectins** increase Cl⁻ permeability in helminth muscle – possibly by a similar mechanism. **Pyrantel** and **levamisole** are agonists at nematode acetylcholine nicotinic receptors on muscle, causing contraction followed by paralysis (Ch. 56).

> **Formed structures of the cell that are targets for chemotherapy**
>
> - The bacterial cell wall may be affected by several classes of antibiotics, such as the β-lactams.
> - The plasma membrane is affected by:
>   - **amphotericin**, which acts as an ionophore in fungal cells
>   - azoles, which inhibit fungal membrane ergosterol synthesis
> - Microtubule function is disrupted by:
>   - benzimidazoles (antihelminthics)
> - Muscle fibres are affected by:
>   - avermectins (antihelminthics), which increase Cl⁻ permeability
>   - **pyrantel** (antihelminthic), which stimulates nematode nicotinic receptors, eventually causing muscle paralysis by depolarising neuromuscular block

RESISTANCE TO ANTIBACTERIAL DRUGS

Since the 1940s, the development of effective and safe drugs to deal with bacterial and other infections has revolutionised medical treatment, and the morbidity and mortality associated with these diseases have been dramatically reduced. Unfortunately, the development of effective antibacterial drugs has been accompanied by the emergence of drug-resistant organisms.

The growing concern about antibiotic resistance has prompted several supra-national and domestic political responses. In addition to the WHO, which has formulated a *Global Action Plan on Antibiotic Resistance* and regularly issues updated fact sheets on the problem, other organisations such as the *Global Antibiotic Resistance Partnership* (GARP) have been monitoring the emergence of resistant strains around the world since 2009 and advising on local treatment strategies. There have been domestic initiatives too: in the United States, a national action plan was announced in 2015 and many other countries have introduced similar, if less formal, strategies to implement the advice arising from the WHO, GARP and other organisations. Developing countries often struggle to introduce such measures and, because they are often burdened with large numbers of immunocompromised patients, lack of access to drugs, poor hygiene and infection control, are faring less well.

▼ So what is the cause of this problem? The prevailing view used to be that antibiotic resistance was a phenomenon unique to our age and which arose largely through human mismanagement of antibiotic resources. This 'anthropogenic' view seemed to be supported by the relative absence of resistance elements in samples of bacteria taken from remote uninhabited islands (such as some of the Galapagos islands) or from ancient samples that predated the antibiotic era. On the other hand, sequencing of recovered DNA from Pleistocene fossils (around 30,000 years old) suggested that at least some of the antibiotic resistance elements had a very ancient origin (see Bhullar et al., 2012). This presumption was dramatically confirmed by (amongst others) the discovery, in New Mexico, of multidrug resistant bacteria in a deep cave system, which had been isolated from human and animal contact for 4–7 million years (Bhullar et al., 2012). A detailed analysis of one of the species recovered, *Paenibacillus*, which is resistant to most clinically used antibiotics, found that these resistance genes in this bacterium had evidently been conserved for millions of years – and incidentally uncovered several hitherto-unknown resistance mechanisms (Pawlowski et al., 2016). Interestingly, whilst resistance to naturally occurring antibiotics (e.g. penicillin) was extensive, little resistance to synthetic drugs such as linezolid was observed. None of these genes were expressed in samples of this bacterium collected from the nearby cave surface, suggesting that the organisms in the cave expressed these under some selection pressure. Findings such as these have led to a reappraisal of the origin and role of the bacterial 'resistome' and the issue of antibiotic resistance in general. It is now clear that we have to take a more nuanced view of the problem.

Many clinically used antibiotics are complex, naturally occurring chemicals derived from soil-dwelling bacteria or fungi. These are released as part of a defensive strategy by these organisms. Obviously, organisms which release antibiotics must protect themselves against the effects of these substances perhaps explaining, at least in part, why the resistome – the pool of genes involved in antibiotic resistance – is so significant in soil-dwelling organisms. In addition, it is now thought that these endogenous antibiotics may also have a more 'physiological' role: perhaps regulating metabolic pathways, acting as communication molecules

or as part of bacterial 'quorum sensing' mechanisms.[5] Many of the resistance genes are located on mobile elements of DNA and transfer between organisms in the soil is by *horizontal gene transfer* (as opposed to the *vertical gene transfer* that occurs during reproduction). This in part explains why the incidence of resistance is high in sites where bacteria proliferate and antibiotic usage is high, such as in agriculture or in hospitals.

The impact of the intense clinical usage of antibiotics has been the stimulus for the accumulation of multiple resistance elements in pathogens under the 'selection pressure' of drug usage. This obviously imposes serious constraints on the options available for the medical treatment of many bacterial infections. Whilst resistance to chemotherapeutic agents can also develop in protozoa and multicellular parasites (and in populations of malignant cells; see Ch. 57), we will confine our discussion here mainly to the mechanisms of resistance in bacteria.

THE SPREAD OF ANTIBIOTIC RESISTANCE

Antibiotic resistance may be *innate* – pre-existing in a particular strain – or *acquired* in some way from other bacterial cells. In either case, *natural selection* works to favour resistant strains when the antibiotic is prevalent in the environment. Fundamental to the whole issue is how bacterial resistance genes are moved around between chromosomal DNA and mobile elements both *within* and *between* bacteria.

Several basic mechanisms have been identified:

1. By transfer of resistance genes between genetic elements *within* bacteria, on transposons.
2. By transfer of resistance genes *between* bacteria by mobile elements (such as plasmids).
3. By transfer of resistant bacteria between people or animals.

An understanding of these mechanisms is crucial for the sensible clinical use of existing medicines ('antibiotic stewardship') as well as in the design of new antibacterial drugs. We look first at the mechanisms whereby genetic information can be exchanged and then at how these transferred genes undermine the activity of antibiotics.

MOVEMENT OF GENETIC INFORMATION
Plasmids and mobile elements

▼ In addition to the chromosome itself, many species of bacteria contain extrachromosomal genetic elements called plasmids that exist free in the cytoplasm. These are also genetic elements that can replicate independently. Structurally, they are closed loops of DNA that may comprise a single gene or as many as 500 or even more. Only a few plasmid copies may exist in the cell but often multiple copies are present, and there may also be more than one type of plasmid in each bacterial cell. Plasmids that carry genes for resistance to antibiotics (r genes) are referred to as *R plasmids*. Much of the drug resistance encountered in clinical medicine is plasmid-determined.

The whole process can occur with frightening speed. *Staphylococcus aureus*, for example, is a past master of the art of antibiotic resistance. Having become completely resistant to penicillin through plasmid-mediated mechanisms, this organism, within only 1–2 years, was able to acquire resistance to its β-lactamase-resistant (see later) descendant, **meticillin** (de Lencastre et al., 2007).

---

[5]Quorum sensing is a mechanism by which bacterial colonies can regulate their gene expression (and other metabolic activity) according to the population density.

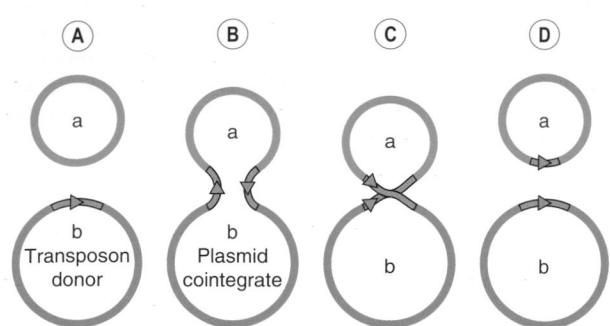

Fig. 51.7 An example of the transfer and replication of a transposon (which may carry genes coding for resistance to antibiotics). (A) Two plasmids, *a* and *b*, with plasmid *b* containing a transposon *(shown in brown)*. (B) An enzyme encoded by the transposon cuts DNA of both donor plasmid and target plasmid *a* to form a cointegrate. During this process, the transposon replicates. (C) An enzyme encoded by the transposon resolves the cointegrate. (D) Both plasmids now contain the transposon DNA.

Transposons

▼ Some stretches of DNA are readily transferred (transposed) from one plasmid to another and also from plasmid to chromosome or vice versa.[6] This is because integration of these segments of DNA, which are called transposons, into the acceptor DNA can occur independently of the normal mechanism of homologous genetic recombination. Unlike plasmids, transposons are not able to replicate independently, although some may replicate during the process of integration (Fig. 51.7), resulting in a copy in both the donor and the acceptor DNA molecules. Transposons may carry one or more resistance genes and can 'hitch-hike' on a plasmid to a new species of bacterium. Even if the plasmid is unable to replicate in the new host, the transposon may integrate into its chromosome or into its indigenous plasmids. This probably accounts for the widespread distribution of certain of the resistance genes on different R plasmids and among unrelated bacteria.

Gene cassettes and integrons

▼ Plasmids and transposons do not complete the tally of mechanisms that natural selection has provided to confound the hopes of the microbiologist/chemotherapist. Resistance – in fact, multidrug resistance – can also be spread by another mobile element, the *gene cassette*, which consists of a resistance gene attached to a small recognition site. Several cassettes may be packaged together in a multicassette array, which can, in turn, be integrated into a larger mobile DNA unit termed an *integron*. The integron (which may be located on a transposon) contains a gene for an enzyme, integrase (recombinase), which inserts the cassette(s) at unique sites into the host DNA. This system – transposon/integron/multiresistance cassette array – allows particularly rapid and efficient transfer of multidrug resistance between genetic elements both within and between bacteria.

THE TRANSFER OF RESISTANCE GENES BETWEEN BACTERIA

▼ Horizontal gene transfer between bacteria of the same, or indeed of different, species is considered the most significant mechanism whereby antibiotic resistance is spread. There are several important mechanisms including conjugation, transduction and transformation with the former being the most significant.

Conjugation

▼ Conjugation involves cell-to-cell contact during which chromosomal or extrachromosomal DNA is transferred from one bacterium to another, and is the main mechanism for the spread of resistance. The ability to conjugate is encoded in *conjugative plasmids*: these are plasmids that contain transfer genes that, in (for example) coliform bacteria, code for the production by the host bacterium of proteinaceous surface tubules termed *sex pili*, which connect the two cells. The conjugative plasmid then passes across from one bacterial cell to another (generally of the same species).

Many gram-negative and some gram-positive bacteria can conjugate. Some promiscuous plasmids can cross the species barrier, adopting one host as readily as another. Many R plasmids are conjugative. Non-conjugative plasmids, if they co-exist in a 'donor' cell with conjugative plasmids, can hitch-hike from one bacterium to the other with the conjugative plasmids. The transfer of resistance by conjugation is particularly significant in populations of bacteria that are normally found at high densities, as in the gut.

Transduction

▼ *Transduction* is a process by which plasmid DNA is enclosed in a virus that infects bacteria (termed a *phage*) and transferred to another bacterium of the same species. It is a relatively ineffective means of transfer of genetic material but is clinically important in the transmission of resistance genes between strains of staphylococci and of streptococci.

Transformation

▼ A few species of bacteria can, under natural conditions, undergo transformation by taking up DNA from the environment and incorporating it into the genome by normal homologous recombination. However, this mechanism is probably not of importance clinically.

There are several other mechanisms through which resistance genes can arise.

CHROMOSOMAL MUTATIONS

The spontaneous mutation rate in bacterial populations for any particular gene is very low, and the probability is that approximately only one cell in 10 million will, on division, give rise to a daughter cell containing a mutation in that gene. However, as there are likely to be very many more cells than this over the course of an infection, the probability of a mutation causing a change from drug sensitivity to drug resistance can be quite high. Fortunately, the presence of a few mutants is not generally sufficient to produce resistance: despite the selective advantage that the resistant mutants possess, the drastic reduction of the population by the antibiotic usually enables the host's natural defences (see Ch. 7) to prevail at least in acute, if not chronic, infections. However, the outcome may not be quite so happy if the primary infection is caused by a drug-resistant strain.

GENE AMPLIFICATION

▼ *Gene duplication* and *amplification* are important mechanisms for resistance in some organisms (Sandegren & Andersson, 2009). According to this idea, treatment with antibiotics can induce an increased number of copies for pre-existing resistance genes such as antibiotic-destroying enzymes and efflux pumps.

BIOCHEMICAL MECHANISMS OF RESISTANCE TO ANTIBIOTICS

Resistance genes are translated into proteins that subvert the action of antibiotics in several ways. Here we discuss several of these, but new mechanisms are still being uncovered (Pawlowski et al., 2016).

---

[6]According to one school of thought, viruses may have arisen as transposons that escaped from cells and continued to ply their trade independently.

Resistance to antibiotics

- Antibiotic resistance is a naturally occurring phenomenon which plays a role in the normal bacterial ecology.
- In many bacterial species, resistance genes (r genes) are of ancient origin and are expressed in the presence of the antibiotic.
- R genes may be moved around between genetic elements within individual bacteria. There are several mechanisms:
  - Plasmids are extrachromosomal genetic elements that can replicate independently and can carry genes coding for resistance to antibiotics (r genes).
  - Transposons are stretches of DNA that can be transposed from one plasmid to another, from a plasmid to a chromosome or vice versa. A plasmid containing an r gene-bearing transposon may code for enzymes that cause the plasmid to be integrated with another. Following their separation, this transposon replicates so that both plasmids then contain the r gene.
- R genes, including *multicassette arrays* of drug resistance genes can also be transferred to other bacteria of the same, or different, species. There are several mechanisms:
  - The main method of transfer of r genes from one bacterium to another is by conjugative plasmids. The bacterium forms a connecting tube with other bacteria through which the plasmids pass.
  - A less common method of transfer is by transduction, i.e. the transmission by a bacterial virus (phage) of a plasmid bearing an r gene into another bacterium.

THE PRODUCTION OF ENZYMES THAT INACTIVATE DRUGS

Inactivation of β-lactam antibiotics

Perhaps the most important example of resistance caused by inactivation is that of the *β-lactam antibiotics*. The enzymes concerned are *β-lactamases*, which cleave the β-lactam ring of penicillins and **cephalosporins** (see Ch. 52). Cross-resistance between the two classes of antibiotic is not complete, because some β-lactamases have a preference for penicillins and some for cephalosporins.

Staphylococci are the principal bacterial species producing β-lactamase, and the genes coding for the enzymes are on plasmids that can be transferred by transduction. In staphylococci, the enzyme is inducible (i.e. it is not expressed in the absence of the drug) and minute, sub-inhibitory, concentrations of antibiotics de-repress the gene and result in a 50- to 80-fold increase in expression. The enzyme passes through the bacterial envelope and inactivates antibiotic molecules in the surrounding medium. The grave clinical problem posed by resistant staphylococci secreting β-lactamase was tackled by developing semisynthetic penicillins (such as meticillin) and new β-lactam antibiotics (the **monobactams** and **carbapenems**), and cephalosporins (such as **cefamandole**), that are less susceptible to inactivation. In addition to acquiring resistance to β-lactams

susceptible to β-lactamase, some strains of *S. aureus* have even become resistant to some antibiotics that are not significantly inactivated by β-lactamase (e.g. meticillin), because they express an additional β-lactam-binding protein coded for by a mutated chromosomal gene. See Lambert (2005) for other examples of this type of action.

▼ Gram-negative organisms can also produce β-lactamases, and this is a significant factor in their resistance to the semisynthetic broad-spectrum β-lactam antibiotics. In these organisms, the enzymes may be coded by either chromosomal or plasmid genes. In the former case, the enzymes may be inducible, but in the latter they are produced constitutively. When this occurs, the enzyme does not inactivate the drug in the surrounding medium but instead remains attached to the cell wall, preventing access of the drug to membrane-associated target sites. Many of these β-lactamases are encoded by transposons, some of which may also carry resistance determinants to several other antibiotics.

Inactivation of chloramphenicol

Chloramphenicol is inactivated by *chloramphenicol acetyltransferase*, an enzyme produced by resistant strains of both gram-positive and gram-negative organisms, the resistance gene being plasmid borne. In gram-negative bacteria, the enzyme is produced constitutively, resulting in levels of resistance five-fold higher than in gram-positive bacteria, in which the enzyme is inducible.

Inactivation of aminoglycosides

Aminoglycosides are inactivated by phosphorylation, adenylation or acetylation, and the requisite enzymes are found in both gram-negative and gram-positive organisms. The resistance genes are carried on plasmids, and several are found on transposons. Many other examples of this kind are given by Wright (2005) and Giedraitiene et al. (2011).

ALTERATION OF DRUG-BINDING SITE

The aminoglycoside-binding site on the 30S subunit of the ribosome may be altered by chromosomal mutation. A plasmid-mediated alteration of the binding site protein on the 50S subunit also underlies resistance to **erythromycin**, and decreased binding of fluoroquinolones because of a point mutation in DNA gyrase A has also been described. An altered DNA-dependent RNA polymerase determined by a chromosomal mutation is reported to be the basis for **rifampicin** resistance.

DECREASED ACCUMULATION OF DRUGS BY BACTERIA

An important example of decreased drug accumulation is the plasmid-mediated resistance to **tetracyclines** encountered in both gram-positive and gram-negative bacteria. In this case, resistance genes in the plasmid code for inducible proteins in the bacterial membrane, which promote energy-dependent efflux of the tetracyclines, and hence resistance. This type of resistance is common and has greatly reduced the therapeutic value of the tetracyclines in human and veterinary medicine. Resistance of *S. aureus* to erythromycin and the other macrolides, and to fluoroquinolones, is also brought about by energy-dependent efflux. Inhibitors of such pumps may be useful adjuncts to antibiotics (Van Bambeke et al., 2006).

There is also recent evidence of plasmid-determined inhibition of *porin* synthesis, which could affect those hydrophilic antibiotics that enter the bacterium through these water-filled channels in the outer membrane. Altered permeability as a result of chromosomal mutations involving the polysaccharide components of the outer membrane of gram-negative organisms may confer enhanced resistance to **ampicillin**. Mutations affecting envelope components have been reported to affect the accumulation of aminoglycosides, β-lactams, chloramphenicol, peptide antibiotics and tetracycline.

ALTERATION OF ENZYME SELECTIVITY

Resistance to trimethoprim is the result of plasmid-directed synthesis of a *dihydrofolate reductase* with low or zero affinity for trimethoprim. It is transferred by transduction and may be spread by transposons.

Sulfonamide resistance in many bacteria is plasmid-mediated and results from the production of a form of *dihydropteroate synthetase* with a low affinity for sulfonamides but no change in affinity for PABA. Bacteria causing serious infections and carrying plasmids with resistance genes to both sulfonamides and trimethoprim have been reported.

Biochemical mechanisms of resistance to antibiotics

The principal mechanisms are as follows:
- *Production of enzymes that inactivate the drug*: for example, β-lactamases, which inactivate **penicillin**; acetyltransferases, which inactivate **chloramphenicol**; kinases and other enzymes, which inactivate aminoglycosides.
- *Alteration of the drug-binding sites*: this occurs with aminoglycosides, **erythromycin**, **penicillin**.
- *Reduction of drug uptake by the bacterium*: for example, tetracyclines.
- *Alteration of enzyme sensitivity*: for example, dihydrofolate reductase becomes insensitive to **trimethoprim**.

CURRENT STATUS OF ANTIBIOTIC RESISTANCE IN BACTERIA

The latest WHO assessment (2016) stresses that antibiotic resistance is now found in every country. Without effective antibiotics, many routine surgical procedures and other medical interventions are impossible. Taking the United Kingdom and the United States together, deaths from infection by resistant strains are in the region of 23,000–25,000 per annum, but in developing countries the mortality figures are at least double those numbers.

It also highlights the following cases as being of special significance:

- *Klebsiella pneumoniae*. Resistance of this organism to 'last resort' antibiotics such as carbapenem drugs has spread around the world and in many countries, treatment fails in about half of all cases.
- *Escherichia coli*. In many countries this organism has become resistant to fluoroquinolone antibiotics and again, treatment fails in about half of the patients in some parts of the world.

- *Neisseria gonorrhoea*. Is now resistant to 'last resort' cephalosporin antibiotics in some 10 countries.
- *Staphylococcus aureus*. There is now widespread resistance to first line drugs and patients with methicillin-resistant *staphylococcus aureus* (MRSA) are more than twice as likely to die following infection. Death rates are declining in the North America and Europe but increasing in developing countries.
- *Enterbacteriaceae spp*. These organisms can cause life threatening infections and recently resistance to the 'last resort' drug colistin has been reported.
- *Mycobacterium tuberculosis*. Multidrug resistant strains (MDR-TB) and *extensively multidrug resistant strains* (XMDR-TB) are increasing and mortality from this hitherto treatable disease is on the increase.

So what is the way forward? Some authors (e.g. Chaudhary, 2016) have advocated tackling the problem at the point of diagnosis and prescription suggesting that bacterial susceptibility testing should be mandatory before the drug is dispensed. Unnecessary prescribing (e.g. for viral infections), inadequate dosing, or inappropriate duration of treatment (which often leads to resistance) should all be scrupulously avoided and more rigorous adherence by patients to antibiotic regimes would help. Therapy using multiple antibiotics acting through different mechanisms can be a useful strategy in some cases. Public health measures such as infection control procedures also play a key role.

Prescribers and consumers must also bear a responsibility for the burgeoning problem of resistance. Indiscriminate use of antibiotics in agriculture, human and veterinary medicine, and their use in animal foodstuffs, has undoubtedly encouraged the spread of resistant strains. Most members of the general public have only a vague notion of the causes of the problem, its likely implications and their role in its development (McCullough et al., 2016). More worryingly, many clinicians, whilst realising the scope of the problem also seem unaware of their crucial role in its spread (McCullough et al., 2015). Some governmental and regulatory bodies (e.g. the European Union) have devised political and social measures to curb such excesses, and these have been at least partly successful. Let us hope that they continue to be so.

Multidrug resistance

Some pathogenic bacteria have developed resistance to many or most commonly used antibiotics. Examples include the following:
- Some strains of staphylococci and enterococci that are resistant to virtually all current antibiotics, the resistance being transferred by transposons and/or plasmids; such organisms can cause serious and virtually untreatable hospital-acquired (so-called nosocomial) infections.
- Some strains of *Mycobacterium tuberculosis* that have become resistant to most antituberculosis agents.

REFERENCES AND FURTHER READING

Amyes, S.G.B., 2001. Magic Bullets, Lost Horizons: The Rise and Fall of Antibiotics. Taylor & Francis, London. (*Thought-provoking book by a bacteriologist with wide experience in bacterial resistance and genetics; he opines that unless the problem of antibiotic resistance is solved within 5 years, 'we are going to slip further into the abyss of uncontrollable infection'*)

Arias, C.A., Murray, B.E., 2012. The rise of the *Enterococcus*: beyond vancomycin resistance. Nat. Rev. Microbiol. 10, 266–278. (*A comprehensive review dealing with many aspects of vancomycin resistance in enterococci and other species. Highly recommended*)

Barrett, C.T., Barrett, J.F., 2003. Antibacterials: are the new entries enough to deal with the emerging resistance problem? Curr. Opin. Biotechnol. 14, 621–626. (*Good general review with some compelling examples and a round-up of new drug candidates*)

Bax, R., Mullan, N., Verhoef, J., 2000. The millennium bugs – the need for and development of new antibacterials. Int. J. Antimicrob. Agents 16, 51–59. (*Excellent review of the problem of resistance and some potential new antibiotics*)

Bhullar, K., Waglechner, N., Pawlowski, A., et al., 2012. Antibiotic resistance is prevalent in an isolated cave microbiome. PLoS ONE 7, e34953. (*The extraordinary discovery of antibiotic resistant bacteria in caves which had been isolated since before hominids walked the earth has changed our understanding of the nature of this important mechanism. See also Pawlowski et al. below*)

Chaudhary, A.S., 2016. A review of global initiatives to fight antibiotic resistance and recent antibiotics discovery. Acta. Pharm. Sin. B 6, 552–556. (*Short but succinct account of the fight back against antibiotic resistance. Easy to read*)

Cox, G., Wright, G.D., 2013. Intrinsic antibiotic resistance: mechanisms, origins, challenges and solutions. Int. J. Med. Microbiol. 303, 287–292. (*This paper reviews general mechanisms of bacterial resistance based upon the notion that resistance is a naturally occurring defence in bacteria. Recommended*)

de Lencastre, H., Oliveira, D., Tomasz, A., 2007. Antibiotic resistant *Staphylococcus aureus*: a paradigm of adaptive power. Curr. Opin. Microbiol. 10, 428–435. (*A little specialised, but worth reading. It details the extraordinary ability of this organism to survive attack by virtually all the drugs in our antibiotic arsenal*)

Giedraitiene, A., Vitkauskiene, A., Naginiene, R., Pavilonis, A., 2011. Antibiotic resistance mechanisms of clinically important bacteria. Medicina 47, 137–146. (*Good review of resistance mechanisms*)

Hawkey, P.M., 1998. The origins and molecular basis of antibiotic resistance. Br. Med. J. 7159, 657–659. (*Succinct overview of resistance; useful, simple diagrams; this is one of 12 papers on resistance in this issue of the journal*)

Knodler, L.A., Celli, J., Finlay, B.B., 2001. Pathogenic trickery: deception of host cell processes. Mol. Cell. Biol. 2, 578–588. (*Discusses bacterial ploys to subvert or block normal host cellular processes: mimicking the ligands for host cell receptors or signalling pathways. Useful list of examples*)

Lambert, P.A., 2005. Bacterial resistance to antibiotics: modified target sites. Adv. Drug Deliv. Rev. 57, 1471–1485. (*Excellent review dealing with this important topic. Numerous examples drawn from studies with many different bacterial species*)

Levy, S.B., 1998. The challenge of antibiotic resistance. Sci. Am. March, 32–39. (*Simple, clear review by an expert in the field; excellent diagrams*)

McCullough, A.R., Rathbone, J., Parekh, S., Hoffmann, T.C., Del Mar, C.B., 2015. Not in my backyard: a systematic review of clinicians' knowledge and beliefs about antibiotic resistance. J. Antimicrob. Chemother. 70, 2465–2473.

McCullough, A.R., Parekh, S., Rathbone, J., Del Mar, C.B., Hoffmann, T.C., 2016. A systematic review of the public's knowledge and beliefs about antibiotic resistance. J. Antimicrob. Chemother. 71, 27–33.

Nesme, J., Simonet, P., 2015. The soil resistome: a critical review on antibiotic resistance origins, ecology and dissemination potential in telluric bacteria. Environ. Microbiol. 17, 913–930. (*An excellent review which deals with the importance of soil dwelling bacteria as the source of resistance genes. Very informative and easy to read. Highly recommended*)

Pawlowski, A.C., Wang, W., Koteva, K., Barton, H.A., McArthur, A.G., Wright, G.D., 2016. A diverse intrinsic antibiotic resistome from a cave bacterium. Nat. Commun. 7, 13803. (*Analyses the resistance genes in a particular bacterium isolated from deep caves and compares it with the surface dwelling species, finding five novel resistance mechanisms. Read in conjunction with Bhullar et al. 2012, above*)

Sandegren, L., Andersson, D.I., 2009. Bacterial gene amplification: implications for the evolution of antibiotic resistance. Nat. Rev. Microbiol. 7, 578–588.

Shlaes, D.M., 2003. The abandonment of antibacterials: why and wherefore? Curr. Opin. Pharmacol. 3, 470–473. (*A good review that explains the reasons underlying the resistance problem and the regulatory and other hurdles that must be overcome before new antibacterials appear on to the market; almost apocalyptic in tone*)

St Georgiev, V., 2000. Membrane transporters and antifungal drug resistance. Curr. Drug Targets 1, 184–261. (*Discusses various aspects of multidrug resistance in disease-causing fungi in the context of targeted drug development*)

Van Bambeke, F., Pages, J.M., Lee, V.J., 2006. Inhibitors of bacterial efflux pumps as adjuvants in antibiotic treatments and diagnostic tools for detection of resistance by efflux. Recent. Pat. Antiinfect. Drug Discov. 1, 157–175.

van Belkum, A., 2000. Molecular epidemiology of methicillin-resistant *Staphylococcus aureus* strains: state of affairs and tomorrow's possibilities. Microb. Drug Resist. 6, 173–187.

Volpato, J.P., Pelletier, J.N., 2009. Mutational 'hot-spots' in mammalian, bacterial and protozoal dihydrofolate reductases associated with antifolate resistance: sequence and structural comparison. Drug Resist. Updat. 12, 28–41.

Walsh, C., 2000. Molecular mechanisms that confer antibacterial drug resistance. Nature 406, 775–781. (*Excellent review outlining the mechanisms of action of antibiotics and the resistance ploys of bacteria; very good diagrams*)

Woodford, N., 2005. Biological counterstrike: antibiotic resistance mechanisms of Gram-positive cocci. Clin. Microbiol. Infect. 3, 2–21. (*A useful reference that classifies antibiotic resistance as one of the major public health concerns of the 21st century and discusses drug treatment for resistant strains*)

Wright, G.D., 2005. Bacterial resistance to antibiotics: enzymatic degradation and modification. Adv. Drug Deliv. Rev. 57, 1451–1470. (*This comprehensive review gives details of the many pathways that have evolved in bacteria to destroy antibiotics. A little complex, but fascinating reading*)

Zasloff, M., 2002. Antimicrobial peptides of multicellular organisms. Nature 415, 389–395. (*Thought-provoking article about the potent broad-spectrum antimicrobial peptides possessed by both animals and plants, which are used to fend off a wide range of microbes; it is suggested that exploiting these might be one answer to the problem of antibiotic resistance*)

Useful web resources

The Global Antibiotic Resistance Partnership (GARP) see https://www.cddep.org/garp/home. (*This, largely charity funded, organisation comprises many national working groups that seek to understand antibiotic usage in countries around the world and make recommendations for sensible and sustainable usage based upon knowledge of local conditions*)

The World Health Organisation (WHO) hosts web pages that deal with the global problem of antibiotics and the regularly-updated *Antibiotic Resistance* Fact Sheet (see http://www.who.int/mediacentre/factsheets/fs194/en) contains definitive information on the current situation around the world.

Antibacterial drugs

52

OVERVIEW

In this chapter we develop the ideas introduced in the previous chapter. A detailed discussion of bacteriology is beyond the scope of this book, but information about some clinically significant pathogens is included to provide necessary context. The major classes of antibacterial[1] drugs are described, along with their mechanism of action, relevant pharmacokinetic properties and adverse effects. We conclude with an overview of new directions in research in this vital area.

INTRODUCTION

In 1928, Alexander Fleming, working at St Mary's Hospital in London, discovered that a culture plate on which staphylococci were being grown had become contaminated with a mould of the genus *Penicillium*. He made the crucial observation that bacterial growth in the vicinity of the mould had been inhibited. He subsequently isolated the mould in pure culture and demonstrated that it produced an antibacterial substance, which he called **penicillin**. This substance was subsequently prepared in bulk, extracted and its antibacterial effects analysed by Florey, Chain and their colleagues at Oxford in 1940. Their experiment showed that it was non-toxic to the host but killed the pathogens in infected mice, and thus ushered in the 'antibiotic era'. Since then, many new types of antibiotics have been discovered and the practice of medicine would be unthinkable without them.

Gram staining and bacterial cell wall structure

Most bacteria are classified as being either *gram-positive* or *gram-negative*, depending on whether they stain with *Gram stain*. This reflects fundamental differences in the structure of their cell walls and has important implications for the action of antibiotics.

The cell wall of gram-positive organisms is a relatively simple structure. It is some 15–50 nm thick and comprises about 50% peptidoglycan (see Ch. 51), 40%–45% acidic polymer together with 5%–10% proteins and polysaccharides. The cell surface is highly polar and negatively charged and this influences the penetration of some antibiotics.

The cell wall of gram-negative organisms is much more complex. From the plasma membrane outwards, it consists of the following:

- A *periplasmic space* containing enzymes and other components.
- A *peptidoglycan layer* 2 nm in thickness, forming 5% of the cell wall mass, which is often linked to outwardly projecting lipoprotein molecules.
- An *outer membrane* consisting of a lipid bilayer, similar in some respects to the plasma membrane, that contains protein molecules and (on its inner aspect) lipoproteins linked to the peptidoglycan. Other proteins form transmembrane water-filled channels, termed *porins*, through which some hydrophilic antibiotics can move freely (see also Ch. 9).
- *Complex polysaccharides* forming important components of the outer surface. These differ between strains of bacteria and are the main determinants of their antigenicity. They are also the source of *endotoxin*, a lipopolysaccharide which, when shed in vivo, triggers various aspects of the inflammatory reaction by activating complement and cytokines, causing fever, etc. (see Ch. 7).

Difficulty in penetrating this complex outer layer explains why some antibiotics are less active against gram-negative than gram-positive bacteria. It is also one reason for the extraordinary antibiotic resistance exhibited by *Pseudomonas aeruginosa*, a pathogen that can cause life-threatening infections in neutropenic patients and those with burns and wounds, as well as chronic bronchial infection in patients with cystic fibrosis. The cell wall lipopolysaccharide is also a major barrier to penetration of some antibiotics, including **benzylpenicillin**, **meticillin**, the macrolides, **rifampicin**, **fusidic acid** and **vancomycin**.

Antibiotics that interfere with bacterial cell wall synthesis (e.g. penicillins) or inhibit crucial enzymes (such as the quinolones) generally kill bacteria (i.e. they are *bactericidal*), while those that inhibit protein synthesis, such as the tetracyclines, tend to be *bacteriostatic*, that is they prevent growth and replication. The distinction is not, however, clinically relevant, as the outcome depends critically on the host response in dealing with compromised bacterial populations.

In discussing the pharmacology of antibacterial drugs, it is convenient to divide them into different groups based upon their mechanism of action.

ANTIBACTERIAL AGENTS THAT INTERFERE WITH FOLATE SYNTHESIS OR ACTION

SULFONAMIDES

In a landmark discovery in the 1930s, prior to the advent of penicillin, Domagk demonstrated that it was possible

---

[1]Strictly speaking, the term 'antibiotic' only applies to antibacterials that are produced by one organism to kill others (e.g. penicillin) in contrast to synthetic compounds such as the sulfonamides. In practice, however, this distinction is often ignored as many antibacterial drugs are 'semi-synthetic' (e.g. flucloxacillin).

- - - Pteridine ring - - -|- - p-Aminobenzoic - -|- -Glutamic acid-
                                   acid (PABA)

H$_2$N

Folic acid

H$_2$N—◯—SO$_2$NH$_2$

Sulfanilamide

H$_2$N—◯—SO$_2$NH—◯

Sulfadiazine

H$_2$N

Trimethoprim (dihydrofolate reductase inhibitor)

Fig. 52.1 **Structures of two representative sulfonamides and trimethoprim.** The structures illustrate the relationship between the sulfonamides and the *p*-aminobenzoic acid moiety in folic acid (*orange box*), as well as between the antifolate drugs and the pteridine moiety (*orange*). Co-trimoxazole is a mixture of sulfamethoxazole and trimethoprim.

Clinical uses of sulfonamides

- Combined with **trimethoprim (co-trimoxazole)** for *Pneumocystis carinii* (now known as *P. jirovecii*), for toxoplasmosis and nocardiasis.
- Combined with **pyrimethamine** for drug-resistant malaria (Table 55.1) and for toxoplasmosis.
- In inflammatory bowel disease: **sulfasalazine** (sulfapyridine–aminosalicylate combination) is used (see Ch. 31).
- For infected burns (silver **sulfadiazine**) given topically

for a drug to suppress a bacterial infection. The drug was a dye called **prontosil**,[2] which proved to be an inactive prodrug that was metabolised in vivo to an active product, **sulfanilamide** (Fig. 52.1). Many sulfonamides have been developed since, but their importance has declined in the face of increasing resistance. The only sulfonamide drugs still commonly used as *systemic* antibacterials are **sulfamethoxazole** (usually in combination with **trimethoprim** as **co-trimoxazole**) and **sulfasalazine** (poorly absorbed in the gastrointestinal (GI) tract, used to treat ulcerative colitis and Crohn's disease; see Chs 27 and 31). Silver **sulfadiazine** is used topically, for example, to treat infected burns. Some drugs with quite different clinical uses (e.g. the antiplatelet drug **prasugrel**, Ch. 25, and the carbonic anhydrase inhibitor **acetazolamide**, Ch. 30), are sulfonamides and share some of the off-target adverse effects of this class.

Mechanism of action

Sulfanilamide is a structural analogue of *p*-aminobenzoic acid (PABA; see Fig. 52.1), which is an essential precursor

in the synthesis of folic acid, required for the synthesis of DNA and RNA in bacteria (see Ch. 51). Sulfonamides compete with PABA for the enzyme *dihydropteroate synthetase*, and the effect of the sulfonamide may be overcome by adding excess PABA. This is why some local anaesthetics, which are PABA esters (such as **procaine**; see Ch. 44), can antagonise the antibacterial effect of these agents.

Sulfonamide action is vitiated in the presence of pus or products of tissue breakdown, because these contain thymidine and purines, which bacteria utilise directly, bypassing the requirement for folic acid. Resistance, which is common, is plasmid-mediated (see Ch. 51) and results from the synthesis of a bacterial enzyme insensitive to the drugs.

▼ *Pharmacokinetic aspects.* Most sulfonamides can be given orally and, apart from sulfasalazine, are well absorbed and widely distributed in the body. There is a risk of sensitisation or allergic reactions when these drugs are given topically. The drugs pass into inflammatory exudates and cross both placental and blood–brain barriers. They are metabolised mainly in the liver, the major product being an acetylated derivative that lacks antibacterial action.

Unwanted effects. Serious adverse effects necessitating cessation of therapy include hepatitis, hypersensitivity reactions (rashes including Stevens–Johnson syndrome and toxic epidermal necrolysis, fever, anaphylactoid reactions – see Ch. 58), bone marrow depression and acute renal failure due to interstitial nephritis or crystalluria. This last effect results from the precipitation of acetylated metabolites in the urine (Ch. 30). Cyanosis caused by methaemoglobinaemia may occur, but is a lot less alarming than it looks. Mild to moderate side effects include nausea and vomiting, headache and mental depression.

TRIMETHOPRIM

Mechanism of action

Trimethoprim is chemically related to the antimalarial drug **pyrimethamine** (Ch. 55), both being folate antagonists. Structurally (see Fig. 52.1), it resembles the pteridine moiety of folate and the similarity is close enough to fool the bacterial dihydrofolate reductase, which is many times more sensitive to trimethoprim than is the equivalent enzyme in humans.

Trimethoprim is active against most common bacterial pathogens as well as protozoa, and is used to treat various urinary, pulmonary and other infections. It is sometimes given in combination with sulfamethoxazole as **co-trimoxazole** (see Fig. 52.1). Because sulfonamides inhibit a different stage on the same bacterial metabolic pathway, they can potentiate the action of trimethoprim (Fig. 52.2).

[2]Domagk believed, wrongly, that the staining property of azo dyes, such as prontosil, was responsible for their antibacterial selectivity. He used prontosil – a red dye – to treat his young daughter for a life-threatening streptococcal infection. She survived, but was left with permanently red-stained skin – testament to its lack of selectivity for the invading bacteria.

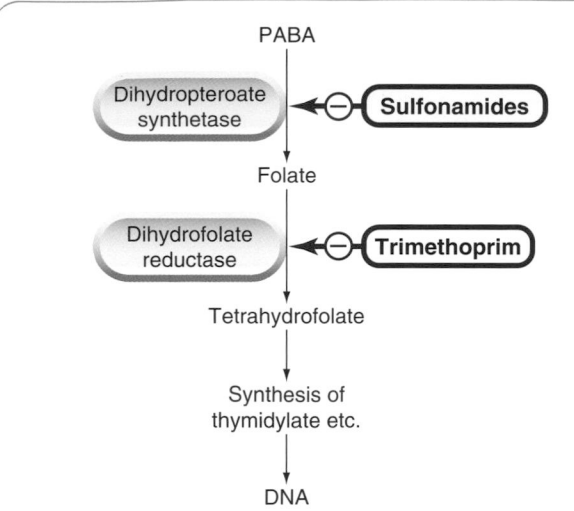

Fig. 52.2 The action of sulfonamides and trimethoprim on bacterial folate synthesis. See Chapter 26 for more detail of tetrahydrofolate synthesis, and Table 51.1 for comparisons of antifolate drugs. *PABA*, *p*-aminobenzoic acid.

In the United Kingdom, the use of co-trimoxazole is generally restricted to the treatment of *Pneumocystis carinii* (now known as *P. jirovecii*) pneumonia (a fungal infection), toxoplasmosis (a protozoan infection) or nocardiasis (a bacterial infection).

▼ *Pharmacokinetic aspects.* Trimethoprim is well absorbed orally, and widely distributed throughout the tissues and body fluids. It reaches high concentrations in the lungs and kidneys, and fairly high concentrations in the cerebrospinal fluid (CSF). When given with sulfamethoxazole, about half the dose of each is excreted within 24 h. Because trimethoprim is a weak base, its elimination by the kidney increases with decreasing urinary pH.

Unwanted effects. Folate deficiency, with resultant megaloblastic anaemia (see Ch. 26) can be caused by long-term administration of trimethoprim. Other unwanted effects include nausea, vomiting, blood disorders and rashes.

Antimicrobial agents that interfere with the synthesis or action of folate

- Sulfonamides are bacteriostatic; they act by interfering with folate synthesis and thus with nucleotide synthesis. Unwanted effects include crystalluria and hypersensitivities.
- **Trimethoprim** is bacteriostatic. It acts by antagonising folate.
- **Co-trimoxazole** is a mixture of **trimethoprim** with **sulfamethoxazole**, which affects bacterial nucleotide synthesis at two points in the pathway.
- **Pyrimethamine** and **proguanil** are also antimalarial agents (see Ch. 55).

β-LACTAM ANTIBIOTICS AND OTHER AGENTS THAT INTERFERE WITH BACTERIAL WALL OR MEMBRANE SYNTHESIS

PENICILLINS

The remarkable antibacterial effects of systemic penicillin in humans were clearly demonstrated in 1941.[3] A small amount of penicillin, extracted laboriously from crude cultures in the laboratories of the Dunn School of Pathology in Oxford, was given to a desperately ill policeman with septicaemia and multiple abscesses. Although sulfonamides were available, they would have had no effect in the presence of pus. Intravenous injections of penicillin were given every 3 h. All of the patient's urine was collected, and each day the bulk of the excreted penicillin was extracted and reused. After 5 days, the patient's condition was vastly improved, and there was obvious resolution of the abscesses. Furthermore, there seemed to be no toxic effects of the drug. Unfortunately, when the supply of penicillin was finally exhausted his condition gradually deteriorated and he died a month later.

Penicillins, often combined with other antibiotics, remain crucially important in antibacterial chemotherapy, but regrettably they are destroyed by bacterial *amidases* and *β-lactamases* (*penicillinases*; Fig. 52.3). This forms the basis of one of the principal types of antibiotic resistance.

Mechanisms of action

All β-lactam antibiotics interfere with the synthesis of the bacterial cell wall peptidoglycan (see Ch. 51, Fig. 51.3). After attachment to *penicillin-binding proteins* on bacteria (there may be seven or more types in different organisms), they inhibit the transpeptidation enzyme that cross-links the peptide chains attached to the backbone of the peptidoglycan.

The final bactericidal event is the inactivation of an inhibitor of autolytic enzymes in the cell wall, leading to lysis of the bacterium. Some organisms, referred to as 'tolerant', have defective autolytic enzymes in which case lysis does not occur in response to the drug. Resistance to penicillin may result from a number of different causes and is discussed in detail in Chapter 51.

Types of penicillin and their antimicrobial activity

The first penicillins were the naturally occurring **benzylpenicillin (penicillin G)** and its congeners, including **phenoxymethylpenicillin (penicillin V)**. Benzylpenicillin is active against a wide range of organisms and is the drug of first choice for many infections (see clinical box). Its main drawbacks are poor absorption in the GI tract (which means it must be given by injection) and its susceptibility to bacterial β-lactamases.

Semisynthetic penicillins, incorporating different side-chains attached to the penicillin nucleus (at R_1 in Fig. 52.3), include *β-lactamase-resistant* penicillins (e.g. **meticillin**,[4] **flucloxacillin**,

---

[3]Although *topical* penicillin had actually been used with success in five patients with eye infections 10 years previously by Paine, a graduate of St Mary's who had obtained some penicillin mould from Fleming.
[4]Meticillin (previous name: methicillin) was the first β-lactamase-resistant penicillin. It is not now used clinically because it was associated with interstitial nephritis, but is remembered in the acronym 'MRSA' – meticillin-resistant *Staphylococcus aureus*, which are resistant to other β-lactamase-resistant penicillins as well as meticillin.

Fig. 52.3 Basic structures of four groups of β-lactam antibiotics and clavulanic acid. The structures illustrate the β-lactam ring *(marked B; outlined in orange)* and the sites of action of bacterial enzymes that inactivate these antibiotics *(A, thiazolidine ring).* Various substituents are added at R₁, R₂ and R₃ to produce agents with different properties. In carbapenems, the stereochemical configuration of the part of the β-lactam ring shown shaded in *orange* here is different from the corresponding part of the penicillin and cephalosporin molecules; this is probably the basis of the β-lactamase resistance of the carbapenems. The β-lactam ring of clavulanic acid is thought to bind strongly to β-lactamase, meanwhile protecting other β-lactams from the enzyme.

Clinical uses of the penicillins

- Penicillins are given by mouth or, in more severe infections, intravenously, and often in combination with other antibiotics.
- Uses are for sensitive organisms and may (but may not: individual sensitivity testing is often appropriate depending on local conditions) include:
  - *bacterial meningitis* (e.g. caused by *Neisseria meningitidis, Streptococcus pneumoniae*): **benzylpenicillin**, high doses intravenously;
  - *bone* and *joint infections* (e.g. with *Staphylococcus aureus*): **flucloxacillin**;
  - *skin* and *soft tissue infections* (e.g. with *Streptococcus pyogenes* or *S. aureus*): **benzylpenicillin, flucloxacillin**; animal bites: **co-amoxiclav**;
  - *pharyngitis* (from *S. pyogenes*): **phenoxymethylpenicillin**;
  - *otitis media* (organisms commonly include *S. pyogenes, Haemophilus influenzae*): **amoxicillin**;
  - *bronchitis* (mixed infections common): **amoxicillin**;
  - *pneumonia*: **amoxicillin**;
  - *urinary tract infections* (e.g. with *Escherichia coli*): **amoxicillin**
  - *gonorrhoea*: **amoxicillin** (plus **probenecid**);
  - *syphilis*: **procaine benzylpenicillin**;
  - *endocarditis* (e.g. with *Streptococcus viridans* or *Enterococcus faecalis*): high-dose intravenous **benzylpenicillin** sometimes with an aminoglycoside;
  - *serious infections with Pseudomonas aeruginosa*: **ticarcillin, piperacillin**.

This list is not exhaustive. Treatment with penicillins is sometimes started empirically, if the likely causative organism is one thought to be susceptible to penicillin, while awaiting the results of laboratory tests to identify the organism and determine its antibiotic susceptibility.

---

temocillin) and *broad-spectrum* penicillins (e.g. **ampicillin, amoxicillin**). *Extended-spectrum* penicillins (e.g. **ticarcillin, piperacillin**) with activity against *Pseudomonas* have gone some way to overcoming the problem of serious infections caused by *P. aeruginosa*. Amoxicillin and ticarcillin are sometimes given in combination with the β-lactamase inhibitor **clavulanic acid** (e.g. **co-amoxiclav**). **Pivmecillinam**

is a prodrug of **mecillinam**, which also has a wide spectrum of action.

▼ *Pharmacokinetic aspects.* Oral absorption of penicillins varies, depending on their stability in acid and their adsorption to foodstuffs in the gut. Penicillins can also be given by intravenous injection. Preparations for intramuscular injection are also available, including slow-release preparations such as benzathine benzylpenicillin which is useful for treating syphilis since *Treponema pallidum* is a very slowly dividing organism. Intrathecal administration of benzylpenicillin (used historically to treat meningitis) is no longer used, as it can cause convulsions.[5]

The penicillins are widely distributed in body fluids, passing into joints; into pleural and pericardial cavities; into bile, saliva and milk and across the placenta. Being lipid-insoluble, they do not enter mammalian cells, and cross the blood–brain barrier only if the meninges are inflamed, in which case they may reach therapeutically effective concentrations in the CSF.

Elimination of most penicillins occurs rapidly and is mainly renal, 90% being through tubular secretion. The relatively short plasma half-life is a potential problem in the clinical use of benzylpenicillin, although because penicillin works by preventing cell wall synthesis in dividing organisms, intermittent rather than continuous exposure to the drug can be an advantage.

Unwanted effects. Penicillins are relatively free from direct toxic effects (other than their proconvulsant effect when given intrathecally). The main unwanted effects are hypersensitivity reactions caused by the degradation products of penicillin, which combine with host protein and become antigenic. Rashes and fever are common; a delayed type of serum sickness occurs infrequently. Much more serious is acute anaphylactic shock which, although rare, may be fatal. When given orally, penicillins, particularly the broad-spectrum type, alter the bacterial flora in the gut. This can be associated with GI disturbances and in some cases with suprainfection by other, penicillin-insensitive, microorganisms leading to problems such as pseudomembranous colitis (caused by *Clostridium difficile*, see later).

CEPHALOSPORINS AND CEPHAMYCINS

Cephalosporins and cephamycins are β-lactam antibiotics, first isolated from fungi. They all have the same mechanism of action as penicillins.

Semisynthetic broad-spectrum cephalosporins have been produced by addition, to the cephalosporin C nucleus, of different side-chains at R_1 and/or R_2 (see Fig. 52.3). These agents are water soluble and relatively acid stable. They vary in susceptibility to β-lactamases. Many cephalosporins and cephamycins are now available for clinical use (see list in Table 52.2). Resistance to this group of drugs has increased because of plasmid-encoded or chromosomal β-lactamase. The latter is present in nearly all gram-negative bacteria and it is more active in hydrolysing cephalosporins than penicillins. In several organisms a single mutation can result in high-level constitutive production of this enzyme. Resistance also occurs when there is decreased penetration of the drug as a result of alterations to outer membrane proteins, or mutations of the binding-site proteins.

▼ *Pharmacokinetic aspects.* Some cephalosporins are given orally, but most are given parenterally, intramuscularly (which may be painful) or intravenously. After absorption, they are widely distributed in the body and some, such as **cefotaxime**, **cefuroxime** and **ceftriaxone**, cross the blood–brain barrier. Excretion is mostly via the kidney, largely by tubular secretion, but 40% of ceftriaxone is eliminated in the bile.

Unwanted effects. Hypersensitivity reactions, very similar to those seen with penicillin, may occur, and there may be some cross-sensitivity; about 10% of penicillin-sensitive individuals will have allergic reactions to cephalosporins. Nephrotoxicity has been reported (especially with cefradine), as has drug-induced alcohol intolerance. Diarrhoea is common and can be due to *C. difficile*.

---

[5]Indeed, penicillins applied topically to the cortex are used to induce convulsions in an animal model of epilepsy (see Ch. 46).

Clinical uses of the cephalosporins

Cephalosporins are used to treat infections caused by sensitive organisms. As with other antibiotics, patterns of sensitivity vary geographically, and treatment is often started empirically. Many different kinds of infection may be treated, including:

- *septicaemia* (e.g. **cefuroxime**, **cefotaxime**)
- *pneumonia* caused by susceptible organisms
- *meningitis* (e.g. **ceftriaxone**, **cefotaxime**)
- *biliary tract infection*
- *urinary tract infection* (especially in pregnancy or in patients unresponsive to other drugs)
- *sinusitis* (e.g. **cefadroxil**)

OTHER β-LACTAM ANTIBIOTICS

Carbapenems and monobactams (see Fig. 52.3) were developed to deal with β-lactamase-producing gram-negative organisms resistant to penicillins.

CARBAPENEMS

Imipenem, an example of a carbapenem, acts in the same way as the other β-lactams (see Fig. 52.3). It has a very broad spectrum of antimicrobial activity, being active against many aerobic and anaerobic gram-positive and gram-negative organisms. However, many of the 'meticillin-resistant' staphylococci are less susceptible, and resistant strains of *P. aeruginosa* have emerged during therapy. Resistance to imipenem was initially low, but is increasing as some organisms now have chromosomal genes that code for imipenem-hydrolysing β-lactamases. The drug is sometimes given together with **cilastatin**, which inhibits its inactivation by renal enzymes. **Meropenem** is similar but is not metabolised by the kidney. **Ertapenem** has a broad spectrum of antibacterial actions but is licensed only for a limited range of indications. Most carbapenems are not orally active, and are used only in special situations.

▼ *Unwanted effects* are generally similar to those seen with other β-lactams, nausea and vomiting being the most frequently seen. Neurotoxicity can occur with high plasma concentrations.

MONOBACTAMS

The main monobactam is **aztreonam** (see Fig. 52.3), which is resistant to most β-lactamases. It is given by injection and has a plasma half-life of 2 h. Aztreonam has an unusual spectrum of activity and is effective only against gram-negative aerobic bacilli such as pseudomonas species, *Neisseria meningitidis* and *Haemophilus influenzae*. It has no action against gram-positive organisms or anaerobes.

▼ *Unwanted effects* are, in general, similar to those of other β-lactam antibiotics, but this agent does not necessarily cross-react immunologically with penicillin and its products, and does not usually cause allergic reactions in penicillin-sensitive individuals.

OTHER ANTIBIOTICS THAT INHIBIT BACTERIAL CELL WALL PEPTIDOGLYCAN SYNTHESIS
GLYCOPEPTIDES

Vancomycin is a glycopeptide antibiotic, and **teicoplanin** is similar but longer lasting. Vancomycin inhibits cell wall synthesis (Ch. 51, Fig. 51.3). It is effective mainly against gram-positive bacteria. Vancomycin is not absorbed from the gut and is only given by the oral route for treatment of GI infection with *C. difficile*.

The main clinical use of vancomycin is the treatment of methicillin-resistant *Staphylococcus aureus* (MRSA). It is often the drug of last resort for this condition, an alarming consideration since vancomycin-resistant *S. aureus*, VRSA, has emerged). It is also valuable in some other serious infections including severe staphylococcal infections in patients allergic to both penicillins and cephalosporins.

▼ *Pharmacokinetic aspects*. For systemic use, it is given intravenously and has a plasma half-life of about 8 h.

Unwanted effects include fever, rashes and phlebitis at the infusion site. Ototoxicity and nephrotoxicity can occur, and hypersensitivity reactions are occasionally seen.

Daptomycin is a relatively new lipopeptide antibacterial with a similar spectrum of actions to vancomycin. It is used, in combination with other drugs, for the treatment of MRSA. **Telavancin** (another lipopeptide) is also active against MRSA and has a longer duration of action than vancomycin.

POLYMIXINS

The polymixin antibiotics comprise **polymixin B** and **colistimethate**. They have cationic detergent properties and disrupt the bacterial outer cell membrane (Ch. 51). They have a selective, rapidly bactericidal action on gram-negative bacilli, especially pseudomonads and coliform organisms.

▼ *Pharmacokinetic aspects*. They are not absorbed from the GI tract. Clinical use of these drugs is limited by their toxicity and is confined largely to gut sterilisation and topical treatment of ear, eye or skin infections caused by susceptible organisms.

Unwanted effects may be serious and include neurotoxicity and nephrotoxicity.

Fosfomycin is a small organic molecule originally found in *Streptomyces*, which blocks peptidoglycan synthesis by inactivating a key enzyme *Mur A*. It has a good spectrum of activity but, currently, fairly limited use for the treatment of urinary tract infections.

ANTIMICROBIAL AGENTS AFFECTING BACTERIAL PROTEIN SYNTHESIS

TETRACYCLINES

The tetracyclines are broad-spectrum antibiotics. The group includes **tetracycline, oxytetracycline, demeclocycline, lymecycline, doxycycline, minocycline** and **tigecycline**.

Mechanism of action
Following uptake into susceptible organisms by active transport, tetracyclines act by inhibiting protein synthesis (see Ch. 51, Fig. 51.4). They are bacteriostatic.

Antibacterial spectrum
The spectrum of antimicrobial activity of the tetracyclines is very wide and includes gram-positive and gram-negative bacteria, *Mycoplasma*, *Rickettsia*, *Chlamydia* spp., spirochaetes and some protozoa (e.g. amoebae). Minocycline is also effective against *N. meningitidis* and has been used to eradicate this organism from the nasopharynx of carriers.

β-Lactam antibiotics

Bactericidal because they inhibit peptidoglycan synthesis.

Penicillins
- The first choice for many infections.
- **Benzylpenicillin**:
  - given by injection, short half-life and is destroyed by β-lactamases;
  - spectrum: gram-positive and gram-negative cocci and some gram-negative bacteria;
  - many staphylococci are now resistant.
- β-Lactamase-resistant penicillins (e.g. **flucloxacillin**):
  - given orally;
  - spectrum: as for benzylpenicillin;
  - many staphylococci are now resistant.
- Broad-spectrum penicillins (e.g. **amoxicillin**):
  - given orally; they are destroyed by β-lactamases;
  - spectrum: as for **benzylpenicillin** (although less potent); they are also active against gram-negative bacteria.
- Extended-spectrum penicillins (e.g. **ticarcillin**):
  - given orally; they are susceptible to β-lactamases;
  - spectrum: as for broad-spectrum penicillins; they are also active against pseudomonads.
- Unwanted effects of penicillins: mainly hypersensitivities.
- A combination of **clavulanic acid** plus **amoxicillin** or **ticarcillin** is effective against many β-lactamase-producing organisms.

Cephalosporins and cephamycins
- Second choice for many infections.
- Oral drugs (e.g. **cefaclor**) are used in urinary infections.
- Parenteral drugs (e.g. **cefuroxime**, which is active against *Staphococcus aureus*, *Haemophilus influenzae*, Enterobacteriaceae).
- Unwanted effects: mainly hypersensitivities.

Carbapenems
- **Imipenem** is a broad-spectrum antibiotic.
- Imipenem is used with **cilastin**, which prevents its breakdown in the kidney.

Monobactams
- **Aztreonam**: active only against gram-negative aerobic bacteria and resistant to most β-lactamases.

However, widespread resistance to these agents has decreased their usefulness. This is transmitted mainly by plasmids and, because the genes controlling resistance to tetracyclines are closely associated with genes for resistance to other antibiotics, organisms may develop resistance to many drugs simultaneously.

▼ *Pharmacokinetic aspects*. The tetracyclines are generally given orally but can also be administered parenterally. Minocycline and doxycycline are well absorbed orally. The absorption of most other tetracyclines is irregular and incomplete but is improved in the absence of food. Because tetracyclines chelate metal ions (calcium, magnesium, iron, aluminium), forming non-absorbable complexes, absorption is decreased in the presence of milk, certain antacids and iron preparations.

Unwanted effects. The commonest unwanted effects are GI disturbances caused initially by direct irritation and later by modification of the gut flora. Vitamin B complex deficiency can occur, as can suprainfection. Because they chelate Ca^{2+}, tetracyclines are deposited in growing bones and teeth, causing staining and sometimes dental hypoplasia and bone deformities. They should therefore not be given to children, pregnant women or nursing mothers. Another hazard to pregnant women is hepatotoxicity. Phototoxicity (sensitisation to sunlight) has also been seen, particularly with demeclocycline. Minocycline can produce vestibular disturbances (dizziness and nausea). High doses of tetracyclines can decrease protein synthesis in host cells, an antianabolic effect that may result in renal damage. Long-term therapy can cause disturbances of the bone marrow.

CHLORAMPHENICOL

Chloramphenicol was originally isolated from cultures of *Streptomyces*. It inhibits bacterial protein synthesis by binding to the 50S ribosomal subunit (see Ch. 51, Fig. 51.4).

Antibacterial spectrum
Chloramphenicol has a wide spectrum of antimicrobial activity, including gram-negative and gram-positive organisms and rickettsiae. It is bacteriostatic for most organisms but kills *H. influenzae*. Resistance, caused by the production of *chloramphenicol acetyltransferase*, is plasmid-mediated.

▼ *Pharmacokinetic aspects.* Given orally, chloramphenicol is rapidly and completely absorbed and reaches its maximum concentration in the plasma within 2 h. It can also be given parenterally. The drug is widely distributed throughout the tissues and body fluids including the CSF. Its half-life is approximately 2 h. About 10% is excreted unchanged in the urine, and the remainder is inactivated in the liver.

Unwanted effects. The most important unwanted effect of chloramphenicol is severe, idiosyncratic depression of the bone marrow, resulting in *pancytopenia* (a decrease in all blood cell elements) – an effect that, although rare, can occur even with low doses in some individuals. Chloramphenicol must be used with great care in newborns, with monitoring of plasma concentrations, because inadequate inactivation and excretion of the drug can result in the 'grey baby syndrome' – vomiting, diarrhoea, flaccidity, low temperature and an ashen-grey colour – which carries 40% mortality. Hypersensitivity reactions can occur, as can GI disturbances secondary to alteration of the intestinal microbial flora.

AMINOGLYCOSIDES

The aminoglycosides are a group of antibiotics of complex chemical structure, resembling each other in antimicrobial activity, pharmacokinetic characteristics and toxicity. The main agents are **gentamicin**, **streptomycin**, **amikacin**, **tobramycin** and **neomycin**.

Mechanism of action
Aminoglycosides inhibit bacterial protein synthesis (see Ch. 51). There are several possible sites of action. Their penetration through the cell membrane of the bacterium depends partly on oxygen-dependent active transport by a polyamine carrier system (which, incidentally, is blocked by chloramphenicol) and they have minimal action against anaerobic organisms. The effect of the aminoglycosides is bactericidal and is enhanced by agents that interfere with cell wall synthesis (e.g. penicillins).

Resistance
Resistance to aminoglycosides is becoming a problem. It occurs through several different mechanisms, the most important being inactivation by microbial enzymes, of which

Table 52.1 Some clinically significant pathogenic bacteria

Genus	Morphology	Species	Disease
Gram-negative			
Bordetella	Cocci	*B. pertussis*	Whooping cough
Brucella	Curved rods	*B. abortus*	Brucellosis (cattle and humans)
Campylobacter	Spiral rods	*C. jejuni*	Food poisoning
Escherichia	Rods	*E. coli*	Septicaemia, wound infections, UTIs
Haemophilus	Rods	*H. influenzae*	Acute respiratory tract infection, meningitis
Helicobacter	Motile rods	*H. pylori*	Peptic ulcers, gastric cancer
Klebsiella	Capsulated rods	*K. pneumoniae*	Pneumonia, septicaemia
Legionella	Flagellated rods	*L. pneumophila*	Legionnaires' disease
Neisseria	Cocci, paired	*N. gonorrhoeae*	Gonorrhoea
Pseudomonas	Flagellated rods	*P. aeruginosa*	Septicaemia, respiratory infections, UTIs
Rickettsiae	Cocci or threads	Several spp.	Tick- and insect-borne infections
Salmonella	Motile rods	*S. typhimurium*	Food poisoning
Shigella	Rods	*S. dysenteriae*	Bacillary dysentery
Yersinia	Rods	*Y. pestis*	Bubonic plague
Vibrio	Flagellated rods	*V. cholera*	Cholera
Gram-positive			
Bacillus	Rods, chains	*B. anthrax*	Anthrax
Clostridium	Rods	*C. tetani*	Tetanus
Corynebacterium	Rod	*C. diphtheria*	Diphtheria
Mycobacterium	Rods	*M. tuberculosis*	Tuberculosis
		M. leprae	Leprosy
Staphylococcus	Cocci, clusters	*S. aureus*	Wound infections, boils, septicaemia
Streptococcus	Cocci, pairs	*S. pneumoniae*	Pneumonia, meningitis
	Cocci, chains	*S. pyogenes*	Scarlet fever, rheumatic fever, cellulitis
Other			
Chlamydia	Gram 'uncertain'	*C. trachomatis*	Eye disease, infertility
Treponema	Flagellated spiral rods	*T. pallidum*	Syphilis

UTI, urinary tract infection.

nine or more are known. Amikacin was designed as a poor substrate for these enzymes, but some organisms can inactivate this agent as well. Resistance as a result of failure of penetration can be largely overcome by the concomitant use of penicillin and/or vancomycin, at the cost of an increased risk of severe adverse effects.

Antibacterial spectrum
The aminoglycosides are effective against many aerobic gram-negative and some gram-positive organisms. They are most widely used against gram-negative enteric organisms and in sepsis. They may be given together with a penicillin in streptococcal infections and those caused by *Listeria* spp. and *P. aeruginosa* (Table 52.1). Gentamicin is the aminoglycoside most commonly used, although tobramycin is the preferred member of this group for *P.*

aeruginosa infections. Amikacin has the widest antimicrobial spectrum and can be effective in infections with organisms resistant to gentamicin and tobramycin.

▼ *Pharmacokinetic aspects.* The aminoglycosides are polycations and therefore highly polar. They are not absorbed from the gastrointestinal tract and are usually given intramuscularly or intravenously. They cross the placenta but do not cross the blood–brain barrier, although high concentrations can be attained in joint and pleural fluids. The plasma half-life is 2–3 h. Elimination is virtually entirely by glomerular filtration in the kidney, 50%–60% of a dose being excreted unchanged within 24 h. If renal function is impaired, accumulation occurs rapidly, with a resultant increase in those toxic effects (such as ototoxicity and nephrotoxicity) that are dose related.
Unwanted effects. Serious, dose-related toxic effects, which may increase as treatment proceeds, can occur with the aminoglycosides, the main hazards being ototoxicity and nephrotoxicity.

Table 52.2 A general overview of antibacterials and their mechanism of action.

Family	Examples	Typical target organism	Cellular target
Sulfonamides	Sulfadiazine, sulfamethoxazole (used together with trimethoprim)	*T. gondii, P. jirovecii*	Bacterial folate synthesis or action. Generally bacteriostatic.
β-lactams	**PENICILLINS** Benzylpenicillin, phenoxymethylpenicillin	Overall, mainly gram-positive spp.; some gram-negative spp.	Bacterial membrane or cell wall /peptidoglycan synthesis. Generally bactericidal.
	Penicillinase-resistant penicillins Flucloxacillin, temocillin	Used for staphylococcal infections	
	Broad-spectrum penicillins Amoxicillin, ampicillin	A wide range of gram-positive and gram-negative spp.	
	Antipseudomonal penicillins Piperacillin, ticarcillin (used with β-lactamase inhibitors)	Selected gram-negative spp., especially *P. aeruginosa*	
	MECILLINAMS Pivmecillinam	Mainly gram-negative spp.	
	CEPHALOSPORINS Cefalcor, cefadroxil, cefalexin, cefixime, cefotaxime, cefradine, ceftaroline, ceftazidime, ceftriaxone, cefuroxime	Broad spectrum of activity against gram-negative and positive spp.	
	CARBAPENEMS Ertapenem, imipenem, meropenem.	Many gram-negative and positive spp. Some anaerobes	
	MONOBACTAMS Aztreonam	Gram-negative aerobes	
Glycopeptides	Vancomycin, teicoplanin, telavancin, daptomycin (actually a lipopeptide)	Many gram-positive spp. Including MRSA.	
Phosphonic acids	Fosfomycin	Many gram-positive and gram-negative spp. Treatment of UTI.	
Polymixins	Colistimethate, polymixin B	Gram-negative spp.	Bacterial outer cell membrane structure
Tetracyclines	Demeclocycline, doxycycline, lymecycline, minocycline, oxytetracycline, tetracycline tigecycline	Broad-spectrum activity against many gram-negative and gram-positive spp.	Bacterial protein synthesis (multiple mechanisms inhibited including initiation, transpeptidation and translocation; see text). Generally bacteriostatic.
Aminoglycosides	Amikacin, gentamicin, neomycin, streptomycin, tobramycin	Many gram-negative, some gram-positive spp.	
Macrolides	Azithromycin, clarithromycin, erythromycin, telithromycin	Similar to penicillin	
Oxazolidinones	Linezolid	Gram-positive spp. including MRSA	
Lincosamides	Clindamycin	Gram-positive spp. Many anaerobes	
Amphenicols	Chloramphenicol	Broad-spectrum activity against gram-negative and gram-positive spp.	
Streptogramins	Quinupristin, dalfopristin	Gram-positive spp.	
Steroidals	Fusidic acid	Narrow spectrum. Gram-positive spp.	
Quinolones	Ciprofloxacin, levofloxacin, moxifloxacin, nalidixic acid, norfloxacin, ofloxacin	Gram-negative and gram-positive spp.	Bacterial DNA synthesis, structure or replication. Generally bacteriostatic.
Macrocyclics	Fidaxomicin	Used to treat *Clostridium difficile*	
Ansamycins	Rifaximin	Traveller's diarrhoea	
Nitroimidazoles	Metronidazole and tinidazole	Treatment of *C. difficile* and other infections.	
Nitrofurans	Nitrofurantoin	Gram-negative UTIs	

Continued

Table 52.2 A general overview of antibacterials and their mechanism of action—cont'd

Family	Examples	Typical target organism	Cellular target
Anti-mycobacterials	Bedaquillone, capreomycin, clofazimine, cycloserine, delamanid, dapsone, ethambutol, isoniazid, pyrazinamide, rifabutin, rifampicin[a]	Most used for mycobacterial infections only	Various unrelated mechanisms (see text)
Miscellaneous	Methenamine	Gram-negative UTIs	Prodrug of formaldehyde (bacteriostatic).

Drug mixtures (e.g. co-fluampicil – flucloxacillin with ampicillin) are not shown.
[a]These drugs are often used in combination.
MRSA, methicillin-resistant staphylococcus aureus; *UTI*, urinary tract infection.

The ototoxicity involves progressive damage to, and eventually destruction of, the sensory cells in the cochlea and vestibular organ of the ear. The result, usually irreversible, may manifest as vertigo, ataxia and loss of balance in the case of vestibular damage, and auditory disturbances or deafness in the case of cochlear damage. Any aminoglycoside may produce both types of effect, but streptomycin and gentamicin are more likely to interfere with vestibular function, whereas neomycin and amikacin mostly affect hearing. Ototoxicity is potentiated by the concomitant use of other ototoxic drugs (e.g. loop diuretics; Ch. 30) and susceptibility is genetically determined via mitochondrial DNA (see Ch. 12).

The nephrotoxicity consists of damage to the kidney tubules and may necessitate dialysis, although function usually recovers if administration ceases as soon as renal toxicity is detected. Nephrotoxicity is more likely to occur in patients with pre-existing renal disease or in conditions in which urine volume is reduced, and concomitant use of other nephrotoxic agents (e.g. first-generation cephalosporins, vancomycin) increases the risk. As the elimination of these drugs is almost entirely renal, this nephrotoxic action can impair their own excretion and a vicious cycle may develop. Plasma concentrations should be monitored regularly and the dose adjusted accordingly.

A rare but serious toxic reaction is paralysis caused by neuromuscular blockade. This is usually seen only if the agents are given concurrently with neuromuscular-blocking agents. It results from inhibition of the Ca²⁺ uptake necessary for the exocytotic release of acetylcholine (see Ch. 14).

MACROLIDES

The term *macrolide* relates to the structure – a many-membered lactone ring to which one or more deoxy sugars are attached. The main macrolide and related antibiotics are **erythromycin**, **clarithromycin** and **azithromycin**. **Telithromycin** is of minor utility.

Mechanism of action

The macrolides inhibit bacterial protein synthesis by an effect on ribosomal translocation (Ch. 51, Fig. 51.4). The drugs bind to the same 50S subunit of the bacterial ribosome as chloramphenicol and **clindamycin**, and any of these drugs may compete if given concurrently.

Antimicrobial spectrum

The antimicrobial spectrum of erythromycin is very similar to that of penicillin, and it is a safe and effective alternative for penicillin-sensitive patients. Erythromycin is effective against gram-positive bacteria and spirochaetes but not against most gram-negative organisms, exceptions being *N. gonorrhoeae* and, to a lesser extent, *H. influenzae*. *Mycoplasma pneumoniae*, *Legionella* spp. and some chlamydial organisms are also susceptible (see Table 52.1). Resistance

can occur and results from a plasmid-controlled alteration of the binding site for erythromycin on the bacterial ribosome (Ch. 51, Fig. 51.4).

Azithromycin is less active than erythromycin against gram-positive bacteria but is considerably more effective against *H. influenzae* and may be more active against *Legionella*. It can be used to treat *Toxoplasma gondii*, as it kills the cysts. Clarithromycin is as active, and its metabolite is twice as active, against *H. influenzae* as erythromycin. It is also effective against *Mycobacterium avium-intracellulare* (which can infect immunologically compromised individuals and elderly patients with chronic lung disease), and it may also be useful in leprosy and against *Helicobacter pylori* (see Ch. 31). Both these macrolides are also effective in *Lyme disease*.

▼ *Pharmacokinetic aspects.* The macrolides are administered orally or parenterally, although intravenous injections can cause local thrombophlebitis. They diffuse readily into most tissues but do not cross the blood–brain barrier, and there is poor penetration into synovial fluid. The plasma half-life of erythromycin is about 90 min; that of clarithromycin is three times longer, and that of azithromycin 8–16 times longer. Macrolides enter and indeed are concentrated within phagocytes – azithromycin concentrations in phagocyte lysosomes can be 40 times higher than in the blood – and they can enhance intracellular killing of bacteria by phagocytes.

Erythromycin is partly inactivated in the liver; azithromycin is more resistant to inactivation, and clarithromycin is converted to an active metabolite. Inhibition of the P450 cytochrome system by these agents can affect the bioavailability of other drugs leading to clinically important interactions, for example, with theophylline (see Ch. 12). The major route of elimination is in the bile.

Unwanted effects. GI disturbances are common and unpleasant but not serious. With erythromycin, the following have also been reported: hypersensitivity reactions such as rashes and fever, transient hearing disturbances and rarely, following treatment for longer than 2 weeks, cholestatic jaundice. Opportunistic infections of the GI tract or vagina can occur.

OXAZOLIDINONES

Originally hailed as the 'first truly new class of antibacterial agents to reach the marketplace in several decades' (Zurenko et al., 2001), the oxazolidinones inhibit bacterial protein synthesis by a novel mechanism: inhibition of N-formylmethionyl-tRNA binding to the 70S ribosome. **Linezolid** is the first member of this new antibiotic family to be introduced. It is active against a wide variety of gram-positive bacteria and is particularly useful for the treatment of drug-resistant bacteria such as MRSA, penicillin-resistant *Streptococcus pneumoniae* and vancomycin-resistant enterococci. The drug is also effective against some anaerobes, such as *C. difficile*. Most common gram-negative organisms are not susceptible to the drug. Linezolid can be used to treat pneumonia, septicaemia, and skin and soft tissue infections. Its use is restricted to serious bacterial infections where other antibiotics have failed, and there have so far been few reports of resistance.

▼ *Unwanted effects* include thrombocytopenia, diarrhoea, nausea and, rarely, rash and dizziness. Linezolid is a non-selective inhibitor of monoamine oxidase, and appropriate precautions need to be observed (see Ch. 48).

FUSIDIC ACID

Fusidic acid is a narrow-spectrum steroidal antibiotic active mainly against gram-positive bacteria. It acts by inhibiting bacterial protein synthesis (Ch. 51, Fig. 51.4), but resistance commonly emerges if it is used as a single agent. It is used in combination with other anti-staphylococcal agents in staphylococcal sepsis, and is used topically for staphylococcal infections (e.g. as eye drops or cream).

▼ *Pharmacokinetic aspects.* As the sodium salt, the drug is well absorbed from the gut and is distributed widely in the tissues. Some is excreted in the bile and some metabolised.

Unwanted effects such as GI disturbances are fairly common. Skin eruptions and jaundice can occur. Resistance occurs if it is used systemically as a single agent so it is always combined with other antibacterial drugs when used systemically.

STREPTOGRAMINS

Quinupristin and **dalfopristin** are cyclic peptides, which inhibit bacterial protein synthesis by binding to the 50S subunit of the bacterial ribosome. Dalfopristin changes the structure of the ribosome so as to promote the binding of quinupristin. Individually, they exhibit only very modest bacteriostatic activity, but combined together as an intravenous injection they are active against many gram-positive bacteria. The combination is used to treat serious infections, usually where no other antibacterial is suitable. For example, the combination is effective against MRSA and vancomycin-resistant *Enterococcus faecium*. They are not currently used in the United Kingdom.

▼ *Pharmacokinetic aspects.* Both drugs undergo extensive first-pass hepatic metabolism and must therefore be given as an intravenous infusion. The half-life of each compound is 1–2 h.

Unwanted effects include inflammation and pain at the infusion site, arthralgia, myalgia and nausea, vomiting and diarrhoea. To date, resistance to quinupristin and dalfopristin does not seem to be a major problem.

CLINDAMYCIN

The lincosamide clindamycin is active against gram-positive cocci, including many penicillin-resistant staphylococci and many anaerobic bacteria such as *Bacteroides* spp. It acts in the same way as macrolides and chloramphenicol (Ch. 51, Fig. 51.4). In addition to its use in infections caused by *Bacteroides* organisms, it is used to treat staphylococcal infections of bones and joints. It is also given topically, as eye drops, for staphylococcal conjunctivitis and as an antiprotozoal drug (see Ch. 55).

▼ *Unwanted effects* consist mainly of GI disturbances, ranging from uncomfortable diarrhoea to potentially lethal pseudomembranous colitis, caused by a toxin-forming *C. difficile*.[6]

---

[6]This may also occur with broad-spectrum penicillins and cephalosporins.

Antimicrobial agents affecting bacterial protein synthesis

- *Tetracyclines* (e.g. **minocycline**). These are orally active, bacteriostatic, broad-spectrum antibiotics. Resistance is increasing. GI disorders are common. They also chelate calcium and are deposited in growing bone. They are contraindicated in children and pregnant women.
- ***Chloramphenicol***. This is an orally active, bacteriostatic, broad-spectrum antibiotic. Serious toxic effects are possible, including bone marrow depression and 'grey baby syndrome'. It should be reserved for life-threatening infections.
- *Aminoglycosides* (e.g. **gentamicin**). These are given by injection. They are bactericidal, broad-spectrum antibiotics (but with low activity against anaerobes, streptococci and pneumococci). Resistance is increasing. The main unwanted effects are dose-related nephrotoxicity and ototoxicity. Serum levels should be monitored. (**Streptomycin** is an antituberculosis aminoglycoside.)
- *Macrolides* (e.g. **erythromycin**). Can be given orally and parenterally. They are bactericidal/bacteriostatic. The antibacterial spectrum is the same as for penicillin. Erythromycin can cause jaundice. Newer agents are **clarithromycin** and **azithromycin**.
- *Lincosamides* (e.g. **clindamycin**). Can be given orally and parenterally. It can cause pseudomembranous colitis.
- *Streptogramins* (e.g. **quinupristin/dalfopristin**). Given by intravenous infusion as a combination. Considerably less active when administered separately. Active against several strains of drug-resistant bacteria.
- ***Fusidic acid***. This is a narrow-spectrum antibiotic that acts by inhibiting protein synthesis. It penetrates bone. Unwanted effects include GI disorders.
- ***Linezolid***. Given orally or by intravenous injection. Active against several strains of drug-resistant bacteria.

Clinical uses of the fluoroquinolones

- Complicated *urinary tract infections* (**norfloxacin, ofloxacin**).
- *Pseudomonas aeruginosa* respiratory infections in patients with cystic fibrosis.
- Invasive external otitis ('malignant otitis') caused by *P. aeruginosa*.
- Chronic gram-negative bacillary osteomyelitis.
- Eradication of *Salmonella typhi* in carriers.
- *Gonorrhoea* (**norfloxacin, ofloxacin**).
- Bacterial *prostatitis* (**norfloxacin**).
- *Cervicitis* (**ofloxacin**).
- *Anthrax*.

Fig. 52.4 A simplified diagram of the mechanism of action of the fluoroquinolones. (A) An example of a quinolone (the quinolone moiety is shown in *orange*). (B) Schematic diagram of *(left)* the double helix and *(right)* the double helix in supercoiled form (see also Fig. 51.6). In essence, the DNA gyrase unwinds the RNA-induced positive supercoil (not shown) and introduces a negative supercoil.

ANTIMICROBIAL AGENTS AFFECTING TOPOISOMERASE

QUINOLONES

The quinolones include the broad-spectrum agents **cipro-floxacin**, **levofloxacin**, **ofloxacin**, **norfloxacin** and **moxi-floxacin** as well as **nalidixic acid**, a narrow-spectrum drug used in urinary tract infections. Most are fluorinated (fluoroquinolones). These agents inhibit topoisomerase II (a bacterial DNA gyrase), the enzyme that produces a negative supercoil in DNA and thus permits transcription or replication (Fig. 52.4).

Antibacterial spectrum and clinical use

Ciprofloxacin is the most commonly used and typical of the group. It is a broad-spectrum antibiotic effective against both gram-positive and gram-negative organisms, including the Enterobacteriaceae (enteric gram-negative bacilli), many organisms resistant to penicillins, cephalosporins and aminoglycosides, and against *H. influenzae*, penicillinase-producing *Neisseria gonorrhoeae*, *Campylobacter* spp. and pseudomonads. Of the gram-positive organisms, streptococci and pneumococci are only weakly inhibited, and there is a high incidence of staphylococcal resistance. Ciprofloxacin should be avoided in MRSA infections. Clinically, the fluoroquinolones are best reserved for infections with

facultative and aerobic gram-negative bacilli and cocci.[7] Resistant strains of *S. aureus* and *P. aeruginosa* have emerged.

▼ *Pharmacokinetic aspects.* Fluoroquinolones are well absorbed following oral administration. The drugs accumulate in several tissues, particularly in the kidney, prostate and lung. All quinolones are concentrated in phagocytes. Most fail to cross the blood–brain barrier, but ofloxacin does so. Aluminium and magnesium antacids interfere with the absorption of the quinolones. Elimination of ciprofloxacin and norfloxacin is partly by hepatic metabolism by P450 enzymes (which they can inhibit, giving rise to interactions with other drugs) and partly by renal excretion. Ofloxacin is excreted in the urine.

Unwanted effects. In hospitals, infection with *C. difficile* may prove hazardous but otherwise unwanted effects are infrequent, usually mild and reversible. The most frequent manifestations are GI disorders and rashes. Arthropathy has been reported in young individuals. Central nervous system (CNS) symptoms – headache and dizziness – have occurred, as have, less frequently, convulsions associated with CNS pathology or concurrent use of theophylline or a non-steroidal anti-inflammatory drug (NSAID) (Ch. 27).

There is a clinically important interaction between ciprofloxacin and theophylline (through inhibition of P450 enzymes), which can lead to theophylline toxicity in asthmatics treated with the fluoroquinolones. The topic is discussed further in Chapter 29. Moxifloxacin prolongs the electrocardiographic QT interval and is used extensively, following FDA guidance, as a positive control in studies in healthy volunteers examining possible effects of new drugs on cardiac repolarisation.

Antimicrobial agents affecting DNA topoisomerase II

- The quinolones interfere with the supercoiling of DNA.
- **Ciprofloxacin** has a wide antibacterial spectrum, being especially active against gram-negative enteric coliform organisms, including many organisms resistant to penicillins, cephalosporins and aminoglycosides; it is also effective against *Haemophilus influenzae*, penicillinase-producing *Neisseria gonorrhoeae*, *Campylobacter* spp. and pseudomonads. There is a high incidence of staphylococcal resistance.
- Unwanted effects include GI tract upsets, hypersensitivity reactions and, rarely, central nervous system disturbances.

MISCELLANEOUS ANTIBACTERIAL AGENTS

Fidaxomicin is a relatively new drug which was originally discovered in actinomycetes. It inhibits bacterial RNA polymerase. It is not used to treat systemic infections as it is poorly absorbed from the gut, but has a role in treating *C. difficile* infections.

METRONIDAZOLE

Metronidazole was introduced as an antiprotozoal agent (see Ch. 55), but it is also active against anaerobic bacteria

[7]When ciprofloxacin was introduced, clinical pharmacologists and microbiologists sensibly suggested that it should be reserved for organisms already resistant to other drugs, to prevent emergence of resistance. However, by 1989 it was already estimated that it was prescribed for 1 in 44 of Americans, so it would seem that the horse had not only left the stable but had bolted into the blue!

such as *Bacteroides*, *Clostridia* spp. and some streptococci. It is effective in the therapy of *pseudomembranous colitis*, and is important in the treatment of serious anaerobic infections (e.g. sepsis secondary to bowel disease). It has a disulfiram-like action (see Ch. 50), so patients must avoid alcohol while taking metronidazole.

NITROFURANTOIN

Nitrofurantoin is a synthetic compound active against a range of gram-positive and gram-negative organisms. The development of resistance in susceptible organisms is rare, and there is no cross-resistance. Its mechanism of action is probably related to its ability to damage bacterial DNA. **Methanamine** has a similar clinical utility to nitrofurantoin and shares several of its unwanted effects. It exerts its effects following slow conversion (in acidic urine) to formaldehyde.

▼ *Pharmacokinetic aspects.* Nitrofurantoin is given orally and is rapidly and totally absorbed from the GI tract and just as rapidly excreted by the kidney. Its use is confined to the treatment of urinary tract infections.

Unwanted effects. GI disturbances are relatively common, and hypersensitivity reactions involving the skin and the bone marrow (e.g. leukopenia) can occur. Hepatotoxicity and peripheral neuropathy have also been reported.

ANTIMYCOBACTERIAL AGENTS

The main mycobacterial infections in humans are tuberculosis (TB) and leprosy, chronic infections caused by *Mycobacterium tuberculosis* and *M. leprae*, respectively. Another mycobacterial infection is *M. avium-intracellulare* (actually two organisms), which can infect some AIDS patients. A particular problem with mycobacteria is that they can survive inside macrophages after phagocytosis, unless these cells are 'activated' by cytokines produced by T-helper (Th)1 lymphocytes (see Chs 7 and 19). Drugs in this section are usually considered separately since some of them are specific for mycobacteria or used only to treat these infections for other reasons.

DRUGS USED TO TREAT TUBERCULOSIS

For centuries, TB was a major killer disease, but the introduction of **streptomycin** in the late 1940s followed by **isoniazid** and, in the 1960s, of **rifampicin** and **ethambutol** revolutionised therapy and TB came to be regarded as an easily treatable condition. Regrettably, this is no longer true. Strains with increased virulence or exhibiting multidrug resistance are now common (Bloom & Small, 1998), and TB now causes more deaths than any other single agent, even though infection rates are slowly falling. It has been estimated that one-third of the world's population (2 billion people) harbour the TB bacillus, 10% of whom will develop the disease at some point in their lifetime. In 2015, the WHO estimated that 10.4 million people (including 1 million children) contracted the disease and some 1.8 million died as a result of the infection. Alarmingly, almost half a million people developed multidrug resistant TB. Poverty-stricken countries in Africa and Asia bear the brunt of the disease, partly because of an ominous synergy between mycobacteria (e.g. *M. tuberculosis*, *M. avium-intracellulare*) and HIV. Infections with the latter increase the risk of catching the disease 20–30 fold and about a quarter of HIV-associated deaths are caused by TB.

Treatment is led by the first-line drugs isoniazid, rifampicin, **rifabutin**, ethambutol and **pyrazinamide**. Second-line drugs include **capreomycin**, **cycloserine**, streptomycin (rarely used now in the United Kingdom), **clarithromycin** and ciprofloxacin. These are used to treat infections likely to be resistant to first-line drugs, or when the first-line agents have to be abandoned because of adverse effects. Two newer drugs, **bedaquiline** and **delamanid**, have recently been introduced for use in multidrug resistant cases of TB, usually in conjunction with other agents.

To decrease the probability of the emergence of resistant organisms, combination drug therapy is usually mandatory. This commonly involves:

- an initial phase of treatment (about 2 months) with a combination of isoniazid, rifampicin and pyrazinamide (plus ethambutol if the organism is suspected to be resistant);
- a second, continuation phase (about 4 months) of therapy, with isoniazid and rifampicin. Longer-term treatment is needed for patients with meningitis, bone/joint involvement or drug-resistant infection.

ISONIAZID

The antibacterial activity of isoniazid is limited to mycobacteria. It halts the growth of resting organisms (i.e. is bacteriostatic) but can also kill dividing bacteria. It passes freely into mammalian cells and is thus effective against intracellular organisms. Isoniazid is a prodrug that must be activated by bacterial enzymes before it can exert its inhibitory activity on the synthesis of *mycolic acids*, important constituents of the cell wall peculiar to mycobacteria. Resistance to the drug, secondary to reduced penetration into the bacterium, may be present, but cross-resistance with other tuberculostatic drugs does not occur.

▼ *Pharmacokinetic aspects.* Isoniazid is readily absorbed from the gastrointestinal tract and is widely distributed throughout the tissues and body fluids, including the CSF. An important point is that it penetrates well into 'caseous' tuberculous lesions (i.e. necrotic lesions with a cheese-like consistency). Metabolism, which involves acetylation, depends on genetic factors that determine whether a person is a slow or rapid acetylator of the drug (see Ch. 12), with slow inactivators enjoying a better therapeutic response. The half-life in slow inactivators is 3 h and in rapid inactivators, 1 h. Isoniazid is excreted in the urine partly as unchanged drug and partly in the acetylated or otherwise inactivated form.

Unwanted effects depend on the dosage and occur in about 5% of individuals, the commonest being allergic skin eruptions. A variety of other adverse reactions have been reported, including fever, hepatotoxicity, haematological changes, arthritic symptoms and vasculitis. Adverse effects involving the central or peripheral nervous systems are largely consequences of pyridoxine deficiency and are common in malnourished patients unless prevented by supplementation of this vitamin. Isoniazid may cause haemolytic anaemia in individuals with glucose 6-phosphate dehydrogenase deficiency, and it decreases the metabolism of the antiepileptics **phenytoin, ethosuximide** and **carbamazepine**, resulting in an increase in the plasma concentration and toxicity of these drugs.

RIFAMPICIN

Rifampicin (also called **rifampin**) acts by binding to, and inhibiting, DNA-dependent RNA polymerase in prokaryotic but not in eukaryotic cells (Ch. 51). It is one of the most active antituberculosis agents known, and is also effective against leprosy and most gram-positive bacteria as well as many gram-negative species. It enters phagocytic cells and kills intracellular tubercle bacilli. Resistance can develop rapidly in a one-step process in which a chromosomal mutation changes its target site on microbial DNA-dependent RNA polymerase (see Ch. 51).

▼ *Pharmacokinetic aspects.* Rifampicin is given orally and is widely distributed in the tissues and body fluids (including CSF), giving an orange tinge to saliva, sputum, tears and sweat. It is excreted partly in the urine and partly in the bile, some of it undergoing enterohepatic cycling. The metabolite retains antibacterial activity but is less well absorbed from the GI tract. The half-life is 1–5 h, becoming shorter during treatment because of induction of hepatic microsomal enzymes.

Unwanted effects are relatively infrequent. The commonest are skin eruptions, fever and GI l disturbances. Liver damage with jaundice has been reported and has proved fatal in a very small proportion of patients, and liver function should be assessed before treatment is started. Rifampicin induces hepatic metabolising enzymes (Ch. 11), increasing the degradation of warfarin, glucocorticoids, narcotic analgesics, oral antidiabetic drugs, **dapsone** and oestrogens, the last effect leading to failure of oral contraception.

ETHAMBUTOL

Ethambutol has no effect on organisms other than mycobacteria. It is taken up by the bacteria and exerts a bacteriostatic effect after a period of 24 h, probably by inhibiting mycobacterial cell wall synthesis. Resistance emerges rapidly if the drug is used alone.

▼ *Pharmacokinetic aspects.* Ethambutol is given orally and is well absorbed. It can reach therapeutic concentrations in the CSF in tuberculous meningitis. In the blood, it is taken up by erythrocytes and slowly released. Ethambutol is partly metabolised and is excreted in the urine.

Unwanted effects are uncommon, the most significant being optic neuritis, which is dose-related and is more likely to occur if renal function is decreased. This results in visual disturbances manifesting initially as red–green colour blindness progressing to a decreased visual acuity. Colour vision should be monitored before and during prolonged treatment.

PYRAZINAMIDE

Pyrazinamide is inactive at neutral pH but tuberculostatic at acid pH. It is effective against the intracellular organisms in macrophages because, after phagocytosis, the organisms are contained in phagolysosomes where the pH is low. The drug probably inhibits bacterial fatty acid synthesis. Resistance develops rather readily, but cross-resistance with isoniazid does not occur.

▼ *Pharmacokinetic aspects.* The drug is well absorbed after oral administration and is widely distributed, penetrating the meninges. It is excreted through the kidney, mainly by glomerular filtration.

Unwanted effects include gout, which is associated with high concentrations of plasma urates. GI upsets, malaise and fever have also been reported. Serious hepatic damage due to high doses was once a problem but is less likely with lower dose/shorter course regimens now used; nevertheless, liver function should be assessed before treatment.

CAPREOMYCIN

Capreomycin is a peptide antibiotic given by intramuscular injection. Its principal mechanism of action is thought to be through binding to the 70S ribosomal unit thereby inhibiting protein synthesis, but it may have other effects on the bacterial cell membrane.

▼ *Unwanted effects* are many and the drug should be used with great caution. They include kidney damage and injury to the auditory

Antituberculosis drugs

To avoid the emergence of resistant organisms, compound therapy is used (e.g. three drugs initially, followed by a two-drug regimen later).

First-line drugs

- **Isoniazid** kills actively growing mycobacteria within host cells. Given orally, it penetrates necrotic lesions, also the cerebrospinal fluid (CSF). 'Slow acetylators' (genetically determined) respond well. It has low toxicity. Pyridoxine deficiency increases risk of neurotoxicity. No cross-resistance with other agents.
- **Rifampicin** is a potent, orally active drug that inhibits mycobacterial RNA polymerase. It penetrates CSF. Unwanted effects are infrequent (but serious liver damage has occurred). It induces hepatic drug-metabolising enzymes. Resistance can develop rapidly.
- **Ethambutol** inhibits growth of mycobacteria. It is given orally and can penetrate CSF. Unwanted effects are uncommon, but optic neuritis can occur. Resistance can emerge rapidly.
- **Pyrazinamide** is tuberculostatic against intracellular mycobacteria. Given orally, it penetrates CSF. Resistance can develop rapidly. Unwanted effects include increased plasma urate and liver toxicity with high doses.

Second-line drugs

- **Capreomycin** is given intramuscularly. Unwanted effects include damage to the kidney and to the auditory nerve.
- **Cycloserine** is a broad-spectrum agent. It inhibits an early stage of peptidoglycan synthesis. Given orally, it penetrates the CSF. Unwanted effects affect mostly the central nervous system.
- **Streptomycin**, an aminoglycoside antibiotic, acts by inhibiting bacterial protein synthesis. It is given intramuscularly. Unwanted effects are ototoxicity (mainly vestibular) and nephrotoxicity.

nerve, with consequent deafness and ataxia. The drug should not be given at the same time as streptomycin or other drugs that may cause deafness.

CYCLOSERINE

Cycloserine is a broad-spectrum antibiotic that inhibits the growth of many bacteria, including coliforms and mycobacteria. It is water-soluble and destroyed at acid pH. It acts by competitively inhibiting bacterial cell wall synthesis. It does this by preventing the formation of D-alanine and the D-Ala-D-Ala dipeptide that is added to the initial tripeptide side-chain on *N*-acetylmuramic acid, i.e. it prevents completion of the major building block of peptidoglycan (Ch. 51, Fig. 51.3). It is absorbed orally and distributed throughout the tissues and body fluids, including CSF. Its use is limited to TB that is resistant to other drugs.

▼ *Pharmacokinetic aspects.* Most of the drug is eliminated in active form in the urine, but approximately 35% is metabolised.

Unwanted effects are mainly on the CNS. A wide variety of disturbances may occur, ranging from headache and irritability to depression, convulsions and psychotic states.

Antileprosy drugs

• For *tuberculoid leprosy*: **dapsone** and **rifampicin** (**rifampin**).
  – **Dapsone** is sulfonamide-like and may inhibit folate synthesis. It is given orally. Unwanted effects are fairly frequent; a few are serious. Resistance is increasing.
  – **Rifampicin** (see *Antituberculosis drugs* box).
• For *lepromatous leprosy*: dapsone, **rifampicin** and **clofazimine**.
  – **Clofazimine** is a dye that is given orally and can accumulate by sequestering in macrophages. Action is delayed for 6–7 weeks, and its half-life is 8 weeks. Unwanted effects include red skin and urine, sometimes GI disturbances.

DRUGS USED TO TREAT LEPROSY

Leprosy is one of the most ancient diseases known to mankind and has been mentioned in texts dating back to 600 BC. The causative organism is *M. leprae*. It is a chronic disfiguring illness with a long latency and, historically, sufferers have been ostracised and forced to live apart from their communities, even though the disease is not particularly contagious. Once viewed as incurable, the introduction in the 1940s of dapsone, and subsequently rifampicin and **clofazimine** in the 1960s, completely changed our perspective on leprosy. It is now generally curable, and the global figures show that the prevalence rates for the disease have dropped by 99% over the last 20 years as a result of public health measures and **M**ulti**d**rug **T**reatment (MDT) regimens (to avoid drug resistance) implemented by WHO and supported by some pharmaceutical companies. The latest (2017) figures from the WHO suggest that the disease has been now eliminated from all but a few small countries. Nevertheless, in 2016, some 210,000 new cases were reported, mainly in Asia and Africa.

There are two forms:

• *Paucibacillary leprosy*, leprosy characterised by one to five numb patches, is mainly *tuberculoid*[8] in type and is generally treated for 6 months with dapsone and rifampicin.
• *Multibacillary leprosy*, characterised by more than five numb skin patches, is mainly *lepromatous* in type and is treated for at least 2 years with rifampicin, dapsone and clofazimine.

DAPSONE

Dapsone is chemically related to the sulfonamides and, because its action is antagonised by PABA, probably acts through inhibition of bacterial folate synthesis. Resistance to the drug has steadily increased since its introduction and treatment in combination with other drugs is now recommended.

▼ *Pharmacokinetic aspects.* Dapsone is given orally; it is well absorbed and widely distributed through the body water and in all tissues. The plasma half-life is 24–48 h, but some drug persists in liver, kidney (and, to some extent, skin and muscle) for much longer periods. There is enterohepatic recycling of the drug, but some is acetylated and excreted in the urine. Dapsone is also used to treat *dermatitis herpetiformis*, a chronic blistering skin condition associated with coeliac disease.

Unwanted effects occur fairly frequently and include haemolysis of red cells (usually not severe enough to lead to frank anaemia), methaemoglobinaemia, anorexia, nausea and vomiting, fever, allergic dermatitis and neuropathy. *Lepra reactions* (an exacerbation of lepromatous lesions) can occur, and a potentially fatal syndrome resembling infectious mononucleosis has occasionally been seen.

CLOFAZIMINE

Clofazimine is a dye of complex structure. Its mechanism of action against leprosy bacilli may involve an action on DNA. It also has anti-inflammatory activity and is useful in patients in whom dapsone causes inflammatory side effects.

▼ *Pharmacokinetic aspects.* Clofazimine is given orally and accumulates in the body, being sequestered in the mononuclear phagocyte system. The plasma half-life may be as long as 8 weeks. The anti-leprotic effect is delayed and is usually not evident for 6–7 weeks.

Unwanted effects may be related to the fact that clofazimine is a dye. The skin and urine can develop a reddish colour and the lesions a blue–black discoloration. Dose-related nausea, giddiness, headache and GI disturbances can also occur.

POSSIBLE NEW ANTIBACTERIAL DRUGS

In contrast to the rapid discoveries and developments that characterised the 'heroic' years of antibiotic research spanning approximately 1950–1980, during which virtually all our existing drugs were produced, the flow has since dried up, with only two completely *novel* antibiotics introduced since 1980 (Jagusztyn-Krynicka & Wysznska, 2008). At the same time, resistance has been increasing, with about half the infection-related deaths in Europe now attributable to drug resistance (Watson, 2008).[9]

Resistance normally appears within 2 years or so of the introduction of a new agent (Bax et al., 2000). In a disquieting review and meta-analysis, Costelloe et al. (2010) concluded that most patients prescribed antibiotics for a respiratory or urinary tract infection develop individual resistance to the drug within a few weeks and that this may persist for up to a year after treatment. Since about half the antibiotic use is for veterinary purposes, it is not just human medicine that is implicated in this phenomenon.

Historically, antibiotics were one of the mainstays of the pharmaceutical industry and the medicines they produced were so successful that, by 1970, it was thought that infectious diseases had been effectively vanquished.[10] Most of the drugs developed since are the result of incremental changes in the structures of a relatively small number of well-known molecular structures, such as the β-lactams,

---

[8]The difference between *tuberculoid* and *lepromatous* disease appears to be that the T cells from patients with the former vigorously produce interferon-γ, which enables macrophages to kill intracellular microbes, whereas in the latter case the immune response is dominated by interleukin-4, which blocks the action of interferon-γ (see Ch. 19).

[9]The worst offenders are sometimes collectively referred to, rather fittingly, as 'ESKAPE pathogens'. The acronym is formed of the initial letters of *E. faecium, S. aureus, K. pneumonia, A. baumanii, P. aeruginosa* and *Enterobacter* spp.
[10]In 1967 the United States Surgeon General announced (in effect) that infectious diseases had been vanquished, and that the researchers should turn their attention to chronic diseases instead.

to which resistance has developed rapidly. Many pharmaceutical companies scaled down their efforts in the area, despite the continuing need for compounds acting by novel mechanisms to keep pace with the adaptive potential of pathogens. The industry was also discouraged by the fear of inadequate returns from antibiotic drugs which may not recoup their initial outlay – evidence of efficacy is difficult to generate and 'success' is rewarded by a product that is used for the shortest duration possible, which physicians will be anxious to restrict in order to minimise the emergence of resistance, for diseases that are most prevalent in poor countries that cannot afford expensive drugs. These and other complex reasons for the failure to develop new antibiotics have been analysed in detail by Coates et al. (2011), who also evaluate many new leads arising from academic and industrial research. Their overall message is rather depressing: they point out that another 20 new classes of antibiotics would need to be discovered in the next 50 years to keep up with the challenges posed by the increasing prevalence of drug resistance.

So the reality is, unfortunately, that the antibiotic pipeline is still far from satisfactory. In the five years leading up to 2016, the FDA only approved eight new antibiotics and some of those were essentially reformulations of existing drugs. Legislation and government initiatives have been introduced in some countries (e.g. United States) which promise fast track FDA approval and extended patent life for those wishing to take the huge financial risks. These, and other potentially useful strategies, have been reviewed in detail by Renwick et al. (2016).

Current approaches include modification of existing drugs (Tillotson, 2016), the isolation and characterisation of new groups of naturally occurring antibiotic substances such as the muramycins (Wiegmann et al., 2016), from plants (Limsuwan et al., 2009) or bacteria (Sit & Vederas, 2008) as well the use of antisense RNA to overcome resistance mechanisms (Ji et al., 2013).

The latest conceptual tools have all been deployed: bioinformatics, utilising information derived from pathogen genome sequencing, is one such approach (Bansal, 2008). The hunt for, and targeting of, bacterial *virulence factors* has shown promise (Escaich, 2008). New types of screening procedures have been devised (Falconer & Brown, 2009) which could reveal novel targets, and sophisticated pharmacodynamic profiling is being brought to bear on the problem (Lister, 2006).

The world awaits developments with bated breath.

REFERENCES AND FURTHER READING

Antibacterial drugs

Allington, D.R., Rivey, M.P., 2001. Quinupristine/dalfopristin: a therapeutic review. Clin. Ther. 23, 24–44.
Ball, P., 2001. Future of the quinolones. Semin. Resp. Infect 16, 215–224. (*Good overview of this class of drugs*)
Blondeau, J.M., 1999. Expanded activity and utility of the new fluoroquinolones: a review. Clin. Ther. 21, 3–15. (*Good overview*)
Duran, J.M., Amsden, G.W., 2000. Azithromycin: indications for the future? Expert Opin. Pharmacother. 1, 489–505.
Greenwood, D. (Ed.), 1995. Antimicrobial Chemotherapy, third ed. Oxford University Press, Oxford. (*Good all-round textbook*)
Lowy, F.D., 1998. *Staphylococcus aureus* infections. N. Engl. J. Med. 339, 520–541. (*Explains the basis of S. aureus pathogenesis of infection, resistance; extensive references; impressive diagrams*)
Perry, C.M., Jarvis, B., 2001. Linezolid: a review of its use in the management of serious gram-positive infections. Drugs 61, 525–551.
Shimada, J., Hori, S., 1992. Adverse effects of fluoroquinolones. Prog. Drug Res. 38, 133–143.
Zurenko, G.E., Gibson, J.K., Shinabarger, D.L., et al., 2001. Oxazolidinones: a new class of antibacterials. Curr. Opin. Pharmacol. 1, 470–476. (*Easy-to-assimilate review that discusses this relatively new group of antibacterials*)

Resistance (see also reading list in Ch. 51)

Bax, R., Mullan, N., Verhoef, J., 2000. The millennium bugs – the need for and development of new antibacterials. Int. J. Antimicrob. Agents 16, 51–59. (*Good review that includes an account of the development of 'resistance' and a round-up of potential new drugs*)
Bloom, B.R., Small, P.M., 1998. The evolving relation between humans and *Mycobacterium tuberculosis*. Lancet 338, 677–678. (*Editorial comment*)
Coates, A.R., Halls, G., Hu, Y., 2011. Novel classes of antibiotics or more of the same? Br. J. Pharmacol. 163, 184–194. (*A comprehensive review that sets out the challenges we face because of antibiotic resistance. Also includes a survey of potential new leads. Easy to read and highly recommended*)
Costelloe, C., Metcalfe, C., Lovering, A., Mant, D., Hay, A.D., 2010. Effect of antibiotic prescribing in primary care on antimicrobial resistance in individual patients: systematic review and meta-analysis. BMJ 340, c2096. (*Details the incidence of resistance following simple antibiotic regimes. Truly depressing*)
Courvalin, P., 1996. Evasion of antibiotic action by bacteria. J. Antimicrob. Chemother. 37, 855–869. (*Covers developments in the understanding of the genetics and biochemical mechanisms of resistance*)
Gold, H.S., Moellering, R.C., 1996. Antimicrobial drug resistance. N. Engl. J. Med. 335, 1445–1453. (*Excellent well-referenced review; covers mechanisms of resistance of important organisms to the main drugs; has useful table of therapeutic and preventive strategies, culled from the literature*)
Iseman, M.D., 1993. Treatment of multidrug-resistant tuberculosis. N. Engl. J. Med. 329, 784–791.
Livermore, D.M., 2000. Antibiotic resistance in staphylococci. J. Antimicrob. Agents 16, S3–S10. (*Overview of problems of bacterial resistance*)
Michel, M., Gutman, L., 1997. Methicillin-resistant *Staphylococcus aureus* and vancomycin-resistant enterococci: therapeutic realities and possibilities. Lancet 349, 1901–1906. (*Excellent review article; good diagrams*)
Nicas, T.I., Zeckel, M.L., Braun, D.K., 1997. Beyond vancomycin: new therapies to meet the challenge of glycopeptide resistance. Trends Microbiol. 5, 240–249.
Watson, R., 2008. Multidrug resistance responsible for half of deaths from healthcare associated infections in Europe. BMJ 336, 1266–1267.

New approaches to antibacterial drug discovery

(*These papers have been provided for those who want to learn more about the work under way to develop novel antibacterial drugs. Some are quite technical in nature*)
Bansal, A.K., 2008. Role of bioinformatics in the development of new antibacterial therapy. Expert Rev. Anti Infect. Ther. 6, 51–65.
Draenert, R., Seybold, U., Grutzner, E., Bogner, J.R., 2015. Novel antibiotics: are we still in the pre-post-antibiotic era? Infection 43, 145–151.
Escaich, S., 2008. Antivirulence as a new antibacterial approach for chemotherapy. Curr. Opin. Chem. Biol. 12, 400–408.
Falconer, S.B., Brown, E.D., 2009. New screens and targets in antibacterial drug discovery. Curr. Opin. Microbiol. 12, 497–504.
Jagusztyn-Krynicka, E.K., Wyszynska, A., 2008. The decline of antibiotic era – new approaches for antibacterial drug discovery. Pol. J. Microbiol. 57, 91–98.
Ji, Y., Lei, T., 2013. Antisense RNA regulation and application in the development of novel antibiotics to combat multidrug resistant bacteria. Sci. Prog. 96, 43–60.
Limsuwan, S., Trip, E.N., Kouwen, T.R., et al., 2009. Rhodomyrtone: a new candidate as natural antibacterial drug from *Rhodomyrtus tomentosa*. Phytomedicine 16, 645–651.
Lister, P.D., 2006. The role of pharmacodynamic research in the assessment and development of new antibacterial drugs. Biochem. Pharmacol. 71, 1057–1065.
Loferer, H., 2000. Mining bacterial genomes for antimicrobial targets. Mol. Med. Today 6, 470–474. (*An interesting article focusing on the way*

in which a better understanding of the bacterial genome may lead to new drugs)

O'Neill, A.J., 2008. New antibacterial agents for treating infections caused by multi-drug resistant Gram-negative bacteria. Expert. Opin. Invest. Drugs 17, 297–302.

Renwick, M.J., Brogan, D.M., Mossialos, E., 2016. A systematic review and critical assessment of incentive strategies for discovery and development of novel antibiotics. J. Antibiot. (Tokyo) 69, 73–88.

Sit, C.S., Vederas, J.C., 2008. Approaches to the discovery of new antibacterial agents based on bacteriocins. Biochem. Cell Biol. 86, 116–123.

Tillotson, G.S., 2016. Trojan horse antibiotics-a novel way to circumvent gram-negative bacterial resistance? Infect. Dis. (Auckl.) 9, 45–52.

Wiegmann, D., Koppermann, S., Wirth, M., Niro, G., Leyerer, K., Ducho, C., 2016. Muraymycin nucleoside-peptide antibiotics: uridine-derived natural products as lead structures for the development of novel antibacterial agents. Beilstein J. Org. Chem. 12, 769–795.

Useful website

http://www.who.int. (*Once again, the World Health Organization website is a mine of information about the demographics and treatment of infectious diseases. The sections on leprosy and tuberculosis are especially worthwhile studying. The site includes photographs, maps and much statistical information, as well as information on drug resistance. Highly recommended*)

53 Antiviral drugs

OVERVIEW

This chapter deals with drugs used to treat infections caused by viruses. We first provide some basic information about viruses, including a simple outline of their structure, a list of the main pathogenic species and a brief summary of the life history of an infectious species. We then continue with a consideration of the host–virus interaction: the defences deployed by the human host against viruses and the strategies employed by viruses to evade these measures. We then discuss the various types of antiviral drugs and their mechanisms of action, with particular reference to the treatment of acquired immunodeficiency syndrome (AIDS), an infection caused by the human immunodeficiency virus (HIV).

BACKGROUND INFORMATION ABOUT VIRUSES

AN OUTLINE OF VIRUS STRUCTURE

Viruses are small (usually in the range 20–30 nm) infective agents that are incapable of reproduction outside their host cells. The free-living virus particle is termed a *virion*, and consists of segments of nucleic acid (either RNA or DNA) enclosed in a protein coat comprised of symmetrical repeating structural units and called a *capsid* (Fig. 53.1). The viral coat, together with the nucleic acid core, is termed the *nucleocapsid*. Some viruses have a further external lipoprotein envelope, which may be decorated with antigenic viral glycoproteins or phospholipids acquired from its host when the nucleocapsid buds through the membranes of the infected cell. Certain viruses also contain enzymes that initiate their replication in the host cell.

Viruses are generally characterised either as *DNA or RNA viruses*, depending on the nature of their nucleic acid content. These two broad categories are conventionally subdivided into subgroups, which classify viruses according to whether they contain single- or double-stranded nucleic acids and how this functions during replication.

EXAMPLES OF PATHOGENIC VIRUSES

Viruses can infect virtually all living organisms, and they are a common cause of disease in humans. Some important examples are as follows:

- *DNA viruses*: poxviruses (smallpox), herpesviruses (chickenpox, shingles, cold sores, glandular fever), adenoviruses (sore throat, conjunctivitis) and papillomaviruses (warts).

- *RNA viruses*: orthomyxoviruses (influenza), paramyxoviruses (measles, mumps, respiratory tract infections), rubella virus (German measles), rhabdoviruses (rabies), picornaviruses (colds, meningitis, poliomyelitis), retroviruses (AIDS, T-cell leukaemia), arenaviruses (meningitis, Lassa fever), hepadnaviruses (serum hepatitis) and arboviruses (various **ar**thropod-**bo**rne illnesses, e.g. encephalitis, yellow fever).

VIRUS FUNCTION AND LIFE HISTORY

Viruses have no metabolic machinery of their own, so to replicate they must first attach to and penetrate a living host cell – animal, plant or bacterial – and hijack the victim's own metabolic processes. The first step in this process is facilitated by polypeptide binding sites on the envelope or capsid which interact with receptors on the host cell. These 'receptors' are normal membrane constituents, for example, receptors for cytokines, neurotransmitters or hormones, ion channels, integral membrane glycoproteins, etc. Some examples are listed in Table 53.1.

Following attachment, the receptor–virus complex enters the cell, often utilising receptor-mediated endocytosis (though some viruses bypass this route). The virus coat is removed by host cell enzymes (often lysosomal in nature) and the virion is dismantled. This is known as the *eclipse phase* of viral infection because virus particles can no longer be detected. Within the host cell the viral nucleic acid is released and then utilises the host cellular machinery to synthesise nucleic acids and proteins. These are subsequently assembled into new virus particles and released from the cell during the *shedding* (or *budding*) phase. The actual way in which this occurs differs between DNA and RNA viruses.

Replication of DNA viruses

Viral DNA enters the host cell nucleus (and may become incorporated into host DNA), where transcription into mRNA occurs catalysed by the host cell *RNA polymerase*. Translation of the mRNA into virus-specific proteins then takes place. Some of these proteins are enzymes which then synthesise more viral DNA, as well as structural proteins comprising the viral coat and envelope. After assembly of coat proteins around the viral DNA, complete virions are released by shedding or after host cell lysis.

Replication of RNA viruses

Enzymes within the virion synthesise its mRNA from the viral RNA template (sometimes the viral RNA serves as its own mRNA). This is translated by the host cell into various enzymes, including *RNA polymerase* (which directs the synthesis of more viral RNA), and also into structural proteins for the virion. Assembly and release of virions

Fig. 53.1 Schematic diagram of the components of a virus particle or virion.

Table 53.1 Some host cell structures that can function as receptors for viruses

Host cell structure[a]	Virus(es)
Helper T lymphocytes CD4 glycoprotein	HIV (causing AIDS)
CCR5 receptor for chemokines MCP-1 and RANTES	HIV (causing AIDS)
CXCR4 chemokine receptor for cytokine SDF-1	HIV (causing AIDS)
Acetylcholine receptor on skeletal muscle	Rabies virus
B lymphocyte complement C3d receptor	Glandular fever virus
T lymphocyte interleukin-2 receptor	T-cell leukaemia viruses
β-Adrenoceptors	Infantile diarrhoea virus
MHC molecules	Adenovirus (causing sore throat and conjunctivitis) T-cell leukaemia viruses

[a]For more detail on complement, interleukin-2, the CD4 glycoprotein on helper T lymphocytes, MHC molecules, etc., see Chapter 7.
MCP-1, monocyte chemoattractant protein-1; *MHC*, major histocompatibility complex; *RANTES*, regulated on activation normal T cell expressed and secreted; *SDF-1*, stromal cell-derived factor-1.

then occurs as explained earlier. The host cell nucleus is not usually involved in replication of RNA viruses, although some (e.g. *orthomyxoviruses*) replicate exclusively within the host nuclear compartment.

Replication in retroviruses
Retroviruses contain RNA but may nevertheless be incorporated in host DNA. To achieve this, the virion in retroviruses[1] contains a unique enzyme, *reverse transcriptase* (virus

---
[1]Viruses that can synthesise DNA from an RNA template – the reverse of the normal situation.

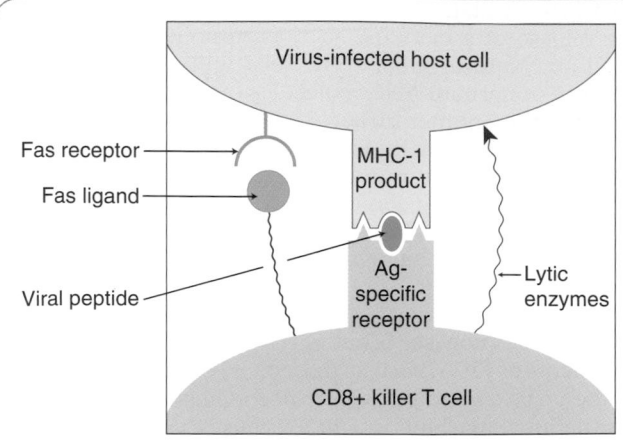

Fig. 53.2 How a CD8+ T cell kills a virus-infected host cell. The virus-infected host cell expresses a complex of virus peptides plus major histocompatibility complex class I product (MHC-I) on its surface. This is recognised by the CD8+ T cell, which then releases lytic enzymes into the virus-infected cell. The killer T cell also expresses a Fas ligand which triggers apoptosis in the infected cell by stimulating its Fas 'death receptor'.

RNA-dependent DNA polymerase), which makes a DNA copy of the viral RNA. This DNA copy can then be integrated into the host genome, and it is then termed a *provirus*. The provirus DNA is transcribed into both new viral genome RNA as well as mRNA for translation in the host into viral proteins, and the completed viruses are again released by budding. Many retroviruses can replicate without killing the host cell.

Like the DNA viruses, some retroviruses remain dormant in the genome being replicated, together with host genetic material. This accounts for the periodic nature of some viral diseases, such as those caused by *herpes labialis* (cold sores) or *varicella zoster* – another type of herpes virus (which causes chickenpox and shingles), which can recur when viral replication is reactivated by some factor (or when the immune system is compromised in some way). Other RNA retroviruses (e.g. the *Rous sarcoma* virus) can transform normal cells into malignant cells (a serious concern with use of retroviral vectors for gene therapy, see Ch. 5).

THE HOST–VIRUS INTERACTION

HOST DEFENCES AGAINST VIRUSES
The host's first line of defence is the simple barrier function of intact skin, which most viruses are unable to penetrate. However, broken skin (e.g. at sites of wounds or insect bites) and mucous membranes are more vulnerable to viral attack. Should the virus gain entry to the body, then the host will deploy both an innate and, subsequently, an adaptive immune response (Ch. 7) to limit the incursion. An infected cell presents viral peptides, complexed with major histocompatibility complex (MHC) class I molecules on its surface. This is recognised by T lymphocytes, which then kill the infected cell (Fig. 53.2). Killing may be accomplished by the release of lytic proteins (such as *perforins*, *granzymes*) or by triggering the apoptotic pathway of the infected cell by activation of its Fas receptor ('death receptor',

see Ch. 6). The latter may also be triggered indirectly through the release of a cytokine such as tumour necrosis factor (TNF)-α. Natural killer (NK) cells will also react to the absence of normal MHC molecules by killing the cell. This is called the 'mother turkey' strategy (kill everything that does not sound exactly like a baby turkey; see Ch. 7). The virus may escape immune detection by cytotoxic lymphocytes by modifying the expression of the peptide–MHC complex (see Ch. 7), but still fall victim to NK cells, though some viruses also have a device for evading NK cells as well (see later).

Within the cell itself, *gene silencing* provides a further level of protection (see Schutze, 2004). Short double-stranded fragments of RNA, such as those that could arise as a result of the virus's attempts to recruit the host's transcription/translational machinery, actually cause the gene coding for the RNA to be 'silenced' – to be switched off. The gene is then no longer able to direct further viral protein synthesis and replication is halted. This mechanism can be exploited for experimental purposes in many areas of biology, and tailored siRNA (*small- or short-interfering RNA*) is a cheap and useful technique to suppress temporarily the expression of a particular gene of interest. Attempts to harness the technique for viricidal purposes have met with some success (see Barik, 2004), and are beginning to find their way into therapeutics (see Ch. 5).

VIRAL PLOYS TO CIRCUMVENT HOST DEFENCES

Viruses have evolved a variety of strategies to ensure successful infection, some entailing redirection of the host's response for the advantage of the virus (discussed by Tortorella et al., 2000). Some examples are discussed later.

Subversion of the immune response

Viruses can inhibit the synthesis or action of cytokines, such as interleukin-1, TNF-α and antiviral interferons (IFNs) that normally coordinate the innate and adaptive immune responses. For example, following infection, some poxviruses express proteins that mimic the extracellular ligand-binding domains of cytokine receptors. These *pseudoreceptors* bind cytokines, preventing them from reaching their natural receptors on cells of the immune system and thus moderating the normal immune response to virus-infected cells. Other viruses that can interfere with cytokine signalling include human cytomegalovirus, Epstein–Barr virus, herpesvirus and adenovirus.

Evasion of immune detection and attack by killer cells

Once within host cells, viruses may also escape immune detection and evade lethal attack by cytotoxic lymphocytes and NK cells in various ways, such as:

- *Interference with the surface protein markers on the infected cells necessary for killer cell recognition and attack.* Some viruses inhibit generation of the antigenic peptide and/or the presentation of MHC–peptide molecules that signals that the cells are infected. In this way, the viruses remain undetected. Examples of viruses that can do this are adenovirus, herpes simplex virus, human cytomegalovirus, Epstein–Barr virus and influenza virus.
- *Interference with the apoptotic pathway.* Adenovirus, human cytomegalovirus and Epstein–Barr virus can subvert this pathway to ensure their own survival.

- *Fooling the 'baby turkey' ploy.* Other viruses (e.g. cytomegalovirus) get round the 'mother turkey strategy' of NK cells by expressing a homologue of MHC class I (the equivalent of a turkey chick's chirping) that is close enough to the real thing to hoodwink NK cells.

It is evident that natural selection has equipped pathogenic viruses with many efficacious tactics for circumventing host defences, and understanding these in more detail is likely to suggest new types of antiviral therapy. Fortunately, the biological arms race is not one-sided, and evolution has also equipped the host with sophisticated countermeasures. In the majority of cases these prevail, and most viral infections eventually resolve spontaneously, except in immunocompromised hosts. The situation does not always end happily though; some viral infections, such as Lassa fever and Ebola virus infection, have a high mortality and we now discuss a further, grave, example: the HIV virus. This emphasis is appropriate because, whilst the infection develops more slowly than (e.g.) Ebola virus, HIV exhibits many of the features common to other viral infections, and the sheer scale of the global AIDS problem has pushed HIV to the top of the list of antiviral targets.

Viruses

- Viruses are small infective agents consisting of nucleic acid (RNA or DNA) enclosed in a protein coat.
- They are not cells and, having no metabolic machinery of their own, are obligate intracellular parasites, utilising the metabolic processes of the host cell to replicate.
- *DNA viruses* (e.g. herpes virus) usually enter the host cell nucleus and direct the generation of new viruses.
- *RNA viruses* (e.g. rubella virus) usually direct the generation of new viruses without involving the host cell nucleus (the influenza virus is an exception).
- *RNA retroviruses* (e.g. HIV, T-cell leukaemia virus) contain an enzyme, reverse transcriptase, which makes a DNA copy of the viral RNA. This DNA copy is integrated into the host cell genome and directs the generation of new virus particles.

HIV AND AIDS

HIV is an RNA retrovirus. Two forms are known: *HIV-1* is the principal organism responsible for human AIDS. The *HIV-2* organism is similar to the HIV-1 virus in that it also causes immune suppression, but it is less virulent. HIV-1 is distributed around the world, whereas the HIV-2 virus is confined to parts of Africa.

▼ The HIV/AIDS epidemic is overwhelmingly centred on sub-Saharan Africa, which accounts for two-thirds of the total global number of infected persons, and where the adult prevalence is over 10 times greater than in Europe. For a review of the pathogenesis (and many other aspects) of AIDS, see Moss (2013).

Thanks to increased availability of effective drug therapy, the global situation is improving and the number of AIDS-related deaths is falling. Even so, recent statistics (UNAIDS, 2016) suggest that over 36 million people are presently living with HIV, including over 2 million children (a particularly horrid thought) and that new infections are appearing at the rate of about 2 million per year.

More optimistically, the overall infection rate amongst adults has declined by more than 10% since 2010 and by almost 50% in the case of children. Global deaths from HIV have also fallen by almost half since 2005 and access to antiretroviral therapy has increased year upon year. Currently some 19 million people are receiving the drugs – approximately half of all those suffering from HIV.

INDUCTION OF THE DISEASE

The interaction of HIV with the host's immune system is complex, and although it involves mainly cytotoxic T lymphocytes (CTLs, CD8+ T cells) and CD4+ helper T lymphocytes (CD4+ cells), other immune cells, such as macrophages, dendritic cells and NK cells, also play a part. Antibodies are produced by the host to various HIV components, but it is the action of the CTLs and CD4+ cells that initially prevents the spread of HIV within the host.

- **Cytotoxic T lymphocytes** (**CTLs**) directly kill virally infected cells and produce and release antiviral cytokines (see Fig. 53.2). The lethal event is lysis of the target cell, but induction of apoptosis by interaction of Fas ligand (see Ch. 6) on the CTL with Fas receptors on the virally infected cell also plays a part.
- **CD4+ cells** have an important role as helper cells and may have a direct role in the control of HIV replication (e.g. lysis of target cells: Norris et al., 2004). It is the progressive loss of these cells that is the defining characteristic of HIV infection (see Fig. 53.4 later).

The priming of naive T cells to become CTL during the induction phase involves interaction of the T-cell receptor complex with antigenic HIV peptide, in association with MHC class I molecules on the surface of antigen-presenting cells (APCs; see Ch. 7). Priming also requires the presence and participation of CD4+ cells. It is thought that both types of cell need to recognise antigen on the surface of the same APC.

The CTLs thus generated are effective during the initial stages of the infection but are not able to stop the progression of the disease. It is believed that this is because they become 'exhausted' and unable to maintain their protective function. Different mechanisms may be involved (see Jansen et al., 2004, and Barber et al., 2006, for further details).

▼ The HIV virion cannily attaches to proteins on the host cell surface to gain entry to the cells. The main targets are CD4 (the glycoprotein marker of a particular group of helper T lymphocytes) and CCR5 (a co-receptor for certain chemokines, including monocyte chemoat-tractant protein-1 and RANTES; see Ch. 7). CD4+ cells normally orchestrate the immune response to viruses, but by entering these cells and using them as virion factories, HIV virtually cripples this aspect of the immune response. Fig. 53.3 shows an HIV virion infecting a CD4+ T cell. Such infected activated cells in lymphoid tissue form the major source of HIV production in HIV-infected individuals; infected macrophages are another source.

As for CCR5, evidence from exposed individuals who somehow evade infection indicates that this surface protein has a central role in HIV pathogenesis. Compounds that inhibit the entry of HIV into cells by blocking CCR5 are now available.

When immune surveillance breaks down, other strains of HIV arise, through spontaneous mutational events, which recognise other host cell surface molecules. A surface glycoprotein, gp120, on the HIV envelope recognises and binds to CD4 and also to the T-cell chemokine co-receptor CXCR4. Another viral glycoprotein, gp41, then causes fusion of the viral envelope with the plasma membrane of the cell (see Fig. 53.3).

PROGRESS OF INFECTION

Once within the cell, the HIV RNA directs synthesis of DNA (the provirus) which is integrated with the host DNA, undergoes transcription and begins to generate new virions. This process, which takes less than 48 h, can lead to the release of a staggering 10^{10} new virus particles each day (see Fig. 53.3). Intracellular HIV can remain silent (latent) for a long time.

Viral replication is highly error prone. Many mutations occur daily at each site in the HIV genome, so HIV soon escapes recognition by the original cytotoxic lymphocytes. Although other cytotoxic lymphocytes arise that recognise the altered virus protein(s), further mutations eventually allow escape from surveillance by these cells too. It is suggested that wave after wave of cytotoxic lymphocytes act against new mutants as they arise, gradually depleting a T-cell repertoire already seriously compromised by the loss of CD4+ helper T cells, until eventually the immune response falters or completely fails.

There is considerable variability in the progress of the disease, but the usual clinical course of an untreated HIV infection is shown in Fig. 53.4. An initial acute influenza-like illness is associated with an increase in the number of virus particles in the blood, their widespread dissemination through the tissues and the seeding of lymphoid tissue with the virion particles. Within a few weeks, this *viraemia* is reduced by the action of cytotoxic lymphocytes as explained earlier.

The acute initial illness is followed by a symptom-free period during which there is reduction in the viraemia accompanied by silent virus replication in the lymph nodes, associated with damage to lymph node architecture and the loss of CD4+ lymphocytes and dendritic cells. Clinical latency (median duration 10 years) comes to an end when the immune response finally fails and the signs and symptoms of AIDS appear – opportunistic infections (e.g. *Pneumocystis* pneumonia or tuberculosis), neurological disease (e.g. confusion, paralysis, dementia), bone marrow depression and malignancies such as lymphoma and *Kaposi's sarcoma*.[2] Chronic gastrointestinal (GI) infections contribute to the severe weight loss. Cardiovascular and kidney damage can also occur. In an untreated patient, death usually follows within 2 years. The advent of effective drug regimens has greatly improved the prognosis in countries that are able to deploy them and patients thus treated may enjoy a near-normal life expectancy.

There is evidence that genetic factors play an important role in determining the susceptibility – or resistance – to HIV (see Flores-Villanueva et al., 2003).

ANTIVIRAL DRUGS

Because viruses hijack many of the metabolic processes of the host cell itself, it is difficult to find drugs that are selective for the pathogen. However, there are some enzymes that are virus-specific and these have proved to be useful drug targets. Most currently available antiviral agents are effective

---

[2]A tumor caused by infection with human herpesvirus 8 (HHV8), also known as Kaposi's sarcoma-associated herpesvirus (KSHV) or KS agent, was originally described by Moritz Kaposi, a Hungarian dermatologist practicing at the University of Vienna in 1872. It became more widely known as one of the AIDS-defining illnesses in the 1980s.

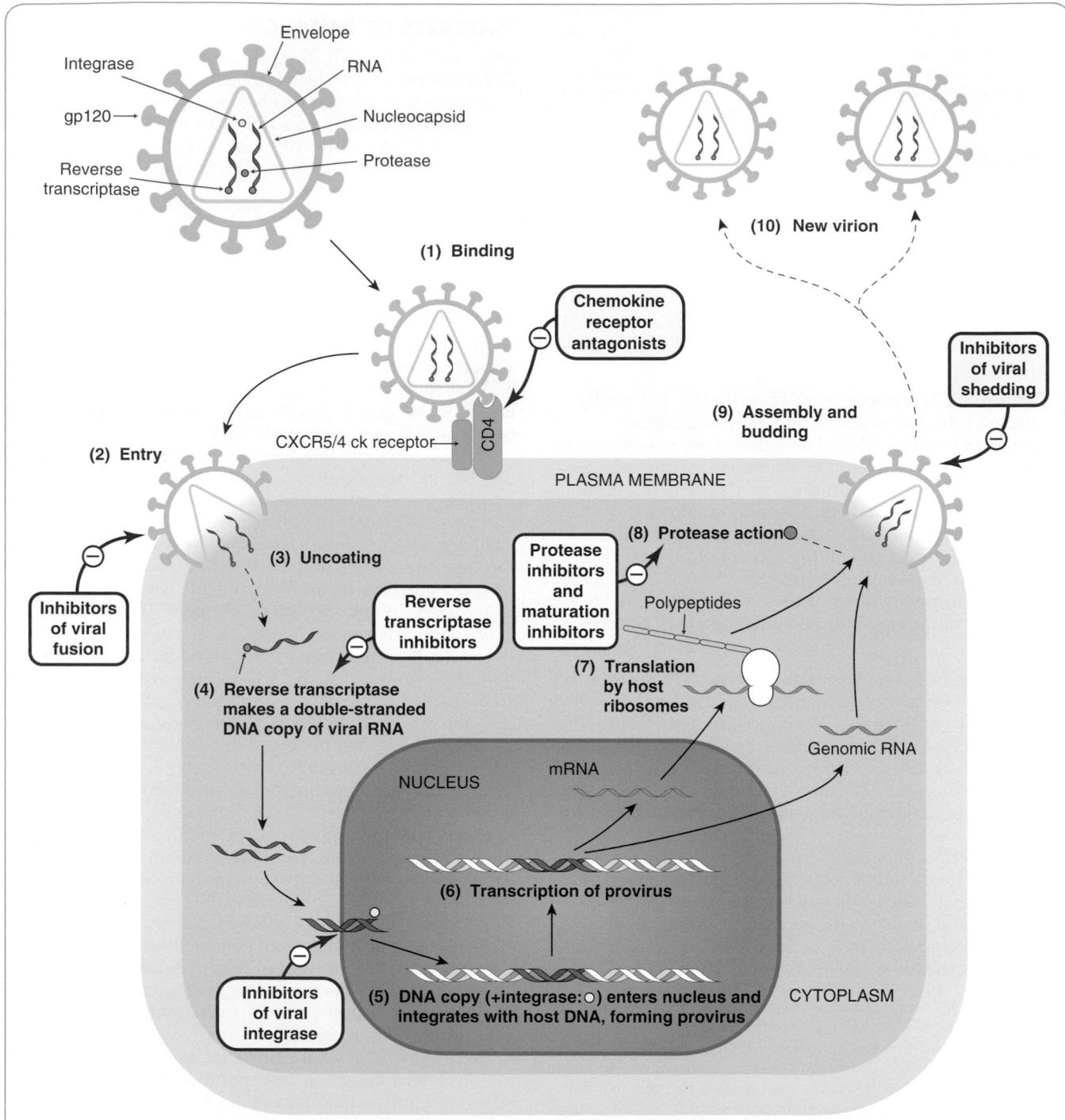

Fig. 53.3 Schematic diagram of infection of a CD4+ T cell by an HIV virion, with the sites of action of the main classes of anti-HIV drugs. The 10 steps of HIV infection, from attachment to the cell to release of new virions, are shown. The virus uses the CD4 co-receptor and the chemokine (ck) receptors CCR5/CXCR4 as binding sites to facilitate entry into the cell, where it becomes incorporated into host DNA *(steps 1–5)*. When transcription occurs *(step 6)*, the T cell itself is activated and the transcription factor nuclear factor κB initiates transcription of both host cell and provirus DNA. A viral protease cleaves the nascent viral polypeptides *(steps 7 and 8)* into enzymes (integrase, reverse transcriptase, protease) and structural proteins for new virions. These are assembled and released from the cells, initiating a fresh round of infection *(steps 9 and 10)*. The sites of action of anti-HIV drugs are shown.

only while the virus is replicating. Because the initial phases of viral infection are often asymptomatic, treatment is often not initiated until the infection is well established. This is unfortunate because, as is often the case with infectious diseases, an ounce of prevention is worth a pound of cure,

hence the importance of pre-exposure prophylaxis wherever possible.

Antiviral drugs, of which many are now available, may be conveniently grouped according to their mechanisms of action. Table 53.2 shows the commonest agents, classified

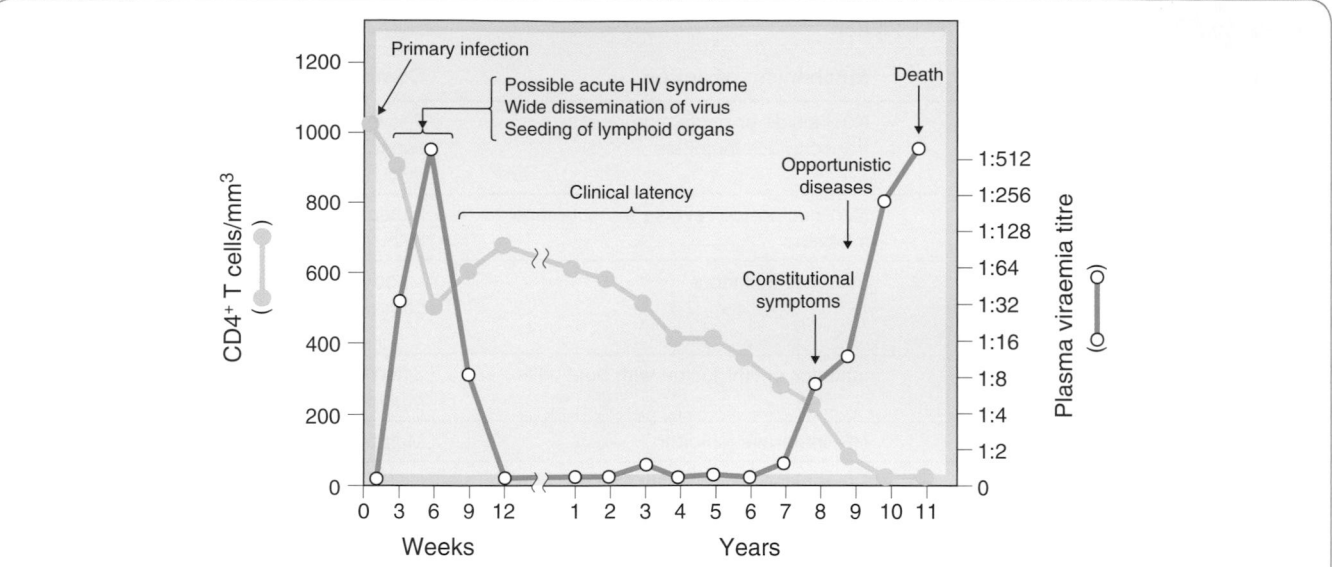

Fig. 53.4 **Schematic outline of the course of HIV infection.** The CD4+ T-cell titre is often expressed as cells/mm³. (Adapted from Pantaleo et al., 1993.)

Table 53.2 Drugs used to treat viral infections

Common use	Drug	Mechanism of action	Comments
Cytomegalovirus	Cidofovir, foscarnet, ganciclovir, valganciclovir	Nucleoside or nucleotide analogues and other drugs that inhibit viral DNA polymerase	Multiple GI and other SE
Hepatitis B	Adefovir, entecavir, lamivudine, telbivudine, tenvofir	Nucleoside or nucleotide analogues that inhibit reverse transcriptase	Multiple GI and other SE common
Hepatitis C	Daclatasvir, ledipasvir, ombitasvir, ritonavir	NS 5A Protease inhibitors	Ritonavir delays metabolism of other drugs and enhances their effects. Multiple SE common. Ledipasvir used as part of a fixed-dose combination with sofosbuvir.
	Boceprevir, paritaprevir, simeprevir, telaprevir	NS 3/4A protease inhibitors	
	Dasabuvir, sofosbuvir	NS 5B RNA polymerase inhibitors	
	Ribavirin	Nucleoside analogue: uncertain mechanism	Also used for other viral infections. Multiple SE common.
Hepatitis B and C	Interferon-α, pegylated interferon-α	Immuno-stimulant	'Flu-like' SE common
Herpes	Aciclovir, famciclovir (PD), idoxuridine, penciclovir, valaciclovir	Nucleoside and other viral DNA polymerase inhibitors	Multiple SE common. Idoxuridine used for topical ocular usage.
	Inosine prabonex	Immunomodulator	Metabolic SE
Influenza A & B	Oseltamivir	Neuraminidase inhibitor	Should be given with 2 days of infection. GI side effects common.
	Zanamivir	Neuraminidase inhibitor	Should be given with 2 days of infection. Used in immunocompetent patients. Common SEs include rash.
	Amantadine	Blocks ion channel in virus	Influenza A only (seldom used today)
Respiratory syncytial virus	Palivizumab	Targets viral protein important for internalisation into cells	Ribavirin also used

GI, gastrointestinal; *PD,* prodrug; *SE,* side effects.
(Data from various sources including BNF 2017.)

Table 53.3 Drugs used to treat HIV infection

Drug	Mechanism of action	Comments
Abacavir, didanosine, emtricitabine, lamivudine, stavudine, tenofovir, zidovudine	Nucleoside or nucleotide reverse transcriptase inhibitors	The first anti-HIV drugs. Multiple SE, especially on GI and metabolic systems (e.g. lactic acidosis), are common.
Efavirenz, etravirine, nevirapine, rilpivirine	Non-nucleoside reverse transcriptase inhibitors	Multiple SE common. Not effective against HIV-2.
Atazanavir, darunavir, fosamprenavir (PD), indinavir, lopinavir, ritonavir, saquinavir, tipranavir	Protease inhibitors	Lipodystrophy and many GI-related SE common
Enfuvirtide	Inhibitor of HIV fusion with host cells	Often used to treat resistant infections Multiple SE common.
Dolutegravir, elvitegravir, raltegravir	HIV integrase inhibitor	Multiple SE common
Maraviroc	Chemokine receptor antagonist (CCR5)	CCR5 dependent HIV. GI SE common.
Cobicistat	Pharmacokinetic enhancer	No antiviral activity but prolongs action of atazanavir and darunavir

These drugs are seldom given singly, being mostly used in combinations which can be changed to avoid toxicity issues, or if the treatment fails or falters.

GI, gastrointestinal; *PD*, prodrug; *SE*, side effects.

(Data from various sources including BNF 2017.)

in this manner together with some of the diseases they are used to treat, whilst Table 53.3 lists the principal agents specifically used to treat HIV.

REVERSE TRANSCRIPTASE INHIBITORS

These include *nucleoside* or *nucleotide analogues*, exemplified by **zidovudine** and **tenofovir**, respectively. Nucleosides are first phosphorylated to the corresponding nucleotides and can then act as false substrates, being further phosphorylated by host cell enzymes and incorporated into the growing DNA chain, but causing chain termination. The γ-DNA polymerase in the host cell mitochondria is also susceptible to inhibition by these agents. Mammalian α-DNA polymerase is relatively resistant but effects may be seen at high doses and inhibition of host polymerase enzymes may be the basis of some unwanted effects. The main utility of these drugs is the treatment of HIV, but a number of them have useful activity against other viruses also (e.g. hepatitis B, which, though not a retrovirus, uses reverse transcriptase for replication).

Zidovudine

Zidovudine (or **azidothymidine**, AZT) was the first drug to be introduced for the treatment of HIV and retains an important place in therapy. It can prolong life in HIV-infected individuals and diminish HIV-associated dementia. Given during pregnancy and then to the newborn infant, it can reduce mother-to-baby transmission by more than 20%. It is generally administered orally 2–3 times each day but can also be given by intravenous infusion. Its plasma half-life is 1 h, but the intracellular half-life of the active trisphosphate is 3 h. The concentration in cerebrospinal fluid (CSF) is 65% of the plasma level. Most of the drug is metabolised to the inactive glucuronide in the liver, only 20% of the active form being excreted in the urine.

Because of rapid mutation, the virus is a constantly moving target, and resistance develops with long-term use of zidovudine, particularly in late-stage disease. Furthermore, resistant strains can be transferred between individuals. Other factors that underlie the loss of efficacy of the drug are decreased activation of zidovudine to the trisphosphate and increased virus load as the host immune response fails.

Unwanted effects include GI disturbances (e.g. nausea, vomiting, abdominal pain), blood disorders (sometimes anaemia or neutropenia) and central nervous system (CNS) effects (e.g. insomnia, dizziness, headache), as well as the risk of lactic acidosis (possibly secondary to mitochondrial toxicity) in some patients; all these effects are shared by this entire group of drugs to a greater or lesser extent.

Other, currently approved, antiviral drugs in this group include **abacavir**, **adefovir**, **dipivoxil**, **didanosine**, **emtricitabine**, **entecavir**, **lamivudine**, **stavudine**, **telbivudine** and **tenofovir** which are used for hepatitis B as well as treatment.

NON-NUCLEOSIDE REVERSE TRANSCRIPTASE INHIBITORS

Non-nucleoside reverse transcriptase inhibitors are chemically diverse compounds that bind to the reverse transcriptase enzyme near the catalytic site and inactivate it. Most are also inducers, substrates or inhibitors, to varying degrees, of the liver cytochrome P450 enzymes (Ch. 10). Currently available drugs include **efavirenz** and **nevirapine**, and the related compounds **etravirine** and **rilpivarine**.

Efavirenz (plasma half-life ~50 h) is given orally, once daily. It is 99% bound to plasma albumin, and its CSF concentration is ~1% of that in the plasma. Nevertheless, its major adverse effects are insomnia, bad dreams and sometimes psychotic symptoms. It is teratogenic.

Nevirapine has good oral bioavailability, and penetrates into the CSF. It is metabolised in the liver, and the metabolite is excreted in the urine. Nevirapine can prevent mother-to-baby transmission of HIV.

Unwanted effects include rash (common) as well as a cluster of other effects.

PROTEASE INHIBITORS

In HIV and many other viral infections, the mRNA transcribed from the provirus is translated into biochemically inert *polyproteins*. A virus-specific protease then converts the polyproteins into various structural and functional proteins by cleavage at the appropriate positions (see Fig. 53.3). Because this protease does not occur in the host, it is a useful target for chemotherapeutic intervention. HIV infection generates two such proteins named *Gag* and *Gag-Pol*. Specific protease inhibitors bind to the site where cleavage occurs, and their use, in combination with reverse transcriptase inhibitors, has transformed the therapy of AIDS. In the case of the hepatitis C virus, two protease targets have also been identified, *non-structural protein (NS) 3*, a serine protease, and *NS 5A*, which appears to act as an accessory protein for NS3. Examples of current protease inhibitors are shown in Tables 53.2 and 53.3.

Darunavir, a typical example, binds tightly to the specific retropepsin proteases from HIV-1 or HIV-2, inactivating the catalytic site. **Ritonavir** acts in a similar way but also inhibits the P450 enzymes that metabolise these drugs potentiating their activity and for this reason is often given in combination with other protease inhibitors (e.g. **lopinavir**).

Unwanted effects that are shared among this group include GI disturbances (e.g. nausea, vomiting, abdominal pain), blood disorders (sometimes anaemia or neutropenia) and CNS effects (e.g. insomnia, dizziness, headache) as well as the risk of hyperglycaemia.

Drug interactions are numerous, clinically important and unpredictable. As with other antiretroviral drugs, it is essential to look up possible interactions before prescribing any other drugs in patients receiving antiretroviral treatment.

DNA POLYMERASE INHIBITORS

Aciclovir

The development of the landmark drug **aciclovir** (see Table 53.2) launched the era of effective selective antiviral therapy. Typical of drugs of this type, it is a guanosine derivative that is converted to the monophosphate by viral thymidine kinase. This viral enzyme is much more effective in carrying out the phosphorylation than the enzyme of the host cell, so aciclovir is predominantly activated in infected cells. The host cell kinases then convert the monophosphate to the trisphosphate, the active form that inhibits viral DNA polymerase, terminating the nucleotide chain. It is 30 times more potent against the herpes virus enzyme than the host enzyme. Aciclovir trisphosphate is inactivated within the host cells, presumably by cellular phosphatases. Resistance caused by changes in the viral genes coding for thymidine kinase or DNA polymerase has been reported, and aciclovir-resistant herpes simplex virus has been the cause of pneumonia, encephalitis and mucocutaneous infections in immunocompromised patients.

Aciclovir can be given orally, intravenously or topically. When it is given orally, only 20% of the dose is absorbed. The drug is widely distributed, and reaches effective concentrations in the CSF. It is excreted by the kidneys, partly by glomerular filtration and partly by tubular secretion.

Unwanted effects are minimal. Local inflammation can occur during intravenous injection if there is extravasation of the solution. Renal dysfunction has been reported when aciclovir is given intravenously; slow infusion reduces the risk. Nausea and headache can occur and, rarely, encephalopathy.

There are now other drugs with a similar action to aciclovir (see list in Table 53.2). **Foscarnet** achieves the same effect through a slightly different mechanism.

> ### Clinical uses of drugs for herpes viruses
>
> - *Varicella zoster* infections (chickenpox, shingles):
>   - orally (e.g. **famciclovir**) including in immunocompetent patients;
>   - intravenously (e.g. in encephalitis, **aciclovir**) including in immunocompromised patients.
> - *Herpes simplex* infections: *genital* herpes (systemic and/ or topical treatment depending on severity, whether immunocompromised and whether or not a first attack), *mucocutaneous* herpes (e.g. aciclovir or, if unresponsive, **foscarnet**) and herpes *encephalitis* (e.g. intravenous aciclovir).
> - Prophylactically:
>   - patients who are to be treated with immunosuppressant drugs or radiotherapy and who are at risk of herpesvirus infection owing to reactivation of a latent virus;
>   - in individuals who suffer from frequent recurrences of genital infection with herpes simplex virus.
> - *Cytomegalovirus* (CMV)
>   - CMV, whilst a herpes virus, is less sensitive to aciclovir than is *Herpes simplex* or *Herpes zoster*. **Valaciclovir** is licensed for prevention of CMV during immunosuppression following organ transplantation. **Ganciclovir** and **valaganciclovir** are more active against CMV than aciclovir, but are more toxic; they are used by specialists for serious problems such as CMV retinitis in patients with AIDS.

NEURAMINIDASE INHIBITORS AND INHIBITORS OF VIRAL COAT DISASSEMBLY

Viral neuraminidase is one of three transmembrane proteins coded by the influenza genome. Infection with these RNA viruses begins with the attachment of the viral haemagglutinin to neuraminic (sialic) acid residues on host cells. The viral particle then enters the cell by endocytosis. The endosome is acidified following influx of H^+ through another viral protein, the *M2 ion channel*. This facilitates the disassembly of the viral structure, allowing the RNA to enter the host nucleus, thus initiating a round of viral replication. Newly replicated virions escape from the host cell by budding from the cell membrane. Viral neuraminidase promotes this by severing the bonds linking the particle coat and host sialic acid.

The neuraminidase inhibitors **oseltamivir** and **zanamivir** are active against both influenza A and B viruses, and are licensed for use at early stages in the infection or when use of the vaccine is impossible. Zanamivir is available as a powder for inhalation, and oseltamivir as an oral preparation. Though oseltamivir has been 'stockpiled' by governments when flu pandemics (e.g. 'swine' flu – H1N1) are forecast, clinical trials suggest that its efficacy in reducing disease severity is very limited.

Unwanted effects of oseltamivir include GI symptoms (nausea, vomiting, dyspepsia and diarrhoea), but these are less frequent and severe in the inhaled preparation. Zanamivir commonly causes a rash.

Amantadine,[3] quite an old drug (1966) and seldom recommended today, effectively blocks viral M2 ion channels, thus inhibiting disassembly. It is active against influenza A virus (an RNA virus) but has no action against influenza B virus. Given orally, amantadine is well absorbed, reaches high levels in secretions (e.g. saliva) and most is excreted unchanged via the kidney. Aerosol administration is feasible.

Unwanted effects are relatively infrequent, occurring in 5%–10% of patients, and are not serious. Dizziness, insomnia and slurred speech are the most common adverse effects.

DRUGS ACTING THROUGH OTHER MECHANISMS

Enfuvirtide inhibits the fusion of HIV with host cells. It is generally given by subcutaneous injection in combination with other drugs to treat HIV when resistance becomes a problem or when the patient is intolerant of other antiretroviral drugs.

Unwanted effects include flu-like symptoms, central effects such as headache, dizziness, alterations in mood, GI effects and, sometimes, hypersensitivity reactions.

Raltegravir and related agents act by inhibiting HIV DNA integrase, the enzyme that splices viral DNA into the host genome when forming the provirus. It is used for the treatment of HIV as part of combination therapy, and is generally reserved for cases that are resistant to other antiretroviral agents.

Maraviroc. CCR5, together with CXCR4, are cell surface chemokine receptors that have been exploited by some strains of HIV to gain entry to the cell (see earlier). In patients who harbour 'R5' strains, the chemokine receptor antagonist maraviroc may be used, in combination with more conventional antiretroviral drugs. This drug represents a novel concept in HIV therapy (see Dhami et al., 2009) and is the only drug of its type currently available. Its use, in combination with other antiretroviral drugs, is currently restricted to CCR5-tropic HIV infection in patients previously treated with other antiretrovirals.

BIOPHARMACEUTICAL ANTIVIRAL DRUGS

Biopharmaceuticals that have been recruited in the fight against virus infections include immunoglobulin preparations, interferons (IFNs) and monoclonal antibodies.

Immunoglobulins

Pooled immunoglobulin contains antibodies against various viruses present in the population. The antibodies are directed against the virus envelope and can 'neutralise' some viruses and prevent their attachment to host cells. If used before the onset of signs and symptoms, it may attenuate or prevent measles, German measles, infectious hepatitis, rabies or poliomyelitis. *Hyperimmune* globulin, specific against particular viruses, is used against hepatitis B, varicella zoster and rabies.

Palivizumab

Related in terms of its mechanism of action to immunoglobulins is **palivizumab**, a monoclonal antibody (see Ch. 5) directed against a glycoprotein on the surface of respiratory syncytial virus. It is used as an intramuscular injection, under specialist supervision, in children at high risk to prevent infection by this organism.

Interferons

IFNs are a family of inducible proteins synthesised by mammalian cells and now generally produced commercially by recombinant DNA technology. There are at least three types, α, β and γ, constituting a family of hormones involved in cell growth and regulation and the modulation of immune reactions. **IFN-γ**, termed *immune interferon*, is produced mainly by T lymphocytes as part of an immunological response to both viral and non-viral antigens, the latter including bacteria and their products, rickettsiae, protozoa, fungal polysaccharides and a range of polymeric chemicals and other cytokines. **IFN-α** and **IFN-β** are produced by B and T lymphocytes, macrophages and fibroblasts in response to the presence of viruses and cytokines. The general actions of the IFNs are described briefly in Chapters 7 and 19.

The IFNs bind to specific ganglioside receptors on host cell membranes. They induce, in host cell ribosomes, the production of enzymes that inhibit the translation of viral mRNA into viral proteins, thus halting viral replication. They have a broad spectrum of action and inhibit the replication of most viruses in vitro. Given intravenously, IFNs have a half-life of 2–4 h. They do not cross the blood–brain barrier.

IFN-α-2a is used for treatment of hepatitis B infections and AIDS-related Kaposi's sarcomas; **IFN-α-2b** is used for hepatitis C (a chronic viral infection which can progress insidiously in apparently healthy people, leading to end-stage liver disease or liver cancer). There are reports that IFNs can prevent reactivation of herpes simplex after trigeminal root section in animals and can prevent spread of herpes zoster in cancer patients. Preparations of IFNs conjugated with polyethylene glycol (pegylated IFNs) have a longer lifetime in the circulation.

Unwanted effects are common and resemble the symptoms of influenza (which are mediated by cytokine release) including fever, lassitude, headache and myalgia. Repeated injections cause chronic malaise. Bone marrow depression, rashes, alopecia and disturbances in cardiovascular, thyroid and hepatic function can also occur.

OTHER AGENTS

Immunomodulators are drugs that act by modulating the immune response to viruses or use an immune mechanism to target a virus or other organism. **Inosine pranobex** may interfere with viral nucleic acid synthesis but also has immunopotentiating actions on the host. It is sometimes used to treat herpes infections of mucosal tissues or skin.

Tribavirin (ribavirin) is a synthetic nucleoside, similar in structure to guanosine. The exact mechanism of action

---

[3]Also used for its mildly beneficial effects in Parkinson's disease (see Ch. 41).

is unclear but it interferes with the synthesis of viral mRNA. While it inhibits a wide range of DNA and RNA viruses, including many that affect the lower airways, it is mainly used in aerosol or tablet form to treat infections with *respiratory syncytial virus* (an RNA paramyxovirus). It has also been shown to be effective in hepatitis C as well as Lassa fever, an extremely serious *arenavirus* infection. When given promptly to victims of the latter disease, it has been shown to reduce to fatality rates (usually about 76%) by approximately eight-fold.

Antiviral drugs

Most antiviral drugs generally fall into the following groups:

- *Nucleoside (or nucleotide) analogues* that inhibit the viral reverse transcriptase enzyme, preventing replication (e.g. **lamivudine, zidovudine**).
- *Non-nucleoside analogues* that have the same effect (e.g. **efavirenz**).
- *Inhibitors of proteases* that prevent viral protein processing (e.g. **saquinavir, indinavir**).
- *Inhibitors of viral DNA polymerase* that prevent replication (e.g. **aciclovir, famciclovir**).
- *Inhibitors of HIV integrase* that prevent the incorporation of viral DNA into the host genome (**ratelgravir**).
- *Inhibitors of viral fusion with cells* (e.g. **enfuvirtide**).
- *Inhibitors of viral entry* that block the use of host cell surface receptors, which are used as entry points by viruses (**maraviroc**).
- *Inhibitors of viral capsule disassembly* (e.g. **amantadine**).
- *Inhibitors of neuraminidase* that prevent viral escape from infected cells (e.g. **oseltamivir**).
- *Immunomodulators* that generally enhance host defences (e.g. interferons and **inosine pranobex**).
- *Immunoglobulin and related preparations* that contain neutralising antibodies to various viruses.

COMBINATION THERAPY FOR HIV

Because the two main classes of antiviral drugs used to treat HIV (reverse transcriptase inhibitors and protease inhibitors) have different mechanisms of action (see Fig. 53.3), they can usefully be deployed in combinations and this has dramatically improved the prognosis of the disease. Such combination treatment is known as **H**ighly **A**ctive **A**ntiretroviral **T**herapy (HAART). A typical HAART three- or four-drug combination would involve two nucleoside reverse transcriptase inhibitors with either a non-nucleoside reverse transcriptase inhibitor or one or two protease inhibitors.

Using a HAART protocol, HIV replication is inhibited, the presence in the plasma of HIV RNA is reduced to undetectable levels and patient survival is greatly prolonged – so much so that near-normal life spans can now be achieved, given prompt diagnosis and treatment and good patient compliance. The latter is a key point – a rate of 95% or more is required to achieve this result and prevent treatment failure. This is difficult to achieve because the daily multiple dosing regimens are complex and these drugs have many unwanted effects. Since lifelong treatment is necessary, 'treatment fatigue' is a real issue.

To circumvent at least some of these problems, several 'once-a-day' formulations have been devised. The first one to be approved, **Atripla**, comprises a fixed-dose mixture of nucleoside and non-nucleoside reverse transcriptase inhibitors (tenofovir, emtricitabine and efavirenz). Several other proprietary combinations have also been approved with different constituent drugs. It is estimated that switching to a 'once' daily' administration doubles the likelihood of maintaining the 95% adherence rate that is crucial to treatment success (see Truong et al., 2015).

Unwelcome interactions can occur between the component drugs of HAART combinations, and there may be inter-individual variations in absorption. Metabolic and cardiovascular complications attend the usage of these drugs and pose a problem to patients requiring lifelong therapy (see Hester, 2012). Some drugs penetrate poorly into the brain, and this could lead to local proliferation of the virus. So far there is little cross-resistance between the three groups of drugs, but the virus has a high mutation rate – so this could be a problem in the future.

The choice of drugs to treat pregnant or breastfeeding women is difficult. The main aims are to avoid damage to the fetus and to prevent transmission of the disease to the neonate. Therapy with zidovudine alone is often used in these cases and although combination therapy is more effective, it increases the chance of fetal toxicity. Another area that requires special consideration is prophylaxis for individuals who may have been exposed to the virus accidentally. Specific guidelines have been developed for both such cases, but they are beyond the scope of this chapter.

The AIDS virus has certainly not yet been vanquished. It is not eradicated by drug treatment, but with any of these treatments, lies latent in the host genome of memory T cells, ready to reactivate if therapy is stopped.

PROSPECTS FOR NEW ANTIVIRAL DRUGS

At the beginning of the 1990s, there were only five drugs available to treat viral infections, but this number has increased some 10-fold during the intervening years. Our understanding of the biology of pathogenic viruses and their actions in the host has grown enormously and this has led to the discovery of new types of antivirals, such as those that prevent CCR5 – and possibly other chemokine receptors – from serving as an entry portal for HIV. Another potentially fruitful lead is *HIV maturation inhibitors* which prevent proteolytic processing of viral proteins by binding to the polypeptide chain rather than the protease itself. Compounds such as **bevirimat** (now discontinued) target the precursor of the Gag polyprotein. Since this is the main structural protein responsible for assembly and budding of virion particles the drug effectively inhibits replication (see Salzwedel et al., 2007). The quest for further novel antivirals continues and computational biology techniques are being deployed to predict resistance to existing drugs based upon the HIV phenotype to enhance the quality of clinical treatment (Zazzi et al., 2016).

The discovery and development of antiviral drugs and the formulation and implementation of HAART therapy has been a triumph in the fight against HIV, transforming the lives of millions of people in a dramatic manner.

However, the ultimate weapon in the fight against HIV would be vaccination. This has proved to be highly effective in the past against diseases such as polio and smallpox, and more recently against influenza (both types), hepatitis B and other pathogens.

Unfortunately, and despite some encouraging results in animal models, the prospect of an imminent introduction of a vaccine against HIV (and sadly many other viruses) still seems rather distant (Pollara et al., 2017). Some success was reported in a vaccine trial (RV144), which tested a combination of two vaccines that had proved ineffective when given separately (see Rerks-Ngarm et al., 2017).

Although the benefits claimed in the trial were later questioned (Desrosiers, 2017), a further trial (HVTN 702) using the same vaccine is currently in progress in South Africa at the time of writing.

Part of the problem in designing vaccines is *antigenic drift*, a process whereby the virus mutates, thus presenting shifting antigenic structures and minimising the chance of an effective and long-lasting immune response. A vaccine which induces *broad neutralising antibody* production by the host is today considered to be a key objective. The problem of HIV vaccines is the subject of numerous reviews (see, for example, Cohen & Frahm, 2017).

Drug mechanisms in HIV infections

- Reverse transcriptase inhibitors (RTIs):
  - *nucleoside (or nucleotide) analogue RTIs* are phosphorylated by host cell enzymes to give the 5'-trisphosphate, which competes with the equivalent host cellular trisphosphates that are essential substrates for the formation of proviral DNA by viral reverse transcriptase (examples are **zidovudine** and **abacavir**); they are used in combination with protease inhibitors.
  - *non-nucleoside RTIs* are chemically diverse compounds that bind to the reverse transcriptase near the catalytic site and denature it; an example is **nevirapine**.
- Protease inhibitors inhibit cleavage of the nascent viral protein into functional and structural proteins. They are often used in combination with RTIs. An example is **saquinavir**.
- Combination therapy is essential in treating HIV; this characteristically comprises two nucleoside RTIs with either a non-nucleoside RTI or one or two protease inhibitors. Other drugs, such as the HIV integrase inhibitor **ratelgravir**, the chemokine receptor antagonist **maraviroc** and the HIV fusion inhibitor **enfuvirtide**, may also be used in such combination therapy regimens. 'Once daily' combination therapies greatly improve patient compliance.

Treatment of HIV/AIDS

- Current treatment (supervised by experienced physicians) is not curative, but aims to optimise quantity and quality of life using highly active antiretroviral treatment (HAART). This consists of combinations of drugs (e.g. of two nucleoside reverse transcriptase inhibitors with either a non-nucleoside reverse transcriptase inhibitor or with a boosted protease inhibitor or with an integrase inhibitor). Drugs with additive or synergistic therapeutic effects are selected to minimise the emergence of resistance, minimise toxicity and optimise adherence to lifelong therapy.
- Plasma viral load and CD4$^+$ cell count are monitored; viral sensitivity is determined before starting treatment and before changing drugs if the viral load increases.
- Treatment is started based on CD4$^+$ cell count and aims to reduce viral load as much as possible for as long as possible.
- Special situations (e.g. prophylaxis following accidental exposure via needle-stick injury, treatment of children and during pregnancy) are best managed by specialists.

REFERENCES AND FURTHER READING

Viral infections in general

Hanazaki, K., 2004. Antiviral therapy for chronic hepatitis B: a review. Curr. Drug Targets Inflamm. Allergy 3, 63–70. (*Reviews the use of IFN and lamivudine, alone or in combination, in the treatment of this viral infection*)

Lauer, G.M., Walker, B.D., 2001. Hepatitis C virus infection. N. Engl. J. Med. 345, 41–52. (*Comprehensive review of pathogenesis, clinical characteristics, natural history and treatment of hepatitis C infection*)

Schmidt, A.C., 2004. Antiviral therapy for influenza: a clinical and economic comparative review. Drugs 64, 2031–2046. (*A useful review of influenza biology, together with a comprehensive evaluation of drug treatments, their mechanisms of action and relative economic costs*)

Whitley, R.J., Roizman, B., 2001. Herpes simplex virus infections. Lancet 357, 1513–1518. (*A concise review of the viral replication cycle and the pathogenesis and treatment of herpes simplex virus infections*)

HIV infections

Barber, D.L., Wherry, E.J., Masopust, D., et al., 2006. Restoring function in exhausted CD8 T cells during chronic viral infection. Nature 439, 682–687. (*Deals with a potential mechanism whereby the exhaustion of T cells may be reversed*)

Jansen, C.A., Piriou, E., Bronke, C., et al., 2004. Characterisation of virus-specific CD8(+) effector T cells in the course of HIV-1 infection: longitudinal analyses in slow and rapid progressors. Clin. Immunol. 11, 299–309.

Levy, J.A., 2001. The importance of the innate immune system in controlling HIV infection and disease. Trends Immunol. 22, 312–316. (*Stresses the role of innate immunity in the response to HIV; clear exposition of the various components of the innate and adaptive immune systems, as well as the role of non-cytotoxic CD8$^+$ cell response to HIV*)

Moss, J.A., 2013. HIV/AIDS review. Radiol. Technol. 84, 247–267. (*This paper was written to update radiologists and radiographers and is therefore* an excellent introduction to all matters related to HIV/AIDS. Highly recommended)

Murphy, P.M., 2001. Viral exploitation and subversion of the immune system through chemokine mimicry. Nat. Immunol. 2, 116–122. (Excellent description of virus–immune system interaction)

Norris, P.J., Moffett, H.F., Brander, C., et al., 2004. Fine specificity and cross-clade reactivity of HIV type 1 Gag-specific CD4+ T cells. AIDS Res. Hum. Retroviruses 20, 315–325.

Pantaleo, G., Graziosi, C., Fauci, A.S., 1993. New concepts in the immunopathogenesis of human immunodeficiency virus infection. N. Engl. J. Med. 328, 327–335.

Schutze, N., 2004. siRNA technology. Mol. Cell. Endocrinol. 213, 115–119. (An article explaining the siRNA concept)

Tortorella, D., Gewurz, B.E., Furman, M.H., et al., 2000. Viral subversion of the immune system. Annu. Rev. Immunol. 18, 861–926. (A comprehensive and clearly written review of the various mechanisms by which viruses elude detection and destruction by the host immune system)

Mechanisms of antiviral drug action

de Clercq, E., 2002. Strategies in the design of antiviral drugs. Nat. Rev. Drug Discov. 1, 13–24. (Outstanding article describing the rationale behind current and future strategies for antiviral drug development)

Hester, E.K., 2012. HIV medications: an update and review of metabolic complications. Nutr. Clin. Pract. 27, 51–64. (Deals with the problems encountered by many patients who may have to take HAART medication for years)

Gubareva, L., Kaiser, L., Hayden, F.G., 2000. Influenza virus neuraminidase inhibitors. Lancet 355, 827–835. (Admirable coverage of this topic; lucid summary and clear diagrams of the influenza virus and its replication cycle; description of the structure and the action of, and resistance to, zanamivir and oseltamivir, and the relevant pharmacokinetic aspects and clinical efficacy)

Combination treatment for HIV

Flexner, C., 2000. Dual protease inhibitor therapy in HIV-infected patients: pharmacologic rationale and clinical benefits. Annu. Rev. Pharmacol. Toxicol. 40, 649–674. (Review emphasising interactions between individual protease inhibitors and the potential benefits and disadvantages of dual therapy)

Richman, D.D., 2001. HIV chemotherapy. Nature 410, 995–1001. (Outstanding article; covers pathogenesis and natural history of HIV infection and the impact on viral dynamics and immune function of antiretroviral therapy; discusses the main antiretroviral drugs, drug resistance of HIV and targets for new drugs; excellent figures and comprehensive references)

Truong, W.R., Schafer, J.J., Short, W.R., 2015. Once-daily, single-tablet regimens for the treatment of HIV-1 infection. P T 40, 44–55.

New leads in antiviral drug therapy

Barik, S., 2004. Control of nonsegmented negative-strand RNA virus replication by siRNA. Virus Res. 102, 27–35. (Interesting article explaining how siRNA technology might be used to inhibit viral replication)

Cohen, K.W., Frahm, N., 2017. Current views on the potential for development of a HIV vaccine. Expert Opin. Biol. Ther. 17, 295–303.

Desrosiers, R.C., 2017. Protection against HIV acquisition in the RV144 Trial. J. Virol. 91, e00905–00917.

Dhami, H., Fritz, C.E., Gankin, B., et al., 2009. The chemokine system and CCR5 antagonists: potential in HIV treatment and other novel therapies. J. Clin. Pharm. Ther. 34, 147–160. (Excellent and easy-to-read review of this area. Helpful diagrams)

Flores-Villanueva, P.O., Hendel, H., Caillat-Zucman, S., et al., 2003. Associations of MHC ancestral haplotypes with resistance/susceptibility to AIDS disease development. J. Immunol. 170, 1925–1929. (A paper that deals with the hereditary component of HIV susceptibility/resistance; interesting, but complex for the non-geneticist)

Kaufman, D.R., Barouch, D.H., 2009. Translational mini-review series on vaccines for HIV: T lymphocyte trafficking and vaccine-elicited mucosal immunity. Clin. Exp. Immunol. 157, 165–173. (This paper, together with the paper by Rhee et al. below, review new research that seeks to design better HIV vaccines through an increased understanding of the innate and adaptive immune systems. They are fairly advanced but worthwhile if you are interested in the topic)

Kilby, J.M., Eron, J.J., 2003. Novel therapies based on mechanisms of HIV-1 cell entry. N. Engl. J. Med. 348, 2228–2238. (Excellent review on this innovative strategy)

Kitabwalla, M., Ruprecht, R.M., 2002. RNA interference: a new weapon against HIV and beyond. N. Engl. J. Med. 347, 1364–1368. (An article in the series 'Clinical implications of basic research')

Moore, J.P., Stevenson, M., 2000. New targets for inhibitors of HIV-1 replication. Nat. Rev. Mol. Cell Biol. 1, 40–49. (Excellent coverage of stages of the viral life cycle that might be susceptible to new drugs. Introduces various potentially promising chemical compounds)

Pollara, J., Easterhoff, D., Fouda, G.G., 2017. Lessons learned from human HIV vaccine trials. Curr. Opin. HIV AIDS 12, 216–221.

Rerks-Ngarm, S., Pitisuttithum, P., Excler, J.L., et al., 2017. Randomized, double-blind evaluation of late boost strategies for HIV-uninfected vaccine recipients in the RV144 HIV vaccine efficacy trial. J. Infect. Dis. 215, 1255–1263.

Rhee, E.G., Barouch, D.H., 2009. Translational mini-review series on vaccines for HIV: harnessing innate immunity for HIV vaccine development. Clin. Exp. Immunol. 157, 174–180. (See review of Kaufman & Barouch above)

Salzwedel, K., Martin, D.E., Sakalian, M., 2007. Maturation inhibitors: a new therapeutic class targets the virus structure. AIDS Rev. 9, 162–172.

Zazzi, M., Cozzi-Lepri, A., Prosperi, M.C., 2016. Computer-aided optimization of combined anti-retroviral therapy for HIV: new drugs, new drug targets and drug resistance. Curr. HIV Res. 14, 101–109.

Books

Pisani, E., 2008. The Wisdom of Whores. Granta Books, London. (An entertaining and informative account of efforts made to pioneer HIV programmes in developing countries and the many bureaucratic and other obstacles that had to be surmounted. See also www.wisdomofwhores.com/ subtitled 'Of sex and science. Elisabeth Pisani's blog about HIV and other sundry things'. Highly recommended)

Useful Web resources

https://www.aidsinfo.nih.gov/. (The official HIV/AIDS site of the US National Institutes of Health. Authoritative and up-to-date information on every aspect of this disease and its treatment, including data on drugs and drug action as well as the results of recent clinical trials and the latest progress in developing a vaccine. Also includes links to downloadable 'Apps' on HIV and its therapy. Superb)

http://www.unaids.org/. (The official site of the United Nations Programme on HIV/AIDS. It focuses on the demographics of the epidemic with various resources that bring home the enormous problems in dealing with this disease. Prepare to be appalled)

54

Antifungal drugs

OVERVIEW

Fungal infections (*mycoses*) are widespread in the population. In temperate climates, such as the United Kingdom, they are generally associated with the skin (e.g. 'athlete's foot') or mucous membranes (e.g. 'thrush').[1] In otherwise healthy people, these infections are mainly minor, being more of a nuisance than a threat. However, they become a more serious problem when the immune system is compromised or when the organism gains access to the systemic circulation. When this occurs, the infection can be fatal. In this chapter, we will briefly review the main types of fungal infections and discuss the drugs that can be used to treat them.

FUNGI AND FUNGAL INFECTIONS

Fungi are non-motile eukaryotic cells. Unlike green plants, they cannot photosynthesise and many are parasitic or saprophytic in nature. Thousands of species have been characterised. Many are of economic importance, either because they are edible (e.g. mushrooms), useful in manufacturing other products (e.g. yeast in brewing and in the production of antibiotics) or because of the damage they cause to other animals, crops or foodstuffs.

Approximately 50 species are pathogenic in humans. These organisms are present in the environment or may co-exist with humans as *commensals* without causing any overt risks to health. However, since the 1970s there has been a steady increase in the incidence of serious secondary systemic fungal infections, causing some 2 million deaths per year, usually in immunologically vulnerable individuals. One of the contributory factors has been the widespread use of broad-spectrum antibiotics, which eradicate the non-pathogenic bacterial populations that normally compete with fungi for nutritional resources. Other causes include the spread of AIDS and the use of immunosuppressant, and cancer chemotherapy agents. The result has been an increased prevalence of *opportunistic infections*, that is, infections that exploit vulnerabilities in host immune systems. Older people, diabetics, pregnant women and burn wound victims are particularly at risk of fungal infections such as *candidiasis*. Primary systemic fungal infections, once rare in the temperate world, are also now encountered more often because of increased international travel.

Clinically important fungi may be classified into four main types on the basis of morphological and other characteristics. Of particular taxonomic significance is the presence of *hyphae* – filamentous projections that can knit together to form a complex *mycelium*, a mat-like structure that is responsible for the characteristic appearance of moulds. Fungi are remarkably specific in their choice of preferred location. The main groups are:

- yeasts (e.g. *Cryptococcus neoformans*)
- yeast-like fungi that produce a structure resembling a mycelium (e.g. *Candida albicans*)
- filamentous fungi with a true mycelium (e.g. *Aspergillus fumigatus*)
- 'dimorphic' fungi which, depending on nutritional constraints, may grow as either yeasts or filamentous fungi (e.g. *Histoplasma capsulatum*[2])

As a general rule, most fungi only cause systemic infections in immunocompromised individuals but the dimorphic fungi can infect healthy individuals.

Another organism, *Pneumocystis carinii* (also known as *P. jirovecii*), described in Ch. 55, shares characteristics of both protozoa and fungi; it is an important opportunistic pathogen in patients with compromised immune systems (e.g. those suffering from AIDS), but is not susceptible to antifungal drugs.

Drugs vary in their efficacy between the different fungal groups. Table 54.1 gives examples of each type of organism and lists some of the diseases they cause and the most common choice of drug.

Superficial fungal infections can be classified into the *dermatomycoses* and *candidiasis*. Dermatomycoses include infections of the skin, hair and nails (*onychomycosis*). They are most commonly caused by *Trichophyton*, *Microsporum* or *Epidermophyton*, giving rise to circular rashes known as 'ringworm' or, generically, *tinea* (not to be confused with genuine helminth infections; see Ch. 56). *Tinea capitis* affects the scalp; *Tinea cruris*, the groin ('dhobie itch'); *Tinea pedis*, the feet ('athlete's foot'); and *Tinea corporis*, the body. Superficial candidiasis, caused by a yeast-like organism, may infect the mucous membranes of the mouth or vagina (thrush), or the skin. Secondary bacterial infections may complicate the course and treatment of these conditions.

Systemic (or 'disseminated') fungal diseases are much more serious than superficial infections. The commonest in the United Kingdom is candidiasis. Other serious conditions include cryptococcal meningitis, endocarditis

---

[1]However, they may also 'infect' buildings too and contribute to the 'sick building syndrome'.

[2]*Histoplasma* is a common asymptomatic infection in the American mid-west. It is carried by bats and hence infects spelunkers (cavers).

Table 54.1 Some clinically significant fungal infections and a typical first choice of antifungal drug therapy

	Organism(s) responsible	Principal disease(s)	Common drug treatments
Yeasts	*Cryptococcus neoformans*	Meningitis	Amphotericin, flucytosine, fluconazole
Yeast-like fungus	*Candida albicans*	Thrush (and other superficial infection)	Fluconazole, itraconazole
		Systemic candidiasis	Echinocandins, amphotericin, fluconazole, other azoles
Filamentous fungi	*Trichophyton* spp. *Epidermophyton floccosum* *Microsporum* spp.	All these organisms cause skin and nail infections and are referred to as tinea or 'ringworm'	Itraconazole, terbinafine, griseofulvin
	Aspergillus fumigatus	Pulmonary aspergillosis	Amphotericin, capsofungin, voriconazole, other azoles
Dimorphic fungi	*Histoplasma capsulatum*	Histoplasmosis	Itraconazole, amphotericin
	Coccidioides immitis	Coccidiomycosis	
	Blastomyces dermatitidis	Blastomycosis	

(particularly of artificial valves), pulmonary aspergillosis, and rhinocerebral mucormycosis. Invasive pulmonary aspergillosis is now a leading cause of death in recipients of bone marrow transplants or those with neutropenia. Colonisation by *Aspergillus* of the lungs of patients with asthma or cystic fibrosis can lead to a condition termed allergic *bronchopulmonary aspergillosis*.

In other parts of the world, systemic fungal infections include blastomycosis, histoplasmosis (which produces characteristic calcifications on chest X-rays), coccidiomycosis and paracoccidiomycosis; these are often *primary* infections, that is, they are not secondary to reduced immunological function or altered commensal microorganisms.

In addition to a free-floating lifestyle, some fungi can develop and grow in *biofilms*, that is, fungal communities attached to the surface of inert (e.g. catheters) or living (e.g. implants) surfaces. Such colonies are highly resistant to stress and to antifungal drugs, making them very difficult to treat.

DRUGS USED TO TREAT FUNGAL INFECTIONS

The current therapeutic agents can be broadly classified into two groups: first, the naturally–occurring antifungal antibiotics such as the *polyenes* and *echinocandins*, and second, synthetic drugs including *azoles* and *fluorinated pyrimidines*. Because many infections are superficial, there are many topical preparations. Many antifungal agents are quite toxic, and when systemic therapy is required this is generally undertaken under strict medical supervision.

Fig. 54.1 shows sites of action of common antifungal drugs.

ANTIFUNGAL ANTIBIOTICS

Amphotericin

Amphotericin (also called **amphotericin B**) is a mixture of antifungal substances derived from cultures of *Streptomyces*. Structurally, these are very large ('macrolide') molecules belonging to the polyene group of antifungal agents.

Like other polyene antibiotics (see Ch. 52), the site of amphotericin action is the fungal cell membrane. The hydrophilic core of the doughnut-shaped amphotericin molecule creates a transmembrane ion channel, causing gross disturbances in ion balance including the loss of intracellular K^+, altering cellular permeability and disrupting transport systems. Amphotericin has a selective action, binding avidly to the membranes of fungi and some protozoa, less avidly to mammalian cells and not at all to bacteria. The basis of this relative specificity is the drug's greater avidity for *ergosterol*, a fungal membrane sterol that is not found in animal cells (where cholesterol is the principal sterol). Amphotericin is active against most fungi and yeasts, and is the gold standard for treating disseminated infections caused by organisms including *Aspergillus* and *Candida*. Amphotericin also enhances the antifungal effect of **flucytosine**, providing a useful synergistic combination.

Pharmacokinetic aspects

Amphotericin is very poorly absorbed when given orally, and this route is used only for treating fungal infections of the upper gastrointestinal (GI) tract. It can be used topically, but for systemic infections it is generally administered, formulated in liposomes or other lipid-containing preparations, by slow intravenous infusion. This improves the pharmacokinetics and reduces the (considerable) burden of side effects.

Amphotericin is very highly protein-bound. It penetrates tissues and membranes poorly, although it is found in fairly high concentrations in inflammatory exudates and may cross the blood–brain barrier quite readily when the meninges are inflamed. Intravenous amphotericin is essential in the treatment of cryptococcal meningitis, often with flucytosine. It is excreted very slowly via the kidney, traces being found in the urine for 2 months or more after administration has ceased.

Unwanted effects

The commonest (indeed almost invariable) adverse effects of amphotericin include rigors, fever, chills and headache during drug infusion; hypotension and anaphylactoid reactions occur in more severely affected individuals. The (considerably more expensive) liposome-encapsulated and lipid-complexed preparations have no greater efficacy than

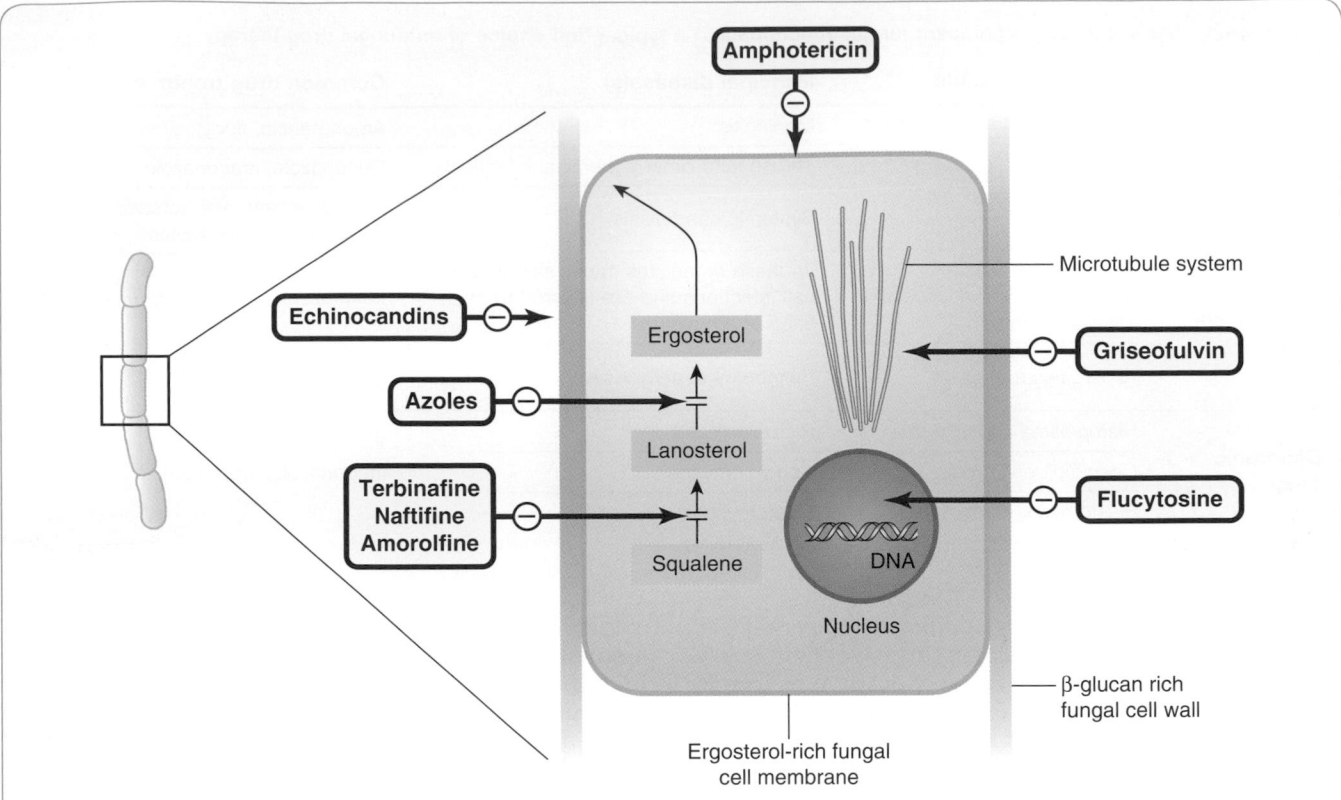

Fig. 54.1 Sites of action of common antifungal drugs. Fungi are morphologically very diverse organisms, and this schematic diagram of a 'typical' fungal cell is not intended to be structurally accurate. The principal sites of action of the main antifungal agents mentioned in this chapter are indicated as shown in *red-bordered boxes*.

the native drug but cause much less frequent and less severe infusion reactions.

The most serious unwanted effect of amphotericin is renal toxicity. Some reduction of renal function occurs in more than 80% of patients receiving the drug; although this generally improves after treatment is stopped, some impairment of glomerular filtration may remain. Hypokalaemia occurs in 25% of patients, due to the primary action of the drug on fungi spilling over into renal tubular cells, causing potassium loss, which often requires potassium chloride supplementation. Hypomagnesaemia also occurs for the same reason. Acid-base disturbance and anaemia can be further problems. Other unwanted effects include impaired hepatic function and thrombocytopenia. The drug is irritant to the endothelium of the veins, and can cause local thrombophlebitis. Intrathecal injections can cause neurotoxicity, and topical applications cause a rash.

Nystatin
Nystatin (also called **fungicidin**) is a polyene macrolide antibiotic similar in structure to amphotericin and with the same mechanism of action. It is given orally, but is not absorbed through mucous membranes or skin, and its use is mainly limited to *Candida* infections of the skin, mucous membranes and the GI tract. *Unwanted effects* may include nausea, vomiting and diarrhoea.

Griseofulvin
Griseofulvin is a narrow-spectrum antifungal agent isolated from cultures of *Penicillium griseofulvum*. It interferes

with mitosis by binding to fungal microtubules. It can be used to treat dermatophyte infections of skin or nails when local administration is ineffective, but treatment needs to be prolonged. It has largely been superseded by other drugs.

Pharmacokinetic aspects
Griseofulvin is given orally. It is poorly soluble in water, and absorption varies with the type of preparation, in particular with particle size. It is taken up selectively by newly formed skin and concentrated in the keratin. The plasma half-life is 24 h, but it is retained in the skin for much longer. It potently induces cytochrome P450 enzymes and causes several clinically important drug interactions.

Unwanted effects
Unwanted effects with griseofulvin use are infrequent, but the drug can cause GI upsets, headache and photosensitivity. Allergic reactions (rashes, fever) may also occur. The drug should not be given to pregnant women.

Echinocandins
Echinocandins comprise a ring of six amino acids linked to a lipophilic side-chain. All drugs in this group are synthetic modifications of **echinocandin B**, which is found naturally in *Aspergillus nidulans*. As a group, the echinocandins are fungicidal for *Candida* and fungistatic for *Aspergillus*. The drugs inhibit the synthesis of 1,3-β-glucan, a glucose polymer that is necessary for maintaining the structure of fungal cell walls. In the absence of this polymer,

fungal cells lose integrity and lyse. Resistance genes have been identified in *Candida* (Chen et al., 2011).

Caspofungin is active in vitro against a wide variety of fungi, and it has proved effective in the treatment of candidiasis and forms of invasive aspergillosis that are refractory to amphotericin. Oral absorption is poor, and it is given intravenously, once daily. **Anidulafungin** is used mainly for invasive candidiasis; again it is given intravenously. The principal side effects of both drugs include nausea, vomiting and diarrhoea, and rash. The relatively new **micafungin** is also mainly used for treating invasive candidiasis. It shares many of the side effects of the group but may also cause serious hepatotoxicity.

SYNTHETIC ANTIFUNGAL DRUGS
AZOLES

The azoles are a group of synthetic fungistatic agents with a broad spectrum of antifungal activity. **Clotrimazole**, **econazole**, **fenticonazole**, **ketoconazole**, **miconazole**, **tioconazole** and **sulconazole** (not United Kingdom) are based on the imidazole nucleus and **itraconazole**, **posaconazole**, **voriconazole** and **fluconazole** are triazole derivatives.

The azoles inhibit the fungal cytochrome P450 3A enzyme, lanosine 14α-demethylase, which is responsible for converting lanosterol to ergosterol, the main sterol in the fungal cell membrane. The resulting depletion of ergosterol alters the fluidity of the membrane, and this interferes with the action of membrane-associated enzymes. The net effect is an inhibition of replication. Azoles also inhibit the transformation of candidal yeast cells into hyphae – the invasive and pathogenic form of the parasite. Depletion of membrane ergosterol reduces the binding of amphotericin.

Ketoconazole

Ketoconazole was the first azole that could be given orally to treat systemic fungal infections. It is effective against several different types of organism (see Table 54.1). It is, however, toxic, and relapse is common after apparently successful treatment. It is well absorbed from the GI tract. It is distributed widely throughout the tissues and tissue fluids but does not reach therapeutic concentrations in the central nervous system unless high doses are given. It is inactivated in the liver and excreted in bile and in urine. Its half-life in the plasma is 8 h.

Unwanted effects

The main hazard of ketoconazole is liver toxicity, which is rare but can prove fatal. Liver function is monitored before and during treatment. Other side effects that occur are GI disturbances and pruritus. Inhibition of adrenocortical steroid and testosterone synthesis has been recorded with high doses, the latter resulting in gynaecomastia in some male patients. There may be adverse interactions with other drugs. **Ciclosporin** and **astemizole** compete with ketoconazole for cytochrome P450 mixed function oxidase enzymes, causing increased plasma concentrations of ketoconazole and often that of the interacting drugs themselves. Histamine H₂-receptor antagonists and antacids decrease the absorption of ketoconazole and **rifampicin** reduces the plasma concentration by induction of metabolising enzymes.

Fluconazole

Fluconazole is well absorbed and can be given orally or intravenously. It reaches high concentrations in the cerebrospinal fluid and ocular fluids, and is used to treat most types of fungal meningitis. Fungicidal concentrations are also achieved in vaginal tissue, saliva, skin and nails. It has a half-life of ~25 h, and is mainly excreted unchanged in the urine.

Unwanted effects

Unwanted effects, which are generally mild, include nausea, headache and abdominal pain. However, exfoliative skin lesions (including, on occasion, Stevens–Johnson syndrome[3]) have been seen in some individuals – primarily in AIDS patients who are being treated with multiple drugs. Hepatitis has been reported, although this is rare, and fluconazole, in the doses usually used, does not inhibit steroidogenesis and hepatic drug metabolism to the same extent as occurs with ketoconazole.

Itraconazole

Itraconazole is active against a range of dermatophytes. It may be given orally but, after absorption (which is variable) undergoes extensive hepatic metabolism. It is highly lipid-soluble (and water-insoluble), and a formulation in which the drug is retained within pockets of β-cyclodextrin is available. In this form, itraconazole can be administered intravenously, thereby overcoming the problem of variable absorption from the GI tract. Administered orally, its half-life is about 36 h, and it is excreted in the urine. It does not penetrate the cerebrospinal fluid.

Unwanted effects

The most serious are hepatoxicity and Stevens–Johnson syndrome. GI disturbances, headache and allergic skin reactions can occur. Inhibition of steroidogenesis has not been reported. Drug interactions as a result of inhibition of cytochrome P450 enzymes occur (similar to ketoconazole).

Miconazole

Miconazole is generally used topically (often as a gel) for oral and other infections of the GI tract or for skin or mucosal fungal infection. If significant systemic absorption occurs, drug interactions can present a problem.

Other azoles

Clotrimazole, econazole, tioconazole and sulconazole are used only for topical application. Clotrimazole interferes with amino acid transport into the fungus by an action on the cell membrane. It is active against a wide range of fungi, including candidal organisms. These drugs are sometimes combined with anti-inflammatory glucocorticoids (see Ch. 27). Posacanazole and voriconazole are used mainly for the treatment of invasive life-threatening infections such as aspergillosis.

OTHER ANTIFUNGAL DRUGS

Flucytosine is a synthetic, orally active antifungal agent that is effective against a limited range (mainly yeasts) of systemic fungal infections. In fungal, but not human, cells it is converted to the antimetabolite 5-fluorouracil which

[3]This is a severe and sometimes fatal condition involving blistering of the skin, mouth, GI tract, eyes and genitalia, often accompanied by fever, polyarthritis and kidney failure.

inhibits thymidylate synthetase and thus DNA synthesis (see Chs 6 and 57). If given alone, drug resistance commonly arises during treatment, so it is usually combined with amphotericin for severe systemic infections such as candidiasis and cryptococcal meningitis.

Flucytosine is usually given by intravenous infusion (because such patients are often too ill to take medicine by mouth) but can also be given orally. It is widely distributed throughout the body fluids, including the cerebrospinal fluid. About 90% is excreted unchanged via the kidneys, and the plasma half-life is 3–5 h. The dosage should be reduced if renal function is impaired.

Unwanted effects include GI disturbances, anaemia, neutropenia, thrombocytopenia and alopecia (possibly due to formation of fluorouracil [Ch. 57] from flucytosine by gut bacteria), but these are usually manageable. Uracil is reported to decrease the toxic effects on the bone marrow without impairing the antimycotic action. Hepatitis has been reported but is rare.

Terbinafine is a highly lipophilic, keratinophilic fungicidal compound active against a wide range of skin pathogens. It is particularly useful against nail infections. It acts by selectively inhibiting the enzyme *squalene epoxidase*, which is involved in the synthesis of ergosterol from squalene in the fungal cell wall. The accumulation of squalene within the cell is toxic to the organism.

When used to treat ringworm or fungal infections of the nails, it is given orally. The drug is rapidly absorbed and is taken up by skin, nails and adipose tissue. Given topically, it penetrates skin and mucous membranes. It is metabolised in the liver by the cytochrome P450 system, and the metabolites are excreted in the urine.

Unwanted effects occur in about 10% of individuals and are usually mild and self-limiting. They include GI disturbances, rashes, pruritus, headache and dizziness. Joint and muscle pains have been reported and, more rarely, hepatitis.

Naftifine (not United Kingdom) is similar in action to terbinafine. Among other developments, a morpholine derivative, **amorolfine**, which interferes with fungal sterol synthesis, is available as a nail lacquer, being effective against onychomycoses.

FUTURE DEVELOPMENTS

Fungal infections are on the rise because of the prevalence of cancer chemotherapy and transplant-associated immunosuppression. Many existing drugs have low efficacy, and problems with toxicity and new strains of commensal-turned-pathogenic fungi are emerging. Furthermore, increasing numbers of fungal strains are becoming resistant to the current antifungal drugs as they develop resistance genes or acquire naturally occurring protective mutations (although, fortunately, drug resistance is not transferable in fungi), and the capacity of some species to develop biofilms exacerbates this problem (although also offering other opportunities for drug design; see de Mello et al., 2017).

There is therefore a pressing need for more antifungals. Encouragingly, new synthetic compounds are in development, including novel azole drugs (see, for example, Zeichner, 2015) as well as some further developments, some with novel mechanisms of action.

The development of new inhibitors of β-glucan has been reviewed by Hector and Bierer (2011); new targets such as V-ATPase are being assessed (Zhang & Rao, 2012) while the prospect of discovering new naturally occurring antifungals (like the antibiotic drugs already mentioned) continues to attract attention (Dhankhar et al., 2012).

An ideal solution would be an antifungal vaccine(s). The idea was first mooted in the 1960s, but has so far met with limited success in animals (see Torosantucci et al., 2005) and none have reached the clinic. A problem in the past has been understanding how the immune system combats fungal infection but recently many issues have now been clarified and this should aid vaccine design in the future. Progress in this area has been reviewed by Medici and Del Poeta (2015), Nanjappa and Klein (2014) and Datta and Hamad (2015).

One problem with this approach is that the development of active vaccine-induced immunity is dependent upon the functioning of the patient's immune system and it is precisely immunocompromised patients who often require treatment.

REFERENCES AND FURTHER READING

Chen, S.C., Slavin, M.A., Sorrell, T.C., 2011. Echinocandin antifungal drugs in fungal infections: a comparison. Drugs 71, 11–41. (*A very comprehensive review of the echinocandin drugs, including comments upon the phenomenon of drug resistance*)

Datta, K., Hamad, M., 2015. Immunotherapy of fungal infections. Immunol. Invest. 44, 738–776. (*A comprehensive paper covering many aspects of fungal immunity and prospects for immunotherapy*)

de Mello, T.P., de Souza Ramos, L., Braga-Silva, L.A., et al., 2017. Fungal biofilm - a real obstacle against an efficient therapy: lessons from Candida. Curr. Top. Med. Chem. (*A paper which deals with the growing problems of fungal biofilms and describes potential novel ways of inhibiting their formation*)

Deepe, G.S., Jr., 2004. Preventative and therapeutic vaccines for fungal infections: from concept to implementation. Expert Rev. Vaccines 3, 701–709. (*An interesting, and optimistic, overview of the quest for antifungal vaccines*)

Denning, D.W., 2003. Echinocandin antifungal drugs. Lancet 362, 1142–1151. (*General review on the echinocandins, focusing on their clinical use*)

Dhankhar, S., Dhankhar, S., Kumar, M., Ruhil, S., Balhara, M., Chhillar, A.K., 2012. Analysis toward innovative herbal antibacterial and antifungal drugs. Recent Pat. Antiinfect. Drug Discov. 7, 242–248. (*The quest for more naturally occurring antifungals continues with the identification of potential new active compounds*)

Dodds, E.S., Drew, R.H., Perfect, J.R., 2000. Antifungal pharmacodynamics: review of the literature and clinical applications. Pharmacotherapy 20, 1335–1355. (*Good review of antifungals used to treat systemic infections; somewhat clinical in tone*)

Gupta, A.K., Tomas, E., 2003. New antifungal agents. Dermatol. Clin. 21, 565–576. (*Quite a comprehensive review that deals mainly with the newer antifungals, their mechanisms of action and resistance*)

Hadrich, I., Makni, F., Neji, S., et al., 2012. Invasive aspergillosis: resistance to antifungal drugs. Mycopathologia 174, 131–141. (*Mainly deals with the mechanisms of resistance of aspergillus to conventional antifungal drugs*)

Hector, R.F., Bierer, D.E., 2011. New beta-glucan inhibitors as antifungal drugs. Expert Opin. Ther. Pat. 21, 1597–1610. (*A review of new patents in the area. Strictly for those who want to go into the subject in depth*)

Lupetti, A., Nibbering, P.H., Campa, M., et al., 2003. Molecular targeted treatments for fungal infections: the role of drug combinations. Trends Mol. Med. 9, 269–276. (*Interesting and accessible article that deals with the use of combination antifungal therapy. Some good diagrams*)

Medici, N.P., Del Poeta, M., 2015. New insights on the development of fungal vaccines: from immunity to recent challenges. Mem. Inst. Oswaldo Cruz 110, 966–973. (*Discusses the need for, and the problems associated with, fungal vaccines. Very readable*)

Nanjappa, S.G., Klein, B.S., 2014. Vaccine immunity against fungal infections. Curr. Opin. Immunol. 28, 27–33. (*This paper reviews developments, our understanding of fungal immunity and how this applies to vaccine design. It also includes a list of vaccine candidates*)

Noel, T., 2012. The cellular and molecular defense mechanisms of the *Candida* yeasts against azole antifungal drugs. J. Mycol. Med. 22, 173–178. (*Another paper that discusses resistance mechanisms, in this case to the azoles*)

Sant, D.G., Tupe, S.G., Ramana, C.V., et al., 2016. Fungal cell membrane-promising drug target for antifungal therapy. J. Appl. Microbiol. 121 (6), 1498–1510. (*Useful review of drug action at the fungal membrane and of potential new targets for pharmacotherapy*)

Thursky, K.A., Playford, E.G., Seymour, J.F., et al., 2008. Recommendations for the treatment of established fungal infections. Intern. Med. J. 38, 496–520. (*A very comprehensive review of the treatment of fungal infections. Clinical in tone*)

Torosantucci, A., Bromuro, C., Chiani, P., et al., 2005. A novel glyco-conjugate vaccine against fungal pathogens. J. Exp. Med. 202, 597–606. (*An experimental paper demonstrating the development of a novel type of vaccine effective against Candida infections in mice*)

Zeichner, J.A., 2015. New topical therapeutic options in the management of superficial fungal infections. J. Drugs Dermatol. 14, s35–s41.

Zhang, Y., Rao, R., 2012. The V-ATPase as a target for antifungal drugs. Curr. Protein Pept. Sci. 13, 134–140. (*The title is self explanatory*)

Useful Web resources

http://www.fungionline.org.uk (*This site is sponsored by the British Mycological Society. It deals with the basic biology of fungi and contains many useful diagrams and images as well as links to other resources and video clips. It doesn't specifically relate to the pathology of fungal infections or drug therapy, but is very interesting for those wishing to delve more deeply into the biology of these unique organisms*)

55

Antiprotozoal drugs

OVERVIEW

Protozoa are motile, unicellular eukaryotic organisms that have colonised virtually every habitat and ecological niche. As a group, the protozoa are responsible for an enormous burden of illness in humans as well as domestic and wild animal populations. Historically, malaria has been one of mankind's greatest afflictions. Even today there are over 200 million cases of malaria each year and some half a million deaths. In this chapter, we will first review some general features of protozoa, discuss the interactions of these parasites with their hosts and then consider the therapy of each group of diseases in turn. In view of its global importance, malaria is the main topic.

BACKGROUND

Protozoa may be conveniently classified into four main groups on the basis of their mode of locomotion: *amoebas*, *flagellates* and *sporozoa* are easily characterised, but the final group comprises *ciliates* and other organisms of uncertain affiliation, such as the *Pneumocystis jirovecii* mentioned in the last chapter. Protozoa have diverse feeding behaviour, with some being parasitic. Many have extremely complex life cycles, sometimes involving several hosts, reminiscent of the helminths discussed in Chapter 56. Table 55.1 lists some of these clinically important organisms, together with the diseases that they cause and an overview of anti-infective drugs.

HOST–PARASITE INTERACTIONS

While mammals have developed very efficient mechanisms for defending themselves against invading parasites, many species have, in turn, evolved sophisticated evasion tactics. One common parasite ploy is to take refuge within the cells of the host, where antibodies cannot reach them. Most protozoa do this, for example, *Plasmodium* species take up residence in red cells, *Leishmania* species infect macrophages exclusively, while *Trypanosoma* species invade many other cell types. The host deals with these intracellular fugitives by deploying cytotoxic CD8[+] T cells and T helper (Th)1 pathway cytokines, such as interleukin (IL)-2, tumour necrosis factor (TNF)-α and interferon-γ. These cytokines (see Ch. 19) activate macrophages, which can then kill the infected cells along with the intracellular parasites.

As we explained in Chapter 7, the Th1 pathway responses can be down-regulated by Th2 pathway cytokines (e.g. transforming growth factor-β, IL-4 and IL-10). Some intracellular parasites have exploited this fact by stimulating the production of Th2 cytokines thus reducing their vulnerability to Th1-driven activated macrophages. For example, the invasion of macrophages by *Leishmania* species induces transforming growth factor-β, IL-10, inactivates complement pathways, and down-regulates many other intracellular defence mechanisms (Singh et al., 2012). Similar mechanisms operate during worm infestations (see Ch. 56).

Toxoplasma gondii has evolved a different gambit – *up-regulation* of host defence responses. The definitive (i.e. where sexual recombination occurs) host of this protozoon is the cat, but humans can inadvertently become intermediate hosts, harbouring the asexual form of the parasite. In humans, *T. gondii* infects numerous cell types and has a highly virulent replicative stage. To ensure that its host survives, it stimulates production of interferon-γ, modulating the host's cell-mediated responses to promote encystment (and thus persistence) of the parasite in the tissues.

MALARIA AND ANTIMALARIAL DRUGS

Malaria[1] is caused by parasites belonging to the genus *Plasmodium*. Four main species infect humans: *P. vivax*, *P. falciparum*, *P. ovale* and *P. malariae*. A related parasite that infects monkeys, *P. knowlesi*, can also infect humans and is causing increasing concern in some regions, such as South-east Asia. The insect vector in all cases is the female *Anopheles* mosquito. This breeds in stagnant water and the disease it spreads is one of the major killers on our planet.

Malaria was eradicated from most temperate countries in the 20th century, and the WHO attempted to eradicate malaria elsewhere using the powerful 'residual' insecticides and the highly effective antimalarial drugs, such as **chloroquine**, which had, by then, become available. By the end of the 1950s, the incidence of malaria had dropped dramatically. However, it was clear by the 1970s that the attempt at eradication had failed, largely because of the increasing resistance of the mosquito to the insecticides, and of the parasite to antimalarial drugs.

Largely because of a massive increase in spending (currently about US$3 billion) on public health campaigns such as the *Roll Back Malaria* programme (which is sponsored by a partnership of transnational organisations including the WHO and the World Bank), the global malaria mortality rate has fallen by approximately a quarter over the last 5 years, with some geographical areas achieving almost 50% reduction (e.g. western Pacific and South-east Asia). Even so, the overall statistics make gloomy reading. According

---

[1]The disease was once considered to arise from marshy land, hence the Latin name '*mal aria*', meaning bad or poisonous air.

Table 55.1. Principal protozoal infections and common drug treatments

Type	Species	Disease	Common drug treatment
Amoeba	*Entamoeba histolytica*	Amoebic dysentery	Metronidazole, tinidazole, diloxanide
Flagellates	*Trypanosoma brucei rhodesiense* *Trypanosoma brucei gambiense*	Sleeping sickness	Suramin, pentamidine, melarpasol, eflornithine, nifurtimox
	Trypanosoma cruzi	Chagas disease	Nifurtimox, benznidazole
	Leishmania tropica *Leishmania donovani* *Leishmania mexicana* *Leishmania braziliensis*	Kala-azar Chiclero's ulcer Espundia Oriental sore	Sodium stibogluconate, amphotericin pentamidine isethionate
	Trichomonas vaginalis	Vaginitis	Metronidazole, tinidazole
	Giardia lamblia	Diarrhoea, steatorrhoea	Metronidazole, tinidazole, mepacrine
Sporozoa	*Plasmodium falciparum*[a] *Plasmodium vivax* *Plasmodium ovale* *Plasmodium malarariae*	Malignant tertian malaria Benign tertian malaria Benign tertian malaria Quartan malaria	Artemether, atovaquone, chloroquine, clindamycin, dapsone, doxycycline, lumefantrine, mefloquine, primaquine, proguanil, pyrimethamine, quinine, sulfadoxine, tafenoquine and tetracycline
	Toxoplasma gondii	Encephalitis, congenital malformations, eye disease	Pyrimethamine–sulfadiazine
Ciliates and others	*Pneumocystis carinii*[b]	Pneumonia	Co-trimoxazole, atovaquone, pentamidine isethionate

[a]See also Table 55.2.
[b]This organism is of uncertain classification. See text for details and Chapter 54 for further comments.

Malaria

- Malaria is caused by various species of plasmodia, which are carried by the female *Anopheles* mosquito. Sporozoites (the asexual form of the parasite) are introduced into the host following insect bite and these develop in the liver into:
  - schizonts (the pre-erythrocytic stage), which liberate merozoites – these infect red blood cells, forming motile trophozoites, which, after development, release another batch of erythrocyte-infecting merozoites, causing fever; this constitutes the *erythrocytic cycle*;
  - dormant hypnozoites, which may liberate merozoites later (the exoerythrocytic stage).
- The main malarial parasites causing tertian ('every third day') malaria are:
  - *P. vivax*, which causes benign tertian malaria;
  - *P. falciparum*, which causes malignant tertian malaria; unlike *P. vivax*, this plasmodium has no exoerythrocytic stage.
- Some merozoites develop into gametocytes, the sexual forms of the parasite. When ingested by the mosquito, these give rise to further stages of the parasite's life cycle within the insect.

to the 2016 WHO report, half the world's population is at risk from the disease and it remains a significant public health problem in more than 100 countries. In 2015, there were an estimated 212 million cases and >400,000 deaths from the disease. More than 90% of these occurred in sub-Saharan Africa, and most of the victims children. Even those who survive may suffer from lasting mental impairment. Other high-risk groups include pregnant women, refugees and labourers entering endemic regions. Malaria also imposes a huge economic burden on countries where the disease is rife.

Also of concern is the fact that malaria has gained a foothold in other countries where it is not normally endemic. In Europe, for example, virtually all reported cases (>6000 in 2014) of the disease are *imported malaria*[2] and this figure has remained fairly constant, unlike the global fall in cases. This phenomenon is partly due to increasing international travel, partly due to immigration from countries where the disease is endemic and (possibly) partly caused by global warming.

The symptoms of malaria include fever, shivering, pain in the joints, headache, repeated vomiting, generalised convulsions and coma. Symptoms become apparent only 7–9 days after being bitten by an infected mosquito. By far the most dangerous parasite is *P. falciparum*.

---

[2]'Airport malaria' is caused by infected mosquitoes in aircraft arriving from areas where the disease is endemic; 'baggage malaria' is caused by their presence in luggage arriving from such areas; and 'runway malaria' has been contracted by unlucky passengers who have stopped in endemic areas, but have not even left the aircraft.

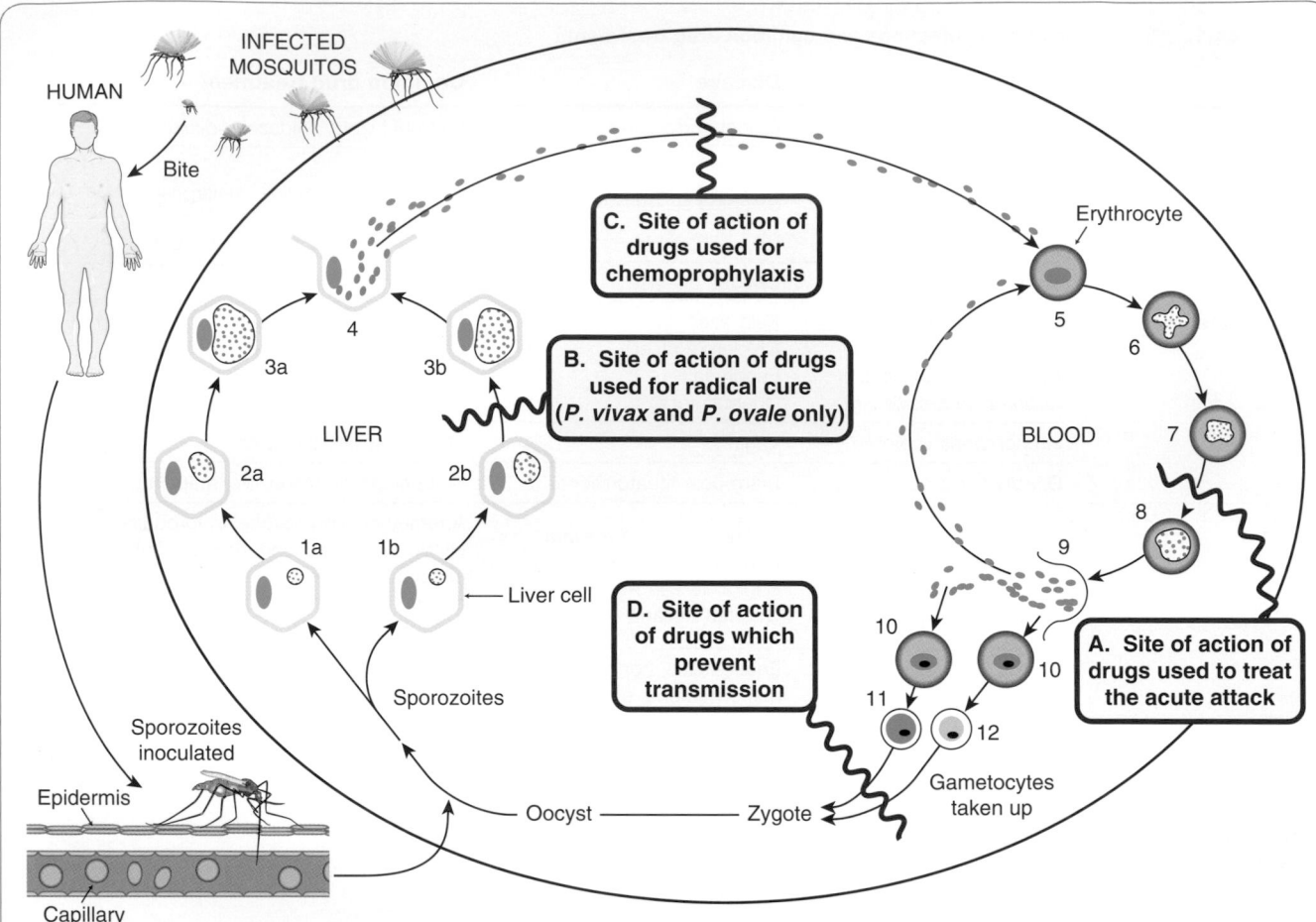

Fig. 55.1 **The life cycle of the malarial parasite and the site of action of antimalarial drugs.** The infection is initiated by the bite of an infected female *Anopheles* mosquito, which introduces the parasite into the blood. This then enters a pre- or exoerythrocytic cycle in the liver and an erythrocytic cycle in the blood: *(1a)* from the blood stream the sporozoite enters into liver cells (the parasite is shown as a small circle containing dots, and the liver cell nucleus as a blue oval); *(2a and 3a)* the schizont develops in the liver cells; *(4)* these eventually rupture releasing merozoites (some may enter further liver cells and become resting forms of the parasite, hypnozoites). *(5)* Merozoites enter into red cells and form motile trophozoites *(6)*; following division and multiplication *(7 and 8)* schizonts develop in red cells that eventually *(9)* rupture releasing further merozoites, most of which parasitise other red cells. Sometimes *(10–12)* merozoites develop into male and female gametocytes in red cells. These can constitute a fresh source of infective material if the blood is then consumed by another mosquito. *(1b)* Resting form of parasite in liver (hypnozoite). *(2b and 3b)* Growth and multiplication of hypnozoites. Sites of drug action are as follows. (A) Drugs used to treat the acute attack (also called 'blood schizonticidal agents' or 'drugs for suppressive or clinical cure'). (B) Drugs that affect the exoerythrocytic hypnozoites and result in a 'radical' cure of *P. vivax* and *P. ovale*. (C) Drugs that block the link between the exoerythrocytic stage and the erythrocytic stage; they are used for chemoprophylaxis (also termed *causal prophylactics*) and prevent the development of malarial attacks. (D) Drugs that prevent transmission and thus prevent increase of the human reservoir of the disease.

THE LIFE CYCLE OF THE MALARIA PARASITE

The life cycle of the parasite consists of a *sexual cycle*, which takes place in the female *Anopheles* mosquito, and an *asexual cycle*, which occurs in humans (Fig. 55.1 and the 'Malaria' box). Therefore the mosquito, not the human, is the *definitive* host for plasmodia. Indeed, it has been said that the only function of humans is to enable the parasite to infect more mosquitoes so that further sexual recombination can occur.

▼ The sexual cycle in the mosquito involves fertilisation of the female *gametocyte* by the male gametocyte, with the formation of a *zygote*, which develops into an *oocyst* (*sporocyst*). A further stage of division and multiplication takes place, leading to rupture of the sporocyst with release of *sporozoites*, which then migrate to the mosquito's salivary glands and thus enter the human host following mosquito bites.

When sporozoites enter the human host they disappear from the bloodstream within 30 min and enter the parenchymal cells of the liver where, during the next 10–14 days, they undergo a *pre-erythrocytic* stage of development and multiplication. The parasitised liver cells then rupture, and a host of fresh *merozoites* are released. These bind to and enter erythrocytes and form motile intracellular parasites termed *trophozoites*. During the *erythrocytic stage*, the parasite remodels the host cell, inserting parasite proteins and phospholipids into the red cell membrane. The host's haemoglobin is transported to the parasite's food vacuole, where it is digested, providing a source of amino acids. Free haem, which would be toxic to the plasmodium, is rendered harmless by polymerisation to *haemozoin*. Some antimalarial drugs act by inhibiting the haem polymerase enzyme responsible for this step.

▼ Following mitotic replication, the parasite in the red cell is termed a *schizont*, and its rapid growth and division, *schizogony*. Another phase of multiplication results in the production of further merozoites, which are released when the red cell ruptures. These merozoites then bind to and enter fresh red cells, and the erythrocytic cycle begins again. In certain forms of malaria, some sporozoites entering the liver cells form *hypnozoites*, or 'sleeping' forms of the parasite, which can be reactivated months or years later to continue an *exoerythrocytic* cycle of multiplication.

Malaria parasites can multiply in the body at a phenomenal rate – a single parasite of *P. vivax* can give rise to 250 million merozoites in 14 days. To appreciate the action required of an antimalarial drug, note that destruction of 94% of the parasites every 48 h will serve only to maintain equilibrium and will not further reduce their number or their propensity for proliferation. Some merozoites, on entering red cells, differentiate into male and female gametocytes. These can complete their cycle only when taken up again by the mosquito, when it sucks the blood from the infected host.

The periodic episodes of fever that characterise malaria result from the synchronised rupture of red cells with release of merozoites and cell debris. The rise in temperature is associated with a rise in the concentration of TNF-α in the plasma. Relapses of malaria are likely to occur with those forms of malaria that have an exoerythrocytic cycle, because the dormant hypnozoite form in the liver may emerge after an interval of weeks or months to start the infection again.

▼ The characteristic clinical presentations of the different forms of human malaria are as follows (see Fig. 55.1 for details):
- *P. falciparum*, which has an erythrocytic cycle of 48 h in humans, produces *malignant tertian malaria* – 'tertian' because the fever was believed to recur every third day (actually it varies), 'malignant' because it is the most severe form of malaria and is responsible for most malaria deaths. The plasmodium induces adhesion molecules on the infected cells, which then stick to uninfected red cells, forming clusters (rosettes), and also adhere to and pack the vessels of the microcirculation, interfering with tissue blood flow and causing organ dysfunction including renal failure and encephalopathy (cerebral malaria). *P. falciparum* does not have an exoerythrocytic stage, so if the erythrocytic stage is eradicated, relapses do not occur.
- *P. vivax* produces *benign tertian malaria*, less severe than falciparum malaria and rarely fatal. Exoerythrocytic forms may persist for years and cause relapses.
- *P. ovale*, which has a 48-h cycle and an exoerythrocytic stage, is the cause of a rare form of malaria.
- *P. malariae* has a 72-h cycle, causes *quartan malaria* and has no exoerythrocytic cycle.

Individuals living in areas where malaria is endemic may acquire a natural immunity, but this may be lost if the individual is absent from the area for more than 6 months. The best way to prevent malaria is to prevent mosquito bites by suitable clothing, insect repellents and bed nets. Bed nets sprayed with insecticides such as permethrin are very effective and form the cornerstone of many public health campaigns.

ANTIMALARIAL DRUGS

Most current drugs are only effective against the erythrocytic phase of the parasitic life cycle (**primaquine** is an exception). Some are used prophylactically to prevent malaria (Table 55.2), while others are directed towards treating acute attacks. In general, antimalarial drugs are classified in terms

Table 55.2 Examples of drug treatment and chemoprophylaxis of malaria[a]

To treat ...	Typical drug choices
Infection with *Plasmodium falciparum*	Quinine followed by doxycycline or clindamycin; Sometimes pyrimethamine with sulfadoxine if appropriate **or** Malarone[b] or Riamet[c]
Infection with unknown or mixed organisms	Quinine, Malarone or Riamet
Infection with *P. malariae*, *P. vivax* or *P. ovale*	Chloroquine (if not in a resistant area) **or** Quinine, Malarone or Riamet (if in a chloroquine-resistant area) possibly followed by primaquine in the case of *P. vivax* or *P. ovale*
Chemoprophylaxis (short-term)	Malarone or doxycycline
Chemoprophylaxis (long-term)	Malarone, mefloquine, doxycycline, chloroquine and proguanil can be used depending upon the duration required

[a]It must be appreciated that this is only a summary, not a definitive guide to prescription, as the recommended drug combinations vary depending on the patient, the area visited, the overall risk of infection, the presence of resistant forms of the disease and so on. This information is based on current UK recommendations *(source: British National Formulary 2017)*.
[b]Malarone is a proprietary fixed-dose combination of atovaquone and proguanil hydrochloride.
[c]Riamet is a proprietary fixed-dose combination of artemether and lumefantrine.

of their action against the different stages of the life cycle of the parasite (see Fig. 55.1). Fig. 55.2 shows chemical structures of some significant agents and Fig. 55.3 summarises what is known about their molecular targets.

The use of drugs for the treatment of malaria has changed considerably during the last half-century, mainly because resistance developed to chloroquine and other successful early drug combinations (see Butler et al., 2010). Where this has occurred, therapy has largely been abandoned in favour of **artemisinin**-based combination regimes (ACT). Only antimalarial drugs in common use are described in this chapter. For a brief summary of currently recommended treatment regimens, see the 'Antimalarial drugs' box and Table 55.2. The WHO 'malaria' page (see reading list) provides links to their latest recommendations covering all areas in the world.

Drugs used to treat the acute attack

Blood schizonticidal agents (see Fig. 55.1, site A) are used to treat the acute attack but also produce a 'suppressive' or 'clinical' cure. They act on the erythrocytic forms of the plasmodium. In the case of *P. falciparum* or *P. malariae*, which have no exoerythrocytic stage, these drugs effect a cure; however, with *P. vivax* or *P. ovale*, the drugs suppress

Pyrimethamine

Proguanil

Artemisinin

Sulfadoxine

Dapsone

Artemether

(A)

(B)

Quinoline-methanols

4-Aminoquinoline

Chloroquine

Quinine

8-Aminoquinoline

Primaquine

Lumefantrine

Mefloquine

(C)

(D)

Fig. 55.2 **Structures of some significant antimalarial drugs.** (A) Drugs that act on the folic acid pathway of the plasmodia. Folate antagonists (pyrimethamine, proguanil) inhibit dihydrofolate reductase; the relationship between these drugs and the pteridine moiety is shown in orange. Sulfones (e.g. dapsone) and sulfonamides (e.g. sulfadoxine) compete with p-aminobenzoic acid for dihydropteroate synthetase (relationship shown in *orange box*; see also Chs 51 and 52). (B) Artemisinin and a derivative artemether. Note the endoperoxide bridge structure *(in orange)* that is crucial to their action. (C) Some quinolone antimalarials. The quinoline moiety is shown in *orange*. (D) The aryl amino alcohol lumefantrine.

Antimalarial therapy and the parasite life cycle

Drugs used in the treatment of malaria are directed at several sites of action because no single agent is able to target all of the parasite's life cycle:
• Drugs used to treat the acute attack of malaria act on the parasites in the blood; these can cure infections with parasites (e.g. *P. falciparum*) that have no exoerythrocytic stage.

• Drugs used for prophylaxis act on merozoites emerging from liver cells.
• Drugs used for 'radical cure' are active against parasites in the liver.
• Some drugs act on gametocytes and prevent transmission by the mosquito.

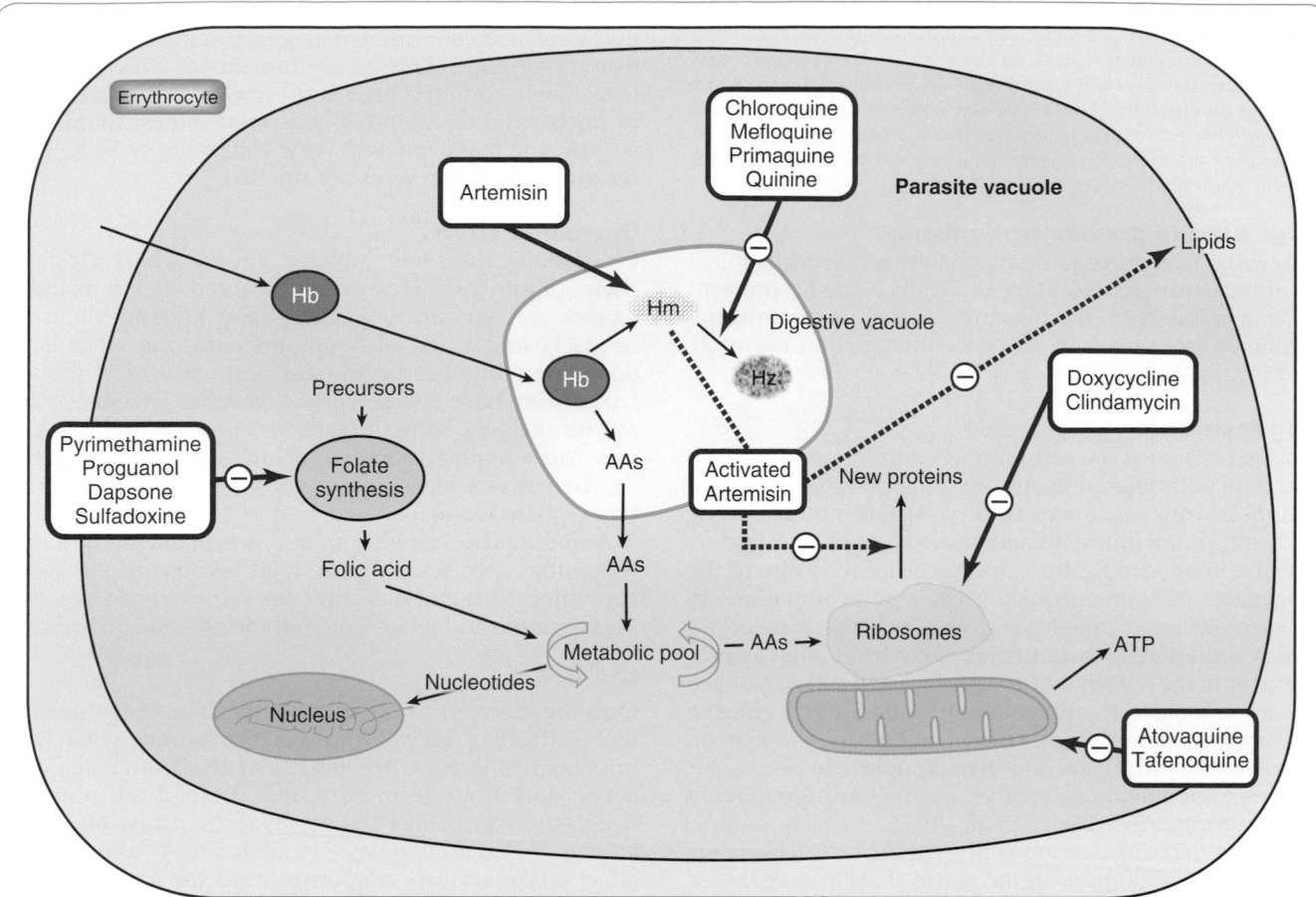

Fig. 55.3 Schematic diagram showing the sites of action of antimalarial drug targets in plasmodia. During the *erythrocytic stage* of infection the parasite lives within erythrocytes in a *parasitophorus vacuole* and feeds on haemoglobin (Hb) which is imported into the *digestive vacuole* where it is metabolised to amino acids (AAs) for use by the parasite. The haem (Hm) residue remaining is toxic to the parasite so this is metabolised to haemozoin (Hz). Some quinolone antimalarials (e.g. chloroquine) prevent the detoxification of haem, thus poisoning the parasite. Other drugs (e.g. pyrimethamine) prevent the synthesis of folic acid which is essential for nucleotide synthesis, target the synthesis of nascent proteins by ribosomes (e.g. antibiotics such as clindamycin) or inhibit mitochondrial function (e.g. atovaquone). Artemisinin and its derivatives enter the digestive vacuole where they are 'activated' by haem to form compounds that react with, and thus damage, proteins and lipids. (After Blasco et al., 2017.)

the actual attack but exoerythrocytic forms can re-emerge later to cause relapses.

This group of drugs includes:

- artemisinin and related compounds derived from the Chinese herb *qinghao*, which are usually used in combination with other drugs;
- the quinoline–methanols (e.g. **quinine** and **mefloquine**) and various 4-aminoquinolines (e.g. chloroquine);
- agents that interfere either with the synthesis of folate (e.g. **dapsone**) or with its action (e.g. **pyrimethamine** and **proguanil**);
- **atovaquone**, which affects mitochondrial function.

Combinations of these agents are frequently used. Some antibiotics, such as the tetracycline **doxycycline** (see Ch. 52), have proved useful when combined with the above agents. They have an antiparasite effect in their own right, but also control other concomitant infections.

Drugs that effect a radical cure

Tissue schizonticidal agents effect a 'radical' cure by eradicating *P. vivax* and *P. ovale* parasites in the liver (see Fig. 55.1, site B). Only the 8-aminoquinolines (e.g. primaquine and **tafenoquine**) have this action. These drugs also destroy gametocytes and thus reduce the spread of infection.

Drugs used for chemoprophylaxis

Drugs used for chemoprophylaxis (also known as *causal prophylactic drugs*) block the link between the exoerythrocytic stage and the erythrocytic stage, and thus prevent the development of malarial attacks. True causal prophylaxis – the prevention of infection by the killing of the sporozoites on entry into the host – is not feasible with present drugs, although it may be possible in the future with vaccines. Clinical attacks can be prevented by chemoprophylactic drugs that kill the parasites when they emerge from the liver after the pre-erythrocytic stage (see Fig. 55.1, site C). The drugs used for this purpose are mainly artemisinin derivatives, chloroquine, **lumefantrine**, mefloquine, proguanil, pyrimethamine, dapsone and doxycycline. They are often used in combinations.

▼ Chemoprophylactic agents are given to individuals who intend travelling to an area where malaria is endemic. Administration should start at least 1 week before entering the area and should be continued throughout the stay and for at least a month afterwards. No chemoprophylactic regimen is 100% effective, and unwanted effects may occur. A further problem is the complexity of some regimens, which require different drugs to be taken at different times, and the fact that different agents may be required for different travel destinations. For a brief summary of currently commonly recommended regimens of chemoprophylaxis, see Table 55.2.

Drugs used to prevent transmission

Some drugs (e.g. primaquine, proguanil and pyrimethamine) can also destroy gametocytes (see Fig. 55.1, site D), preventing transmission by the mosquito and thus diminishing the human reservoir of the disease, although they are rarely used for this action alone.

Drug resistance

Parasite resistance is a serious and ongoing problem with almost all antimalarial drugs, with the possible exception of lumefantrine. In many cases, resistant strains of the parasite appear within a decade, or even less, of the introduction of a novel drug. Most of the resistance is due to the appearance of spontaneously arising point mutations in (for example) target proteins such as dihydrofolate reductase (which confers resistance to antifolate drugs such as proguanil) or in the mitochondrial cytochrome B subunit (which confers resistance to atovaquone). Mutations in parasite transporters that facilitate entry, or control the exit of, quinolone drugs into the digestive vacuoles can also confer resistance and mutations in other enzymes are also thought to be important (see Blasco et al., 2017).

A rather alarming development is the increase in *multidrug resistance* in certain parts of the world. This may be linked to poor compliance, poor drugs or local variations in host immune responses to infection

CHLOROQUINE

The 4-aminoquinoline chloroquine dates from the 1940s but is still widely used as a blood schizonticidal agent (see Fig. 55.1, site A), effective against the erythrocytic forms of all four plasmodial species (where resistance is not an issue), but it does not have any effect on sporozoites, hypnozoites or gametocytes. It is uncharged at neutral pH and can therefore diffuse freely into the parasite lysosome. At the acid pH of the lysosome, it is converted to a protonated, membrane-impermeable form and is 'trapped' inside the parasite. Its chief antimalarial action derives from an inhibition of *haem polymerase*, the enzyme that polymerises toxic free haem to haemozoin. This poisons the parasite and prevents it from utilising the amino acids from haemoglobin proteolysis. Chloroquine is also used as a disease-modifying antirheumatoid drug (Ch. 27) and also has some quinidine-like actions on the heart (Ch. 22).

Resistance

P. falciparum is now resistant to chloroquine in most parts of the world. Resistance appears to result from enhanced efflux of the drug from parasitic vesicles as a result of mutations in plasmodia transporter genes (Baird, 2005). Resistance of *P. vivax* to chloroquine is also a growing problem.

Administration and pharmacokinetic aspects

Chloroquine is generally administered orally, but severe falciparum malaria may be treated by frequent intramuscular or subcutaneous injection of small doses, or by slow continuous intravenous infusion. Following oral dosing, it is

completely absorbed, extensively distributed throughout the tissues and concentrated in parasitised red cells. Release from tissues and infected erythrocytes is slow. The drug is metabolised in the liver and excreted in the urine, 70% as unchanged drug and 30% as metabolites. Elimination is slow, the major phase having a half-life of 50 h, and a residue persists for weeks or months.

Unwanted effects

Chloroquine has few adverse effects when given for chemoprophylaxis. However, unwanted effects, including nausea and vomiting, dizziness and blurring of vision, headache and urticarial symptoms, can occur when larger doses are administered to treat acute attacks of malaria. Large doses have also sometimes resulted in retinopathies and hearing loss. Bolus intravenous injections of chloroquine may cause hypotension and, if high doses are used, fatal dysrhythmias. Chloroquine is considered to be safe for use by pregnant women.

Amodiaquine has very similar action to chloroquine. It was withdrawn several years ago because of the risk of agranulocytosis, but has now been reintroduced in several areas of the world where chloroquine resistance is endemic.

QUININE

Quinine, derived from cinchona bark, has been used for the treatment of 'fevers' since the 16th century, when Jesuit missionaries brought the bark, and the knowledge of its action, to Europe from Peru. It is a blood schizonticidal drug effective against the erythrocytic forms of all four species of *Plasmodium* (see Fig. 55.1, site A), but it has no effect on exoerythrocytic forms or on the gametocytes of *P. falciparum*. Its mechanism of action is the same as that of chloroquine, but quinine is not so extensively concentrated in the plasmodium as chloroquine, so other mechanisms could also be involved. With the emergence and spread of chloroquine resistance, quinine is now the main chemotherapeutic agent for *P. falciparum* in certain parts of the world. Pharmacological actions on host tissue include a depressant action on the heart, a mild oxytocic effect on the uterus in pregnancy, a slight blocking action on the neuromuscular junction and a weak antipyretic effect.

Resistance

Some degree of resistance to quinine has developed because of increased expression of plasmodial drug efflux transporters.

Pharmacokinetic aspects

Quinine is well absorbed and is usually administered orally as a 7-day course, but it can also be given by slow intravenous infusion for severe *P. falciparum* infections and in patients who are vomiting. A loading dose may be required, but bolus intravenous administration is contraindicated because of the risk of cardiac dysrhythmias. The half-life of the drug is 10 h; it is metabolised in the liver and the metabolites are excreted in the urine within about 24 h.

Unwanted effects

Quinine has a bitter taste, and oral compliance is often poor.[3] It is irritant to the gastric mucosa and can cause

---

[3]Hence the invention of palatable drinks containing the drug, including, of course, the famous 'tonic' drunk together with gin, vodka and other beverages.

nausea and vomiting. 'Cinchonism' – characterised by nausea, dizziness, tinnitus, headache and blurring of vision – is likely to occur if the plasma concentration exceeds 30–60 µmol/L. Excessive plasma levels may also cause hypotension, cardiac dysrhythmias and severe central nervous system (CNS) disturbances such as delirium and coma.

Other, infrequent, unwanted reactions that have been reported are bone marrow depression (mainly thrombocytopenia) and hypersensitivity reactions. Quinine can stimulate insulin release. Patients with marked falciparum parasitaemia can have low blood sugar for this reason and also because of glucose consumption by the parasite. This can make a differential diagnosis between a coma caused by cerebral malaria and hypoglycaemia difficult. A rare result of treating malaria with quinine, or of erratic and inappropriate use of quinine, is *Blackwater fever*, a severe and often fatal condition in which acute haemolytic anaemia is associated with renal failure.

MEFLOQUINE

Mefloquine (see Fig. 55.2) is a blood schizonticidal compound active against *P. falciparum* and *P. vivax* (see Fig. 55.1, site A); however, it has no effect on hepatic forms of the parasites, so treatment of *P. vivax* infections should be followed by a course of primaquine to eradicate the hypnozoites. Mefloquine acts in the same way as quinine, and is frequently combined with pyrimethamine.

Resistance

P. falciparum is resistant to mefloquine in some areas – particularly in South-East Asia – and is thought to be caused, as with quinine, by increased expression in the parasite of drug efflux transporters.

Pharmacokinetic aspects and unwanted effects

Mefloquine is given orally and is rapidly absorbed. It has a slow onset of action and a very long plasma half-life (up to 30 days), which may be the result of enterohepatic cycling or tissue storage.

When mefloquine is used for treatment of the acute attack, about 50% of subjects complain of gastrointestinal (GI) disturbances. Transient CNS side effects – giddiness, confusion, dysphoria and insomnia – can occur, and there have been a few reports of aberrant atrioventricular conduction and serious, but rare, skin diseases. Rarely, mefloquine may provoke severe neuropsychiatric reactions. Mefloquine is contraindicated in pregnant women or in those liable to become pregnant within 3 months of stopping the drug, because of its long half-life and uncertainty about its teratogenic potential. When used for chemoprophylaxis, the unwanted actions are usually milder, but the drug should not be used in this way unless there is a high risk of acquiring chloroquine-resistant malaria.

LUMEFANTRINE

This aryl amino alcohol drug is related to an older compound, **halofantrine**, which is now seldom used. Lumefantrine is never used alone but in combination with **artemether**. Its mode of action is probably to prevent parasite detoxification of haem. The pharmacokinetics of the combination is complex and the reader is referred to Ezzet et al. (1998) for more details. Unwanted effects of the combination may include GI and CNS symptoms.

DRUGS AFFECTING FOLATE METABOLISM

Sulfonamides and sulfones, used as antibacterial drugs (see Ch. 52), inhibit the synthesis of folate in plasmodia by competing with p-aminobenzoic acid. Pyrimethamine and proguanil inhibit dihydrofolate reductase, which prevents the utilisation of folate in DNA synthesis. Used together, they block the folate pathway at different points, and thus act synergistically.

The main sulfonamide used in malaria treatment is **sulfadoxine**, and the only sulfone used is dapsone. Details of these drugs are given in Chapter 52. The sulfonamides and sulfones are active against the erythrocytic forms of *P. falciparum* but are less active against those of *P. vivax*; they have no activity against the sporozoite or hypnozoite forms of the plasmodia. Pyrimethamine–sulfadoxine has been extensively used for chloroquine-resistant malaria, but unfortunately resistance to this combination has developed in many areas.

Pyrimethamine is similar in structure to the antibacterial drug **trimethoprim** (see Ch. 52). Proguanil has a slightly different structure but its (active) metabolite can assume a similar configuration. Both drugs have a greater affinity for the plasmodium enzyme than for the human enzyme. They have a slow action against the erythrocytic forms of the parasite (see Fig. 55.1, site A), and proguanil is believed to have an additional effect on the initial hepatic stage (see 1a to 3a in Fig. 55.1) but not on the hypnozoites of *P. vivax* (see Fig. 55.1, site B). Pyrimethamine is used only in combination with either a sulfone or a sulfonamide.

Resistance

Point mutations in the enzymes of the folate synthesis pathway confer resistance to these drugs.

Pharmacokinetic aspects

Both pyrimethamine and proguanil are given orally and are well, although slowly, absorbed. Pyrimethamine has a plasma half-life of 4 days, and effective 'suppressive' plasma concentrations may last for 14 days; it is taken once a week. The half-life of proguanil is 16 h. It is a prodrug and is metabolised in the liver to its active form, *cycloguanil*, which is excreted mainly in the urine. It must be taken daily.

Unwanted effects

These drugs have few untoward effects in therapeutic doses. Larger doses of the pyrimethamine–dapsone combination can cause serious reactions such as haemolytic anaemia, agranulocytosis and lung inflammation. The pyrimethamine–sulfadoxine combination can cause serious skin reactions, blood dyscrasias and allergic alveolitis; it is no longer recommended for chemoprophylaxis. In high doses, pyrimethamine may inhibit mammalian dihydrofolate reductase and cause a *megaloblastic anaemia* (see Ch. 26) and folic acid supplements should be given if this drug is used during pregnancy. Resistance to antifolate drugs arises from single-point mutations in the genes encoding parasite dihydrofolate reductase.

PRIMAQUINE

Primaquine is an 8-aminoquinoline drug, which is (almost uniquely among clinically available antimalarial drugs) active against liver hypnozoites (see Fig. 55.2). **Etaquine** and tafenoquine are more active and slowly metabolised analogues of primaquine. These drugs can effect a radical cure of *P. vivax* and *P. ovale* malaria in which the parasites have a dormant stage in the liver. Primaquine does not affect sporozoites and has little if any action against the erythrocytic stage of the parasite. However, it has a gametocidal action and is the most effective antimalarial drug for preventing transmission of all four species of plasmodia. It is almost invariably used in combination with another drug, usually chloroquine. The pharmacology of primaquine and similar drugs has been reviewed by Shanks et al. (2001).

Resistance

Resistance to primaquine is (happily) scarce, although evidence of a decreased sensitivity of some *P. vivax* strains has been reported.

Pharmacokinetic aspects

Primaquine is given orally and is well absorbed. Its metabolism is rapid, and very little drug is present in the body after 10–12 h. The half-life is 3–6 h. Tafenoquine is metabolised much more slowly and therefore has the advantage that it can be given on a weekly basis.

Unwanted effects

Primaquine has few unwanted effects in most patients when used in normal therapeutic dosage. Dose-related GI symptoms can occur, and large doses may cause methaemoglobinaemia with cyanosis.

Primaquine can however cause haemolysis in individuals with the X chromosome-linked genetic metabolic condition, *glucose 6-phosphate dehydrogenase deficiency*, in red cells (Ch. 12). When this deficiency is present, the red cells are not able to regenerate NADPH, which is depleted by the oxidant metabolic derivatives of primaquine. As a consequence, the metabolic functions of the red cells are impaired and haemolysis occurs. The deficiency of the enzyme occurs in up to 15% of black males and is also fairly common in some other ethnic groups. Glucose 6-phosphate dehydrogenase activity should be estimated before giving primaquine.

ARTEMISININ AND RELATED COMPOUNDS

The importance of this group is that they are often the only drugs that can currently effectively treat resistant *P. falciparum*. These sesquiterpene lactones are derived from *sweet wormwood, qinghao*, a traditional Chinese remedy for fevers. The scientific name, conferred on the herb by Linnaeus, is *Artemisia*.[4] **Artemisinin**, a poorly soluble chemical extract from *Artemisia*, is a fast-acting blood schizonticide effective in treating the acute attack of malaria (including chloroquine-resistant and cerebral malaria). In randomised trials, artemisinins have cured attacks of malaria, including cerebral malaria, more rapidly and with fewer unwanted effects than other antimalarial agents. Artemisinin and

derivatives are effective against multidrug-resistant *P. falciparum* in sub-Saharan Africa and, combined with mefloquine, against multidrug-resistant *P. falciparum* in South-east Asia.

Pharmacokinetic aspects

Derivatives of artemisinin, which include **artesunate** (a water-soluble derivative available in some countries) and **artemether**, have higher activity and are better absorbed. The compounds are concentrated in parasitised red cells and, entering the digestive vacuoles, their unusual 'endoperoxide bridge' is activated by haem iron, giving rise to highly reactive oxygen containing compounds. These cause irreversible damage to parasite proteins, lipid membranes and other targets. These drugs are without effect on liver hypnozoites. Artemisinin can be given orally, intramuscularly or by suppository, artemether orally or intramuscularly, and artesunate intramuscularly or intravenously. They are rapidly absorbed and widely distributed, and are converted in the liver to the active metabolite dihydroartemisinin. The half-life of artemisinin is about 4 h, of artesunate, 45 min and of artemether, 4–11 h.

Unwanted effects are few. Transient heart block, decrease in blood neutrophil count and brief episodes of fever have been reported. In animal studies, artemisinin causes an unusual injury to some brain stem nuclei, particularly those involved in auditory function; however, there have been no reported incidences of neurotoxicity in humans.

In rodent studies, artemisinin potentiated the effects of mefloquine, primaquine and tetracycline, was additive with chloroquine and antagonised the sulfonamides and the folate antagonists. For this reason, artemisinin derivatives are frequently used in combination with other antimalarial drugs as part of ACT regimes; for example, artemether is often given in combination with lumefantrine.

Resistance

Initially resistance was not a major problem but, alarmingly, reports that the parasite in some areas of the world (e.g. South-east Asia) was becoming less sensitive to these drugs – either alone or in ACT combinations – began to appear about a decade ago (Blasco et al., 2017). The situation is monitored very carefully.

ATOVAQUONE

Atovaquone is a hydroxynaphthoquinone drug used prophylactically to prevent malaria, and to treat cases resistant to other drugs. It acts primarily to inhibit the parasite's mitochondrial electron transport chain, possibly by mimicking the natural substrate ubiquinone. Atovaquone is usually used in combination with the antifolate drug proguanil, because they act synergistically. The mechanism underlying this synergism is not known, but it is specific for this particular pair of drugs, because other antifolate drugs or electron transport inhibitors have no such synergistic effect. When combined with proguanil, atovaquone is highly effective and well tolerated. Few unwanted effects of such combination treatment have been reported, but abdominal pain, nausea and vomiting can occur. Pregnant or breastfeeding women should not take atovaquone.

Resistance

Resistance to atovaquone alone is rapid and results from a single-point mutation in the gene for cytochrome B.

---

[4]*Artemisia* extracts have been used for thousands of years in China for treating 'fevers'. *Artemisia*, was the wife and sister of the 4th-century king of Halicarnassus. She was so distraught at his death that she mixed his ashes with whatever she drank to make it bitter. Since sweet wormwood is noted for its extreme bitterness it was named in her honour. The biologically active compound artemisinin was isolated by Chinese chemists in 1972. This was ignored in the West for more than 10 years, until the WHO recognised its importance and, in 2002, placed it on their list of 'essential drugs' for malaria treatment. In 2015, the Chinese pharmacologist Yoyou Tu was awarded the Nobel Prize for her role in developing this drug.

Resistance to combined treatment with atovaquone and proguanil is less common.

POTENTIAL NEW ANTIMALARIAL DRUGS

Malaria has been dubbed a 're-emerging disease', largely because of the increasing appearance of resistant strains of the parasite. No new *synthetic* drug has been discovered for over 40 years and so progress has become a matter of some urgency. Successes, both in the search for new entities (see Thota, 2016; Mishra et al., 2017) and new targets (e.g. Achieng et al., 2017; Deu, 2017), coupled with a better understanding of the pharmacokinetic aspects of current drugs (Na-Bangchang & Karbwang, 2009; Basore et al., 2015), should enable better treatment regimes. Held et al. (2015) have reviewed novel antimalarials in phase II development.

But perhaps the most significant advance has come through the application of synthetic biology to solve the problem of artemisinin production. Artemisinin is notoriously difficult to synthesise by conventional chemical techniques and awkward to harvest in large amounts. Using genetically modified yeast transfected with genes from *Artemisia* it has been possible to produce large amounts of the precursor *artemisinic acid*, which can be easily converted into artemisinin (Paddon et al., 2013), thus relieving the desperate shortage of the drug.

The prospects for an effective malaria vaccine have also increased dramatically over the last decade and some candidate vaccines (especially for *P. falciparum*) are undergoing field trials organised by the WHO and others. Discussion is beyond the scope of this chapter but the reader is referred to Hoffman et al. (2015) and Matuschewski (2017) for more information.

AMOEBIASIS AND AMOEBICIDAL DRUGS

Amoebiasis is caused by infection with one or more strains of *Entamoeba* organisms. Infection may be asymptomatic or provoke a range of GI symptoms, some of which may be serious. The main organism of concern is *Entamoeba histolytica*, the causative agent of amoebiasic dysentery, which can produce a severe colitis (dysentery) and, sometimes, liver abscesses.

▼ The infection is encountered around the world, but more often in warmer climates and is associated with poor sanitation. Approximately 500 million people are thought to harbour the disease, with 40,000–100,000 deaths occurring each year as a result. It is considered to be the second-leading cause of death from parasitic diseases worldwide.

The organism has a simple life cycle, and humans are the chief hosts. Infection, generally spread by poor hygiene, follows the ingestion of the mature cysts in water or food that is contaminated with human faeces. The infectious cysts pass into the colon, where they develop into trophozoites. These motile organisms adhere to colonic epithelial cells, utilising a galactose-containing lectin on the host cell membrane. Here, the trophozoites feed, multiply, encyst and eventually pass out in the faeces, thus completing their life cycle. Some individuals are symptomless 'carriers' and harbour the parasite without developing overt disease, but cysts are present in their faeces and they can infect other individuals. The cysts can survive outside the body for at least a week in a moist and cool environment.

The trophozoite lyses the colonic mucosal cells (hence 'histolytica') using proteases, *amoebapores* (peptides that form pores in cell membranes) or by inducing host cell apoptosis. The organism then invades the submucosa, where it secretes factors to modify the host response

Antimalarial drugs

- **Chloroquine** is a blood schizonticide that is concentrated in the parasite and inhibits the haem polymerase. Orally active; half-life 50 h. *Unwanted effects*: gastrointestinal (GI) disturbances, dizziness and urticaria. Bolus intravenous injections can cause dysrhythmias. Resistance is now common.
- **Quinine** is a blood schizonticide. It may be given orally or intravenously; half-life 10 h. *Unwanted effects*: GI tract disturbances, tinnitus, blurred vision and, in large doses, dysrhythmias and central nervous system disturbances. It is usually given in combination therapy with:
  - **pyrimethamine**, a folate antagonist that acts as a slow blood schizonticide (orally active; half-life 4 days), and either
  - **dapsone**, a sulfone (orally active; half-life 24–48 h), or
  - **sulfadoxine**, a long-acting sulfonamide (orally active; half-life 7–9 days).
- **Proguanil**, a folate antagonist, is a slow blood schizonticide with some action on the primary liver forms of *P. vivax*. Orally active; half-life 16 h.
- **Mefloquine** is a blood schizonticidal agent active against *P. falciparum* and *P. vivax*, and acts by inhibiting the parasite haem polymerase. Orally active; half-life 30 days. The onset of action is slow. *Unwanted effects*: GI disturbances, neurotoxicity and psychiatric problems.
- **Primaquine** is effective against the liver hypnozoites and is also active against gametocytes. Orally active; half-life 36 h. *Unwanted effects*: GI tract disturbances and, with large doses, methaemoglobinaemia. Erythrocyte haemolysis in individuals with genetic deficiency of glucose 6-phosphate dehydrogenase.
- **Artemisinin** derivatives are now widely used particularly in combination with other drugs such as **lumefantrine**. They are fast-acting blood schizonticidal agents that are effective against both *P. falciparum* and *P. vivax*.
- **Artesunate** is water-soluble and can be given orally or by intravenous, intramuscular or rectal administration. Side effects are rare. Resistance is so far uncommon.
- **Atovaquone** (in combination with **proguanil**) is used for prevention, and for the treatment of, acute uncomplicated *P. falciparum* malaria. The drug combination is effective orally. It is given at regular intervals over 3 to 4 days. *Unwanted effects*: diarrhoea, nausea and vomiting. Resistance to **atovaquone** develops rapidly if it is given alone.

which would otherwise prove lethal to the parasite. It is this process that produces the characteristic bloody diarrhoea and abdominal pain, although a chronic intestinal infection may be present in the absence of dysentery. In some patients, an *amoebic granuloma* (amoeboma) may be present in the intestinal wall. The trophozoites may also migrate through the damaged intestinal tissue into the portal blood and hence the liver, giving rise to the most common extra-intestinal symptom of the disease – amoebic liver abscesses.

The use of drugs to treat this condition depends largely on the site and type of infection. The drugs of choice for the various forms of amoebiasis are:

- **metronidazole** (or **tinidazole**) followed by **diloxanide** for acute invasive intestinal amoebiasis resulting in acute severe amoebic dysentery;
- diloxanide for chronic intestinal amoebiasis;
- metronidazole followed by diloxanide for hepatic amoebiasis;
- diloxanide for the asymptomatic 'carrier' state.

These agents are often used in combination.

METRONIDAZOLE

Metronidazole kills the trophozoites of *E. histolytica* but has no effect on the cysts. It is the drug of choice for invasive amoebiasis of the intestine or the liver, but it is less effective against organisms in the lumen of the gut. Metronidazole is activated by anaerobic organisms to a compound that damages DNA, leading to parasite apoptosis.

Metronidazole is usually given orally and is rapidly and completely absorbed. Rectal and intravenous preparations are also available. It is distributed rapidly throughout the tissues, reaching high concentrations in the body fluids, including the cerebrospinal fluid. Some is metabolised, but most is excreted in urine.

Unwanted effects are mild. The drug has a metallic, bitter taste in the mouth but causes few unwanted effects in therapeutic doses. Minor GI disturbances have been reported, as have CNS symptoms (dizziness, headache, sensory neuropathies). Metronidazole causes a disulfiram-like reaction to alcohol (see Ch. 50), which should be strictly avoided. Metronidazole should not be used in pregnancy.

Tinidazole is similar to metronidazole in its mechanism of action and unwanted effects, but is eliminated more slowly, having a half-life of 12–14 h.

DILOXANIDE

Diloxanide or, more commonly, an insoluble ester, diloxanide furoate, are the drugs of choice for the asymptomatic infected patient, and are often given as a follow-up after the disease has been reversed with metronidazole. Both drugs have a direct amoebicidal action, affecting the parasites before encystment. Diloxanide furoate is given orally, and acts without being absorbed. Unwanted GI or other effects may be seen but it has an excellent safety profile.

Other drugs that are sometimes used include the antibiotic **paromomycin** (see reading list for further information).

TRYPANOSOMIASIS AND TRYPANOCIDAL DRUGS

Trypanosomes belong to the group of pathogenic flagellate protozoa. Two subtypes of *Trypanosoma brucei* (*rhodesiense* and *gambiense*) cause sleeping sickness in Africa (also called *HAT* – Human African Trypanosomiasis). In South America, another species *Trypanosoma cruzi*, causes *Chagas disease* (also known as American trypanosomiasis).

Almost eliminated by 1960, HAT re-emerged but, thanks to concerted public health campaigns, the number of cases is now falling again. In 2017, WHO reported less than 20,000 cases out of some 65 million people at risk of contracting sleeping sickness. The disease caused by *T. b. rhodesiense* is the more aggressive form albeit less widespread. Civil

unrest, famine and AIDS encourage the spread of the disease by reducing the chances of distributing medication or because patients are immunocompromised. Related trypanosome infections also pose a major risk to livestock and thus have a secondary impact on human health and well-being. In the case of Chagas disease, some 7 million people are believed to harbour the infection.

> ### Drugs used in amoebiasis
>
> Amoebiasis is caused by infection with *Entamoeba histolytica*, which causes dysentery and liver abscesses. The organism may be present in motile invasive form or as a cyst. The main drugs are:
>
> - **Metronidazole** given orally (half-life 7 h). Active against the invasive form in gut and liver but not the cysts. Unwanted effects (rare); gastrointestinal (GI) disturbances and central nervous system symptoms. **Tinidazole** is similar. Follow-on treatment directed at the GI lumen is needed to ensure eradication.
> - **Diloxanide** is a luminal agent given orally with no serious unwanted effects. It is active, while unabsorbed, against the non-invasive form in the GI tract.

▼ The vector of HAT is the tsetse fly. In both types of the disease, there is an initial local lesion at the site of entry, which may (in the case of *T. b. rhodesiense*) develop into a painful *chancre* (ulcer or sore). This is followed by bouts of parasitaemia and fever as the parasite enters the haemolymphatic system. The parasites and the toxins they release during the second phase of the disease cause organ damage. This manifests as 'sleeping sickness' when parasites reach the CNS causing somnolence and progressive neurological breakdown. Left untreated, such infections are fatal.

T. cruzi is spread through other blood-sucking insects, including the 'kissing bugs'. The initial phases of the infection are similar but parasites damage the heart, muscles and sometimes liver, spleen, bone and intestine. Many people harbour chronic infections. The cure rate is good if treatment begins immediately after infection, but is less successful if delayed.

The main drugs used for HAT are **suramin**, with **pentamidine** as an alternative, in the haemolymphatic stage of the disease, and the arsenical **melarsoprol** for the late stage with CNS involvement and **eflornithine** (see Burchmore et al., 2002; Burri & Brun, 2003). All have toxic side effects. **Nifurtimox**, eflornithine and **benznidazole** are used in Chagas disease: however, there is no totally effective treatment for this form of trypanosomiasis.

SURAMIN

Suramin was introduced into the therapy of trypanosomiasis in 1920. The drug binds firmly to host plasma proteins, and the complex enters the trypanosome by endocytosis, and is then liberated by lysosomal proteases. It inhibits key parasite enzymes inducing gradual destruction of organelles, such that the organisms are cleared from the circulation after a short interval.

The drug is given by slow intravenous injection. The blood concentration drops rapidly during the first few hours and then more slowly over the succeeding days. A residual concentration remains for 3–4 months. Suramin tends to accumulate in mononuclear phagocytes, and in the cells of the proximal tubule in the kidney.

Unwanted effects are common. Suramin is relatively toxic, particularly in malnourished patients, the main organ affected being the kidney. Many other slowly developing adverse effects have been reported, including optic atrophy, adrenal insufficiency, skin rashes, haemolytic anaemia and agranulocytosis. A small proportion of individuals have an immediate idiosyncratic reaction to suramin injections, which may include nausea, vomiting, shock, seizures and loss of consciousness.

PENTAMIDINE

Pentamidine has a direct trypanocidal action in vitro. It is rapidly taken up into parasites by a high-affinity energy-dependent carrier and is thought to interact with their DNA. The drug is administered intravenously or by deep intra-muscular injection, usually daily for 10–15 days. After absorption from the injection site, it binds strongly to tissues (especially in the kidney) and is eliminated slowly, only 50% of a dose being excreted over 5 days. Fairly high concentrations of the drug persist in the kidney, the liver and the spleen for several months, but it does not penetrate the blood–brain barrier. It is also active in *Pneumocystis* pneumonia (Ch. 52). Its usefulness is limited by its unwanted effects – an immediate decrease in blood pressure, with tachycardia, breathlessness and vomiting, and later serious toxicity, such as kidney damage, hepatic impairment, blood dyscrasias and hypoglycaemia.

MELARSOPROL

▼ This is an organic arsenical compound that is used mainly when the CNS is involved. It is given intravenously and enters the CNS in high concentrations, where it is able to kill the parasite. It is a highly toxic drug that produces many unwanted effects including encephalopathy and, sometimes, immediate fatality. As such, it is only administered under strict supervision.

EFLORNITHINE

▼ Eflornithine inhibits the parasite ornithine decarboxylase enzyme. It shows good activity against *T. b. gambiense* and is used as a back-up for melarsoprol, although unfortunately it has limited activity against *T. b. rhodesiense*. Side effects are common and may be severe, but are readily reversed when treatment is discontinued. Combined therapy with nifurtimox and eflornithine has yielded promising results in patients with late-stage disease.

There is an urgent need for new agents to treat trypanosome infections, partly because of the toxicity of existing drugs and partly because of developing drug resistance. There is some cause for optimism and new agents, as well as new treatment modalities, are under investigation (Barrett, 2010; Brun et al., 2011).

OTHER PROTOZOAL INFECTIONS AND DRUGS USED TO TREAT THEM

LEISHMANIASIS

Leishmania organisms are flagellate protozoa and *leishmaniasis*, the infection that they cause, is spread by the sandfly. According to the WHO (2017 figures) between 0.7 and 1.0 million new cases and 20,000–30,000 deaths are recorded each year. With increasing international travel, leishmaniasis is being imported into new areas and opportunistic infections are now being reported (particularly in AIDS patients).

▼ The vector is the female sandfly. The parasite exists in a flagellated form (*promastigote*) in the gut of the infected insect, and a non-flagellated intracellular form (*amastigote*) in the mononuclear phagocytes of the infected mammalian host. Within these cells, the parasites thrive in modified phagolysosomes. By deploying an array of countermeasures (Singh et al., 2012), they promote the generation of Th2 cytokines and subvert the macrophage's microbiocidal systems to ensure their survival. The amastigotes multiply, and eventually the infected cell releases a new crop of parasites into the haemolymphatic system, where they can infect further macrophages and possibly other cells.

Different species of *Leishmania* exist in different geographical areas and cause distinctive clinical manifestations (see Table 55.1). Typical presentations include:

- a *cutaneous form*, which presents as an unpleasant chancre ('oriental sore', 'Chiclero's ulcer' and other names) that may heal spontaneously but can leave scarring. This is the most common form and is found in the Americas, some Mediterranean countries and parts of central Asia;
- a *mucocutaneous form* ('espundia' and other names), which presents as large ulcers of the mucous membranes of the mouth, nose and throat; most cases are seen in South America;
- a serious *visceral form* ('kala-azar' and other names), where the parasite spreads through the bloodstream causing hepatomegaly, splenomegaly, anaemia and intermittent fever. This manifestation is encountered mainly in the Indian subcontinent and West Africa.

The main drugs used in visceral leishmaniasis are pentavalent antimony compounds such as **sodium stibogluconate** and pentamidine as well as **amphotericin** (see Ch. 54), which is sometimes used as a follow-up treatment. **Miltefosine**, an antitumour drug, is also used in some countries (not United Kingdom), as is **meglumine antimoniate**.

Sodium stibogluconate is given intramuscularly or by slow intravenous injection in a 10-day course. It is rapidly eliminated in the urine, 70% being excreted within 6 h. More than one course of treatment may be required. The mechanism of action of sodium stibogluconate is not clear, but the drug may increase production of toxic oxygen free radicals in the parasite.

Unwanted effects include anorexia, vomiting, bradycardia and hypotension. Coughing and substernal pain may occur during intravenous infusion. Reversible hepatitis and pancreatitis are common.

Miltefosine (hexadecylphosphocholine) is also effective in the treatment of both cutaneous and visceral leishmaniasis. The drug may be given orally and is well tolerated. Side effects are mild and include nausea and vomiting. In vitro, the drug induces DNA fragmentation and apoptosis in the parasites

Other drugs, such as antibiotics and antifungals, may be given concomitantly with the above agents. They may have some action on the parasite in their own right, but their main utility is to control the spread of secondary infections.

Resistance to current drugs, particularly the pentavalent antimonials (possibly caused by increased expression of an antimonial efflux pump), is a serious problem and there is no immediate prospect of a vaccine. The pharmacology of current drugs and prospects for new agents have been reviewed by Singh et al. (2012).

TRICHOMONIASIS

The principal *Trichomonas* organism that produces disease in humans is *T. vaginalis*. Virulent strains cause inflammation of the vagina and sometimes of the urethra in males. The main drug used in therapy is metronidazole (Ch. 52), although resistance to this drug is on the increase. High doses of tinidazole are also effective, with few side effects.

GIARDIASIS

Giardia lamblia colonises the upper GI tract in its trophozoite form, and the cysts pass out in the faeces. Infection is then spread by ingestion of food or water contaminated with faecal matter containing the cysts. It is encountered worldwide, and epidemics caused by bad sanitation are not uncommon. Metronidazole is the drug of choice, and treatment is usually very effective. Tinidazole or **mepacrine** may be used as an alternative.

TOXOPLASMOSIS

The cat is the definitive host of *Toxoplasma gondii*, a pathogenic member of this group of organisms (i.e. it is the only host in which the sexual cycle can occur). It expels the infectious cysts in its faeces; humans can inadvertently become intermediate hosts, harbouring the asexual form of the parasite. Ingested oocysts develop into sporozoites, then to trophozoites, and finally encyst in the tissues. In most individuals, the disease is asymptomatic or self-limiting, although intrauterine infections can severely damage the developing fetus and it may cause fatal generalised infection in immunosuppressed patients or those with AIDS, in whom *toxoplasmic encephalitis* may occur. In humans, *T. gondii* infects numerous cell types and has a highly virulent replicative stage.

The treatment of choice is pyrimethamine–sulfadiazine (to be avoided in pregnant patients); trimethoprim–**sulfamethoxazole** (co-trimoxazole, see Ch. 52) or combinations of pyrimethamine with **clindamycin**, clarithromycin or **azithromycin** (see Ch. 52) have shown promise.

PNEUMOCYSTIS

First recognised in 1909, *Pneumocystis carinii* (now known as *P. jirovecii*; see also Ch. 54) shares structural features with both protozoa and fungi, leaving its precise classification uncertain. Previously considered to be a widely distributed but largely innocuous microorganism, it is now recognised as an important cause of opportunistic infections in immunocompromised patients. It is common in AIDS, where *P. carinii* pneumonia is often the presenting symptom as well as a leading cause of death.

High-dose **co-trimoxazole** (Chs 51 and 52) is the drug of choice in serious cases, with parenteral pentamidine as an alternative. Treatment of milder forms of the disease (or prophylaxis) can be effected with atovaquone, trimethoprim–dapsone, or clindamycin–primaquine combinations.

FUTURE DEVELOPMENTS

Antiprotozoal pharmacology is a huge global challenge, with each species posing its own distinct problems to the would-be designer of new antiprotozoal drugs. But it is not simply a lack of new drugs that is the problem: for economic reasons, the countries and populations most affected often lack an efficient infrastructure for the distribution and safe administration of the drugs that we already possess. Cultural attitudes, civil wars, famine, the circulation of counterfeit or defective drugs, drought and natural disasters also exacerbate this problem.

REFERENCES AND FURTHER READING

Host–parasite interactions

Brenier-Pinchart, M.P., Pelloux, H., Derouich-Guergour, D., et al., 2001. Chemokines in host–parasite interactions. Trends Parasitol. 17, 292–296. (*Good review of role of immune system*)

Langhorne, J., Duffy, P.E., 2016. Expanding the antimalarial toolkit: targeting host-parasite interactions. J. Exp. Med. 213, 143–153. (*Thought-provoking paper exploring opportunities for antimalarial drug discovery offered by insights into host-parasite interactions. A little technical*)

Malaria

Achieng, A.O., Rawat, M., Ogutu, B., et al., 2017. Antimalarials: molecular drug targets and mechanism of action. Curr. Top. Med. Chem. 17, 2114–2128. (*A comprehensive review dealing largely with the identification of new chemical target compounds for drug development*)

Baird, J.K., 2005. Effectiveness of antimalarial drugs. N. Engl. J. Med. 352, 1565–1577. (*An excellent overview covering many aspects of drug therapy, drug resistance and the socioeconomic factors affecting the treatment of this disease – thoroughly recommended*)

Basore, K., Cheng, Y., Kushwaha, A.K., Nguyen, S.T., Desai, S.A., 2015. How do antimalarial drugs reach their intracellular targets? Front. Pharmacol. 6, 91.

Blasco, B., Leroy, D., Fidock, D.A., 2017. Antimalarial drug resistance: linking *Plasmodium falciparum* parasite biology to the clinic. Nat. Med. 23, 917–928.

Butler, A.R., Khan, S., Ferguson, E., 2010. A brief history of malaria chemotherapy. J. R. Coll. Physicians Edinb. 40, 172–177. (*Deals with the subject from a historical perspective beginning with the discovery of quinine and including recent developments in artemisinin synthesis. Good overview*)

Deu, E., 2017. Proteases as antimalarial targets: strategies for genetic, chemical, and therapeutic validation. FEBS J. 284 (16), 2604–2628. (*The malarial parasite needs to digest haemoglobin, and obviously proteases are important for this. The author reviews new approaches to target these to develop new drugs. Some good diagrams*)

Ezzet, F., Mull, R., Karbwang, J., 1998. Population pharmacokinetics and therapeutic response of CGP 56697 (artemether + benflumetol) in malaria patients. Br. J. Clin. Pharmacol. 46, 553–561. (*Deals with the pharmacokinetics of this increasingly important combination therapy*)

Fidock, D.A., Rosenthal, P.J., Croft, S.L., et al., 2004. Antimalarial drug discovery: efficacy models for compound screening. Nat. Rev. Drug Discov. 3, 509–520. (*Useful review dealing with mechanisms of antimalarial drug action and new concepts for screening future candidates*)

Foley, M., Tilley, L., 1997. Quinoline antimalarials: mechanisms of action and resistance. Int. J. Parasitol. 27, 231–240. (*Good, short review; useful diagrams*)

Greenwood, B.M., Fidock, D.A., Kyle, D.E., et al., 2008. Malaria: progress, perils, and prospects for eradication. J. Clin. Invest. 118, 1266–1276. (*Good overview of the disease, its current and future treatment*)

Gorobets, N.Y., Sedash, Y.V., Singh, B.K., et al., 2017. An overview of currently available antimalarials. Curr. Top. Med. Chem. 17, 2143–2157.

Held, J., Jeyaraj, S., Kreidenweiss, A., 2015. Antimalarial compounds in Phase II clinical development. Expert Opin. Investig. Drugs 24, 363–382.

Hoffman, S.L., Vekemans, J., Richie, T.L., Duffy, P.E., 2015. The march toward malaria vaccines. Am. J. Prev. Med. 49, S319–S333. (*Deals with the development of malaria vaccines. Some useful information and good diagrams, but a bit technical in places*)

Lanteri, C.A., Johnson, J.D., Waters, N.C., 2007. Recent advances in malaria drug discovery. Recent. Pat. Antiinfect. Drug Discov. 2, 95–114. (*This comprehensive review focuses mainly upon chemical leads but also has a good section on drug targets and ways of optimising existing therapies*)

Matuschewski, K., 2017. Vaccines against malaria-still a long way to go. FEBS J. 284 (16), 2560–2568. (*An excellent, and cool headed, update on the vaccine issue. Straightforward reading*)

Mishra, M., Mishra, V.K., Kashaw, V., et al., 2017. Comprehensive review on various strategies for antimalarial drug discovery. Eur. J.

Med. Chem. 125, 1300–1320. (*Good review of many aspects of malaria and its treatment. Recommended*)

Muregi, F.W., Wamakima, H.N., Kimani, F.T., 2012. Novel drug targets in malaria parasite with potential to yield antimalarial drugs with long useful therapeutic lives. Curr. Pharm. Des. 18, 3505–3521. (*Good account of anti-malarial pharmacology and how their usage might be improved*)

Na-Bangchang, K., Karbwang, J., 2009. Current status of malaria chemotherapy and the role of pharmacology in antimalarial drug research and development. Fundam. Clin. Pharmacol. 23, 387–409. (*Excellent overview of the whole area stressing the contribution that pharmacology makes to the development of new drugs. Highly recommended*)

O'Brien, C., 1997. Beating the malaria parasite at its own game. Lancet 350, 192. (*Clear, succinct coverage of mechanisms of action and resistance of current antimalarials and potential new drugs; useful diagram*)

Paddon, C.J., Westfall, P.J., Pitera, D.J., et al., 2013. High-level semi-synthetic production of the potent antimalarial artemisinin. Nature 25, 528–532. (*The use of synthetic biology techniques to produce artemisinic acid in yeast so that the global supply of artemisinin can be increased. A real tour de force*)

Shanks, G.D., Kain, K.C., Keystone, J.S., 2001. Malaria chemoprophylaxis in the age of drug resistance. II. Drugs that may be available in the future. Clin. Infect. Dis. 33, 381–385. (*A useful look ahead to new drugs*)

Thota, S., Yerra, R., 2016. Drug discovery and development of antimalarial agents: recent advances. Curr. Protein Pept. Sci. 17, 275–279. (*Excellent review of the rather alarming development of resistance to antimalarials. Also includes a lot of useful information about how these drugs act. Some excellent diagrams. Highly recommended*)

Amoebiasis

Haque, R., Huston, C.D., Hughes, M., et al., 2003. Amebiasis. N. Engl. J. Med. 348, 1565–1573. (*Good review; concentrates on the pathogenesis of the disease but has a useful table of drugs and their side effects*)

Stanley, S.L., 2001. Pathophysiology of amoebiasis. Trends Parasitol. 17, 280–285. (*A good account of the human disease that incorporates some results from animal models also easy-to-read*)

Stanley, S.L., 2003. Amoebiasis. Lancet 361, 1025–1034. (*Comprehensive and easy-to-read account of this disease, covering all aspects from diagnosis to treatment. Excellent*)

Trypanosomiasis

Aksoy, S., Gibson, W.C., Lehane, M.J., 2003. Interactions between tsetse and trypanosomes with implications for the control of trypanosomiasis. Adv. Parasitol. 53, 1–83. (*A very substantial and comprehensive article covering the biology of the tsetse fly, which also discusses alternative methods from controlling the insect population. Less good on drug therapy, but if you are interested in the biology of the insect vector of trypanosomiasis, then this is for you*)

Barrett, M.P., 2010. Potential new drugs for human African trypanosomiasis: some progress at last. Curr. Opin. Infect. Dis. 23, 603–608. (*An account of the pharmacology of current trypanicides and ways in which their usage might be improved. Discusses how new agents might be developed using (for example) a systems biology approach*)

Brun, R., Don, R., Jacobs, R.T., Wang, M.Z., Barrett, M.P., 2011. Development of novel drugs for human African trypanosomiasis. Future Microbiol. 6, 677–691.

Burchmore, R.J., Ogbunude, P.O., Enanga, B., Barrett, M.P., 2002. Chemotherapy of human African trypanosomiasis. Curr. Pharm. Des. 8, 256–267. (*Very good concise article; nice discussion of future therapeutic possibilities*)

Burri, C., Brun, R., 2003. Eflornithine for the treatment of human African trypanosomiasis. Parasitol. Res. 90 (Suppl. 1), S49–S52. (*The title is self-explanatory*)

Denise, H., Barrett, M.P., 2001. Uptake and mode of action of drugs used against sleeping sickness. Biochem. Pharmacol. 61, 1–5. (*Good coverage of drug therapy*)

Gehrig, S., Efferth, T., 2008. Development of drug resistance in *Trypanosoma brucei rhodesiense* and *Trypanosoma brucei gambiense*. Treatment of human African trypanosomiasis with natural products (Review). Int. J. Mol. Med. 22, 411–419. (*Good overview of drug therapy including sections on mechanisms of drug resistance*)

Keiser, J., Stich, A., Burri, C., 2001. New drugs for the treatment of human African trypanosomiasis: research and development. Trends Parasitol. 17, 42–49. (*Excellent review of a devastating disease*)

Leishmaniasis

Handman, E., Bullen, D.V.R., 2002. Interaction of *Leishmania* with the host macrophage. Trends Parasitol. 18, 332–334. (*Very good article describing how this parasite colonises macrophages and evades intracellular killing; easy to read*)

Mishra, J., Saxena, A., Singh, S., 2007. Chemotherapy of leishmaniasis: past, present and future. Curr. Med. Chem. 14, 1153–1169. (*Self-explanatory title!*)

Singh, N., Kumar, M., Singh, R.K., 2012. Leishmaniasis: current status of available drugs and new potential drug targets. Asian Pac. J. Trop. Med. 5, 485–497. (*Excellent article dealing with the use of drugs to combat leishmaniasis. Also deals with resistance mechanisms in some detail. Highly recommended*)

Pneumocystis pneumonia

Warren, E., George, S., You, J., Kazanjian, P., 1997. Advances in the treatment and prophylaxis of *Pneumocystis carinii* pneumonia. Pharmacotherapy 17, 900–916.

Useful Web resources

http://malaria.who.int/. (*The WHO home page containing the major information on malaria – a terrific starting point for further investigation. Other useful sites cover trypanosomiasis, leishmaniasis and other important protozoal diseases*)

http://www.mmv.org/. (*The Web page of the Medicines for Malaria Venture, a private–public partnership established to bring together funding and expertise from a number of sources to tackle malaria*)

56 Antihelminthic drugs

OVERVIEW

Some 1.5 billion people around the world suffer from *helminthiasis* **– infection with various species of parasitic** *helminths* **(worms). Inhabitants of tropical or subtropical low-income countries are most at risk; children often become infected at birth (polyparasitaemia is common) and may remain so throughout their lives. The clinical consequences of helminthiasis vary: for example, threadworm infections mainly cause discomfort but infection with** *schistosomiasis* **(***bilharzia***) or hookworm is associated with serious morbidity. Anaemia, nutritional problems and cognitive impairment are common in helminth-infected children. Helminthiasis is often co-endemic with malaria, tuberculosis and HIV/AIDS, adding to the disease burden as well as interfering with vaccination campaigns. Helminth infections are an even greater concern in veterinary medicine, affecting both domestic pets and farm animals leading to significant loss of livestock. Because of its prevalence and economic significance, the pharmacological treatment of helminthiasis is therefore of great practical therapeutic importance.**

HELMINTH INFECTIONS

The helminths comprise two major groups: the *nemathelminths* (nematodes, roundworms) and the *platyhelminths* (flatworms). The latter group is subdivided into the *trematodes* (flukes) and the *cestodes* (tapeworms). Almost 350 species of helminths have been found in humans, and most colonise the gastrointestinal (GI) tract. The global range and occurrence of helminthiasis has been reviewed by Lustigman et al. (2012).

Helminths have a complex life cycle, often involving several host species. Infection may occur in many ways, with poor hygiene a major contributory factor. Humans are generally the *primary* (or *definitive*) host for helminth infections, in the sense that they harbour the sexually mature reproductive form. Direct ingestion is common: eggs or larvae in the faeces of infected humans, enter the soil and subsequently are ingested and infect the *secondary* (*intermediate*) host. In some cases, the eggs or larvae may persist in the human host and become *encysted*, covered with granulation tissue, giving rise to *cysticercosis*. Encysted larvae may lodge in the muscles and viscera or, more seriously, in the eye or the brain.

Approximately 20 helminth species are considered to be clinically significant and used fall into two main categories – those in which the worm lives in the host's alimentary canal, and those in which the worm lives in other tissues of the host's body.

The main examples of intestinal worms are:

- *Tapeworms*: *Taenia saginata*, *Taenia solium*, *Hymenolepis nana* and *Diphyllobothrium latum*. Some 85 million people in Asia, Africa and parts of America harbour one or other of these tapeworm species. Only the first two are likely to be seen in the United Kingdom. Cattle and pigs are the usual intermediate hosts of the most common tapeworms (*T. saginata* and *T. solium*). Humans become infected by eating raw or undercooked meat containing the larvae, which have encysted in the animals' muscle tissue. *H. nana* may exist as both the adult (the intestinal worm) and the larval stage in the same host, which may be human or rodent, although some insects (fleas, grain beetles) can also serve as intermediate hosts. The infection is usually asymptomatic. *D. latum* has two sequential intermediate hosts: a freshwater crustacean and a freshwater fish. Humans become infected by eating raw or incompletely cooked fish containing the larvae.

- *Intestinal roundworms*: *Ascaris lumbricoides* (common roundworm), *Enterobius vermicularis* (threadworm, called pinworm in the United States), *Trichuris trichiura* (whipworm), *Strongyloides stercoralis* (threadworm in the United States), *Necator americanus* and *Ancylostoma duodenale* (hookworms). Again, undercooked meat or contaminated food is an important cause of infection by roundworm, threadworm and whipworm, whereas hookworm is generally acquired when their larvae penetrate the skin. Intestinal blood loss is a common cause of anaemia in regions where hookworm is endemic.

The main examples of worms that live elsewhere in host tissues are:

- *Flukes*: *Schistosoma haematobium*, *Schistosoma mansoni* and *Schistosoma japonicum*. These cause schistosomiasis (bilharzia). The adult worms of both sexes live and mate in the veins or venules of the bladder or the gut wall. The female lays eggs that pass into the bladder or gut, triggering inflammation in these organs. This results in haematuria in the former case and, occasionally, loss of blood in the faeces in the latter. The eggs hatch in water after discharge from the body and thus enter the secondary host – in this case a particular species of snail. After a period of development in this host, free-swimming *cercariae* emerge. These are capable of infecting humans by penetration of the skin. About 200 million people are infected with schistosomes in this manner.

- *Tissue roundworms: Trichinella spiralis, Dracunculus medinensis* (guinea worm) and the *filariae*, which include *Wuchereria bancrofti, Loa loa, Onchocerca volvulus* and *Brugia malayi*. The adult filariae live in the lymphatics, connective tissues or mesentery of the host and produce live embryos or *microfilariae*, which find their way into the bloodstream and may be ingested by mosquitoes or other biting insects. After a period of development within this secondary host, the larvae pass into the mouth parts of the insect and thus infect the next victim. Major filarial diseases are caused by *Wuchereria* or *Brugia*, which cause obstruction of lymphatic vessels, producing *elephantiasis* – hugely swollen legs. Other related diseases are *onchocerciasis* (in which the presence of microfilariae in the eye causes 'river blindness' – a leading preventable cause of blindness in Africa and Latin America) and *loiasis* (in which the microfilariae cause inflammation in the skin and other tissues). *Trichinella spiralis* causes trichinosis; the larvae from the viviparous female worms in the intestine migrate to skeletal muscle, where they become encysted. In *guinea worm disease,*[1] larvae of *D. medinensis* released from crustaceans in wells and waterholes are ingested and migrate from the intestinal tract to mature and mate in the tissues; the gravid female then migrates to the subcutaneous tissues of the leg or the foot, and may protrude through an ulcer in the skin. The worm may be up to a metre in length and must be removed surgically or by slow mechanical winding of the worm on to a stick over a period of days, to ensure that the worm does not break, because the remains would putrefy.
- *Hydatid tapeworm.* These are cestodes of the *Echinococcus* species for which dogs are the primary hosts, and sheep the intermediate hosts. The primary, intestinal stage does not occur in humans, but under certain circumstances humans can function as the intermediate host, in which case the larvae develop into *hydatid cysts* within the tissues, sometimes with fatal consequences.

Some nematodes that generally live in the GI tract of animals may infect humans and penetrate tissues. A skin infestation, termed *creeping eruption* or *cutaneous larva migrans*, is caused by the larvae of dog and cat hookworms which often enter through the foot. Visceral larva migrans is caused by larvae of cat and dog roundworms of the *Toxocara* genus.

ANTIHELMINTHIC DRUGS

The first effective antihelminthic drugs (also known as anthelmintics) were discovered in the 20th century and incorporated toxic metals such as arsenic (*atoxyl*) or antimony (*tartar emetic*). They were used to treat trypanosome and schistosome infestations.

Current antihelminthic drugs generally act by paralysing the parasite (e.g. by preventing muscular contraction), by

damaging the worm such that the host immune system can eliminate it, or by altering parasite metabolism (e.g. by affecting microtubule function). Because the metabolic requirements of these parasites vary greatly from one species to another, drugs that are highly effective against one type of worm may be ineffective against others.

To bring about its action, the drug must penetrate the tough exterior cuticle of the worm or gain access to its alimentary tract. This may present difficulties, because helminths have different lifestyles with some worms being exclusively *haemophagous* ('blood-eating'), while others are best described as 'tissue grazers'. A further complication is that many helminths possess active drug efflux pumps that reduce the concentration of the drug in the parasite. The route of administration and dose of antihelminthic drugs are therefore important. In a reversal of the normal order of things, several antihelminthic drugs used in human medicine were originally developed for veterinary use.

Some individual antihelminthic drugs are described briefly below and indications for their use are given in Table 56.1. Many of these drugs are unlicensed in the United Kingdom but are used on a 'named patient' basis[2]: in some cases (e.g. mebendazole) restricted dosage forms are available from pharmacies.

BENZIMIDAZOLES

This group includes **mebendazole**, **tiabendazole** and **albendazole**, which are widely used broad-spectrum antihelminthics. They are thought to act by inhibiting the polymerisation of helminth β-tubulin, thus interfering with microtubule-dependent functions such as glucose uptake. They have a selective inhibitory action, being 250–400 times more effective in producing this effect in helminth, than in mammalian, tissue. However, the effect takes time to develop and the worms may not be expelled for several days. Cure rates are generally between 60% and 100% with most parasites.

Only 10% of mebendazole is absorbed after oral administration, but a fatty meal increases absorption. It is rapidly metabolised, the products being excreted in the urine and the bile within 24–48 h. It is generally given as a single dose for threadworm, and twice daily for 3 days for hookworm and roundworm infestations. Tiabendazole is rapidly absorbed from the GI tract, very rapidly metabolised and excreted in the urine in conjugated form. It may be given twice daily for 3 days for guinea worm and *Strongyloides* infestations, and for up to 5 days for hookworm and roundworm infestations. Albendazole is also poorly absorbed but, as with mebendazole, absorption is increased by food, especially fats. It is metabolised extensively by presystemic metabolism to sulfoxide and sulfone metabolites. The former is likely to be the pharmacologically active species.

Unwanted effects are few with albendazole or mebendazole, although GI disturbances can occasionally occur. Unwanted effects with tiabendazole are more frequent but usually transient, the commonest being GI disturbances, although

---

[1]Now, happily, eliminated from many parts of the world. There are no effective drug treatments for *guinea worm disease*, but clean drinking water or filtering larval-contaminated water through nylon mesh tights have helped reduce global infection from 3.5 million to 5 in only 30 years – the first globally-eradicated parasitic disease.

[2]A situation in which the physician seeks access to an unlicensed drug from a pharmaceutical company to use in a named individual. The drug is either a 'newcomer' that has shown promise in clinical trials but has not yet been licensed or, as in these instances, an established drug that has not been licensed because the company has not applied for a product license for this indication (possibly for commercial reasons).

Table 56.1 Principal drugs used in helminth infections and some common indications

	Helminth	Principal drug(s) used
Threadworm (pinworm)	*Enterobius vermicularis*	Mebendazole, piperazine (not United Kingdom).
	Strongyloides stercoralis (threadworm in the United States)	Ivermectin, albendazole, mebendazole
Common roundworm	*Ascaris lumbricoides*	Levamisole, mebendazole, piperazine (not United Kingdom)
Other roundworm (filariae)	Lymphatic filariasis 'elephantiasis'. (*Wuchereria bancrofti*, *Brugia malayi*)	Diethylcarbamazine, ivermectin
	Subcutaneous filariasis 'eyeworm' (*Loa loa*)	Diethylcarbamazine
	Onchocerciasis 'river blindness' (*Onchocerca volvulus*)	Ivermectin
	Guinea worm (*Dracunculus medinensis*)	Praziquantel, mebendazole
	Trichiniasis (*Trichinella spiralis*)	Tiabendazole, mebendazole
	Cysticercosis (infection with larval *Taenia solium*)	Praziquantel, albendazole
	Tapeworm (*Taenia saginata*, *Taenia solium*)	Praziquantel, niclosamide
	Hydatid disease (*Echinococcus granulosus*)	Albendazole
	Hookworm (*Ancylostoma duodenale*, *Necator americanus*)	Mebendazole, albendazole, Levamisole
	Whipworm (*Trichuris trichiura*)	Mebendazole, albendazole, diethylcarbamazine
Blood flukes (*Schistosoma* spp.)	Bilharziasis: *S. haematobium*, *S. mansoni*, *S. japonicum*	Praziquantel
Cutaneous larva migrans	*Ancylostoma caninum*	Albendazole, tiabendazole, ivermectin
Visceral larva migrans	*Toxocara canis*	Albendazole, tiabendazole, diethylcarbamazine

headache, dizziness and drowsiness have been reported and allergic reactions (fever, rashes) may also occur. Mebendazole is considered unsuitable for pregnant women or children less than 2 years old.

PRAZIQUANTEL

Praziquantel is a highly effective broad-spectrum antihelminthic drug that was introduced over 20 years ago. It is the drug of choice for all forms of schistosomiasis and is the agent generally used in large-scale schistosome eradication programmes. It is also effective in cysticercosis. The drug affects not only the adult schistosomes but also the immature forms and the cercariae – the form of the parasite that infects humans by penetrating the skin.

Praziquantel disrupts Ca^{2+} homeostasis in the parasite by binding to consensus protein kinase C-binding sites in a β subunit of schistosome voltage-gated calcium channels (Greenberg, 2005). This induces an influx of Ca^{2+}, a rapid and prolonged contraction of the musculature, and eventual paralysis and death of the worm. Praziquantel also disrupts the tegument of the parasite, unmasking novel antigens, and may thus make the worm more susceptible to the host's normal immune responses.

Given orally, praziquantel is well absorbed; much of the drug is rapidly metabolised to inactive metabolites on first passage through the liver, and the metabolites are excreted in the urine. The plasma half-life of the parent compound is 60–90 min.

Praziquantel has minimal side effects in therapeutic dosage. Such unwanted effects as do occur are usually transitory and rarely of clinical importance. Effects may be more marked in patients with a heavy worm load because of products released from the dead worms. Praziquantel is considered safe for pregnant and lactating women, an important property for a drug that is commonly used in national disease control programmes. Some resistance has developed to the drug.

PIPERAZINE

Piperazine (discontinued in United Kingdom) can be used to treat infections with the common roundworm (*A. lumbricoides*) and the threadworm (*E. vermicularis*). It reversibly inhibits neuromuscular transmission in the worm, probably by mimicking GABA (Ch. 39), at GABA-gated chloride channels in nematode muscle. The paralysed worms are expelled alive by normal intestinal peristaltic movements. It is administered with a stimulant laxative such as **senna** (Ch. 31) to facilitate expulsion of the worms.

Piperazine is given orally and some, but not all, is absorbed. It is partly metabolised, and the remainder is eliminated, unchanged, via the kidney. The drug has little pharmacological action in the host. When used to treat roundworm, piperazine is effective in a single dose. For threadworm, a longer course (7 days) at lower dosage is necessary.

Unwanted effects may include GI disturbances, urticaria and bronchospasm. Some patients experience dizziness, paraesthesia, vertigo and incoordination. The drug should not be given to pregnant patients or to those with compromised renal or hepatic function.

DIETHYLCARBAMAZINE

Diethylcarbamazine is a piperazine derivative that is active in filarial infections caused by *B. malayi*, *W. bancrofti* and *L. loa*. Diethylcarbamazine rapidly removes the microfilariae from the blood circulation and has a limited effect on the adult worms in the lymphatics, but it has little action on microfilariae in vitro. It may act by changing the parasite such that it becomes susceptible to the host's normal immune responses or by interfering with helminth arachidonate metabolism.

The drug is absorbed following oral administration and is distributed throughout the cells and tissues of the body, excepting adipose tissue. It is partly metabolised, and both the parent drug and its metabolites are excreted in the urine, being cleared from the body within about 48 h.

Unwanted effects are common but transient, subsiding within a day or so even if the drug is continued. Side effects from the drug itself include GI disturbances, joint pain, headache and a general feeling of weakness. Allergic side effects referable to the products of the dying filariae are common and vary with the species of worm. In general, these start during the first day's treatment and last 3–7 days; they include skin reactions, enlargement of lymph glands, dizziness, tachycardia, and GI and respiratory disturbances. When these symptoms disappear, larger doses of the drug can be given without further problem. The drug is not used in patients with onchocerciasis, in whom it can have serious unwanted effects.

NICLOSAMIDE

Niclosamide is widely used for the treatment of tapeworm infections together with praziquantel. The *scolex* (the head of the worm that attaches to the host intestine) and a proximal segment are irreversibly damaged by the drug, such that the worm separates from the intestinal wall and is expelled. For *T. solium*, the drug is given in a single dose after a light meal, usually followed by a purgative 2 h later in case the damaged tapeworm segments release ova, which are not affected by the drug. For other tapeworm infections, this precaution is not necessary. There is negligible absorption of the drug from the GI tract.

Unwanted effects: nausea, vomiting, pruritus and light-headedness may occur but generally such effects are few, infrequent and transient.

LEVAMISOLE

Levamisole is effective in infections with the common roundworm (*A. lumbricoides*). It has a nicotine-like action (Ch. 14), stimulating and subsequently blocking the neuromuscular junctions. The paralysed worms are then expelled in the faeces. Ova are not killed. Given orally the drug is rapidly absorbed and is widely distributed crossing the blood–brain barrier. It is metabolised in the liver to inactive metabolites, which are excreted via the kidney. Its plasma half-life is 4 h. It has immunomodulatory effects and has in the past been used to treat various solid tumours.

It can cause central nervous system (CNS) and GI disturbances as well as several other unwanted effects, including agranulocytosis. The drug has been withdrawn from North American markets.

IVERMECTIN

First introduced in 1981 as a veterinary drug, **ivermectin** is a safe and highly effective broad-spectrum antiparasitic in humans. It is frequently used in global public health campaigns,[3] and is the first choice of drug for the treatment of many filarial infections. It yields good results against *W. bancrofti*, which causes elephantiasis. A single dose kills the immature microfilariae of *O. volvulus* but not the adult worms. Ivermectin is also the drug of choice for onchocerciasis, which causes river blindness and reduces the incidence of this disease by up to 80%. It is also active against some roundworms: common roundworms, whipworms, and threadworms of both the UK (*E. vermicularis*) and US (*S. stercoralis*) variety, but not hookworms.

Chemically, ivermectin is a semisynthetic agent derived from a group of natural substances, the *avermectins*, obtained from an actinomycete organism. The drug is given orally and has a half-life of 11 h. It is thought to kill the worm either by opening glutamate-gated chloride channels (found only in invertebrates) and increasing Cl^- conductance; by binding to GABA receptors or by binding to a novel allosteric site on the acetylcholine nicotinic receptor to cause an increase in transmission, leading to motor paralysis.

Unwanted effects include skin rashes and itching but in general the drug is very well tolerated. One interesting exception in veterinary medicine is the CNS toxicity seen in Collie dogs.[4]

RESISTANCE TO ANTIHELMINTHIC DRUGS

Resistance to antihelminthic drugs is a widespread and growing problem affecting not only humans but also the animal health market. Understanding of the mechanisms of helminth mutations in drug-resistant forms is not as well understood or researched, as with other microbes. During the 1990s, helminth infections in sheep (and, to a lesser extent, cattle) developed varying degrees of resistance to a number of different drugs. Parasites that develop such resistance pass this ability on to their offspring, leading to treatment failure. The widespread use of antihelminthic agents in farming has been blamed for the spread of resistant species.

There are probably several molecular mechanisms that contribute to drug resistance. The presence of the P-glycoprotein transporter (Ch. 10) in some species of nematode has already been mentioned, and agents such as **verapamil** that block the transporter in trypanosomes can partially reverse resistance to the benzimidazoles. However, some aspects of benzimidazole resistance may be attributed to alterations in their high-affinity binding to parasite β-tubulin. Likewise, resistance to levamisole is associated with changes in the structure of the target acetylcholine nicotinic receptor.

Of great significance is the way in which helminths evade the host's immune system. Even though they may reside in immunologically exposed sites such as the lymphatics or the bloodstream, many are long-lived and may co-exist with their hosts for many years without seriously affecting their health, or in some cases without even being noticed. It is striking that the two major families of helminths, while

---

[3]Ivermectin is supplied by the manufacturers free of charge in countries where river blindness is endemic. Because the worms develop slowly, a single annual dose of ivermectin is sufficient to prevent the disease.
[4]A multidrug-resistance (MDR) gene (see Ch. 3) coding for a transporter that expels ivermectins from the CNS, is mutated to an inactive form in Collie dogs.

evolving separately, deploy similar strategies to evade destruction by the immune system. Clearly, this must be of major survival value for the species.

▼ In addition to rapidly changing external antigens, which hamper immune recognition, it appears that many helminths secrete immunomodulatory products that steer the host's immune system away from a local Th1 response (see Ch. 7), which would damage the parasite, and instead promote a modified systemic Th2 type of response. This is associated with the production by the host of 'anti-inflammatory' cytokines such as interleukin-10 and is favourable to, or at least better tolerated by, the parasites. The immunology underlying this is fascinating but complex (see e.g. Harris, 2011; Harnett, 2014; McNeilly & Nisbet, 2014).

Ironically, the ability of helminths to modify the host immune response in this way may confer some survival value on the hosts themselves. For example, in addition to the local anti-inflammatory effect exerted by helminth infections, rapid wound healing is also seen. Clearly, this is of advantage to parasites that must penetrate tissues without killing the host, but may also be beneficial to the host as well. It has been proposed that helminth infections may mitigate some forms of malaria and other diseases, possibly conferring survival advantages in populations where these diseases are endemic. The deliberate, 'therapeutic' ingestion of helminths by patients has been evaluated as an (admittedly unappealing) strategy to induce remission of inflammatory diseases such as Crohn's disease, ulcerative colitis and even multiple sclerosis (see Ch. 31; Summers et al., 2005 a & b; Heylen et al., 2014; Benzel et al., 2012; Peon & Terrazas, 2016), although their effectiveness in clinical trials is mixed.

On the basis that Th2 responses reciprocally inhibit the development of Th1 diseases, it has also been hypothesised that the comparative absence of Crohn's disease, as well as some other autoimmune diseases, in the developing world may be associated with the high incidence of parasite infection, and that the rise of these disorders in the West is associated with superior sanitation and reduced helminth infection! This type of argument is generally known as the 'hygiene hypothesis'.

On the negative side however, helminth infections may undermine the efficacy of tuberculosis and other vaccination programmes that depend upon a vigorous Th1 response (see, for example, Elias et al., 2006 and Apiwattanakul et al., 2014).

VACCINES AND OTHER NOVEL APPROACHES

Despite the enormity of the clinical (and economic) problems associated with helminth infection, there are few novel antihelminthic drugs in development, possibly because the similarity between helminth and mammalian targets makes achieving selective toxicity difficult. New candidates such as **tribendimidine** are being assessed in a range of human infections and have shown promise in liver fluke infection (Duthaler et al., 2016) and some new veterinary drugs (e.g. **derquantel**) also tested in humans (see Prichard et al., 2012). The identification of new parasite metabolic enzymes as targets may help with future drug design (Timson, 2016).

Public health measures to eliminate helminth infections depend upon promoting better sanitation and mass drug administration programmes (e.g. McCarty et al., 2014). The development of effective anti-helminth vaccines would be a major step forward in this endeavour. Using surface protein and glycoprotein antigens as immunogens, some success has been achieved with veterinary vaccines (e.g. Sciutto et al., 2013; Bassetto & Amarante, 2015). The use of sophisticated tools such as genomics, transcriptomics, proteomics, metabolomics, lipidomics (collectively known as 'OMICS') to identify novel antigens may facilitate progress (Loukas et al., 2011).

REFERENCES AND FURTHER READING

General papers on helminths and their diseases

Boatin, B.A., Basanez, M.G., Prichard, R.K., et al., 2012. A research agenda for helminth diseases of humans: towards control and elimination. PLoS Negl. Trop. Dis. 6, e1547. (*Discussion of the overall strategies that would be required to eliminate helminth infections*)

Horton, J., 2003. Human gastrointestinal helminth infections: are they now neglected diseases? Trends Parasitol. 19, 527–531. (*Accessible review on helminth infections and their treatments*)

Lustigman, S., Prichard, R.K., Gazzinelli, A., et al., 2012. A research agenda for helminth diseases of humans: the problem of helminthiases. PLoS Negl. Trop. Dis. 6, e1582. (*Another paper in this series, dealing mainly with the distribution of helminth diseases around the world*)

McCarty, T.R., Turkeltaub, J.A., Hotez, P.J., 2014. Global progress towards eliminating gastrointestinal helminth infections. Curr. Opin. Gastroenterol. 30, 18–24.

Antihelminthic drugs

Burkhart, C.N., 2000. Ivermectin: an assessment of its pharmacology, microbiology and safety. Vet. Hum. Toxicol. 42, 30–35. (*Useful paper that focuses on ivermectin pharmacology*)

Croft, S.L., 1997. The current status of antiparasite chemotherapy. Parasitology 114, S3–S15. (*Rather dated but provides a comprehensive coverage of many drugs still in current use*)

Geary, T.G., Sangster, N.C., Thompson, D.P., 1999. Frontiers in anthelmintic pharmacology. Vet. Parasitol. 84, 275–295. (*Thoughtful account of the difficulties associated with drug treatment. A little dated but still relevant*)

Greenberg, R.M., 2005. Are Ca²⁺ channels targets of praziquantel action? Int. J. Parasitol. 35, 1–9. (*Interesting review on praziquantel action*)

Prichard, R., Tait, A., 2001. The role of molecular biology in veterinary parasitology. Vet. Parasitol. 98, 169–194. (*Excellent review of the application of molecular biology to understanding the problem of drug resistance and to the development of new antihelminthic agents*)

Prichard, R.K., Basanez, M.G., Boatin, B.A., et al., 2012. A research agenda for helminth diseases of humans: intervention for control and elimination. PLoS Negl. Trop. Dis. 6, e1549. (*Another providing a useful review of new antihelminthic drugs*)

Robertson, A.P., Bjorn, H.E., Martin, R.J., 2000. Pyrantel resistance alters nematode nicotinic acetylcholine receptor single channel properties. Eur. J. Pharmacol. 394, 1–8. (*A research paper describing the interactions of praziquantel and levamisole with the nematode nicotinic receptor and a proposed mechanism of drug resistance*)

Timson, D.J., 2016. Metabolic enzymes of helminth parasites: potential as drug targets. Curr. Protein Pept. Sci. 17, 280–295. (*A paper describing attempts to identify further targets form selectively toxic drugs. Describes the advantages and pitfalls of current approaches*)

Antihelminthic vaccines

Bassetto, C.C., Amarante, A.F., 2015. Vaccination of sheep and cattle against haemonchosis. J. Helminthol. 89, 517–525. (*Reviews the progress and setbacks associated with vaccination against gastrointestinal nematodes and the importance of the choice of antigens used*)

Harris, N.L., 2011. Advances in helminth immunology: optimism for future vaccine design? Trends Parasitol. 27, 288–293. (*An easy-to-read paper reviewing the latest advances in helminth vaccine immunology. Some good diagrams*)

Loukas, A., Gaze, S., Mulvenna, J.P., et al., 2011. Vaccinomics for the major blood feeding helminths of humans. OMICS 15, 567–577. (*Describes how parasite genomics and proteomics is assisting in the hunt for new vaccine targets in hookworms and schistosomes. A little technical*)

Sciutto, E., Fragoso, G., Hernandez, M., et al., 2013. Development of the S3Pvac vaccine against porcine *Taenia solium* cysticercosis: a historical review. J. Parasitol. 99, 686–692. (*Review of a successful experimental vaccine. Mainly of interest because of the way that the vaccine was prepared using a mixture of peptides. A little technical*)

Immune evasion by helminths and therapeutic exploitation

Apiwattanakul, N., Thomas, P.G., Iverson, A.R., McCullers, J.A., 2014. Chronic helminth infections impair pneumococcal vaccine responses. Vaccine 32, 5405–5410. (*The title is pretty explanatory*)

Benzel, F., Erdur, H., Kohler, S., et al., 2012. Immune monitoring of *Trichuris suis* egg therapy in multiple sclerosis patients. J. Helminthol. 86, 339–347. (*An interesting account of a small study with MS patients describing how whipworm eggs modulated their immunological profile*)

Duthaler, U., Sayasone, S., Vanobbergen, F., et al., 2016. Single-ascending-dose pharmacokinetic study of tribendimidine in opisthorchis viverrini-infected patients. Antimicrob. Agents Chemother. 60, 5705–5715. (*Deals with the development of a new drug for treatment of opisthorchiasis, a parasitic disease caught from undercooked fish in SE Asia. Mainly pharmaceutical in tone*)

Elias, D., Akuffo, H., Britton, S., 2006. Helminths could influence the outcome of vaccines against TB in the tropics. Parasite Immunol. 28, 507–513. (*Easy-to-read introduction to this phenomenon for those who want to follow up this topic*)

Harnett, W., 2014. Secretory products of helminth parasites as immunomodulators. Mol. Biochem. Parasitol. 195, 130–136. (*An interesting account of the isolation and identification of immunomodulatory products secreted by helminths and how these caould be used to treat gastrointestinal diseases*)

Heylen, M., Ruyssers, N.E., Gielis, E.M., et al., 2014. Of worms, mice and man: an overview of experimental and clinical helminth-based therapy for inflammatory bowel disease. Pharmacol. Ther. 143, 153–167. (*Good overview of the whole area of 'helminth therapy' and easy to follow. Recommended*)

McNeilly, T.N., Nisbet, A.J., 2014. Immune modulation by helminth parasites of ruminants: implications for vaccine development and host immune competence. Parasite 21, 51. (*The authors highlight evidence suggesting that helminth infections can affect the ability of cattle to control other disease as well as interfering with vaccination campaigns*)

Peon, A.N., Terrazas, L.I., 2016. Immune-regulatory mechanisms of classical and experimental multiple sclerosis drugs: a special focus on helminth-derived treatments. Curr. Med. Chem. 23, 1152–1170. (*Reviews the immunomodulatory action of many drug treatments for MS and compares the action of helminth-derived immunomodulators. Includes a substantial amount of information about the immunology of MS*)

Summers, R.W., Elliott, D.E., Urban, J.F., Jr., Thompson, R., Weinstock, J.V., 2005a. *Trichuris suis* therapy in Crohn's disease. Gut 54, 87–90. (*This paper and the one below, by the same authors, describe the action of therapeutic whipworm administration in small scale trials of Crohn's and ulcerative colitis. Interesting reading*)

Summers, R.W., Elliott, D.E., Urban, J.F., Jr., Thompson, R.A., Weinstock, J.V., 2005b. *Trichuris suis* therapy for active ulcerative colitis: a randomized controlled trial. Gastroenterology 128, 825–832.

57 Anticancer drugs

OVERVIEW

Cancer is one of the great challenges for pharmacology. A wealth of new drugs have been brought onto the market, due in part to the often terminal nature of the disease and the willingness of a sufferer to try a novel treatment in the hope of extending their life. Many of the toxicities associated with cancer treatments are tolerated in the hope of a cure. Companies continually strive to improve cancer drug effectiveness without increasing toxicity, resulting in a range of new anticancer therapies that have evolved and improved over recent decades. In this chapter, we consider cancer in general and anticancer drug therapy. We discuss first the pathogenesis of cancer and then describe the drugs that can be used to treat malignant disease. Finally, we consider the extent to which our new knowledge of cancer biology is leading to new therapies.

INTRODUCTION

'Cancer' is characterised by uncontrolled multiplication and spread of abnormal forms of the body's own cells. It is second only to cardiovascular disease as cause of death in developed nations and one in every two people born after 1960 will be diagnosed with some form of cancer during their lifetime. According to Cancer Research UK (2016), over 356,000 new cases were reported in the United Kingdom in 2014 and mortality was in excess of 163,000 (global figure, 8.8 million). Cancer is responsible for approximately 30% of all deaths in the United Kingdom. Lung and bowel cancer are the commonest malignancies, closely followed by breast and prostate cancer. Statistics from most other countries in the developed world tell much the same story.

A comparison of the incidence of cancer over the past 100 years or so gives the impression that the disease is increasing in developed countries, but this is not so. Cancer occurs mainly in later life and, with advances in public health and medical science, many more people now live to an age where malignancy is common.[1]

The terms *cancer*, *malignancy* and *malignant tumour* are often used synonymously.[2] Both benign and malignant tumours manifest uncontrolled proliferation, but the latter are distinguished by their capacity for *de-differentiation*, their *invasiveness* and their ability to *metastasise* (spread to other parts of the body). The appearance of these abnormal characteristics reflects altered patterns of gene expression in the cancer cells, resulting from inherited or acquired mutations.

There are three main approaches to treating established cancer – *surgical excision*, *irradiation* and *drug therapy* (previously often called *chemotherapy*, but now often including hormonal and biological agents as described below and in Chs 5 and 36) – and the relative value of each of these approaches depends on the disease and the stage of its development. Drug therapy may be used on its own or as an adjunct to other forms of therapy.

Compared with that of bacterial diseases, cancer chemotherapy presents a difficult conceptual problem. Microorganisms differ qualitatively from human cells (see Ch. 51), but cancer cells and normal cells are so similar in most respects that it is more difficult to find general, exploitable, biochemical differences between them. Conventional *cytotoxic drugs* act on all cells and rely on a small margin of selectivity to be useful as anticancer agents, but the scope of cancer therapy has now broadened to include drugs that affect either the hormonal regulation of tumour growth, or the defective cell cycle controls that underlie malignancy (see Ch. 6 and Weinberg et al., 1996; Croce, 2008). Numerous biopharmaceuticals including monoclonal antibodies (see Ch. 5), as well as other novel immunomodulators, have transformed the chemotherapeutic landscape.

THE PATHOGENESIS OF CANCER

It is important to consider the pathobiology in more detail to understand how anticancer drugs work and may be improved on in future.

Cancer cells manifest, to varying degrees, four characteristics that distinguish them from normal cells. These are

- *Uncontrolled proliferation*
- *De-differentiation and loss of function*
- *Invasiveness*
- *Metastasis*

---

[1]Cancer in general is a disease of older age – you have to be around long enough for all the mutations to accumulate in a cell and create a cancer phenotype that escapes the body's immune surveillance system. Clinical oncologists are gradually improving their treatment. Their goal is to keep you alive long enough so that you die of something other than cancer: a measure of their success.

[2]Blood cell malignancies – lymphomas and leukaemias – are non tumour-forming, and at times not referred to as cancers. Along with myelomas, they are generally classed as 'blood cancers'. In this account, 'cancer' is used to cover all malignancy types.

THE GENESIS OF A CANCER CELL

A normal cell turns into a cancer cell because of one or, more often, several mutations in its DNA. These can be inherited or acquired, usually through exposure to viruses or *carcinogens* (e.g. tobacco products, ultraviolet radiation, asbestos). A good example is breast cancer; women who inherit a single defective copy of either of the tumour suppressor genes *BRCA1* and *BRCA2* have a significantly increased *risk* of developing breast cancer. However, carcinogenesis is a complex multistage process, usually involving more than one genetic change as well as other, *epigenetic* factors (hormonal, co-carcinogen and tumour promoter effects – see later) that do not themselves produce cancer but which increase the *likelihood* that the genetic mutation(s) will eventually result in cancer. These mutations accumulate and lead to '*genomic instability*', which is a hallmark of carcinogenesis.

There are two main categories of relevant genetic change:

1. The activation of *proto-oncogenes* to *oncogenes*. Proto-oncogenes are genes that normally control cell division, apoptosis and differentiation (see Ch. 6), but which can be converted by viruses or carcinogens to oncogenes that induce malignant change.
2. The inactivation of *tumour suppressor genes*. Normal cells contain genes that suppress malignant change – termed tumour suppressor genes (*anti-oncogenes*) – and mutations of these genes are commonly involved in many different cancers. The loss of function of tumour suppressor genes can be the critical event in carcinogenesis.

About 30 tumour suppressor genes and 100 dominant oncogenes have been identified. The changes that lead to malignancy are a result of point mutations, gene amplification or chromosomal translocation (see Hanahan & Weinberg, 2011).

THE SPECIAL CHARACTERISTICS OF CANCER CELLS
UNCONTROLLED PROLIFERATION

It is not generally true that cancer cells proliferate faster than normal cells. Many healthy cells, in the bone marrow and the epithelium of the gastrointestinal (GI) tract (for example), undergo continuous rapid division. Some cancer cells multiply slowly (e.g. those in plasma cell tumours) and some much more rapidly (e.g. the cells of *Burkitt's lymphoma*). The significant issue is that cancer cells *have escaped from the mechanisms that normally regulate cell division and tissue growth; the normal brakes on cell division, present in a healthy cell, have been cut*. It is this, rather than their rate of proliferation, that distinguishes them from normal cells.

What are the changes that lead to the uncontrolled proliferation of tumour cells? Inactivation of tumour suppressor genes or transformation of proto-oncogenes into oncogenes can confer autonomy of growth on a cell and thus result in uncontrolled proliferation by producing changes in cellular systems (Fig. 57.1), including:

- *growth factors*, their receptors and signalling pathways;
- the *cell cycle transducers*, for example, cyclins, cyclin-dependent kinases (cdks) or the cdk inhibitors;
- the *apoptotic machinery* that normally disposes of abnormal cells;

- *telomerase expression;*
- *local blood supply*, resulting from tumour-directed angiogenesis.

Potentially all the genes coding for the above components could be regarded as oncogenes or tumour suppressor genes (Fig. 57.2), although not all are equally prone to malignant transformation and malignant transformation of several components is needed for the development of cancer.

Resistance to apoptosis
Apoptosis is programmed cell death (Ch. 6), and mutations in antiapoptotic genes are usually a prerequisite for cancer; indeed, resistance to apoptosis is a hallmark of malignant disease. It can be brought about by inactivation of proapoptotic factors or by activation of antiapoptotic factors.

Telomerase expression
Telomeres are specialised structures that cap the ends of chromosomes – like the small metal tubes on the end of shoelaces – protecting them from degradation, rearrangement and fusion with other chromosomes. Furthermore, DNA polymerase cannot easily duplicate the last few nucleotides at the ends of DNA, and telomeres prevent loss of these 'end' genes. With each round of cell division, a portion of the telomere is eroded, so that eventually it becomes non-functional. At this point, DNA replication ceases and the cell becomes senescent.[3]

Healthy stem cells express *telomerase*, a *terminal transferase* enzyme that maintains and elongates telomere ends. While it is absent from most fully differentiated somatic cells, about 95% of late-stage malignant tumours express telomerase enzymes to continuously rebuild the telomere end and extend the cell's replicative ability, thus elongating the telomere ends and effectively conferring 'immortality' on cancer cells (see Buys, 2000; Keith et al., 2004).

The control of tumour-related blood vessels
The factors described above lead to the uncontrolled proliferation of individual cancer cells, but other factors, particularly blood supply, determine the actual growth of a solid tumour. Tumours 1–2 mm in diameter can obtain nutrients by diffusion, but their further expansion requires *angiogenesis*, the development of new blood vessels in response to growth factors produced by the growing tumour itself (see Griffioen & Molema, 2000).

DE-DIFFERENTIATION AND LOSS OF FUNCTION

The multiplication of normal cells in a tissue begins with division of the undifferentiated stem cells giving rise to two *daughter cells*, one of which differentiates to become a mature non-dividing cell, ready to perform functions appropriate to that differentiated tissue. One of the main

---

[3]Once eroded down, telomere ends signal cells to stop replicating forever, which is why we humans have a limited life-span. Cancer cells however express telomerases to constantly build upon the telomere-end, and as such have lost this 'end replication' signal to limit their lifetime – some cancer cell lines have been replicating in the laboratory for many decades. The entire weight of an individual tumour line grown in all laboratories worldwide, means that the original single cancer cell has now amassed many, many tonnes of itself in total – much heavier than the individual tumour it was derived from. The patient may have mouldered in the grave, but their cancer cells go marching on – theoretically forever!

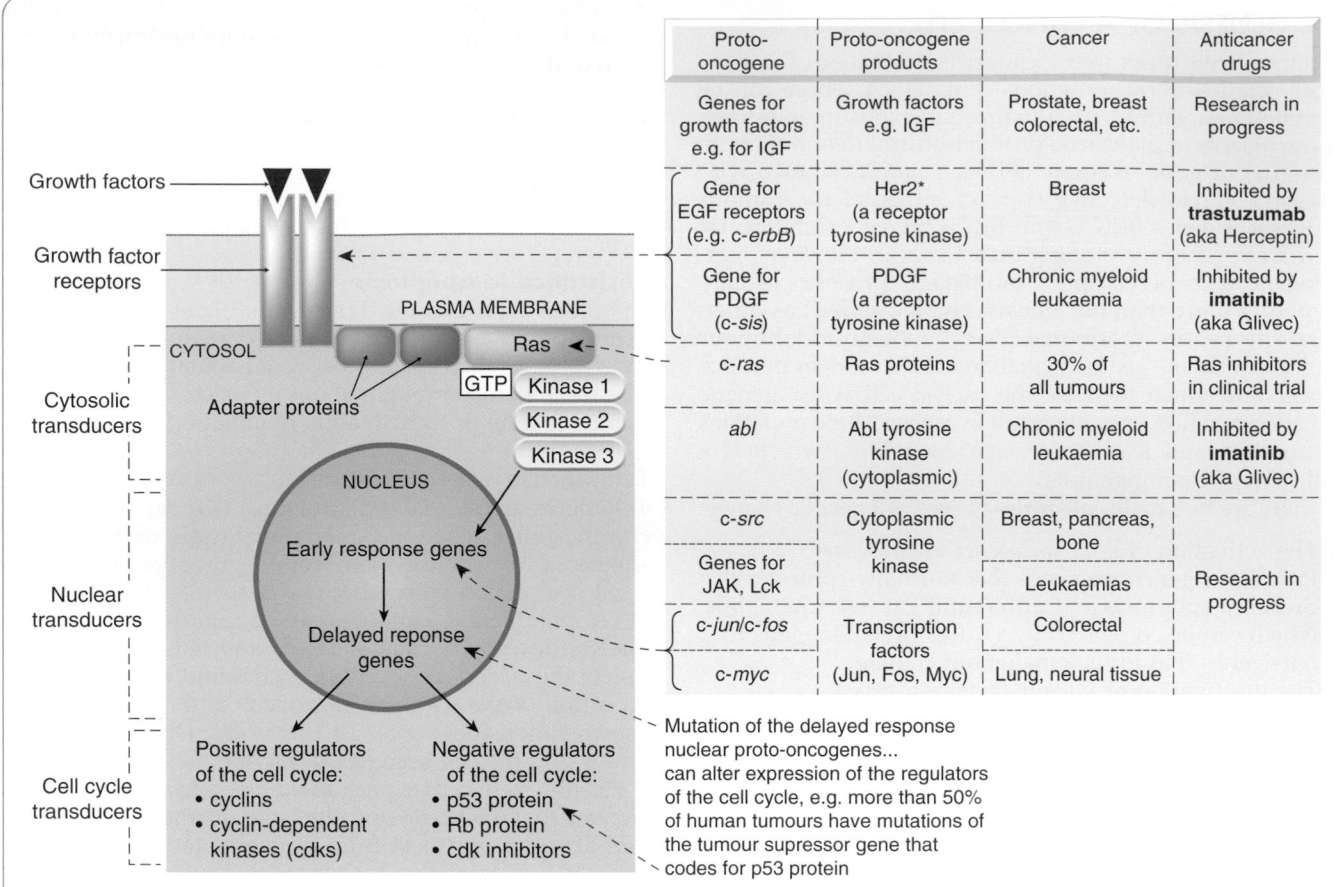

Proto-oncogene	Proto-oncogene products	Cancer	Anticancer drugs
Genes for growth factors e.g. for IGF	Growth factors e.g. IGF	Prostate, breast colorectal, etc.	Research in progress
Gene for EGF receptors (e.g. c-erbB)	Her2* (a receptor tyrosine kinase)	Breast	Inhibited by **trastuzumab** (aka Herceptin)
Gene for PDGF (c-sis)	PDGF (a receptor tyrosine kinase)	Chronic myeloid leukaemia	Inhibited by **imatinib** (aka Glivec)
c-ras	Ras proteins	30% of all tumours	Ras inhibitors in clinical trial
abl	Abl tyrosine kinase (cytoplasmic)	Chronic myeloid leukaemia	Inhibited by **imatinib** (aka Glivec)
c-src	Cytoplasmic tyrosine kinase	Breast, pancreas, bone	
Genes for JAK, Lck		Leukaemias	Research in progress
c-jun/c-fos	Transcription factors (Jun, Fos, Myc)	Colorectal	
c-myc		Lung, neural tissue	

Fig. 57.1 **Signal transduction pathways initiated by growth factors and their relationship to cancer development.** A few examples of proto-oncogenes and the products they code for are given in the table, with examples of the cancers that are associated with their conversion to oncogenes. Many growth factor receptors are receptor tyrosine kinases, the cytosolic transducers including adapter proteins that bind to phosphorylated tyrosine residues in the receptors. Ras proteins are guanine nucleotide-binding proteins and have GTPase action; decreased GTPase action means that Ras remains activated. *EGF*, epidermal growth factor; *IGF*, insulin-like growth factor; *PDGF*, platelet-derived growth factor. **Her2 is also termed her2/neu.*

characteristics of cancer cells is that they de-differentiate to varying degrees. In general, poorly differentiated cancers carry a worse prognosis than well-differentiated cancers.

INVASIVENESS

Normal cells, other than those of the blood and lymphoid tissues, are not generally found outside their 'designated' tissue of origin. This is because, during differentiation and tissue or organ growth, they develop certain spatial relationships with respect to each other. These relationships are maintained by various tissue-specific survival factors that prevent apoptosis (see Ch. 6). In this way, any cells that escape accidentally lose these survival signals and die.

For example, whilst the cells of the normal mucosal epithelium of the rectum proliferate continuously as the lining is shed, they remain as a lining epithelium. A cancer of the rectal mucosa, in contrast, invades other surrounding tissues. Cancer cells have not only lost, through mutation, the restraints that act on normal cells, but also secrete enzymes (e.g. metalloproteinases; see Ch. 6) that break down the extracellular matrix, enabling them to move around.

METASTASIS

Metastases are *secondary tumours* ('secondaries') formed by cells that have been released from the initial or *primary tumour* and which have reached other sites through blood vessels or lymphatics, by transportation on other cells or as a result of being shed into body cavities. Often, the primary tumour is asymptomatic and it is not until the cancer spreads that the secondary tumours cause symptoms leading to diagnosis of illness. As such, metastases are the principal cause of mortality and morbidity in most solid tumours and constitute a major problem for cancer therapy[4] (see Chambers et al., 2002).

As discussed earlier, displacement or aberrant migration of normal cells would lead to programmed cell death as a result of withdrawal of the necessary antiapoptotic factors. Cancer cells that metastasise have undergone a series of

---

[4]Although not widely accepted, there is a school of thought that maintaining the primary tumour's integrity and stopping it spreading would prolong life in the cancer sufferer. It may seem anathema to nurture a tumour to keep it happy and avoid stressing it, to prevent any metastatic behaviour.

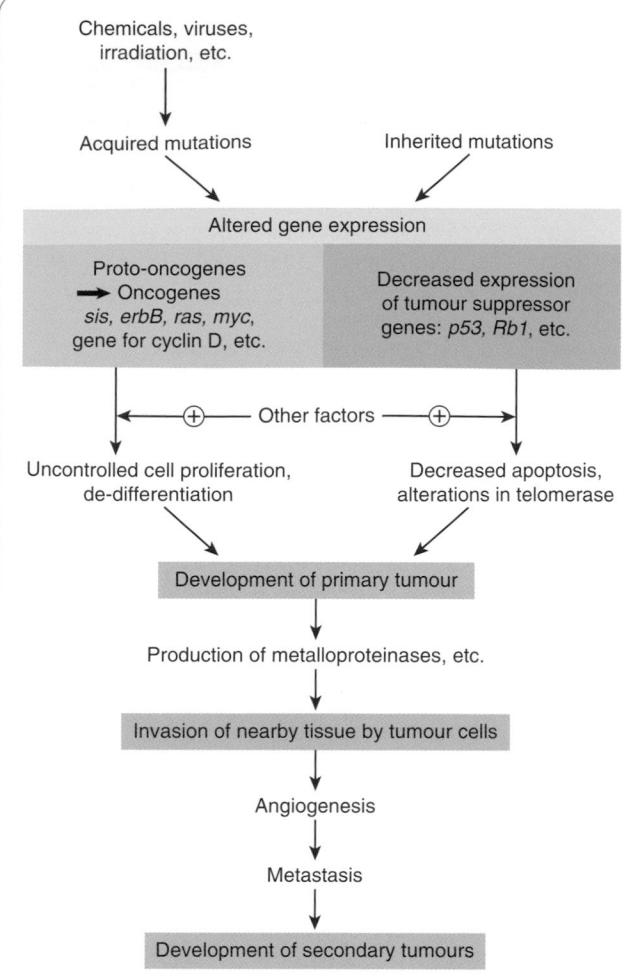

Fig. 57.2 Simplified outline of the genesis of cancer. The diagram summarises the information given in the text. The genesis of cancer is usually multifactorial, involving more than one genetic change. 'Other factors', as specified above, may involve the actions of promoters, co-carcinogens, hormones, etc. which, while not themselves carcinogenic, increase the likelihood that genetic mutation(s) will result in cancer.

GENERAL PRINCIPLES OF CYTOTOXIC ANTICANCER DRUGS

In experiments with rapidly growing transplantable leukaemias in mice, it has been found that a given therapeutic dose of a cytotoxic drug[5] destroys a constant fraction of the malignant cells. If used to treat a tumour with 10^{11} cells, a dose of drug that kills 99.99% of cells will still leave 10 million (10^7) viable malignant cells. As the same principle holds for fast-growing tumours in humans, schedules for chemotherapy are aimed at producing as near a total cell kill as possible because, in contrast to the situation that occurs in microorganisms, little reliance can be placed on the host's immunological defence mechanisms against the remaining cancer cells. If a tumour is removed (or at least *de-bulked*) surgically, any remaining *micro-metastases* are now more accessible to chemotherapy, hence its use as adjuvant therapy in these circumstances.

One of the major difficulties in treating cancer is that tumour growth is usually far advanced before cancer is diagnosed. Let us suppose that a tumour arises from a single cell and that the growth is exponential, as it may well be during the initial stages. 'Doubling' times vary, being, for example, approximately 24 h with Burkitt's lymphoma, 2 weeks in the case of some leukaemias, and 3 months with mammary cancers. Approximately 30 doublings would be required to produce a cell mass with a diameter of 2 cm, containing 10^9 cells. Such a tumour is within the limits of diagnostic procedures, although it could easily go unnoticed. A further 10 doublings would produce 10^{12} cells, a tumour mass that is likely to be lethal, and which would measure about 20 cm in diameter if it were one solid mass.

However, continuous exponential growth of this sort does not usually occur. In the case of most solid tumours, as opposed to *leukaemias* (tumours of white blood cells), the growth rate falls as the neoplasm grows. This is partly because the tumour outgrows its blood supply, and partly because not all the cells proliferate continuously. The cells of a solid tumour can be considered as belonging to three compartments:

1. *Compartment A* consists of dividing cells, possibly being continuously in the cell cycle.
2. *Compartment B* consists of resting cells (G_0 phase) which, although not dividing, are potentially able to do so.
3. *Compartment C* consists of cells that are no longer able to divide but which contribute to the tumour volume.

Essentially, only cells in *compartment A*, which may form as little as 5% of some solid tumours, are susceptible to the main current cytotoxic drugs. The cells in *compartment C* do not constitute a problem, but the existence of *compartment B* makes cancer chemotherapy difficult, because these cells are not very sensitive to cytotoxic drugs and are liable to re-enter *compartment A* following chemotherapy.

Benign tumours can still grow (often more slowly) but are characteristically unable to metastasise and spread, and are thus considered much less dangerous to the individual. One example of such is basal cell carcinoma (BCC) skin cancer

genetic changes that alter their responses to the regulatory factors that control the cellular architecture of normal tissues, enabling them to establish themselves 'extraterritorially'. Tumour-induced growth of new blood vessels locally favours metastasis.

Secondary tumours occur more frequently in some tissues than in others. For example, metastases of mammary cancers are often found in brain, lung, bone and liver. The reason for this is that breast cancer cells express chemokine receptors such as CXCR4 (see Ch. 19) on their surfaces, and chemokines that recognise these receptors are expressed at high level in these tissues but not in others (e.g. kidney), facilitating the selective accumulation of cells at these sites, providing a microenvironmental niche for them to reside and thrive. Similarly, lung cancer most commonly spreads to brain, bone and adrenal gland; malignant melanoma to brain; colorectal and ovarian tumours most commonly spread to liver and pancreatic cancer typically to liver and lung.

[5]The term *cytotoxic drug* applies to any drug that can damage or kill cells. In practice, it is used more restrictively to refer to drugs that inhibit cell division and are therefore potentially useful in cancer chemotherapy.

which continues to expand but will not metastasise; unlike malignant melanoma skin cancer, which readily metastasises to threaten critical organs, such as the brain. BCC still has the potential to transform from its benign form into a malignant form, and kill. Conversely, malignant tumours may senesce to become benign. Either way, it is always prudent to remove benign tumours in case they develop into a malignant form and gain any potential to metastasise.

Most current anticancer drugs, particularly cytotoxic agents, affect only one characteristic aspect of cancer cell biology – cell division – but have no specific inhibitory effect on invasiveness, the loss of differentiation or the tendency to metastasise. In many cases, the antiproliferative action results from an action during S phase of the cell cycle, and the resultant damage to DNA initiates apoptosis. Furthermore, because their main target is cell division, they will affect all rapidly dividing normal tissues, and therefore are likely to produce, to a greater or lesser extent, the following general toxic effects:

- *bone marrow toxicity* (myelosuppression) with decreased leukocyte production and thus decreased resistance to infection;
- *impaired wound healing*;
- *loss of hair* (alopecia);
- damage to GI *epithelium* (including oral mucous membranes);
- *depression of growth* in children;
- *sterility*;
- *teratogenicity*;
- *carcinogenicity* – because many cytotoxic drugs are mutagens.

Rapid cell destruction also entails extensive purine catabolism, and urates may precipitate in the renal tubules and cause kidney damage. Finally, in addition to specific toxic effects associated with individual drugs, virtually all cytotoxic drugs produce severe nausea and vomiting, an 'inbuilt deterrent' now thankfully largely overcome by modern antiemetic drug prophylaxis (Ch. 31).

Cytotoxic drugs, along with surgery and radiotherapy, remain the mainstay of cancer treatment, but newer treatments based on targeting the specific malfunctions of cell cycle control that characterise cancer cells, and on increasing their susceptibility to immunological attack, are becoming increasingly important. These include hormone antagonists, kinase inhibitors and monoclonal antibodies – drugs that are not cytotoxic in the conventional sense, and have a different range of side effects. Described later, they herald a significant shift in pharmacological approaches to cancer treatment. Often these newer types of therapy are guided by the genomic profile of the cancer they target – a principle that is coming more and more into reality for most drugs aimed at treating cancer.

ANTICANCER DRUGS

The main anticancer drugs can be divided into the following general categories:

- *Cytotoxic drugs.* These include:
  - *alkylating agents* and related compounds, which act by forming covalent bonds with DNA and thus impeding replication;

Cancer pathogenesis and cancer chemotherapy: general principles

- Cancer arises as a result of a series of genetic and epigenetic changes, the main genetic lesions being:
  - inactivation of tumour suppressor genes;
  - the activation of oncogenes (mutation of the normal genes controlling cell division and other processes).
- Cancer cells have four characteristics that distinguish them from normal cells:
  - uncontrolled proliferation;
  - loss of function because of lack of capacity to differentiate;
  - invasiveness;
  - the ability to metastasise.
- Cancer cells have uncontrolled proliferation often because of changes in:
  - growth factors and/or their receptors;
  - intracellular signalling pathways, particularly those controlling the cell cycle and apoptosis;
  - telomerase expression.
- Proliferation may be supported by tumour-related angiogenesis.
- Most anticancer drugs are antiproliferative – most damage DNA and thereby initiate apoptosis. They also affect rapidly dividing normal cells and are thus likely to depress bone marrow, impair healing and depress growth. Most cause nausea, vomiting, sterility, hair loss and teratogenicity.

- *antimetabolites*, which block or subvert one or more of the metabolic pathways involved in DNA synthesis;
- *cytotoxic antibiotics*, i.e. substances of microbial origin that prevent mammalian cell division;
- *plant derivatives* (e.g. vinca alkaloids, taxanes, camptothecins): most of these specifically affect microtubule function and hence the formation of the mitotic spindle.
- *Hormones*, especially steroids and their antagonists (Chs 34 and 36).
- *Protein kinase inhibitors* which inhibit growth factor receptor signal transduction (see Krause & van Etten, 2005) and other non-proliferative effects of tyrosine kinases, such as cell adhesion.
- *Monoclonal antibodies.*
- *Miscellaneous agents.*

The clinical use of anticancer drugs is the province of the specialist, who selects treatment regimens appropriate to the patient with the objective of curing, prolonging life or providing palliative therapy.[6] There are over 80 drugs available in the United Kingdom for this purpose and they are often used in combination. The principal treatments are listed in Table 57.1. For reasons of space, we restrict our discussion of mechanisms of action to common examples from each group. A textbook (Airley, 2009) provides detailed information.

---

[6]You will have gathered that many anticancer drugs are toxic. 'To be an oncologist,' one practitioner commented, 'one has to hate cancer more than one loves life.'

Table 57.1 An overview of anticancer drugs

Type	Group	Examples	Main mechanism
Alkylating, and related, agents	Nitrogen mustards	Bendamustine, chlorambucil, cyclophosphamide, estramustine,[a] ifosfamide, melphalan	Intrastrand cross-linking of DNA
	Nitrosoureas	Carmustine, lomustine	
	Platinum compounds	Carboplatin, cisplatin, oxaliplatin	
	Other	Busulfan, dacarbazine, hydroxycarbamide, mitobronitol, procarbazine treosulfan, thiotepa, temozolomide	
Antimetabolites	Folate antagonists	Methotrexate, pemetrexed, raltitrexed	Blocking the synthesis of DNA and/or RNA
	Pyrimidine pathway	Azacitidine, capecitabine, cytarabine, decitabine, fluorouracil gemcitabine, tegafur	
	Purine pathway	Cladribine, clofarabine, fludarabine, mercaptopurine, nelarabine, pentostatin, tioguanine	
Cytotoxic antibiotics	Anthracyclines	(Amsacrine), daunorubicin, doxorubicin, epirubicin, idarubicin, (mitoxantrone)	Multiple effects on DNA/RNA synthesis and topoisomerase action
	Other	Bleomycin, dactinomycin, mitomycin, trabectedin	
Plant derivatives and similar compounds	Taxanes	Cabazitaxel, docetaxel, paclitaxel	Microtubule assembly; prevents spindle formation
	Vinca alkaloids	Vinblastine, vincristine, vindesine, vinflunine, vinorelbine (eribulin).	
	Campothecins	Irinotecan, topotecan	Inhibition of topoisomerase
	Other	Etoposide	
Hormones/ antagonists	Hormones/analogues	Buserelin, diethylstilboestrol, ethinyloestradiol, goserelin, histrelin, lanreotide, leuprorelin, medroxyprogesterone, megesterol, norhisterone, triptorelin, octreotide, pasreotide	Act as physiological agonists, antagonists or hormone synthesis inhibitors to disrupt hormone-dependent tumour growth
	Antagonists	Bicalutamide, cyproterone, degarelix, flutamide, fulvestrant, mitotane, tamoxifen, toremifene	
	Aromatase inhibitors	Anastrozole, exemastine, letrozole	
Protein kinase inhibitors	Tyrosine, or other kinase, inhibitors	Acalabrutinib, axitinib, crizotinib, dasatinib, erlotinib, gefitinib, ibrutinib, imatinib, lapatinib, nilotinib, pazopanib, ponatinib, ruxolitinib, sunitinib, vandetanib, vemurafenib	Inhibition of kinases involved in growth factor receptor transduction
	Pan-kinase inhibitors	Everolimus, sorafenib, temsirolimus	
Monoclonal antibodies	Anti-EGF, EGF-2	Panitumumab, trastuzumab	Blocks cell proliferation
	Anti-CD20/CD30/ CD52	Brentuximab, ofatumumab, rituximab	Inhibition of lymphocyte proliferation
	Anti-CD3/EpCAM	Catumaxomab	Binds adhesion molecules promoting cell killing
	Anti-PD-1/PD-L1 or CTLA4	Nivolumab, pembrolizumab, atezolizumab, ipilimumab	Immune checkpoint inhibitors that prevent immune cell suppression
	Anti-VEGF	Bevacizumab	Prevents angiogenesis
Miscellaneous	Retinoid X receptor antagonist	Bexarotene	Inhibits cell proliferation and differentiation
	Proteasome inhibitor	Bortezomib	Activation of programmed cell death
	Enzyme	Cristantaspase	Depletes asparagine
	Photoactivated cytotoxics	Porfimer, temoporfin	Accumulate in cells and kills them when activated by light

[a]A combination of oestrogen and chlormethine. Drugs in parentheses have similar pharmacological actions but are not necessarily chemically related.
CD, cluster of differentiation; *EGF,* epidermal growth factor; *EpCAM,* epithelial cell adhesion molecule; *PD,* programmed cell death protein; *VEGF,* vascular endothelial growth factor.

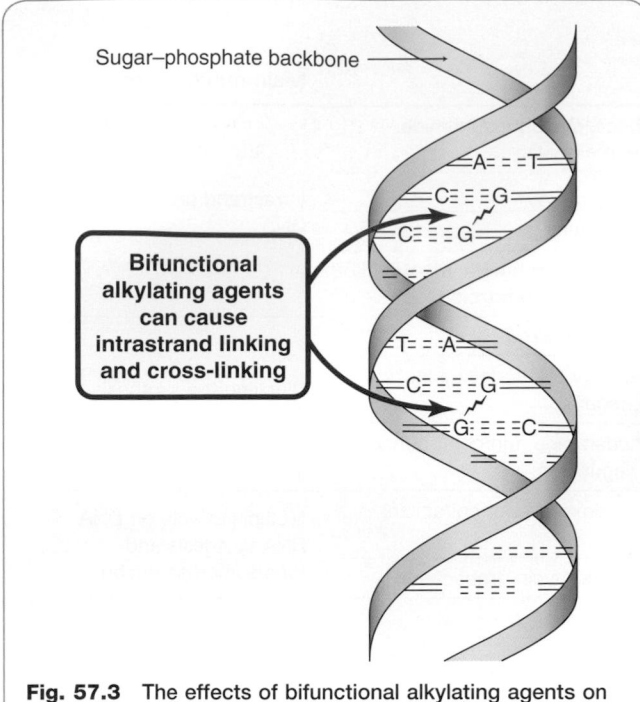

Fig. 57.3 The effects of bifunctional alkylating agents on DNA. Note the cross-linking of two guanines. *A*, adenine; *C*, cytosine; *G*, guanine; *T*, thymine.

Fig. 57.4 An example of alkylation and cross-linking of DNA by a nitrogen mustard. A bis(chloroethyl)amine *(1)* undergoes intramolecular cyclisation, forming an unstable ethylene immonium cation *(2)* and releasing Cl⁻, the tertiary amine being transformed to a quaternary ammonium compound. The strained ring of the ethylene immonium intermediate opens to form a reactive carbonium ion *(in yellow box) (3)*, which reacts immediately with N7 of guanine *(in green circle)* to give 7-*alkylguanine (bond shown in blue)*, the N7 being converted to a quaternary ammonium nitrogen. These reactions can then be repeated with the other $-CH_2CH_2Cl$ to give a cross-link.

ALKYLATING AGENTS AND RELATED COMPOUNDS

Alkylating agents and related compounds contain chemical groups that can form covalent bonds with particular nucleophilic substances in the cell (such as DNA). With alkylating agents themselves, the first step is the formation of a *carbonium ion* – a carbon atom with only six electrons in its outer shell. Such ions are highly reactive and react instantaneously with an electron donor such as an amine, hydroxyl or sulfhydryl group. Most of the cytotoxic anticancer alkylating agents are *bifunctional*, i.e. they have two alkylating groups (Fig. 57.3).

▼ The nitrogen at position 7 (N7) of guanine, being strongly nucleophilic, is probably the main molecular target for alkylation in DNA (see Fig. 57.3), although N1 and N3 of adenine and N3 of cytosine may also be affected. A bifunctional agent, by reacting with two groups, can cause intra- or inter-chain cross-linking. This interferes not only with transcription, but also with DNA replication, which is probably the critical effect of anticancer alkylating agents.

All alkylating agents depress bone marrow function and cause hair loss and diarrhoea. Depression of gametogenesis, leading to sterility, and an increased risk of a second malignancy occur with prolonged use.

Alkylating agents are among the most commonly employed of all anticancer drugs. Only a few commonly used examples will be dealt with here.

Nitrogen mustards

Nitrogen mustards are related to the 'mustard gas' used during the First World War,[7] their basic formula (R-*N-bis*-[2-chloroethyl]) is shown in Fig. 57.4. In the body, each 2-chloroethyl side-chain undergoes an intramolecular cyclisation with the release of a Cl⁻. The highly reactive *ethylene immonium* derivative so formed can interact with DNA (see Figs 57.3 and 57.4) and other molecules.

Cyclophosphamide is probably the most commonly used alkylating agent. It is inactive until metabolised in the liver by the P450 mixed function oxidases (see Ch. 10). It has a pronounced effect on lymphocytes and can also be used as an immunosuppressant (see Ch. 27). It is given orally or by intravenous injection. Important toxic effects are nausea and vomiting, bone marrow depression and haemorrhagic cystitis. This last effect (which also occurs with the related drug **ifosfamide**) is caused by the metabolite acrolein and can be ameliorated by increasing fluid intake and administering compounds that are sulfhydryl donors, such as **N-acetylcysteine** or **mesna** (sodium-2-mercaptoethane sulfonate). These agents react with acrolein, forming a non-toxic compound. (See also Chs 10 and 58.)

▼ Other nitrogen mustards used include **bendamustine**, ifosfamide, **chlorambucil** and **melphalan**. Estramustine is a combination of **chlormethine** (mustine) with an oestrogen. It has both cytotoxic and hormonal action, and is used for the treatment of prostate cancer.

---

[7]It was the clinical insight of Alfred Goodman and Louis Gilman that led to the testing of (what became the first effective anticancer drug) mustine, a modified and stable version of 'mustard gas', to treat lymphomas. They also wrote what was to become a famous textbook of pharmacology.

Nitrosoureas

Examples include **lomustine** and **carmustine**. As they are lipid soluble and cross the blood–brain barrier, they are used to treat tumours of the brain and meninges. However, most nitrosoureas have a severe cumulative depressive effect on the bone marrow that starts 3–6 weeks after initiation of treatment.

Other alkylating agents

Busulfan has a selective effect on the bone marrow, depressing the formation of granulocytes and platelets in low dosage and of red cells in higher dosage. It has little or no effect on lymphoid tissue or the GI tract. It is used in chronic granulocytic leukaemia.

Dacarbazine, a prodrug, is activated in the liver, and the resulting compound is subsequently cleaved in the target cell to release an alkylating derivative. Unwanted effects include myelotoxicity and severe nausea and vomiting. **Temozolomide** is a related compound with a restricted usage (malignant glioma).

Procarbazine inhibits DNA and RNA synthesis and interferes with mitosis at interphase. Its effects may be mediated by the production of active metabolites. It is given orally, and its main use is in Hodgkin's disease. It causes **disulfiram**-like actions with alcohol (see Ch. 50), exacerbates the effects of central nervous system depressants and, because it is a weak monoamine oxidase inhibitor, can produce hypertension if given with certain sympathomimetic agents (see Ch. 48). Other alkylating agents in clinical use include **hydroxycarbamide**, **mitobronitol**, **thiotepa** and **treosulfan**.

Platinum compounds

Cisplatin is a water-soluble planar coordination complex containing a central platinum atom surrounded by two chlorine atoms and two ammonia groups. Its action is analogous to that of the alkylating agents. When it enters the cell, Cl⁻ dissociates, leaving a reactive complex that reacts with water and then interacts with DNA. It causes intrastrand cross-linking, probably between N7 and O6 of adjacent guanine molecules, which results in local denaturation of DNA.

Cisplatin has revolutionised the treatment of solid tumours of the testes and ovary. Therapeutically, it is given by slow intravenous injection or infusion. It is seriously nephrotoxic, and strict regimens of hydration and diuresis must be instituted. It has low myelotoxicity but causes very severe nausea and vomiting. The 5-HT₃ receptor antagonists (e.g. **ondansetron**; see Chs 16, 31 and 40) are very effective in preventing this and have transformed cisplatin-based chemotherapy. Tinnitus and hearing loss in the high-frequency range may occur, as may peripheral neuropathies, hyperuricaemia and anaphylactic reactions.

▼ **Carboplatin** is a derivative of cisplatin. Because it causes less nephrotoxicity, neurotoxicity, ototoxicity, nausea and vomiting than cisplatin (although it is more myelotoxic), it is sometimes given on an outpatient basis. **Oxaliplatin** is another platinum-containing compound with a restricted application.

ANTIMETABOLITES

Folate antagonists

The main folate antagonist in cancer chemotherapy is **methotrexate** (see also Ch. 27 for its use as an immunosuppressant in rheumatology). Folates are essential for the synthesis of purine nucleotides and thymidylate, which in

---

Anticancer drugs: alkylating agents and related compounds

- Alkylating agents have groups that form covalent bonds with cell substituents; a carbonium ion is the reactive intermediate. Most have two alkylating groups and can cross-link DNA. This causes defective replication and chain breakage.
- Their principal effect occurs during DNA synthesis and the resulting damage triggers apoptosis.
- Unwanted effects include myelosuppression, sterility and risk of non-lymphocytic leukaemia.
- The main alkylating agents are:
  - nitrogen mustards, for example **cyclophosphamide**, which is converted to phosphoramide mustard (the cytotoxic molecule); **cyclophosphamide** myelosuppression affects particularly the lymphocytes.
  - nitrosoureas, for example **lomustine**, may act on non-dividing cells, can cross the blood–brain barrier and cause delayed, cumulative myelotoxicity.
- Platinum compounds (e.g. **cisplatin**) cause intrastrand linking in DNA. **Cisplatin** has low myelotoxicity but causes severe nausea and vomiting, and can be nephrotoxic. It has revolutionised the treatment of germ cell tumours.

---

turn are essential for DNA synthesis and cell division. (This topic is also dealt with in Chs 26, 51 and 55.) The main action of the folate antagonists is to interfere with thymidylate synthesis. Folates consist of three elements: a pteridine ring, p-aminobenzoic acid and glutamic acid; methotrexate is structurally closely related (Fig. 57.5). Its effect on thymidylate synthesis is summarised in Fig. 57.6.

Methotrexate is usually given orally but can also be given intramuscularly, intravenously or intrathecally. It has low lipid solubility and thus does not readily cross the blood–brain barrier. It is, however, actively taken up into cells by the folate transport system and is metabolised to polyglutamate derivatives, which are retained in the cell for weeks or months even in the absence of extracellular drug. Resistance to methotrexate may develop in tumour cells by a variety of mechanisms.

Unwanted effects include depression of the bone marrow and damage to the epithelium of the GI tract. Pneumonitis can occur. In addition, high-dose regimens – doses 10 times greater than the standard doses, sometimes used in patients with methotrexate resistance – can lead to nephrotoxicity. This is caused by precipitation of the drug or a metabolite in the renal tubules. High-dose regimens must be followed by 'rescue' with folinic acid (a form of FH₄).

Also chemically related to folate are **raltitrexed**, which inhibits thymidylate synthetase, and **pemetrexed**, which inhibits thymidylate transferase.

Pyrimidine analogues

Fluorouracil, an analogue of uracil, also interferes with 2'-deoxythymidylate (dTMP) synthesis (see Fig. 57.6). It is converted into a 'fraudulent' nucleotide, *fluorodeoxyuridine monophosphate* (FdUMP). This interacts with thymidylate

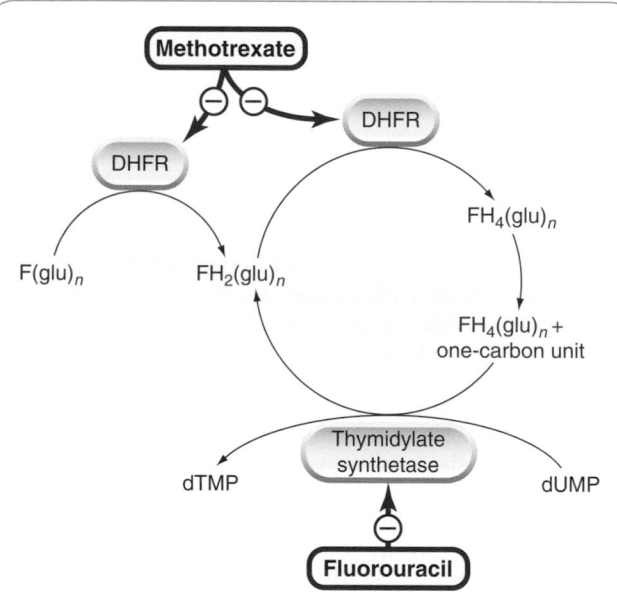

Folic acid

Methotrexate

Fig. 57.5 **Structure of folic acid and methotrexate.** Both compounds are shown as polyglutamates. In tetrahydrofolate, one-carbon groups (R, *in orange box*) are transported on N5 or N10 or both *(shown dotted)*. The points at which methotrexate differs from endogenous folic acid are shown in the *blue boxes*.

Fig. 57.6 Simplified diagram of action of methotrexate and fluorouracil on thymidylate synthesis. Tetrahydrofolate polyglutamate $FH_4(glu)_n$ functions as a carrier of a one-carbon unit, providing the methyl group necessary for the conversion of 2′-deoxyuridylate (dUMP) to 2′-deoxythymidylate (dTMP) by thymidylate synthetase. This one-carbon transfer results in the oxidation of $FH_4(glu)_n$ to $FH_2(glu)_n$. Fluorouracil is converted to FdUMP, which inhibits thymidylate synthetase. *DHFR*, dihydrofolate reductase.

synthetase but cannot be converted into DTMP. The result is inhibition of DNA but not RNA or protein synthesis.

Fluorouracil is usually given parenterally. The main unwanted effects are GI epithelial damage and myelotoxicity. Cerebellar disturbances can also occur. Two other drugs, **capecitabine** and **tegafur**, are metabolised to fluorouracil.

Cytarabine (cytosine arabinoside [ara-C]) is an analogue of the naturally occurring nucleoside 2′-deoxycytidine. The

drug enters the target cell and undergoes the same phosphorylation reactions as the endogenous nucleoside to give cytosine arabinoside trisphosphate, which inhibits DNA polymerase (Fig. 57.7). The main unwanted effects are on the bone marrow and the GI tract.

Gemcitabine, an analogue of cytarabine, has fewer unwanted actions, the main ones being an influenza-like syndrome and mild myelotoxicity. It is often given in combination with other drugs such as cisplatin. **Azacitidine** and **decitabine** inhibit DNA methylase.

Purine analogues

The main anticancer purine analogues include **cladribine**, **clofarabine, fludarabine, pentostatin, nelarabine, mercaptopurine** and **tioguanine**.

Fludarabine is metabolised to the trisphosphate and inhibits DNA synthesis by actions similar to those of cytarabine. It is myelosuppressive. Pentostatin has a different mechanism of action. It inhibits adenosine deaminase, the enzyme that transforms adenosine to inosine. This action interferes with critical pathways in purine metabolism and can have significant effects on cell proliferation. Cladribine, mercaptopurine and tioguanine are used mainly in the treatment of leukaemia.

CYTOTOXIC ANTIBIOTICS

This is a widely used group of drugs that mainly produce their effects through direct action on DNA. As a rule, they should not be given together with radiotherapy, as the cumulative burden of toxicity is very high.

Doxorubicin and the anthracyclines

Doxorubicin, idarubicin, daunorubicin and **epirubicin** are widely used anthracycline antibiotics; **mitoxantrone** (**mitozantrone**) is a derivative.

Doxorubicin has several cytotoxic actions. It binds to DNA and inhibits both DNA and RNA synthesis, but its main cytotoxic action appears to be mediated through an effect on topoisomerase II (a DNA gyrase; see Ch. 51), the activity of which is markedly increased in proliferating cells. During replication of the DNA helix, reversible swivelling needs to take place around the replication fork

Fig. 57.7 The mechanism of action of cytarabine (cytosine arabinoside). For details of DNA polymerase action, see Fig. 51.5. Cytarabine is an analogue of cytosine.

Anticancer drugs: antimetabolites

Antimetabolites block or subvert pathways of DNA synthesis.
- *Folate antagonists*. **Methotrexate** inhibits dihydrofolate reductase, preventing generation of tetrahydrofolate interfering with thymidylate synthesis.
- *Pyrimidine analogues*. **Fluorouracil** is converted to a 'fraudulent' nucleotide and inhibits thymidylate synthesis. **Cytarabine** in its trisphosphate form inhibits DNA polymerase. They are potent myelosuppressives.
- *Purine analogues*. **Mercaptopurine** is converted into fraudulent nucleotide. **Fludarabine** in its trisphosphate form inhibits DNA polymerase and is myelosuppressive. **Pentostatin** inhibits adenosine deaminase – a critical pathway in purine metabolism.

---

in order to prevent the daughter DNA molecule becoming inextricably entangled during mitotic segregation. The 'swivel' is produced by topoisomerase II, which 'nicks' both DNA strands and subsequently reseals the breaks. Doxorubicin intercalates in the DNA, and its effect is, in essence, to stabilise the DNA–topoisomerase II complex after the strands have been nicked, thus halting the process at this point.

Doxorubicin is given by intravenous infusion. Extravasation at the injection site can cause local necrosis. In addition to the general unwanted effects, the drug can cause cumulative, dose-related cardiac damage, leading to dysrhythmias

and heart failure. This action may be the result of generation of free radicals. Marked hair loss frequently occurs.

Dactinomycin
Dactinomycin intercalates in the minor groove of DNA between adjacent guanosine–cytosine pairs, interfering with the movement of RNA polymerase along the gene and thus preventing transcription. There is also evidence that it has a similar action to that of the anthracyclines on topoisomerase II. It produces most of the toxic effects outlined previously, except cardiotoxicity. It is mainly used for treating paediatric cancers.

Bleomycins
The bleomycins are a group of metal-chelating glycopeptide antibiotics that degrade preformed DNA, causing chain fragmentation and release of free bases. This action is thought to involve chelation of ferrous iron and interaction with oxygen, resulting in the oxidation of the iron and generation of superoxide and/or hydroxyl radicals. **Bleomycin** is most effective in the G_2 phase of the cell cycle and mitosis, but it is also active against non-dividing cells (i.e. cells in the G_0 phase; Ch. 6, Fig. 6.4). It is often used to treat germline cancer. In contrast to most anticancer drugs, bleomycin causes little myelosuppression: its most serious toxic effect is pulmonary fibrosis, which occurs in 10% of patients treated and is reported to be fatal in 1%. Allergic reactions can also occur. About half the patients manifest mucocutaneous reactions (the palms are frequently affected), and many develop hyperpyrexia.

Mitomycin
Following enzymic activation, **mitomycin** functions as a bifunctional alkylating agent, binding preferentially at O6 of the guanine nucleus. It cross-links DNA and may also degrade DNA through the generation of free radicals. It causes marked delayed myelosuppression and can also cause kidney damage and fibrosis of lung tissue.

Anticancer drugs: cytotoxic antibiotics

- **Doxorubicin** inhibits DNA and RNA synthesis; the DNA effect is mainly through interference with topoisomerase II action. Unwanted effects include nausea, vomiting, myelosuppression and hair loss. It is cardiotoxic in high doses.
- **Bleomycin** causes fragmentation of DNA chains. It acts on non-dividing cells. Unwanted effects include fever, allergies, mucocutaneous reactions and pulmonary fibrosis. There is virtually no myelosuppression.
- **Dactinomycin** intercalates in DNA, interfering with RNA polymerase and inhibiting transcription. It also interferes with the action of topoisomerase II. Unwanted effects include nausea, vomiting and myelosuppression.
- **Mitomycin** is activated to give an alkylating metabolite.

PLANT DERIVATIVES

Several naturally occurring plant products exert potent cytotoxic effects and have a use as anticancer drugs.

Vinca alkaloids

The vinca alkaloids are derived from the Madagascar periwinkle (*Catharanthus roseus*). The principal members of the group are **vincristine**, **vinblastine** and **vindesine**. **Vinflunine**, a fluorinated vinca alkaloid, and **vinorelbine** are semisynthetic vinca alkaloids with similar properties. The drugs bind to tubulin and inhibit its polymerisation into microtubules, preventing spindle formation in dividing cells and causing arrest at metaphase. Their effects become manifest only during mitosis. They also inhibit other cellular activities that require functioning microtubules, such as leukocyte phagocytosis and chemotaxis, as well as axonal transport in neurons.

The adverse effects of vinca alkaloids differ from other anticancer drugs. Vincristine has very mild myelosuppressive activity but is neurotoxic and commonly causes *paraesthesia* (sensory changes), abdominal pain and weakness. Vinblastine is less neurotoxic but causes leukopenia, while vindesine has both moderate myelotoxicity and neurotoxicity. All members of the group can cause reversible hair loss.

Paclitaxel and related compounds

These *taxanes* are derived from a naturally occurring compound found in the bark of the Pacific yew tree (*Taxus* spp.). The group includes **paclitaxel** and the semisynthetic derivatives **docetaxel** and **cabazitaxel**. These agents act on microtubules, stabilising them (in effect 'freezing' them) in the polymerised state, achieving a similar effect to that of the vinca alkaloids. These drugs are usually given by intravenous infusion. They are generally used to treat breast and lung cancer and paclitaxel, given with carboplatin, is the treatment of choice for ovarian cancer.

Unwanted effects, which can be serious, include bone marrow suppression and cumulative neurotoxicity. Resistant fluid retention (particularly oedema of the legs) can occur with docetaxel. Hypersensitivity to these compounds is common and requires pretreatment with corticosteroids and antihistamines.

Camptothecins

The camptothecins **irinotecan** and **topotecan**, isolated from the stem of the tree *Camptotheca acuminata*, bind to and inhibit topoisomerase I, high levels of which are present throughout the cell cycle. Diarrhoea and reversible bone marrow depression occur but, in general, these alkaloids have fewer unwanted effects than most other anticancer agents.

Etoposide

Etoposide is derived from mandrake root (*Podophyllum peltatum*). Its mode of action is not clearly known, but it may act by inhibiting mitochondrial function and nucleoside transport, as well as having an effect on topoisomerase II similar to doxorubicin. *Unwanted effects* include nausea and vomiting, myelosuppression and hair loss.

▼ **Compounds from marine sponges.** Eribulin is a naturally occurring compound from marine sponges. Its main inhibitory action on cell division is through inhibition of microtubule function. **Trabectedin**, another compound derived from marine sponges, also disrupts DNA but utilises a superoxide-related mechanism.

Anticancer drugs: plant derivatives

- **Vincristine** (and related alkaloids) inhibit mitosis at metaphase by binding to tubulin. It is relatively non-toxic but can cause unwanted neuromuscular effects.
- **Etoposide** inhibits DNA synthesis by an action on topoisomerase II and also inhibits mitochondrial function. Common unwanted effects include vomiting, myelosuppression and alopecia.
- **Paclitaxel** (and other taxanes) stabilise microtubules, inhibiting mitosis; it is relatively toxic and hypersensitivity reactions occur.
- **Irinotecan** and **topotecan** inhibit topoisomerase I; They have relatively few toxic effects.

HORMONES

Tumours arising in hormone-sensitive tissues (e.g. breast, uterus, prostate gland) may be *hormone-dependent*, an effect related to the presence of hormone receptors in the malignant cells, gauged by the receptors present in screened biopsy samples. Their growth can be inhibited by hormone agonists or antagonists, or by agents that inhibit the synthesis of the hormone.

Hormones or their analogues that have inhibitory actions on target tissues can be used in treatment of tumours of those tissues. Such procedures alone rarely effect a cure but do retard tumour growth and mitigate the symptoms of the cancer, and thus play an important part in the clinical management of sex hormone-dependent tumours.

Glucocorticoids

Glucocorticoids such as **prednisolone** have marked inhibitory effects on lymphocyte proliferation (see Chs 27 and 34) and are used in the treatment of leukaemias and lymphomas. The ability of **dexamethasone** to lower raised intracranial pressure is exploited in treating patients with brain tumours. Glucocorticoids mitigate some of the side effects of anticancer drugs, such as nausea and vomiting, making them useful as supportive therapy when treating other cancers, as well as in palliative care.

Oestrogens

Diethylstilboestrol and **ethinyloestradiol** are still occasionally used in the palliative treatment of androgen-dependent prostatic tumours. These tumours can also be treated with gonadotrophin-releasing hormone analogues (see Ch. 34).

Progestogens

Progestogens such as **megestrol**, **norehisterone** and **medroxyprogesterone** have a role in treatment of endometrial cancer.

Gonadotrophin-releasing hormone analogues

As explained in Chapter 36, analogues of the gonadotrophin-releasing hormones, such as **goserelin**, **buserelin**, **leuprorelin** and **triptorelin**, can, when administered chronically, inhibit gonadotrophin release. These agents are therefore used to treat advanced breast cancer in premenopausal women and prostate cancer. The effect of the transient surge of testosterone secretion that can occur in patients treated in this way for prostate cancer must be prevented by an antiandrogen such as **cyproterone**. **Degaralix** is a gonadotrophin-releasing hormone antagonist used for the treatment of prostate cancer.

Somatostatin analogues

Analogues of somatostatin such as **octreotide** and **lanreotide** (see Ch. 34) are used to relieve the symptoms of neuroendocrine tumours, including hormone-secreting tumours of the GI tract such as VIPomas, glucagonomas, carcinoid tumours and gastrinomas. These tumours express somatostatin receptors, activation of which inhibits cell proliferation as well as hormone secretion.

HORMONE ANTAGONISTS

In addition to the hormones themselves, hormone antagonists can also be effective in the treatment of several types of hormone-sensitive tumours.

Antioestrogens

An antioestrogen, **tamoxifen**, is remarkably effective in some cases of hormone-dependent breast cancer and may have a role in preventing these cancers. In breast tissue, tamoxifen competes with endogenous oestrogens for the oestrogen receptors and therefore inhibits the transcription of oestrogen-responsive genes. Tamoxifen has less disruptive effects due to it being a partial agonist at the oestrogen receptor types found in endometrium, bone and the cardiovascular system. Tamoxifen is also reported to have cardioprotective effects, partly by virtue of its ability to protect low-density lipoproteins against oxidative damage, or by inhibition of cholesterol esterification and foam cell formation (Ch. 24). Other oestrogen receptor antagonists include **toremifene** and **fulvestrant**.

Unwanted effects are similar to those experienced by women following the menopause. Potentially more serious are hyperplastic events in the endometrium, which may progress to malignant changes, and the risk of thromboembolism.

Aromatase inhibitors such as **anastrozole**, **letrozole** and **exemestane**, which suppress the synthesis of oestrogen from androgens in the adrenal cortex (but not in the ovary), are also effective in the treatment of breast cancer in postmenopausal (but not in premenopausal) women, in whom they are somewhat more effective than tamoxifen.

Antiandrogens

The androgen antagonists **flutamide**, **cyproterone** and **bicalutamide** may be used either alone or in combination with other agents to treat tumours of the prostate. They are also used to control the testosterone surge ('flare') that is seen when treating patients with gonadorelin analogues. Degarelix does not cause this flare.

MONOCLONAL ANTIBODIES

Monoclonal antibodies (see Ch. 5) are relatively recent additions to the anticancer armamentarium. In some cases, binding of the antibody to its target activates the host's immune mechanisms and the cancer cell is killed by complement-mediated lysis or by killer T cells (see Ch. 7). Other monoclonal antibodies attach to and inactivate growth factors or their receptors on cancer cells, thus inhibiting the survival pathway and promoting apoptosis (Ch. 6, Fig. 6.5). Unlike most of the cytotoxic drugs described above, they offer the prospect of highly targeted therapy without many of the side effects of conventional chemotherapy.

Anticancer agents: hormones

Hormones or their antagonists are used in hormone-sensitive tumours:
- **Glucocorticoids** for leukaemias and lymphomas.
- **Tamoxifen** for breast tumours.
- **Gonadotrophin-releasing hormone analogues** for prostate and breast tumours.
- **Antiandrogens** for prostate cancer.
- **Aromatase inhibitors** for postmenopausal breast cancer.

This advantage is offset in most instances as they are often given in combination with more traditional drugs. Several monoclonals are in current clinical use. Their high cost is a significant problem.

Rituximab

Rituximab is a monoclonal antibody that is used (in combination with other chemotherapeutic agents) for treatment of certain types of *lymphoma*, including non-Hodgkin's lymphoma. It lyses B lymphocytes by binding to the calcium-channel forming CD20 protein and activating complement. It also sensitises resistant cells to other chemotherapeutic drugs. It provides progression-free survival in 40%–50% of cases when combined with standard chemotherapy (R-CHOP; rituximab–cyclophosphamide, hydroxydaunorubicin [doxorubicin], oncovin [vincristine] plus prednisolone).

The drug is given by infusion, and its plasma half-life is approximately 3 days when first given, increasing with each administration to about 8 days by the fourth administration.

Unwanted effects include hypotension, chills and fever during the initial infusions and subsequent hypersensitivity reactions. A cytokine release reaction can occur and has been fatal. The drug may exacerbate cardiovascular disorders.

▼ **Alemtuzumab** is another monoclonal antibody that lyses B lymphocytes, and is used in the treatment of resistant chronic lymphocytic leukaemia. It may also cause a similar cytokine release reaction to that with rituximab. **Ofatumumab** is similar. **Brentuximab** additionally targets T cells but in a different manner. It is a conjugate of a cytotoxic drug attached to an antibody that binds to CD30 on malignant cells. It is used to treat *Hodgkin's lymphoma*.

Trastuzumab

Trastuzumab (Herceptin) is a humanised murine monoclonal antibody that binds to an oncogenic protein termed *HER2* (the human epidermal growth factor receptor 2), a member of the wider family of receptors with integral tyrosine kinase activity (see Fig. 57.1). There is some evidence that, in addition to inducing host immune responses, trastuzumab induces cell cycle inhibitors p21 and p27 (Ch. 6, Fig. 6.2). Tumour cells, in about 25% of breast cancer patients, overexpress this receptor and the cancer proliferates rapidly. Early results show that trastuzumab given with standard chemotherapy has resulted in a 79% 1-year survival rate in treatment-naive patients with this aggressive form of breast cancer. The drug is often given with a taxane such as docetaxel. Unwanted effects are similar to those with rituximab.

▼ Two mechanically related compounds are **panitumumab** and **cetuximab**, which bind to epidermal growth factor (EGF) receptors (also overexpressed in a high proportion of tumours). They are used for the treatment of colorectal cancer usually in combination with other agents.

Bevacizumab

Bevacizumab is a humanised monoclonal antibody that is used for the treatment of colorectal cancer and now used in a wide range of other cancers. It neutralises *VEGF* (vascular endothelial growth factor), thereby preventing the angiogenesis that is crucial to tumour survival. It is administered by intravenous infusion and is generally combined with other agents. A closely related preparation is also given by direct injection into the eye to retard the progress of *acute macular degeneration* (AMD), a common cause of blindness associated with increased retinal vascularisation.

Catumaxomab

Catumaxomab attaches to an epithelial adhesion molecule, EpCAM, which is overexpressed in some malignant cells. It is given by intraperitoneal injection to treat malignant ascites, a collection of fluid and cancer cells in the peritoneal cavity. The antibody binds to this adhesion molecule and also to T lymphocytes and antigen-presenting cells, thus facilitating the action of the immune system in clearing the cancer.

Nivolumab

Nivolumab is a fully humanised monoclonal antibody (mAb) against **P**rogrammed cell **D**eath protein-1 (PD-1) which is a cell surface receptor that dampens down the immune system to promote self-tolerance and suppress T-cell activation. Its ligand is PD-L1. Nivolumab has been used to re-prime the immune system so that it will recognise and destroy cancer cells that have previously evaded immunosurveillance. It has been approved for the treatment of metastatic melanoma, lymphoma, lung, kidney and head and neck cancers. **Pembrolizumab** is another approved variant of a PD-1 mAb. **Atezolizumab** is a mAb against PD-L1 approved in 2016 for the treatment of bladder cancer.

Ipilimumab

Approved in 2011 for the treatment of melanoma, **ipilimumab** targets the immune checkpoint system known as cytotoxic T-lymphocyte-associated protein 4 (CTLA-4) which functions similarly to the PD-1 system to 'stand down' the immune system. Cancers often employ both these mechanisms to evade immunodetection. Inhibitors of both systems are called 'immune *checkpoint inhibitors*'. Ipilimumab has been used in the treatment of melanoma, with efficacy shown in combating lung and pancreatic cancers. Trials combining both PD-1 and CTLA-4 inhibitors have proven that combined therapy of these checkpoint inhibitors will be a useful strategy to reactivate our immune systems and target it against cancer cells in general.

PROTEIN KINASE INHIBITORS

Imatinib

Hailed as a conceptual breakthrough in targeted chemotherapy, **imatinib** (see Savage & Antman, 2002) is a small-molecule inhibitor of signalling pathway kinases. It inhibits an oncogenic cytoplasmic kinase (Bcr/Abl, see Fig. 57.1. and Fig. 57.8), considered to be a unique factor in the pathogenesis of chronic myeloid leukaemia (CML). It

has transformed the (hitherto poor) prognosis of patients with CML. It also inhibits platelet-derived growth factor receptor (a receptor tyrosine kinase; see Fig. 57.1) and the c-kit receptor (CD117) whose ligand is stem cell factor (SCF), and is licensed for the treatment of c-kit positive **G**astro**I**ntestinal **S**tromal **T**umours (GISTs), not susceptible to surgery.

The drug is given orally. The half-life is about 18 h, and the main site of metabolism is in the liver, where approximately 75% of the drug is converted to a metabolite that is also biologically active. The bulk (81%) of the metabolised drug is excreted in the faeces.

Unwanted effects include GI symptoms (pain, diarrhoea, nausea), fatigue, headaches and sometimes rashes. Resistance to imatinib, resulting from mutation of the kinase gene, is a growing problem. It results in little or no cross-resistance to other kinase inhibitors. Various second (**nilotinib**, **dasatinib**, **bosutinib**) and third (**ponatinib**) generation Bcr/Abl tyrosine kinase inhibitors have been developed to combat, to varying degrees, a typical drug-resistant mutation in Bcr/Abl (T315I) occurring in imatinib-treated CML patients.

▼ Many similar tyrosine kinase inhibitors have recently been developed, including **axitinib**, **crizotinib**, **erlotinib**, **gefitinib**, **imatinib**, **lapatinib**, **pazopanib**, **sunitinib** and **vandentanib**. **Ruxolitinib** inhibits the JAK1 and JAK2 kinases and **vemurafenib** inhibits BRAF kinase. **Sorafenib**, **everolimus** and **temsirolimus** are pan-kinase inhibitors with a similar utility. Ibrutinib and acalabrutinib inhibit Bruton's Tyrosine Kinase (BTK) (see Ch. 7). They covalently modify residue C481 on BTK and irreversibly inhibit its cellular actions, which include chemotaxis and secretion of factors necessary for adhesion to the microenvironment. Interestingly their effectiveness in B lymphoid leukaemias and lymphomas, derives from the ability to prevent migration and adhesion of these cancer cells to their resident tissues. Lymphocytosis (the extrusion of B cells from lymph nodes, spleen and bone marrow into the peripheral blood) is one of the first effects of these drugs, and is a marker of their chemotherapeutic effect. Thus, such anticancer drugs with cellular responses other than simple cytotoxic actions, represent a new approach to chemotherapeutics.

Anticancer drugs: monoclonal antibodies and protein kinase inhibitors

- Many tumours overexpress growth factor receptors that therefore stimulate cell proliferation and tumour growth. This can be inhibited by:
  - monoclonal antibodies, which bind to the extracellular domain of the epidermal growth factor (EGF) receptor (e.g. **panitumumab**), the oncogenic receptor human epidermal growth factor 2 [HER2] receptor (e.g. **trastuzumab**), or which neutralise the growth factors themselves (e.g. vascular endothelial growth factor [VEGF]; **bevacizumab**);
  - protein kinase inhibitors, which prevent downstream signalling triggered by growth factors by inhibiting specific oncogenic kinases (e.g. **imatinib**; bcr/abl) or by inhibiting specific receptor tyrosine kinases (e.g. EGF receptor; **erlotinib**) or several receptor-associated kinases (e.g. **sorafenib**).
- Some monoclonals act directly on lymphocyte cell surface proteins to cause lysis (e.g. **rituximab**), thereby preventing proliferation.

Fig. 57.8 **The mechanism of action of anticancer monoclonal antibodies and protein kinase inhibitors.** Many tumours overexpress growth factor receptors such as epidermal growth factor receptor (EGFR), the proto-oncogene human epidermal growth factor 2 (HER2) or vascular endothelial growth factor receptor (VEGFR). Therapeutic monoclonals can prevent this by interacting directly with the receptor itself (e.g. trastuzumab, cetuximab) or with the ligand (e.g. bevacizumab). An alternate way of reducing this drive on cell proliferation is by inhibiting the downstream signalling cascade. The receptor tyrosine kinases are good targets as are some oncogenic kinases such as bcr/abl. *K*, kinase domain in receptor; *P-*, phosphate group; *PDGFR*, platelet-derived growth factor receptor.

MISCELLANEOUS AGENTS

Crisantaspase

▼ **Crisantaspase** is a preparation of the enzyme *asparaginase*, given by injection. It converts asparagine to aspartic acid and ammonia, and is active against tumour cells, such as those of acute lymphoblastic leukaemia, that have lost the capacity to synthesise asparagine and therefore require an exogenous source. As most normal cells are able to synthesise asparagine, the drug has a fairly selective action and has very little suppressive effect on the bone marrow, the mucosa of the GI tract or hair follicles. It may cause nausea and vomiting, central nervous system depression, anaphylactic reactions and liver damage.

Hydroxycarbamide

▼ **Hydroxycarbamide** (hydroxyurea) is a urea analogue that inhibits ribonucleotide reductase, thus interfering with the conversion of ribonucleotides to deoxyribonucleotides. It is mainly used to treat *polycythaemia rubra vera* (a myeloproliferative disorder of the red cell lineage) and (in the past) chronic myelogenous leukaemia. Its use (in somewhat lower dose) in sickle cell anaemia is described in Chapter 25. It has the familiar spectrum of unwanted effects, bone marrow depression being significant.

Bortezomib

▼ **Bortezomib** is a boron-containing tripeptide that inhibits cellular proteasome function. For some reason, rapidly dividing cells are more sensitive than normal cells to this drug, making it a useful anticancer agent. It is mainly used for the treatment of myeloma (a clonal malignancy of plasma cells).

Thalidomide

▼ Investigations of the notorious teratogenic effect of **thalidomide** showed that it has multiple effects on gene transcription, angiogenesis and proteasome function, leading to trials of its efficacy as an anticancer drug.[8] In the event, it proved efficacious in myeloma, for which it is now widely used. The main adverse effect of thalidomide, apart from teratogenesis (irrelevant in myeloma treatment), is peripheral neuropathy, leading to irreversible weakness and sensory loss. It also increases the incidence of thrombosis and stroke.

A thalidomide derivative **lenalidomide** is thought to have fewer adverse effects, but unlike thalidomide, can cause bone marrow depression and neutropenia.

Biological response modifiers and others

▼ Agents that enhance the host's response are referred to as *biological response modifiers*. Some, for example **interferon-α** (and its pegylated derivative), are used in treating some solid tumours and lymphomas, and **aldesleukin** (recombinant interleukin-2) is used in some cases of renal tumours. **Tretinoin** (a form of vitamin A; see Ch. 28) is a powerful inducer of differentiation in leukaemic cells and is used as an adjunct to chemotherapy to induce remission. A related compound is **bexarotene**, a retinoid X receptor antagonist (see Ch. 3) that inhibits cell proliferation and differentiation.

Porfimer and **temoporfin** are haematoporphyrin photosensitising agents. They accumulate in cells and kill them when excited by the appropriate wavelength light. They are usually used in cases where the light source can be selectively aimed at the tumour (e.g. in the case of obstructing oesophageal tumours).

RESISTANCE TO ANTICANCER DRUGS

The resistance that neoplastic cells manifest to cytotoxic drugs is said to be *primary* (present when the drug is first

---

[8]Thalidomide had earlier been found, unexpectedly when used as a sedative, to cause shrinkage of the cutaneous swellings of leprosy (Ch. 52), and is approved for this indication as well as for myeloma.

given) or *acquired* (developing during treatment with the drug). Acquired resistance may result from either *adaptation* of the tumour cells or *mutation*, with the emergence of cells that are less susceptible or resistant to the drug and consequently have a selective advantage over the sensitive cells. The following are examples of various mechanisms of resistance. See Mimeault et al. (2008) for a critical appraisal of this issue.

- *Decreased accumulation of cytotoxic drugs* in cells as a result of the increased expression of cell surface, energy-dependent drug transport proteins. These are responsible for multidrug resistance to many structurally dissimilar anticancer drugs (e.g. doxorubicin, vinblastine and dactinomycin; see Gottesman et al., 2002). An important member of this transporter group is *P-glycoprotein* (P-gp/MDR1; see Ch. 9). P-glycoprotein protects cells against environmental toxins. It functions as a hydrophobic 'vacuum cleaner', picking up foreign chemicals, such as drugs, as they enter the cell membrane and expelling them. Non-cytotoxic agents that reverse multidrug resistance are being investigated as potential adjuncts to treatment.
- *A decrease in the amount of drug taken up by the cell* (e.g. in the case of methotrexate).
- *Insufficient activation of the drug*. Some drugs require metabolic activation to manifest their antitumour activity. If this fails, they may no longer be effective. Examples include conversion of fluorouracil to FdUMP, phosphorylation of cytarabine and conversion of mercaptopurine to a fraudulent nucleotide.
- *Increase in inactivation* (e.g. cytarabine and mercaptopurine).
- *Increased concentration of target enzyme* (methotrexate).
- *Decreased requirement for substrate* (crisantaspase).
- *Increased utilisation of alternative metabolic pathways* (antimetabolites).
- *Rapid repair of drug-induced DNA damage* (alkylating agents).
- *Altered activity of target*, for example modified topoisomerase II (doxorubicin).
- *Mutations in various genes*, giving rise to resistant target molecules. For example, the *p53* gene, C481S mutation in BTK gene developing in ibrutinib resistance, and overexpression of the *Bcl-2* gene family (several cytotoxic drugs).

COMBINATION THERAPIES

Treatment with combinations of anticancer agents increases the cytotoxicity against cancer cells without necessarily increasing the general toxicity. For example, methotrexate, which mainly has myelosuppressive toxicity, may be used in a regimen with vincristine, which has mainly neurotoxicity. The few drugs we possess with low myelotoxicity, such as cisplatin and bleomycin, are good candidates for combination regimens. Treatment with combinations of drugs also decreases the possibility of the development of resistance to individual agents. Drugs are often given in large doses intermittently in several courses, with intervals of 2–3 weeks between courses, rather than in small doses continuously, because this permits the bone marrow to regenerate during the intervals. Furthermore, it has been shown that the same total dose of an agent is more effective when given in one or two large doses than in multiple small doses.

CONTROL OF EMESIS AND MYELOSUPPRESSION
EMESIS

The nausea and vomiting induced by many cancer chemotherapy agents are a serious deterrent to patient compliance (see also Ch. 31). It is a particular problem with cisplatin but also complicates therapy with many other compounds, such as the alkylating agents. 5-hydroxytryptamine (HT)$_3$-receptor antagonists such as **ondansetron** or **granisetron** (see Chs 16 and 31) are effective against cytotoxic drug-induced vomiting and have revolutionised cisplatin chemotherapy. Of the other antiemetic agents available, **metoclopramide**, given intravenously in high dose, has proved useful and is often combined with dexamethasone (Ch. 34) or **lorazepam** (Ch. 45), both of which further mitigate the unwanted effects of chemotherapy. As metoclopramide commonly causes extrapyramidal side effects in children and young adults, **diphenhydramine** (Ch. 27) can be used instead.

MYELOSUPPRESSION

Myelosuppression limits the use of many anticancer agents. Regimens contrived to surmount the problem have included removal of some of the patient's own bone marrow prior to treatment, purging it of cancer cells (using specific monoclonal antibodies) and replacing it after cytotoxic therapy is finished. A protocol in which aliquots of stem cells, harvested from the blood following administration of the growth factor **molgramostim**, which increases their abundance in blood, are expanded in vitro using further haemopoietic growth factors (Ch. 26) is now frequently used. The use of such growth factors after replacement of the marrow has been successful in some cases. A further possibility is the introduction, into the extracted bone marrow, of the mutated gene that confers multidrug resistance, so that when replaced, the marrow cells (but not the cancer cells) will be resistant to the cytotoxic action of the anticancer drugs. **Folinic acid** may be given as a supplement to prevent anaemia or as a 'rescue' after high-dose methotrexate.

FUTURE DEVELOPMENTS

As the reader will have judged by now, our current approach to cancer chemotherapy embraces an eclectic mixture of drugs – some very old and some very new – in an attempt to target cancer cells selectively. Real therapeutic progress has been achieved, although 'cancer' as a disease (actually many different diseases with a similar outcome) remains a massive challenge for future generations of researchers. In this therapeutic area, probably more than in any other, the debate about the risk–benefit of treatment and the patient quality of life issues has taken centre stage and remains a major area of concern (see Duric & Stockler, 2001; Klastersky & Paesmans, 2001).

Of the recent advances in drug therapy, the tyrosine kinase inhibitors and the biopharmaceuticals have arguably been the most innovative advances. Further drugs of the kinase inhibitor type are under active investigation (see Vargas et al., 2013), as are anti-angiogenic drugs (similar to bevacizumab; see Ferrarotto & Hoff, 2013). Novel drugs targeting HER2-receptor in breast cancer have been reviewed by Abramson and Arteaga (2011). Warner and Gustafsson (2010) have highlighted the opportunities afforded by the discovery of a further isoform of the oestrogen receptor for the treatment of hormone-dependent breast and other cancers. Additionally, recent advances in BTK inhibitors primarily targeting non-cytotoxic signalling mechanisms, plus the use of immune checkpoint inhibitors to reset our immune systems so it can once more recognise and destroy cancer cells, are interesting paradigms for the future of intelligent cancer drug design. Moreover, the use of genetically-modified cells as 'living drug' anticancer therapies are becoming a reality. For example, chimaeric antigen receptor T cells (CAR-T cells) have been approved for the treatment of acute lymphoblastic leukaemia, with trials underway for other cancer types. These cells express modified antigens that target and kill cancer cells. Advances in gene-editing technology (e.g. CRISPR-Cas9 and TALENs) have made it possible for patients to receive cancer-killing altered T cells generated from either their own T cells or from a donor (Delhove & Qasim, 2017). Impressive breakthroughs have been seen with these 'living drugs' in cancer patients whose previous treatment failed using standard chemotherapy.

▼ For years, epidemiological and experimental evidence has been accumulating, which suggests that chronic use of cyclo-oxygenase (COX) inhibitors (see Ch. 27) protects against cancer of the GI tract and possibly other sites as well. The COX-2 isoform is overexpressed in about 85% of cancers, and prostanoids originating from this source may activate signalling pathways that enable cells to escape from apoptotic death. The literature has been controversial but the balance of evidence now favours the notion that COX-2 may be a potentially important target for anticancer drug development (see Khan et al., 2011). COX-2 inhibitors could therefore be useful in the treatment of some cancers, either alone or in combination with conventional chemotherapeutic agents (Ghosh et al., 2010; Kraus et al., 2013). Ironically, some authors (Gurpinar et al., 2013) argue that the mechanism of action of these inhibitors in cancer models is unrelated to COX inhibition. No doubt these apparent paradoxes will be resolved with the passage of time.

Much work is going into genotyping of tumour tissue as a guide to selecting the best drug combination to use in treating an individual patient, based on the particular genetic abnormality present in the tumour cells (see Patel et al., 2013; Dagogo-Jack & Shaw, 2018 for reviews). This approach, still in its early stages, is an example of personalised medicine (see Ch.12), and is beginning to yield promising approaches to optimising treatment, tailored to individual cases of a variety of cancers, such as melanoma and lung cancer, and is expected to develop rapidly. Analysis of circulating tumour DNA in blood is a possibility, obviating the need for biopsies.

REFERENCES AND FURTHER READING

General textbook
Airley, R., 2009. Anticancer Drugs. Wiley-Blackwell, Chichester. (*Recent textbook covering all aspects from basic pharmacology to clinical use*)

Mechanisms of carcinogenesis
Buys, C.H.C.M., 2000. Telomeres, telomerase and cancer. N. Engl. J. Med. 342, 1282–1283. (*Clear, concise coverage*)

Chambers, A.F., Groom, A.C., MacDonald, I.C., 2002. Dissemination and growth of cancer cells in metastatic sites. Nat. Rev. Cancer 2, 563–567. (*Review; stresses the importance of metastases in most cancer deaths, discusses the mechanisms involved in metastasis and raises the possibility of targeting these in anticancer drug development*)

Croce, C.M., 2008. Oncogenes and cancer. N. Engl. J. Med. 358, 502–511. (*Good review of the most significant oncogenes involved in carcinogenesis*)

Griffioen, A., Molema, G., 2000. Angiogenesis: potentials for pharmacologic intervention in the treatment of cancer, cardiovascular diseases and chronic inflammation. Pharmacol. Rev. 52, 237–268. (*Comprehensive review covering virtually all aspects of angiogenesis and the potential methods of modifying it to produce an antineoplastic effect*)

Hanahan, D., Weinberg, R.A., 2011. Hallmarks of cancer: the next generation. Cell 144, 646–674. (*Excellent review on the mechanisms underlying carcinogenesis, cancer development and metastasis*)

Mimeault, M., Hauke, R., Batra, S.K., 2008. Recent advances on the molecular mechanisms involved in the drug resistance of cancer cells and novel targeting therapies. Clin. Pharmacol. Ther. 83, 673–691. (*Comprehensive review covering all aspects of this field*)

Weinberg, R.A., 1996. How cancer arises. Sci. Am. 275 (3), 62–70. (*Simple, clear overview, listing main oncogenes, tumour suppressor genes and the cell cycle; excellent diagrams*)

Anticancer therapy
Gottesman, M.M., Fojo, T., Bates, S.E., 2002. Multidrug resistance in cancer: role of ATP-dependent transporters. Nat. Rev. Cancer 2, 48–56. (*Outlines cellular mechanisms of resistance; describes ATP-dependent transporters, emphasising those in human cancer; considers resistance reversal strategies*)

Krause, D.S., Van Etten, R., 2005. Tyrosine kinases as targets for cancer therapy. N. Engl. J. Med. 353, 172–187. (*Excellent review on tyrosine kinases as targets; good diagrams and tables as well as a highly readable style*)

Savage, D.G., Antman, K.H., 2002. Imatinib mesylate – a new oral targeted therapy. N. Engl. J. Med. 346, 683–693. (*Review with detailed coverage of this drug for chronic myelogenous leukaemia; very good diagrams*)

New directions and miscellaneous
Abramson, V., Arteaga, C.L., 2011. New strategies in HER2-overexpressing breast cancer: many combinations of targeted drugs available. Clin. Cancer Res. 17, 952–958. (*Deals mainly with ways in which the use of existing biologics can be optimized, but also discusses several new therapeutic directions*)

Dagogo-Jack, I., Shaw, A.T., 2018. Tumour heterogeneity and resistance to cancer therapies. Nat. Rev. Clin. Oncol. 15, 81–94. (*Excellent review of tumour heterogeneity and personalizing therapy*)

Delhove, J.M.K.M., Qasim, W., 2017. 2017 genome-edited T Cell therapies. Curr. Stem Cell Rep. 3 (2), 124–136.

Duric, V., Stockler, M., 2001. Patients' preferences for adjuvant chemotherapy in early breast cancer. Lancet Oncol. 2, 691–697. (*The title is self-explanatory; deals with patients' assessment of quality of life issues*)

Ferrarotto, R., Hoff, P.M., 2013. Antiangiogenic drugs for colorectal cancer: exploring new possibilities. Clin. Colorectal Cancer 12, 1–7. (*Good review of this field, clinical in tone and content*)

Ghosh, N., Chaki, R., Mandal, V., Mandal, S.C., 2010. COX-2 as a target for cancer chemotherapy. Pharmacol. Rep. 62, 233–244. (*Excellent review of this, often controversial, area*)

Gurpinar, E., Grizzle, W.E., Piazza, G.A., 2013. COX-independent mechanisms of cancer chemoprevention by anti-inflammatory drugs. Front. Oncol. 3, 1–81. (*A contrarian viewpoint on the target of action of COX-2 inhibitors in cancer. Interesting reading*)

Keith, W.N., Bilsland, A., Hardie, M., Evans, T.R., 2004. Drug insight: cancer cell immortality – telomerase as a target for novel cancer gene therapies. Nat. Clin. Pract. Oncol. 1, 88–96.

Khan, Z., Khan, N., Tiwari, R.P., Sah, N.K., Prasad, G.B., Bisen, P.S., 2011. Biology of COX-2: an application in cancer therapeutics. Curr. Drug Targets 12, 1082–1093.

Klastersky, J., Paesmans, M., 2001. Response to chemotherapy, quality of life benefits and survival in advanced non-small lung cancer: review of literature results. Lung Cancer 34, S95–S101. (*Another paper that addresses quality of life issues surrounding chemotherapy*)

Kraus, S., Naumov, I., Arber, N., 2013. COX-2 active agents in the chemoprevention of colorectal cancer. Recent Results Cancer Res. 191, 95–103.

Patel, L., Parker, B., Yang, D., Zhang, W., 2013. Translational genomics in cancer research: converting profiles into personalized cancer medicine. Cancer Biol. Med. 10, 214–220. (*Discusses prospects for personalised cancer therapy based on genotyping*)

Tookman, L., Roylance, R., 2010. New drugs for breast cancer. Br. Med. Bull. 96, 111–129. (*Easy-to-read account of the use and actions of biologics in breast cancer and a review of some promising new leads in the field. Recommended*)

Vargas, L., Hamasy, A., Nore, B.F., Smith, C.I., 2013. Inhibitors of BTK and ITK: state of the new drugs for cancer, autoimmunity and inflammatory diseases. Scand. J. Immunol. 78, 130–139. (*An excellent account of this area together with a discussion of 'loss of function' mutations in these kinases that may predispose towards cancer. Good diagrams*)

Warner, M., Gustafsson, J.A., 2010. The role of estrogen receptor beta (ERbeta) in malignant diseases – a new potential target for antiproliferative drugs in prevention and treatment of cancer. Biochem. Biophys. Res. Commun. 396, 63–66. (*The title is self explanatory. A thought-provoking paper if you have an interest in oestrogen receptors and cancer*)

Useful Web resources

http://www.cancer.org/. (*The US equivalent of the website below. The best sections for you are those marked* Health Information Seekers *and* Professionals)

http://www.cancerresearchuk.org/. (*The website of Cancer Research UK, the largest cancer charity in the UK. Contains valuable data on the epidemiology and treatment of cancer, including links to clinical trials. An excellent resource*)

Harmful effects of drugs

OVERVIEW

This chapter addresses harmful effects of drugs, both in the context of therapeutic use – so-called adverse drug reactions – and of deliberate or accidental overdose. We are concerned here with serious harm, sometimes life-threatening or irreversible, distinct from the minor side effects that virtually all drugs produce, as described throughout this book. The classification of adverse drug reactions is considered, followed by aspects of drug toxicity, namely toxicity testing in drug development, mechanisms of toxin-induced cell damage, mutagenesis and carcinogenicity, teratogenesis and allergic reactions.

INTRODUCTION

Paracelsus, a 16th-century alchemist, is credited with the aphorism that all drugs are poisons: '… the dosage makes it either a poison or a remedy'. Today, toxic effects of drugs remain clinically important in the context of overdose (self-poisoning accounts for approximately 10% of the workload of emergency medicine departments in the United Kingdom; by contrast, homicidal poisoning is extremely uncommon). Some susceptible individuals may experience dose-related toxicity even during therapeutic dosing and some of this susceptibility is genetically determined. There are now a wide range of genetic tests for identification and risk prediction of susceptible individuals, although relatively few of these tests are routinely used in current clinical practice (Ch. 12).

Rigorous toxicity testing in animals (see p. 740), including tests for carcinogenicity, teratogenicity and organ-specific toxicities, is carried out on potential new drugs during development (see Ch. 60), often leading to abandonment of the compound before it is tested in humans. These toxicity studies form part of the package of information routinely submitted to regulatory agencies by drug companies seeking approval to market a new drug. Nevertheless, harmful effects are often encountered after a drug is marketed for human use, due to the emergence of adverse effects not detected in animals. These harms are usually referred to as 'adverse drug reactions' (ADRs) and are of great concern to drug regulatory authorities, which are charged with establishing the safety, as well as the efficacy, of drugs. Unpredictable events are of particular concern. Some ADRs are predictable as a consequence of the main pharmacological effect of the drug and are relatively easily recognised, but some (e.g. immunological reactions), are unpredictable, sometimes serious, and likely to occur only in some patients.

Clinically important ADRs are common, costly and often avoidable (see Pirmohamed et al., 2004).[1] Any organ can be the principal target, and several organ systems can be involved simultaneously. The symptoms and signs sometimes closely shadow drug administration and discontinuation, but in other cases adverse effects only occur during prolonged use (*osteoporosis* during continued high-dose glucocorticoid therapy [Ch. 34], or *tardive dyskinesia* during continuous use of antipsychotic drugs [Ch. 47], for example). Some adverse effects occur on ending treatment, either within a few days (e.g. tachycardia on abrupt discontinuation of β-adrenoceptor blockade) or after a delay, first appearing months or years after treatment is discontinued, as in the case of some second malignancies following successful chemotherapy. Consequently, anticipating, avoiding, recognising and responding to ADRs are among the most challenging and important parts of clinical practice. Evaluation of harm from unexpected or rare adverse reactions after long periods of therapy is especially problematic. Precise estimates of risk are seldom obtainable in such circumstances.

CLASSIFICATION OF ADVERSE DRUG REACTIONS

Harmful effects of drugs may or may not be related to the known mechanism of action of the drug. In either case, individual variation (see Ch. 12) is a major factor in determining the response of a particular patient and their susceptibility to harm. Aronson and Ferner (2003) have suggested that ADRs are described according to the **do**se, **t**ime course and **s**usceptibility (DoTS). Potential susceptibility factors such as age and co-morbid conditions are thereby explicitly considered.

ADVERSE EFFECTS RELATED TO THE KNOWN PHARMACOLOGICAL ACTION OF THE DRUG

Many adverse effects related to the known pharmacological actions of the drug are predictable, at least if these actions are well understood. They are sometimes referred to as type A ('augmented') adverse reactions in the Rawlins and Thomson classification, and are related to dose and individual susceptibility (Lee, 2005). Many such reactions have been described in previous chapters. For example, postural hypotension occurs with α₁-adrenoceptor antagonists,

---

[1] Of hospital admissions in the United Kingdom, 6.5% were due to ADRs, at a projected annual cost of £466 million. Antiplatelet drugs, diuretics, non-steroidal anti-inflammatory drugs and anticoagulants between them accounted for 50% of the ADRs, and 2.3% of the patients died. Most events were avoidable.

bleeding with anticoagulants, sedation with anxiolytics and so on. In many instances, this type of unwanted effect is reversible, and the problem can often be dealt with by adjusting the dose to obtain a more favourable balance between efficacy and safety. Such effects are sometimes serious (e.g. intracerebral bleeding caused by anticoagulants, hypoglycaemic coma from insulin), and occasionally they are not easily reversible, for example, drug dependence produced by opioid analgesics (see Ch. 50).

Some adverse effects related to the main action of a drug result in discrete events rather than graded symptoms, and can be difficult to detect. For example, drugs that block cyclo-oxygenase (COX)-2 (including 'coxibs', for example, **rofecoxib**, **celecoxib**, and **valdecoxib**, as well as conventional non-steroidal anti-inflammatory drugs [NSAIDs]), increase the risk of myocardial infarction in a dose-dependent manner (Ch. 27). This potential was predictable from the ability of these drugs to inhibit prostacyclin biosynthesis and increase arterial blood pressure, and early studies gave a hint of such problems. The effect was difficult to prove because of the high background incidence of coronary thrombosis, and it was only when placebo-controlled trials were performed for another indication (in the hope that COX-2 inhibitors could prevent bowel cancer) that this effect was confirmed unequivocally.

ADVERSE EFFECTS UNRELATED TO THE KNOWN PHARMACOLOGICAL ACTION OF THE DRUG

Adverse effects unrelated to the main pharmacological effect may be predictable when a drug is taken in excessive dose, for example, **paracetamol** hepatotoxicity (see later) or **aspirin**-induced tinnitus; or when susceptibility is increased, for example, during pregnancy or by a predisposing disorder such as glucose 6-phosphate dehydrogenase deficiency or a mutation in the mitochondrial DNA that predisposes to aminoglycoside ototoxicity (Ch. 12).

Unpredictable reactions unrelated to the main effect of the drug (sometimes termed *idiosyncratic reactions*, or type B for Bizarre in the Rawlins and Thomson classification) are often initiated by a chemically reactive metabolite rather than the parent drug. Examples of such ADRs, which are often immunological in nature, include drug-induced hepatic or renal damage, bone marrow suppression, carcinogenesis and disordered fetal development. Uncommon but severe unpredictable adverse effects that have been mentioned in earlier chapters include aplastic anaemia from **chloramphenicol** and anaphylaxis in response to **penicillin**. They are usually severe – otherwise they would go unrecognised – and their existence is important in establishing the safety of medicines. The unpredictable nature of such reactions means that adjustment of the recommended therapeutic regimen (e.g. using a lower dose) may not prevent them.

Meyler's Side Effects of Drug is a comprehensive source of regularly updated and detailed textbook coverage of ADRs and their clinical manifestations (Aronson, 2015).

DRUG TOXICITY

TOXICITY TESTING

Toxicity testing in animals is carried out on new drugs to identify potential hazards before they are administered to humans. It involves the use of a wide range of tests in different species, with long-term administration of the drug, regular monitoring for physiological or biochemical abnormalities, and a detailed postmortem examination at the end of the trial to detect any gross or histological abnormalities. Toxicity testing is performed with doses well above the expected therapeutic range, and establishes which tissues or organs are likely 'targets' of toxic effects of the drug. Recovery studies are performed to assess whether toxic effects are reversible, and particular attention is paid to irreversible changes such as carcinogenesis or neurodegeneration. The basic premise is that toxic effects caused by a drug are similar in humans and other animals. There are, however, wide interspecies variations, especially in drug-metabolising enzymes; consequently, a toxic metabolite formed in one species may not be formed in another, and so toxicity testing in animals is not always a reliable guide. **Pronethalol**, the first β-adrenoceptor antagonist synthesised, was not developed because it caused carcinogenicity in mice; it subsequently emerged that carcinogenicity occurred only in the one strain tested – but by then other β blockers were already in development.

Toxic effects can range from negligible to so severe as to preclude further development of the compound. Intermediate levels of toxicity are more acceptable in drugs intended for severe illnesses (e.g. AIDS or cancers), and decisions on whether or not to continue development are often difficult. If development does proceed, safety monitoring can be concentrated on the system 'flagged' as a potential target of toxicity by the animal studies.[2] *Safety* of a drug (as distinct from toxicity) can be established only during use in humans.

> ### Types of drug toxicity
>
> - Toxic effects of drugs can be:
>   - related to the principal pharmacological action (e.g. bleeding with anticoagulants), and can usually be predicted from knowledge of the target sites;
>   - unrelated to the principal pharmacological action (e.g. liver damage with **paracetamol**), This can be difficult to predict, and is sometimes referred to as 'off-target', collateral, or bystander damage.
> - Some adverse reactions that occur with ordinary therapeutic dosage are initially unpredictable, serious and uncommon (e.g. agranulocytosis with **carbimazole**). Such reactions (termed idiosyncratic) are almost inevitably detected only after widespread use of a new drug. It is sometimes possible to develop a test to exclude susceptible subjects from drug exposure (e.g. mitochondrial DNA variants/increased susceptibility to aminoglycoside ototoxicity).
> - Adverse effects unrelated to the main action of a drug are often caused by reactive metabolites and/or immunological reactions.

[2]The value of toxicity testing is illustrated by experience with **triparanol**, a cholesterol-lowering drug marketed in the United States in 1959. Three years later, a team from the FDA, acting on a tip-off, paid the manufacturer a surprise visit that revealed falsification of toxicology data demonstrating cataracts in rats and dogs. The drug was withdrawn, but some patients who had been taking it for a year or more did develop cataracts. Regulatory authorities now require that toxicity testing is performed under a tightly defined code of practice (Good Laboratory Practice), which incorporates many safeguards to minimise the risk of error or fraud.

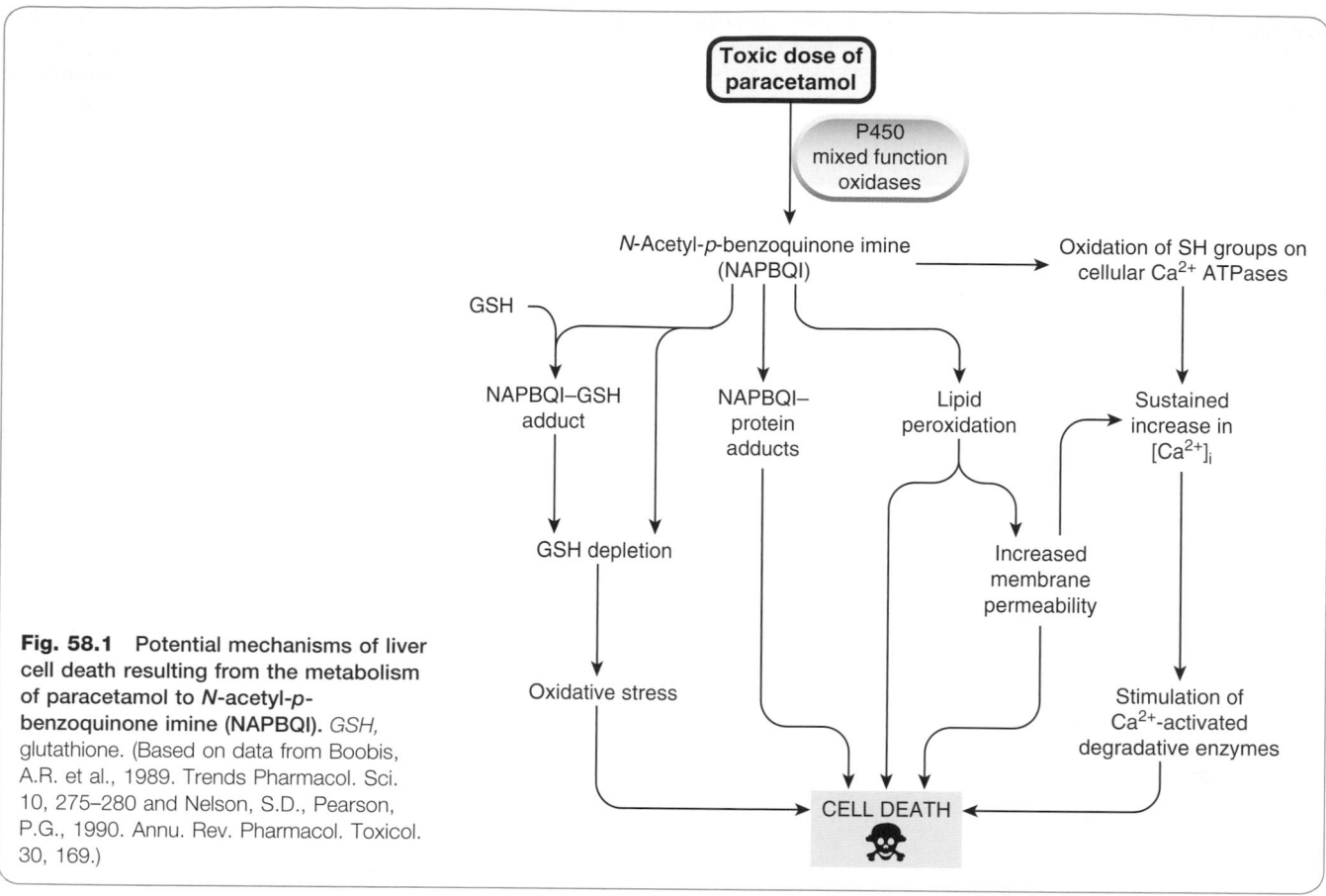

Fig. 58.1 Potential mechanisms of liver cell death resulting from the metabolism of paracetamol to *N*-acetyl-*p*-benzoquinone imine (NAPBQI). *GSH, glutathione.* (Based on data from Boobis, A.R. et al., 1989. Trends Pharmacol. Sci. 10, 275–280 and Nelson, S.D., Pearson, P.G., 1990. Annu. Rev. Pharmacol. Toxicol. 30, 169.)

GENERAL MECHANISMS OF TOXIN-INDUCED CELL DAMAGE AND CELL DEATH

Toxic concentrations of drugs or drug metabolites can cause necrosis; however, programmed cell death (apoptosis; see Ch. 6) is increasingly recognised to be of equal or greater importance, especially in chronic toxicity.

Chemically reactive drug metabolites can form covalent bonds with target molecules, or can damage tissue by non-covalent mechanisms. The liver is of great importance in drug metabolism (Ch. 10), and hepatocytes are exposed to high concentrations of nascent metabolites. Drugs and their polar metabolites are concentrated in renal tubular fluid as water is reabsorbed, so renal tubules are exposed to higher concentrations than are other tissues. Several hepatotoxic drugs (e.g. paracetamol) are also nephrotoxic. Consequently, hepatic or renal damage are common reasons for abandoning development of drugs during toxicity testing and chemical pathology tests of hepatic damage (usually levels of transaminase enzymes measured in blood plasma or serum) and renal function (usually creatinine concentration) are routine.

NON-COVALENT INTERACTIONS

▼ Reactive metabolites of drugs are implicated in several potentially cytotoxic, non-covalent processes, including:

- lipid peroxidation
- generation of toxic reactive oxygen species
- depletion of reduced glutathione (GSH)
- modification of sulfhydryl groups

Lipid peroxidation

▼ Peroxidation of unsaturated lipids can be initiated either by reactive metabolites or by reactive oxygen species (Fig. 58.1). Lipid peroxyradicals (ROO•) can produce lipid hydroperoxides (ROOH), which produce further lipid peroxyradicals. This chain reaction – a peroxidative cascade – may eventually affect much of the membrane lipid. Defence mechanisms, for example GSH peroxidase and vitamin E, protect against this. Cell damage results from alteration of membrane permeability or from reactions of the products of lipid peroxidation with proteins.

Reactive oxygen species

▼ Reduction of molecular oxygen to superoxide anion ($O_2^{-•}$) may be followed by enzymic conversion to hydrogen peroxide (H_2O_2), hydroperoxyl (HOO•) and hydroxyl (OH•) radicals or singlet oxygen. These reactive oxygen species are cytotoxic, both directly and through lipid peroxidation, and are important in excitotoxicity and neurodegeneration (Ch. 41, Fig. 41.2).

Depletion of glutathione

▼ The GSH redox cycle protects cells from oxidative stress. GSH can be depleted by accumulation of normal oxidative products of cell metabolism, or by the action of toxic chemicals. GSH is normally maintained in a redox couple with its disulfide, GSSG. Oxidising species convert GSH to GSSG, GSH being regenerated by NADPH-dependent GSSG reductase. When cellular GSH falls to about 20%–30% of normal, cellular defence against toxic compounds is impaired and cell death can result.

Modification of sulfhydryl groups

▼ Modification of sulfhydryl groups can be produced either by oxidising species that alter sulfhydryl groups reversibly or by covalent interaction. Free sulfhydryl groups have a critical role in the catalytic activity of many enzymes. Important targets for sulfhydryl modification by reactive metabolites include the cytoskeletal protein actin GSH reductase and Ca^{2+}-transporting ATPases in the plasma membrane and endoplasmic reticulum. These maintain cytoplasmic Ca^{2+} concentration at approximately 0.1 µmol/L in the face of an extracellular Ca^{2+} concentration of more than 1 mmol/L. A sustained rise in cell Ca^{2+} occurs with inactivation of these enzymes (or with increased membrane permeability; see earlier), and this compromises cell viability. Lethal processes leading to cell death after acute Ca^{2+} overload include activation of degradative enzymes (neutral proteases, phospholipases, endonucleases) and protein kinases, mitochondrial damage and cytoskeletal alterations (e.g. modification of association between actin and actin-binding proteins).

COVALENT INTERACTIONS

Targets for covalent interactions include DNA, proteins/peptides, lipids and carbohydrates. Covalent bonding to DNA is a basic mechanism of mutagenic chemicals; this is dealt with later. Several non-mutagenic chemicals also form covalent bonds with macromolecules, but the relationship between this and cell damage is incompletely understood. For example, the cholinesterase inhibitor paraoxon (the active metabolite of the insecticide parathion) binds acetylcholinesterase at the neuromuscular junction (Ch. 14) and causes necrosis of skeletal muscle. One toxin from an exceptionally poisonous toadstool, *Amanita phalloides*, binds actin, and another binds RNA polymerase, interfering with actin depolymerisation and protein synthesis, respectively.

General mechanisms of cell damage and cell death

- Drug-induced cell damage/death is usually caused by reactive metabolites of the drug, involving non-covalent and/or covalent interactions with target molecules. Cell death often occurs by apoptosis.
- Non-covalent interactions include:
  – lipid peroxidation via a chain reaction;
  – generation of cytotoxic reactive oxygen species;
  – depletion of reduced glutathione;
  – modification of sulfhydryl groups on key enzymes (e.g. Ca^{2+}-ATPase) and structural proteins.
- Covalent interactions, for example adduct formation between a metabolite of **paracetamol** (NAPBQI: *N*-acetyl-*p*-benzoquinone imine) and cellular macromolecules (see Fig. 58.1). Covalent binding to protein can produce an immunogen; binding to DNA can cause carcinogenesis and teratogenesis.

HEPATOTOXICITY

Many therapeutic drugs cause liver damage, manifested clinically as hepatitis or (in less severe cases) only by laboratory tests (e.g. increased activity of plasma aspartate transaminase, an enzyme released from damaged liver cells). **Paracetamol** and **halothane** cause hepatotoxicity by the mechanisms of cell damage outlined above. Genetic differences in drug metabolism (see Ch. 12) have been implicated in some instances (e.g. **isoniazid**, **phenytoin**). Mild drug-induced abnormalities of liver function are not

uncommon, but the mechanism of liver injury is often uncertain (e.g. *statins*; Ch. 24). It is not always necessary to discontinue a drug when such mild laboratory abnormalities occur, but the occurrence of cirrhosis as a result of long-term low-dose **methotrexate** treatment for arthritis or psoriasis (see Chs 27 and 28) argues for caution. Hepatotoxicity of a different kind, namely reversible obstructive jaundice, occurs with **chlorpromazine** (Ch. 47) and androgens (Ch. 36).

Hepatotoxicity caused by **paracetamol** overdose remains a common cause of death following self-poisoning. An outline is given in Chapter 27. Paracetamol poisoning exemplifies many of the general mechanisms of cell damage outlined previously. With toxic doses of paracetamol, the enzymes catalysing the normal conjugation reactions are saturated, and mixed-function oxidases instead convert the drug to the reactive metabolite *N*-acetyl-*p*-benzoquinone imine (NAPBQI). As explained in Chapter 10, paracetamol toxicity is increased in patients in whom P450 enzymes have been induced, for instance by chronic excessive consumption of alcohol. NAPBQI initiates several of the covalent and non-covalent interactions described previously and illustrated in Fig. 58.1. Oxidative stress from GSH depletion is important in leading to cell death. Regeneration of GSH from GSSG depends on the availability of cysteine, the intracellular availability of which can be limiting. *Acetylcysteine* or *methionine* can substitute for cysteine, increasing GSH availability; they are used to treat patients with paracetamol poisoning.

Liver damage can also be produced by immunological mechanisms (see p. 741), which have been particularly implicated in halothane hepatitis (see Ch. 42).

Hepatotoxicity

- Hepatocytes are exposed to reactive metabolites of drugs as these are formed by P450 enzymes.
- Liver damage is produced by several mechanisms of cell injury; **paracetamol** exemplifies many of these (see Fig. 58.1).
- Some drugs (e.g. **chlorpromazine**, co-amoxiclav) can cause reversible cholestatic jaundice.
- Immunological mechanisms are sometimes implicated (e.g. **halothane**).

NEPHROTOXICITY

Drug-induced nephrotoxicity is a common clinical problem: NSAIDs (Table 58.1) and angiotensin-converting enzyme (ACE) inhibitors are among the commonest precipitants of acute renal failure, usually caused by the principal pharmacological actions of these drugs. Chronic kidney disease, associated with renal tubular or papillary damage, may be caused by a wide range of drugs, including aminoglycoside antibiotics, antiviral drugs and lithium. Nephrotoxic drugs are often well tolerated in healthy people, but can cause renal failure in old people or children, or those with concurrent renal disease.

MUTAGENESIS AND ASSESSMENT OF GENOTOXIC POTENTIAL

Drug-induced mutagenesis is one important cause of carcinogenesis and teratogenesis. Registration of pharmaceuticals

Table 58.1 Adverse effects of non-steroidal anti-inflammatory drugs on the kidney

Cause	Adverse effects
Principal pharmacological action (i.e. inhibition of prostaglandin biosynthesis)	Acute ischaemic renal failure Sodium retention (leading to or exacerbating hypertension and/or heart failure) Water retention Hyporeninaemic hypoaldosteronism (leading to hyperkalaemia)
Unrelated to principal pharmacological action (allergic-type interstitial nephritis)	Renal failure Proteinuria
Unknown whether or not related to principal pharmacological action (analgesic nephropathy)	Papillary necrosis Chronic renal failure

(Adapted from Murray & Brater, 1993.)

Nephrotoxicity

- Renal tubular cells are exposed to high concentrations of drugs and metabolites as urine is concentrated.
- Renal damage can cause papillary and/or tubular necrosis.
- Inhibition of prostaglandin synthesis by non-steroidal anti-inflammatory drugs causes vasoconstriction and lowers glomerular filtration rate.

requires a comprehensive assessment of their genotoxic potential. Because no single test is adequate, the usual approach is to carry out a battery of in vitro and in vivo tests for genotoxicity, usually comprising tests for gene mutation in bacteria, in vitro and in vivo tests for chromosome damage, and in vivo tests for reproductive toxicity and carcinogenicity (see later).

BIOCHEMICAL MECHANISMS OF MUTAGENESIS

Chemical agents cause mutation by covalent modification of DNA. Certain mutations result in carcinogenesis, because the affected DNA sequence codes for a protein that regulates cell growth. It usually requires more than one mutation in a cell to initiate the changes that result in malignancy, mutations in proto-oncogenes (which regulate cell growth) and tumour suppressor genes (which code for products that inhibit the transcription of oncogenes) being particularly implicated (see Chs 6, 12 and 57).

▼ Most chemical carcinogens act by modifying bases in DNA, particularly guanine, the O6 and N7 positions of which readily combine covalently with reactive metabolites of chemical carcinogens. Substitution at the O6 position is the more likely to produce a permanent mutagenic effect, because N7 substitutions are usually quickly repaired.

The accessibility of bases in DNA to chemical attack is greatest when DNA is in the process of replication (i.e. during cell division). The likelihood of genetic damage by many mutagens is therefore related to the frequency of cell division. The developing fetus is particularly susceptible, and mutagens are also potentially teratogenic for this reason (see p. 739). This is also important in relation to mutagenesis of germ cells, particularly in girls, because in humans the production of primary oocytes occurs by a rapid succession of mitotic divisions very early in embryogenesis. Each primary oocyte then undergoes only two further divisions much later in life, at the time of ovulation. It is consequently during early pregnancy that germ cells of the developing female embryo are most likely to undergo mutagenesis, the mutations being transmitted to progeny conceived many years later. In the male, germ cell divisions occur throughout life, and sensitivity of germ cells to mutagens is continuously present.

Mutagenesis and carcinogenicity

- Mutagenesis involves modification of DNA.
- Mutation of proto-oncogenes or tumour suppressor genes leads to carcinogenesis. More than one mutation is usually required.
- Drugs are relatively uncommon (but not unimportant) causes of birth defects and cancers.

CARCINOGENESIS

Alteration of DNA is the first step in carcinogenesis (see Chs 6 and 57). Carcinogenic compounds can interact directly with DNA (genotoxic carcinogens) or act at a later stage to increase the likelihood that mutation will result in a tumour (epigenetic carcinogens; Fig. 58.2).

MEASUREMENT OF MUTAGENICITY AND CARCINOGENICITY

Much effort has gone into developing assays to detect mutagenicity and carcinogenicity. In vitro tests for *mutagenicity* are used to screen large numbers of compounds but are unreliable as predictors of carcinogenicity. Whole-animal tests for carcinogenicity are expensive and time-consuming but are usually required by regulatory authorities before a new drug is licensed for use in humans. The main limitation of this kind of study is that there are important species differences, mainly to do with the metabolism of the foreign compound and the formation of reactive products.

The widely used *Ames test* for mutagenicity measures the effect of substances on the rate of back-mutation (i.e. reversion from mutant to wild-type form) in *Salmonella typhimurium*.

▼ The wild-type strain can grow in a medium containing no added amino acids, because it can synthesise all the amino acids it needs. A mutant form of the organism cannot make histidine in this way and therefore grows only on a medium containing this amino acid. The Ames test involves growing the mutant form on a medium containing a small amount of histidine, plus the drug to be tested. After several divisions, the histidine becomes depleted, and the only cells that continue dividing are those that have back-mutated to the wild type. A count of colonies following subculture on plates deficient in histidine gives a measure of the mutation rate.

Primary carcinogens cause mutation by a direct action on bacterial DNA, but most carcinogens have to be converted to an active metabolite (see Fig. 58.2). Therefore it is necessary to include, in the culture, enzymes that catalyse the necessary conversion. An extract of liver from a rat treated with **phenobarbital** to induce liver enzymes is usually employed. There are many variations based on the same principle.

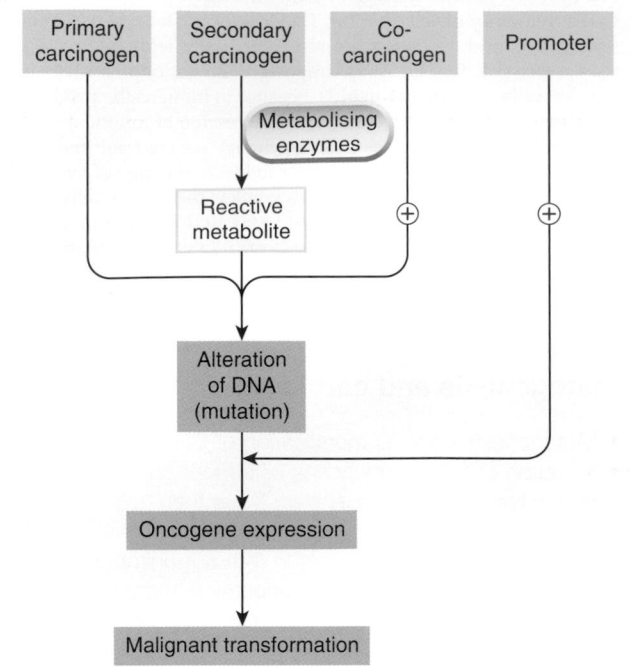

Fig. 58.2 Sequence of events in mutagenesis and carcinogenesis. Alterations to methylation and acetylation patterns of DNA and histones in an epigenetic manner can change gene expression during transcription, translation or even after translation, to increase the likelihood of carcinoma formation.

Carcinogens

- Carcinogens can be:
  - genotoxic, i.e. causing mutations directly (primary carcinogens) or after conversion to reactive metabolites (secondary carcinogens);
  - epigenetic, i.e. increasing the possibility that a mutagen will cause cancer, although not themselves mutagenic.
- New drugs are tested for mutagenicity and carcinogenicity.
- The Ames test for mutagenicity measures back-mutation, in histidine-free medium, of a mutant *Salmonella typhimurium* (which, unlike the wild type, cannot grow without histidine) in the presence of:
  - the chemical to be tested;
  - a liver microsomal enzyme preparation for generating reactive metabolites.
- Colony growth indicates that mutagenesis has occurred. The test is rapid and inexpensive, but some false-positives and false-negatives occur.
- Carcinogenicity testing:
  - involves chronic dosing of groups of animals;
  - is expensive and time-consuming;
  - does not readily detect epigenetic carcinogens.

Other short-term in vitro tests for genotoxic chemicals include measurements of mutagenesis in mouse lymphoma cells, and assays for chromosome aberrations and sister chromatid exchanges in Chinese hamster ovary cells. However, all the in vitro tests give some false-positive and some false-negative results.

In vivo tests for carcinogenicity entail detection of tumours in groups of test animals. Carcinogenicity tests are inevitably slow, because there is usually a latency of months or years before tumours develop. Furthermore, tumours can develop spontaneously in control animals, and the results often provide only equivocal evidence of carcinogenicity of the test drug, making it difficult for industry and regulatory authorities to decide on further development and possible licensing of a product. None of the tests so far described can reliably detect epigenetic carcinogens. To do this, tests that measure the effect of the substance on tumour formation in the presence of a threshold dose of a separate genotoxic agent are being evaluated.

Few therapeutic drugs in clinical use are known to increase the risk of cancer, the most important groups being drugs that act on DNA, i.e. cytotoxic and immunosuppressant drugs (Chs 57 and 27, respectively), and sex hormones (e.g. *oestrogens*, Ch. 36).

TERATOGENESIS AND DRUG-INDUCED CONGENITAL ANOMALIES

Teratogenesis signifies the production of gross structural malformations during fetal development, in distinction from other kinds of drug-induced fetal damage such as growth retardation, dysplasia (e.g. iodide-associated goitre)

or the asymmetrical limb reduction resulting from vaso-constriction caused by **cocaine** (see Ch. 50) in an otherwise normally developing limb.

Other congenital anomalies may relate to neurobehavioural function. For instance, many psychoactive drugs (see Ch. 46) administered during pregnancy are known, or suspected, to increase the risk of cognitive and behavioural problems in offspring. Examples of drugs that affect fetal development adversely are given in Table 58.2.

The importance of X irradiation and rubella infection as causes of fetal malformation was recognised early in the 20th century, but it was not until 1960 that drugs were implicated as causative agents in teratogenesis: the shocking experience with **thalidomide** led to a widespread reappraisal of many other drugs in clinical use, and to the setting up of drug regulatory bodies in many countries. Most birth defects (about 70%) occur with no recognisable causative factor. Drug or chemical exposure during pregnancy is estimated to account for only approximately 1% of all fetal malformations. Fetal malformations are common, so the absolute numbers of children affected are substantial.

MECHANISM OF TERATOGENESIS

The timing of the teratogenic insult in relation to fetal development is critical in determining the type and extent of damage. Mammalian fetal development passes through three phases (Table 58.3):

1. Blastocyst formation
2. Organogenesis
3. Histogenesis and maturation of function

Cell division is the main process occurring during blastocyst formation. During this phase, drugs can kill the embryo by inhibiting cell division, but provided the embryo survives, its subsequent development does not generally seem to be

Table 58.2 Some drugs reported to have adverse effects on human fetal development

Agent	Effect(s)	Risk of congenital anomaly[a]	See chapter
Thalidomide	Phocomelia, heart defects, gut atresia, etc.	K	This chapter
Warfarin	Saddle nose; retarded growth; defects of limbs, eyes, central nervous system	K	25
Corticosteroids	Cleft palate and congenital cataract – rare	—	34
Androgens	Masculinisation in female	—	36
Oestrogens	Testicular atrophy in male	—	36
Stilbestrol	Vaginal adenosis in female fetus, also vaginal or cervical cancer	20+ years later	36
Phenytoin	Cleft lip/palate, microcephaly, mental retardation	K	46
Valproate	Neural tube defects (e.g. spina bifida, facial anomalies)	K	46
Carbamazepine	Retardation of fetal head growth	S	46
Cytotoxic drugs (especially folate antagonists)	Hydrocephalus, cleft palate, neural tube defects, etc.	K	57
Aminoglycosides	Deafness	—	52
Tetracycline	Staining of bones and teeth, thin tooth enamel, impaired bone growth	S	52
Ethanol	Fetal alcohol syndrome	K	50
Nicotine	Altered neurological function	K	49
Retinoids	Hydrocephalus, etc.	K	28
Angiotensin-converting enzyme inhibitors	Oligohydramnios, renal failure	K	23

[a]K, known to carry a high risk of congenital anomaly (in experimental animals and/or humans); S, suspected of causing or increasing risk of congenital anomaly (in experimental animals and/or humans).

Table 58.3 The nature of drug effects on fetal development

Stage	Gestation period in humans	Main cellular process(es)	Affected by
Blastocyst formation	0–16 days	Cell division	Cytotoxic drugs, ? alcohol
Organogenesis	17–60 days approximately	Division Migration Differentiation Death	Teratogens Teratogens Teratogens Teratogens
Histogenesis and functional maturation	60 days to term	As above	Miscellaneous drugs (e.g. alcohol, nicotine, antithyroid drugs, steroids)

compromised. Ethanol is an exception, affecting development even at this very early stage (Ch. 50).

Drugs can cause gross malformations if administered during organogenesis (days 17–60 in humans). The structural organisation of the embryo occurs in a well-defined sequence: eye and brain, skeleton and limbs, heart and major vessels, palate, genitourinary system. The type of malformation produced thus depends on the time of exposure to the teratogen.

The cellular mechanisms by which teratogenic substances produce their effects are not at all well understood. There is a considerable overlap between mutagenicity and teratogenicity. In one large survey, among 78 compounds, 34 were both teratogenic and mutagenic, 19 were negative in both tests and 25 (among them thalidomide) were positive in one but not the other. Damage to DNA is important but not the only factor. The control of morphogenesis is poorly understood; vitamin A derivatives (retinoids) are involved and are potent teratogens (see p. 741 and Ch. 28). Known teratogens also include several drugs (e.g. **methotrexate** and **phenytoin**) that do not react directly with DNA but which inhibit its synthesis by their effects on folate metabolism (see Ch. 26). Administration of **folate** during pregnancy reduces the frequency of both spontaneous and drug-induced malformations, especially neural tube defects.

The fetus depends on an adequate supply of nutrients during the final stage of histogenesis and functional maturation, and development is regulated by a variety of hormones. Gross structural malformations do not arise from exposure to mutagens at this stage, but drugs that interfere with the supply of nutrients or with the hormonal milieu may have deleterious effects on growth and development. Exposure of a female fetus to androgens at this stage can cause masculinisation. **Stilbestrol** (a synthetic oestrogen, now seldom used, licensed to treat breast or prostate cancer) was commonly given to pregnant women with a history of recurrent miscarriage during the 1950s (for unsound reasons). Used in this way it caused dysplasia of the vagina of female infants and an increased incidence of carcinoma of the vagina, a rare malignancy with almost no background incidence, in such offspring in their teens and twenties. Angiotensin II plays an important part in the later stages of fetal development and in renal function in the fetus, and ACE inhibitors and angiotensin receptor antagonists (Ch. 23) cause oligohydramnios and renal failure if administered during later stages of pregnancy, and fetal malformations if given earlier.

TESTING FOR TERATOGENICITY

The thalidomide disaster dramatically brought home the need for teratogenicity studies on new therapeutic drugs. Detection of drug-induced teratogenesis in humans is a particularly difficult problem because the 'spontaneous' malformation rate is high (3%–10%, depending on the definition of a significant malformation) and highly variable between different regions, age groups and social classes. Large-scale long-term studies are required, and the results are often inconclusive.

▼ Studies using embryonic stem cells in assessing developmental toxicity are showing some promise. In vitro methods, based on the culture of cells, organs or whole embryos, have, however, not so far been developed to a level where they satisfactorily predict teratogenesis in vivo, and most regulatory authorities require teratogenicity testing in a rodent and a non-rodent species (e.g. rabbit). Pregnant females are dosed at various levels during the critical period of organogenesis, and the fetuses are examined for structural abnormalities. However, poor cross-species correlation means that tests of this kind are not reliably predictive in humans, and it is usually recommended that new drugs are not used in pregnancy unless it is essential.

SOME DEFINITE AND PROBABLE HUMAN TERATOGENS

Although many drugs have been found to be teratogenic in varying degrees in experimental animals, relatively few are known to be teratogenic in humans (see Table 58.2). Some of the more important ones are discussed later.

Thalidomide

Thalidomide is almost unique in producing, at therapeutic dosage, virtually 100% malformed infants when taken in the first 3–6 weeks of gestation. It was introduced in 1957 as a hypnotic and sedative with the special feature that it was much less hazardous in overdosage than barbiturates, and it was even recommended specifically for use in pregnancy (with the advertising slogan 'the safe hypnotic'). It had been subjected to toxicity testing only in mice, which are resistant

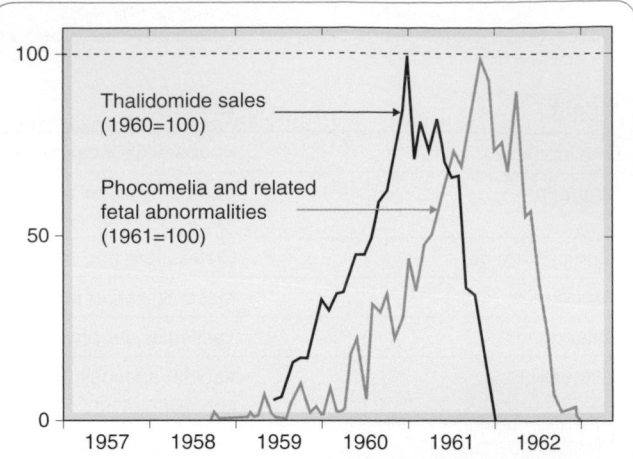

Fig. 58.3 Incidence of major fetal abnormalities in Western Europe following the introduction and withdrawal of thalidomide, linked to sales data for thalidomide.

Table 58.4 Thalidomide teratogenesis

Day of gestation	Type of deformity
21–22	Malformation of ears Cranial nerve defects
24–27	Phocomelia of arms
28–29	Phocomelia of arms and legs
30–36	Malformation of hands Anorectal stenosis

to thalidomide teratogenicity. Thalidomide was marketed energetically and successfully, and the first suspicion of its teratogenicity arose early in 1961 with reports of a sudden increase in the incidence of phocomelia ('seal limbs', an absence of development of the long bones of the arms and legs) that had hitherto been virtually unknown. At this time, a million tablets were being sold daily in West Germany. Reports of phocomelia came simultaneously from Hamburg and Sydney, and the connection with thalidomide was made.[3] The drug was withdrawn late in 1961, by which time an estimated 10,000 malformed babies had been born (Fig. 58.3 illustrates the use of data linkage in detecting delayed ADRs). Epidemiological investigation showed very clearly the correlation between the time of exposure and the type of malfunction produced (Table 58.4). Though the mechanism is not clearly understood, inhibition

---

[3]A severe peripheral neuropathy, leading to irreversible paralysis and sensory loss, was reported within a year of the drug's introduction and subsequently confirmed in many reports. The drug company responsible was less than punctilious in acting on these reports (see Sjöström & Nilsson, 1972), which were soon eclipsed by the discovery of teratogenic effects, but the neurotoxic effect was severe enough in its own right to have necessitated restriction of the drug from general use. Today, use of thalidomide has had a resurgence related to several highly specialised applications. It is prescribed by specialists (in dermatology, oncology and in HIV infection, among others) under tightly controlled and restricted conditions.

of blood vessel formation (angiogenesis) is thought to be involved.

Cytotoxic drugs

Many alkylating agents (e.g. **chlorambucil** and **cyclophosphamide**) and antimetabolites (e.g. **azathioprine** and **mercaptopurine**) cause malformations when used in early pregnancy but more often lead to abortion (see Ch. 57). Folate antagonists (e.g. **methotrexate**) produce a much higher incidence of major malformations, evident in both liveborn and stillborn fetuses.

Retinoids

Etretinate, a retinoid (i.e. vitamin A derivative) with marked effects on epidermal differentiation, is a known teratogen and causes a high proportion of serious abnormalities (notably skeletal deformities) in exposed fetuses. Dermatologists use retinoids to treat skin diseases, including several, such as acne and psoriasis, that are common in young women. Etretinate accumulates in subcutaneous fat and is eliminated extremely slowly, detectable amounts persisting for many months after chronic dosing is discontinued. Because of this, women should avoid pregnancy for at least 2 years after treatment. **Acitretin** is an active metabolite of etretinate. It is equally teratogenic, but tissue accumulation is less pronounced and elimination may be more rapid.

Heavy metals

Lead, *cadmium* and *mercury* all cause fetal malformation in humans. The main evidence comes from *Minamata disease*, named after the locality in Japan where an epidemic occurred when the local population ate fish contaminated with methylmercury that had been used as an agricultural fungicide. This impaired brain development in exposed fetuses, resulting in cerebral palsy and mental retardation, often with microcephaly. Mercury, like other heavy metals, inactivates many enzymes by forming covalent bonds with sulfhydryl and other groups, and this is believed to be responsible for these developmental abnormalities.

Antiepileptic drugs (see Ch. 46)

Congenital malformations are increased two- to three-fold in babies of epileptic mothers, especially of mothers treated with two or more antiepileptic drugs during the first trimester, and in association with above-therapeutic plasma concentrations. Many antiepileptic drugs have been implicated, including **phenytoin** (particularly cleft lip/palate), **valproate** (neural tube defects) and **carbamazepine** (spina bifida and hypospadias, a malformation of the male urethra) (Ch. 46). The relative risks attributable to different antiepileptic drugs are not well defined, but valproate is considered to be particularly harmful (rate of congenital anomalies of about 10%, compared with 2%–3% in the general population), and is contraindicated in women of childbearing age.

Warfarin

Administration of **warfarin** (Ch. 25) in the first trimester is associated with nasal hypoplasia and various central nervous system abnormalities, affecting roughly 25% of exposed babies. In the last trimester, it must not be used because of the risk of intracranial haemorrhage in the baby during delivery.

Teratogenesis and drug-induced fetal damage

- Teratogenesis means production of gross structural malformations of the fetus (e.g. the absence of limbs after **thalidomide**). Less comprehensive damage can be produced by several drugs (see Table 58.2). Less than 1% of congenital fetal defects are attributed to drugs given to the mother.
- Gross malformations are produced only if teratogens act during organogenesis. This occurs during the first 3 months of pregnancy but after blastocyst formation. Drug-induced fetal damage is rare during blastocyst formation (exception: fetal alcohol syndrome) and after the first 3 months (exception: angiotensin-converting enzyme [ACE] inhibitors and sartans).
- The mechanisms of action of teratogens are not clearly understood, although DNA damage is a factor.

IMMUNOLOGICAL REACTIONS TO DRUGS

Biological agents (Ch. 5) may provoke an immune response; antidrug antibodies to insulin are common in diabetic patients, though they seldom cause problems (Ch. 32), but antidrug antibodies to erythropoietin and thrombopoietin can have serious consequences for patients treated with these agents (see Ch. 26). Measurement of antidrug antibodies is now routine during development of biological products. Seemingly trivial differences in manufacturing process (e.g. between different batches, or when a new manufacturer makes a copy of a biological product after it is no longer protected by patent – so-called biosimilar products) can result in marked changes in immunogenicity.

Allergic reactions of various kinds are a common form of adverse drug reaction. Low molecular-weight drugs are not immunogenic in themselves. A drug or its metabolites can, however, act as a *hapten* by interacting with protein to form a stable immunogenic conjugate (Ch. 7). The immunological basis of some allergic drug reactions has been well worked out, but often it is inferred from the clinical characteristics of the reaction, and direct evidence of an immunological mechanism is lacking. The existence of an allergic reaction is suggested by its delayed onset, or occurrence only after repeated exposure to the drug. Allergic reactions are generally unrelated to the main action of the drug, and conform to syndromes associated with types I, II, III and IV of the Gell and Coombs classification (see later and Ch. 7).

The overall incidence of allergic drug reactions is variously reported as being between 2% and 25%. Most are minor skin eruptions. Serious reactions (e.g. anaphylaxis, haemolysis and bone marrow depression) are rare. Penicillins, which are the commonest cause of drug-induced anaphylaxis, produce this response in an estimated 1 in 50,000 patients exposed. Rashes can be severe, and fatalities occur with Stevens–Johnson syndrome (provoked, for example, by sulfonamides), and toxic epidermal necrolysis (TEN, which can be caused, for example, by **allopurinol**). The association between **carbamazepine**-induced TEN and the gene for a particular human leukocyte antigen (HLA) allele *HLAB*1502* in people of Asian ancestry is mentioned in Chapter 12. Susceptibility to severe rashes in response to **abacavir** is closely linked to the variant *HLAB*5701* and this forms the basis of a clinically useful genomic test (Ch. 12).

IMMUNOLOGICAL MECHANISMS

The formation of an immunogenic conjugate between a small molecule and an endogenous protein requires covalent bonding. In most cases, reactive metabolites, rather than the drug itself, are responsible. Such reactive metabolites can be produced during drug oxidation or by photoactivation in the skin. They may also be produced by the action of toxic oxygen metabolites generated by activated leukocytes. Rarely (e.g. in drug-induced lupus erythematosus), the reactive moiety interacts to form an immunogen with nuclear components (DNA, histone) rather than proteins. Conjugation with a macromolecule is usually essential, although penicillin is an exception because it can form sufficiently large polymers in solution to elicit an anaphylactic reaction in a sensitised individual even without conjugation to protein, although penicillin–protein conjugates can also act as the immunogen.

CLINICAL TYPES OF ALLERGIC RESPONSE TO DRUGS

Hypersensitivity reactions of types I, II and III (Ch. 7) are antibody-mediated reactions, while type IV is cell mediated. Unwanted reactions to drugs involve both antibody- and cell-mediated reactions. The more important clinical manifestations of hypersensitivity include anaphylactic shock, haematological reactions, allergic liver damage and other hypersensitivity reactions.

ANAPHYLACTIC SHOCK

Anaphylactic shock – see also Chapters 7 and 29 – is a type I hypersensitivity response. It is a sudden and life-threatening reaction that results from the release of histamine, leukotrienes and other mediators. The main features include urticarial rash, swelling of soft tissues, bronchoconstriction and hypotension.

Penicillins account for about 75% of anaphylactic deaths, reflecting the frequency with which they are used in clinical practice. Other drugs that can cause anaphylaxis include enzymes, such as **asparaginase** (Ch. 57); therapeutic monoclonal antibodies (Ch. 5); hormones, for example, **corticotropin** (Ch. 34); **heparin** (Ch. 25); dextrans; radiological contrast agents; vaccines; and other serological products. Anaphylaxis with local anaesthetics (Ch. 44), the antiseptic chlorhexidine and with many other drugs (sometimes as a consequence of contaminants such as latex used to seal reusable vials or of excipients and colouring agents rather than the drug itself) can occur. Treatment of anaphylaxis is mentioned in Chapter 29.

It is sometimes feasible to carry out a skin test for the presence of hypersensitivity, which involves injecting a minute dose intradermally. A patient who reports that she or he is allergic to a drug such as penicillin may actually be allergic to fungal contaminants, which were common in early preparations, rather than to penicillin itself. The use of penicilloylpolylysine as a skin test reagent for penicillin allergy is an improvement over the use of penicillin itself, because it bypasses the need for conjugation of the test substance, thereby reducing the likelihood of a false

negative. Other specialised tests are available to detect the presence of specific immunoglobulin E in the plasma, or to measure histamine release from the patient's basophils, but these are not used routinely.

HAEMATOLOGICAL REACTIONS

Drug-induced haematological reactions can be produced by type II, III or IV hypersensitivity. Type II reactions can affect any or all of the formed elements of the blood, which may be destroyed by effects either on the circulating blood cells themselves or on their progenitors in the bone marrow. They involve antibody binding to a drug–macromolecule complex on the cell surface membrane. The antigen–antibody reaction activates complement, leading to lysis, or provokes attack by killer lymphocytes or phagocytic leukocytes (Ch. 7). *Haemolytic anaemia* has been most commonly reported with sulfonamides and related drugs (Ch. 52) and with an antihypertensive drug, **methyldopa** (Ch. 15), which is still widely used to treat hypertension during pregnancy. With methyldopa, significant haemolysis occurs in less than 1% of patients, but the appearance of antibodies directed against the surface of red cells is detectable in 15% by the Coombs test. The antibodies are directed against Rh antigens, but it is not known how methyldopa produces this effect.

Drug-induced *agranulocytosis* (complete absence of circulating neutrophils) is usually delayed 2–12 weeks after beginning drug treatment but may then be sudden in onset. It often presents with mouth ulcers, a severe sore throat or other infection. Serum from the patient lyses leukocytes from other individuals, and circulating anti-leukocyte antibodies can usually be detected immunologically. Drugs associated with agranulocytosis include NSAIDs, especially **phenylbutazone**, **carbimazole** (Ch. 35) and **clozapine** (Ch. 47) and **sulfonamides** and related drugs (e.g. *thiazides* and *sulfonylureas*). Agranulocytosis is rare but life-threatening. Recovery when the offending drug is stopped is often slow or absent. Antibody-mediated leukocyte destruction must be distinguished from the direct effect of cytotoxic drugs (see Ch. 56), which cause granulocytopenia that is rapid in onset, predictably related to dose and reversible.

Thrombocytopenia (reduction in platelet numbers) can be caused by type II reactions to **quinine** (Ch. 55), **heparin** (Ch. 25) and thiazide diuretics (Ch. 30).

Some drugs (notably **chloramphenicol**) can suppress all three haemopoietic cell lineages, giving rise to *aplastic anaemia* (anaemia with associated agranulocytosis and thrombocytopenia).

The distinction between type III and type IV hypersensitivity reactions in the causation of haematological reactions is not clear cut, and either or both mechanisms can be involved.

ALLERGIC LIVER DAMAGE

Most drug-induced liver damage results from the direct toxic effects of drugs or their metabolites, as described above. However, hypersensitivity reactions are sometimes involved, a particular example being **halothane**-induced hepatic necrosis (see Ch. 42). *Trifluoroacetylchloride*, a reactive metabolite of halothane, couples to a macromolecule to form an immunogen. Most patients with halothane-induced liver damage have antibodies that react with halothane–carrier conjugates. Halothane–protein antigens can be expressed on the surface of hepatocytes. Destruction of the cells occurs by type II hypersensitivity reactions involving killer T cells, and type III reactions can also contribute.

OTHER HYPERSENSITIVITY REACTIONS

The clinical manifestations of type IV hypersensitivity reactions are diverse, ranging from minor skin rashes to generalised autoimmune disease. Fever may accompany these reactions. Rashes can be antibody mediated but are usually cell mediated. They range from mild eruptions to fatal exfoliation. Stevens–Johnson syndrome is a very severe generalised rash that extends into the alimentary tract and carries an appreciable mortality. In some cases, the lesions are photosensitive, probably because ultraviolet light converts the drug to reactive products.

▼ Some drugs (notably **hydralazine** and **procainamide**) can produce an autoimmune syndrome resembling systemic lupus erythematosus. This is a multisystem disorder in which there is immunological damage to many organs and tissues (including joints, skin, lung, central nervous system and kidney) caused particularly, but not exclusively, by type III hypersensitivity reactions. The prodigious array of antibodies directed against 'self' components has been termed an 'autoimmune thunderstorm'. The antibodies react with determinants shared by many molecules, for example, the phosphodiester backbone of DNA, RNA and phospholipids. In drug-induced systemic lupus erythematosus, the immunogen may result from the reactive drug moiety interacting with nuclear material, and joint and pulmonary damage is common. The condition usually resolves when treatment with the offending drug is stopped.

> ### Allergic reactions to drugs
>
> - Drugs or their reactive metabolites can bind covalently to proteins to form immunogens. **Penicillin** (which can also form immunogenic polymers) is an important example.
> - Drug-induced allergic (hypersensitivity) reactions may be antibody mediated (types I, II, III) or cell mediated (type IV). Important clinical manifestations include the following:
>   - anaphylactic shock (type I): many drugs can cause this, and most deaths are caused by **penicillin**;
>   - haematological reactions (type II, III or IV): including haemolytic anaemia (e.g. **methyldopa**), agranulocytosis (e.g. **carbimazole**), thrombocytopenia (e.g. **quinine**) and aplastic anaemia (e.g. **chloramphenicol**);
>   - hepatitis (types II, III): for example, **halothane**, **phenytoin**;
>   - rashes (type I, IV): are usually mild but can be life-threatening (e.g. Stevens–Johnson syndrome);
>   - drug-induced systemic lupus erythematosus (mainly type II): antibodies to nuclear material are formed (e.g. **hydralazine**).

REFERENCES AND FURTHER READING

Adverse drug reactions

Aronson, J.K., Ferner, R.E., 2003. Joining the DoTS: a new approach to classifying adverse drug reactions. Br. Med. J. 327, 1222–1225. (*Description of ADRs in terms of dose, time course and susceptibility*)

Aronson, J.K. (Ed.), 2015. Meyler's Side Effects of Drugs: The International Encyclopedia of Adverse Drug Reactions and Interactions, sixteenth ed. Elsevier Science.

Lee, A. (Ed.), 2005. Adverse Drug Reactions, second ed. Pharmaceutical Press, London, pp. 12–38. (*Good reference text covering classification and adverse reactions according to organ system*)

Pirmohamed, M., James, S., Meakin, S., et al., 2004. Adverse drug reactions as cause of admission to hospital: prospective analysis of 18820 patients. Br. Med. J. 329, 15–19. (*A sobering analysis, emphasising the frequency and cost of adverse drug reactions, most of which were avoidable. Drugs most commonly implicated were aspirin and other NSAIDs, diuretics, warfarin; the most common reaction was gastrointestinal bleeding*)

Talbot, J., Aronson, J.K. (Eds.), 2012. Stephens' Detection and Evaluation of Adverse Drug Reactions, sixth ed. Wiley–Blackwell, Oxford. (*Invaluable reference book that is also readable*)

Drug toxicity: general and mechanistic aspects

Bhogal, N., Grindon, C., Combes, R., Balls, M., 2005. Toxicity testing: creating a revolution based on new technologies. Trends Biotechnol. 23, 299–307. (*Reviews current and likely future value of new technologies in relation to toxicological evaluation*)

Timbrell, J.A., 2009. Principles of Biochemical Toxicity. Informa Healthcare, New York.

Walker, D.K., 2004. The use of pharmacokinetic and pharmacodynamic data in the assessment of drug safety in early drug development. Br. J. Clin. Pharmacol. 58, 601–608. (*Pharmacokinetic profile is a factor in assessing safety during early drug development, especially in relation to safety parameters such as QT interval prolongation, where free plasma concentrations are predictive; procedures are available that allow this on the microdose scale – potential limitations are discussed*)

Wobus, A.M., Loser, P., 2011. Present state and future perspectives of using pluripotent stem cells in toxicology research. Arch. Toxicol. 85, 79–117. (*Describes methods for selection and differentiation of cardiac and hepatic cells from human pluripotent stem cells*)

Drug toxicity: carcinogenesis, teratogenesis

Briggs, G.G., Freeman, R.K., Towers, C.V., Forinash, A.V., 2017. Drugs in Pregnancy and Lactation, eleventh ed. Lippincott, Williams & Wilkins, Philadelphia. (*Invaluable reference guide to fetal and neonatal risk for clinicians caring for pregnant women*)

Sjöström, H., Nilsson, R., 1972. Thalidomide and the Power of the Drug Companies. Penguin Books, London.

Drug toxicity: organ involvement

Murray, M.C., Brater, D.C., 1993. Renal toxicity of the nonsteroidal anti-inflammatory drugs. Annu. Rev. Pharmacol. Toxicol. 33, 435–465.

Park, B.K., Kitteringham, N.R., Maggs, J.L., et al., 2005. The role of metabolic activation in drug-induced hepatotoxicity. Annu. Rev. Pharmacol. Toxicol. 45, 177–202. (*Reviews evidence for reactive metabolite formation from hepatotoxic drugs such as paracetamol, tamoxifen, diclofenac and troglitazone, and the current hypotheses of how this leads to liver injury*)

Ritter, J.M., Harding, I., Warren, J.B., 2009. Precaution, cyclooxygenase inhibition, and cardiovascular risk. Trends Pharmacol. Sci. 30, 503–514.

Svensson, C.K., Cowen, E.W., Gaspari, A.A., 2001. Cutaneous drug reactions. Pharmacol. Rev. 53, 357–380. (*Covers epidemiology, clinical morphology and mechanisms. Assesses current knowledge of four types of cutaneous drug reaction: immediate-type immune mediated, delayed-type immune mediated, photosensitivity and autoimmune. Also reviews the role of viral infection as predisposing factor*)

Valentin, J.P., 2010. Reducing QT liability and proarrhythmic risk in drug discovery and development. Br. J. Pharmacol. 159, 5–11. (*See also accompanying articles in this themed section on QT safety*)

59

Lifestyle and drugs in sport

OVERVIEW

The term *lifestyle* denotes that such drugs are used for non-medical purposes. It is a diverse group that includes drugs of abuse, drugs used to enhance athletic or other performance, as well as those taken for cosmetic purposes or for purely social reasons. Many lifestyle drugs have dual uses and are also employed as conventional therapeutics for other indications; their pharmacology is described elsewhere in this book. In this chapter we present an overall summary of lifestyle drugs and discuss some of the social and medico-legal problems associated with their growing use.

Drugs used to enhance sporting performance, while being officially prohibited, represent a special category of lifestyle drugs. Once again, many types of substances are used for this purpose, including some established medicines. We discuss specific issues relating to their use in competitive sports.

WHAT ARE LIFESTYLE DRUGS?

This is a question that is sometimes difficult to answer. Here we define them as drugs or medicines that are taken by choice to give pleasure (e.g. cannabis, alcohol, cocaine), to improve performance (e.g. drugs in sport, cognition-enhancing drugs) or to improve appearance (e.g. **botox**, slimming aids for the non-obese), in other words, to satisfy an aspiration or a non-health-related goal rather than to treat a clinical condition. Put simply, they are drugs taken by choice by people who are not ill, and a better term might be *lifestyle uses* as many are conventional therapeutic agents. Examples include the use of the antihypertensive **minoxidil** for treating baldness. Oral contraceptives, which clearly lie in the domain of mainstream medicine, could also be considered lifestyle drugs. Also included are food supplements and other related preparations (sometimes referred to as *nutraceuticals*) that are consumed because of some claimed benefit – even though there is often no good evidence that they are effective.

CLASSIFICATION OF LIFESTYLE DRUGS

The lifestyle category covers lifestyle *uses* of a wide variety of drugs and medicines and cuts across the pharmacological classification used throughout this book. The scheme in Table 59.1 is based largely on the work of Gilbert et al. (2000) and Young (2003). It embraces drugs that have been used for lifestyle choices based on historical precedent,

such as oral contraceptives, as well as agents used to manage potentially debilitating *lifestyle illnesses* such as addiction to smoking (e.g. **bupropion**; see Ch. 50). It also includes drugs such as **caffeine** and **alcohol** that are consumed on a massive scale around the world, and drugs of abuse such as cocaine as well as nutritional supplements.

Particularly topical is the controversial use of 'neuro-enhancers', such as **modafinil** and **methylphenidate** (Ch. 49) which, under some circumstances can improve intellectual performance (see Sahakian & Morein-Zamir, 2007; Sahakian & LaBuzetta, 2015, for example).[1] The use of drugs that improve cognitive defects in conditions such as dementia (Ch. 41), schizophrenia (Ch. 47) and depression (Ch. 48) is generally seen as desirable even though current drugs are only marginally effective. But watch this space! (see Chs. 41 and 49). Extending the use of existing and future drugs to give healthy people an advantage in competitive situations is much more controversial. The possibility, not yet realised, of finding drugs able to prolong life by retarding the functional and degenerative changes characteristic of old age, is another social and ethical minefield.

For a more complete discussion of human enhancement by pharmacological means, see Buchanan (2011) and Flower (2012).

Over time, drugs can switch between 'lifestyle' and 'clinical' categories. For example, **cocaine** was used as a lifestyle drug by South American Indians. Early explorers commented that it 'satisfies the hungry, gives new strength to the weary and exhausted and makes the unhappy forget their sorrows'. Originally adopted into European medicine as a local anaesthetic (Ch. 44), it is now largely returned to lifestyle drug status and, regrettably, is the basis of an illegal multimillion dollar international drugs industry. Cannabis is another good example of a drug that has been considered (in the West at least) as a purely recreational drug but which is now (as a plant extract containing **tetrahydrocannabinol** and **cannabidiol**) licensed for various clinical uses (see Chs 20, 43 and 50). There are many other examples (Flower, 2004).

Many widely used lifestyle 'drugs' or 'sports supplements' consist of natural products (e.g. *Ginkgo* extracts, melatonin, St John's wort, *Cinchona* extracts), the manufacture and sale of which have historically not been regulated.[2] Their composition is therefore highly variable, and their efficacy

---

[1] Drugs intended to give a competitive advantage in sport are, of course, considered unfair, banned and very actively policed. Will there come a time when taking drugs to improve examination performance will become illegal, with similar surveillance methods and sanctions? See Bostrom and Sandberg (2009) for a discussion of this ethical minefield.
[2] Happily, this is changing. Since 2014, the United Kingdom Medicines and Healthcare Products Regulatory Agency has a Herbal Medicines Advisory Committee designed to fulfil this demanding role.

Table 59.1 Some examples of lifestyle drugs and medicines (excluding drugs in sport)

Category	Example(s)	Primary clinical use	'Lifestyle' use	Chapter
Medicines approved for specific indications but which also have other 'lifestyle' uses.	Sildenafil[a]	Erectile dysfunction	Erectile enhancement	36
	Oral contraceptives	Preventing conception	Preventing conception	36
	Orlistat	Obesity	Weight loss	33
	Sibutramine	Anorectic agent (withdrawn in Europe)	Weight loss	33
Medicines approved for specific indications which can also be used to satisfy 'lifestyle choices' or to treat 'lifestyle diseases'	Minoxidil	Hypertension	Regrowth of hair	23
	Methylphenidate	ADHD	Improving academic performance	49
	Modafinil	Treatment of ADHD	Cognitive enhancement	49
	Opiates	Analgesia	'Recreational' usage	43, 50
Drugs that have only minor, or no, current clinical use but which fall into the lifestyle category	Alcohol	None as such	Widespread component of drinks	50
	Botulinum toxin	Relief of muscle spasm	Cosmetic alteration	14
	Caffeine	Migraine treatment	Widespread component of drinks	16, 49
	Cannabis	Managing chronic pain, nausea and possibly muscle spasm	'Recreational' usage	20, 50
Drugs (generally illegal) that have no clinical utility but which are used to satisfy lifestyle requirements[b]	Methylenedioxy-methamphetamine (MDMA, 'ecstasy')	None	'Recreational' usage	49
	Tobacco (nicotine)	Nicotine preparations for tobacco addiction	'Recreational' usage	50
	Cocaine (some formulations)	Local anaesthesia (largely obsolete)	'Recreational' usage	43

[a]Obviously only in men. However, in some countries, **flibanserin** is used to increase female sexual desire and may turn out to be a new addition to this category.
[b]In addition, there are countless herbal preparations and other natural products, largely unregulated, which are marketed as health-promoting, life-enhancing and beneficial for many disorders, despite lack of rigorous evidence of therapeutic efficacy. Examples include numerous vitamin preparations, fish oils, melatonin, ginseng, *Echinacea*, *Ginkgo* and much besides.
ADHD, attention deficit hyperactivity disorder.

(From Flower, 2004, after Gilbert et al., 2000 and Young, 2003.)

and safety generally untested. Many contain active substances that, like synthetic drugs, can produce harmful as well as beneficial effects.

DRUGS AND SEX

A myriad of foods and natural products have been claimed to have aphrodisiac properties but the validity of such claims remain largely unsubstantiated. Enhanced libido may be a therapeutically useful outcome, e.g. **pramipexole**, a dopamine receptor agonist, is sometimes used to counteract the decrease in libido induced by serotonin-selective reuptake inhibitor (SSRI) antidepressant drugs. From a lifestyle perspective, drugs associated with sexual activity are used not only to enhance performance and/or pleasure but also to prevent negative consequences such as unwanted pregnancies and HIV infection. Table 59.2 provides a resume of various lifestyle drugs associated with sexual activity.

Chemsex – having sex often with multiple partners under the influence of a combination of psychoactive drugs in sessions lasting several hours or days – has become increasingly popular amongst certain gay men (see McCall et al., 2015 for a fuller description). The drugs commonly taken include **mephedrone**, γ-hydroxybutyrate (GHB), and **methamphetamine** (see Chs 39 and 49).

DRUGS IN SPORT

The use of drugs to enhance performance ('doping') in elite sporting competitions such as the Olympic games is evidently widespread, although officially prohibited. The World Anti-Doping Agency (WADA: http://www.wada-ama.org), which was established partly in response to some high-profile doping cases and drug-induced deaths among athletes, publishes an annually updated list of prohibited substances that may not be used by sportsmen or

Table 59.2 Drugs associated with sexual activity

Drug	Function	Notes
Oestrogens and progestogens (Ch. 36)	Contraception	—
Levonorgestrel (Ch. 36)	Postcoital contraception	The morning after pill taken to avoid conception by women after unprotected sex
Sildenafil (Chs 21 and 36)	Maintain erection	To enhance male sexual function
Benzocaine (Ch. 44)	Delay ejaculation	Contained in condoms for topical application to the penis
Flibanserin	Enhance female sexual pleasure	Not yet available in United Kingdom
Antiretroviral drugs (Ch. 53)	Prophylactic treatment for HIV infection	For gay men following unprotected sex
Amyl nitrite	Anal sphincter relaxation	Primarily used by gay men
Methamphetamine (crystal meth)	Increase libido and cause frequent or prolonged erections	Occurs with high doses Taken along with mephedrone and GHB in chemsex

GHB, γ-hydroxybutyrate.

sportswomen either in, or out of, competition. Drug testing is based mainly on analysis of blood or urine samples according to strictly defined protocols. The chemical analyses, which rely mainly on gas chromatography/mass spectrometry or immunoassay techniques, must be carried out by approved laboratories.

Lifestyle drugs

- More accurately called *lifestyle uses*, these comprise a group of drugs and medicines taken mainly for non-medical reasons.
- Include prescription drugs such as **sildenafil** and **methylphenidate**, substances such as **alcohol** and **caffeine**, drugs of abuse and various nutritional preparations.
- Are linked to the concepts of 'self-diagnosis' and 'non-disease'.
- Are a growing sector of the pharmaceutical market.
- Are often brought to the consumer's attention through the internet or direct marketing.

Despite these precautions, there have been many instances where these rules have been flouted both by individual athletes or, in some cases, by entire teams. The American cyclist Lance Armstrong was a national hero who, having overcome testicular cancer, went on to win the Tour de France on no less than seven occasions. Persistent accusations of drug abuse were strenuously denied until January 2013, when Armstrong admitted having used a cocktail of drugs to enhance his performance over the course of many years.[3] It prompted one commentator (Sparling, 2013) to despair of the 'charade of drug-free sport'.

In 2016, WADA published the results of an investigation in Russia, concluding that a large-scale state-sponsored doping programme had taken place, leading to a ban on the Russian team's participation in the subsequent Summer Olympics and other events.

Table 59.3 summarises the main classes of drugs currently banned by WADA. While athletes are easily persuaded of the potential of a wide variety of drugs to increase their chances of winning, controlled trials of such claims are difficult. In many cases these agents probably produce little or no effect although of course, marginal improvements in performance (often 1% or less), which are difficult to measure experimentally, may make the difference between winning and losing, and the competitive instincts of athletes and their trainers generally carry more weight than scientific evidence.

A brief account of some of the more important drugs in common use follows. For a broader and more complete coverage, see British Medical Association (2002), Reardon and Creado (2014) and Mottram (2005). Gould (2013) has reviewed the potential use of gene therapy in promoting athletic performance. Another potential nightmare for the regulators!

ANABOLIC STEROIDS

Anabolic steroids (Ch. 36) include a large group of compounds with testosterone-like effects, including about 50 named compounds on the prohibited list. New chemical derivatives ('designer steroids'), such as **tetrahydrogestrinone** (THG), are regularly developed and offered illicitly to athletes, posing a continuing problem to the authorities charged with detecting and identifying them. A further problem is that some of these drugs are endogenous compounds or their metabolites and their concentration can vary dramatically for physiological reasons. This makes it difficult to prove that the substance had been administered illegally. Isotope ratio techniques, based on the fact that endogenous and exogenous steroids have slightly different $^{12}C:^{13}C$ ratios, may enable the two to be distinguished analytically. Since anabolic steroids produce long-term effects and are normally used throughout training, rather than during the event itself, out-of-competition testing is essential.

When given in combination with training and high protein intake, anabolic steroids undoubtedly increase muscle mass

---

[3]Apparently including steroids, growth hormone and erythropoietin. He was later stripped of all his sporting honours.

Table 59.3 Some examples of drugs used in sport

Drug class	Example(s)	Effects	Detection	Notes
Anabolic agents	Androgenic steroids (testosterone, nandrolone and many others; Ch. 36)	Increased muscle development, aggression and competitiveness Serious long-term side effects	Urine or blood samples	Many are endogenous hormones, so results significantly above normal range are required
	Clenbuterol (Ch. 15)	Combined anabolic and agonist action on β_2 adrenoceptors may increase muscle strength	—	Human chorionic gonadotrophin is sometimes used to increase androgen secretion
Hormones and related substances	Erythropoietin (Ch. 26)	Increased erythrocyte formation and oxygen transport. Increased blood viscosity causes hypertension and risk of strokes and coronary attacks Used mainly for endurance sports[a]	Plasma half-life is short, so detection is difficult	Use of other plasma markers indicating erythropoietin administration may be possible
	Human growth hormone (Ch. 34)	Increased lean body mass and reduced fat May accelerate recovery from tissue injury. Causes cardiac hypertrophy, acromegaly, liver damage and increased cancer risk	Blood testing	Distinguishing endogenous (highly variable) from exogenous human growth hormone can be difficult
	Insulin (Ch. 32)	Sometimes used (with glucose so as to avoid hypoglycaemia) to promote glucose uptake and energy production in muscle Probably ineffective in improving performance	Plasma samples	—
β_2-Adrenoceptor agonists	Salbutamol and others (Ch. 15)	Used by runners, cyclists, swimmers, etc. to increase oxygen uptake (by bronchodilatation) and increased cardiac function. Controlled studies show no improvement in performance	Urine samples	—
β-Adrenoceptor antagonists	Propranolol, etc. (Ch. 15)	Used to reduce tremor and anxiety in 'precision' sports (e.g. shooting, gymnastics, diving)	Urine samples	Not banned in most sports, where they actually impair performance
CNS 'stimulants'	Ephedrine and derivatives; amphetamines, cocaine, caffeine (Ch. 49)	Many trials show slight increase in muscle strength and performance in non-endurance events (sprint, swimming, field events, etc.)	Urine samples	The most widely used group, along with anabolic steroids
Diuretics	Thiazides, furosemide (Ch. 30)	Used mainly to achieve rapid weight loss before 'weighing in'. Also used to 'mask' the presence of other agents in urine by dilution	Urine samples	—
Narcotic analgesics	Codeine, morphine, etc. (Ch. 43)	Used to mask injury-associated pain	Urine samples	—

[a]'Blood doping' (removal of 1–2 L of blood well ahead of the competition, followed by re-transfusion immediately prior to the event) has a similar effect and is even more difficult to detect. Training at altitude or in a hypoxic environment achieves a similar effect and is not banned.

and strength but probably not other parameters of sporting performance. However, they have serious long-term effects, including male infertility, female masculinisation, liver and kidney tumours, hypertension and increased cardiovascular risk, and (in adolescents) premature skeletal maturation causing irreversible cessation of growth. Anabolic steroids produce a feeling of physical well-being, increased competitiveness and aggressiveness, sometimes progressing to actual psychosis. Depression is common when the drugs are stopped, sometimes leading to long-term psychiatric problems. In attempt to circumvent the rules, other drugs that release androgens, for example, **human chorionic** gonadotrophin (hCG, Ch. 36) or modify their action, such as androgen receptor modulators (Ch. 4), are increasingly used.

Clenbuterol, is a β-adrenoceptor agonist (see Ch. 15). Through an unknown mechanism of action, it produces anabolic effects similar to those of androgenic steroids, with apparently fewer adverse effects. It can be detected in urine and its use in sport is banned.

HUMAN GROWTH HORMONE

The use of **human growth hormone** (hGH; see Ch. 34) by athletes followed the availability of the recombinant form of hGH, used to treat endocrine disorders. It is given by injection and its effects appear to be similar to those of anabolic steroids. hGH is also reported to produce a similar feeling of well-being, although without the accompanying aggression and changes in sexual development and behaviour. It increases lean body mass, reduces fat and improves sprint capacity, but its effects on other aspects of athletic performance are unclear. It is claimed to increase the rate of recovery from tissue injury, allowing more intensive training routines. The main adverse effect of hGH is the development of acromegaly, causing overgrowth of the jaw and thickening of the fingers (Ch. 34), but it may also lead to cardiac hypertrophy and cardiomyopathy, and possibly also an increased cancer risk.

Detection of hGH administration is difficult because physiological secretion is pulsatile, so normal plasma concentrations vary widely. The plasma half-life is short (20–30 min), and only trace amounts are excreted in urine. However, secreted hGH consists of three isoforms varying in molecular weight, whereas recombinant hGH contains only one, so measuring the relative amounts of the isoforms can be used to detect the exogenous material. Growth hormone acts partly by releasing insulin-like growth factor (**IGF**) from the liver, and this hormone itself is sometimes used by athletes.

Another hormone, **erythropoietin**, which increases erythrocyte production (see Ch. 26), is given by injection for days or weeks to increase the erythrocyte count and hence boost the O_2-carrying capacity of blood. The development of recombinant erythropoietin has made it widely available, and detection of its use is difficult. It carries a risk of hypertension, neurologic disease and thrombosis.

STIMULANT DRUGS

The main drugs of this type used by athletes and officially prohibited are: **ephedrine** and **methylephedrine**; various amphetamines and similar drugs, such as **fenfluramine** and methylphenidate[4]; cocaine; and a variety of other central nervous system stimulants such as **nikethamide**, **amiphena-zole** (no longer used clinically) and **strychnine** (see Ch. 49). Caffeine is also used: some commercially available 'energy drinks' contain taurine as well as caffeine. However, taurine is an agonist at glycine and extrasynaptic $GABA_A$ receptors (see Ch. 40). Its effects on the brain are therefore likely to be inhibitory rather than stimulatory. In this regard, taurine may be responsible for the post-energy-drink low that is experienced once the stimulatory effect of caffeine has worn off.

In contrast to steroids, some trials have shown stimulant drugs to improve performance in events such as sprinting, and under experimental conditions they increase muscle strength and reduce muscle fatigue significantly. The psychological effect of stimulants is probably as important as their physiological effects. Surprisingly, caffeine appears to be more consistently effective in improving muscle performance than other more powerful stimulants and is amongst a few drugs (including nicotine and alcohol) that are not prohibited.

Several deaths have occurred among athletes taking amphetamines and ephedrine-like drugs in endurance events. The main causes are coronary insufficiency, associated with hypertension; hyperthermia, associated with cutaneous vasoconstriction; and dehydration.

Drug use by athletes for bona fide clinical reasons is allowed under the 'Therapeutic Use Exemptions' scheme. According to this scheme, which was introduced in the 1990s, an athlete may use a medicine (say, glucocorticoids for asthma) if it is determined clinically that this exemption is justified. Clearly, this system could be open to abuse.

The financial and reputational inducements for athletes taking performance enhancing drugs are great whilst the chance of getting caught is quite small, fuelling the search for better and less detectable agents. This in turn poses further analytical problems for the regulators who must devise screening tests to monitor an increasing range of agents, some of which are difficult to assay. The contest continues as new 'designer' drugs, *masking agents* (which make it more difficult to detect a particular substance in the blood or urine) or procedures are devised by ingenious chemists and physicians.

Doping is banned in professional sports because it constitutes an unfair advantage for the athletes who 'cheat'. However, many other factors are important in determining why one athlete may have an advantage over another – genetic makeup, for example – so there is no real 'level playing field' to begin with. Indeed some argue that athletes should have unrestricted access to performance enhancing drugs with the proviso that they do not impair the athlete's health (see Savulescu et al., 2004), but this view is unlikely to gain public acceptance in the near future.

CONCLUSION

The lifestyle drug phenomenon is one aspect of a broader debate about what actually constitutes 'disease' and how far medical science should go to satisfy the aim of human enhancement and the needs and aspirations of otherwise healthy individuals, or to alleviate human distress and dysfunction in the absence of pathology. Discussion of these issues is beyond the scope of this book but can be found in articles cited at the end of this chapter (see Flower, 2004; 2012).

There are several reasons why these drugs – no matter how we choose to define them – are of increasing concern. The increasing availability of drugs (some counterfeit) from 'e-pharmacies', coupled with the direct advertising by the pharmaceutical industry to the public that occurs in some countries, will ensure that demand is kept buoyant. Most sales are in the developed world and the pharmaceutical industry will undoubtedly develop more lifestyle agents to cater for this lucrative market. The lobbying power of patients advocating particular drugs, regardless of the potential costs or proven utility, causes major problems for drug regulators and those who set healthcare priorities for state-funded systems of social medicine.

[4]Also used to improve academic performance!

Drugs in sport

- Many drugs of different types are commonly used by athletes with the aim of improving performance in competition.
- The main types used are:
  - anabolic agents, mainly androgenic steroids and **clenbuterol**;
  - hormones, particularly **erythropoietin** and **human growth hormone**;
  - stimulants, mainly **amphetamine** and **ephedrine** derivatives and caffeine;
  - β-adrenoceptor antagonists, to reduce anxiety and tremor in 'precision' sports.

- The use of drugs in sport is officially prohibited – in most cases, in or out of competition.
- Detection depends mainly on analysis of the drug or its metabolites in urine or blood samples. Detection of abuse is difficult in the case of endogenous hormones such as **erythropoietin**, **growth hormone** and **testosterone**.
- Controlled trials have mostly shown that drugs produce little improvement in sporting performance. Anabolic agents increase body weight and muscle volume without clearly increasing strength. The effect of stimulants is often psychological rather than physiological.

REFERENCES AND FURTHER READING

Bostrom, N., Sandberg, A., 2009. Cognitive enhancement: methods, ethics, regulatory challenges. Sci. Eng. Ethics 15, 343–349. (*Interesting discussion of a complex problem which will soon have to be faced*)

Flower, R.J., 2004. Lifestyle drugs: pharmacology and the social agenda. Trends Pharmacol. Sci. 25, 182–185. (*Accessible review that enlarges on some of the issues raised in this chapter*)

Flower, R., 2012. The Osler Lecture 2012: pharmacology 2.0, medicines, drugs and human enhancement. QJM 105, 823–830. (*Discusses 'human enhancement' from a pharmacologist's viewpoint. Easy to read*)

Gilbert, D., Walley, T., New, B., 2000. Lifestyle medicines. BMJ 321, 1341–1344. (*Short but focused review dealing mainly with the clinical implications of the 'lifestyle medicine' phenomenon*)

McCall, H., Adams, N., Mason, D., Willis, J., 2015. What is chemsex and why does it matter? BMJ 351, h5790. (*Brief description of the use of various drugs in chemsex sessions*)

Sahakian, B., LaBuzetta, J., 2015. Bad Moves: How Decision Making Goes Wrong, and the Ethics of Smart Drugs. OUP Oxford, Oxford. p. 192. (*A very interesting book which deals at length with the ethics of neuroenhancement using a decision-making model to illustrate their effects. Fascinating reading*)

Sahakian, B., Morein-Zamir, S., 2007. Professor's little helper. Nature 450, 1157–1159. (*Interesting 'commentary' of the use of neuroenhancers, especially by academics, and the ethical questions that this raises. Recommended*)

Walley, T., 2002. Lifestyle medicines and the elderly. Drugs Aging 19, 163–168. (*Excellent review of the whole area and its relevance to the treatment of the elderly*)

Young, S.N., 2003. Lifestyle drugs, mood, behaviour and cognition. J. Psychiatry Neurosci. 28, 87–89.

Drugs in sport

British Medical Association, 2002. Drugs in Sport: The Pressure to Perform. BMJ Publications, London. (*Useful coverage of the whole topic*)

Buchanan, A., 2011. Better Than Human. The Promise and Perils of Enhancing Ourselves. Oxford University Press Inc., New York. p. 199. (*Fascinating book which explores the whole topic of human enhancement including genetic and pharmacological approaches. Recommended for the serious reader*)

Gould, D., 2013. Gene doping: gene delivery for Olympic victory. Br. J. Clin. Pharmacol. 76, 292–298. (*Discusses what must surely be the next challenge to the WADA: deliberately introducing into athletes genes that could boost performance*)

Mottram, D.R. (Ed.), 2005. Drugs in Sport, fourth ed. Routledge, London. (*Comprehensive description of pharmacological and regulatory aspects of drugs in sport, with balanced discussion of evidence relating to efficacy and risk*)

Munby, J., 2010. Drugs in sport. Scott. Med. J. 55, 29–30. (*Brief review of the use of drugs in sport – both professional and amateur – written from the point of view of a physician*)

Reardon, C.L., Creado, S., 2014. Drug abuse in athletes. Subst. Abuse Rehabil. 5, 95–105. (*A good review of drug abuse in sports and notes about the main types of agents used*)

Sparling, P.B., 2013. The Lance Armstrong saga: a wake-up call for drug reform in sports. Curr. Sports Med. Rep. 12, 53–54. (*Brief commentary on the Lance Armstrong affair*)

Savulescu, J., Foddy, B., Clayton, M., 2004. Why we should allow performance enhancing drugs in sport. Br. J. Sports Med. 38, 666–670. (*The authors put forward a compelling argument for allowing access to performance enhancing drugs, but concentrating more on health of the athletes*)

Spedding, M., Spedding, C., 2008. Drugs in sport: a scientist-athlete's perspective: from ambition to neurochemistry. Br. J. Pharmacol. 154, 496–501. (*Very accessible review written by two brothers, one of whom is an Olympic athlete and the other a pharmacologist. Unique insights. Highly recommended*)

60 Drug discovery and development

OVERVIEW

With the development of the pharmaceutical industry towards the end of the 19th century, drug discovery became a highly focused and managed process and moved from the domain of inventive doctors to that of scientists hired for the purpose. The bulk of modern therapeutics, and of modern pharmacology, is based on drugs that originated from the laboratories of these pharmaceutical companies, without which neither the practice of therapeutics nor the science of pharmacology would be more than a pale fragment of what they have become.

In this chapter, we outline the main stages of the process, namely (i) the discovery phase, i.e. the identification of a new chemical entity as a potential therapeutic agent; and (ii) the development phase, during which the compound is tested for safety and efficacy in one or more clinical indications, and suitable formulations and dosage forms devised. The aim is to achieve registration by one or more regulatory authorities, to allow the drug to be marketed legally as a medicine for human use.

Our account is necessarily brief and superficial, and more detail can be found elsewhere (Hill & Rang, 2013).

THE STAGES OF A PROJECT

Fig. 60.1 shows in an idealised way the stages of a 'typical' project, aimed at producing a marketable drug that meets a particular medical need (e.g. to retard the progression of Parkinson's disease or cardiac failure, or to treat drug-resistant infections).

Broadly, the process can be divided into three main components:

1. *Drug discovery*, during which candidate molecules are chosen on the basis of their pharmacological properties.
2. *Preclinical development*, during which a wide range of non-human studies (e.g. toxicity testing, pharmacokinetic/pharmacodynamic analysis and formulation) are performed.
3. *Clinical development*, during which the selected compound is tested for efficacy, side effects and potential dangers in volunteers and patients.

These phases do not necessarily follow in strict succession, as indicated in Fig. 60.1, but generally overlap.

THE DRUG DISCOVERY PHASE

Given the task of planning a project to discover a new drug to treat – say, Parkinson's disease – where does one start? Assuming that we are looking for a novel drug rather than developing a slightly improved 'me-too' version of a drug already in use,[1] we first need to choose a new molecular target.

TARGET SELECTION

As discussed in Chapter 2, drug targets are, with few exceptions, functional proteins (e.g. receptors, enzymes, transport proteins). Although, in the past, drug discovery programmes were often based – successfully – on measuring a complex response in vivo, such as prevention of experimentally induced seizures, lowering of blood sugar or suppression of an inflammatory response, without the need for prior identification of a drug target, nowadays this is rare, and the first step is *target identification*. This most often comes from biological intelligence. It was known, for example, that inhibiting angiotensin-converting enzyme lowers blood pressure by suppressing angiotensin II formation, so it made sense to look for antagonists of the vascular angiotensin II receptor – hence the successful 'sartan' series of antihypertensive drugs (Ch. 23). Similarly, the knowledge that breast cancer is often oestrogen-sensitive led to the development of aromatase inhibitors such as **anastrozole**, which prevents oestrogen synthesis. A recent survey of 1194 FDA-approved human medicines (Santos et al., 2017) noted that they acted at a total of 893 targets, of which 667 were human proteins (comprising 549 small molecule and 146 biopharmaceutical drug targets) and a further 189 were pathogen protein targets. However, there are many other proteins that are thought to play a role in disease (estimates range from a few hundred to several thousand: see Betz, 2005; http://www.guidetopharmacology.org/lists.jsp) for which we still have no cognate drug. Many of these represent potential starting points for drug discovery and await therapeutic exploitation. Selecting *valid* and 'druggable' targets from this plethora is a major challenge.

Conventional biological wisdom, drawing on a rich fund of knowledge of disease mechanisms and chemical signalling

---

[1]Many commercially successful drugs have in the past emerged from exactly such 'me-too' projects; examples are the many β-adrenoceptor-blocking drugs developed in the wake of propranolol, and the 'triptans' that followed the introduction of sumatriptan to treat migraine. Quite small improvements (e.g. in pharmacokinetics or side effects), coupled with aggressive marketing, have often proved enough, but the barriers to registration are getting higher, so the emphasis has shifted towards developing innovative (first in class) drugs aimed at novel molecular targets.

Fig. 60.1 The stages of development of a 'typical' new drug, i.e. a synthetic compound being developed for systemic use. Only the main activities undertaken at each stage are shown, and the details vary greatly according to the kind of drug being developed.

pathways, coupled with genomic data, is the basis on which novel targets are most often chosen. Disciplines such as genomics, bioinformatics, proteomics and systems analysis are playing an increasing role by revealing new proteins involved in chemical signalling, new genes involved in disease and new models of disease progression. Space precludes discussion here of this burgeoning area; interested readers are referred to more detailed accounts (Lindsay, 2003; Kramer & Cohen, 2004; Hill & Rang, 2013; Cutler & Voshol, 2015; Kuepfer & Schuppert, 2016).

Overall, it is evident that in the foreseeable future there is ample biological scope in terms of novel drug targets for therapeutic innovation. What limits innovation is not the biology and primary pharmacology, but other factors, such as poor target selection or the emergence of unforeseen adverse effects during clinical testing, as well as the cost and complexity of drug discovery and development in relation to healthcare economics and increasingly rigorous regulatory hurdles.

LEAD FINDING

When the biochemical target has been decided and the feasibility of the project has been assessed, the next step is to find *lead compounds*. Here we focus on lead compounds derived from synthetic chemistry. The development of biopharmaceuticals is described below and in Ch. 5. Commonly, lead finding involves cloning and expression of the target protein – normally the human form, because the sequence variation among species is often associated with pharmacological differences, and it is essential to optimise for activity in humans. An assay system must then be developed, allowing the functional activity of the target protein to be measured. This could be a cell-free enzyme assay, a membrane-based binding assay or a cellular response assay. It must be engineered to run automatically,

if possible with an optical read-out (e.g. fluorescence or optical absorbance), and in a miniaturised multiwell plate format (96-, 384-, 1536- or 3456-well versions are available) for reasons of speed and economy. Robotically controlled assay facilities capable of testing tens of thousands of compounds per day[2] in several parallel assays are now commonplace in the pharmaceutical industry, and have become the standard starting point for most drug discovery projects. For details on high-throughput screening, see Hüser (2006).

To keep such hungry monsters running requires very large *compound libraries*. Large companies will typically maintain a growing collection of a million or more synthetic compounds, which will be routinely screened whenever a new assay is set up. Whereas, in the past, compounds were generally synthesised and purified one by one, often taking a week or more for each, the use of combinatorial chemistry allows large families of related compounds to be made simultaneously. By coupling such high-speed chemistry to high-throughput assay systems, the time taken over the initial lead-finding stage of projects has been reduced to a few months in most cases, having previously often taken several years. Increasingly, use is being made of X-ray crystallography and other techniques to provide knowledge of the three-dimensional structure of the target protein, and computer-based molecular modelling to identify possible lead structures within the compound library, in order to reduce the number of compounds to be screened. Molecular modelling can also be used to screen huge numbers of hypothetical – not yet synthesised – molecules to provide pointers for synthesis and screening of new

[2]Testing up to 100,000 compounds per day is possible, and is known as ultra-high throughput screening.

compound families. Refined in this way, screening is often successful in identifying lead compounds that have the appropriate pharmacological activity and are amenable to further chemical modification.

'Hits' detected in the initial screen often turn out to be molecules that have features undesirable in a drug, such as excessive molecular weight or polarity, or possession of groups known to be associated with toxicity. Computational 'prescreening' of compound libraries is often used to eliminate such compounds.

The hits identified from the primary screen are used as the basis for preparing sets of homologues by combinatorial chemistry to establish the critical structural features necessary for binding selectively to the target. Several such iterative cycles of synthesis and screening are usually needed to identify one or more lead compounds for the next stage.

Natural products as lead compounds

Historically, natural products, derived mainly from fungal and plant sources, have proved to be a fruitful source of new therapeutic agents, particularly in the field of anti-infective, anticancer and immunosuppressant drugs. Familiar examples include **penicillin**, **streptomycin** and many other antibiotics; vinca alkaloids; **paclitaxel**; **ciclosporin** and **sirolimus** (**rapamycin**). These substances presumably serve a specific protective function, having evolved to recognise, with great precision, vulnerable target molecules in an organism's enemies or competitors. The surface of this resource has barely been scratched, and many companies are actively engaged in generating and testing natural product libraries for lead-finding purposes. Fungi and other microorganisms are particularly suitable for this, because they are ubiquitous, highly diverse and easy to collect and grow in the laboratory. They have also had aeons of evolution to devise an armoury of effective substances fit for specific functions (e.g. anti-bacterial) which can sometimes be utilised as a starting compound in the search for our desired drug. However, compounds obtained from plants, animals or marine organisms are much more troublesome to produce commercially. Their main disadvantage as lead compounds is that they are often complex molecules that are difficult to synthesise or modify by conventional synthetic chemistry, so that *lead optimisation* may be difficult and commercial production very expensive.

LEAD OPTIMISATION

Lead compounds found by screening are the basis for the next stage, lead optimisation, where the aim (usually) is to increase the potency of the compound on its target and to optimise it with respect to other characteristics, such as selectivity and pharmacokinetic properties. In this phase, the tests applied include a broader range of assays in different systems, including studies to measure the activity and time course of the compounds in vivo (where possible in animal models mimicking aspects of the clinical condition; see Ch. 8), and checking for unwanted effects in animals, evidence of genotoxicity and usually oral availability. The objective of the lead optimisation phase is to identify one or more *drug candidates* suitable for further development.

As shown in Fig. 60.1, only about one project in five succeeds in generating a drug candidate, and it can take up to 5 years. The most common problem is that lead optimisation proves to be impossible; despite much ingenious and back-breaking chemistry, the lead compounds,

like antisocial teenagers, refuse to give up their bad habits. In other cases, the candidate leads, although they produce the desired effects on the target molecule and have no other obvious defects, fail to produce the expected effects in animal models of the disease, implying that the target probably would not be a useful one in humans either. The virtuous minority of drugs proceed to the next phase, preclinical development.

PRECLINICAL DEVELOPMENT

The aim of preclinical development is to satisfy all the requirements that have to be met before a new compound is deemed ready to be tested for the first time in humans. The work falls into four main categories:

1. Pharmacological testing to check that the drug does not produce any obviously hazardous acute effects, such as bronchoconstriction, cardiac dysrhythmias, blood pressure changes and ataxia (lacking coordinated muscle movement). This is termed *safety pharmacology*.
2. Preliminary toxicological testing to eliminate genotoxicity and to determine the maximum non-toxic dose of the drug (usually when given daily for 28 days, and tested in two species). As well as being checked regularly for weight loss and other gross changes, the animals so treated are examined minutely *post mortem* at the end of the experiment to search for histological and biochemical evidence of tissue damage (see also Ch. 58).
3. Pharmacokinetic and pharmacodynamic (PK/PD) testing,[3] including studies on the absorption, metabolism, distribution and elimination (*ADME studies*) in the species of laboratory animals used for toxicology testing, to link the pharmacological and toxicological effects to plasma concentration and drug exposure.
4. Chemical and pharmaceutical development to assess the feasibility of large-scale synthesis and purification, to assess the stability of the compound under various conditions and to develop a formulation suitable for clinical studies.

Much of the work of preclinical development, especially that relating to safety issues, is done under a formal operating code, known as *Good Laboratory Practice* (GLP), which covers such aspects as record-keeping procedures, data analysis, instrument calibration and staff training. The aim of GLP is to eliminate human error as far as possible and to ensure the reliability of the data submitted to the regulatory authority, and laboratories are regularly monitored for compliance to GLP standards. The strict discipline involved in working to this code is generally ill-suited to the creative research needed in the earlier stages of drug discovery, so GLP standards are not usually adopted until projects get beyond the discovery phase.

Roughly half the compounds identified as drug candidates fail during the preclinical development phase; for the rest, a detailed dossier (the 'investigator brochure') is prepared for submission alongside specific study protocols to the regulatory authority, such as the European Medicines Agency or the US FDA, the permission of which is required

---

[3]Pharmacokinetics is the ways in which the organism changes the drug, whereas pharmacodynamics is the how the drug affects the organism.

to proceed with studies in humans.[4] This is not lightly given, and the regulatory authority may refuse permission or require further work to be done before giving approval.

Non-clinical development work continues throughout the clinical trials period, when much more data, particularly in relation to long-term and reproductive toxicity in animals, has to be generated. Failure of a compound at this stage is very costly, and considerable efforts are made to eliminate potentially toxic compounds much earlier in the drug discovery process using in vitro, or even in silico, methods.

CLINICAL DEVELOPMENT

Clinical development proceeds through four distinct but overlapping phases of clinical trials (see Ch. 8). For detailed information, see Friedman et al. (2010).

- *Phase I studies* are performed on a small group (normally 20–80) of volunteers – often healthy young men but sometimes patients, and their aim is to check for signs of any potentially *dangerous effects*, for example on cardiovascular,[5] respiratory, hepatic or renal function; *tolerability* (does the drug produce any unpleasant symptoms, for example, headache, nausea, drowsiness?); and *pharmacokinetic properties* (is the drug well absorbed? Is absorption affected by food? What is the time course of the plasma concentration? Is there evidence of accumulation or non-linear kinetics?). Phase I studies may also test for pharmacodynamic effects in volunteers, sometimes called 'proof-of-concept' studies (e.g. does a novel analgesic compound block experimentally induced pain in humans? How does the desired effect vary with dose?). Just as the regulatory authorities require GLP studies, clinical trials need to be performed under equally strict *Good Clinical Practice* (GCP) conditions.
- *Phase II studies* are performed on groups of patients (normally 100–300) and are designed to determine clinically beneficial pharmacodynamic effects in patients, and if this is confirmed, to establish the dose regimen to be used in the definitive phase III study. Often, such studies will cover several distinct clinical disorders (e.g. depression, anxiety states and phobias) to identify the possible therapeutic indications for the new compound and the dose required. When new drug targets are being studied, it is not until these phase II trials are completed that the team finds out whether or not its initial hypothesis was correct, and lack of the expected effect is a common reason for failure.
- *Phase III studies* are the definitive double-blind, randomised trials, commonly performed as multicentre trials on thousands of patients, aimed at comparing the new drug with commonly used alternatives or placebos. These are extremely costly,

difficult to organise and often take years to complete, particularly if the treatment is designed to retard the progression of a chronic disease. It is not uncommon for a drug that seemed highly effective in the limited patient groups tested in phase II to look much less impressive under the more rigorous conditions of phase III trials.

▼ As mentioned earlier, the conduct of trials has to comply with an elaborate code known as GCP, covering every detail of the patient group, data collection methods, recording of information, statistical analysis and documentation.[6]

Increasingly, phase III trials are now required to include a *pharmacoeconomic analysis* (see Ch. 1), such that not only clinical but also economic benefits of the new treatment are assessed.

At the end of phase III, the drug will be submitted to the relevant regulatory authority for licensing. The dossier required for this is a massive and detailed compilation of preclinical and clinical data. Evaluation by the regulatory authority normally takes a year or more, and further delays often arise when aspects of the submission must be clarified or more data are required. Eventually, about two-thirds of submissions gain marketing approval. Overall, only 11.5% of compounds entering phase I are eventually approved (see Munos, 2009). Increasing this proportion by better compound selection at the laboratory stage is one of the main challenges for the pharmaceutical industry.

- *Phase IV studies* comprise the obligatory post-marketing surveillance designed to detect any rare or long-term adverse effects resulting from the use of the drug in a clinical setting in many thousands of patients. Such events may necessitate limiting the use of the drug to particular patient groups, or even withdrawal of the drug.[7]

Disclosure and publication of trials data

Recently, concern has been expressed that clinical trials showing negative or inconclusive results are less likely to be published than those giving positive results, so creating a more favourable impression of a new drug's clinical efficacy than would be the case if every trial was published. To ensure that all data, good and bad, is published and available to regulatory authorities and researchers, it is now mandatory to register the initiation of any trial in humans and to publish the results in full when the trial is completed. The difficult question of whether to require all past trials of currently registered drugs is under discussion. The accessibility of past data, much of it in the form of paper records in dusty repositories, and the cost of this exercise, are serious problems.

BIOPHARMACEUTICALS

'Biopharmaceuticals', i.e. therapeutic agents produced by biotechnology rather than conventional synthetic chemistry, are discussed in Chapter 5. Such therapeutic agents now

---

[4]The rules that will govern the licencing of drugs in the United Kingdom 'post-Brexit', when it leaves the European Union's EMA, are yet to be decided.
[5]QT prolongation, a sign of potentially dangerous cardiac arrhythmias (see Ch. 22), is a common cause of failure in early development, and regulators demand extensive – and expensive – studies to test for this risk. Today, such studies are usually performed on cells expressing the hERG (human Ether-à-go-go-Related Gene – no, seriously!) that produces the $K_v11.1$ potassium channel. Drugs that inhibit hERG channel activity are routinely screened out, as this implies a fatal QT prolongation side effect.

[6]Similar strict codes must be followed in laboratory tests to determine safety (Good Laboratory Practice; see text) and drug manufacture (Good Manufacturing Practice; GMP).
[7]Recent high-profile cases include the withdrawal of rofecoxib (a cyclo-oxygenase-2 inhibitor; see Ch. 27) when it was found (in a phase III trial for a new indication) to increase the frequency of heart attacks, and of cerivastatin (Ch. 24), a cholesterol-lowering drug found to cause severe muscle damage in a few patients.

comprise about 30% of new products registered each year. The principles underlying the development and testing of biopharmaceuticals are basically the same as for synthetic drugs. In practice, biopharmaceuticals generally run into fewer toxicological problems than synthetic drugs,[8] but more problems relating to production, quality control, immunogenicity and drug delivery. Walsh (2003) and Revers and Furzcon (2010) cover this specialised field in more detail. In 2017 the first gene therapy products (for amyotrophic lateral sclerosis) and cell-based therapies for advanced cancer (see Ch. 57) were approved – a significant milestone.

COMMERCIAL ASPECTS

Fig. 60.1 shows the approximate time taken for such a project and the attrition rate (at each stage and overall) based on recent data from several large pharmaceutical companies. The key messages are (i) that it is a high-risk business, with only about one drug discovery project in 50 and one development compound in 10 reaching the goal of putting a new drug on the market, (ii) that it takes a long time – about 12 years on average and (iii) that it costs a lot of money to develop one drug – estimated at a mind-boggling US$3–4 billion per drug (see Munos, 2009; DiMasi et al., 2016).[9] For any one project, the costs escalate rapidly as development proceeds, phase III trials and long-term toxicology studies being particularly expensive. The time factor is crucial, because the new drug has to be patented, usually at the end of the discovery phase, and the period of exclusivity (20 years in most countries) during which the company is free from competition in the market starts on that date. After 20 years, the patent expires, and other companies, which have not supported the development costs, are free to make and sell the drug much more cheaply, so the revenues for the original company decrease rapidly thereafter. Many profitable drugs will reach the end of their patent lives before 2018, adding to the industry's problems. Reducing the development time after patenting is a major concern for all companies, but so far it has remained stubbornly fixed at around 10 years, partly because the regulatory authorities are demanding more clinical data before they will grant a licence. In practice, only about one drug in three that goes on the market brings in enough revenue to cover its development costs. Success for the company relies on this one drug generating enough profit to pay for the rest.[10]

FUTURE PROSPECTS

Since about 1990, the drug discovery process has been in the throes of a substantial methodological revolution, following the rapid ascendancy of molecular biology,

genomics and informatics, amid high expectations that this would bring remarkable dividends in terms of speed, cost and success rate. High-throughput screening has undoubtedly emerged as a powerful lead-finding technology, but overall the benefits are not yet clear: costs have risen steadily, the success rate has not improved and development times have not decreased.

Fig. 60.2 illustrates the trend in the number of new drugs launched in the major markets worldwide, which had until recently declined steadily despite escalating costs and improved technology, causing serious worries to the industry. There was much speculation as to the causes of the decline, the optimistic view being that fewer but better drugs were being introduced, and that the genomics revolution had yet to make its impact. This optimism may be well founded, for as Fig. 60.2 shows, the number of approvals has shown an encouraging upturn in recent years.

If the new drugs that are being developed improve the quality of medical care, there is room for optimism. In recent ('pre-revolutionary') years, synthetic drugs aimed at new targets (e.g. selective serotonin reuptake inhibitors, statins, kinase inhibitors and several monoclonal antibodies) have made major contributions to patient care. The ability of new technologies to make new targets available to the drug discovery machine is beginning to have a real effect on patient care. Creativity remains high, despite the rising costs and declining profits that remain a challenge to the pharmaceutical industry.

Trends to watch include the growing armoury of biopharmaceuticals. Recent successful examples include monoclonal antibodies such as **trastuzumab** (an antibody directed against human epidermal growth factor receptor 2 – HER2 – which is used to treat breast cancers that overexpress this receptor; see Ch. 57) and **infliximab** (a tumour necrosis factor antibody used to treat inflammatory disorders; see Ch. 27); many similar drugs are now available and more are in the pipeline. Another likely change will be the use of genotyping to 'individualise' drug treatments, to reduce the likelihood of administering drugs to 'non-responders' (see Evans & Relling, 2004; and Ch. 12, which summarises the current status of 'personalised medicine'). The implications for drug discovery will be profound, for the resulting therapeutic compartmentation (or *stratification* as it is sometimes known) of the patient population will mean that markets will decrease in size, ending the reliance on the 'blockbusters' referred to earlier. At the same time, clinical trials will become more complex (and expensive), as different genotypic groups will have to be included in the trial design. The hope is that therapeutic efficacy will be improved, not that it will be a route to developing drugs more cheaply and quickly. However, there is general agreement that the current modus operandi is commercially unsustainable (see Munos, 2009). Costs and regulatory requirements are continuing to rise, and the anticipated use of genomics to define subgroups of patients likely to respond to particular therapeutic agents (see Ch. 12) will mean fragmentation of the market, as we move away from the 'one-drug-suits-all' approach that encouraged companies to focus their efforts on blockbuster drugs. More niche products targeted at smaller patient groups will be needed, though each costs as much to develop as a blockbuster and carries a similar risk of failure, and in a more limited market – factors that necessitate higher prices than in the past.

---

[8]The serious toxicity caused to human volunteers in the 2006 phase I trials of the monoclonal antibody TGN 1412 (see Ch. 5) showed that this general principle could not be relied on, and led to substantial tightening of standards (and a temporary slowdown of the development of biopharmaceuticals).

[9]These cost estimates have been strongly challenged by commentators (see Angell, 2004) who argue that the pharmaceutical companies overestimate their costs several-fold to justify high drug prices.

[10]Actually, companies spend at least as much on marketing and administration as on research and development.

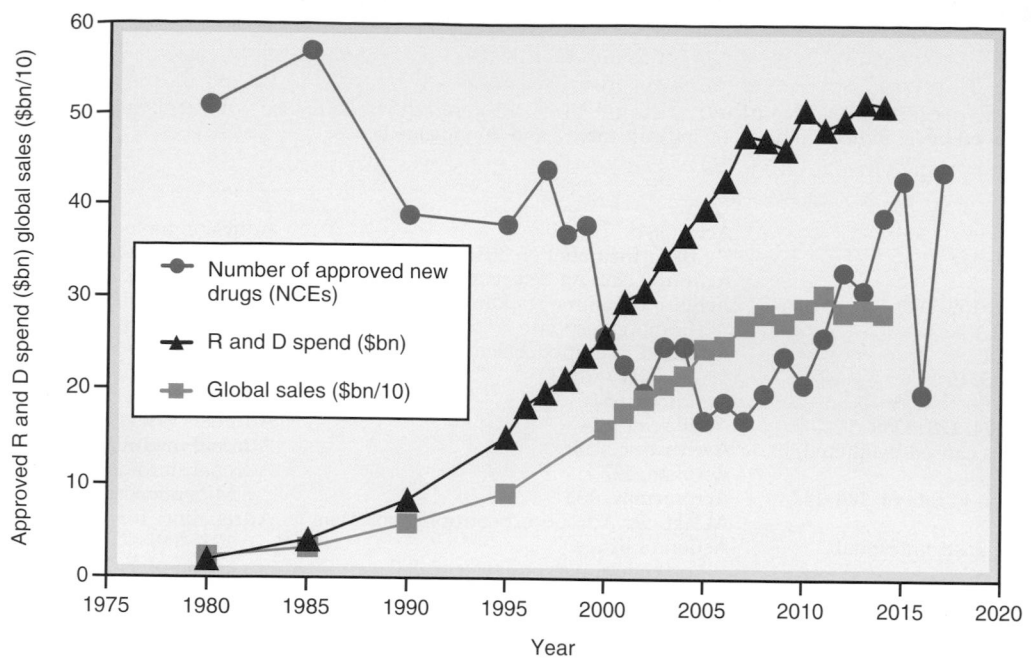

Fig. 60.2 Research and development (R&D) spend, sales and new drug registrations, 1980–2017. Registrations refer to new chemical entities (including biopharmaceuticals, excluding new formulations and combinations of existing registered compounds). The decline in registrations up to 2010 has since seen some reversal in more recent years. (Data from various sources, including the Centre for Medicines Research, Pharmaceutical Research and Manufacturers Association of America.)

A FINAL WORD

The pharmaceutical industry in recent years has attracted much adverse publicity, some of it well deserved, concerning drug pricing and profits, non-disclosure of adverse clinical trials data, reluctance to address major global health problems such as tuberculosis and malaria, aggressive marketing practices and much else (see Angell, 2004; Goldacre, 2012). It needs to be remembered though that, despite its faults, the industry has been responsible for most of the therapeutic advances of the past half-century, without which medical care would effectively have stood still. Innovation has by no means dried up. Over the last 5 years, about 30% of newly approved drugs are 'first-in-class', meaning that they act in new ways on molecular targets not previously addressed – ample scope for future pharmacologists.

REFERENCES AND FURTHER READING

Angell, M., 2004. The Truth About the Drug Companies. Random House, New York. (*A powerful broadside directed against the commercial practices of pharmaceutical companies*)

Betz, U.A.K., 2005. How many genomics targets can a portfolio afford? Drug Discov. Today 10, 1057–1063. (*Interesting analysis – despite its odd title – of approaches to target identification in drug discovery programmes*)

Cutler, P., Voshol, H., 2015. Proteomics in pharmaceutical research and development. Proteomics Clin. Appl. 9, 643–650. (*Recounts the history of proteomics and follows its development into a useful – or even essential-tool for drug discovery*)

DiMasi, J.A., Grabowski, H.G., Hansen, R.W., 2016. Innovation in the pharmaceutical industry: new estimates of R&D costs. J. Health Econ. 47, 20–33.

Evans, W.E., Relling, M.V., 2004. Moving towards individualised medicine with pharmacogenomics. Nature 429, 464–468. (*Good review article discussing the likely influence of pharmacogenomics on therapeutics*)

Friedman, L.M., Furberg, C.D., DeMets, D.L., 2010. Fundamentals of Clinical Trials, fourth ed. Mosby, St Louis. (*Standard textbook*)

Goldacre, B., 2012. Bad Pharma. Fourth Estate, London. (*An outspoken polemic, flawed in places, that exposes malpractice in the industry*)

Hill, R.G., Rang, H.P. (Eds.), 2013. Drug Discovery and Development, second ed. Elsevier, Amsterdam. (*Short textbook describing the principles and practice of drug discovery and development in the modern era*)

Hüser, J. (Ed.), 2006. High Throughput Screening in Drug Discovery, vol. 35. Methods and Principles in Drug Discovery. Wiley–VCH,

Weinheim. (*Comprehensive textbook covering all aspects of this technology*)

Kramer, R., Cohen, D., 2004. Functional genomics to new drug targets. Nat. Rev. Drug Discov. 3, 965–972. (*Describes the various approaches for finding new drug targets, starting from genomic data*)

Kuepfer, L., Schuppert, A., 2016. Systems medicine in pharmaceutical research and development. Methods Mol. Biol. 1386, 87–104. (*A little technical and mainly of interest if you want to dig deep into the subject*)

Lindsay, M.A., 2003. Target discovery. Nat. Rev. Drug Discov. 2, 831–836. (*Well-balanced discussion of the application of genomics approaches to discovering new drug targets; more realistic in its stance than many*)

Munos, B., 2009. Lessons from 60 years of pharmaceutical innovation. Nat. Rev. Drug Discov. 8, 959–968. (*Informative summary of the current status of the drug discovery industry, making clear that the modus operandi that has been successful in the past is no longer sustainable*)

Santos, R., Ursu, O., Gaulton, A., et al., 2017. A comprehensive map of molecular drug targets. Nat. Rev. Drug Discov. 16, 19–34. (*A very comprehensive survey of drugs and their targets. A mine of useful data*)

Revers, L., Furczon, E., 2010. An introduction to biologics and biosimilars. Part II: subsequent entry biologics: biosame or biodifferent? Can. Pharm. J. 143, 184–191.

Walsh, G., 2003. Biopharmaceuticals, second ed. Wiley, Chichester. (*Comprehensive textbook covering all aspects of discovery, development and applications of biopharmaceuticals*)

Index

Page numbers followed by 'f' indicate figures, 't' indicate tables, and 'b' indicate boxes.

A

Abacavir, 684, 684t
  HLAB*5701 and, 159, 160f
Abatacept, 355, 356t
ABC transporters, 24
Abciximab, 85, 330, 331b
Abecarnil, 572–573
Absorption, drug, 124–128, 128b
  drug interactions caused by altered, 130
  effect of variation in rate of, 146–147, 148f
  factors affecting gastrointestinal, 125–126
  from intestine, 124–125, 125f
  methods for delaying, 128
Abstinence syndrome, 644
Acamprosate, for alcohol dependence, 647b
Acarbose, for insulin secretion, 418
Aceclofenac, 344t
Acemetacin, 344t
Acetaldehyde, 638–639
Acetazolamide, 119, 127, 183t, 391, 661–662
Acetylation, drug, 158
Acetylcholine, 165–167, 165f, 266, 506–508
  in central nervous system, 508b
  effect on blood pressure, 175, 176f
  functional aspects of, 507–508
  gastric acid secretion and, 396
  muscarinic action of, 175
  nicotinic action of, 175
  pathways, in CNS, 507
  release of, 178–180
    drugs inhibiting, 191–192
  synthesis of, 178–180
    drugs inhibiting, 190–191
  vomiting and, 400
Acetylcholine antagonists, 527
Acetylcholine receptors, 175, 178b, 507
  muscarinic. See Muscarinic acetylcholine receptors
  nicotinic. See Nicotinic acetylcholine receptors
Acetylcholinesterase (AChE), 170, 192
  inhibitors, 522b
Acetylcysteine, 736
N-Acetylcysteine, 722
N-Acetyl-p-benzoquinone imine (NAPBQI), 350, 736
Acetyltransferase, 158
Aciclovir, 655b, 685, 685b, 687b
  action/effects of, 131, 654
Acid-base balance, 387
Acidic drugs
  binding of, 121–122
  excretion of, 140
  ionisation of, 140
  pKa values for, 121f
  weak, 119, 120f
Acidic phospholipid, exposure of, 328
Acidosis, lactic, biguanides and, 416
Acid-sensing ion channels (ASICs), 59f
Acitretin, 368
Aclidinium, 377

Acne, 364
  drug treatment of, 363t
Acquired clotting defects, 322
Acquired immune response. See Adaptive immune response
Acquired immunodeficiency syndrome. See HIV/AIDS
Acridines, 654
Acriflavine, 654
Acrolein, 137
Acrivastine, 358t
Acromegaly, 435
ACTH. See Adrenocorticotrophic hormone
Action of drugs
  on central nervous system, 480
  sites of, 173
Action potential, 55, 58
  drugs and toxins in channels involved in, 60f
  electrical and ionic events in, 57–58
Activated partial thromboplastin time (APTT), 324
Activation, 280
Activation function 1 (AF1), 44
Activation function 2 (AF2), 44
Acute dystonias, 599
Acute intermittent porphyria, 158
Acute-phase proteins, 103
Adalimumab, 355, 356t, 367, 406
Adapalene, 368
Adapter protein (AP), 85, 86f
Adaptive immune response, 93, 98–103, 100b
  antibody-mediated (humoural), 100–102
  cell-mediated, 99f, 102–103
  effector phase of, 100–103
  induction phase of, 99–100, 101f
Addict, term, 643t
Addison's disease, 439
Adefovir, 684
Adeno-associated virus, 77
Adenohypophysis, 432
Adenosine, 274–276, 280t, 282–283, 283b, 288b, 302b
  in asthma, 231
  cardiovascular system and, 230–231
  in CNS, 231
  in inflammation, 231
  as mediator, 228–231
  pain and, 548
  receptors of, 228, 230t
Adenosine deaminase, 228–230
Adenosine diphosphate (ADP), as mediator, 231
Adenosine ($P2Y_{12}$) receptor antagonists, 329–330
Adenosine triphosphate (ATP)
  co-transmission and, 170, 171f
  in inflammation, 232
  as mediator, 231–232
  NANC transmission and, 170, 172t
  as neurotransmitter, 231–232
  in nociception, 232
Adenylyl cyclase, 33–34, 34f
Adhesion, 327

Adhesion molecules, 94–95
Adhesive proteins, 84
Adipose tissue, autonomic nervous system effects on, 166t
Administration, routes of, 124–128, 125f
ADP. See Adenosine diphosphate
Adrafinil, 626
Adrenal cortex, 432–447
Adrenal medulla, 165
Adrenal steroids, 437b. See also Mineralocorticoids
Adrenaline, 163, 197, 277, 280t, 307, 308b, 408, 409t
  action of, 7, 204t
  for allergic emergencies, 379
  clinical uses of, 568b
  delaying drug absorption of, 128
  hyperglycaemia and, 207
  local anaesthesia and, 566
Adrenoceptor agonists, 207–209, 209b
  actions of, 204t
  clinical uses of, 209b
β-Adrenoceptor agonists, 375–376, 376b
  unwanted effects of, 376
β₂-Adrenoceptor agonists, 203–207
Adrenoceptor antagonists, 205t, 209–213
α-Adrenoceptor antagonists, 209–210, 210b
  action of, 205t
  clinical uses of, 210, 210b
  non-selective, 209–210
  unwanted effects of, 210
α₁-Adrenoceptor antagonists, 203–207
  for systemic hypertension, 304t
α₂-Adrenoceptor antagonists, 611
β-Adrenoceptor antagonists, 210–213, 212b, 280–282, 286–287
  actions of, 205t, 211–212, 211f
  clinical uses of, 212, 212b
    for anxiety, 571
  for systemic hypertension, 303, 304t
  for thyroid, 453
  unwanted effects of, 212–213
β₁-Adrenoceptor antagonists, 203–207
Adrenoceptor polymorphisms, 49–50
Adrenoceptors
  characteristics of, 199t
  classification of, 197–198, 198b
  distribution and actions of, 199t
  drugs acting on, 202–213
α-Adrenoceptors, 167
α₂-Adrenoceptors, 611
β-Adrenoceptors, 167, 306
β₁-Adrenoceptors, down regulation of, 611
Adrenocorticotrophic hormone (ACTH), 433, 436, 437b, 604
  actions of, 436, 436f
  receptors, mutated, 49–50
Adrenomedullin, 40, 292
Adsorbents, 405–406
Aducanumab, 522
Adult stem cells (AS cells), 90
Advanced glycation end products (AGE), 414

Cough reflex, depression of, opioids and, 552
Counter-ligands, of neutrophils, 96
Coxibs, 350
C-peptide, 410
Cranial nerve, 165
Cranial outflow, 165
C-reactive protein, 103
Creeping eruption, 710
Creutzfeldt-Jakob disease (CJD), 69
    growth hormone and, 435
    protein misfolding and aggregation, 515t
Crisantaspase, 729
Crizotinib, 728
CRLR. See Calcitonin receptor-like receptor
Crohn's disease, 406, 633
Cromoglicate, 375
    for asthma, 378
    for diarrhoea, 406
Cromones, 251
Crotamiton, 367
Cryptococcus neoformans, 691t
Cryptosporidium spp., 405
Crystal meth. See Methamphetamine
CTOP, 551t
Curare, 124–125, 163, 186–187
Cushing's syndrome, 433, 439–440, 443f
Cutaneous administration, 127
Cutaneous larva migrans, 710, 712t
C-X-C chemokines, 249
CXCR4, 681, 686
Cyanide poisoning, 286
Cyclase activation, 298
Cyclic ADP-ribose (cADPR), 55
Cyclic endoperoxides, 235
Cyclic nucleotides, drugs acting via, 298
Cyclin-dependent kinase 5 (CDK5), 521
Cyclin-dependent kinases (cdks), 82–83
    activation of, 83f
    in cell cycle, 84f
Cyclins, 82–83
    in cell cycle, 84f
Cyclizine, 358t, 401–403
Cyclo-oxygenase
    binding sites of, 346f
    COX-1, 343
    COX-2, 343, 734
Cyclo-oxygenase (COX) inhibitors, 343–350
    comparison of, 344t
    therapeutic effects of, 345b
    unwanted effects of, 348b
    on uterine contraction, 466–467
Cyclopentolate, 184–185
Cyclophilin, 354
Cyclophosphamide, 355, 722
    action of, 131
    adverse effects of, 741
    bladder toxicity of, 137
    stereoselectivity of, 135–136
Cycloplegia, 184–185
Cyclopropane, 532
Cycloserine, 673–674
    effects of, 652
        unwanted, 674
    pharmacokinetic aspects of, 674
Cyclothiazide, 493
CYP2C9 + VKORC1 genotyping, 161, 161f
Cyproheptadine, 225, 358t, 359
Cyproterone, 462b, 726–727
Cyproterone acetate, 368
CysLT₁ receptor, 239t
CysLT₂ receptor, 239t
Cystathionase (CSE), 268
Cystathionine β-synthase (CBS), 268
Cysteinyl leukotrienes, 372–373

Cysteinyl leukotriene receptor antagonists, 377
Cystic fibrosis, 74
Cystic fibrosis transmembrane conductance regulator (CFTR), 67–68, 68b, 75
Cytarabine, 251b, 724, 725b
    action of, 725f
Cytokines, 233, 248–251, 250t, 251b, 355–356, 482t
    in atherogenesis, 311
    in bone remodelling, 472
    synthesis or action of, 680
Cytokine receptors, 40, 41f
'Cytokine storm', 74, 251
Cytomegalovirus (CMV), 685b
Cytoplasm, 650
Cytoprotective agents, 400
Cytosolic PLA₂ (cPLA₂), 235
Cytotoxic drugs, 716, 719–720
    adverse effects of, 739t, 741
    antibiotics, 720, 721t, 724–725, 725b
Cytotoxic hypersensitivity, antibody dependent, 104
Cytotoxic T cells, 102
Cytotoxic T lymphocytes (CTLs), 681

D

D cells, 396
Dabigatran, 325, 327b
Dabigatran etexilate, 325
Dacarbazine, 723
Daclizumab, 355, 356t
Dactinomycin, 725, 725b
Daidzin, 639–640
Dalfopristin, 671, 671b
Dalteparin, 324
DAMGO, 551t
D-amino acid oxidase (DAAO), 593
Danaparoid, 324–325
Danazol, 379, 462, 462f, 463b
    actions of, 463
    pharmacokinetics of, 463
Dantrolene, 55, 190, 591
Dantron, 404
Dapagliflozin, for insulin secretion, 418
Dapsone, 675, 705b
    metabolism of, 158–159
    pharmacokinetic aspects of, 675
    structure, 700f
    unwanted effects of, 675
Daptomycin, 666
Darbepoetin, 339–340
Darifenacin, 178, 185
DARPP-32 (cAMP-regulated phosphoprotein), 502
Darunavir, 684t, 685
Dasatinib, 728
    BCR-ABL1 and, 161
Daunorubicin, 724
DDT, 568
Deadly nightshade, 183–184
Death receptors, 87
Debrisoquin, 213
Decamethonium, 187t
Decitabine, 724
Defensins, 93
Deferiprone, 336–337
Degarelix, 726–727
Degludec, insulin, 415
3β-Dehydrogenase, 440
Delamanid, 673
Delayed after depolarisation, 273, 273f
Delayed hypersensitivity, 104

Delivery systems
    for gene therapy, 75t
    special drug, 131
Demeclocycline, 387, 438, 667b
Dementia, clinical use of drugs in, 522b
N-Demethylation, 615
Dendritic cells
    in innate immune response, 98
    TLRs and, 94
Denervation supersensitivity, 8–9, 171–173
5′-Deoxyadenosylcobalamin (ado-B 12), 338
Depolarisation block, 180–181, 181f
Depolarisation-induced suppression of inhibition (DSI), 257
Depolarising blocking agents, 189–190
Depressant drugs, 635–640, 635t
Depression, 480, 603
    animal models of, 607–611
    bipolar disorder, 603
    clinical uses of drugs in, 619b
    endogenous, 603
    human tests, 611
    monoamine theory of, 603–604, 604t
    nature of, 603
    pathophysiology of, 606f
    reactive, 603
    theories of, 603–606, 607b
    unipolar, 603
Dermatomycoses, 690
Dermis, 364
Dermoepidermal junction, 362–364
Dermographia, 365
Des-Arg9 bradykinin, 547–548
Descending inhibitory controls, 545, 545f
Desensitisation, of drug, 18–19
Desferrioxamine, 336–337
Desflurane, 537t, 539–540, 540b
Desipramine, 559, 606, 608t–610t, 613
Desloratadine, 358t
N-Desmethyldiazepam, 575
Desmopressin, 393, 438
Desmosomes, 362–364
Desogestrel, 459
Desvenlafaxine, 606, 615, 616b
Detemir, insulin, 415
Development, human. See also Growth
    thyroid hormones on, 451
Dexamethasone, 403, 444, 726
Dexamphetamine, 624t, 626b
Dexfenfluramine, 225, 307, 625
    for obesity, 428–429
Dexibuprofen, 344t
Dexies. See Dextroamphetamine
Dexketoprofen, 344t
Dextroamphetamine, 623
Dextromethorphan, 519, 552, 560
    for cough, 381
Dhobie itch, 690
Diabetes Control and Complications Trial, 415
Diabetes insipidus
    drug responsiveness and, 155
    nephrogenic, antidiuretic hormone and, 387
    thiazide diuretics in, 390
    vasopressin and, 437
Diabetes mellitus, 408, 413–419
    animal models for, 110
    treatment of, 419
        with drugs, 408–421, 420b
        type 1, 413
        type 2, 413
Diabetic neuropathy, 414
Diacetyl morphine, 131
Diacylglycerol, 36

Pyrethrins, 568
Pyridostigmine, 190*t*, 193
Pyrimethamine, 662
 clinical uses of, malaria, 655*b*, 705*b*
 effect of, 651
 structure, 700*f*
Pyrimethamine-sulfadiazine, 708
Pyrimidine
 analogues, 654, 723–724, 725*b*
 fluorinated, 691
PYY3-36, 424*t*
PZM21, 549

Q

Qsymia, for obesity, 429
'Quality-adjusted life years' (QALYs), 114, 115*b*
Quaternary ammonium compounds, 186–187
Quetiapine, 571, 572*b*, 577, 595*b*, 598
 action of, 599
 characteristics of, 596*t*–597*t*
 clinical use of, bipolar disorder, 620–621, 621*b*
Quiescent (G0) cells, 82
Quinagolide, 436
Quinidine, 130–131, 280–281
Quinine, 702–703, 705*b*
 allergic response to, 742
 excretion of, 388
 pharmacokinetic aspects of, 702
 resistance, 702
 structure, 700*f*
 unwanted effects of, 702–703
Quinoline-methanols, 700*f*
Quinolones, 672
 antibacterial spectrum and clinical use of, 672
 mechanism of action, 669*t*–670*t*
 pharmacokinetic aspects of, 672
 unwanted effects of, 672
Quinupristin, 671, 671*b*

R

R plasmids, 656
Rabeprazole, 398–399
Racecadotril, for diarrhoea, 405
Radioiodine, 452, 454*b*
Raloxifene, 459, 460*b*, 476
 unwanted effects of, 476
Raltegravir, 684*t*, 686, 687*b*
Raltitrexed, 723
Ramelteon, 577
Ramipril, 302*b*, 306*b*, 307
RAMPs. *See* Receptor activity-modifying proteins
Randomised controlled clinical trial, 111–112
Ranibizumab, intravitreal injection of, 128
Ranitidine, 398, 398*b*
Ranolazine, 284
RANTES receptor. *See* Regulated on activation normal T cell expressed and secreted (RANTES) receptor
Rapamycin, as lead compounds, 752
Rapid depolarisation, in cardiac action potential, 271
Ras signalling complex, 412
Rasagiline, 524, 526
Rasburicase, 358
Ras/Raf pathway, 42
Raynaud's disease, vasoactive drugs for, 307

Rb protein, 84
Reactive depression, 603
Reactive oxygen species, 516, 735
Rebound hyperglycaemia, 415
Reboxetine, 606, 608*t*–610*t*, 616
Receptors, 23, 24*f*
 activation of, 8, 8*f*
  constitutive, 14
 antagonists. *See* Antagonists
 binding of drugs to, 8–9, 21*b*
 change in, 18–19
 classification of, 8
 cloning of, 25
 control of expression of, 49
 death, 87*f*
 desensitisation of, 18*f*
 disease and, 49–50
 drug, 6–7
 drug interactions with, 8–10
  quantitative aspects of, 19–21
 heterogeneity of, 27
 ionotropic. *See* Ligand-gated ion channels
 kinase-linked. *See* Kinase-linked receptors
 metabotropic. *See* G protein-coupled receptors
 molecular structure of, 28–29, 28*f*, 32*f*
 nuclear. *See* Nuclear receptors
 orphan, 23, 25
 in physiological systems, 7
 proteins, 25–46
 spare, 10
 subtypes of, 27
 translocation of, 19
 two-state model of, 14, 15*f*
 types of, 25–26, 26*t*
Receptor activator of nuclear factor kappa B (NF-κB), 472
Receptor activity-modifying proteins (RAMPs), 40
Receptor occupancy, 11–13
Receptor serine/threonine kinases, 40
Receptor tyrosine kinases (RTKs), 40, 94
Receptor-effector linkage, types of, 26*f*
'Receptor-operated channels', 54–55
Receptor-response linkage, block of, 18
Recombinant protein, 70
Recreational drug use, term, 643*t*
Rectal administration, 127
Rectangular hyperbola, 20, 20*f*
Red blood cells, 334
Re-entry, 273, 273*f*
Refractoriness, of drug, 18
Regadenoson, 230–231, 282–283, 285
Regeneration, 89*b*, 90
Regulated on activation normal T cell expressed and secreted (RANTES) receptor, 97, 250*t*
Regulators of G-protein signalling (RGS) proteins, 33
Relapse, 645
Relative potency, 107–108
Remifentanil, 554, 555*t*–556*t*, 557
Renal clearance, 139
Renal failure, drugs used in, 393
Renal tubular function, 387*b*
Renal tubule, diffusion across, 140, 140*t*, 141*f*
Renin, 383
Renin inhibitors, 299*t*, 300
Renin-angiotensin system, 295–296, 295*f*
Renin-angiotensin-aldosterone system, 305
 drugs inhibiting, 299*t*
Repaglinide, for insulin secretion, 417
Repair, 89, 89*b*

Repolarisation, in cardiac action potential, 272
Reproductive system, 455–469
 drugs affecting, 458–463
 endocrine control of, 455–458
 female, neurohormonal control of, 455–457, 456*f*, 457*b*
 male, neurohormonal control of, 457–458, 457*f*
Reserpine, 200, 213, 302–303, 607*b*
 action of, 205*t*, 593
Resistance arteries, 165
Reslizumab, for asthma, 378
Resolvins, 241–242
Respiration
 afferent pathways and, 372
 control of, 371
 efferent pathways and, 371–372
 physiology of, 371–372
 regulation of musculature, blood vessels and glands of airways in, 371–372, 372*b*
 sensory receptors and, 372
Respiratory depression, due to opioids, 552
Respiratory distress syndrome, 380
Respiratory syncytial virus, 686–687
Respiratory system, 371–381
 effect of muscarinic antagonists on, 186*b*
 general anaesthetic agents on, 533–534
 leukotriene in, 241
'Resting' cell, 57
 ionic balance of, 57*f*
Reteplase, 331, 332*b*
Reticular layer, 364
Retinoblastoma (Rb) gene, 84*f*
Retinoblastoma (Rb) protein, 84
Retinoic acid receptor, 46*t*
Retinoid X receptor (RXR), 44, 46*t*
Retinoids, 368–369, 368*f*
 adverse effects of, 739*t*, 741
 unwanted effects of, 369
Retroviral integrase, 76
Retroviruses, 654
 replication in, 679
Reverse transcriptase, 654
Reverse transcriptase enzyme, 679
Reverse transcriptase inhibitors, 684*t*, 688*b*
Reward pathways, 644
Reye's syndrome, 349
Rhabdomyolysis, 315–316
Rheumatoid joint damage, 351*f*
Rho A/Rho kinase system, 34
Rho/Rho kinase system, 36
Ribavirin, 251*b*
Ribonucleotide reductase, 341
Ribosomes, 652
Rickets, 475
Rifabutin, 464, 673
Rifampicin, 326, 464, 654, 661, 673–674
 drug interactions of, 377
 effect of, 138, 138*f*
 excretion of, 139
 in induction of microsomal enzymes, 136
 pharmacokinetic aspects of, 468, 674
 resistance to, 658
 unwanted effects of, 674
Rifampin, 673–674
Rifamycin, 654
Rikettsiae, 668*t*
Rilmenidine, 500
Rilpivirine, 684, 684*t*
Riluzole, 516
Rimonabant, 257–258
 for obesity, 429

783